To Barbara

and

David, Deborah, Douglas, Derek, and Denise

Table of Contents

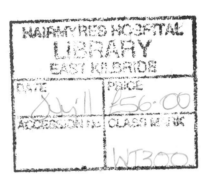

RENAL AND
Electrolyte Disorders

Seventh Edition

Edited by

Robert W. Schrier, MD

Professor of Medicine
University of Colorado Denver
Aurora, Colorado

Wolters Kluwer | Lippincott Williams & Wilkins
Health

Philadelphia · Baltimore · New York · London
Buenos Aires · Hong Kong · Sydney · Tokyo

Acquisitions Editor: Sonya Seigafuse
Product Manager: Kerry Barrett
Production Manager: Alicia Jackson
Senior Manufacturing Manager: Benjamin Rivera
Marketing Manager: Kim Schonberger
Design Coordinator: Doug Smock
Production Service: MPS Limited

Library of Congress Cataloging-in-Publication Data

Renal and electrolyte disorders / edited by Robert W. Schrier.—7th ed.
　　p. ; cm.
　Includes bibliographical references and index.
　ISBN 978-1-60831-072-2 (alk. paper)
　1. Kidneys—Diseases.　2. Water-electrolyte imbalances.　I. Schrier, Robert W.
　[DNLM: 1. Kidney Diseases—physiopathology.　2. Water-Electrolyte Imbalance—physiopathology.　WJ 300 R391 2010]
　RC903.R47 2010
　616.6'1—dc22
2009042586

Care has been taken to confirm the accuracy of the information presented and to describe generally accepted practices. However, the authors, editors, and publisher are not responsible for errors or omissions or for any consequences from application of the information in this book and make no warranty, expressed or implied, with respect to the currency, completeness, or accuracy of the contents of the publication. Application of the information in a particular situation remains the professional responsibility of the practitioner.

The authors, editors, and publisher have exerted every effort to ensure that drug selection and dosage set forth in this text are in accordance with current recommendations and practice at the time of publication. However, in view of ongoing research, changes in government regulations, and the constant flow of information relating to drug therapy and drug reactions, the reader is urged to check the package insert for each drug for any change in indications and dosage and for added warnings and precautions. This is particularly important when the recommended agent is a new or infrequently employed drug.

Some drugs and medical devices presented in the publication have Food and Drug Administration (FDA) clearance for limited use in restricted research settings. It is the responsibility of the health care provider to ascertain the FDA status of each drug or device planned for use in their clinical practice.

To purchase additional copies of this book, call our customer service department at **(800) 638-3030** or fax orders to **(301) 223-2320**. International customers should call **(301) 223-2300**.

Visit Lippincott Williams & Wilkins on the Internet: at LWW.com. Lippincott Williams & Wilkins customer service representatives are available from 8:30 am to 6 pm, EST.

10 9 8 7 6 5 4 3 2 1

Contributing Authors

Matthew K. Abramowitz, MD
Assistant Professor
Department of Medicine
Division of Nephrology
Albert Einstein College of Medicine
Bronx, New York

Tomas Berl, MD
Professor
Department of Medicine
University of Colorado
Aurora, Colorado

Laurence Chan, MD, DPhil (Oxon), FRCP (London & Edin), FACP
Professor of Medicine
Division of Renal Diseases and Hypertension
University of Colorado Health Sciences Center
Denver, Colorado

Michel B. Chonchol, MD
Associate Professor of Medicine
Division of Renal Diseases and Hypertension
Department of Medicine
University of Colorado Denver Health Sciences Center
Aurora, Colorado

Kirk P. Conrad, MD
Professor
Departments of Physiology and Functional
    Genomics, and Obstetrics and Gynecology
University of Florida College of Medicine
Gainesville, Florida

Burl R. Don, MD, FASN
Professor of Medicine
Division of Nephrology
Department of Medicine
University of California
Director, Clinical Nephrology
Department of Medicine
University of California Davis Medical Center
Sacramento, California

Thomas D. DuBose Jr., MD
Tinsley R. Harrison Professor and Chair
Department of Internal Medicine
Wake Forest University School of Medicine
Winston Salem, North Carolina

Charles L. Edelstein, MD, PhD, FAHA
Professor of Medicine
Attending Physician
Director of Renal Hypertension Clinic
Division of Renal Diseases and Hypertension
University of Colorado Denver
Aurora, Colorado

Ryan J. Goldberg, MD
Fellow
Department of Medicine
Division of Renal Diseases and Hypertension
University of Colorado Denver
Aurora, Colorado

Kevin P. G. Harris, MD, FRCP
Reader
Infection, Immunity and Inflammation
University of Leicester
Honorary Consultant Nephrologist
John Walls Renal Unit
University Hospitals of Leicester
Leicester, United Kingdom

Thomas H. Hostetter, MD
Professor and Director of Nephrology
Department of Medicine
Albert Einstein College of Medicine
Bronx, New York

Arun Jeyabalan, MD
Assistant Professor
Department of Obstetrics, Gynecology and
    Reproductive Sciences
University of Pittsburgh School of Medicine
Pittsburgh, Pennsylvania

William D. Kaehny, MD
Professor of Medicine
Department of Medicine
Division of Renal Diseases and Hypertension
University of Colorado Denver
Denver, Colorado

George A. Kaysen, MD, PhD
Professor of Medicine
Chief, Division of Nephrology
Professor and Acting Chairman of Biochemistry
    and Molecular Medicine

Departments of Internal Medicine, Biochemistry and
    Molecular Medicine
University of California Davis
Davis/Sacramento, California
Chief, Renal Division
Department of Medicine
Division of Nephrology
UC Davis Medical Center
Department of Veterans Affairs Northern California
Sacramento/Mather, California

Charles R. Nolan, MD
Professor
Departments of Medicine and Surgery
University of Texas Health Sciences Center
Medical Director, Kidney Transplantation
Organ Transplant Section
University Hospital
San Antonio, Texas

Biff F. Palmer, MD
Professor of Internal Medicine
Renal Fellowship Program Director
Department of Internal Medicine
Division of Nephrology
University of Texas Southwestern Medical Center
Dallas, Texas

Manish P. Ponda, MD
Clinical Instructor
Department of Medicine
Division of Nephrology
NYU School of Medicine
New York, New York

Mordecai M. Popovtzer, MD, FASN, FACP
Professor of Clinical Medicine
Department of Medicine
Section of Nephrology
University of Arizona
Tucson, Arizona

Shobha Ratnam, MD, PhD
Assistant Professor
University of Toledo Health Science Campus
Department of Medicine
University of Toledo Medical Center
Toledo, Ohio

Robert W. Schrier, MD
Professor of Medicine
Department of Medicine
University of Colorado Denver
Aurora, Colorado

Joseph I. Shapiro, MD
Professor
Department of Medicine
University of Toledo Health Science Campus
Chairman, Department of Medicine
University of Toledo Medical Center
Toledo, Ohio

David M. Spiegel, MD, FACP
Professor of Medicine
Division of Renal Diseases and Hypertension
University of Colorado Denver Health Sciences
    Center
Attending Physician
Department of Medicine
University of Colorado Hospital
Aurora, Colorado

Joshua M. Thurman, MD
Associate Professor
Department of Medicine
Division of Renal Diseases and Hypertension
University of Colorado Denver
Aurora, Colorado

Preface

The seventh edition of *Renal and Electrolyte Disorders* has been an exciting challenge to update because of the many advances that have occurred in the various areas of renal pathophysiology over the past seven years. We are in a revolutionary era of biomedical science. Since the kidney is responsible for maintaining the milieu intérieur in health and disease, it is very difficult for any physician to practice state-of-the-art medicine without an up-to-date knowledge of renal physiology and pathophysiology.

For 35 years, virtually thousands of medical students, house officers, and fellows have been introduced to the intricacies of renal physiology and pathophysiology by reading and studying *Renal and Electrolyte Disorders*. This is both a remarkable tradition and a demanding responsibility to which a brilliant group of authors have responded in the seventh edition of *Renal and Electrolyte Disorders*.

The recent developments in disorders of water homeostasis have been very exciting and are discussed by Tomas Berl and Robert Schrier. The vasopressin receptor has been cloned, as have several water channels (aquaporins) including the collecting duct water channel which responds to vasopressin. This has allowed the delineation of mutation defects causing congenital nephrogenic diabetes insipidus. Now there are nonpeptide, orally active vasopressin antagonists that are clinically available as "aquaretics," that is, drugs that increase only solute-free water, but not electrolyte, excretion. These agents can treat the hyponatremia associated with the syndrome of inappropriate antidiuretic hormone secretion (SIADH), cirrhosis, and cardiac failure. A detailed understanding of the afferent and efferent mechanisms of renal sodium retention in edematous disorders, including the optimal use of diuretics, is discussed in the context of body fluid volume regulation in health and disease.

The acid–base disorders have been updated by Joseph Shapiro and William Kaehny, both long-standing experts in the field. This complex area is written in a lucid and understandable manner. Biff Palmer and Thomas DuBose have added substantial new information in their potassium chapter including the advances in genetic hypokalemic and hyperkalemic disorders.

Mordecai M. Popovtzer provides the most up-to-date information on calcium, phosphorus, vitamin D, and parathyroid hormone activity, an area where the recent advances in our molecular knowledge have been remarkable. David Spiegel has updated and dedicated his magnesium chapter to the late Allen Alfrey. Thomas Hostetter, an international expert, has written with his associates an exciting chapter dealing with the genomic and nongenomic effects of angiotensin and aldosterone in renal and cardiovascular disease. Charles R. Nolan, a premier clinician-educator, discusses in a very erudite manner the pivotal role of the kidney in the pathogenesis of hypertensive states. Kirk Conrad, a highly respected expert about the physiology and pathophysiology of pregnancy, with Arun Jeyabalan, has included the recent advances in understanding the state of preeclampsia and eclampsia in their chapter.

There has been substantial new knowledge regarding the mechanisms of vascular and epithelial kidney injury during ischemia, which is discussed by Charles Edelstein and Robert Schrier relative to the pathophysiology of acute kidney injury. Kevin Harris has followed in the excellent tradition of his mentor, Saulo Klahr, in discussing the physiology and pathophysiology of urinary tract obstruction. Michel Chonchol and Lawrence Chan have written about the renal advances in chronic kidney disease in understanding and treating this growing problem. George A. Kaysen has been a major contributor to our understanding of proteinuric states and he shares with Don Burl that pioneering knowledge in the nephrotic syndrome chapter. The advances in our understanding of the glomerulopathies and vasculitides have never been greater and Joshua Thurman and Ryan Goldberg have completely and authoritatively written this chapter.

In the nearly 35 years of *Renal and Electrolyte Disorders*, there has never been an edition with so much new knowledge as this seventh edition. We are very fortunate to have these distinguished authors provide this exciting seventh edition for our readers. I also want to thank Jan Darling for her excellent editorial support.

Robert W. Schrier

CHAPTER 1

Disorders of Water Homeostasis

TOMAS BERL AND ROBERT W. SCHRIER

Historical and Evolutionary Aspects of Renal Concentrating and Diluting Processes

In *From Fish to Philosopher*, Homer Smith (1) suggested that the concentrating capacity of the mammalian kidney may have played an important role in the evolution of various biologic species, including Homo sapiens. He suggested that the earliest protovertebrates resided in a saltwater environment that had a composition similar to their own extracellular fluid (ECF); therefore, these species could ingest freely from the surrounding sea without greatly disturbing the composition of their own *milieu interieur*. However, when these early vertebrates migrated into freshwater streams, the evolution of a relatively water-impermeable integument was mandatory to avoid fatal dilution from their hyposmotic, freshwater environment. Thus a vascular tuft—which we now call the glomerulus—developed, enabling the fish to filter the excess fluid from their blood.

The proximal tubule, which reabsorbed isotonic fluid, evolved in response to the need for salt preservation. However, this did not allow the excretion of hypotonic urine, which is mandatory for organisms ingesting hypotonic fluid from their freshwater environment. This need was met by the development of the distal tubule, which could dilute urine. In this portion of the nephron, salt was reabsorbed without water, because the distal tubular epithelium was relatively impermeable to water. The fish then could excrete the excess solute-free water they had obtained from their freshwater environment without concomitantly losing their body salts.

Vertebrates began to reside on dry land several million years later. The problem of salt conservation persisted in this terrestrial environment, but the excretion of large volumes of fluid was no longer necessary; paradoxically, conservation of fluid was of primary importance in the new arid environment. The kidneys of reptiles, birds, and mammals, however, had glomeruli, which filtered large amounts of fluid and salt, even though excretion of only minute amounts of these substances was needed to maintain daily balance. In reptiles and birds, the kidneys responded to this challenge by a decrease in the number of capillary loops in their glomerular tufts. Aglomerular kidneys actually evolved in some fish, such as the sea horse and pipefish, which may have been the first vertebrates to return to the sea. Tubular secretory systems evolved in the nephron also to allow elimination of nitrogenous wastes without the need for extremely large filtered volumes of fluid. Last, a relatively insoluble nitrogenous end product, uric acid, was produced that could be excreted in supersaturated solutions with a minimal amount of water loss.

The high-pressure glomerular filters were maintained in mammals; however, the countercurrent mechanism developed for concentrating urine. Mammals, along with birds, are unique among vertebrates in possessing loops of Henle and in their ability to compensate for water deficits by elaborating urine more concentrated than blood.

Countercurrent Concentrating Mechanism

By analogy with heat exchangers, the functional significance of the loops of Henle was proposed when Kuhn and Ryffel of the physical chemistry department at the University of Basel, Switzerland, originated the concept of the countercurrent multiplier system for urine concentration in 1942 (2). The hypothesis states that a small difference in osmotic concentration (single effect, or *einzeln Effekt*) at any point between fluid flowing in opposite directions in two parallel tubes connected in hairpin manner can be multiplied many times along the length of the tubes. In the kidney, a small, 200 mOsm gradient, results in a large osmolar concentration difference between the corticomedullary junction and the hairpin loop at the tip of the papilla. Since then, numerous experiments have confirmed the operation of a countercurrent multiplier in the kidney, with the thick ascending limb of Henle as the water-impermeable site of active solute reabsorption (3).

URINARY CONCENTRATION AND DILUTION

As disturbances in the capacity of the kidney to concentrate and dilute the urine are central to the pathogenesis of disorders of water balance, we will briefly review the components of the diluting and concentrating process in the mammalian kidney. These are depicted in Figures 1.1(**A**) and 1.1(**B**), respectively. It is important to emphasize that many of these processes are the same whether the final excreted urine is hypotonic or hypertonic to plasma.

Glomerular Filtration Rate and Proximal Tubular Reabsorption

The rates of glomerular filtration and proximal tubular reabsorption are important primarily in determining the rate of sodium and water delivery to the more distal portions of the nephron, where the renal concentrating and diluting mechanisms are operative. Fluid reabsorption in the proximal tubule is

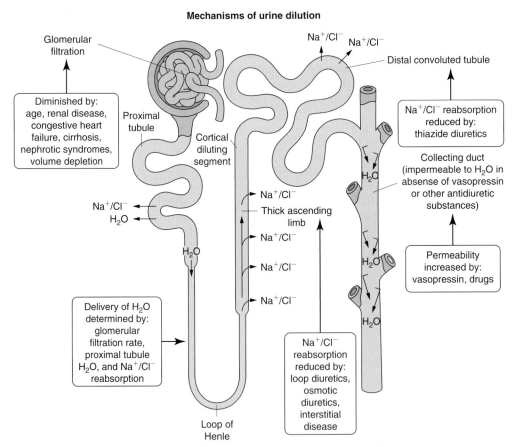

■ **Figure 1.1A** Urinary dilution mechanisms. Normal determinants of urinary dilution and disorders causing hyponatremia. (From Parikh C, Berl T. Disorders of water metabolism. In: London MI, ed. *Comprehensive Clinical Nephrology*. 4 ed. In press, with permission.)

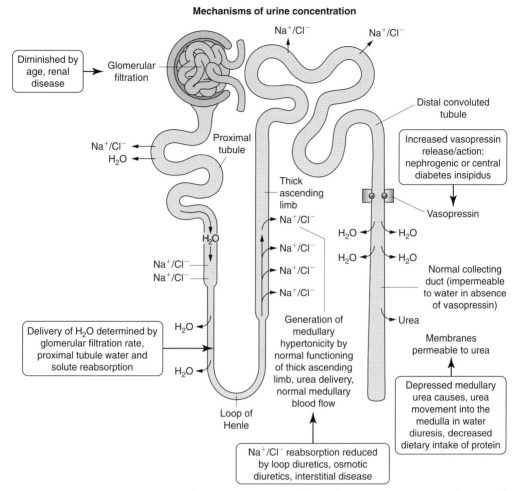

Mechanisms of urine concentration

■ **Figure 1.1B** Urinary concentrating mechanisms. Determinants of normal urinary concentrating mechanism and disorders causing hypernatremia. (From Parikh C, Berl T. Disorders of water metabolism. In: London MI, ed. *Comprehensive Clinical Nephrology*. 4 ed. In press, with permission.)

isosmotic because of the water permeability of tubular epithelium; therefore, tubular fluid is neither concentrated nor diluted in the proximal portion of the nephron. Rather, after approximately 70% of glomerular filtrate is reabsorbed in the proximal tubules, the remaining 30% of fluid entering the loop of Henle is still isotonic to plasma. The removal of sodium chloride is mediated by the Na^+/H^+ 3 transporter while the isotonic removal of water is facilitated by the robust expression of the water channel aquaporin 1 (AQP_1), depicted in Figure 1.2. A decrease in glomerular filtration rate (GFR) or an increase in proximal tubular reabsorption, or both, may diminish the amount of fluid delivered to the distal nephron and thus limit the renal capacity to excrete water. Similarly, a diminished GFR and increased proximal tubular reabsorption may limit the delivery of sodium chloride to the ascending limb, where the tubular transport of these ions without water initiates the formation of the hypertonic medullary interstitium. With diminished delivery of sodium chloride to the ascending limb, the resultant lowering of medullary hypertonicity impairs maximal renal concentrating capacity by limiting the osmotic gradient for passive water movement from the collecting duct.

Descending and Ascending Limbs of the Loops of Henle, Distal Tubule, and Collecting Ducts

The first nephron segment actually involved in urinary concentration is the descending limb of loop of Henle, because the urine that emerges from the proximal tubule is isosmotic. There are two types of

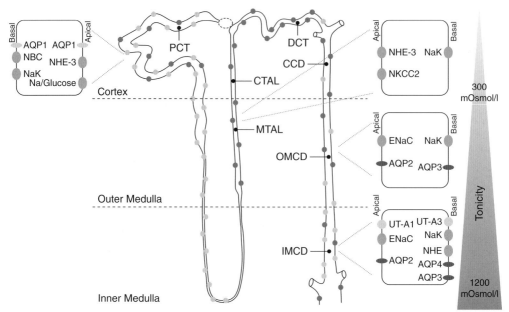

■ **Figure 1.2** Schematic representation of key elements of the kidney tubule that mediate water reabsorption. Direct mediators are those involved in sodium (*depicted as red circles*), urea (*green circles*), and water (*blue circles*) transport. PCT, proximal convoluted tubule; CTAL, cortical thick ascending limb; MTAL, medullary thick ascending limb; DCT, distal convoluted tubule; CCD, cortical collecting duct; OMCD outer medullary collecting duct; IMCD, inner medullary collecting duct; AQP, aquaporin; NHE, NA^+/H^+ exchanger; Na/Glucose, sodium-glucose cotransporter; NBC, sodium bicarbonate cotransporter; NaK, Na^+, K^+-ATPase; NKCC2, Na^+2Cl-K^+ cotransporter; ENaC, epithelial sodium channel: UT-A, urea transporter A isoform. (From Hasler U, Leroy V, Martin P-Y, et al. Aquaporin-2 abundance in the renal collecting duct: new insights from cultured cell models. *Am J Physiol Renal Physiol.* 2009 at http://www.ncbi.nlm.nih.gov/pubmed/19244407, with permission.)

descending limbs. The short loops originate in superficial and midcortical glomeruli and turn in the outer medulla. The long loops originate in deep cortical and juxtamedullary glomeruli and penetrate variable distances into the inner medulla. Short and long descending limbs are anatomically distinct; the long limbs in particular display considerable interspecies variability (4). It is interesting that no correlation is apparent between a species' maximal concentrating ability and the ratio of short and long loops. In fact, in rodents with highest urinary concentrations, the number of short loops is considerably greater than the number of long loops. Approximately 15% of nephrons possess long loops in the human kidney; the other 85% of nephrons have short loops. The descending thin limb is very water permeable as it also has abundant expression of AQP_1 (5). Thus tubular fluid is concentrated as it descends primarily, but probably not exclusively, by the extraction of water.

Somewhat proximal to the hairpin turn, there is a transition from the descending limb to the ascending thin limb of loop of Henle. This segment, as well as the remainder of ascending limb, is water impermeable. Whether the movement of solute out of this thin segment is passive or active remains controversial. Active sodium transport has not been demonstrated convincingly, and this segment's morphologic appearance with few mitochondria does not suggest active metabolic work.

The thick ascending limb of loop of Henle appears both structurally and functionally distinct from its thin counterpart. The epithelium is remarkably uniform among species with tall, heavily interdigitating cells with large mitochondria. The observation that fluid emerges into the early distal tubule hypotonic (about 100 mOsm/kg H_2O) supports the view that active sodium chloride transport out of this water-impermeable segment provides the single effect required for the operation of the countercurrent multiplier. The primary mechanism of chloride absorption in the thick ascending limb is mediated by an electroneutral sodium, potassium, and chloride (Na^+:K^+:$2Cl^-$) cotransport (Fig. 1.2).

The distal convoluted tubule is the segment between the macula densa and collecting ducts. This is a morphologically heterogenous segment (4) that is also water impermeable and unresponsive to

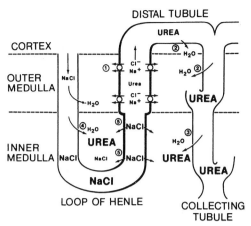

DISTAL TUBULE

■ **Figure 1.3** Schematic representation of the passive urinary concentrating mechanism. Both the thin ascending limb in the inner medulla and the thick ascending limb in the outer medulla, as well as the first part of the distal tubule, are impermeable to water, as indicated by the thickened lining. In the thick ascending limb, active sodium, chloride, and potassium cotransport: renders the tubule fluid dilute and the outer medullary interstitium hyperosmotic (*1*). In the last part of the distal tubule and the collecting tubule in the cortex and outer medulla, water is reabsorbed down its osmotic gradient (*2*), increasing the concentration of urea that remains behind. In the inner medulla, both water and urea are reabsorbed from the collecting duct (*3*). Some urea reenters the loop of Henle (not shown). This medullary recycling of urea, in addition to trapping of urea by countercurrent exchange in the vasa recta (not shown) causes urea to accumulate in large quantities in the medullary interstitium (indicated by Urea), where it osmotically extracts water from the descending limb (*4*) and thereby concentrates sodium chloride in descending limb fluid. When the fluid rich in sodium chloride enters the sodium chloride-permeable (but water impermeable) thin ascending limb, sodium chloride moves passively down its concentration gradient (*5*), rendering the tubule fluid relatively hyposmotic to the surrounding interstitium. (From Jamison RL, Maffly RH. The urinary concentrating mechanism. *N Engl J Med*. 1976;295:1059, with permission.)

vasopressin. The collecting ducts are formed in the cortex by the confluence of several distal tubules. They descend through the cortex and outer medulla individually, but successively fuse together on entering the inner medulla. In humans, a terminal inner medullary collecting duct draws from as many as 7,800 nephrons. The collecting ducts possess vasopressin-sensitive adenylate cyclase in all species studied; they are virtually impermeable to water in the absence of the hormone. The vasopressin-sensitive water channel AQP_2 mediates water reabsorption in this segment of the nephron in concert with AQP_3 and AQP_4 (5). The collecting duct in its cortical and medullary segments is also impermeable to urea, but in response to the vasopressin-sensitive urea transporter, UT 1, the inner medullary collecting duct is rendered urea permeable (6).

Kokko and Rector (7) have proposed a model of urinary concentration that is in concert with the anatomic features and the permeability characteristics of the various segments of the system, while limiting the active transport of solute to the thick portion of the ascending limb of loop of Henle in the outer medulla. The components of the mechanism are as follows, as depicted in Figure 1.3:

1. The water-impermeable thick ascending limb of loop of Henle actively cotransports sodium, chloride, and potassium, thereby increasing the tonicity of the surrounding interstitium and delivering hypotonic fluid to the distal tubule. Urea is poorly reabsorbed and therefore retained in the tubule.
2. Under the influence of vasopressin in the cortical and outer medullary collecting ducts, tubular fluid equilibrates with the isotonic and hypertonic interstitium, respectively. Low urea permeability in this portion of the nephron allows its concentration to further increase.
3. The inner medullary collecting duct is more permeable to urea. Therefore, in this segment of nephron, in addition to water reabsorption, urea is reabsorbed as it diffuses passively along its concentration gradient into the interstitium, where it constitutes a significant component of the medullary interstitial tonicity.

4. The resulting increase in interstitial tonicity creates the osmotic gradient that abstracts water from a highly water permeable and solute impermeable descending limb of loop of Henle. This process elevates the concentration of sodium chloride in the tubular fluid. When tubular fluid arrives at the bend of the loop, its tonicity is the same as that of the surrounding interstitium. However, the sodium chloride concentration of the tubular fluid is higher and the urea concentration lower than that of the interstitium.

5. Tubular fluid then enters the thin ascending limb, which is more permeable to sodium than urea. The sodium gradient provides for passive removal of sodium chloride from this segment into the interstitium.

To prevent urea removal from the inner medulla to the cortex, the ascending and descending vasa recta act as a countercurrent exchanger and "trap" urea in the inner medulla. The ascending vasa recta also may deposit urea into adjacent descending thin limbs of a short loop of Henle, thereby recycling it to the inner medullary collecting tubule. The descending limbs of short loops do not enter the inner medulla; thus, the addition of urea to these loops does not interfere with the removal of water from the descending thin limb in the inner medulla, a step that is so crucial to the concentrating process.

This model of urinary concentration has a number of attractive features, and many of its aspects have been experimentally supported (7). Furthermore, the single effect in the ascending limb of loop of Henle so critical to the operation of the countercurrent system and urinary concentration also serves to dilute the urine. In the absence of vasopressin, and thus with water impermeability of the collecting ducts, the continued reabsorption of solute in the remainder of the distal nephron results in a maximally dilute urine (50 mOsm/kg). Thus, it should be apparent that impairment of sodium, chloride, and potassium cotransport in the ascending limb of the loop of Henle will limit the renal capacity both to concentrate and to dilute the urine.

Medullary Blood Flow

Medullary blood flow, whose rate can be regulated independently of whole kidney blood flow, may also affect the renal capacity both to concentrate and dilute the urine, because the preservation of the medullary hypertonicity in the interstitium is dependent on the countercurrent exchange mechanism in the vasa recta (8). Although medullary blood flow constitutes only 5% to 10% of total renal blood flow, this flow is still several times more rapid than the tubular flow. The vasa recta posses AQP_1 and serve as a countercurrent exchanger that permits the preservation of interstitial tonicity. Blood that enters the descending vasa recta becomes increasingly concentrated as water diffuses out of and solutes diffuse into this portion of the nephron. The hairpin configuration of the vasa recta, however, does not allow the solute-rich blood to leave the medulla. In the ascending portion of the vasa recta, water diffuses into the vasa recta and solute moves out, thus maintaining interstitial hypertonicity. Even with an intact countercurrent exchange system in the vasa recta, circumstances that increase medullary blood flow may "wash out" the medullary concentration gradient and thereby diminish renal concentrating capacity. Moreover, even in the absence of vasopressin, the collecting duct is not completely water impermeable; therefore, a further decrease in the hypertonic medullary interstitium during an increase in medullary blood flow may decrease the vasopressin-independent osmotic water movement from the collecting duct and thereby increase water excretion.

Distal Solute Load

The rate of solute delivery to the collecting duct is a known determinant of renal concentrating capacity. As depicted in Figure 1.4, in spite of maximal levels of vasopressin, urinary osmolality in normal humans progressively diminishes as solute excretion increases. At high rates of solute excretion, urinary osmolality may reach isotonicity in humans, even though supraphysiologic doses of vasopressin are infused. An increase in solute excretion even may be associated with hypotonic urine with the infusion of submaximal doses of vasopressin in patients with pituitary diabetes insipidus. At least two factors may be responsible for this effect of solute excretion on renal concentrating capacity. First, a solute diuresis generally is associated with an increase in medullary blood flow, which could lower the medullary solute concentration profile. Second, the rapid rate of tubular flow through the medullary

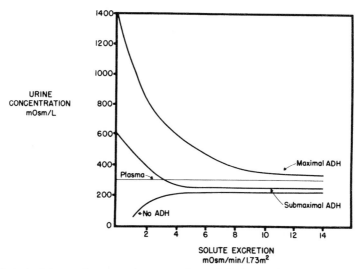

■ Figure 1.4 Effect of solute excretion on renal concentration and diluting mechanisms. The submaximal response to ADH may result from the presence of submaximal amounts of ADH or the diminished response of the collecting duct to maximal amounts of ADH. ADH, antidiuretic hormone. (From de Wardener HE, del Greco F. Influence of solute excretion rate on production of hypotonic urine in man. *Clin Sci.* 1955;14:715, with permission.)

collecting duct could shorten contact time sufficiently so that complete osmotic equilibrium of fluid would not be allowed between the collecting duct and medullary interstitium, even though vasopressin had made the collecting duct membrane maximally permeable to water.

Antidiuretic Hormone

The renal concentrating and diluting processes are ultimately, and most importantly, dependent on the presence or absence, respectively, of arginine vasopressin (AVP) to modulate the water permeability of the collecting duct (9). AVP, a cyclic hexapeptide (mol wt 1,099) with a tail of three amino acids, is the antidiuretic hormone (ADH) in humans (Fig. 1.5). The presence of a basic amino acid (arginine or lysine) in the middle of the intact hormone at position 8 is crucial for antidiuresis, as is the asparagine at position 5. Arginine vasopressin is synthesized in the supraoptic and paraventricular magnocellular nuclei in the hypothalamus. In these nuclei, a biologically inactive macromolecule is cleaved into the smaller, biologically active AVP. Both oxytocin and AVP are encoded in human chromosome 20 in close proximity to each other, depicted in Figure 1.6. The prohormone gene is approximately 2,000 base pairs in length and comprises three exons (Fig. 1.6). Arginine vasopressin is encoded in the first exon following a signal peptide. Although spanning all three exons, the binding protein neurophysin is primarily encoded in exon B and the terminal glycoprotein in exon C. The promoter has *cis*-acting elements, including a glucocorticoid response element, a cyclic adenosine monophosphate (cAMP) response element, and four AP-2 binding sites (10). The precursor prohormone, called propressophysin, is cleaved by removal of the signal peptide after translation. Vasopressin, with its binding protein neurophysin II, and the glycoprotein are transported in neurosecretory granules down the axons and stored in nerve terminals in the pars nervosa. There is no known physiologic role of the neurophysins, but they neutralize the negative charge of vasopressin. The release of stored peptide hormone and its neurophysin into the systemic or hypophyseal portal circulation occurs by an exocytosis. With increased

Arginine-vasopressin
$$\text{Cys-Tyr-Phe-Glu(NH}_2\text{)-Asp(NH}_2\text{)-Cys-Pro-Arg-Gly-NH}_2$$

■ Figure 1.5 Structure of the human antidiuretic hormone, arginine vasopressin. (From Schrier RW, Miller PD. Water metabolism in diabetes insipidus and the syndrome of inappropriate antidiuretic hormone secretion. In: Kurtzman NA, Martinez Maldonado M, eds. *Pathophysiology of the Kidney.* Springfield, IL: Charles C Thomas; 1977, with permission.)

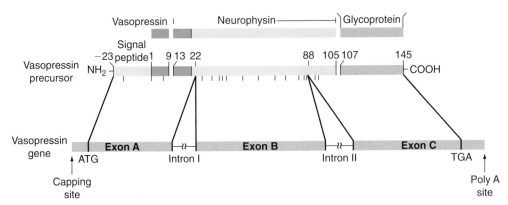

■ **Figure 1.6** The arginine vasopressin (AVP) gene and its protein products. The three exons encode a 145-amino acid prohormone with an NH-2-terminal signal peptide. The prohormone is packaged into neurosecretory granules of magnocellular neurons. During axonal transport of the granules from the hypothalamus to the posterior pituitary, enzymatic cleavage of the prohormone generates the final products: AVP, neurophysin, and a COOH-terminal glycoprotein. When afferent stimulation depolarizes the AVP-containing neurons, the three products are released into capillaries of the posterior pituitary. (From Brenner BM, ed. *The Kidney*. Philadelphia, PA: Saunders Elsevier, 2008, with permission.)

plasma osmolality, electrical impulses travel along the axons and depolarize the membrane of the terminal axonal bulbs. The membrane of the secretory granules fuses with the plasma membrane of the axonal bulbs, and the peptide contents are then extruded into the adjacent capillaries. The Brattleboro rat, a strain with an autosomal recessive defect that causes AVP deficiency is afflicted by a single base deletion in exon B. This leads to a shift in the reading frame, with loss of the translational stop code. Although transcribed and translated in the hypothalamus, the translational product is neither transported nor processed in these mutant rats.

The regulation of AVP release from the posterior pituitary is dependent primarily on two mechanisms: osmotic and nonosmotic pathways (Fig. 1.7).

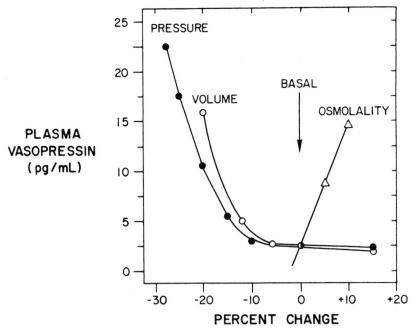

■ **Figure 1.7** Osmotic and nonosmotic stimulation of arginine vasopressin release. (From Robertson GL, Berl T. Pathophysiology of water metabolism. In: Brenner BM, ed. *The Kidney,* 6th ed. Philadelphia, PA: WB Saunders; 2000:875, with permission.)

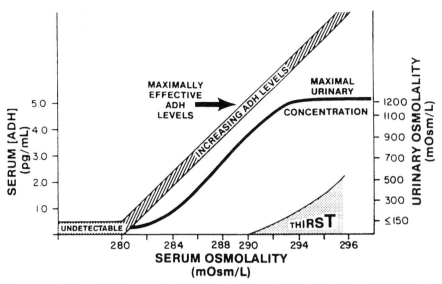

■ **Figure 1.8** Antidiuretic hormone levels, urinary osmolality, and thirst as functions of serum osmolality. (From Narins RG, Krishna GC. Disorders of water balance. In: Stein JH, ed. *Internal Medicine.* Boston: Little Brown, 1987:794, with permission.)

Osmotic Release of Vasopressin

The osmotic regulation of AVP is dependent on "osmoreceptor" cells in the anterior hypothalamus in proximity but separate from supraoptic nuclei. These cells, most likely by altering their cell volume, recognize changes in ECF osmolality. Cell volume is decreased most readily by substances that are restricted to the ECF, such as hypertonic saline or hypertonic mannitol, and thus enhance osmotic water movement from cells; these substances are very effective in stimulating AVP release. Since the effects of saline and mannitol are comparable, this supports the view that the response is due to changes in effective osmolality rather than to sodium per se. In contrast, urea moves readily into cells and therefore does not alter cell volume; hypertonic urea does not effectively stimulate AVP release. The effects of increased osmolality on vasopressin release are associated with measurable (twofold to fivefold) increases in vasopressin precursor messenger RNA (mRNA) in the hypothalamus. The osmoreceptor cells are very sensitive to changes in ECF osmolality. An increase of ECF osmolality by 1% stimulates AVP release, whereas water ingestion causing a 1% decrease in ECF osmolality suppresses AVP release (Fig. 1.8). A close correlation between AVP and plasma osmolality has been demonstrated in subjects with various states of hydration, although there are considerable genetically determined individual variations in both the threshold and sensitivity (Fig. 1.8). In humans the osmotic threshold for vasopressin release is between 280 and 290 mOsm/kg. The system is so efficient that plasma osmolality usually does not vary more than 1% to 2% despite great variations in water intake. There is also a close correlation between AVP and urinary osmolality, allowing for the maintenance of tonicity of body fluids.

Nonosmotic Release of Vasopressin

Vasopressin release can occur in the absence of changes in plasma osmolality (9). Although a number of such nonosmotic stimuli exist, physical pain, emotional stress, and a decrement in blood pressure or volume are the most prominent ones. A 7% to 10% decrement in either blood pressure or blood volume causes the prompt release of vasopressin (Fig. 1.7). Because the integrity of the circulatory volume takes precedence over mechanisms that maintain tonicity, activation of these nonosmotic pathways overrides any decline in the osmotic stimulus that otherwise would suppress the hormone's release. This process accounts for the pathogenesis of hyponatremia in various pathophysiologic states, including cirrhosis, heart failure, and several endocrine disorders.

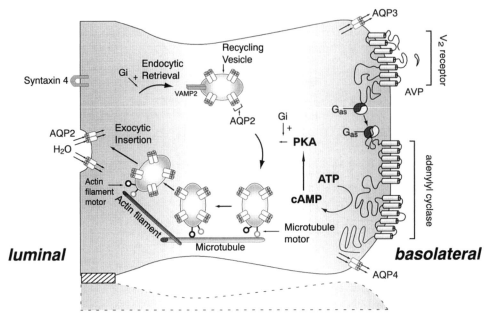

■ **Figure 1.9** Schematic representation of the cellular action of vasopressin. The binding of vasopressin to the V_2 receptor in the basolateral membrane initiates a cascade of events resulting in AQP_2 insertion in the luminal membrane, see text for details. (From Bichet D. Nephrogenic and central diabetes insipidus. In: Schrier RW, ed. *Diseases of the Kidney and Urinary Tract,* 7th ed., vol. 3. New York, NY: Lippincott Williams & Wilkins; 2000:2553, with permission.)

There is considerable evidence for the existence of baroreceptor sensors in the low-pressure (venous) areas of the circulation, particularly in the atria. Atrial distention causes a decrease in plasma AVP levels, and a water dieresis; this reflex is mediated by the vagus nerve. Alternatively, arterial baroreceptors in the aorta and carotid sensors send impulses through the vagus and glossopharyngeal nerves to the nucleus tractus solitarii of the medulla. Unloading of these arterial baroreceptors decreases tonic inhibition and leads to the nonosmotic release of vasopressin. Denervation of these arterial baroreceptors have been shown to abolishes the nonosmotic release of AVP.

It is possible that angiotensin II is a mediator of AVP release in these states because many of the pathophysiologic states associated with nonosmotic AVP release are characterized by enhanced plasma renin activity and therefore increased angiotensin II levels. The experimental results in this regard are however conflicting. Activation of the sympathetic nervous system seemed be involved in the nonosmotic stimulation of AVP. In this regard, the supraoptic nuclei are heavily innervated by noradrenergic neurons. Other pathways that could stimulate the nonosmotic secretion of AVP have been proposed; for example, the antidiuresis associated with nausea, vomiting, and pain has been ascribed to an emetic and cerebral pain center, respectively. A role for baroreceptor pathways, however, has not been convincingly excluded even in these settings. Other biogenic amines, polypeptides, and even cytokines have been implicated as modulators of AVP release in addition to catecholamines.

Cellular Action of Vasopressin

Once released from the posterior pituitary, vasopressin exerts its biologic action on water excretion by binding to V_2 receptors in the basolateral membrane of the collecting duct (Fig. 1.9) (11). The receptors to which vasopressin binds have been cloned and fully described. The V_1 receptor on blood vessels and elsewhere is a 394 amino acid protein with seven transmembrane domains (12). The 370 amino acid V_2 receptor, which is only in the kidney and has a similar configuration, has been cloned for both rat (13) and humans (14). Although the V_1 receptor messenger is plentiful in the glomerulus, it is detected also in the collecting duct, where the V_2 message predominates.

Binding of AVP to its V_2 receptor results in increased adenylate cyclase activity, which catalyzes the formation of cyclic adenosine 3^1-, 5^1-monophosphate from adenosine triphosphate. The V_2 receptor is coupled to the catalytic unit of adenylate cyclase by the stimulatory guanine nucleotide binding regulatory protein, Gs. This is a heterotrimeric protein whose α-subunit binds and hydrolyzes guanosine triphosphate (GTP). The AVP stimulated increase in adenylate cyclase activity results in heightened cAMP formation, which ultimately causes the apical (luminal) cell membrane of the principal cell of the collecting duct to become more permeable to water (11). cAMP activates protein kinase A (PKA), which in turn phosphorylates serine and threonines. The activation of protein kinase A brings about the phosphorylation of the water channel aquaporin 2 (AQP_2) at serine 256 in intracellular vesicles, a critical event to increase the trafficking of the water channel to the luminal membrane (15). AQP_2 is a member of an increasingly large family of water channels (5) whose archetypal member, AQP_1, cloned by Agre et al. (16) is, as mentioned previously, abundant in the proximal tubule and descending limb of Henle (5). In contrast, AQP_2 is limited to the vasopressin-sensitive principal cell of the collecting duct and particularly to the cytoplasm and luminal membrane (5). Vasopressin also is involved in the long-term regulation of the expression of AQP_2 (17). AQP_3 and AQP_4 are widely distributed (5,17), including the collecting duct principal cell, where they are localized at the basolateral membrane. In this basolaterial they serve as conduits for water exit from the cell. Other aquaporins 6–8 also are expressed in the kidney. AQP_6 is present in intercalated cells, AQP_7 in the S_3 segment of the proximal tubules, AQP_8 in proximal tubules and collecting ducts, and AQP 11 in the proximal tubule (17). There, physiological roles of this water channels in the kidney are not clear. The cytoskeleton also plays an important role in the trafficking of the AQP_2 water channel to the luminal membrane, a process involving both exocytic insertion associated with AVP stimulation and endocytic retrieval associated with suppression of AVP action.

Quantitation of Renal Water Excretion

The quantitation of water excretion has been facilitated by the concept that urine flow (V) is divisible into two components. One component is the urine volume needed to excrete solutes at the concentration of solutes in plasma. This isotonic component has been termed "osmolar clearance" (C_{osm}). The other component is called solute-free water clearance (C_{H_2O}) and is the theoretic volume of solute-free water that has been added to (positive C_{H_2O}) or reabsorbed from (negative C_{H_2O} or $T^c_{H_2O}$) the isotonic portion of urine (C_{osm}) to create with hypotonic or hypertonic urine, respectively. These terms are calculated as follows:

$$V = C_{osm} + C_{H_2O}$$
$$C_{H_2O} = V - C_{osm}$$

Because,
$$C_{osm} = \frac{\text{Urine osmolality } (U_{osm}) \times \text{urine flow (V)}}{\text{plasma osmolality } (P_{osm})}$$
(1.1)

$$C_{H_2O} = V - \frac{U_{osm} + V}{P_{osm}}$$
$$C_{H_2O} = V \left(1 - \frac{U_{osm}}{P_{osm}} \right)$$

Further inspection of these relationships will reveal the following:

1. When U_{osm} equals P_{osm} (isotonic urine), V equals C_{osm}; therefore, C_{H_2O} is zero.
2. When U_{osm} is greater than P_{osm} (hypertonic urine), C_{osm} is greater than V; therefore, C_{H_2O} is negative (also denoted as $T^c_{H_2O}$).
3. When U_{osm} is less than P_{osm} (hypotonic urine), C_{osm} is less than V, and C_{H_2O} is positive.

This relationship is depicted further in Figure 1.10.

The excretion of a hypertonic urine has the net effect of returning solute-free water to the organism and thereby dilutes body fluids. In contrast, the excretion of a hypotonic urine has the net effect of ridding the organism of solute-free water and thus concentrating body fluids. The urine osmolality alone

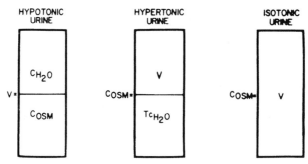

■ **Figure 1.10** Relationship between urine flow (V), C_{osm}, CH_2O, and $T^c_{H_2O}$ in hypotonic, hypertonic, and isotonic urine.

does not give the volume of water added to or removed from the organism; the calculation of C_{H_2O} or $T^c_{H_2O}$ better allows the quantitation of water balance.

A limitation of the equation is that it fails to predict clinically important alterations in tonicity and serum sodium concentration because it factors in urea. Urea is an important component of urine osmolality, but does not establish transcellular osmotic gradients because it readily crosses cell membranes. Consequently, urea influences neither the serum sodium concentration nor the release of vasopressin, and its inclusion in urine osmolality does not predict changes in serum sodium. This is better reflected if specifically electrolyte-free water clearance ($C_{H_2O}^e$) is measured. In this formulation, the serum osmolality is replaced by serum sodium and urine osmolality by $U_{Na} + U_K$.

Therefore:

$$C_{H_2O}\ (e) = V \left(1 - \frac{U_{NA} + U_K}{P_{NA}} \right) \tag{1.2}$$

If a patient's $U_{Na} + U_K < P_{Na}$, then $C_{H_2O}(e)$ is positive, a process that will raise the plasma concentration of sodium. Conversely, if $U_{Na} + U_K > P_{Na}$, then $C_{H_2O}(e)$ is negative, a process that tends to lower the serum concentration of sodium.

RELATIONSHIP AMONG DAILY SOLUTE LOAD, RENAL CONCENTRATING CAPACITY, AND DAILY URINE VOLUME

A person ingesting a diet containing average amounts of sodium and protein has to dispose of approximately 600 mOsm of solutes per day. The daily volume of urine in which this solute is excreted depends on the fluid intake. The 600 mOsm can be excreted in 6 L of urine with an osmolality of 100 mOsm/kg H_2O if the daily fluid intake is generous. If water ingested is limited and renal concentrating capacity is intact, then the 600 mOsm solute load can be excreted in 500 mL of urine with an osmolality 1,200 mOsm/kg H_2O.

This flexibility in daily urine volumes for a given solute load is limited if renal concentrating ability is impaired. For example, if the maximal renal concentrating ability is reduced to 300 mOsm/kg H_2O, then the 600 mOsm of solute obligates 2 L of urine per day to maintain total body solute. The 600 mOsm of daily solute requires 10 L of urine per day with a more severe concentrating defect that does not allow urine to be concentrated above 60 mOsm/kg H_2O, that is, diabetes insipidus.

In terms of water conservation, the kidney's ability to increase urine osmolality from 60 to 300 mOsm/kg H_2O is quantitatively more important than its ability to increase urine osmolality from 300 to 1,200 mOsm/kg H_2O. For example, with a daily solute load of 600 mOsm, a decrease in maximal urine osmolality from 1,200 to 300 mOsm/kg H_2O increases obligatory urine flow from .5 to 2.0 L/day. Thus, severe polydipsia and polyuria should not be observed even in the complete absence of the renal capacity to concentrate urine above plasma. However, for the same solute load, a further decrease in maximal urinary concentration from 300 to 60 mOsm/kg H_2O requires the excretion to increase from 2 to 10 L of urine/day. This degree of defect in water conservation obviously is associated with overt polyuria and polydipsia. In this setting, a severe water deficit and hypernatremia occur in the absence of an intact thirst mechanism and a large intake of water.

RENAL CAPACITY TO REABSORB SOLUTE FREE ($T^c_{H_2O}$) VERSUS CAPACITY TO EXCRETE SOLUTE-FREE WATER (C_{H_2O})

In quantitative terms, the normal kidney's ability to reabsorb $T^c_{H_2O}$ is more limited than its ability to excrete C_{H_2O}. With maximal urine osmolality of 1,200 mOsm/kg H_2O and a daily urine volume of 500 mL, $T^c_{H_2O}$ can be calculated as follows:

$$C_{osm} = \frac{UV}{P} \ or \ C_{osm} = \frac{1,200 \text{ mOsm/kg } H_2O \times 500 \text{ mL/day}}{300 \text{ mOsm/kg } H_2O}$$

$$C_{osm} = 200 \text{ mL/day}$$

$$T^c_{H_2O} = C_{osm} - V \tag{1.3}$$

$$T^c_{H_2O} = 2,000 - 500 \text{ mL/day}$$

$$T^c_{H_2O} = 1,500 \text{ mL/day}$$

Thus, only 1,500 mL of solute-free water is returned to body fluids during this maximal antidiuresis. In contrast, with the same daily solute load of 600 mOsm, a minimal urine osmolality of 60 mOsm/kg H_2O, and a daily urine volume of 10 L, the renal capacity to excrete C_{H_2O} is much greater than the capacity to return solute-free water ($T^c_{H_2O}$) to the body. More specifically,

$$C_{osm} = \frac{UV}{P} \ or \ \frac{60 \text{ mOsm/kg}}{300 \text{ mOsm/kg}} \times 10 = 2 \text{ L/day} \tag{1.4}$$

$$C_{H_2O} = V - C_{osm} \ or \ 10 \text{ L} - 2 \text{ L} = 8 \text{ L/day}$$

Thus, with comparable solute loads and relatively maximal and minimal urine osmolalities, the $T^c_{H_2O}$ of 1.5 L/day is substantially less than the C_{H_2O} of 8 L/day.

Thus, prevention of a total body water deficit is largely dependent on water intake as modulated by thirst. The thirst center appears to be closely associated anatomically with the osmoreceptor in the region of the hypothalamus. Defects in thirst response may involve either organic or generalized central nervous system (CNS) lesions and can lead to severe water deficit even in the presence of a normal concentrating mechanism. Of course, the water deficit occurs more promptly if renal concentrating ability is impaired as well.

Clinical Disorders of Urinary Concentration Causing Hypernatremic States

The renal concentrating mechanism represents the first defense against water depletion and hyperosmolality. A perturbation in any component of the concentrating mechanism, shown in Figure 1.1(**B**) culminates in an inability to maximally concentrate urine. Renal concentrating defects ensue when there is impairment in the generation of medullary hypertonicity either as a consequence of decreased delivery of solutes to the loop (diminished GFR) or inability to reabsorb NaCl in the loop of Henle (loop diuretics). Likewise, failure to render the collecting duct permeable to water because vasopressin is absent or the tubule is unresponsive to vasopressin also results in a renal concentrating defect. Thirst becomes a very effective mechanism for preventing further increases in serum sodium when renal concentration is impaired (18,19). The plasma osmolality threshold for thirst appears to be approximately 10 mOsm/kg H_2O above that of vasopressin release (Fig. 1.8). In fact, thirst is so effective that even patients with complete diabetes insipidus avoid hypernatremia by fluid intake in excess of 10 L/day. Therefore, hypernatremia supervenes only when hypotonic fluid losses occur in combination with a disturbance in water intake (20). This is most commonly seen in the aged (with an alteration in level of consciousness), the very young (with inadequate access to water), or a rare subject (with a primary disturbance in thirst).

Hypernatremia can develop with either low, normal, or, more rarely, high total body sodium, as shown in Figure 1.11 (21).

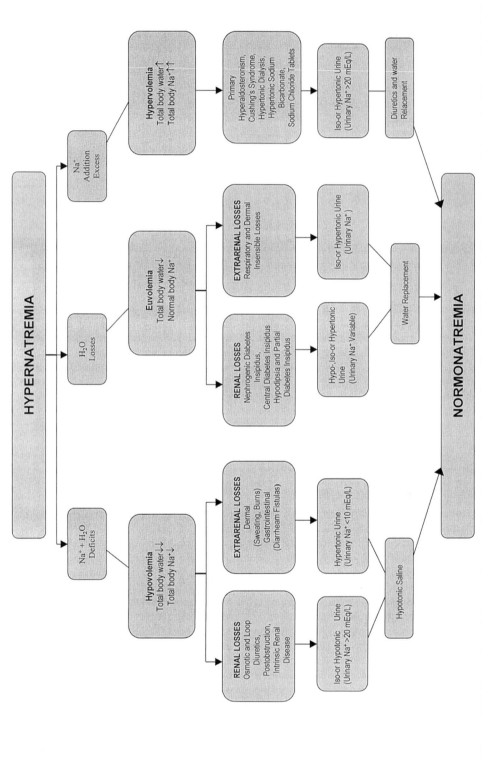

■ **Figure 1.11** Diagnostic and therapeutic approach to the hypernatremic patient. (From Berl T, Kumar S. Disorders of water balance. In: Johnson RJ, Feehally J, eds. *Comprehensive Clinical Nephrology.* St. Louis: CV Mosby; 2000:3–9, with permission.)

HYPERNATREMIA IN PATIENTS WITH LOW TOTAL BODY SODIUM

Patients who sustain losses of both sodium and water but with a relatively greater loss of water are classified as having hypernatremia with low total body sodium. Such patients exhibit the signs of hypovolemia such as orthostatic hypotension, tachycardia, flat neck veins, poor skin turgor, and dry mucous membranes. The causes that underlie the hypovolemic state are similar to those that cause hypovolemic hyponatremia. The effect on serum sodium is determined by the failure to ingest water (hypernatremia) or excessive free water intake (hyponatremia). Extrarenal loss of hypotonic fluid can occur either through the skin because of profuse sweating in a hot and/or humid environment or, more frequently, from the gastrointestinal tract in the form of diarrhea. Lactulose-induced diarrhea leading to hypernatremia appears to be common, although primarily recognized in children. Urine osmolality is high (usually >800 mOsm/kg H_2O) and urinary sodium concentration is low (<10 mEq/L) because the renal water and sodium conserving mechanisms operate normally in these patients. Hypotonic losses also can occur by the renal route during a loop diuretic–induced hypotonic diuresis or an osmotic diuresis with either mannitol, glucose, or as is not uncommon, urea in the setting of excessive protein supplementation. Elderly patients with partial urinary tract obstruction can excrete large volumes of hypotonic urine. The urine with such obstruction is hypotonic or isotonic, and the urinary sodium concentration is >20 mEq/L. Since glucose and mannitol enhance osmotic water movement from the intracellular fluid to the ECF compartment, these patients may have a normal or even low serum sodium concentration in spite of serum hypertonicity.

HYPERNATREMIA IN PATIENTS WITH NORMAL TOTAL BODY SODIUM

Loss of water without sodium does not lead to clinically significant volume contraction unless the water losses are massive. Therefore, patients with hypernatremia secondary to water loss appear to be euvolemic with a normal total body sodium. The extrarenal sources of such water losses are the skin and respiratory tract. A high environmental temperature as well as a febrile or hypermetabolic state can cause considerable water losses. Hypernatremia supervenes if such hypotonic losses are not accompanied by appropriate water intake. Urine osmolality is very high, reflecting an intact osmoreceptor–vasopressin–renal response. Urinary sodium concentration varies according to the patient's sodium intake.

More frequently the losses of water are of renal origin, as in diabetes insipidus. Diabetes insipidus is a polyuric disorder characterized by high rates of electrolyte-free water excretion. Hypernatremia supervenes when these losses are not appropriately replaced. Depending on whether the water losses are caused by a failure to secrete vasopressin or renal resistance to the hormone, the diabetes insipidus is designated as being central or nephrogenic, respectively.

Central Diabetes Insipidus

Failure to normally synthesize or secrete vasopressin limits maximal urinary concentration and causes varying degrees of polyuria and polydipsia, depending on the severity of the disease. The causes of central diabetes insipidus are listed in Table 1.1.

In a survey of 79 children and young adults, the disease was idiopathic in 52%, with a significant number having tumors and Langerhans cell histiocytosis. Most had magnetic resonance imaging (MRI) findings and some had thickening of the pituitary stalk that may reflect lymphocytic infiltration as part of an autoimmune process. The probability of also developing anterior pituitary hormone deficiency was 80% in the group who had tumors, compared with 50% in subjects with idiopathic diabetes insipidus (22,23). The disease may rarely be inherited. Families with an autosomal dominant inheritance pattern have been described (24). Mutations in the coding region of the gene in all three exons have been described affecting one allele. These mutations are in the signal protein and neurophysin. Most are missense mutation, but other mutations have been described as well (24). What is peculiar about this inherited form of central diabetes insipidus is that the onset of symptoms are delayed for several months after birth and sometimes even longer. It appears that the mutant hormone forms complexes with the native hormone and the accumulation of these complexes in the endoplasmic reticulum causes

TABLE 1.1 CAUSES OF CENTRAL DIABETES INSIPIDUS

Hereditary
Autosomal dominant
Autosomal recessive (Wolfram syndrome)

Acquired
Head trauma, skull fracture, and orbital trauma
Posthypophysectomy
Suprasellar and intrasellar tumors
   Primary (suprasellar cyst, craniopharyngioma, pinealoma, meningioma, and glioma)
   Metastatic (breast or lung cancer, leukemia, and lymphomas)

Granulomas
   Sarcoid
   Wegener granulomatosis
   Tuberculosis
   Syphilis

Histiocytosis
   Eosinophilic granuloma
   Hand–Schüller–Christian disease

Infections
   Encephalitis
   Meningitis
   Guillain–Barré syndrome

Vascular
   Cerebral aneurysm
   Cerebral thrombosis or hemorrhage
   Sickle cell disease
   Postpartum necrosis (Sheehan syndrome)
   Pregnancy (transient)

From Levi M, Berl T. Water metabolism. In: Gonick HC, ed. *Current Nephrology,* vol. 5. Chicago: Year Book Medical Publishers; 1982:23, with permission.

progressive loss of vasopressin producing neurons (25). There is also a rare inherited autosomal recessive form of central diabetes insipidus that occurs in association with diabetes mellitus, optic atrophy, and deafness (Wolfram syndrome). The syndrome appears to result from mutations in region PC 16 of chromosome 4, which codes form a protein expressed in various tissues (26).

Head trauma, hypophysectomy, and neoplasms, either primary or metastatic (mainly from lung and breast tumors), constitute most of the other causes. Other etiologic factors include encephalitis, sarcoidosis, eosinophilic granuloma, and histiocytosis. Finally, central diabetes insipidus has been described following development of cerebral edema in 11 postoperative hyponatremic women (27).

Clinical Features

Polyuria and polydipsia are the hallmarks of central diabetes insipidus and must be considered in the differential diagnosis of any patient who presents with such symptoms. As illustrated in Figure 1.10, polyuria can occur from a solute diuresis, in which case C_{osm} is increased and the urine osmolality is >300 mOsm/kg. A diagnosis of central (vasopressin deficient) diabetes insipidus should be considered when polyuria is caused by an increase in C_{H_2O} and urine osmolality is <150 mOsm/kg. Urine flow can range between 3 and 15 L/day, depending on the severity of the disease. The disorder frequently has an abrupt onset and occurs with equal frequency in both sexes. Although the time of onset is extremely variable, it is rare in infancy and is most frequent in the 10- to 20-year age group. Patients with central diabetes insipidus often have a predilection for cold water. Nocturia frequently is marked because there is little diurnal variation in the polyuria. Bladder capacity may be increased in untreated patients, however; consequently, nocturia may not be a prominent symptom. Nevertheless, nocturia is frequent generally, and sleep deprivation commonly leads to fatigue and irritability. Patients with central diabetes insipidus do not develop hypernatremia if the thirst mechanism is intact and water is available; thus, they have no symptoms except for the inconvenience associated with marked polyuria and polydipsia. However, severe and even life-threatening hypernatremia can supervene with concomitant hypodipsia, no access to water, or an illness that precludes adequate water intake.

Diagnosis

The development of severe polyuria and polydipsia (>6 to 8 L/day) in an adult patient who does not have diabetes mellitus (the most common cause of a solute diuresis) indicates the possibility of either a failure of vasopressin release, that is, central diabetes insipidus or excessive water intake, that is, compulsive water drinking (perhaps better termed "dipsogenic diabetes insipidus" or primary polydipsia). Profound polyuria in childhood is more likely to be congenital nephrogenic diabetes insipidus, a disorder that is discussed later.

The differential diagnosis between central diabetes insipidus and primary polydipsia drinking may be very difficult. Plasma vasopressin levels are diminished in both circumstances. This is caused by impaired synthesis or secretion of vasopressin in central diabetes insipidus. Thus, these patients have polydipsia secondary to impaired renal water conservation in the absence of AVP. In contrast, the patient with primary polydipsia ingests large amounts of fluids, which physiologically suppress endogenous AVP release, resulting in the urinary excretion of the large volume of ingested water. Thus, the patient with central diabetes insipidus has polydipsia because of polyuria, whereas the individual with primary polydipsia has polyuria because of polydipsia. Abnormalities in the hypothalamic-pituitary region can be seen in a majority of patients with central diabetes insipidus with the use of the computed tomography (CT) scan MRI may improve the sensitivity further (22). Normally on T1-weighted images, the posterior pituitary produces a bright signal that is indistinguishable from fatty tissue, but this signal is lost in patients with central diabetes insipidus (28).

The patient's history can be helpful in making the differential diagnosis. Whereas the patient with central diabetes insipidus has an abrupt onset of polyuria and polydipsia, the patient with primary polydipsia has a more vague history of the onset of these symptoms. The latter patients also may have a history of considerable variation in water intake and urine output on an hour-to-hour or day-to-day basis, whereas the patient with central diabetes insipidus has a very consistent need for water intake. Large variations in water intake, in the patient whose intakes and outputs are measured, therefore are a clue to the diagnosis of compulsive water drinking. Nocturia is more severe and frequent in subjects with central diabetes insipidus. Finally, the previously noted preference for ice water usually is not described by subjects with primary polydipsia. These patients also may have a history of psychiatric disorders and not infrequently are women during menopause. A plasma osmolality below 270 mOsm/kg H_2O strongly suggests primary polydipsia because the modest positive fluid balance while the patient with central diabetes insipidus is generally in modest negative fluid balance. Thus, a sodium >143 mm/L or plasma osmolality above 295 mOsm/kg H_2O essentially excludes primary polydipsia and suggests central diabetes insipidus. Although the differentiation between central and dipsogenic diabetes insipidus in their classic forms may pose no difficulties, the correct diagnosis is frequently difficult to make when the defect in vasopressin release is partial. A fluid deprivation test may provide the most reliable information regarding the assessment of these polyuric disorders (Fig. 1.12) (9). Fluid deprivation must be instituted with careful monitoring of body weight and vital signs, because the patient with central diabetes insipidus may rapidly develop a severe negative fluid balance. The test is stopped when body weight decreases by >3%, the patient develops orthostatic blood pressure changes, the serum sodium is >145 mmol/L, or the urine osmolality reaches a plateau in three consecutive hourly collections. This period of fluid deprivation is followed by the injection of 5 U of aqueous vasopressin or 1 μg of 1-desamino-D-arginine vasopressin or desmopressin acetate (brand name dDAVP) subcutaneously. Normal subjects require 16 to 18 hours to achieve a mean maximum urine osmolality of approximately 1,000 to 1,200 mOsm/kg and the administration of vasopressin causes no further increase in their urine osmolality. This suggests that the dehydration test has maximally stimulated endogenous vasopressin release. One might surmise, therefore, that fluid deprivation readily discriminates between those with a normal neurohypophyseal system, such as those with primary polydipsia, and the patient with central diabetes insipidus. As illustrated in Figure 1.12, this is not always the case. Observations of normal subjects who have drunk large daily volumes of water, however, have demonstrated a blunted response to vasopressin (29). A decrease in medullary tonicity occurs, previously occurs a result of an increase in

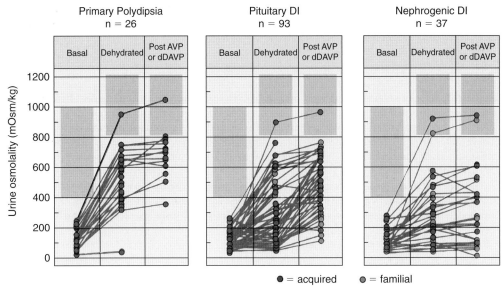

● = acquired   ● = familial

■ **Figure 1.12** Effects of fluid deprivation and subsequent AVP (Pitressin) administration on urine osmolality in 156 patients with polyuria of diverse causes. The shaded area indicate the range of values in healthy adults. Note that, although AVP responses tended to be greater in patients with central (neurogenic) DI, the overlap between the three groups is significant. (From Brenner BM; *The Kidney*; Philadelphia, PA: Saunders Elsevier; 2008, with permission.)

medullary blood flow, is associated with the diminution in renal concentrating capacity. For this reason, patients with primary polydipsia may demonstrate submaximal concentrating ability after fluid deprivation, but their urine osmolality still generally exceeds 300 mOsm/kg. There is, however, no further increase with exogenous vasopressin because endogenous vasopressin secretion is maximal with fluid deprivation. This serves to differentiate such patients from those with central diabetes insipidus, whose urine osmolality substantially increases (>10%) following the administration of vasopressin Figure 1.12. The recognition of patients who have only a partial defect in AVP secretion is of particular importance. Urine osmolalities in these patients and those with primary polydipsia may be similar after fluid deprivation, but only the patient with partial diabetes insipidus will respond further to exogenous vasopressin. If exogenous vasopressin increases urine osmolality by >10% after fluid deprivation, a defect in AVP release is probably present. Only patients with complete diabetes insipidus may demonstrate overt clinical symptoms of polyuria and polydipsia, whereas patients with partial central diabetes insipidus may remain asymptomatic. The measurement of urinary aquaporins has been suggested to differentiate various forms of diabetes insipidus (30) and more specifically to differentiate psychogenic polydipsia for central diabetes insipidus (31). Urinary AQP_2 was decreased in subjects with central deficiency AVP, but not in those with psychogenic polydipsia. The clinical applicability of this test is limited at this time.

The above described water deprivation test followed by exogenous AVP administration is useful in the differential diagnosis of polyuric disorders in 95% of cases; it is time consuming and requires considerable patient cooperation. Occasionally the diagnosis of central diabetes insipidus needs to be made more promptly or in acutely ill subjects. An examination of the relationship between plasma osmolality (excluding glucose and urea) and urine osmolality can be helpful. The finding of a low urine osmolality as plasma tonicity rises during a brief period of water withdrawal suggests the diagnosis of central diabetes insipidus.

Measurements of circulating AVP can serve as a valuable adjunct to the water deprivation test and in large measure confirmed the diagnosis reached by the dehydration test in most patients. The incorporation of vasopressin measurements by a sensitive radioimmunoassay may complement and refine the accuracy of previously available tests in the differential diagnosis of polyuric syndromes, but is not essential to the establishment of the various diagnosis and is not routinely measured.

TABLE 1.2 THERAPEUTIC REGIMENS FOR THE TREATMENT OF DIABETES INSIPIDUS

	Drug	Dose
Complete central diabetes insipidus	dDAVP	10–20 μg intranasally q q 12–24 h
	Oral	100–800 μg/d
Partial central diabetes insipidus	dDAVP	As above
	Aqueous vasopressin	5–10 U SQ q 4–6 h
	Chlorpropamide	250–500 mg/day
	Clofibrate	500 mg t.i.d.–q.i.d.
	Carbamazepine	400–600 mg/day
Nephrogenic diabetes insipidus	Thiazide diuretics	
	Amiloride (for lithium-related NDI)	5 mg q.i.d.
Gestational diabetes insipidus	dDAVP	As above

dDAVP, desmopressin acetate; NDI, nephrogenic diabetes insipidus; NSAID, nonsteroidal antiinflammatory drug.

From Thurman J, Berl T. Therapy in nephrology and hypertension. In: Wilcox CS, ed. *Therapy in Nephrology and Hypertension.* 3 ed. Phialdelphia, PA: WB Saunders; 2008:337–352, with permission.

Treatment

Patients with central diabetes insipidus do not develop hypernatremia if the thirst mechanism is intact and water is available; thus, they have no symptoms except for the inconvenience associated with marked polyuria and polydipsia. AVP replacement and pharmacologic agents both are available for the treatment of central diabetes insipidus (Table 1.2). In acute settings, such as after hypophysectomy, the aqueous vasopressin (Pitressin) preparation is preferable. Its short duration of action allows for more careful monitoring and decreases the likelihood of complications such as water intoxication.

A modification of the natural vasopressin molecule to form dDAVP has resulted in a compound with prolonged antidiuretic activity (6 to 24 hours) and virtual elimination of V_1 vasopressor receptor activity (antidiuretic to pressor ratio of approximately 2,000:1) as compared with the natural hormone AVP (duration of action of 2 to 4 hours and antidiuretic to pressor ratio of approximately 1:1) (32). Substitution D-arginine for L-arginine at position 8 resulted in a peptide DAVP with diminished vasopressor activity, and deamination of the hemicysteine at position 1 gave rise to a second peptide, with enhanced antidiuretic pressor activity and prolonged duration of action. dDAVP is administered intranasally in a dosage ranging from 10 to 20 μg every 8 to 12 hours. The drug has eliminated the need for previously employed long-acting vasopressin in oil. There are considerable individual variations in the required dosage, but most patients require twice daily administration for good control of polyuria. It can be also administered intravenously or subcutaneously during periods of respiratory illness or surgery in doses between 1 μg and 4 μg. It is active orally at large doses also (between 50 and 800 μg) (33).

Large doses of dDAVP may cause transient headaches, nausea, and a slight increase in blood pressure; these symptoms disappear if the dosage is reduced. Nasal congestion, mild abdominal cramps, and vulval pain have occurred rarely. These patients need careful monitoring of water intake and serum sodium to avoid development of hyponatremia. In fact, there are increasing reports of cases of hyponatremia in patients on these agents, particularly when used for other indications such as von Willebrand disease (34) and enuresis (35).

Intranasal dDAVP currently is the treatment of choice for partial or complete central diabetes insipidus. However, alternatives to hormone replacement may be helpful at times. With dilute urine of fixed low osmolality, the urine volume is determined by the solute load requiring excretion. A reduction of salt and protein in the diet therefore will reduce the major urinary solutes and thus the volume of urine necessary to accommodate their excretion. Moreover, a number of pharmacologic agents with antidiuretic properties are used; the hypoglycemic agent chlorpropamide (Diabinese) is the most commonly employed. Its antidiuretic effects are manifested only if some vasopressin is present; therefore, it is useful only in partial diabetes insipidus. A trial of 250 mg every day or twice a day may be offered to patients with partial central diabetes insipidus and at least 7 days allowed for an effect to occur. The anticonvulsant carbamazepine (Tegretol) has caused antidiuresis in subjects with central diabetes insipidus. A combination of chlorpropamide and carbamazepine has been found to provide an effect that could be synergistic (32). Clofibrate also has been used to treat partial central diabetes insipidus. At present, however, none of these approaches can be recommended over intranasal dDAVP.

Congenital Nephrogenic Diabetes Insipidus

Congenital nephrogenic diabetes insipidus is a rare hereditary disorder in which the renal tubule is insensitive to vasopressin (36). The disease has been described in various patterns, including the X-linked form, and autosomal recessive and even an autosomal dominant form. The most common variety is the X-linked whose complete form manifests itself in males, with females expressing variable degrees of polyuria and polydipsia. In 85% of patients the disease is a consequence of mutations on the V_2 receptor, resulting in a loss of function (37). To date, >180 mutations of the V_2 receptor in chromosome region Xq28, have been identified (38). Half are missense mutations but other types of mutations occur as well. A significant number of the mutant receptors have defective intracellular trafficking (36). The autosomal recessive form of congenital nephrogenic diabetes insipidus is due to a mutation in the AQP_2 water channel and accounts for approximately 15% of disease (39). To date, at least 30 disease causing mutations have been identified, most of them of the missense type. As was the case with the V_2 receptor mutant, misrouting of the AQP_2 mutant protein has been described in the setting (40). Finally, it appears that mutations at the *C*-terminal of AQP_2 can cause a rare autosomal dominant form of congenital nephrogenic diabetes insipidus (41). A modest concentrating defect is present also in humans deficient in the AQP_1 water channel (42). Finally, knockout mice lacking AQP_3 and/or AQP_4 also fail to maximally concentrate their urine (43).

Clinical Manifestations

Distinct phenotype differences among the various genotypes have not been completely described. The most complete clinical description is available for the X-linked form. Although the disease is most probably inborn, the diagnosis of this form of congenital nephrogenic diabetes insipidus is usually not made until the infant presents with a hypoosmolar urine in the face of severe dehydration, hypernatremia, vomiting, and fever. Unlike some of the females, who have partial responsiveness to vasopressin, males with the full-blown complete form of this disorder do not elaborate a hypertonic urine even in the face of severe dehydration. The impaired growth and occasional mental retardation that occurs in these cases, if not treated with adequate fluids, are most likely the result of repeated episodes of dehydration and hypernatremia rather than being integral components of the disease. Hydronephrosis is common in these patients perhaps because of voluntary retention of large volumes of urine with subsequent vesicoureteral reflux.

Treatment

Neither vasopressin nor other pharmacologic agents that potentiate its action or stimulate its release (e.g., chlorpropamide) are effective in concentrating the urine of patients with congenital nephrogenic diabetes insipidus. Consequently, an intact thirst mechanism is indispensable for the maintenance of good hydration in children with this disorder, as is careful monitoring of fluid balance. Children with this disorder who need rehydration should receive hypotonic (2.5%) rather than isotonic (5%) glucose solutions because the excretion of solute requires further water losses. Glucosuria may occur with the latter solution and thus aggravate fluid losses.

Limitation of oral solute intake (low-sodium diet) also may lead to a decrease in urine flow in patients with nephrogenic diabetes insipidus. Thiazide diuretics, which inhibit sodium reabsorption in the cortical diluting segment of the nephron, have met with some success in the management of these patients. The ability of thiazides to diminish sodium reabsorption in this water-impermeable portion of the nephron would by itself decrease C_{H_2O} but not urine flow. It seems most likely that the decrease in urine flow is secondary to the sodium loss and ECF volume contraction. ECF volume depletion in turn decreases GFR and increases proximal tubular sodium and water reabsorption. These secondary effects of the diuretic agent then decrease urine flow. The ECF volume contraction can be maintained with a low-sodium intake after discontinuance of the diuretic, so that the therapy still remains effective. The addition of amiloride to hydrochlorothiazide may provide added benefit. Nonsteroidal antiinflammatory drugs have been found to be effective, and in this regard, tolmetin appears to be particularly well tolerated in children. It should be noted that none of these modalities results in the elaboration of a hypertonic urine. Even an increase in urine osmolality from 50 to 200 mOsm/kg H_2O is very important, however, because it significantly reduces obligatory urine loss from 10 to 12 L/day to a tolerable 3 to 4 L/day. Such a change in urine flow also minimizes the dilatation of the urinary tract. An intriguing new approach involves the use of cell-permeable vasopressin antagonists as chaperones that facilitate the folding of the mutant protein retained in the endoplasmic reticulum and increase the expression of the cell surface (44). In one study of subjects with nephrogenic diabetes insipidus this approach resulted in a decrease in urine flow from 12 to 8 L with a modest increase in urinary osmolality (45).

Acquired Nephrogenic Diabetes Insipidus

The acquired form of nephrogenic diabetes insipidus is much more common than the congenital form of the disease, but it is rarely severe. In fact, although maximal concentrating ability is impaired in this disorder, the ability to elaborate a hypertonic urine usually is preserved. Nocturia, polyuria, and polydipsia may occur in this acquired form of nephrogenic diabetes insipidus, but the urine volumes generally are less (<3 to 4 L/day) than those observed with complete central diabetes insipidus, psychogenic water drinking, or congenital nephrogenic central diabetes insipidus. The more common causes of acquired nephrogenic diabetes insipidus are listed in Table 1.3.

TABLE 1.3 CAUSES OF ACQUIRED NEPHROGENIC DIABETES INSIPIDUS

Chronic Renal Disease
Polycystic disease
Medullary cystic disease
Ureteral obstruction
Amyloidosis
Advanced renal failure of any etiology

Electrolyte Disorders
Hypokalemia
Hypercalcemia

Drugs
Alcohol
Phenytoin
Lithium
Demeclocycline
Acetohexamide
Tolazamide
Glyburide
Propoxyphene
Amphotericin
Foscarnet
Methoxyflurane
Norepinephrine
Vinblastine
Colchicine
Gentamicin
Methicillin
Isophosphamide
Angiographic dyes
Osmotic diuretics
Furosemide and ethacrynic acid

Sickle Cell Disease

Dietary Abnormalities
Excessive water intake
Decreased sodium chloride intake
Decreased protein intake

Miscellaneous
Gestational diabetes insipidus

Chronic Renal Failure

A defect in renal concentrating capacity is a consistent accompaniment of most forms of advanced renal failure. Thus, chronic renal failure constitutes a form of acquired nephrogenic diabetes insipidus. Advanced renal insufficiency of any cause can cause a vasopressin resistance associated with hypotonic urine (46).

In some forms of kidney disease, listed in Table 1.3, vasopressin unresponsiveness can occur at a stage when GFR is not markedly diminished. The occurrence of a profound diuresis in association with a concentrating defect in glomerular diseases of the kidney is rare, and in general, a close correlation exists between GFR and maximal urine osmolality.

The causes of the defect in renal concentrating capacity associated with chronic renal failure are probably multiple. These include: (a) a disruption of inner medullary structures or local alterations in medullary blood flow as is seen in tubulointerstitial diseases, sickle cell disease, and analgesic nephropathy; (b) an impairment in sodium chloride transport out of the thick ascending limb of loop of Henle, a process that limits maximal interstitial tonicity; and (c) an increase in solute excretion in the remaining few functioning nephrons, an adaptive response to the need to excrete the same solute load as the normal kidney. Solute diuresis in normal humans may cause isotonic urine in the presence of maximal amounts of vasopressin. However, none of these pathogenic mechanisms alone can explain the observation that vasopressin resistant hypotonic urine may be found in patients with advanced renal failure (46). If the assumption is made that even in the absence of a countercurrent system the tonicity of the renal medulla is never less than that of plasma, a failure of complete osmotic equilibration between the collecting duct and medullary interstitium must occur to explain vasopressin resistant hypotonic urine. One possibility is that the response to AVP of the collecting duct membranes in the damaged kidney is submaximal as a result from a selective downregulation of the V_2 receptor (47). In a model of 5/6 nephrectomy induced renal failure, a decrease in collecting duct AQP_2 and AQP_3 expression was reported (48). A similar decrement in AQP_2 has been described in obstructive uropathy and during recovery from acute tubular necrosis (Fig. 1.13).

Recognition of the renal concentration defect is foremost in the therapeutic approach. If the maximal renal concentrating capacity of a patient with chronic renal failure is 300 mOsm/kg H_2O and the daily solute load is 600 mOsm, a urine volume of 2 L/day is necessary to excrete the solute load. The patient's fluid intake, including 500 mL for insensible losses, must therefore be at least 2,500 mL/day. Thus, if the patient is ill and cannot ingest fluids for several days, severe water depletion can occur because of the failure of the kidney to concentrate the urine. Recognition of the subclinical concentrating defect, which can emerge as an important clinical problem during an acute illness, therefore is pivotal in the long-term management of patients with chronic renal failure.

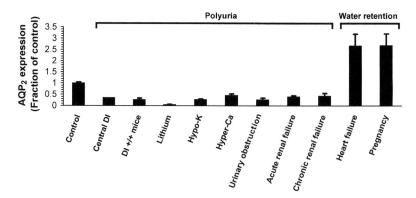

■ **Figure 1.13** Changes in AQP_2 expression seen in association with different water balance disorders. Levels are expressed as a percentage of control levels *(leftmost bar)*. AQP_2 expression is reduced, sometimes dramatically, in a wide range of hereditary and acquired forms of diabetes insipidus characterized by different degrees of polyuria. Conversely, congestive heart failure and pregnancy are conditions associated with increased expression of AQP_2 levels and excessive water retention. (From Neilsen S, Knepper MA, Kwon T-H, et al. Urine concentration and dilution. In: Schrier RW, ed. *Diseases of the Kidney and Uurinary Tract,* 7th ed., vol. 1. New York, NY: Lippincott Williams & Wilkins; 2000:128, with permission.)

Electrolyte Abnormalities

Hypokalemia of any cause has long been known to cause polyuria and a reversible form of a vasopressin-resistant renal concentrating defect. The pathogenesis is multifacotrial. Hypokalemia stimulates water intake and reduces interstitial tonicity, as a consequence of a decreased Na^+/Cl^- reabsorption in the thick ascending limb. Hypokalemia also decreases intracellular cAMP accumulation and causes a reduction in vasopressin-sensitive AQP_2 expression (49) (see Fig. 1.13).

Hypercalcemia also impairs urinary concentrating ability, resulting in mild polydipsia. The pathophysiology is also multifactorial and includes a reduction in medullary interstitial tonicity caused by decreased vasopressin-stimulated adenylate cyclase in the thick ascending limb and a defect in adenylate cyclase activity with decreased AQP_2 expression in the collecting duct (50,51) (Fig. 1.13).

Pharmacologic Agents

Various pharmacologic agents also have been found to impair the renal capacity to concentrate urine (Table 1.3). By virtue of its widespread use in the treatment of affective disorders, lithium has emerged as perhaps the most common cause of congenital nephrogenic diabetes insipidus, affecting as many as 50% of patients on the drug. Lithium decreases vasopressin-stimulated water transport in the perfused cortical collecting duct. This is most likely a consequence of inhibition of adenylate cyclase and cAMP generation (36). A marked downregulation AQP_2 and AQP_3 has been described in lithium treated rats (52). Lithium may also increase the expression of cyclooxygenase 2 a lead to increasing renal prostaglandins that contribute to the polyuira (53). The concentrating defect may be persistent and not entirely reversible.

Demeclocycline is another drug that causes nephrogenic diabetes insipidus. Because it is better tolerated than lithium, it is a better choice agent to treat the syndrome of inappropriate AVP release now, however, the recently approved orally active Tolvaptan, maybe preferable treatment for SIADH. The precise cellular mechanism whereby demeclocycline causes this effect has not been elucidated.

Sickle Cell Anemia

A renal concentrating defect is a common accompaniment of sickle cell anemia and sickle cell trait. Sickling of red blood cells in the hypertonic medullary interstitium with occlusion of the vasa recta appears to cause inner medullary and papillary damage. Microradioangiographic studies have failed to demonstrate vasa recta blood flow in patients with sickle cell disease. The resultant medullary ischemia may impair sodium chloride transport in the ascending limb and thus diminish medullary tonicity. Transfusions of normal blood have been shown to restore renal concentrating capacity in children, thus indicating that the sickled red blood cells have a role in the defect. Medullary infarcts occur with more prolonged disease, and the concentrating defect is no longer reversible with transfusions. The diminished maximal urine osmolality also occurs in sickle cell anemia in association with papillary edema, thus providing a situation analogous to experimental papillectomy.

Dietary Abnormalities

As noted in the discussion of primary polydipsia, excessive water intake culminates in an impairment of maximal urinary concentration. In a recent experimental study primary polydipsya did not decrease medullary interstitial tonicity, but an alteration in the cellular action of vasopressin was shown to be associated with downregulation of AQP_2 (54). A marked restriction in sodium chloride intake also impairs the urinary concentrating mechanism. A similar defect is encountered in states of severe protein restriction. Because urea and sodium chloride account for virtually all interstitial tonicity, their decreased availability may account in large part for the observed defect. A defect in water reabsorption related to decrement in aquaporin expression has been invoked (55).

Gestational Diabetes Insipidus

An acquired form of diabetes insipidus has been described in pregnancy that is AVP unresponsive. An increase in circulating vasopressinase, leading to excessive catabolism explains the vasopressin

TABLE 1.4 THERAPEUTIC HYPERTONIC SOLUTIONS

Solute	Molecular Weight	Concentration (mg/dL)	Osmolality (mOsm/kg H_2O)	Typical Container Size (mL)	Use
Sodium chloride	58.5	3	1,026	500	Emergency treatment of hypotonic states; intraamniotic instillation for therapeutic abortion
		5	1,711	500	
		20	6,845	250	
Sodium bicarbonate	84.0	5	1,190	500	Treatment of metabolic acidosis, hyperkalemia, cardiopulmonary arrest
		7.5	1,786	50	

From Morrison G, Singer I. Hyperosmolal states. In: Narins RG, ed. *Clinical Disorders of Fluid and Electrolyte Metabolism.* New York, NY: McGraw-Hill; 1994:646, Part I, with permission.

resistance (56). Such patients can develop severe hypernatremia. However, because dDAVP is not affected by vasopressinase, this agent can reduce urine flow and can serve as a diagnostic tool of this entity.

HYPERNATREMIA IN PATIENTS WITH INCREASED TOTAL BODY SODIUM

Hypernatremia with increased total body sodium is the least common type of hypernatremia and is usually caused by exogenous administration of hypertonic sodium containing solutes (Table 1.4). Hypernatremia supervenes during resuscitative efforts with hypertonic sodium bicarbonate, inadvertent intravascular infusion of hypertonic saline in therapeutic abortions, inadvertent dialysis against a high sodium concentration dialysate, seawater drowning, and even after ingestion of large quantities of sodium chloride tablets. Patients with primary hyperaldosteronism and Cushing syndrome have slight, clinically unimportant elevations in serum sodium concentration. As expected, patients with hypernatremia and high total body sodium excrete generous quantities of the cation in the urine concentrate of their urine (Fig. 1.11).

Signs and Symptoms of Hypernatremia

Hypernatremia always reflects a hyperosmolar state. The most prominent manifestations of hyperosmolar disorders are of a neurologic nature. These follow movement of water out of cells, resulting in a cellular dehydration, particularly in the brain. The signs and symptoms of hypernatremia are listed in Table 1.5. Restlessness, irritability, depression of sensorium, lethargy, muscular twitching, hyperreflexia, and spasticity may occur and culminate in coma, seizures, and death. The morbidity and mortality of hypernatremia, particularly in the acute forms, are very high. In children, the mortality of acute

TABLE 1.5 SIGNS AND SYMPTOMS OF HYPERNATREMIA

Depression of sensorium
Irritability
Seizures (unusual in adults)
Focal neurologic deficits
Muscle spasticity (unusual in adults)
Signs of volume depletion (variable)
Fever
Nausea or vomiting
Labored respiration
Intense thirst

From Lanese D, Teitelbaum I. Hypernatremia. In: Jacobson HR, Striker GE, Klahr S, eds. *The Principles and Practice of Nephrology,* 2nd ed. St. Louis: Mosby; 1995:896, with permission.

hypernatremia ranges between 10% and 70%, with a mean of approximately 45%. Unfortunately, neurologic sequelae are common even in survivors, affecting as many as two-thirds of the children. Mortality in chronic hypernatremia is approximately 10%. In adults, acute elevation of serum sodium above 160 mEq/L is associated with 75% mortality, whereas the mortality in chronic cases is approximately 60%. It must be pointed out, however, that hypernatremia frequently occurs in the adult in the setting of serious underlying diseases, which may be the primary cause of the high mortality. The sequelae of hypernatremia in adults have not been studied systematically.

The signs and symptoms of hypernatremia are most likely related to a variety of anatomic derangements. The loss of volume and shrinkage of brain cells associated with the hyperosmolar states cause tearing of cerebral vessels. In addition to these gross anatomic changes, the brain sustains alterations in the composition of water and solutes that may be of great importance in the pathophysiology of the symptoms of hypernatremia (57). These are responses designed to regulate volume and restore cell size; thus, the water losses are not as severe as would be predicted. In the early phase, the entry of sodium and chloride into brain cells greatly mitigates the loss of water that would otherwise occur from ideal osmotic behavior. After 7 days of hypernatremia, brain water has returned to control levels because brain osmolality remains elevated. At this time, newly generated idiogenic osmoles account for as much as 60% of the increase in intracellular osmolality. Some of these idiogenic osmoles result from an increase in intracellular amino acids, particularly taurine. In addition, accumulation of osmolytes such as urea, glutamine, glycerophosphorylcholine, and myoinositol has been documented in hypernatremic rats (58).

Prevention of Hypernatremia

Because hypernatremia occurs in predictable clinical settings, early recognition may allow prevention or decreased severity of injury. Elderly persons, hospitalized patients receiving hypertonic infusions, those suffering increased insensible losses or undergoing osmotic losses, diabetic patients, and patients with previous symptoms of polydipsia and polyuria should invoke a high index of suspicion when displaying neurologic alterations.

Compared with younger individuals, geriatric patients have impaired thirst responses, decreased urinary concentrating ability, and lower baseline levels of total body water. As a result, elderly patients are the group most likely to develop severe hypernatremia in the outpatient setting, and hypernatremia in the elderly accounts for 1% to 2% of all hospital admissions. The most common scenario is that of a debilitated patient with a febrile illness. Increased insensible losses are not compensated because of impaired access to solute-free water. Recognition of mental status changes in settings of increased insensible losses should prompt close attention to the serum sodium and increased administration of solute-free water.

Hospitalized patients also are susceptible to the development of hypernatremia. Compared with outpatients, individuals developing hypernatremia during a hospital admission are more likely to be younger and to have an iatrogenic etiology (59). Inpatients with high insensible losses (e.g., patients on mechanical ventilators) develop hypernatremia because of restricted access to water and inadequate fluid prescriptions. Hypertonic fluid administration (e.g., sodium bicarbonate) and osmotic diuretics including mannitol and urea also may result in hypertonicity. Hyperosmolar tube feedings may induce diarrhea and gastrointestinal water losses, and the large daily osmolar load may lead to increased electrolyte-free water losses. Palevsky et al. (59) noted that despite frequent serum sodium measurements, treatment of hypernatremia was often delayed. Fifty percent of patients with serum sodiums >150 mM/L did not receive hypotonic fluid within 24 hours of becoming hypernatremic, and only 36% were corrected within 72 hours. The development of hypernatremia in the intensive care setting is associated with prolonged hospitalization and increased mortalilty (60). This is clearly a preventable complication.

Therapy of Hypernatremia

The primary goal in the treatment of hypernatremia is the restoration of serum tonicity. The specific approach depends on the patient's ECF volume (Fig. 1.11). The following principles are useful (61):

1. Isotonic sodium chloride should be given until systemic hemodynamics are stabilized when the patient has low total body sodium, as evidenced by circulatory manifestations (e.g., orthostatic hypotension). Thereafter, the hypernatremia can be treated with .45% sodium chloride or 5% dextrose.

TABLE 1.6 GENERAL GUIDELINES FOR THE TREATMENT OF SYMPOTOMATIC HYPERNATREMIA

Correct at rate of 2 mEq/L/h
Replace half calculated water deficit over first 12–24 h
Replace remaining deficit over the next 24 h
Perform serial neurological examinations; prescribed rate of correction can be decreased with improvement in symptoms
Perform measurements of serum and urine electrolytes every 1–2 h

From Thurman J, Berl T. Therapy in nephrology and hypertension. In: Wilcox CS, ed. *Therapy in Nephrology and Hypertension.* 3 ed. Phialdelphia, PA: WB Saunders; 2008:337–352, with permission.

2. When the patient is hypervolemic and hypernatremic, the removal of excess sodium is the goal, which can be achieved either by administration of diuretics along with 5% dextrose or, if renal function is impaired, by dialysis.
3. The euvolemic hypernatremic patient who has sustained pure water losses requires water replacement as a 5% dextrose infusion. The water deficit in this setting can be calculated on the basis of the serum sodium concentration and on the assumption that 60% of the body's weight is water. It can be expressed by the equation:

$$Water deficit = 0.6 \times bodyweight\ (kg) \times P_{NA}/140 - 1 \qquad (1.5)$$

Thus, in a patient who weighs 75 kg and presents with a serum sodium of 154 mEq/L, the water deficit can be calculated as

$$0.6 \times 75 \times (154/140 - 1)$$
$$45 \times (1.1 - 1)$$
$$45 \times 0.1 = 4.5\ L \qquad (1.6)$$
$$154/140 \times 45\ L = 49.5\ L$$
$$49.5 - 45.0 = 4.5\ L$$

This represents the water deficit and is the net positive water balance necessary to correct the hypernatremia. In addition ongoing losses of free water require replacement as well to achieve normonatremia.

The general guidelines for the treatment of symptomatic hypernatremia are listed in Table 1.6 (61). The rapidity with which the correction should be made has been a matter of some controversy, primarily as concerns the pediatric population (62). In children, two studies suggest a correction rate of <0.5 mEq/L/h because no seizures occurred in treated children, whereas 20% of those treated more rapidly had seizures (62,63). Most feel that even in adults correction should be achieved in >48 hours and at a rate not >2 mEq/h. It is likely that the described cerebral adjustments to hypernatremia, whereby brain water content is corrected and new solutes are generated, increases the risk for seizures during the correction phase. As extracellular osmolality is rapidly decreased, an osmotic gradient may develop between brain and plasma. This would result in net movement of water into the brain, causing cerebral edema. A slower rate of correction probably can prevent this sequence of events by allowing idiogenic osmoles time to be dissipated.

In patients with essential hypernatremia and the elderly with hypodipsia, 1 to 2 L of water per day may need to be administered as a prescription. Chlorpropamide itself augments thirst, and its use in conjunction with dDAVP in patients with adipsia has been proposed.

Clinical Disorders of Renal Diluting Capacity: Hyponatremic States

While the disorders of renal concentrating capacity described in this chapter may be associated with water depletion and hypernatremia, disorders of renal diluting capacity most frequently present with hyponatremia. Sodium and its accompanying anions account for nearly all the osmotic activity of plasma (64).

TABLE 1.7 RELATIONSHIP BETWEEN SERUM TONICITY AND SODIUM CONCENTRATION IN THE PRESENCE OF OTHER SUBSTANCES

Condition of Substance	Serum Tonicity	Serum Sodium
Hyperglycemia	↑	↓
Mannitol, maltose, glycine	↑	↓
Anzotemia (high blood urea)	↑	↔
Ingestion of ethanol, methanol, ethylene glycol	↑	↔
Elevated serum lipid and/or protein	↔	↓[a]

[a]As measured by flame photometer.

From Berl T., Robertson GL. Pathology of water metabolism. In: Brenner BM, Rector FC Jr, eds. *The Kidney*, 6th ed. Philadelphia, PA: WB Saunders, 2000:894, with permission.

Calculated serum osmolality $= (2Na^+ +$ blood urea nitrogen $(mg/dl)/2.8 +$ glucose $(g/dl)/18)$.

An increase in serum sodium always reflects hyperosmolality, hyponatremia usually is associated with hypoosmolality, and the most common setting in which the serum sodium does not reflect serum osmolality occurs when there is an additional osmolyte such as ethanol, methanol, or ethylene glycol in the ECF. An osmolar gap is said to be present when the preceding calculated serum osmolality is >10 mOsm lower than the osmolality directly measured by the osmometer. It must be noted also that the nature of the solute determines whether there is an increase only in measured osmolality, but not effective osmolality and whether the serum sodium concentration is altered (Table 1.7). Solutes that are permeable across cell membranes such as urea, methanol, ethanol, and ethylene glycol increased measured but not effective osmolality. Thus, they do not cause water movement from cells, therefore hypertonicity occurs without causing cellular dehydration. There is therefore no alteration in serum sodium concentration. A high blood urea nitrogen (BUN) and ethanol intoxication are the most common settings in which this occurs. In contrast, glucose, in the insulinopenic state, is not permeable and establishes an effective osmotic gradient for water to leave the cell and move into the ECF compartment. This process lowers the serum sodium concentration, and hyponatremia can coexist with a normal or even elevated tonicity. Conceptually, this can be viewed as "translocational" hyponatremia, as an alteration in the plasma sodium concentration level does not reflect a change in total body water but rather reflects water movement from the intracellular to the extracellular space. This effect of hyperglycemia must be considered in the interpretation of the serum sodium, and an appropriate correction must be made. The decrease in plasma sodium is approximately 1.6 mEq/L for every 100 mg/dL increase in plasma glucose, but this calculation may somewhat underestimate the decrement in serum sodium (65). The serum sodium concentration returns to normal without specific intervention as the plasma glucose is lowered. Similar decrements in serum sodium concentration following the infusion of other osmotically active substance such as, mannitol, or the absorption of glycine during transurethral prostate resection or hysterectomies.

Pseudohyponatremia occurs when the solid phase of plasma (normally 6% to 8%) is markedly increased by large increments in serum lipids or protein, because the flame photometer measures sodium concentration of the entire plasma and not just the liquid phase concentrations. The use of a direct ion selective electrode, measuring only the sodium concentration of the liquid phase, eliminates this problem. Only a direct potentiometry measurement (undiluted sample) gives an accurate determination in this setting. The impact of specific increments in lipids and protein on measured serum sodium have recently been experimentally quantified (66). Plasma water content (%) $= 99.1 - (0.1 \times L) - (0.07 \times P)$.

Where L and P refer to the total lipid and protein concentration in gram per liter, respectively. For example, if the formula reveals that plasma water is 90% of the plasma sample rather than the normal 93% (which yields a serum sodium of 140 mmol/L as $150 \times 0.93 = 140$), the concentration of measured sodium would be expected to decrease to 135 mmol/L (150×0.90).

Hyponatremia is among the most common electrolyte disorders seen in clinical practice. Hyponatremia may be associated with decreased, increased, or near-normal amounts of total body sodium (67,68). This section attempts to discuss and categorize the disorders of renal diluting capacity and associated hyponatremia in relationship to total body sodium and ECF volume status. In each instance, the pathogenetic mechanisms that may be involved are considered.

Disorders of diluting capacity, depicted in Figure 1(**A**) are caused by (a) the continued secretion of AVP in spite of the presence of serum hypoosmolality, which does not allow the collecting duct to remain water impermeable; or (b) intrarenal factors, such as a decrease in GFR or proximal tubular fluid and sodium reabsorption, or both, which diminish the delivery of fluid to the distal diluting segments of the nephron. A defect in sodium chloride transport out of the water-impermeable portions of the nephron, including the cortical and medullary ascending limb of the loop of Henle, and particularly in the distal convoluted tubule is another intrarenal factor that impairs the nephron's capacity to dilute tubular fluid and urine.

In Figure 1.14 are summarized the diagnostic and therapeutic approach to hyponatremia discussed in this chapter. After the patient's hyponatremia is shown to reflect a truly hypotonic state, a thorough history and physical examination are essential in order to assess the volume status of the patient with hyponatremia. The diagnostic possibilities are narrowed once the patient is placed in one of three categories (edematous states, hypovolemic states, or neither). Examination of the urinary sodium concentration provides supportive evidence for the diagnosis. This diagnostic approach to hyponatremia also makes the appropriate therapy easy to define (61,68).

HYPONATREMIA ASSOCIATED WITH LOW TOTAL BODY SODIUM

In addition to hypothalamic osmoreceptors, another "physiologic" control of AVP release is the person's volume status as sensed by arterial baroreceptors (Fig. 1.7). As discussed, when the osmoreceptor and arterial barorecteptors for control of AVP receive opposing stimuli, the effect of the baroreceptors on AVP release generally predominates. Thus, in the presence of hypovolemia, AVP release is stimulated and water is retained, even at the expense of the occurrence of hypoosmolality. The glossopharyngeal and vagal afferent pathways from the aortic arch and carotid sinus are normally inhibited by the nonosmotic AVP stimulation. With a decrease in arterial pressure these baroreceptors are unloaded and AVP release is stimulated independent of osmolality. Receptors in the left atrium that are also present may modulate vagal afferent tone and AVP release. In the presence of volume depletion, a fall in pressure at the level of both the arterial baroreceptors and left atrium may inhibit afferent neural tone, an effect known to stimulate AVP release. Thus, the baroreceptor-stimulated secretion of vasopressin, coupled with high water intake (either oral or parenteral) culminates in hyponatremia.

Gastrointestinal and Third-Space Losses

The presence of hypovolemia, as judged by weight loss, orthostatic hypotension and tachycardia, and decreased central venous pressure, in association with hyponatremia, raises the question as to the source of the fluid and electrolyte losses. There are primarily two main sources for such losses, the kidney and gastrointestinal tract. In the presence of gastrointestinal losses (through either vomiting or diarrhea), the kidney responds by conserving sodium chloride. A similar pattern is observed with sequestration of fluids into third spaces, as in the peritoneal cavity in peritonitis and pancreatitis, or the bowel lumen with ileus and burns. In these entities, the urinary sodium concentration should be <10 mEq/L if renal function is normal. The urine osmolality also should be in the hyperosmolar range. Vomiting and metabolic alkalosis, in which bicarbonaturia is present, are exceptions. The urinary bicarbonate anion obligates cations and consequently may be associated with a urinary sodium concentration >20 mEq/L. However, the urinary chloride concentration is <10 mEq/L.

Diuretics

The kidney sometimes may be the source of the fluid and electrolyte losses. Excessive use of diuretics is one of the most common situations in which hyponatremia is associated with hypovolemia (69). Advanced age in underweight women appears to be an important risk factor. Hyponatremia occurs almost exclusively with thiazide rather than loop diuretics, presumably because the former do not impair urinary concentration but the latter does. Hyponatremia supervenes within 14 days of initiating diuretic therapy. Diuretics cause hyponatremia by at least three mechanisms: (a) volume depletion, which results in impaired water excretion by both an enhanced AVP release and decreased fluid delivery to the diluting segment; (b) a direct effect of diuretics on the diluting segment; and (c) potassium depletion. The mechanism whereby potassium depletion itself leads to hyponatremia is not entirely understood. However, it appears that it can occur independent of the sodium depletion that frequently

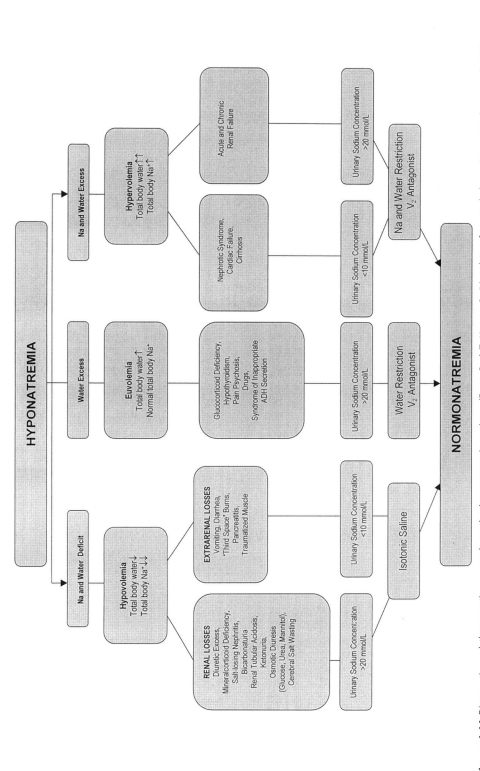

■ **Figure 1.14** Diagnostic and therapeutic approach to the hyponatremic patient. (From Berl T, Kumar S. Disorders of water balance in comprehensive clinical nephrology. In: Johnson RJ, Feehally J, eds. *Comprehensive Clinical Nephrology*. St. Louis: CV Mosby; 2000:3–9.7, with permission.)

accompanies diuretic use. An effect of hypokalemia to stimulate thirst and therefore increase water intake could aggravate any of the aforementioned mechanisms. It must be noted that the concomitant administration of potassium-sparing diuretics does not prevent the development of hyponatremia. Although the diagnosis of diuretic-induced hyponatremia frequently is obvious, surreptitious diuretic abuse is being increasingly recognized and should be considered in patients whose other electrolyte abnormalities such as hypokalemic metabolic alkalosis, and high urinary chloride excretions suggest this possibility.

Salt-Losing Nephritis

Salt losing nephritis is another condition with which hyponatremia and hypovolemia may be associated. In most circumstances, salt losing nephritis is associated with advanced chronic renal failure (GFR <20 mL/min). Nevertheless, salt losing nephritis may occur with less severe renal impairment with certain diseases, such as medullary cystic disease, polycystic disease, analgesic nephropathy, obstructive nephropathy, and chronic pyelonephritis.

Certain patients with renal tubular acidosis, particularly those with the proximal type II variety may exhibit sodium and potassium wastage despite only modest decreases in GFR. These patients have prominent bicarbonaturia because of a defect in the proximal tubule affecting the reclamation of bicarbonate (Chapter 3). As mentioned, bicarbonate is a relatively impermeant anion that obligates the renal excretion of cations, including primarily sodium and potassium. In this setting of renal tubular acidosis, the bicarbonaturia obligates the excretion of sodium, so that a minimal urinary sodium concentration is not achieved despite the presence of hypovolemia.

Mineralocorticoid Deficiency

A finding of hyponatremia and ECF volume depletion also suggests the possibility of primary adrenal insufficiency, particularly in the presence of a urinary sodium concentration higher than minimal, that is, >20 mEq/L. Because of the mineralocorticoid deficiency, a diminished urinary excretion of potassium and hyperkalemia is an indication that primary adrenal insufficiency is the cause of the hyponatremia. It is worthy of mention that urinary sodium concentration may become minimal when hypopituitarism is associated with hyponatremia because the renin–angiotensin–aldosterone pathway is intact.

The mechanisms whereby adrenal insufficiency impairs renal water excretion have been the subject of considerable debate and the effects of mineralocorticoid and glucocorticoid deficiency need to be considered separately. Studies in experimental animals suggest that mineralocorticoid deficiency and an associated negative sodium balance are at least partially responsible for impaired water excretion and hyponatremia as AVP secretion mediates this effect of sodium depletion on renal water excretion. AQP_2 and AQP_3 expressions are increased but the $Na^+/K^+/2Cl^-$ transporter in the outer medulla is decreased in mineralocorticoid deficient animals (70). ECF volume depletion with increased AVP and diminished renal hemodynamics mediate the effect of mineralocorticoid deficiency to cause hyponatremia.

OSMOTIC DIURESIS

An osmotic diuresis can lead to urinary losses of sodium and water, volume depletion, and hyponatremia in the face of either oral or parenteral water intake. The uncontrolled diabetic patient with glucosuria, and the patient with a urea diuresis after relief of urinary tract obstruction or undergoing a mannitol diuresis are examples of such causes of hyponatremia. The urinary sodium concentration generally is >20 mEq/L because the osmotic diuresis obligates cation excretion in spite of concomitant volume depletion. In patients with diabetes, the urinary sodium wasting caused by the glycosuria can be accentuated by ketonuria as hydroxybutyrate and acetoacetate, which also obligate urinary electrolyte losses. Ketonuria may contribute to the renal sodium wasting and hyponatremia seen in starvation and alcoholic ketoacidosis.

CEREBRAL SALT WASTING

Urinary sodium also exceeds 20 mEq/L despite hypovolemia in cerebral salt wasting, a syndrome primarily described in patients with subarachnoid bleeds. The mechanism is not fully understood and the hyponatremia can frequently not be reliably differentiated from the SIADH secretion, since the secretion of the hormone is critical to the development of the hyponatremia and the presence of hypovolemia is not always fully supported (71,72).

HYPONATREMIA ASSOCIATED WITH INCREASED TOTAL BODY SODIUM

Hyponatremia perhaps is observed most frequently in the edematous disorders. In this setting, both total body sodium and total body water are increased, but total body water is increased to a greater extent (Fig. 1.14). Because diuretics are used frequently in edematous disorders, hyponatremia presents a diagnostic dilemma as to whether the impairment in water excretion is owing to the diuretic therapy or primary disease. This is because the edematous disorders—including cirrhosis, cardiac failure, and nephrotic syndrome—may impair renal water excretion and be associated with hyponatremia in the absence of diuretic use.

Congestive Heart Failure

The common association between congestive heart failure and sodium and water retention is well established (38,73). The hyponatremia may be mediated by either a decreased delivery of tubular fluid to the distal nephron or an increased release of vasopressin, or both.

The decrement in "effective arterial blood volume" (74) with the decrease in arterial filling, secondary to a low cardiac output that is sensed by aortic and carotid sinus baroreceptors, causes nonosmotic stimulation of vasopressin release. This stimulation must supersede the inhibition in AVP release that usually accompanies acute distention of the left atrium that occurs with cardiac failure. Experiments using an AVP antagonist in a model of low cardiac output also point to an important role for the hormone in abnormal urinary dilution.

Following the development of a radioimmunoassay for vasopressin, several studies demonstrated elevated plasma AVP levels in patients with heart failure. It is most likely that nonosmotic pathways, whose activation is suggested by the increase in sympathetic activity seen in congestive heart failure, are the mediator of the hormone's release. Thus, an improvement of cardiac function with afterload reduction decreased AVP levels and improved water excretion in such patients. A decrease in plasma AVP levels also accompanied improvement of cardiac function by hemofiltration. It is of note that the V_2 antagonist lixivaptan decreased urinary osmolality, increased solute-free water excretion and increased serum sodium concentration in patients with New York Heart Association II and III heart failure (75–77). AQP_2 expression is increased in experimental heart failure (78) (Fig. 1.13). Furthermore, the V_2 antagonist lowers AQP_2 excretion, whose expression is enhanced in heart failure (78). Finally, it must be noted that the degree of hyponatremia is a powerful prognostic factor in patients with heart failure.

Hepatic Failure

Patients with advanced cirrhosis and ascites frequently present with hyponatremia as a consequence of their inability to excrete a water load (38). Early in cirrhosis, the increase in portal pressure increases splanchnic blood flow leading to a decrease in systemic vascular resistance. This in turn leads to arterial underfilling and activation of neurohumoral pathways including norepinephrine, the renin–angiotensin system and the nonosmotic release of vasopressin. In fact vasopressin levels have been found to be elevated in patients with cirrhosis and ascites. A predominant role for AVP secretion in the pathogenesis of the disorder has been demonstrated in experimental animals (79) and in humans (80). However, a vasopressin-independent intrarenal mechanism may contribute to the defect in water excretion as well. Nitric oxide (NO) may be an important mediator of the vasodilatation in this disorder (81), as inhibition of nitric oxide corrects the arterial hyporesponsiveness to vasodilators (82) and the abnormal water excretion in cirrhotic rats (81). As in heart failure, AQP_2 expression is increased in cirrhotic rats (83).

Nephrotic Syndrome

The incidence of hyponatremia in the nephrotic syndrome is lower than in either congestive heart failure or cirrhosis. An elevated level of plasma vasopressin also has been shown to occur in patients with nephrotic syndrome. In view of the alterations in Starling forces that accompany hypoalbuminemia and allow transudation of salt and water across capillary membranes into the interstitial space, many patients with the nephrotic syndrome have been considered to have intravascular volume contraction. Excretion leading to nonosmotic release of vasopressin. While this mechanism is most likely operant in minimal change disease and those with normal GFR, it may be less applicable to other patients with the nephrotic syndrome. Some of these patients have been shown to have increased plasma volumes with suppressed plasma renin activity and aldosterone levels. Such patients usually have decrements in GFR and a primary renal sodium–retaining disorder. In contrast to the increased AQP_2 found in the described sodium retaining disorders, the expression of the water channels is decreased in models of the nephrotic syndrome (84). The animals did not have hyponatremia and most likely had volume expansion to explain the discrepancy.

Advanced Chronic Renal Failure

The combination of hyponatremia and edema also may occur in patients with advanced renal failure, whether resulting from acute or chronic renal failure (85). Unlike subjects with edematous disorders, these patients do not have a minimal urinary sodium concentration because of the accompanying tubular dysfunction. The chronically diseased kidney also may exhibit a profound increase in fractional sodium excretion in an effort to maintain sodium balance despite its reduced number of functioning nephrons. Generally, edema develops because larger intakes of sodium are ingested than can be excreted by the diseased kidneys, which are filtering only a fraction of the amount of sodium filtered by normal kidneys. For example, at a GFR of 100 mL/min (144 L/day) and a plasma sodium concentration of 140 mEq/L, the daily filtered load of sodium (GFR × plasma sodium concentration) is 20,160 mEq. With a reduction in GFR to 5 mL/min, the daily amount of sodium filtered is only 1,008 mEq. The fractional excretion of sodium necessary to maintain sodium balance is much greater in the latter circumstance.

The narrow range of water handling by the diseased kidney is probably also caused in large part to the smaller volumes of fluid that are filtered daily by the diseased kidney. At a GFR of 5 mL/min, only 7.2 L of filtrate is formed daily, and perhaps 30%, or 2.2 L, of this filtered fluid will reach the diluting segment of the nephron. Thus, even with total suppression of AVP and water impermeability of the collecting duct, a maximum of 2.2 L of solute-free water could be excreted daily. If the daily water intake exceeds this volume, plus insensible losses, then a positive water balance and hyponatremia occur. Thus, in advanced chronic renal failure, the volume of fluid filtered and delivered to the diluting segment is of paramount importance to the renal capacity to excrete water. Although most patients with advanced renal failure (GFR < 10 mL/min) have little capacity to concentrate urine, some capacity to dilute urine may be preserved. As should be apparent from the foregoing discussion, however, the capacity to maintain water balance is dependent not only on the ability to dilute urine but also on the quantitative capacity of the kidney to excrete C_{H_2O}. With acute renal failure, the near absence of GFR provides a sufficient explanation for the virtual absence of the kidney to respond to a water load.

HYPONATREMIA WITH NORMAL TOTAL BODY SODIUM

In Figure 1.14 are listed the causes of euvolemic hyponatremia.

Glucocorticoid Deficiency

Glucocorticoid deficiency is important in the impaired water excretion of primary and secondary adrenal insufficiency. The mechanism is distinct form the one described for mineralocorticoid deficiency as there is no negative sodium balance and hypovolemia (38). An elevation of plasma AVP levels accompanies the water excretory defect of patients' anterior pituitary insufficiency (86) and glucocorticoid-deficient animals. Vasopressin antagonists reverse the water retaining disorder (87). AQP_2 expression is also increased in the medullary tissue of such animals (87). A direct effect of glucocorticoids in magnocellular neurons that are endowed with receptors for hormone also has been proposed (88). It seems clear, however, that ADH-independent factors also are involved in impaired water excretion with glucocorticoid deficiency. Whereas the AVP-dependent component may be observed in adrenalectomized, mineralocorticoid-replaced rats deprived of glucocorticoid hormone for 24 hours, AVP-independent impairment in water excretion occurs after 2 weeks of glucocorticoid deficiency in AVP-deficient

Brattleboro rats. The AVP-independent effect is associated with impaired renal hemodynamics and decreased distal fluid delivery to the diluting segment of the nephron.

Hypothyroidism

Hyponatremia may develop in some patients with advanced hypothyroidism, even in the absence of cardiac failure but it is so unusual that some have questioned the association (89). This is most likely owing to the fact that the impaired water excretion occurs only in severe hypothyroidism. Several mechanisms have been proposed to explain this impaired diluting capacity with hypothyroidism. Studies in hypothyroid humans and rats have demonstrated elevated radioimmunoassayable titers of plasma vasopressin, thus implicating AVP in the impaired water excretion associated with thyroid hormone deficiency. On the other hand, studies of osmoregulation in hypothyroid patients have found that both the threshold and sensitivity of the vasopressin response are intact (90). Such an observation incriminates an intrarenal hemodynamic disturbance. A recent study in rats with severe hypothyroidism revealed an almost complete reversal of the water excretory defect when given a V_2 vasopressin receptor antagonist, suggesting a minor role for an AVP independent mechanisms (91). These rats also had elevated AQP_2 expression in the inner medulla that was also normalized with the V_2 receptor antagonist.

Psychosis: Primary Polydipsia

Acutely psychotic patients, particularly those with schizophrenia, are at risk of developing hyponatremia (92). Polydipsia occurs in approximately 20% of psychiatric patients. The elucidation of the mechanism has been confounded, because possible pharmacologic agents, such as nicotine, thiazides, and carbamazepine, frequently are implicated (93). Psychiatric medications also cause dry mouth and stimulate thirst. However, reports of psychotic patients with water intoxication who are not taking medications also exist. The mechanism of the hyponatremia associated with psychosis thus appears to be multifactorial (94). Thirst perception is increased, there is a nonosmotic stimulus that causes AVP to be secreted at lower osmolality, and the renal response to AVP may be enhanced. Although each derangement alone would be insufficient to cause overt hyponatremia, their combination very well may cause overt hyponatremia (94). The combination of low solute intake with high water intake makes those subjected more prone to develop hyponatremia (95).

Postoperative Hyponatremia

The incidence of hospital-acquired, particularly postoperative, hyponatremia is increased in adults (96) as well as children (97). Most of the patients are euvolemic and have measurable plasma AVP levels (96). The hyponatremia is asymptomatic in most of the patients, but there is a subgroup of postoperative women with cerebral edema who have seizures and hypoxia with catastrophic neurologic events (98).

Pharmacologic Agents

Drugs associated with water retention are listed in Table 1.8. Drug-induced hyponatremia is becoming the most common cause of hyponatremia (69). Thiazide diuretics are the most common cause, probably followed by selective serotonin uptake inhibitors (SSRI). Hyponatremia can be mediated by vasopressin analogs such as dDAVP, drugs that enhance vasopressin release, and agents potentiating the action of vasopressin. In other instances, the mechanism is unknown. The increased use of desmopressin for nocturia in the elderly and enuresis in the young has resulted in a marked increase of reported cases of hyponatremia in these subjects (99). The increasing use of intravenous immunoglobulin (IVIG) as a therapeutic modality in many disorders, cases of hyponatremia associated with its use have been described (100). The mechanism of IVIG associated hyponatremia is multifactorial involving pseudohyponatremia as the protein concentration increases, translocation because of the sucrose present in the solution, and true dilutional hyponatremia related to retention of water, particularly in those with associated acute kidney injury. An increasing number of antipsychotic agents have been associated with hyponatremia, and they are frequently implicated in an explanation for the water intoxication in psychotic patients. The role of the drugs in the etiology of the impaired water excretion in patients receiving the agents has not been

TABLE 1.8 DRUGS ASSOCIATED WITH HYPONATREMIA

Antidiuretic Hormone Analogs

Deamino-D-arginine vasopressin
Oxytocin

Drugs That Enhance Antidiuretic Hormone Release

Chlorpropamide
Clofibrate
Carbamazepine–oxycarbazepine
Vincristine
Nicotine
Narcotics (μ-opioid receptors)
Antipsychotic/antidepressants
Ifosfamide

Drugs That Potentiate Renal Action of Antidiuretic Hormone

Chlorpropamide
Cyclophosphamide
Nonsteroidal antiinflammatory drugs
Acetaminophen

Drugs That Cause Hyponatremia by Unknown Multiple Mechanisms

Haloperidol
Fluphenazine
Amitriptyline
Serotonin uptake inhibitors
"Ecstasy" (amphetamine related)
IVIG

From Veis JH, Berl T. Hyponatremia. In: Jacobson HR, Striker GE, Klahr S, eds. *The Principles and Practice of Nephrology,* 2nd ed. St. Louis: Mosby; 1995:890, with permission.

dissociated, in most cases, from the role of the underlying psychiatric disorder for which the patient is receiving the drug. Therefore, although the clinical association between antipsychotic drugs and hyponatremia frequently is encountered, the pharmacologic agents themselves may not be the primary factors responsible for the water retention. Of particular interest is the frequent occurrence of hyponatremia in elderly subjects receiving SSRI drugs. The incidence has been reported to be as high as 22% to 28% in some studies (101). An increasing number of cases of hyponatremia reports have appeared after the use of the recreational drug 3,4-methylenedioxymethamphetamine ("ecstasy") (102).

Exercise-Induced Hyponatremia

Hyponatremia is increasingly seen in long distance runners. A study at a marathon race associated increased risk of hyponatremia with body mass index (BMI) <20 kg/m^2, running time exceeding 4 hours and greatest weight gain (103). A study in ultramarathon runners showed elevated vasopressin despite normal or low serum sodium (104).

Syndrome of Inappropriate Antidiuretic Hormone Secretion

Pathophysiology

The chronic administration of AVP when accompanied with intake of water culminates in the development of hyponatremia (105). As depicted in Figure 1.15, the continued administration of AVP is accompanied by a decline in the hydroosmotic effect of the hormone as urine osmolality falls and serum sodium stabilizes, a phenomenon denoted as vasopressin escape. A downregulation of receptors, possibly by activation of an inhibitory G protein, has been suggested. This may explain the decrement in cAMP generation and the decrease in AVP-stimulated water permeability during vasopressin escape (106). This is also associated with downregulation of AQP$_2$ but not AQP$_3$ (107). Hypotonic volume expansion also is necessary to achieve vasopressin escape.

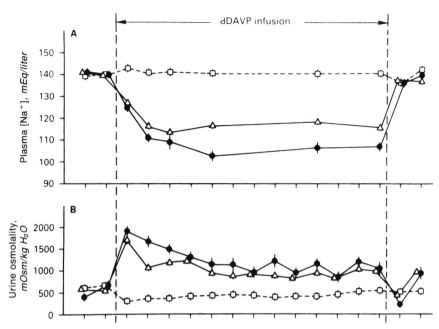

■ **Figure 1.15** Effects of pitressin and water administration. Note that urine flow increases, urine osmolality decreases, and serum sodium stabilizes. dDAVP, desmopressin acetate. (From Verbalis JG, Drutarosky M. Adaptation to chronic hypoosmolality in rats. *Kidney Int.* 1988; 34:351, with permission.)

Clinical Settings

The diagnosis SIADH is made primarily by excluding other causes of hyponatremia. A diagnosis of SIADH should be considered in the absence of hypovolemia, edematous disorders, endocrine dysfunction (including primary and secondary adrenal insufficiency and hypothyroidism), renal failure, and drugs, all of which may impair water excretion. In Table 1.9 are summarized the diagnostic criteria for the syndrome and Table 1.10 lists various diseases in which SIADH may occur. These associated diseases generally fall into three categories: malignancies, pulmonary disorders, and CNS disorders. Idiopathic causes are unusual, except in elderly patients (108). In this elderly population, no cause is found suggesting abnormal AVP secretion in as many as 10% of the patients. The urine is concentrated despite the presence of hyponatremia in patients with SIADH. The urinary sodium concentration generally is

TABLE 1.9 DIAGNOSTIC CRITERIA FOR THE SYNDROME OF INAPPROPRIATE ADH RELEASE

Essential Diagnostic Criteria

Decreased extracellular fluid effective osmolality (<mOsm/kg H_2O)

Innapropriate urinary concentration (>100 mOsm/kg H_2O)

Clinical euvolemia

Elevated urinary Na^+ concentration under conditions of normal salt and water intake

Absence of adrenal, thyroid, pituitary, or renal insufficiency or diuretic use

Supplemental Criteria

Abnormal water-load test (inability to excrete at least 90% of a 20-mL/kg water load in 4 h and/or failure to dilute urine osmolality to <100 mOsm/kg)

Plasma vasopressin level inappropriately elevated relative to the plasma osmolality

No significant correction of plasma Na^+ level with volume expansion, but improvement after fluid restriction

From Parikh C, Berl T. Disorders of water metabolism. In: London MI, ed. *Comprehensive Clinical Nephrology*. 4 ed. In press, with permission.

TABLE 1.10 DISORDERS ASSOCIATED WITH THE SYNDROME OF INAPPROPRIATE ANTIDIURETIC HORMONE SECRETION

Carcinomas	Pulmonary Disorders	Central Nervous System Disorders	Other
Bronchogenic carcinoma	Pneumonia (viral or bacterial)	Encephalitis (viral or bacterial)	AIDS
Carcinoma of the duodenum	Pulmonary abscess	Meningitis (viral, bacterial, tuberculosis, and fungal)	Prolonged exercise
Carcinoma of the pancreas	Tuberculosis	Carcinoma of the ureter	Idiopathic (in elderly)
Thymoma	Aspergillosis	Head trauma	
Carcinoma of the stomach	Positive pressure breathing	Brain abscess	
Lymphoma	Asthma	Guillain–Barré syndrome	
Ewing sarcoma	Pneumothorax	Acute intermittent porphyria	
Carcinoma of the bladder	Mesothelioma	Subarachnoid hemorrhage or subdural hematoma	
Prostatic carcinoma	Cystic fibrosis	Cerebellar and cerebral atrophy	
Oropharyngeal tumor		Cavernous sinus thrombosis	
		Neonatal hypoxia	
		Shy–Drager syndrome	
		Rocky Mountain spotted fever	
		Delirium tremens	
		Cerebrovascular accident (cerebral thrombosis or hemorrhage)	
		Acute psychosis	
		Peripheral neuropathy	
		Multiple sclerosis	

From Levi M, Berl T. Water metabolism. In: Gonick HC, ed. *Current Nephrology,* vol. 5. Chicago: Year Book Medical Publishers; 1982:45, with permission.

>20 mEq/L; however, the urinary sodium concentration may decrease to <1 mEq/L if patients are placed on a low-sodium diet or become volume depleted.

It has become apparent now that most patients with SIADH have a defect in the osmoregulation of vasopressin. Robertson et al. (109) reported plasma vasopressin measurements in 106 patients who fulfiled the clinical criteria for the diagnosis of SIADH before the correction of their hyponatremia. In the vast majority, plasma vasopressin concentration was inadequately suppressed relative to the hypoosmolalitly present. Interestingly, plasma vasopressin was between 1 and 10 pg/mL in most patients, the same range as in normonatremic hydrated, healthy adults, which indicates that nonosmotic AVP secretion can best be demonstrated under hypotonic conditions. As seen in Figure 1.16, four patterns are evident. Type A, is associated with large and erratic fluctuations in plasma vasopressin, which bore no relationship to the rise in plasma osmolality. This pattern was found in six of 25 patients studied who had acute respiratory failure, bronchogenic carcinoma, pulmonary tuberculosis, schizphrenia, and rheumatoid arthritis. This pattern indicates that the secretion of vasopressin either had been totally divorced from osmoreceptor control or was responding to some periodic nonosmotic stimulus. A completely different

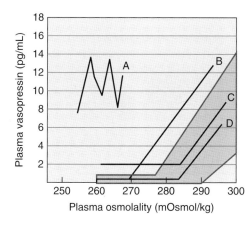

■ **Figure 1.16** Plasma vasopressin as a function of plasma osmolality during the infusion of hypertonic saline in four groups of patients with clinical SIADH. The shaded area indicates the range of normal value. SIADH, syndrome of inappropriate antidiuretic hormone. (From Verbalis J, Berl T. Disorders of water balance. In: *The Kidney*. 8th ed. Philadelphia, PA: Saunders Elsevier; 2008:493, With permission.)

type of osmoregulatory defect is exemplified by type B response, as seen in Figure 1.16. The infusion of hypertonic saline resulted in a prompt and progressive rise in plasma osmolality. Regression analysis showed the precision and sensitivity of this response to be essentially the same as in healthy subjects but the intercept or threshold value at 253 mOsm/kg to be well below the normal range. This pattern, which reflects the "resetting of the osmoreceptor," was found in nine of the 25 patients who had the diagnosis of bronchogenic carcinoma, cerebrovascular disease, tuberculous meningitis, acute respiratory disease, and carcinoma of the pharynx. Another patient with hyponatremia and acute idiopathic polyneuritis had an identical pattern to a hypertonic saline infusion and was determined to have resetting of the osmoreceptor. This and other patients with a reset osmostat have been able to dilute their urine maximally and sustain a urine flow sufficient to prevent a further increase in body water. Thus, an abnormality in AVP regulation can exist in spite of the ability to dilute the urine maximally and excrete a water load, a situation reminiscent of the hypotonicity seen in pregnancy. This was demonstrated, however, with an acute 20 mL/kg water load that lowers plasma osmolality much more rapidly than seen clinically.

As seen in Figure 1.16, in the type C response, plasma vasopressin was elevated initially but did not change during the infusion of hypertonic saline until plasma osmolality reached the normal range. At that point, plasma AVP began to rise appropriately, indicating a normally functioning osmoreceptor mechanism. This response was found in eight of the 25 patients with the diagnosis of CNS disease, bronchogenic carcinoma, carcinoma of the pharynx, pulmonary tuberculosis, and schizophrenia. Its pathogenesis is unknown, but it was speculated that this variety of SIADH might result from a constant, nonsuppressible leak of AVP despite otherwise normal osmoregulatory function. Unlike type II, or the resetting type of defect, it results in impaired urinary dilution and water excretion.

As seen in the type IV response, the osmoregulation of vasopressin appeared to be completely normal despite the marked inability to excrete a water load. The plasma AVP was appropriately suppressed under hypotonic conditions and did not rise until plasma osmolality reached the normal threshold level. When this procedure was reversed by water loading, plasma osmolality and plasma AVP again fell normally, but urinary dilution did not occur and the water load was not excreted (Pattern D in Fig. 1.16). This was seen in 10% of the studied patients. Thus these patients had no detectable AVP when they were hyponatremic. It is possible that at least some of these patients have a recently described defect in the V_2 receptor that renders it constitutively active (110). This has been termed "nephrogenic syndrome of inappropriate antidiuresis."

SIGNS AND SYMPTOMS OF HYPONATREMIA

The most common signs and symptoms of hyponatremia are listed in Table 1.11. Most patients with hyponatremia are asymptomatic. Although gastrointestinal complaints occur early, the most manifestations of hyponatremia are of a neuropsychiatric nature and include lethargy, psychosis, seizures, and coma. These symptoms reflect the brain edema that accompanies the osmotic water shift. This is denoted as hyponatremic encephalopathy (67,111). The water movement may be mediated by AQP_4,

TABLE 1.11 SYMPTOMS AND SIGNS THAT MAY BE ASSOCIATED WITH HYPONATREMIA

Symptoms	Signs
Lethargy, apathy	Abnormal sensorium
Disorientation	Depressed deep tendon reflexes
Muscle cramps	Cheyne–Stokes respiration
Anorexia, nausea	Hypothermia
Agitation	Pathologic reflexes
	Pseudobulbar palsy
	Seizures

From Berl T, Anderson RJ, McDonald KM, et al. Clinical disorders of water metabolism. *Kidney Int.* 1976; 10:117.

since animals with knockout of this water channel seem protected from brain swelling (112) and those that over express it are prone to brain edema (113). In the most severe form, hyponatremia encephalopathy can cause brainstem compression leading to respiratory failure and pulmonary edema leading to hypoxia (114). Elderly patients and young children with hyponatremia are most likely to become symptomatic. Also, it has become apparent that neurologic complications occur more frequently in menstruating women. In a case control study, despite approximately equal incidence of postoperative hyponatremia in males and females, 97% of those with permanent brain damage were women and 75% of them were menstruant (115). The severity of symptoms is dependent on the rate at which serum sodium concentration is lowered as well. There is considerable disagreement as to the mortality of acute hyponatremia. This has been reported to be as high as 50% and as low as 3%. There is general agreement that the mortality of chronic hyponatremia in hospitalized patients is 10% to 27%. However, the deaths are generally caused by the underlying disorder rather than the hyponatremia per se. The mortality is lower with chronic hyponatremia because brain volume regulatory responses protect against cerebral edema over time. Studies in rats demonstrate a loss of both electrolyte and organic osmolytes after the onset of hyponatremia. Although some of the osmolyte losses occur within 24 hours, the loss of such solutes becomes more marked in subsequent days and account for almost complete restoration of cerebral water volume. The electrolytes and other osmolytes lost in the adaptation to hyponatremia are shown in Figure 1.17. The rate at which the brain restores the lost electrolytes and osmolytes when hyponatremia is corrected is of great pathophysiologic importance. Sodium and chloride recover quickly and even overshoot. However, the reaccumulation of osmolytes is considerably delayed. This process is likely to account for the more marked cerebral dehydration that accompanies the rapid correction in previously adapted animals with chronic hyponatremia as well as alteration in the blood–brain barrier that may underlie the development of demyelinating lesions (116).

THERAPY OF HYPONATREMIA

The treatment of hyponatremia has been the subject of considerable interest and controversy (61,117,118). The strategy is dictated by the underlying cause, clinical severity, and timing of hyponatremia development. Unfortunately, the identification of the underlying pathology is not evident

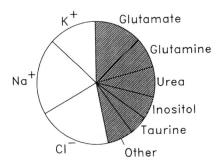

■ **Figure 1.17** Relative decreases in individual osmolytes during adaptation to chronic hyponatremia. The category "other" represents glycerol phosphorylcholine, urea, and several other amino acids. (From Gullans SR, Verbalis JG. Control of brain volume during hyperosmolar and hypoosmolar conditions. *Annu Rev Med.* 1993;44:289–301, with permission.)

immediately. Management should be based on whether the patient is or is not symptomatic and whether the disorder is acute or chronic.

Symptomatic Hyponatremia

Acute

Neurologic symptoms of acute hyponatremia are most commonly seen in premenopausal females in the postoperative state (98), elderly persons on thiazide diuretics, and patients with psychogenic polydipsia (119). It is generally agreed that these patients should be treated promptly. In this setting, the risks of cerebral edema and seizures outweigh any risk of rapid correction. The mortality rate in these patients is considerable, and those who survive frequently have residual neurological signs and symptoms. The female preponderance of the syndrome is not fully understood. The volume-adaptive response whereby the brain decreases its volume in acute hyponatremia may be inhibited by female hormones. A contribution of hypoxia also may be important, because when hypoxia is combined with hyponatremia in experimental animals; the volume-adaptive response is abrogated, resulting in brain edema and increased mortality (120). Because the neurological complications associated with acute symptomatic hyponatremia are devastating, these patients require prompt treatment with 3% NaCl (61,121,122).

Chronic

Patients in whom the adaptive process to hyponatremia has occurred (>48 hours) are at risk of developing a demyelinating syndrome when treated rapidly. If the hyponatremia has taken >48 hours to evolve or if the duration is not known, correction should be undertaken with caution. Controversy exists over whether it is the rate of correction or the magnitude of correction of hyponatremia that predisposes to neurologic complications. In clinical practice, it is difficult to dissociate these two variables since a rapid correction rate is usually accompanied by a greater absolute magnitude of correction over a given period of time. There are important principles to guide treatment (61).

- Increase the serum Na^+ level by 10% or by approximately 10 mmol/L because cerebral water is increased only by approximately 10% in severe chronic hyponatremia.
- Do not exceed a correction rate of 1.0 to 1.5 mmol/L in any given hour.
- Do not increase the serum Na^+ by >8 to 12 mmol/L/24 h.

It is important to take into account the rate and electrolyte content of infused fluids and the rate of production and electrolyte content of urine. Once the desired increment in serum Na^+ concentration is obtained, treatment should consist of water restriction.

If correction has proceeded more rapidly than desired (usually because of excretion of hypotonic urine), the risk of osmotic demyelination may be decreased by relowering serum Na^+ with IV or SQ desmopressin and/or administration of 5% dextrose (123).

The rapid increase in serum osmolality leads to a greater degree of cerebral water loss than a previously normonatremic brain (117) and makes the development of a demyelinating process more likely. Although small demyelinating lesions produce minimal symptoms, patients with more extensive diseases have flaccid quadriplegia, dysphagia, and dysarthria. The factors that predispose to this neurologic complication have not been fully delineated. Patients with underlying liver disease, alcoholism receiving thiazide diuretics, malnutrition, severe hypokalemia, and serum Na <105 mEq/L are more prone to this complication. Formulas have been devised to determine the increment in serum Na that follow the administration of various Na-containing solutions (67). These assume, however, that there are no ongoing losses and are prone to overcorrection if electrolyte-free water is concomitantly excreted (122,124).

Asymptomatic

Patients with asymptomatic hyponatremia invariably have a chronic component to their disease. While many may appear to be asymptomatic, formal neurological testing frequently reveals subtle impairments including gait disturbances comparable to those seen in subjects with toxic levels of alcohol, that reverse upon correction of the hyponatremia (125). This results in an increased risk for falls and fractures (125,126).

TABLE 1.12 NONPEPTIDE ARGININE VASOPRESSIN RECEPTOR ANTAGONISTS

	Tolvaptan	Lixivaptan	Stavaptan	Conivaptan
Receptor	V_2	V_2	V_2	V_1a/V_2
Route of administration	Oral	Oral	Oral	IV
Urine volume	↑	↑	↑	↑
Urine osmolality	↓	↓	↓	↓
Na excretion	↔	↔ Low dose, ↑ High dose	↔	↔
Manufacturer	Otsuka	CardioKine	Sanofi-Aventis	Astellas

From Thurman J, Berl T. Therapy in nephrology and hypertension. In: Wilcox CS, ed. *Therapy in Nephrology and Hypertension.* 3 ed. Philadelphia, PA: WB Saunders; 2008:337–352, with permission.

Water restriction, has been the cornerstone of the treatment of "asymptomatic" hyponatremic patients. The degree of the restriction depends on the severity of the diluting impairment, which can be assessed by urinary electrolyte measurements (127). When the diluting defect is severe, as reflected by a ratio of urinary Na plus urinary potassium to plasma sodium that is >1, almost no amount of fluid restriction will be affective. Furthermore, water restriction is difficult to enforce over a long time; therefore, agents that antagonize the renal action of AVP have been employed. Demeclocycline is more effective and safer than lithium in the treatment of SIADH, but is frequently accompanied by gastrointestinal intolerance. Moreover, in hyponatremic subjects with cirrhosis demeclocycline causes nephrotoxicity and thus should be avoided.

Urine flow and thereby water excretion can be increase by increasing solute excretion (128). A dose of 30 to 60 g of urea per day can successfully treat the syndrome. A similar benefit occurs with the use of furosemide (40 mg/day) with a high salt intake (200 mEq/day).

The development of orally active, nonpeptide antagonists of the hydroosmotic effect of AVP (Vaptans) provide an exciting potential therapeutic tool in the management of patients with water excess and hyponatremia (129). A number of antagonists of the hydroosmotic effect of AVP (V_2 receptor antagonists) have been developed, listed in Table 1.12. Several studies have demonstrated that they can induce a water diuresis and increase serum sodium in patients with SIADH (130–133) as well as with cirrhosis (132,134–136) and congestive heart failure (76,132,137). Although they differ in their relative V_1/V_2 selectivity, they all lower urinary osmolality, and have no effect on sodium and potassium excretion. Conivaptan, a V_1/V_2 antagonist is presently FDA approved for intravenous use (138) for the treatment of hospitalized patients with euvolemic or hypervolemic hyponatremia. Its use is limited to 4 days because it is a potent CYP3A4 inhibitor. In view of its V_1 antagonistic properties its use in patients with liver disease is probably not advisable. The oral antagonist Tolvaptan has received FDA approval and should be available for long-term use. Whether the oral V_2 receptor antagonists can produce an effective and sustained increase in serum sodium and osmolality in patients with high circulating levels of AVP remains to be determined. To date there have been no cases of osmotic demyelination, but caution still needs to be exercised to avoid rapid correction with these agents. V_2 receptor antagonists are an attractive alternative to water restriction and are likely to emerge as the agents of choice in the treatment of hyponatremia.

REFERENCES

1. Smith H. *From Fish to Philosopher: The Story of Our Internal Environment.* Boston, MA: Little Brown; 1953.
2. Kuhn W, Ryffel K. Herstellung konzentrierter Losungen aus verdunnten durch blosse Membranwirkung: ein Modellversuch zur der Niere. *Z Physiol Chem.* 1942:145–180.
3. Knepper MA, Hoffert JD, Packer RK, et al. Urine concentration and dilution. In: Brenner BM, ed. *The Kidney.* 8th ed. Philadelphia, PA: WB Saunders;2008:308–329.
4. Kriz W. Structural organization of the renal medullary counterflow system. *Fed Proc.* 1983;42:2379–2385.
5. Nielsen S, Frokiaer J, Marples D, et al. Aquaporins in the kidney: from molecules to medicine. *Physiol Rev.* 2002;82:205–244.
6. Bagnasco SM, Peng T, Nakayama Y, et al. Differential expression of individual UT-A urea transporter isoforms in rat kidney. *J Am Soc Nephrol.* 2000;11:1980–1986.
7. Sands JM, Kokko JP. Countercurrent system. *Kidney Int.* 1990;38:695–699.

8. Chou SY, Porush JG, Faubert PF. Renal medullary circulation: hormonal control. *Kidney Int.* 1990;37: 1–13.

9. Verbalis J, Berl T. Disorders of water balance. In: Brenner BM, ed. *The Kidney.* 8th ed. Philadelphia: WB Saunders;2008:459–504.

10. Mohr E, Richter D. Sequence analysis of the promoter region of the rat vasopressin gene. *FEBS Lett.* 1990;260:305–308.

11. Brown DN, S. Cell Biology in vasopressin. In: Brenner BM, ed. *The Kidney.* 8th ed. Philadelphia, PA: WB Saunders; 2008:280–307.

12. Morel A, O'Carroll AM, Brownstein MJ, et al. Molecular cloning and expression of a rat V1a arginine vasopressin receptor. *Nature.* 1992;356:523–526.

13. Lolait SJ, O'Carroll AM, McBride OW, et al. Cloning and characterization of a vasopressin V$_2$ receptor and possible link to nephrogenic diabetes insipidus. *Nature.* 1992;357:336–339.

14. Birnbaumer M, Seibold A, Gilbert S, et al. Molecular cloning of the receptor for human antidiuretic hormone. *Nature.* 1992;357:333–335.

15. Nielsen S, Chou CL, Marples D, et al. Vasopressin increases water permeability of kidney collecting duct by inducing translocation of aquaporin-CD water channels to plasma membrane. *Proc Natl Acad Sci U S A.* 1995;92:1013–1017.

16. Agre P, Sasaki S, Chrispeels MJ. Aquaporins: a family of water channel proteins. *Am J Physiol.* 1993;265:F461.

17. Nielsen SK, Knepper MK, Kwon T-H, et al. Regulation of water balance: urine concentration and dilution. In: Schrier RW, ed. *Diseases of the Kidney and Urinary Tract.* 8th ed: New York, NY: Lippincott Williams & Wilkins; 2007: 96–123.

18. Stricker EM, Verbalis JG. Water intake and body fluids. In: Zigmond MJ. Bloom FE, Landis SC. Roberts JL, Squire LR, eds. *Fundamental Neuroscience.* San Diego; 1999:111–126.

19. Fitzsimons JT. Angiotensin, thirst, and sodium appetite. *Physiol Rev.* 1998;78:583–686.

20. Perez GO, Oster JR, Robertson GL. Severe hypernatremia with impaired thirst. *Am J Nephrol.* 1989;9:421–434.

21. Berl T, Anderson RJ, McDonald KM, et al. Clinical disorders of water metabolism. *Kidney Int.* 1976;10: 117–132.

22. Maghnie M, Cosi G, Genovese E, et al. Central diabetes insipidus in children and young adults. *N Engl J Med.* 2000;343:998–1007.

23. Kaltsas GA, Powles TB, Evanson J, et al. Hypothalamo-pituitary abnormalities in adult patients with langerhans cell histiocytosis: clinical, endocrinological, and radiological features and response to treatment. *J Clin Endocrinol Metab.* 2000;85:1370–1376.

24. Rittig S, Robertson GL, Siggaard C, et al. Identification of 13 new mutations in the vasopressin-neurophysin II gene in 17 kindreds with familial autosomal dominant neurohypophyseal diabetes insipidus. *Am J Hum Genet.* 1996;58: 107–117.

25. Russell TA, Ito M, Yu RN, et al. A murine model of autosomal dominant neurohypophyseal diabetes insipidus reveals progressive loss of vasopressin-producing neurons. *J Clin Invest.* 2003;112:1697–1706.

26. Hardy C, Khanim F, Torres R, et al. Clinical and molecular genetic analysis of 19 Wolfram syndrome kindreds demonstrating a wide spectrum of mutations in WFS1. *Am J Hum Genet.* 1999;65: 1279–1290.

27. Fraser CL, Arieff AI. Fatal central diabetes mellitus and insipidus resulting from untreated hyponatremia: a new syndrome. *Ann Intern Med.* 1990;112: 113–119.

28. Kurokawa H, Fujisawa E, Nakano Y, et al. Posterior lobe of the pituitary gland: correlation between signal intensityon T1-weighted MR images and vasopressin concentration. *Radiology.* 1998:79–83.

29. De Wardener HE, Herxheimer A. The effect of a high water intake on the kidney's ability to concentrate the urine in man. 1957. *J Am Soc Nephrol.* 2000;11:980–987.

30. Kanno K, Sasaki S, Hirata Y, et al. Urinary excretion of aquaporin-2 in patients with diabetes insipidus. *N Engl J Med.* 1995;332:1540–1545.

31. Saito T, Higashiyama M, Nakamura T, et al. Urinary excretion of the aquaporin-2 water channel exaggerated in pathological states of impaired water excretion. *Clin Endocrinol (Oxf).* 2001;55:217–221.

32. Seck JR DD. Diabetes insipidus: current treatment recommendation. *Drugs.* 1992:216–224.

33. Fjellestad-Paulsen A, Tubiana-Rufi N, Harris A, et al. Central diabetes insipidus in children. Antidiuretic effect and pharmacokinetics of intranasal and peroral 1-deamino-8-D-arginine vasopressin. *Acta Endocrinol (Copenh).* 1987;115: 307–312.

34. Dunn AL, Powers JR, Ribeiro MJ, et al. Adverse events during use of intranasal desmopressin acetate for haemophilia A and von Willebrand disease: a case report and review of 40 patients. *Haemophilia.* 2000;6:11–14.

35. Robson WL, Norgaard JP, Leung AK. Hyponatremia in patients with nocturnal enuresis treated with DDAVP. *Eur J Pediatr.* 1996;155:959–962.

36. Bichet DG. Nephrogenic and central diabetes insipidus. In: Schrier RW, ed. *Diseases of the Kidney and Urinary Tract.* 8th ed. New York, NY: Lippincott Williams & Wilkins; 2007:2249–2269.

37. Fujiwara TM, Bichet DG. Molecular biology of hereditary diabetes insipidus. *J Am Soc Nephrol.* 2005;16:2836–2846.

38. Schrier RW. Body water homeostasis: clinical disorders of urinary dilution and concentration. *J Am Soc Nephrol.* 2006;17:1820–1832.

39. Deen PM, Croes H, van Aubel RA, et al. Water channels encoded by mutant aquaporin-2 genes in nephrogenic diabetes insipidus are impaired in their cellular routing. *J Clin Invest.* 1995;95: 2291–2296.

40. Tamarappoo BK, Verkman AS. Defective aquaporin-2 trafficking in nephrogenic diabetes insipidus and correction by chemical chaperones. *J Clin Invest.* 1998;101:2257–2267.

41. Kuwahara M, Iwai K, Ooeda T, et al. Three families with autosomal dominant nephrogenic diabetes insipidus caused by aquaporin-2 mutations in the C-terminus. *Am J Hum Genet.* 2001;69:738–748.

42. King LS, Choi M, Fernandez PC, et al. Defective urinary-concentrating ability due to a complete deficiency of aquaporin-1. *N Engl J Med.* 2001; 345:175–179.

43. Ma T, Song Y, Yang B, et al. Nephrogenic diabetes insipidus in mice lacking aquaporin-3 water channels. *Proc Natl Acad Sci USA.* 2000;97: 4386–4391.

44. Bouley R, Hasler U, Lu HA, et al. Bypassing vasopressin receptor signaling pathways in nephrogenic diabetes insipidus. *Semin Nephrol.* 2008;28:266–278.

45. Bernier V, Morello JP, Zarruk A, et al. Pharmacologic chaperones as a potential treatment for X-linked nephrogenic diabetes insipidus. *J Am Soc Nephrol.* 2006;17:232–243.

46. Tannen RL, Regal EM, Dunn MJ, et al. Vasopressin-resistant hyposthenuria in advanced chronic renal disease. *N Engl J Med.* 1969;280: 1135–1141.

47. Teitelbaum I, McGuinness S. Vasopressin resistance in chronic renal failure. Evidence for the role of decreased V_2 receptor mRNA. *J Clin Invest.* 1995;96:378–385.

48. Kwon TH, Frokiaer J, Knepper MA, et al. Reduced AQP1, -2, and -3 levels in kidneys of rats with CRF induced by surgical reduction in renal mass. *Am J Physiol.* 1998;275: F724–F741.

49. Marples D, Frokiaer J, Dorup J, et al. Hypokalemia-induced downregulation of aquaporin-2 water channel expression in rat kidney medulla and cortex. *J Clin Invest.* 1996;97:1960–1968.

50. Sands JM, Flores FX, Kato A, et al. Vasopressin-elicited water and urea permeabilities are altered in IMCD in hypercalcemic rats. *Am J Physiol.* 1998; 274:F978–F985.

51. Earm JH, Christensen BM, Frokiaer J, et al. Decreased aquaporin-2 expression and apical plasma membrane delivery in kidney collecting ducts of polyuric hypercalcemic rats. *J Am Soc Nephrol.* 1998;9:2181–2193.

52. Marples D, Christensen S, Christensen EI, et al. Lithium-induced downregulation of aquaporin-2 water channel expression in rat kidney medulla. *J Clin Invest.* 1995;95:1838–1845.

53. Rao R, Zhang MZ, Zhao M, et al. Lithium treatment inhibits renal GSK-3 activity and promotes cyclooxygenase 2-dependent polyuria. *Am J Physiol Renal Physiol.* 2005;288: F642–F649.

54. Cadnapaphornchai MA, Summer SN, Falk S, et al. Effect of primary polydipsia on aquaporin and sodium transporter abundance. *Am J Physiol Renal Physiol.* 2003;285:F965–F971.

55. Sands JM, Naruse M, Jacobs JD, et al. Changes in aquaporin-2 protein contribute to the urine concentrating defect in rats fed a low-protein diet. *J Clin Invest.* 1996;97:2807–2814.

56. Durr JA, Hoggard JG, Hunt JM, et al. Diabetes insipidus in pregnancy associated with abnormally high circulating vasopressinase activity. *N Engl J Med.* 1987;316:1070–1074.

57. Adrogue HJ, Madias NE. Hypernatremia. *N Engl J Med.* 2000;342:1493–1499.

58. Lien YH, Shapiro JI, Chan L. Effects of hypernatremia on organic brain osmoles. *J Clin Invest.* 1990;85:1427–1435.

59. Palevsky PM, Bhagrath R, Greenberg A. Hypernatremia in hospitalized patients. *Ann Intern Med.* 1996;124:197–203.

60. Polderman KH, Schreuder WO, Strack van Schijndel RJ, et al. Hypernatremia in the intensive care unit: an indicator of quality of care? *Crit Care Med.* 1999;27:1105–1108.

61. Thurman J, Berl T. Therapy in nephrology and hypertension. In: Wilcox CS, ed. *Therapy in Nephrology and Hypertension.* 3 ed. Philadelphia, PA: WB Saunders; 2008:337–352

62. Blum D, Brasseur D, Kahn A, et al. Safe oral rehydration of hypertonic dehydration. *J Pediatr Gastroenterol Nutr.* 1986;5:232–235.

63. Kahn A, Brachet E, Blum D. Controlled fall in natremia and risk of seizures in hypertonic dehydration. *Intensive Care Med.* 1979;5:27–31.

64. Kumar S, Berl T. Sodium. *Lancet.* 1998;352:220–228.

65. Hillier TA, Abbott RD, Barrett EJ. Hyponatremia: evaluating the correction factor for hyperglycemia. *Am J Med.* 1999;106:399–403.

66. Nguyen MK, Ornekian V, Butch AW, Kurtz I. A new method for determining plasma water content: application in pseudohyponatremia. *Am J Physiol Renal Physiol.* 2007;292:F1652–1656.

67. Adrogue HJ, Madias NE. Hyponatremia. *N Engl J Med.* 2000;342:1581–1589.

68. Parikh C, Berl T. Disorders of water metabolism. In: London MI, ed. *Comprehensive Clinical Nephrology.* 4 ed. In press.

69. Liamis G, Milionis H, Elisaf M. A review of drug-induced hyponatremia. *Am J Kidney Dis.* 2008;52: 144–153.

70. Ohara M, Cadnapaphornchai MA, Summer SN, et al. Effect of mineralocorticoid deficiency on ion and urea transporters and aquaporin water channels in the rat. *Biochem Biophys Res Commun.* 2002;299:285–290.

71. Palmer BF. Hyponatraemia in a neurosurgical patient: syndrome of inappropriate antidiuretic hormone secretion versus cerebral salt wasting. *Nephrol Dial Transplant.* 2000;15:262–268.

72. Sterns RH, Silver SM. Cerebral salt wasting versus SIADH: what difference? *J Am Soc Nephrol.* 2008;19:194–196.

73. Schrier RW, Abraham WT. Hormones and hemodynamics in heart failure. *N Engl J Med.* 1999;341:577–585.

74. Schrier RW, Gurevich AK, Cadnapaphornchai MA. Pathogenesis and management of sodium and water retention in cardiac failure and cirrhosis. *Semin Nephrol.* 2001;21:157–172.

75. Martin PY, Abraham WT, Lieming X, et al. Selective V2-receptor vasopressin antagonism decreases urinary aquaporin-2 excretion in patients with chronic heart failure. *J Am Soc Nephrol.* 1999;10:2165–2170.

76. Abraham WT, Shamshirsaz AA, McFann K, et al. Aquaretic effect of lixivaptan, an oral, non-peptide, selective V_2 receptor vasopressin antagonist in New York Heart Association functional class II and III chronic heart failure patients. *J Am Coll Cardiol.* 2006;47:1615–1621.

77. Sica DA. Hyponatremia and heart failure—pathophysiology and implications. *Congest Heart Fail*. 2005;11:274–277.

78. Xu DL, Martin PY, Ohara M, et al. Upregulation of aquaporin-2 water channel expression in chronic heart failure rat. *J Clin Invest*. 1997;99:1500–1505.

79. Claria J, Jimenez W, Arroyo V, et al. Blockade of the hydroosmotic effect of vasopressin normalizes water excretion in cirrhotic rats. *Gastroenterology*. 1989;97:1294–1299.

80. Inoue T, Ohnishi A, Matsuo A, et al. Therapeutic and diagnostic potential of a vasopressin-2 antagonist for impaired water handling in cirrhosis. *Clin Pharmacol Ther*. 1998;63:561–570.

81. Martin PY, Ohara M, Gines P, et al. Nitric oxide synthase (NOS) inhibition for one week improves renal sodium and water excretion in cirrhotic rats with ascites. *J Clin Invest*. 1998;101:235–242.

82. Weigert AL, Martin PY, Niederberger M, et al. Endothelium-dependent vascular hyporesponsiveness without detection of nitric oxide synthase induction in aortas of cirrhotic rats. *Hepatology*. 1995;22:1856–1862.

83. Fernandez-Llama P, Jimenez W, Bosch-Marce M, et al. Dysregulation of renal aquaporins and Na-Cl cotransporter in CCl4-induced cirrhosis. *Kidney Int*. 2000;58:216–228.

84. Apostol E, Ecelbarger CA, Terris J, et al. Reduced renal medullary water channel expression in puromycin aminonucleoside—induced nephrotic syndrome. *J Am Soc Nephrol*. 1997;8:15–24.

85. Gross PR, Rascher W. Vasopressin and hyponatremia in renal insufficiency. *Contrib Nephrol*. 1986:54.

86. Celkjers W. Hyponatremia and inappropriate secretion of vasopressin (antidiuretic hormone) in patients with hypopituitarism. *N Engl J Med*. 1989:492–496.

87. Wang W, Li C, Summer SN, et al. Molecular analysis of impaired urinary diluting capacity in glucocorticoid deficiency. *Am J Physiol Renal Physiol*. 2006;290:F1135–F1142.

88. Berghorn KA, Knapp LT, Hoffman GE, et al. Induction of glucocorticoid receptor expression in hypothalamic magnocellular vasopressin neurons during chronic hypoosmolality. *Endocrinology*. 1995;136:804–807.

89. Hanna FW, Scanlon MF. Hyponatraemia, hypothyroidism, and role of arginine-vasopressin. *Lancet*. 1997;350:755–756.

90. Iwasaki Y, Oiso Y, Yamauchi K, et al. Osmoregulation of plasma vasopressin in myxed-ema. *J Clin Endocrinol Metab*. 1990;70:534–539.

91. Chen YC, Cadnapaphornchai MA, Yang J, et al. Nonosmotic release of vasopressin and renal aquaporins in impaired urinary dilution in hypothyroidism. *Am J Physiol Renal Physiol*. 2005;289:F672–678.

92. Riggs AT, Dysken MW, Kim SW, et al. A review of disorders of water homeostasis in psychiatric patients. *Psychosomatics*. 1991;32:133–148.

93. de Leon J, Verghese C, Tracy JI, et al. Polydipsia and water intoxication in psychiatric patients: a review of the epidemiological literature. *Biol Psychiatry*. 1994;35:408–419.

94. Berl T. Psychosis and water balance. *N Engl J Med*. 1988;318:441–442.

95. Musch W, Xhaet O, Decaux G. Solute loss plays a major role in polydipsia-related hyponatraemia of both water drinkers and beer drinkers. *QJM*. 2003;96:421–426.

96. Anderson RJ, Chung HM, Kluge R, et al. Hyponatremia: a prospective analysis of its epidemiology and the pathogenetic role of vasopressin. *Ann Intern Med*. 1985;102:164–168.

97. Hoorn EJ, Geary D, Robb M, et al. Acute hyponatremia related to intravenous fluid administration in hospitalized children: an observational study. *Pediatrics*. 2004;113:1279–1284.

98. Arieff AI. Permanent neurological disability from hyponatremia in healthy women undergoing elective surgery. *Ann Intern Med*. 1986;102:164.

99. Palmer B, Sterns, RH. Fluid, electrolytes, and acid-base disturbances. *NephSAP*. 2009:70–167.

100. Daphnis E, Stylianou K, Alexandrakis M, et al. Acute renal failure, translocational hyponatremia and hyperkalemia following intravenous immunoglobulin therapy. *Nephron Clin Pract*. 2007;106:c143–c148.

101. Bouman WP, Pinner G, Johnson H. Incidence of selective serotonin reuptake inhibitor (SSRI) induced hyponatraemia due to the syndrome of inappropriate antidiuretic hormone (SIADH) secretion in the elderly. *Int J Geriatr Psychiatry*. 1998;13:12–15.

102. Holmes SB, Banerjee AK, Alexander WD. Hyponatraemia and seizures after ecstasy use. *Postgrad Med*. J 1999;75:32–33.

103. Almond CS, Shin AY, Fortescue EB, et al. Hyponatremia among runners in the Boston Marathon. *N Engl J Med*. 2005;352:1550–1556.

104. Hew-Butler T, Jordaan E, Stuempfle KJ, et al. Osmotic and nonosmotic regulation of arginine vasopressin during prolonged endurance exercise. *J Clin Endocrinol Metab*. 2008;93: 2072–2078.

105. Verbalis JG. Pathogenesis of hyponatremia in an experimental model of the syndrome of inappropriate antidiuresis. *Am J Physiol*. 1994;267:R1617–1625.

106. Ecelbarger CA, Chou CL, Lee AJ, et al. Escape from vasopressin-induced antidiuresis: role of vasopressin resistance of the collecting duct. *Am J Physiol*. 1998;274:F1161–1166.

107. Ecelbarger CA, Nielsen S, Olson BR, et al. Role of renal aquaporins in escape from vasopressin-induced antidiuresis in rat. *J Clin Invest*. 1997;99: 1852–1863.

108. Miller M. Hyponatremia: age-related risk factors and therapy decisions. *Geriatrics*. 1998;53:32–42.

109. Zerbe R, Stropes L, Robertson G. Vasopressin function in the syndrome of inappropriate antidiuresis. *Annu Rev Med*. 1980;31:315–327.

110. Decaux G, Vandergheynst F, Bouko Y, et al. Nephrogenic syndrome of inappropriate antidiuresis in adults: high phenotypic variability in men and women from a large pedigree. *J Am Soc Nephrol*. 2007;18:606–612.

111. Verbalis J. SIADH and other hypoosmolar. In: Schrier RW, ed. *Diseases of the Kidney and Urinary Tract*. 8th ed. New York, NY: Lippincott Williams & Wilkins;2007:2214.

112. Papadopoulos MC, Verkman AS. Aquaporin-4 and brain edema. *Pediatr Nephrol.* 2007;22:778–784.

113. Yang B, Zador Z, Verkman AS. Glial cell aquaporin-4 overexpression in transgenic mice accelerates cytotoxic brain swelling. *J Biol Chem.* 2008;283:15280–15286.

114. Ayus JC, Varon J, Arieff AI. Hyponatremia, cerebral edema, and noncardiogenic pulmonary edema in marathon runners. *Ann Intern Med.* 2000;132:711–714.

115. Ayus JC, Wheeler JM, Arieff AI. Postoperative hyponatremic encephalopathy in menstruant women. *Ann Intern Med.* 1992;117:891–897.

116. Gross P. Treatment of severe hyponatremia. *Kidney Int.* 2001;60:2417–2427.

117. Berl T. Treating hyponatremia: damned if we do and damned if we don't. *Kidney Int.* 1990;37: 1006–1018.

118. Sterns RH. The treatment of hyponatremia: first, do no harm. *Am J Med.* 1990;88:557–560.

119. Cheung J, Zikos D, Spokicki H, et al. Long term neurologic outcome in psychogenic water drinkers with severe symptomatic hyponatremia: the effect of rapid correction. *Am J Med.* 1990:561.

120. Vexler ZS, Ayus JC, Roberts TP, et al. Hypoxic and ischemic hypoxia exacerbate brain injury associated with metabolic encephalopathy in laboratory animals. *J Clin Invest.* 1994;93:256–264.

121. Hew-Butler T, Ayus JC, Kipps C, et al. Statement of the Second International Exercise-Associated Hyponatremia Consensus Development Conference, New Zealand, 2007. *Clin J Sport Med.* 2008;18:111–121.

122. Mohmand HK, Issa D, Ahmad Z, et al. Hypertonic saline for hyponatremia: risk of inadvertent overcorrection. *Clin J Am Soc Nephrol.* 2007;2:1110–1117.

123. Perianayagam A, Sterns RH, Silver SM, et al. DDAVP is effective in preventing and reversing inadvertent overcorrection of hyponatremia. *Clin J Am Soc Nephrol.* 2008;3:331–336.

124. Berl T. The Adrogue-Madias formula revisited. *Clin J Am Soc Nephrol.* 2007;2:1098–1099.

125. Renneboog B, Musch W, Vandemergel X, et al. Mild chronic hyponatremia is associated with falls, unsteadiness, and attention deficits. *Am J Med.* 2006;119:71 e1–e8.

126. Gankam Kengne F, Andres C, Sattar L, et al. Mild hyponatremia and risk of fracture in the ambulatory elderly. *QJM.* 2008;101:583–588.

127. Furst H, Hallows KR, Post J, et al. The urine/plasma electrolyte ratio: a predictive guide to water restriction. *Am J Med Sci.* 2000;319:240–244.

128. Berl T. Impact of solute intake on urine flow and water excretion. *J Am Soc Nephrol.* 2008;19: 1076–1078.

129. Greenberg A, Verbalis JG. Vasopressin receptor antagonists. *Kidney Int.* 2006;69:2124–2130.

130. Decaux G. Long-term treatment of patients with inappropriate secretion of antidiuretic hormone by the vasopressin receptor antagonist conivaptan, urea, or furosemide. *Am J Med.* 2001;110: 582–584.

131. Saito T, Ishikawa S, Abe K, et al. Acute aquaresis by the nonpeptide arginine vasopressin (AVP) antagonist OPC-31260 improves hyponatremia in patients with syndrome of inappropriate secretion of antidiuretic hormone (SIADH). *J Clin Endocrinol Metab.* 1997;82:1054–1057.

132. Schrier RW, Gross P, Gheorghiade M, et al. Tolvaptan, a selective oral vasopressin V2-receptor antagonist, for hyponatremia. *N Engl J Med.* 2006;355:2099–2112.

133. Soupart A, Gross P, Legros JJ, et al. Successful long-term treatment of hyponatremia in syndrome of inappropriate antidiuretic hormone secretion with satavaptan (SR121463B), an orally active nonpeptide vasopressin V2-receptor antagonist. *Clin J Am Soc Nephrol.* 2006;1:1154–1160.

134. Gerbes AL, Gulberg V, Gines P, et al. Therapy of hyponatremia in cirrhosis with a vasopressin receptor antagonist: a randomized double-blind multicenter trial. *Gastroenterology.* 2003;124: 933–939.

135. Wong F, Blei AT, Blendis LM, et al. A vasopressin receptor antagonist (VPA-985) improves serum sodium concentration in patients with hyponatremia: a multicenter, randomized, placebo-controlled trial. *Hepatology.* 2003;37:182–191.

136. Gines P, Wong F, Watson H, et al. Effects of satavaptan, a selective vasopressin V(2) receptor antagonist, on ascites and serum sodium in cirrhosis with hyponatremia: a randomized trial. *Hepatology.* 2008;48:204–213.

137. Gheorghiade M, Niazi I, Ouyang J, et al. Vasopressin V2-receptor blockade with tolvaptan in patients with chronic heart failure: results from a double-blind, randomized trial. *Circulation.* 2003;107:2690–2696.

138. Zeltser D, Rosansky S, van Rensburg H, et al. Assessment of the efficacy and safety of intravenous conivaptan in euvolemic and hypervolemic hyponatremia. *Am J Nephrol.* 2007;27:447–457.

CHAPTER 2

Renal Sodium Excretion, Edematous Disorders, and Diuretic Use

ROBERT W. SCHRIER

An understanding of body fluid volume regulation, as modulated by renal sodium and water excretion, is critical for the practice of clinical medicine. Knowledge of the intrarenal and extrarenal factors affecting renal sodium excretion is important to comprehend the mechanism of body fluid volume regulation in health and disease because the sodium ion is the primary determinant of extracellular fluid (ECF) volume. In this regard, the edematous disorders—cardiac failure, liver disease, and the nephrotic syndrome—present a particular challenge to our understanding of body fluid volume regulation. In normal humans, if the ECF volume is expanded by the administration of isotonic saline, then the kidney excretes the excess amount of sodium and water in the urine, thus returning the ECF volume to normal. However, in these edematous states, avid renal sodium and water retention persists despite expansion of ECF volume and the presence of total body sodium and water excess. In circumstances where advanced kidney disease is present and renal function and excretory capacity are diminished (e.g., acute or chronic intrinsic renal failure), it is obvious why the decreased glomerular filtration rate (GFR) may be associated with retention of sodium and water to the point of pulmonary and/or peripheral edema. However, it is clear that the integrity of the kidney as the ultimate effector organ of body fluid volume regulation is intact in patients with heart failure or liver disease and some patients with the nephrotic syndrome. Thus, the kidney must be responding to extrarenal signals from the afferent limb of a volume regulatory system in these edematous disorders. The study of these edematous disorders has led to our proposal of a unifying hypothesis of body fluid volume regulation that applies to both health and disease (1–8). The purpose of this chapter is to review the afferent and efferent mechanisms that determine renal sodium and water handling, particularly in the context of the edematous disorders, and discuss the treatment of edema with diuretic agents.

Sodium Ion as Determinant of Extracellular Fluid Volume

Sodium ions reside primarily in the ECF compartment, to which they are extruded from cells by active transport mechanisms. These transport processes result in an intracellular sodium concentration of 10 mEq/L and an ECF sodium concentration of 145 mEq/L. The sodium ion and its major anions, chloride and bicarbonate, constitute >90% of the total solute in the ECF space. Thus, total body sodium and its accompanying anions are the osmotically active solutes that are the major determinants of ECF volume. In turn, the regulation of sodium balance is determined by the relationship among sodium intake, extrarenal sodium loss, and renal sodium excretion. Practically, renal sodium excretion may be considered to be the primary determinant of sodium balance, because the kidney is able to excrete virtually sodium-free urine as well as rapidly excrete large sodium loads in response to diminished or increased sodium intakes, respectively.

A positive sodium balance is associated with increased amounts of sodium, located predominantly in the ECF compartment. Because cellular membranes are freely permeable to water, the osmotic gradient created by the addition of ECF sodium causes water to move from cells into the ECF compartment, thus expanding ECF volume. In addition, an increase in ECF osmolality stimulates the hypothalamic thirst center and leads to increased fluid intake and also releases arginine vasopressin (AVP) from the posterior pituitary, which decreases renal water excretion by increasing the water permeability of collecting duct epithelium (9). The latter two effects of an increased ECF osmolality result in a positive water balance, and the combined influence of positive sodium and water balances leads to further expansion of ECF volume. If this expansion of ECF is of sufficient magnitude, then an alteration of the Starling forces that govern the transfer of fluid from the vascular compartment to the surrounding interstitial spaces occurs and edema results (10). Conversely, a negative sodium balance results in a depletion of ECF volume. A decrease in ECF volume may result in a parallel decline in plasma volume. Maintenance of ECF volume and plasma volume is necessary for adequate circulation and survival of the organism. Thus, renal sodium and water retention clearly is appropriate in situations of ECF volume depletion. However, in edematous disorders, continued renal sodium and water retention despite total body sodium and water excess defines a paradoxical clinical situation.

It is worth mentioning that the osmolality of ECF is regulated by the AVP–thirst–renal axis (as discussed in depth in Chapter 1). However, the osmolality of the ECF is not a reliable index of ECF volume. ECF volume and its determinant total body sodium are best assessed by physical examination and determination of urinary sodium concentration. For example, a finding of generalized edema suggests an expanded ECF volume and increased total body sodium. Conversely, orthostatic tachycardia and/or hypotension, flat neck veins, and decreased skin turgor suggest depletion of ECF volume and decreased total body sodium. In fact, alterations in the osmolality of the ECF can occur in association with normal, increased, or decreased ECF volume (Chapter 1).

In summary, the control of ECF volume is dependent on the regulation of sodium balance. The kidneys play the pivotal role in the regulation of sodium balance and therefore of ECF volume homeostasis. In certain edema-forming states associated with a normal GFR, the kidney retains sodium and water despite expansion of the ECF volume and total body sodium and water. A knowledge of the afferent ("sensor") and efferent ("effector") mechanisms of sodium and water retention associated with the edematous disorders forms the basis of our understanding of body fluid volume regulation.

Afferent Mechanisms Involved in Body Fluid Volume Regulation

THE CONCEPT OF "EFFECTIVE BLOOD VOLUME" OR WHAT COMPARTMENT IS SENSED?

If the afferent receptors of body fluid volume regulation primarily sense total blood volume, then the kidneys of edematous patients should increase their excretion of sodium and water since their total blood volumes are increased. However, as mentioned, this does not occur in patients with advanced cardiac failure, liver disease, or the nephrotic syndrome. Thus, there must be some body fluid compartment that is still "underfilled"—even in the presence of expansion of total ECF and blood volumes—and comprises the afferent limb of renal sodium and water retention in patients with edematous disorders. In 1948, Peters coined the enigmatic term "effective blood volume" as a reference to such an underfilled body fluid compartment (11). Accordingly, extrarenal signals must be initiated by this decrease in effective blood volume, which enhances tubular sodium and water reabsorption by the otherwise normal kidney. In this regard, it is clear that renal sodium and water retention can occur in patients with cardiac failure or cirrhosis and in some patients with the nephrotic syndrome prior to any diminution in GFR.

Borst and deVries (12) first suggested cardiac output as the primary modulator of renal sodium and water excretion. In this context, the level of cardiac output would constitute the effective blood volume and thus serve as the primary stimulus for renal sodium and water retention in patients with edematous disorders. Although this concept is appealing, substantial renal sodium and water retention may occur in the presence of an increase in cardiac output. For example, a significant elevation in cardiac output may occur in the presence of avid renal sodium and water retention and expansion of ECF volume in association with cirrhosis, pregnancy, arteriovenous (AV) fistulae, and other causes of high-output cardiac failure, such as thyrotoxicosis and beriberi. Consequently, there must exist some other or additional determinant(s) of effective blood volume.

PRIMACY OF THE ARTERIAL CIRCULATION IN VOLUME REGULATION

The unifying hypothesis of body fluid volume regulation in health and disease states that the fullness of the arterial vascular compartment or the so-called effective *arterial* blood volume (EABV) is the primary determinant of renal sodium and water excretion (1–8). In a 70-kg man, total body water approximates 42 L, of which only 0.7 L (1.7% of total body water) resides in the arterial circulation. From a teleologic viewpoint, it is attractive to propose that the primacy for regulation of renal sodium and water excretion, and body fluid volume homeostasis, is modulated by the smallest body fluid compartment—thus endowing the system with exquisite sensitivity to relatively small changes in body fluid volume. Another advantage of the integrity of the arterial circulation constituting the main afferent sensing compartment for body fluid volume regulation is that perfusion of the vital organs is dependent on the arterial circulation. As a result, total ECF, interstitial fluid, or total intravascular volumes are not primary determinants of renal sodium and water excretion, and the venous component of intravascular volume likewise is excluded as the primary determinant of sodium and water excretion, because all of these body fluid compartments may be expanded while the renal sodium and water retention persists in edematous patients. It is acknowledged, however, that there are experimental and clinical circumstances in which selective rises in right and left atrial pressure stimulate the release of atrial natriuretic peptide (ANP) (13) or suppression of AVP (14), respectively, which may enhance sodium and water excretion. These events, however, must be subservient to the more potent determinants of the arterial circulation, because the patient with advanced left or right ventricular dysfunction, or both, exhibits avid sodium and water retention despite markedly elevated atrial and ventricular pressures.

CARDIAC OUTPUT AND SYSTEMIC ARTERIAL RESISTANCE AS THE DETERMINANTS OF THE FULLNESS OF THE ARTERIAL CIRCULATION AND RENAL SODIUM AND WATER EXCRETION

The EABV is a measure of the adequacy of arterial blood volume to "fill" the capacity of the arterial circulation. Normal arterial filling exists when the ratio of cardiac output to systemic vascular resistance maintains venous return and cardiac output at normal levels. Thus, arterial underfilling may be initiated by either a decrease in cardiac output or a fall in systemic arterial resistance (i.e., arterial vasodilatation, which increases the holding capacity of the arterial vascular tree). Arterial underfilling results in unloading of high-pressure baroreceptors with subsequent activation of the three major neurohormonal vasoconstrictor systems—namely, the sympathetic nervous system, the renin–angiotensin–aldosterone system, and the nonosmotic release of AVP—which diminish renal hemodynamics and promote renal sodium and water retention. This hypothesis accounts for the initiation of sodium and water retention in low- and high-output cardiac failure, liver disease, and other states of arterial underfilling (Figs. 2.1 and 2.2).

AFFERENT VOLUME RECEPTORS

As mentioned, the afferent volume receptors for such a volume regulatory system must reside in the arterial vascular tree, such as the high-pressure baroreceptors in the carotid sinus, aortic arch, left ventricle, and juxtaglomerular apparatus. Although the low-pressure volume receptors of the thorax (cardiac atria, right ventricle, and pulmonary vessels) must be of some importance to the volume regulatory system (15,16), there is considerable evidence that arterial receptors can predominate over low-pressure receptors in volume control in mammals.

High-Pressure Volume Receptors

In humans, the presence of volume-sensitive receptors in the arterial circulation was first suggested by Epstein et al. (17) based on observations made in patients with traumatic AV fistulae. Closure of traumatic AV fistulae was associated with an immediate increase in renal sodium excretion independent of concomitant changes in either GFR or renal blood flow (RBF) (17). Closure of AV fistulae is associated with a decreased rate of emptying of the arterial blood into the venous circulation, as demonstrated by

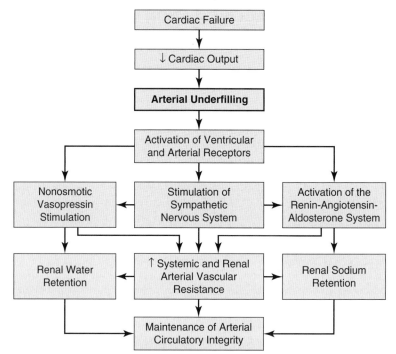

■ **Figure 2.1** Clinical conditions in which a decrease in cardiac output causes arterial underfilling with resultant neurohumoral activation and renal sodium and water retention. (From Schrier RW. Decreased effective blood volume in edematous disorders: what does this mean? *J Am Soc Nephrol.* 2007;18(7):2028–2031, with permission.)

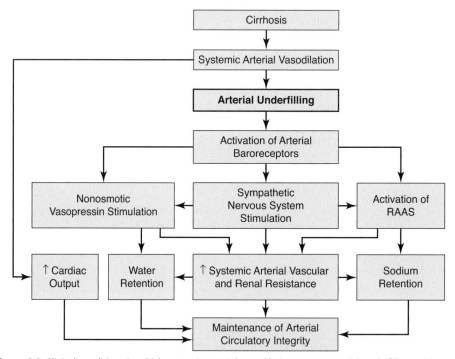

■ **Figure 2.2** Clinical conditions in which systemic arterial vasodilation causes arterial underfilling with resultant neurohumoral activation and renal sodium and water retention. (From Schrier RW. Decreased effective blood volume in edematous disorders: what does this mean? *J Am Soc Nephrol.* 2007;18(7):2028–2031, with permission.)

closure-induced increases in diastolic arterial pressure and decreases in cardiac output (17). Further evidence implicating the relative "fullness" of the arterial vascular tree as being the major sensor in modulating renal sodium excretion can be found in denervation experiments. In these studies, surgical or pharmacologic interruption of sympathetic efferent neural pathways emanating from high-pressure areas inhibited the natriuretic response to volume expansion (18–20). Moreover, reduction of pressure or stretch at the carotid sinus, similar to that produced by decreased cardiac output or arterial hypotension, has been shown to activate the sympathetic nervous system and promote renal sodium and water retention (21). High-pressure baroreceptors also appear to be important factors in regulating nonosmotic release of AVP and thus renal water excretion (22). One of the best-defined high-pressure receptors that are known to act in an appropriate manner to maintain constancy of the EABV is the renal afferent arteriolar baroreceptor (i.e., juxtaglomerular apparatus). This baroreceptor is an important factor in the control of renal renin secretion and consequently angiotensin II formation and aldosterone synthesis and release (23). The vasoconstrictor and sodium-retaining effects of angiotensin II and sodium-retaining effect of aldosterone then act to restore the fullness of the arterial circulation.

Low-Pressure Volume Receptors

Low-pressure sensors also may have an important role to play in body fluid volume regulation because the more compliant venous side of the circulation contains up to 85% of the total blood volume at any given time (Table 2.1). In fact, a variety of maneuvers that decrease thoracic venous return, such as prolonged standing (24), lower-extremity tourniquets (25,26), and positive pressure breathing (27), are associated with diminished renal sodium excretion. Conversely, maneuvers that augment venous filling, such as recumbency (28) and negative pressure breathing (29), are associated with increased renal sodium excretion. Moreover, a direct correlation between renal sodium excretion and left atrial pressure has been demonstrated in the dog, suggesting a role for an atrial receptor as one type of intrathoracic sensor (30). Immersion in water to the neck or so-called head-out water immersion results in a pressure gradient from 80 mm Hg at the foot to 0 mm Hg at water level. This maneuver increases venous return to the heart. In response to head-out water immersion, a profound increase in renal excretion of salt and water occurs independent of major changes in either GFR or renal hemodynamics (31). As first suggested by Gauer et al. (29) and Henry et al. (32), physiologically significant left atrial receptors have been shown to contribute to ECF volume regulation by exerting nonosmotic control over AVP secretion and thus over renal water excretion. In addition, the atria have been demonstrated to be the site for synthesis, storage, and release of vasoactive and natriuretic humoral agents (33,34).

Thus, increased filling of the thoracic vascular and cardiac atria would be expected to signal the kidney to increase urinary sodium excretion in order to return the blood volume to normal. However, in the setting of chronic heart failure, renal sodium and water retention occur despite increased atrial pressure, which loads the low-pressure baroreceptors. Thus, in low-output chronic heart failure, diminished cardiac output must exert the predominant effect via unloading of high-pressure arterial baroreceptors. Chronic studies in animals employing experimental tricuspid insufficiency (35) further support this hypothesis. The increase in right atrial pressure was associated with avid renal sodium retention in these animal models. However, a concomitant fall in cardiac output likely explains the sodium retention.

TABLE 2.1 BODY FLUID DISTRIBUTION

Compartment	Amount	Volume in 70-kg Man (L)
Total body fluid	60% of body weight	42
Intracellular fluid	40% of body weight	28
Extracellular fluid	20% of body weight	14
Interstitial fluid	Two thirds of extracellular fluid	9.4
Plasma fluid	One third of extracellular fluid	4.6
Venous fluid	85% of plasma fluid	3.9
Arterial fluid	15% of plasma fluid	0.7

Zucker et al. (36) have demonstrated that the inhibition of renal sympathetic nerve activity that is seen during acute left atrial distention is lost during chronic heart failure in the dog. Moreover, a decrease in cardiac preload fails to produce the expected parasympathetic withdrawal and sympathetic activation in humans with heart failure (37). These findings also are consistent with the observation of a strong positive correlation between left atrial pressure and coronary sinus norepinephrine, a marker of cardiac adrenergic activity, in patients with chronic heart failure (38). Taken together, these findings suggest that the normal inhibitory control of sympathetic activation accompanying increased atrial pressures is lost in heart failure patients and somehow may even be converted to a stimulatory signal.

In summary, the afferent or sensor mechanisms for sodium and water excretion may be preferentially located on the arterial side of the circulation where diminished fullness of the arterial vascular tree owing to decreased cardiac output or systemic arterial vasodilation results in unloading of high-pressure receptors and subsequent renal sodium and water retention. Reflexes from low-pressure volume receptors also may be altered so as to influence renal sodium and water handling. In any event, changes in systemic and renal hemodynamics and activation of various neurohormonal systems largely comprise the efferent limb of the volume regulatory system.

Efferent Mechanisms Involved in Body Fluid Volume Regulation

THE NEUROHORMONAL RESPONSE TO ARTERIAL UNDERFILLING

Arterial underfilling secondary to a diminished cardiac output or systemic arterial vasodilation elicits a number of compensatory neurohormonal responses that act to maintain the integrity of the arterial circulation by promoting systemic vasoconstriction as well as expansion of the ECF volume through renal sodium and water retention. As noted, the three major neurohormonal vasoconstrictor systems activated in response to arterial underfilling are the sympathetic nervous system, renin–angiotensin–aldosterone system, and nonosmotic release of AVP. Baroreceptor activation of the sympathetic nervous system appears to be the primary integrator of the hormonal vasoconstrictor systems involved in the volume control system, because the nonosmotic release of AVP involves sympathetic stimulation of the supraoptic and paraventricular nuclei in the hypothalamus (39), and activation of the renin–angiotensin–aldosterone system involves renal β-adrenergic stimulation (40). Thus, in low-output cardiac failure, diminished integrity of the arterial circulation as determined by decreased cardiac output causes unloading of arterial baroreceptors in the carotid sinus and aortic arch. Systemic arterial vasodilation produces unloading of these arterial baroreceptors in the setting of high-output cardiac failure, cirrhosis, and other states of arterial underfilling. This baroreceptor inactivation results in diminution of the tonic inhibitory effect of afferent vagal and glossopharyngeal pathways to the central nervous system (CNS) and initiates an increase in sympathetic efferent adrenergic tone with subsequent activation of the renin–angiotensin–aldosterone system. Various counterregulatory, vasodilatory hormones also may be activated in heart failure, including natriuretic peptides and vasodilating renal prostaglandins. Activation of these various neurohormonal vasoconstrictor and vasodilator systems substantially determines renal sodium and water handling in the edematous disorders and comprises a major part of the efferent limb of body fluid volume regulation. The pathogenesis of sodium and water retention associated with cardiac failure, liver disease, and the nephrotic syndrome are now reviewed in the context of the unifying arterial underfilling hypothesis of body fluid volume regulation.

PATHOGENESIS OF SODIUM AND WATER RETENTION IN CARDIAC FAILURE

Sodium and water retention and resultant edema formation are cardinal features of chronic cardiac failure. In fact, the inability to excrete a sodium load has been used as an index of the presence of heart failure (41), and a defect in water excretion is encountered routinely in such patients (42). Two theories have been proposed to explain the renal response to cardiac failure. The "backward" theory of heart failure, proposed in 1832, suggests that increased venous hydrostatic pressure owing to increased ventricular filling pressures causes edema by promoting transudation of fluid from the intravascular to the interstitial compartment, resulting in edema formation (43). The reduced intravascular volume then signals the kidneys to retain sodium and water, further exacerbating the venous hypertension and formation of edema. The alternative "forward" theory of cardiac failure suggests that a primary decrease in cardiac output activates afferent and efferent pathways and results in renal sodium retention (44). As pointed out by Smith (26), these theories are not mutually exclusive, and both are operant in the pathophysiology of heart failure, because both central venous hypertension and arterial underfilling are implicated in the afferent limb of body fluid volume regulation. Nevertheless, the dominant signal for sodium and water retention in cardiac failure appears to occur in the arterial circulation. Decreased cardiac output is the cause of the arterial underfilling in the case of low-output heart failure, whereas systemic arterial vasodilation initiates the afferent limb of sodium and water retention in high-output cardiac failure (Fig. 2.1).

Renal Hemodynamics in Cardiac Failure

Glomerular Filtration Rate

Many early investigators believed that the cause of sodium retention in heart failure was a decrease in GFR; however, studies failed to confirm such a correlation. In fact, GFR often is normal in early heart failure and may even be elevated in states of high-output cardiac failure. It is acknowledged, however, that the contribution of GFR to sodium balance is difficult to evaluate because very minute changes in GFR could lead to substantial changes in sodium excretion if absolute sodium reabsorption remained unchanged. Nevertheless, although GFR may be diminished in patients with advanced heart failure, an increase in tubular sodium reabsorption undoubtedly is an important cause of sodium and water retention in cardiac failure.

Renal Blood Flow

Heart failure commonly is associated with an increase in renal vascular resistance and a decrease in RBF. In general, RBF decreases in proportion to the decrease in cardiac output. Some investigators also have shown a redistribution of RBF from outer cortical nephrons to juxtamedullary nephrons in experimental heart failure (45). It was proposed that deeper nephrons with longer loops of Henle reabsorb sodium more avidly; thus, the redistribution of blood flow to these nephrons with heart failure would result in renal sodium retention. However, other investigators have not been able to demonstrate such a redistribution of blood flow in other models of cardiac failure (46). Thus, the role of redistribution of RBF in the sodium retention of cardiac failure remains uncertain.

Filtration Fraction

Filtration fraction is often increased in heart failure because RBF falls as cardiac output decreases and GFR is preserved. An increase in filtration fraction results in increased protein concentration and oncotic pressure in the efferent arterioles and peritubular capillaries that surround the proximal tubules. Such an increase in peritubular oncotic pressure has been proposed to increase sodium and water reabsorption in the proximal tubule. These changes in renal hemodynamics and filtration fraction, which favor proximal tubular sodium reabsorption, are primarily a consequence of constriction of the efferent arterioles within the kidney. These renal hemodynamic changes are mediated mainly by activation of neurohormonal vasoconstrictor systems, because both activation of renal nerves and increased circulating norepinephrine and angiotensin II have been implicated in efferent arteriolar vasoconstriction (47,48). In addition, decreased activity of such substances as vasodilating renal prostaglandins also may play a role in renal vasoconstriction (49).

Of note, micropuncture studies in dogs with vena caval constriction and AV fistulae have demonstrated the importance of distal nephron sites of increased sodium reabsorption. Increased filtration fraction primarily affects proximal tubular sodium reabsorption. Thus, although clearance and micropuncture studies in animals with heart failure have demonstrated increased sodium reabsorption in the proximal tubule (50), distal sodium reabsorption also seems to be involved. Furthermore, changes in filtration fraction have been observed in heart failure long before changes in sodium balance occur, therefore questioning the dominance of peritubular factors and proximal reabsorption in the sodium retention of cardiac failure.

The Sympathetic Nervous System in Cardiac Failure

The sympathetic nervous system is unquestionably activated in patients with heart failure. Various studies have demonstrated elevated peripheral venous plasma norepinephrine concentrations in heart failure patients. Using tritiated norepinephrine in patients with advanced heart failure, Davis et al. (51) and Hasking et al. (52) have shown that both increased norepinephrine secretion and decreased norepinephrine clearance contribute to the high venous plasma norepinephrine concentrations seen in these patients, suggesting that increased sympathetic activity is at least partially responsible for the elevated circulating plasma norepinephrine. We have demonstrated that the initial rise in plasma norepinephrine in heart failure is solely caused by increased norepinephrine secretion, providing evidence of increased sympathetic nervous system activity early in the course of cardiac failure (53). Moreover, plasma norepinephrine is increased in patients with asymptomatic left ventricular dysfunction (i.e., prior to the onset of overt heart failure) (54). Finally, studies employing peroneal nerve microneurography to directly assess sympathetic nerve activity to muscle have confirmed the presence of increased sympathetic activity in heart failure patients (55). Significantly, the degree of activation of the sympathetic nervous system—as assessed by the peripheral venous plasma norepinephrine concentration—has been correlated with poor prognosis in heart failure (56).

Activation of Renal Nerves

Renal nerves also are activated in human heart failure (52). Enhanced renal sympathetic activity may contribute to the avid sodium and water retention in heart failure by promoting renal vasoconstriction, stimulation of the renin–angiotensin–aldosterone system, and direct effects on the proximal tubule epithelium. Indeed, intrarenal adrenergic blockade has been shown to cause a natriuresis in experimental heart failure (57). In addition, in the rat, renal nerve stimulation has been demonstrated to produce approximately a 25% reduction in sodium excretion and urine volume (58). The diminished renal sodium excretion that accompanies renal nerve stimulation may be mediated by at least two mechanisms. As already discussed, studies performed in rats have demonstrated that norepinephrine-induced efferent arteriolar constriction alters peritubular hemodynamic forces in favor of increased tubular sodium reabsorption (47). In addition, renal nerves have been shown to exert a direct influence on sodium reabsorption in the proximal convoluted tubule (58).

Bello-Reuss et al. (58) have demonstrated this direct effect of renal nerve activation to enhance proximal tubular sodium reabsorption in whole-kidney and individual nephron studies in the rat. In these animals, renal nerve stimulation produced an increase in the tubular fluid to plasma inulin concentration ratio in the late proximal tubule, an outcome of increased fractional sodium and water reabsorption in this segment of the nephron. Hence, increased renal nerve activity may promote sodium retention by a mechanism independent of changes in renal hemodynamics. On the other hand, sodium retention persists in dogs with denervated transplanted kidneys and chronic vena caval constriction. Moreover, renal denervation does not prevent ascites in the dog with chronic vena caval constriction (59). Thus, renal nerves probably contribute but do not fully account for the avid sodium retention of heart failure.

The Renin–Angiotensin–Aldosterone System in Cardiac Failure

The renin–angiotensin–aldosterone system also is activated in heart failure, as assessed by plasma renin activity (PRA) (60). Renin acts on angiotensinogen to produce angiotensin I, which is then converted by angiotensin-converting enzyme (ACE) to angiotensin II. In heart failure, the resultant increased plasma concentration of angiotensin II exerts important circulatory effects, including peripheral arterial and venous vascular constriction, renal vasoconstriction, and cardiac inotropism. Activation of angiotensin receptors on the proximal tubule epithelium directly stimulates the Na^+/H^+ exchanger 3 and thereby increases sodium reabsorption (61). Angiotensin II also acts to promote the secretion of the sodium-retaining hormone aldosterone by the adrenal cortex and in positive-feedback stimulation of the sympathetic nervous system. Activation of this hormonal system may promote sodium retention in the kidney via several mechanisms, as discussed next. Moreover, like adrenergic activation, stimulation of the renin–angiotensin–aldosterone system is associated with an unfavorable prognosis in heart failure (62).

Renal Effects of Increased Angiotensin II and Aldosterone

Angiotensin II may contribute to the sodium and water retention in heart failure through direct and indirect effects on proximal tubular sodium reabsorption and, as mentioned, by stimulating the release of aldosterone from the adrenal gland. Angiotensin II causes preferential renal efferent arteriolar constriction, resulting in decreased RBF and an increased filtration fraction. As with renal nerve stimulation, this results in increased peritubular capillary oncotic pressure and reduced peritubular capillary hydrostatic pressure, which favors the reabsorption of sodium and water in the proximal tubule (48). Moreover, as noted, angiotensin II has been shown to enhance sodium reabsorption in the proximal tubule (63). In a study of the rat proximal tubule, Liu and Cogan (63) demonstrated increased tubular sodium chloride reabsorption during the infusion of angiotensin II, whereas the angiotensin II receptor antagonist, saralasin, decreased proximal tubular sodium chloride reabsorption. Finally, in a report from Abassi et al. (64), the administration of the angiotensin II receptor antagonist, losartan, to decompensated sodium-retaining rats with heart failure secondary to AV fistulae produced a marked natriuresis. Although proximal tubular sodium handling was not examined in this investigation, the observation that losartan restored renal responsiveness to ANP is consistent with a losartan-induced increase in the delivery of sodium to the distal tubular site of ANP action. The role of distal tubular sodium delivery in the renal sodium retention of heart failure is discussed later.

Watkins et al. (65) studied a conscious dog model of heart failure in order to define more precisely the role of the renin–angiotensin–aldosterone axis in cardiac failure. Using either partial constriction of the pulmonary artery or thoracic inferior vena cava (TIVC), these workers acutely produced a low cardiac output state characterized by reduced blood pressure, increased PRA and aldosterone concentrations, and renal sodium retention. As plasma volume and body weight increased over several days, the aforementioned variables all returned toward control levels. During the initial hyperreninemic period, a single injection of an ACE inhibitor significantly lowered blood pressure. Also, chronic administration of the converting enzyme inhibitor prevented a rise in aldosterone and prevented 30% of the sodium retention and subsequent volume expansion. These studies lend support to the hypothesis that aldosterone is an important factor in the pathogenesis of cardiac edema and suggest that angiotensin II plays an important physiologic role in heart failure by supporting blood pressure because of its vasoconstrictor effect and maintaining blood volume secondary to the sodium-retaining effects of angiotensin II and aldosterone. It likewise becomes clear that, depending on the status of cardiac decompensation and plasma volume, the patient with heart failure may have a high or normal PRA and aldosterone level. This may explain some of the controversy that existed regarding the levels of these hormones in patients with heart failure.

A further role for renin–angiotensin–aldosterone system activation in the sodium retention of human heart failure is supported by the finding that urinary sodium excretion inversely correlates with PRA and urinary aldosterone excretion in heart failure patients (66). However, the administration of an ACE inhibitor (ACEI) during heart failure does not consistently increase urinary sodium excretion in spite of a consistent fall in plasma aldosterone concentration (67). The simultaneous fall in blood pressure caused by decreased circulating concentrations of angiotensin II, however, may activate hemodynamic and neurohormonal mechanisms that could obscure the natriuretic response to lowered angiotensin II and aldosterone concentrations. Support for this hypothesis comes from the study performed by Hensen et al. (68). We examined the effect of the specific aldosterone antagonist, spironolactone, on urinary sodium excretion in patients with heart failure who were withdrawn from all medications prior to study. Avid sodium retention occurred in all patients throughout the period prior to aldosterone antagonism. During therapy with spironolactone (200 mg b.i.d.), all heart failure patients exhibited a significant increase in urinary sodium excretion and reversal of the positive sodium balance (Fig. 2.3). Moreover, the urinary sodium to potassium concentration ratio significantly increased during spironolactone administration, consistent with a decrease in aldosterone action in the distal nephron. Of note, PRA and norepinephrine increased and ANP decreased during the administration of spironolactone. Thus, this investigation demonstrates reversal of the sodium retention of heart failure with the administration of an aldosterone antagonist, despite further activation of various antinatriuretic influences, including stimulation of the renin–angiotensin and sympathetic nervous systems, and supports a role for aldosterone in the renal

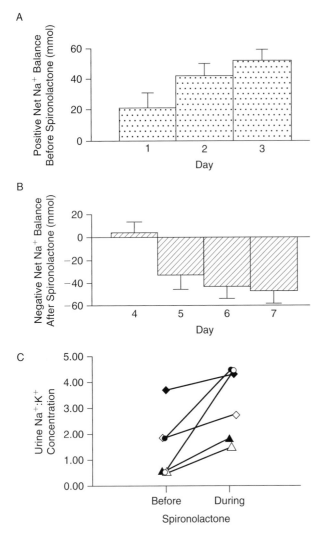

■ **Figure 2.3** Diuretics, digoxin, and ACEI were withdrawn 4 days prior to admission to General Clinical Research Center. The subjects were placed on a constant daily diet of 100 mEq sodium and 60 mEq potassium. **(A)** Upper panel (*dotted bars*) demonstrates the positive cumulative sodium balance in the six patients (four ischemic heart disease, one idiopathic cardiomyopathy, and one aortic valvular disease). **(B)** Middle panel (*cross hatch*) demonstrates in the same patients the significant negative cumulative sodium balance during 200 mg b.i.d. spironolactone ($p < 0.01$). **(C)** Lower panel demonstrates the increase in urine $Na^+:K^+$ concentration ratio during spironolactone in all six patients ($p < 0.05$), a finding compatible with aldosterone antagonism. Mean plasma potassium increased from 3.86 ± 0.2 to 4.1 ± 0.2 mEq/L during spironolactone treatment ($p < 0.05$). Mean systolic blood pressure (112 ± 7 mm Hg vs. $110 \pm$ mm Hg, NS) and creatinine clearance (87 ± 7 mL/min vs. 87.2 ± 8 mL/min, NS) did not change with spironolactone treatment. Plasma hANP decreased significantly with spironolactone (147 ± 58 mg/L vs. 83 ± 30 mg/L, $p < 0.05$). Fluid intake was not restricted and a mean of 2 kg weight loss occurred. (With permission from Bansal S, Lindenfeld J, Schrier RW. Sodium retention in heart failure and cirrhosis: potential role of natriuretic doses of mineralocorticoid antagonist? *Circ Heart Fail.* 2009;2: 370–376.)

sodium retention. A prospective trial, Randomized Aldactone Evaluation Study (RALES), has shown improved survival of heart failure patients receiving 25 mg/day of spironolactone (a competitive inhibitor of aldosterone) (69). This effect of spironolactone in the RALES investigation was found to be independent of any change in sodium balance. An effect of spironolactone to block the effect of aldosterone-mediated cardiac fibrosis has been suggested as the mediator of this improved survival response. Natriuretic doses of spironolactone rarely have been used in patients with heart failure. One study was performed in congestive heart failure (CHF) patients receiving low-dose ACEIs who had diuretic resistance. These patients demonstrated a natriuresis with a daily dose of 100 mg of spironolactone (70).

In the Acute Decompensated Heart Failure Registry (ADHERE), decompensated CHF patients resistant to oral diuretics were hospitalized and 90% were given intravenous diuretics. Forty-two percent of these patients were discharged with unresolved symptoms, 50% lost ≤5 lb and 20% actually gained weight. Approximately 25% to 30% of CHF patients become resistant to diuretics and, as discussed later, secondary hyperaldosteronism is an important factor in such diuretic resistance (71).

Nevertheless, natriuretic doses of mineralocorticoid antagonists are not part of the therapeutic armamentarium for heart failure, primarily because of the danger of hyperkalemia (72). Many of these CHF patients are receiving ACEIs or angiotensin receptor blockers (ARBs) and/or β-blockers, which predispose to hyperkalemia. Whether low-potassium diet, sodium polystyrene sulfonate (Kayexalate), and

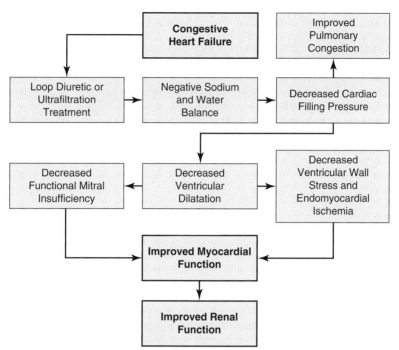

■ **Figure 2.4** Mechanisms in congestive heart failure whereby negative sodium and water balance by loop diuretics or ultrafiltration therapy may improve myocardial and renal function. (From Schrier RW. Role of diminished renal function in cardiovascular mortality: marker or pathogenetic factor? *J Am Coll Cardiol.* 2006;47(1):1–8, with permission.)

potassium-losing diuretics would avoid the occurrence of hyperkalemia during use of natriuretic doses of mineralocorticoid antagonists has not been studied. Given the problem with treating cardiac patients with acute decompensation, as noted in the ADHERE registry, inhibiting the secondary hyperaldosteronism in sodium-retaining CHF patients who are diuretic resistant needs to be studied. Isotonic removal of sodium in CHF patients with ultrafiltration is another therapeutic approach that needs to be studied in a prospective, randomized manner. Fluid removal in CHF patients with ultrafiltration or diuretics can improve cardiac and renal function in addition to treating pulmonary congestion and edema. The mechanisms are shown in Figure 2.4 (73).

The Nonosmotic Release of Arginine Vasopressin in Cardiac Failure

Plasma AVP often is elevated in patients with CHF and correlates in general with the clinical and hemodynamic severity of disease and the serum sodium level. Using a sensitive radioimmunoassay for AVP, Szatalowicz et al. (74) initially showed that plasma AVP was detectable in 30 of 37 patients with cardiac failure and hyponatremia. It was concluded that the nonosmotic AVP release in these patients was the result of baroreceptor stimulation secondary to diminished cardiac output, because these patients had sufficient hyponatremia and hypoosmolality, which would normally suppress maximally the osmotic release of AVP. Riegger et al. (75) also have reported that several patients with heart failure had inappropriately high plasma AVP levels. Cardiac output increased and plasma AVP levels normalized when two of these patients were treated with hemofiltration to remove excess body fluid. Other studies have also incriminated AVP in hyponatremic CHF patients (76,77). Taken together, these observations demonstrate enhanced nonosmotic AVP release in response to a decrease in cardiac output (i.e., arterial underfilling).

Renal Effects of Arginine Vasopressin

AVP, via stimulation of its renal or V_2 receptor subtype, enhances water reabsorption in the distal nephron, namely the cortical and medullary collecting ducts. The evidence supporting a role for AVP in the water retention of heart failure comes from studies using selective peptide and nonpeptide antagonists of the V_2 receptor of AVP in several animal models of cardiac failure. For example, Ishikawa et al. (78) have assessed the antidiuretic effect of plasma AVP in a low-output model of cardiac failure secondary to vena caval constriction in the rat. Plasma AVP concentrations were increased in these animals, and an antagonist of the antidiuretic effect of AVP reversed the defect in water excretion. An orally active non-peptide V_2 receptor AVP antagonist, OPC-31260, was originally described in 1992 (79). The intravenous administration of OPC-31260 during a dose-ranging study in normal human subjects was shown to increase urine output to a similar extent as 20 mg of furosemide given intravenously (80). Virtually simultaneous publications by Xu et al. (81) from our laboratory and Nielsen et al. (82) demonstrated the upregulation of aquaporin 2 (AQP2) water channels in coronary-ligated rats with CHF. The latter group also demonstrated that AQP1 and AQP3 were not upregulated in this CHF model and that increased trafficking of the AQP2 to the apical membrane occurred. Our group further showed that a V_2 vasopressin antagonist reversed the upregulation of the AQP2 protein in the renal cortex and medulla of the CHF rats (81). This effect of the nonosmotic release of AVP to cause water retention in cardiac failure recently has been associated with increased transcription of messenger RNA (mRNA) for the AVP pre-prohormone in the rat hypothalamus (83).

In a study by Bichet et al. (84), the effect of the ACEI captopril and the α_1-adrenergic blocker prazosin to reverse the abnormality in water retention in patients with class III and IV heart failure was examined. The resultant cardiac afterload reduction and increased cardiac output with either agent were associated with improved water excretion and significant suppression of AVP in response to an acute water load. A role of angiotensin II in modulating the effect of AVP in heart failure was unlikely, because captopril and prazosin had divergent effects on the renin–angiotensin system; yet their effects to suppress plasma AVP and improve water excretion were comparable. In this regard, it is important to note that in this study by Bichet et al. (84), the average decrease in mean arterial pressure was 5 mm Hg, a decrement that is <7% to 10% necessary to activate the nonosmotic release of AVP (85). Thus, these results are compatible with the suggestion that a decrease in stroke volume and cardiac output, rather than a fall in mean arterial pressure, may sometimes be the primary stimulus for the nonosmotic release of AVP in low-output cardiac failure. The association of improved cardiac output and water excretion during afterload reduction is compatible with unloading of high-pressure baroreceptors leading to increased AVP release.

The most recent advance relative to the nonosmotic release of AVP in CHF is the FDA approval of vasopressin receptor antagonists for clinical use in the United States. Conivaptan, a combined V_1 and V_2 receptor antagonist, has been approved for treatment of hyponatremia in cardiac failure. This antagonist can be used inhospital by intravenous administration for 4 days. The potential effect of the combined V_1 and V_2 antagonist properties in heart failure is shown in Figure 2.5 (73). Recently, the first orally active V_2 receptor antagonist, tolvaptan, has been approved for use in cardiac failure, cirrhosis, and the syndrome of inappropriate antidiuretic hormone (SIADH) (86). In association with the increase in plasma sodium concentration in hyponatremic CHF patients, the self-reported SF12 demonstrated a significant improvement in mental status in these patients. There are other V_2 receptor antagonists in phase 3 trials. Taken together, these agents are known as "aquaretics" to emphasize that the resultant increase in solute-free water excretion occurs in the absence of a change in electrolyte excretion. This is the major difference with diuretics that increase urinary sodium chloride and other electrolyte excretion. These aquaretic agents can correct plasma sodium concentration in the absence of fluid restriction. In chronic hyponatremia, the correction of plasma sodium concentration with an aquaretic should not exceed 8 mmol over 8 hours or 10 to 12 mmol over 24 hours in order to avoid osmotic demyelination.

Altered renal hemodynamics may contribute to water retention in heart failure in addition to persistent AVP secretion. Decreased RBF and increased filtration fraction would be expected to increase proximal reabsorption of sodium and water, thereby diminishing fluid delivery to distal diluting segments. Increasing distal fluid delivery by administration of furosemide has improved the diluting ability of patients with heart failure (87).

In summary, activation of the sympathetic nervous system, the renin–angiotensin–aldosterone system, and the nonosmotic release of AVP by exerting direct (tubular) and indirect (hemodynamic) effects on the kidneys are implicated in the renal sodium and water retention of heart failure. These neuroendocrine mechanisms appear to be activated in response to arterial underfilling and suppressed by

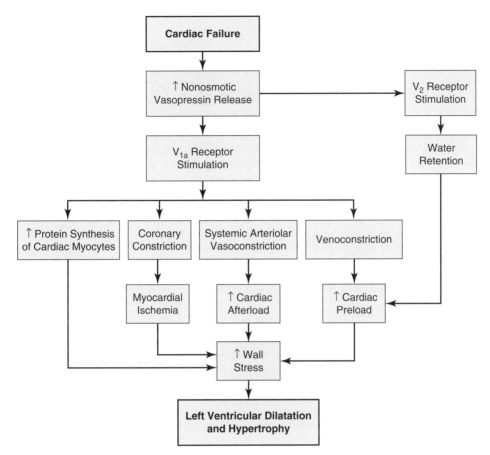

■ **Figure 2.5** Pathways whereby vasopressin stimulation of V_2 and V_{1a} receptors can contribute to events that worsen cardiac function. (From Schrier RW. Role of diminished renal function in cardiovascular mortality: marker or pathogenetic factor? *J Am Coll Cardiol.* 2006;47(1):1–8, with permission.)

maneuvers that restore the integrity of the arterial circulation toward normal. In addition, the effects of these neurohormonal vasoconstrictor systems may be counterbalanced by endogenous vasodilatory and natriuretic hormones.

Natriuretic Peptides in Cardiac Failure

The natriuretic peptides, including ANP and brain natriuretic peptide (BNP), circulate at increased concentrations in patients with heart failure (88,89). These peptide hormones possess natriuretic, vasorelaxant, and renin-, aldosterone-, and sympatho-inhibiting properties (90). Both ANP and BNP appear to be released primarily from the heart in response to increased atrial or ventricular end-diastolic or transmural pressures. We demonstrated that increased ANP production rather than decreased metabolic clearance was the major factor contributing to the elevated plasma ANP concentrations in a study of ANP kinetics in patients with cardiac failure (91). This finding is consistent with the observed increase in expression of both ANP and BNP mRNA in the cardiac ventricles of humans and animals with heart failure (92,93). BNP has been shown to reduce pulmonary capillary wedge pressure (PCWP) and increase cardiac index in acute CHF (94). In a coronary ligation model of heart failure in the rat, the infusion of a monoclonal antibody shown to specifically block endogenous ANP in vivo caused a significant rise in right atrial pressure, left ventricular end-diastolic pressure, and systemic vascular resistance (95). Thus, natriuretic peptides appear to attenuate to some degree the arterial and venous vasoconstriction of heart failure.

Renal Effects of the Natriuretic Peptides

In normal humans, ANP and BNP increase GFR and urinary sodium excretion with no change or only a slight fall in RBF (96). These changes in renal hemodynamics are likely mediated by afferent arteriolar vasodilation with constriction of the efferent arterioles. However, in addition to increasing GFR and filtered sodium load as a mechanism of their natriuretic effect, ANP and BNP are specific inhibitors of sodium reabsorption in the collecting tubule (97). An important role for endogenous ANP in the renal sodium balance of heart failure has been demonstrated by Lee et al. (98). Similar decreases in cardiac output were induced in two groups of dogs by constriction of the TIVC or acute rapid ventricular pacing. Sodium retention paralleled the activation of the renin–angiotensin–aldosterone system in the TIVC constriction group. Atrial pressures and plasma ANP were not increased in this group of dogs. In comparison, the ventricular pacing group did not experience sodium retention or activation of the renin–angiotensin–aldosterone system. This group had similar reductions in cardiac output and arterial pressure as the TIVC constriction group but, unlike the TIVC constriction group, had increased atrial pressures and circulating endogenous ANP levels. In a third group, exogenous ANP was administered to TIVC constriction dogs to increase plasma ANP levels to those observed in the pacing model. The ANP infusion prevented the sodium retention and activation of the renin–angiotensin–aldosterone system.

Unfortunately, the administration of synthetic ANP to patients with low-output heart failure results in a much smaller increase in renal sodium excretion and less significant changes in renal hemodynamics compared to normal subjects (99). Like ANP, the natriuretic effect of BNP is blunted in rats with high-output heart failure produced by AV fistulae (100). In a trial of BNP, 127 patients with a PCWP of 18 mm Hg or higher and a cardiac index of 2.7 L per minute per square meter of body surface area or less were randomly assigned to double-blind treatment with placebo or BNP (nesiritide) infused at a rate of 0.015 or 0.030 μg/kg of body weight per minute for 6 hours (94). BNP significantly decreased PCWP and resulted in improvements in global clinical status in most patients (i.e., reduced dyspnea and fatigue). The most common side effect was dose-related hypotension, which usually was asymptomatic. Therefore, intravenous nesiritide may be useful for the short-term treatment of patients hospitalized with decompensated CHF (94). A recent retrospective report, however, demonstrated an increase in serum creatinine and mortality in heart failure patients receiving BNP (101).

The possible mechanism of the relative renal resistance to natriuretic peptides in heart failure remains controversial.

1. Downregulation of renal ANP receptors
2. Secretion of inactive immunoreactive ANP
3. Enhanced renal neutral endopeptidase activity limiting the delivery of ANP to receptor sites
4. Hyperaldosteronism causing increased sodium reabsorption in the distal renal tubule
5. Diminished delivery of sodium to the distal renal tubule site of ANP action

A strong positive correlation between plasma ANP and urinary cGMP (the second messenger for the natriuretic effect of ANP and BNP in vivo) has been shown in sodium-retaining patients with heart failure (102). This observation supports the active biologic responsiveness of renal ANP receptors in heart failure and thus suggests that diminished distal tubular sodium delivery may explain the natriuretic peptide resistance observed in patients with cardiac failure. In cirrhosis, another edematous disorder associated with renal ANP resistance, increased distal tubular sodium delivery with mannitol has been shown to reverse the ANP resistance (103). Moreover, in heart failure, the administration of an angiotensin II receptor antagonist or furosemide, which are expected to increase distal tubular sodium delivery, also improves the renal response to ANP (64,104). Finally, studies in rats with experimental heart failure have demonstrated that renal denervation reverses the ANP resistance (105), an effect likely mediated by increased distal tubular sodium delivery. In Figure 2.6 is shown the proposed role of diminished distal tubular sodium delivery in natriuretic peptide resistance and impaired aldosterone escape in states of arterial underfilling.

Renal Prostaglandins in Cardiac Failure

Renal prostaglandins do not regulate renal sodium excretion or renal hemodynamics to any significant degree in normal subjects and intact animals. However, prostaglandin activity is increased in patients with heart failure and has been shown to correlate with the severity of disease as assessed by the degree

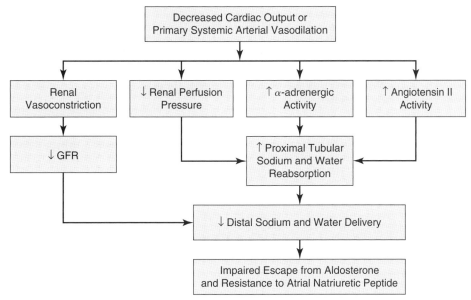

■ **Figure 2.6** Proposed mechanism of natriuretic peptide resistance and impaired aldosterone escape in states of arterial underfilling. GFR, glomerular filtration rate. (From Schrier RW, Better OS. Pathogenesis of ascites formation: mechanism of impaired aldosterone escape in cirrhosis. *Eur J Gastroenterol Hepatol.* 1991;3:721, with permission.)

of hyponatremia (106). Moreover, it has been well documented that the administration of a cyclooxygenase inhibitor in heart failure patients may result in acute reversible renal failure, an effect proposed to result from inhibition of renal prostaglandins (107). An investigation in patients with moderate heart failure and a normal sodium intake demonstrated that the administration of acetylsalicylic acid in doses that decrease the synthesis of renal prostaglandin E_2 results in a significant reduction in urinary sodium excretion (108). These observations support a role for prostaglandins in attenuating the renal vasoconstriction and sodium retention in patients with heart failure.

PATHOGENESIS OF SODIUM AND WATER RETENTION IN CIRRHOSIS

Two earlier theories have attempted to explain the pathogenesis of sodium and water retention in cirrhosis (109,110). The classic "underfill hypothesis" suggested that ascites formation secondary to portal hypertension leads to decreased plasma volume, which secondarily increases renal sodium and water retention (109). However, results of animal studies have shown that sodium and water retention precedes ascites formation in cirrhotic animals, thus contradicting the hypothesis (110). Moreover, plasma volume is increased, not decreased, in cirrhosis. An alternative hypothesis was therefore proposed in which primary renal sodium and water retention occurs secondary to a hepatorenal reflex. This would lead to plasma volume expansion of both the venous and arterial compartments and cause overflow ascites (110). This "overfill hypothesis" of ascites formation in cirrhotic patients, however, did not explain the progressive stimulation of the neurohumoral profile as cirrhotic patients progress from compensated to decompensated with ascites to hepatorenal syndrome. Against this background, we have suggested a primary role for systemic arterial vasodilation for the initiation of renal sodium and water retention in cirrhosis (Fig. 2.2) (111,112). This theory encompasses the entire range of cirrhosis from compensated to decompensated to hepatorenal syndrome and explains the progressive increases in both plasma volume and neurohormonal activation that occur as cirrhosis worsens.

Systemic Arterial Vasodilation Hypothesis

Splanchnic arterial vasodilation occurs early in cirrhosis, and the resultant arterial underfilling stimulates sodium and water retention with plasma volume expansion prior to ascites formation. The normal plasma hormone concentrations in compensated cirrhotic patients are relatively increased for the degree of sodium and water retention and plasma volume expansion. The mediators of the early splanchnic vasodilation in cirrhosis may include the opening of existing shunts, activation of vasodilating hormones, and ultimately the development of collaterals. Vasodilation may occur at other sites including the skin, muscle, and lung as cirrhosis progresses. However, although the presence of splanchnic arterial vasodilation is well documented in experimental and human cirrhosis, the development of arterial vasodilation involving other vascular territories is less certain.

Increased synthesis and release of the potent vasodilator nitric oxide, perhaps owing to increased circulating levels of endotoxin in cirrhosis, have been proposed to account for the arterial vasodilation and hyperdynamic circulation seen in cirrhotic patients (113–116). Although nitric oxide activity is difficult to assess in vivo, indirect evidence supports this hypothesis. For example, urinary cGMP, the second messenger of nitric oxide, is increased in patients with cirrhosis prior to the development of ascites and in some patients prior to an increase in circulating ANP concentrations (117). Markedly increased cGMP concentrations in aortic tissue from rats have been demonstrated in experimental cirrhosis (115). In these animals, aortic cGMP concentrations correlated inversely with arterial pressure ($r = -0.54$, $p < 0.0001$). Significantly, the chronic administration of the nitric oxide synthesis (NOS) inhibitor N^G-nitro-L-arginine-methyl-ester (L-NAME, 10 mg/kg/day for 7 days) induced a marked reduction in aortic cGMP concentration and an increase in arterial blood pressure in cirrhotic rats to similar levels obtained in L-NAME–treated control animals. This indicated that the high aortic cGMP content and decreased arterial blood pressure in cirrhotic rats were due to an increased NOS (115). Normalization of vascular nitric oxide production by chronic NOS inhibition corrects the systemic hemodynamic abnormalities in cirrhotic rats with ascites (116). Furthermore, chronic L-NAME treatment in drinking water for 10 days normalized mean arterial pressure, cardiac output, and systemic vascular resistance in these cirrhotic animals (118). The neurohumoral response in cirrhotic rats was also normalized as PRA, aldosterone, and AVP returned to control levels after 7 days of NOS inhibition (118). These hemodynamic and neurohumoral alterations during NOS inhibition were associated with profound reversal of the sodium and water retention in these cirrhotic rats. Moreover, Guarner et al. (114) have demonstrated elevated serum nitrite and nitrate levels—a crude index of in vivo nitric oxide generation—in 51 cirrhotic patients. Of note, in these patients, the elevated serum nitrite and nitrate levels significantly correlated with plasma endotoxin levels and decreased in response to a reduction in plasma endotoxin concentration following the administration of the antibiotic colistin (114). In addition, an enhanced sensitivity to mediators of endothelium-dependent vasodilation has been demonstrated in human cirrhosis (119). Taken together, these observations are compatible with the presence of nitric oxide–induced arterial vasodilation in cirrhosis. Endogenous opioids also may contribute to the peripheral vasodilation and renal sodium and water retention in cirrhosis, as the administration of opioid antagonists (e.g., naloxone or naltrexone) increased sodium and water excretion after water loading in cirrhotic subjects (120). Other factors that have been proposed to mediate the splanchnic vasodilation in cirrhosis include vasodilating prostaglandins, glucagon, calcitonin gene–related peptide, platelet-activating factor, substance P, and vasoactive intestinal peptide; however, definitive proof is lacking for these potential medications. As with cardiac failure, pretreatment hyponatremia and high plasma concentrations of renin, norepinephrine, and aldosterone portend a poor prognosis in the cirrhotic patient. The highest plasma concentrations of these hormones and the lowest blood pressures occur as the decompensated cirrhotic patient with ascites progresses toward the hepatorenal syndrome.

Nephron Sites of Sodium Retention in Cirrhosis

There is indirect evidence for both enhanced proximal and distal tubular reabsorption in human cirrhotic subjects. The following findings support enhanced proximal tubular reabsorption in hepatic cirrhosis: (a) maneuvers that expand plasma volume and increase distal nephron delivery of fluid (i.e., neck immersion and infusion of saline or mannitol) result in increased renal sodium excretion and solute-free water formation independent of changes in GFR (121); (b) in some water-loaded cirrhotic patients with ascites and minimal urine osmolalities, urine flow rates (an index of distal delivery of tubular fluid under these circumstances) are lower than in normal subjects (122); and (c) enhanced proximal reabsorption of tubular fluid has been found in micropuncture studies with chronic bile duct ligation (123).

Evidence for enhanced distal nephron sodium reabsorption is based on the following observations: (a) water-loaded patients with sodium retention and cirrhosis with minimal urine osmolalities often have urine flow rates comparable to normal controls (124); (b) water-loaded cirrhotic patients with minimal urine osmolalities have increased calculated distal fractional sodium reabsorption after receiving hypotonic saline infusions (124); (c) acetazolamide, a diuretic acting at the proximal tubule, produces a significant natriuresis in cirrhotic subjects only when there is concomitant distal nephron blockade of sodium reabsorption with ethacrynic acid (125); and (d) micropuncture studies in the dimethylnitrosamine and bile duct ligation models of cirrhosis demonstrate enhanced distal nephron sodium reabsorption (126,127).

In summary, clinical and experimental studies suggest that both proximal and distal nephron sites participate in enhanced renal tubular sodium reabsorption in cirrhosis. As in cardiac failure, neurohormonal activation appears to play a major role in the sodium and water retention of cirrhosis. The mechanisms responsible for enhanced sodium and water reabsorption in cirrhosis are no doubt multifactorial. A decrease in GFR may not be observed in some sodium-retaining cirrhotic patients, suggesting that sodium retention can occur independently of a decrease in GFR. An increase in renal vascular resistance and filtration fraction often is seen in decompensated cirrhosis. Thus, peritubular physical forces (decreased hydrostatic pressure and increased oncotic pressure) may act to enhance proximal tubular sodium reabsorption in advanced cirrhosis.

The Sympathetic Nervous System in Cirrhosis

Elevated plasma levels of norepinephrine have been observed in cirrhotic patients with ascites. Plasma norepinephrine levels correlate positively with plasma AVP concentrations and PRA and negatively with urinary sodium excretion (121). Moreover, norepinephrine spillover rates in cirrhotic patients have been shown to be increased compared to normal controls, whereas norepinephrine clearance rates were comparable between the two groups (128). Floras et al. (129), using the technique of peroneal nerve microneurography to directly measure sympathetic nerve activity to muscle, also have demonstrated adrenergic activation in cirrhotic patients. Finally, Ring-Larsen et al. (130) have demonstrated normal hepatic norepinephrine clearances and increased renal norepinephrine release in cirrhotic patients. Taken together, these findings are compatible with the presence of systemic and renal adrenergic activation in cirrhosis.

These findings indicate that increased activity of the sympathetic nervous system and renal nerves may result in enhanced renal sodium reabsorption in cirrhosis. As mentioned, renal adrenergic stimulation has been shown to increase proximal tubular sodium reabsorption. In addition, a negative correlation between plasma norepinephrine and urinary sodium excretion has been shown in cirrhotic patients (131). Ring-Larsen et al. (132) have demonstrated an inverse correlation between plasma norepinephrine and RBF. Moreover, in the report from Floras et al. (129), muscle sympathetic nerve activity was inversely correlated with urinary sodium excretion.

Role of Aldosterone in Cirrhosis

In a study by Gregory et al. (133), 16 out of 21 cirrhotic patients exhibited disappearance of ascites with spironolactone treatment over 3 to 4 weeks; sometimes, a loop diuretic furosemide was added. Thus, the near-uniform natriuretic response to spironolactone in cirrhotic patients, when given in adequate doses (100 to 400 mg/day), suggests that the increased levels of aldosterone contribute to the increased distal sodium reabsorption. Since exogenous aldosterone administration does not cause edema in normal subjects and absence of edema is a hallmark of primary hyperaldosteronism, the major problem in cirrhotic patients appears to be related to a failure to escape from the sodium-retaining effect of aldosterone as occurs in normal subjects. Aldosterone escape in normal subjects is associated with increased sodium delivery to the distal collecting duct site of aldosterone action. In cirrhosis the increased neurohumoral activation, particularly angiotensin and α-adrenergic stimulation, enhances proximal tubular sodium reabsorption and diminishes distal sodium delivery. This sequence of events appears to be the main cause for the failure of cirrhotic patients to escape from the sodium-retaining effect of aldosterone. Because of the elevated endogenous plasma level of aldosterone, mineralocorticoid antagonists, such as spironolactone, need to be given in higher doses. Diuretic resistance in cirrhosis is therefore defined as absence of a natriuresis with daily spironolactone doses of 400 mg and furosemide of 160 mg. On this background, mineralocorticoid antagonists are established as the diuretic of first choice in cirrhotic patients, followed by a loop diuretic if necessary.

The Nonosmotic Release of Vasopressin in Cirrhosis

Hyponatremia with impaired ability to excrete a water load occurs in a substantial number of patients with cirrhosis of the liver, thereby demonstrating an impairment in urinary dilution in these patients (134,135). Decompensated cirrhotic patients with ascites and/or edema have an abnormal response to water administration, whereas cirrhotic patients without ascites or edema usually excrete water normally (135). There are two potential mechanisms for this inability to excrete solute-free water in decompensated cirrhotic patients with ascites: (a) a derangement in renal hemodynamics with decreased fluid delivery to the distal nephron; and (b) an extrarenal mechanism involving nonosmotic AVP release. Volume expansion maneuvers that improve distal fluid delivery of ascitic fluid (136,137), as well as head-out water immersion (121), improve urinary dilution and water excretion in cirrhosis. These maneuvers also increase central blood volume and could improve water excretion by suppressing baroreceptor-mediated nonosmotic AVP release.

Studies of patients with cirrhosis also implicate the nonosmotic release of AVP as a major factor responsible for water retention in cirrhosis. Bichet et al. (138) studied 26 cirrhotic patients who received a standard water load (20 mL/kg). Patients could be separated into two groups on the basis of their ability to excrete this water load: those able to excrete >80% of the water load in 5 hours ("excretors") and those unable to excrete a water load normally ("nonexcretors"). Nonexcretors had lower serum sodium concentrations and higher plasma AVP levels after the water load. These nonexcretors also were found to have higher pulse rates, lower plasma albumin concentrations, higher PRA and aldosterone concentrations, and higher plasma norepinephrine levels than normonatremic cirrhotic patients with normal water excretion (138). A greater increase in systemic arterial vasodilatation in the nonexcretors is supported by these studies. Thus, arterial underfilling may provide the nonosmotic stimulus for AVP release in hyponatremic cirrhotic patients. Enhancement of central blood volume by water immersion to the neck suppressed AVP release and improved, but did not normalize, water excretion in subsequent experiments (121). However, a comparable suppression of AVP with head-out water immersion and norepinephrine infusion normalized water excretion in decompensated cirrhotic patients (139). The increment in water excretion with this combined maneuver, which increases renal perfusion pressure, would be expected to increase distal fluid delivery.

Studies performed in rats made cirrhotic by exposure to carbon tetrachloride and phenobarbital supported AVP hypersecretion as the predominant mechanism of the impairment of water excretion, because the administration of a V_2 vasopressin antagonist normalized water excretion in 9 of the 10 rats studied (140). Moreover, using the orally active nonpeptide V_2 receptor AVP antagonist OPC-31260, Tsuboi et al. (141) normalized the defect in solute-free water excretion in this animal model of cirrhosis. Additional experimental data supporting a primary role for AVP in the impaired water excretion in cirrhosis were reported by Fujita et al. (142). These investigators examined the effect of experimental cirrhosis on expression of the mRNA for the AVP-dependent collecting duct water channel, AQP2, in the rat. Binding of AVP to the V_2 receptor initiates a chain of intracellular signaling events that leads to the insertion of AQP2 water channels into the apical membrane of collecting duct cells, thus rendering these cells permeable to water. In the cirrhotic rats studied by Fujita et al. (142), AQP2 mRNA was markedly increased as compared to control animals. Moreover, an oral water load (30 mL/kg) did not reduce AQP2 mRNA expression, but the blockade of AVP action by the V_2 receptor AVP antagonist OPC-31260 significantly diminished its expression in the cirrhotic animals. Nonpeptide V_2 receptor antagonists have been shown to increase plasma sodium concentration in hyponatremic cirrhotic patients and improve urinary dilution (143,144).

Natriuretic Peptides in Cirrhosis

As with other edematous states associated with arterial underfilling, the neurohumoral responses to the systemic arterial vasodilation of cirrhosis are associated with factors that diminish distal sodium delivery. The impaired aldosterone escape (145) and resistance to ANP (146) that occur in cirrhosis, therefore, are most likely mediated by diminished distal sodium delivery to the collecting duct site of these hormonal actions. As with experimental cardiac failure, renal denervation has been shown to reverse the resistance to ANP in experimental cirrhosis (147). This finding supports a role of diminished distal sodium delivery in the ANP resistance. Moreover, Skorecki et al. (146) have demonstrated a normal increase in urinary cGMP but no natriuresis in some cirrhotic patients infused with ANP. Since cGMP is the secondary messenger of ANP, this finding supports the biologic responsiveness of renal ANP receptors in these patients. An increased distal sodium delivery with mannitol (as assessed by lithium clearance) has been shown to reverse resistance to exogenous ANP.

Renal Prostaglandins in Cirrhosis

Zambraski and Dunn (148) demonstrated that prostaglandins with vasodilator properties are necessary to maintain RBF and GFR in dogs with cirrhosis secondary to bile duct ligation. Similar conclusions about the importance of prostaglandins have been obtained in cirrhotic humans. Inhibition of prostaglandin synthesis in decompensated cirrhotic patients decreases RBF, GFR, sodium excretion, and solute-free water excretion and impairs the natriuretic response to diuretic agents (149,150). Infusion of prostaglandin has been shown to reverse the diminutions in RBF and GFR observed after prostaglandin inhibition in cirrhotic patients (150). Moreover, inhibition of prostaglandin synthesis may cause a syndrome that mimics the hepatorenal syndrome (149). Vasodilating renal prostaglandins may also play an important counterregulatory role in early or well-compensated cirrhosis (151).

In summary, numerous afferent and efferent mechanisms are involved in the abnormal sodium and water excretion seen in patients with liver disease. These mechanisms appear to be initiated by arterial underfilling caused by primary systemic arterial vasodilation. The sympathetic nervous system, renin–angiotensin–aldosterone axis, and the nonosmotic release of AVP are the major effector components of this increased sodium and water reabsorption, which also may be modulated by the release of natriuretic peptides and renal prostaglandins.

PATHOGENESIS OF SODIUM AND WATER RETENTION IN THE NEPHROTIC SYNDROME

Two views of the pathogenesis of edema formation in the nephrotic syndrome are illustrated in Figure 2.7. According to the "underfill" theory, urinary loss of albumin occurs as a consequence of an increase in

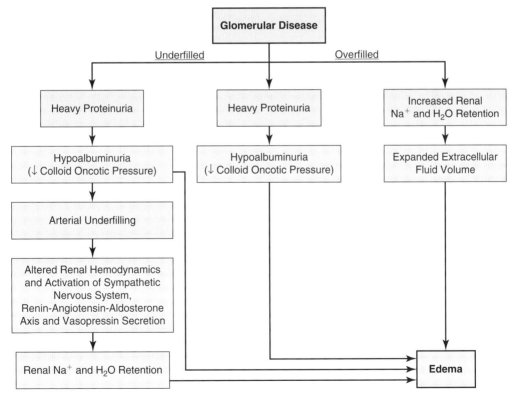

■ **Figure 2.7** Proposed underfilled and overfilled mechanisms of sodium and water retention in the nephrotic syndrome. (From Bansal S, Lindenfeld J, Schrier RW. Sodium retention in cardiac failure and cirrhosis: potential role of natriuretic doses of mineralocorticoid antagonist? *Circ Heart Fail.* In press, with permission.)

glomerular capillary permeability and results in hypoalbuminemia. This decline in serum albumin lowers intravascular colloid oncotic pressure, thereby increasing transudation of plasma from the intravascular to the interstitial space. It is this decrease in plasma volume that causes arterial underfilling and serves as the stimulus for renal sodium and water retention. Ultimately, the decrease in intravascular colloid oncotic pressure and the increase in interstitial hydrostatic pressure secondary to edema formation come into balance, and the edematous state stabilizes. Thus, the diminution in total plasma volume is the critical afferent stimulus in inducing renal sodium and water retention and should be observed in the initiating phase of formation. Several lines of evidence support this traditional underfill theory of edema formation in the nephrotic syndrome (152): (a) plasma volume may be modestly decreased in some nephrotic patients in the absence of diuretic therapy; (b) systemic arterial hypotension and diminished cardiac output, correctable by plasma volume expansion, have been observed in some patients with nephrotic syndrome; (c) some nephrotic patients have humoral markers of arterial underfilling such as elevated plasma levels of PRA, aldosterone, and catecholamines; and (d) head-out water immersion and intravascular infusion of albumin, maneuvers that increase plasma volume, may result in substantial increases in GFR and in fractional excretion of sodium chloride and water in these patients.

Usberti et al. (153) have described two groups of nephrotic syndrome patients distinguished on the basis of their plasma albumin concentrations. Patients in group 1 had a plasma albumin concentration of <1.7 g/dL associated with low blood volumes and plasma ANP levels, elevated plasma angiotensin II concentrations, and increased proximal tubular reabsorption of sodium (determined by lithium clearance). In contrast, group 2 patients had a plasma albumin concentration >1.7 g/dL and exhibited normal blood volumes and plasma hormone concentrations. In all patients, blood volume was positively correlated with the plasma albumin concentration, and PRA was inversely correlated with both blood volume and plasma albumin concentration. Of note, GFR was not different between group 1 and 2 patients (100 ± 25 mL/min vs. 101 ± 22 mL/min, $p =$ NS), whereas urinary sodium excretion was substantially lower in group 1 patients (4.88 ± 5.53 mEq/4 hr vs. 29.9 ± 9.3 mEq/4 hr, $p < 0.001$). Moreover, the acute expansion of blood volume in group 1 patients normalized PRA, plasma angiotensin II and aldosterone concentrations, fractional sodium excretion, and lithium clearance, whereas circulating ANP concentrations increased. Taken together, these observations support the traditional underfill view of the pathogenesis of edema formation in the nephrotic syndrome.

To further explore the state of arterial filling in patients with the nephrotic syndrome, sympathetic nervous system activity was evaluated in six edematous patients with the nephrotic syndrome of various parenchymal etiologies and in six normal control subjects (154). As mentioned, increased adrenergic activity occurs in states of arterial underfilling and may be the earliest sign. Sympathetic nervous system activity was assessed by determining plasma norepinephrine secretion and clearance rates using a whole-body steady-state radionuclide tracer method. Patients were withdrawn from all medications 7 days prior to study. Mean creatinine clearances and serum creatinine concentrations were normal in both the nephrotic syndrome patients and controls. However, the nephrotic syndrome patients exhibited significant hypoalbuminemia (2.0 ± 0.4 g/dL vs. 3.8 ± 0.1 g/dL, $p < 0.01$). The supine plasma norepinephrine levels were elevated in the patients with the nephrotic syndrome as compared to controls. More significantly, the secretion rate of norepinephrine was significantly increased in nephrotic patients, whereas the clearance rate of norepinephrine was similar in the two groups (Fig. 2.8). PRA and plasma aldosterone, AVP, and ANP concentrations were not different in nephrotic syndrome patients compared to controls. These observations indicate that the sympathetic nervous system is activated in patients with the nephrotic syndrome prior to a significant fall in GFR or a marked activation of either the renin–angiotensin–aldosterone system or the nonosmotic release of AVP. These data also support the presence of arterial underfilling in the nephrotic syndrome.

Several investigators, however, have challenged this traditional underfill model based on the following observations: (a) several studies of plasma and/or blood volume in edematous nephrotic patients have reported either normal or elevated values (155); (b) hypertension and low PRA, two indices suggesting volume expansion, have been reported in some patients with nephrotic syndrome (156); (c) hypoalbuminemia in animal studies as well as in patients with analbuminemia do not necessarily lead to edema formation (157); and (d) a low filtration fraction is often observed in patients with the nephrotic syndrome (158), in contrast to the increased filtration fraction usually associated with states of arterial underfilling. Thus, the "overfill" hypothesis has been proposed to account for nephrotic edema formation in some patients. According to this view, the renal retention of sodium and water

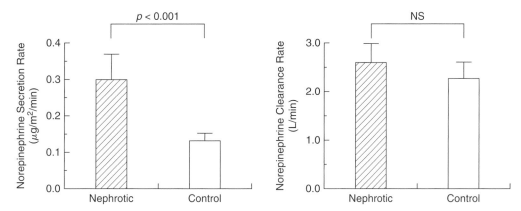

■ **Figure 2.8** Plasma norepinephrine secretion and clearance rates in patients with the nephrotic syndrome and normal glomerular filtration rates and in normal control subjects. The findings of increased norepinephrine secretion and normal norepinephrine clearance in the nephrotic syndrome patients are consistent with early activation of the sympathetic nervous system in the nephrotic syndrome. (From Rahman SN, Abraham WT, Van Putten VJ, et al. Increased norepinephrine secretion in patients with the nephrotic syndrome and normal glomerular filtration rates: evidence for primary sympathetic activation. *Am J Nephrol.* 1993;13:266, with permission of S. Karger AG [Basel].)

occurs as a primary intrarenal phenomenon independent of systemic factors. In this setting, renal sodium and water retention produces an expanded plasma volume, and the overfilled plasma volume then leaks into the interstitium and induces edema formation. The hypoalbuminemia and decreased plasma oncotic pressure serve to enhance the formation of edema.

A possible explanation for the variable volume and humoral results obtained in patients with the nephrotic syndrome is that the afferent stimulus may not be attributed to a single mechanism. Specifically, patients with the nephrotic syndrome are heterogeneous with regard to type of renal lesion, GFR, presence of underlying systemic disease, degree of hypoalbuminemia, and diuretic usage. In rat studies, aminonucleoside-induced nephrosis was characterized by a decreased plasma volume, as well as a well-maintained GFR, and edema could be prevented by adrenalectomy. In contrast, nephrotic syndrome induced by nephrotoxic serum was characterized by increased plasma volume and a very low GFR, and edema occurred independently of the adrenal glands. In this regard, the studies of Meltzer et al. (156) also are of note. In 1979, these investigators characterized a group of patients with the nephrotic syndrome associated with volume depletion and stimulation of the renin–angiotensin–aldosterone system and described a second group with low or normal PRA and aldosterone concentrations and hypervolemia. The "hypovolemic" group was characterized by minimal change disease and well-preserved GFRs. These patients fit nicely into the traditional underfill schema depicted in the left panel in Figure 2.7. The "hypervolemic" patients were characterized by having chronic glomerulopathy and reduced GFR (mean, 53 mL/min) in addition to suppressed plasma concentrations of renin and aldosterone, findings consistent with intrarenal mechanisms contributing to the renal sodium and water retention and thus the overfill theory.

Nephron Sites of Sodium Retention in the Nephrotic Syndrome

The nephron site of enhanced renal sodium retention in the nephrotic syndrome has been studied predominantly in animal models of glomerulonephritis. Bernard et al. (159) used micropuncture and clearance methodology to study the nephron site of increased sodium reabsorption in saline-loaded rats with autologous immune complex nephritis. These rats developed heavy proteinuria, hypoalbuminemia, and hypercholesterolemia. Etiopathologic examination of kidneys from these animals revealed slight thickening of basement membranes, uniform finely granular deposits of IgG and complement distributed along the basement membranes of all glomeruli, and electron-dense subepithelial deposits.

These findings are similar to those observed in human idiopathic membranous nephropathy. Arterial blood pressure, hematocrit, GFR, and renal plasma flow were comparable in control and experimental animals. Proximal tubular sodium reabsorption was decreased in nephrotic rats as compared to controls (35% vs. 44%, $p < 0.05$). Absolute sodium reabsorption along the loop of Henle and in the distal convoluted tubule was comparable in nephrotic and control animals. Despite comparable sodium delivery to sites beyond the late distal convoluted tubule, the fractional excretion of sodium was significantly lower in nephrotic (2.2%) than in control (4.0%) animals. From these results, the authors conclude that nephron sites beyond the late distal convoluted tubule are primarily responsible for the enhanced sodium reabsorption seen in this nephrotic model. Alternatively, it remains possible that enhanced sodium reabsorption by deep nephrons not accessible to micropuncture also could contribute to the diminished sodium excretion.

Different results were reported by Kuroda et al. (160) using a rat nephrotoxic serum model of nephrotic syndrome. Proteinuria, hypoalbuminemia, and hypercholesterolemia also occurred in these studies. Histologic examination of the kidneys revealed mild glomerular hypercellularity, widely dilated proximal tubules, diffuse glomerular linear immunofluorescence, and electron-dense subepithelial deposits. In contrast to the study by Bernard et al. (159), these animals were actively retaining sodium. In micropuncture studies, single-nephron GFR was decreased, and the percentage of filtered water reabsorbed prior to late proximal and distal tubular convolutions was increased in the nephrotic rats.

Two clearance studies have been undertaken in nephrotic patients in an attempt to clarify the nephron site of enhanced sodium reabsorption (161,162). Both of these studies were undertaken in patients with a wide variety of primary renal diseases and GFRs. Usberti et al. (162) measured tubular reabsorption of glucose in 21 patients with glomerulonephritis. Tubular glucose reabsorption was used as a marker for proximal tubular sodium reabsorption. The threshold for glucose reabsorption was reduced in 10 nephrotic patients, suggesting diminished proximal tubular reabsorption. A similar conclusion was reached by Grausz et al. (161) in studies undertaken in five nephrotic patients. Blockade of distal tubular nephron sites of sodium reabsorption with ethacrynic acid and chlorothiazide was used to assess proximal sodium reabsorption in these clearance studies. With this approach, proximal sodium reabsorption was found to be lower in nephrotic patients than in normal and cirrhotic patients. However, the more recent study of Usberti et al. (153) demonstrated increased proximal tubular sodium reabsorption—using the more precise technique of lithium clearance—in nephrotic syndrome patients with low albumin concentrations and blood volumes and elevated PRA.

In summary, it appears from experimental and clinical studies that distal nephron sites are primarily involved in the avid sodium retention of the nephrotic syndrome. However, it is likely that increased proximal tubular sodium reabsorption also may be operative in selected cases, depending on the nature of the underlying renal disease, the blood volume status, and the phase of sodium retention.

Mechanisms of Enhanced Tubular Sodium Reabsorption

Several studies have been undertaken to identify the mechanism underlying the enhanced renal tubular sodium reabsorption in the nephrotic syndrome. Many nephrotic patients with a normal GFR avidly retain sodium, although a reduced GFR frequently is observed in nephrotic patients. Thus, factors in addition to a reduced filtered load of sodium are important in many nephrotic patients. Based on both experimental and clinical studies, however, nephrotic patients with the lowest GFR often demonstrate the greatest degree of sodium retention (156).

Peritubular capillary physical forces (oncotic and hydrostatic pressures) are believed to exert a modulating influence on renal sodium and water reabsorption. This influence is most likely exerted at the level of the proximal convoluted tubule. However, the low filtration fraction, high renal plasma flow, and normal renal vascular resistance frequently observed in nephrotic patients suggest that factors other than peritubular capillary physical forces are responsible for enhanced tubular sodium reabsorption.

The Renin–Angiotensin–Aldosterone System in the Nephrotic Syndrome

A potential role for the renin–angiotensin–aldosterone system in the pathogenesis of nephrotic sodium retention has been studied in detail. Two early experimental studies strongly supported a role for aldosterone in nephrotic edema (163, 164). In rats made nephrotic with aminonucleoside, Tobian et al. (163) found an increase in juxtaglomerular cell granularity during sodium retention. Moreover, Kalant and collaborators (164) found that adrenalectomy prevented the sodium retention of aminonucleoside nephrosis. In one study, aminonucleoside was administered into one renal artery. Proteninuria, a reduced GFR, and sodium retention were observed only in the kidney that received aminonucleoside (165).

Several studies have measured components of the renin–angiotensin–aldosterone system in nephrotic humans (152). In general, studies have been carried out in heterogeneous patient populations at a variety of stages during the patients' illness. A wide range of values varying from very high to very low have been observed. However, PRA values tend to be highest in patients demonstrating characteristics of arterial underfilling and lowest in overfilled patients.

Brown et al. (166) have undertaken clinical studies to examine the physiologic significance of activation of the renin–angiotensin–aldosterone system in sodium-retaining nephrotic patients. Eight of 16 patients had high PRA. Administration of the ACEI captopril to these eight patients did not induce a diuresis despite a significant reduction in plasma aldosterone to normal values. Mean arterial pressure, however, fell in these patients during converting enzyme inhibition. These results suggested that additional factors are responsible for the avid renal sodium retention even in nephrotic patients with high plasma aldosterone. Aldosterone antagonism studies are more definitive, however, because no fall in blood pressure secondary to diminished angiotensin II, as occurs with ACE inhibition, would occur. In this regard, we have demonstrated reversal of the positive sodium balance in patients with the nephrotic syndrome owing to a variety of glomerular diseases treated with the aldosterone antagonist spironolactone (167).

Natriuretic Peptides in the Nephrotic Syndrome

Plasma ANP and BNP concentrations may be elevated in humans and animals with the nephrotic syndrome (168,169); however, the hemodynamic and renal responses to exogenous ANP or BNP have been found to be blunted in experimental nephrosis (169) and in patients with the nephrotic syndrome (168). Perico and Remuzzi (170) have proposed tubular insensitivity to ANP as an initiating factor in the formation of edema in the nephrotic syndrome. According to their hypothesis, renal unresponsiveness to ANP results in distal tubular sodium and water retention with subsequent edema formation. Any ANP cellular resistance may result from a postreceptor, rather than receptor, mechanism, because urinary cGMP responds appropriately to ANP infusion in nephrotic animals (171). Alternatively, this blunted natriuretic response to ANP and BNP may be secondary to neurohormonal activation. The observed sympathetic activation in edematous patients with the nephrotic syndrome supports this possibility (154). Moreover, Koepke and DiBona (105) have shown that renal denervation, which is known to increase distal sodium delivery, reversed the blunted diuretic and natriuretic responses to ANP in a rat model of the nephrotic syndrome.

Other humoral factors (e.g., kinins and prostaglandins) may modulate renal sodium reabsorption in nephrotic patients. Specifically, inhibitors of prostaglandin synthesis have been reported to reduce GFR in patients with the nephrotic syndrome and may precipitate renal insufficiency (172). Thus, prostaglandins may attenuate factors in nephrotic syndrome that decrease GFR and cause sodium retention.

Renal Water Retention in the Nephrotic Syndrome

The nephrotic syndrome is less frequently associated with hyponatremia, in contrast with the two previously described clinical edematous disorders, heart failure and cirrhosis. In fact, serum sodium concentration usually is normal unless it is influenced by vigorous diuretic measures or during an acute water load (173,174). Furthermore, high serum lipid levels may cause pseudohyponatremia in nephrotic patients unless serum sodium concentration is measured by a direct ion-specific electrode. Nevertheless, abnormal water excretion was clearly demonstrated by Gur et al. (175) in six nephrotic children, because their solute-free water clearance during water loading was negative as compared to a positive value after remission of their disease. Head-out water immersion induced an increase in solute-free water clearance in patients with the nephrotic syndrome (176,177), and this improvement may have been secondary to the suppression of the nonosmotic release of AVP. Alternatively, water immersion might improve intrarenal hemodynamics, increase the amount of fluid delivered to the distal diluting nephron, and thereby improve water excretion. Plasma AVP concentrations have been found to be elevated in nephrotic subjects (174,178–180) and to correlate best with blood volume (180). Water immersion and hyperoncotic albumin infusion reduced plasma levels of AVP and induced a water diuresis in nephrotic patients (178–180). Studies by Shapiro et al. (181) have shown a close correlation between decrements in GFR and water excretion during an acute water load in patients with nephrotic syndrome. Therefore, analysis of these studies indicates that the impaired water excretion in nephrotic patients may be related both to intrarenal factors involving a fall in GFR and diminished distal fluid delivery and to extrarenal factors that primarily involve the nonosmotic release of AVP.

In summary, it appears that the effector mechanisms for sodium and water retention in the nephrotic syndrome may involve a fall in GFR and activation of the sympathetic nervous system, the renin–angiotensin–aldosterone system, and the nonosmotic release of AVP. Enhanced renal tubular sodium and water reabsorption observed in nephrotic patients also may involve a diminution in ANP sensitivity.

Treatment of Edematous Disorders

Given the preceding background discussion of the pathophysiology of sodium and water retention in the edematous disorders, the approach to the treatment of cardiac failure, liver disease, and the nephrotic syndrome is now considered. The general principles for such therapy are described in Table 2.2.

EVALUATION OF THE ADEQUACY OF TREATMENT OF THE PRIMARY DISEASE RESPONSIBLE FOR EDEMA

In cardiac failure, cirrhosis, and the nephrotic syndrome, the initiation of sodium and water retention involves the arterial underfilling caused by these diseases. Initial therapeutic attempts should be directed toward treatment of the primary disease. In low-output cardiac failure, the restoration of cardiac output to normal levels abolishes the arterial underfilling and thus the initiating event for renal sodium retention. The use of positive inotropic agents (e.g., digoxin) and afterload-reducing agents (e.g., ACEIs, ARB, arterial vasodilators) to improve cardiac output should be aggressively pursued in heart failure patients. This approach may alleviate the need for inhibiting tubular reabsorption with diuretics, a maneuver that may further decrease cardiac output and worsen the arterial underfilling. In this regard, it should be noted that the clinical practice guidelines for the treatment of heart failure from the Agency for Health Care Policy and Research recommend ACE inhibition as first-line therapy in nonedematous patients with heart failure (182). In the nephrotic syndrome, particularly of the nil disease or lipoid nephrosis variety, administration of corticosteroids may diminish or eliminate the proteinuria and thereby correct the hypoalbuminemia (183). In addition, treatment with ACEIs (184,185) or an ARB (186) has been shown to reduce the urinary protein loss associated with human nephrotic syndrome. In contrast, the administration of albumin solutions is of very little lasting value in the nephrotic syndrome, because the concomitant increase in blood volume is associated with increased urinary clearance of albumin, and thus

TABLE 2.2 GENERAL PRINCIPLES IN THE TREATMENT OF EDEMATOUS DISORDERS

Evaluation of the adequacy of treatment of the primary disease responsible for edema
Evaluation of level of salt and water intake
Mobilization of edema: bed rest and supportive stockings
Evaluation of indications for use of diuretics
Impaired respiratory function
Incipient or overt pulmonary edema
Elevated diaphragms with ascites, associated with incipient or overt atelectasis
Impaired cardiovascular function secondary to fluid overload
Excess fluid limiting physical activity and causing discomfort
To avoid further sodium retention and yet allow the ingestion of palatable (sodium-containing) diet
Cosmetic effect: marginal indication

only a transient increase in plasma albumin concentration occurs. In extreme states of hypoalbuminemia, however, an infusion of albumin may be a lifesaving treatment for a hypotensive episode. Albumin solutions also may be of value for patients with cirrhosis, hypoalbuminemia, and edema, particularly when there is evidence of intravascular volume depletion, such as diminished central venous pressure and a fall in orthostatic blood pressure. The administered albumin is excreted less readily in cirrhotic patients because they have no defect in glomerular capillary permeability and frequently have lower levels of GFR. However, a potential complication of such albumin infusions is the resulting increase in portal hypertension with increased bleeding from esophageal varices and the precipitation of hepatic encephalopathy because of the protein load. In some patients with acute alcoholic hepatitis accompanying cirrhosis, corticosteroid therapy may improve liver function in those with elevated bilirubin and prolonged prothrombin times.

EVALUATION OF THE LEVEL OF SODIUM AND WATER INTAKE

The level of sodium and water intake of edematous patients should be evaluated. However, it should be realized that although sodium restriction alone is effective in preventing further accumulation of edema, it may not induce a negative sodium balance. Patients who are edematous may be maximally retaining sodium (<10 mEq excretion per day). Thus, at best, "sodium-free" diets that contain 10 to 20 mEq of sodium merely prevent a further increase in positive sodium balance. The diuresis that may be observed in cardiac and cirrhotic patients who are hospitalized and placed on low-sodium diets may relate to the salutary consequences of bed rest on cardiac output in the former and improvement in the primary liver disease in the latter, rather than to sodium restriction per se.

The level of fluid intake also must be assessed, because most patients with edematous disorders have a defect in renal water excretion, as has been discussed, as well as in sodium excretion (Chapter 1 and the prior discussion). If the patient is hyponatremic, then the daily fluid intake should be adjusted to equal insensible losses (500 to 700 mL/day) plus daily urinary losses. However, severe fluid restriction often is difficult to accomplish in these patients, because increased angiotensin II and baroreceptor activation may stimulate CNS thirst centers.

MOBILIZATION OF EDEMA

Bed rest alone may lead to a diuresis, particularly in patients with cardiac failure. Furthermore, patients who are resistant to diuretic agents administered on an outpatient basis may become responsive to the same or smaller doses of diuretic agents with hospitalization and bed rest. The use of professionally fitted supportive stockings also may be of value in the mobilization of edema fluid. The mechanism of the supine position or supportive stockings, or both, in mobilizing edema fluid probably is related to the diminished peripheral venous pooling and thus to a more normal central arterial filling and renal perfusion. Finally, because upright posture in the normal person is associated with activation of the sympathetic nervous system and renin–angiotensin–aldosterone axis, the supine position may ameliorate to some extent overactivity of these neurohormonal vasoconstrictor mechanisms.

EVALUATION OF INDICATIONS FOR USE OF DIURETICS

If edema persists despite adequate treatment of the primary disease, then diuretics should be used only for definite indications (Table 2.2). The presence of edema alone is not an absolute indication for diuretic treatment, and any cosmetic value must be weighed against the potential deleterious effect of the drug. In general, the use of diuretic agents should be limited primarily to those situations in which impairment of respiratory or cardiac function, or both, or physical discomfort is secondary to fluid accumulation. An exception to this rule is the patient who will not restrict sodium intake; diuretics given to such patients may prevent edema accumulation despite dietary salt indiscretion. When patients find a low-salt diet unpalatable, diuretics can be used to allow them to include sodium in their diet.

There are two cardinal rules to follow in estimating the optimal rate of diuresis once the decision is made to use diuretic agents to treat an edematous disorder. In general, the daily diuresis should approximate the rate of accumulation of the edema fluid. Thus, acute pulmonary edema necessitates induction of a rapid diuresis, whereas chronic heart failure is best treated with a more gradual diuresis. In either case, the rate of diuresis should be such that the rate of movement of interstitial fluid into the vascular compartment will not be exceeded to any large extent. If renal excretion does exceed the rate of mobilization of interstitial fluid, intravascular volume depletion and hypotension can result, even though ECF volume is still expanded. Careful clinical monitoring of intravascular volume (i.e., neck veins, orthostatic blood pressure, pulse, etc.), therefore, is extremely important, particularly during the induction of an acute diuresis. Intermittent diuretic therapy, such as alternate-day therapy, may be of value in avoiding intravascular volume depletion as well.

DIURETIC THERAPY

The judicious use of diuretic agents necessitates a knowledge of their site of action, potency, and side effects. In Table 2.3 are listed the primary sites of action of the available diuretic agents, but it should be emphasized that several of these diuretics also have secondary sites of action.

Site of Action of Diuretics

Filtration Diuretics

The so-called filtration diuretics are primarily aminophylline and glucocorticoids. In addition, plasma volume expansion or an increase in cardiac output secondary to use of cardiac glycosides or inotropic agents such as dopamine, dobutamine, or the phosphodiesterase inhibitors (e.g., amrinone, milrinone) may enhance GFR. Infusions of metaraminol and angiotensin II also have been shown to increase GFR in patients with cirrhosis, although these vasoconstrictor agents decrease filtration rates in normal subjects (122).

Proximal Tubular Diuretics

Diuretics that act primarily to decrease proximal tubular sodium reabsorption include osmotic diuretics (e.g., mannitol) and carbonic anhydrase inhibitors (acetazolamide). The filtration and proximal tubular diuretics are not very effective when administered alone. Although the largest portion of glomerular

TABLE 2.3 CLASSIFICATION OF DIURETICS BY NEPHRON SITE OF ACTION

Filtration Diuretics

Aminophylline
Glucocorticoids

Proximal Tubular Diuretics

Mannitol
Acetazolamide

Loop of Henle Diuretics

Ethacrynic acid
Furosemide
Bumetanide
Torsemide

Distal Tubular Diuretics

Potassium-losing
Thiazides
Chlorthalidone
Metolazone
Portassium-retaining
Triamterene
Spironolactone
Amiloride
Eplerenone

Collecting Duct Diuretics

Lithium
Demeclocycline
Vasopressin antagonists

filtrate is reabsorbed isosmotically in the proximal tubule (50% to 70%), the distal nephron (particularly the ascending limb of the loop of Henle) has the capacity to increase its rate of sodium reabsorption significantly (187). Thus, an increase in glomerular filtration or depression of proximal tubular reabsorption alone may not be associated with a significant diuresis, because the increased distal sodium and fluid delivery may be reabsorbed at more distal nephron sites. Therefore, the filtration and proximal tubular diuretics are best used in conjunction with a diuretic that acts on the distal nephron, particularly when the patient has shown resistance to distally acting diuretics.

Loop of Henle Diuretics

The loop diuretics—ethacrynic acid, furosemide, bumetanide, and torsemide—are the most potent diuretic agents available. The inhibition by these agents of active sodium chloride transport in the medullary ascending limb of the loop of Henle generally exceeds the rate-limited sodium chloride reabsorption in the more distal nephron, and a maximal diuretic effect equivalent to 20% to 25% of the filtered load of sodium may be achieved.

The loop diuretics limit maximal renal diluting capacity because the reabsorption of tubular sodium chloride without water in the ascending limb is inhibited by these agents. It has been shown, however, that the administration of the loop diuretic furosemide may actually increase solute-free water excretion in edematous patients, who already have impaired diluting capacity (86). It has been proposed that the rapid rate of distal fluid delivery limits the osmotic equilibration between the collecting duct and interstitium, because this diuretic-induced water diuresis is unaffected by exogenous AVP administration. Alternatively, the diuretic may interfere with the action of AVP on the collecting duct, particularly because thiazide diuretics increase and furosemide decreases urine osmolality in the presence of exogenous AVP at comparable solute excretion rates (188). Sodium chloride reabsorption in the ascending limb is also the major factor in the countercurrent concentrating mechanism that generates the hypertonicity in the medullary interstitium. Thus, loop diuretics also impair the renal capacity to concentrate the urine and conserve water. Finally, in contrast to other diuretics that may cause renal vasoconstriction, such as the thiazides, the loop diuretics cause renal vasodilatation, an effect that partially may contribute to their diuretic effect (189).

Distal Tubular Diuretics

The distal tubular diuretics can be classified into two groups: potassium-losing and potassium-retaining diuretics. The thiazide diuretics, chlorthalidone and metolazone, have similar diuretic effects although they are chemically different. These distal tubular diuretics inhibit only urinary diluting capacity and not concentrating capacity, because they decrease sodium reabsorption in the cortical, but not medullary, portion of the ascending limb as well as the distal convoluted tubule. As with the loop diuretics, the use of distal tubular diuretics, which also act proximal to the distal site of potassium secretion, is associated not only with a natriuresis but also with an increase in urinary potassium excretion. As discussed in Chapter 5, this effect of increased sodium delivery on potassium excretion has been shown to be linked to enhanced sodium reabsorption. Thus, an increase in distal sodium delivery may alter potassium excretion by modulating potassium secretion in the collecting duct (190).

The clinically available potassium-conserving diuretics include triamterene, amiloride, and the aldosterone antagonists spironolactone and eplerenone. Although the action of aldosterone antagonists is dependent on the presence of the adrenal cortex and circulating aldosterone, the ability of triamterene and amiloride to block potassium secretion is independent of adrenal function. The effect of amiloride appears to result from inhibition of sodium entry into the cell from luminal fluid by blocking the epithelial sodium channel. Frequently, these diuretics are not potent enough alone, but they may be used to avoid the potassium-losing effects of diuretics that act at more proximal nephron sites, such as the thiazide and loop diuretics.

Collecting Duct Diuretics

In contrast to all the diuretics mentioned, two diuretics act at the level of the collecting duct and induce a water diuresis rather than a natriuresis. These agents, demeclocycline and lithium, impair the ability of AVP to increase the water permeability of the renal collecting duct epithelium, thereby antagonizing the hydroosmotic effect of AVP (191). These agents have been given only to hyponatremic, edematous patients because they induce a water diuresis. Both agents are capable of inducing significant adverse effects; however, one study demonstrated superior effect with less toxicity when demeclocycline was compared with lithium in the treatment of the syndrome of inappropriate AVP secretion (191). Nonetheless, demeclocycline has been shown to be nephrotoxic in hyponatremic cirrhotic patients and thus should be avoided in the presence of liver disease (192), including heart failure with hepatic hypoperfusion and congestion. V_2 receptor AVP antagonists, which directly antagonize the renal effects of AVP, are now available (193). Conivaptan is a nonpeptide, combined V_1/V_2 receptor antagonist that has been approved to treat hyponatremia in euvolemic conditions (e.g., SIADH) and heart failure inhospital. The drug causes an increase in solute-free water excretion without an increase in electrolyte excretion. As noted earlier, conivaptan has been approved for intravenous use for a maximum of 4 days inhospital to increase plasma sodium concentration. The first orally active, nonpeptide V_2 antagonist, tolvaptan, has been approved to treat hyponatremia in euvolemic (e.g., SIADH) and hypervolemic states (heart failure and cirrhosis). Hyponatremia in heart failure and cirrhosis is a major risk factor for increased mortality in these conditions. The major side effects of these aquaretic agents include dry mouth, increased thirst, and polyuria. In chronic hyponatremia, the increase in plasma sodium concentration should not exceed 10 to 12 Eq/L over 24 hours, because more rapid changes may cause osmotic demyelination (see Chapter 1).

Potency of Diuretics

All the thiazide-like drugs have reasonably comparable effects in optimal doses with the exception of metolazone, which is more potent than the others. The other thiazide diuretics differ from each other primarily in duration of action. Thiazide diuretics are probably the agent of choice when an oral agent of moderate potency is desired.

In optimal doses, the loop diuretics (ethacrynic acid, furosemide, bumetanide, and torsemide) are some six to eight times more potent than the thiazide diuretics. This greater potency is expected, because several times more sodium chloride is reabsorbed in the loop of Henle than in the distal convoluted tubule. Because of their potency, the loop but not the thiazide diuretics are effective in patients with advanced renal failure (GFR <25 mL/min). Metolazone also has been shown to be effective in patients with a GFR of <25 mL/min and can enhance the effects of loop diuretics. The thiazide and loop diuretics both can be administered intravenously as well as orally.

Hemodynamic Effects of Diuretics

The hemodynamic actions of diuretics have been examined in normal humans, anephric subjects, patients with heart failure, and experimental animals. In 1973, Dikshit et al. (194) reported the effects of intravenous furosemide (0.5 to 1.0 mg/kg) in 20 patients with left heart failure complicating acute myocardial infarction. These patients exhibited a marked decrease in left ventricular filling pressure, from 20.4 to 14.8 mm Hg, occurring between 5 and 15 minutes after furosemide administration. This effect anteceded the diuretic and natriuretic effect of the drug and was associated with a 52% increase in mean calf venous capacitance, thus demonstrating the venodilating effect of furosemide. This early venodilating effect of furosemide has been confirmed by other workers and also has been observed in normal subjects and experimental animals. The clinical importance of this early increase in venous capacitance and diminished left ventricular filling pressure resides in the resultant early beneficial effects of furosemide on acute pulmonary edema and explains the improved clinical symptoms of pulmonary congestion that may occur with furosemide prior to the onset of the drug's diuretic response. The acute venodilation associated with furosemide administration in these patients may be mediated by vasodilating prostaglandins, because the administration of the prostaglandin synthetase inhibitor, indomethacin, has been shown to abolish the increase in venous capacitance initiated by furosemide in normal volunteers and anephric subjects consuming a low-sodium diet (195).

In contrast to the early venodilation observed in patients with acute left ventricular failure, intravenous furosemide has been shown to induce an acute vasoconstrictor response in patients with decompensated chronic class III and IV heart failure (195). In these patients with advanced heart failure, intravenous furosemide (1.3 mg/kg of body weight) caused a significant increase in mean arterial pressure and systemic vascular resistance, associated with a fall in stroke volume index and a rise in left ventricular filling pressure, 20 minutes after furosemide administration. This acute increase in cardiac afterload was associated with, and presumably resulted from, the accompanying rapid rise in circulating concentrations of three vasoconstrictor hormones, namely plasma norepinephrine, angiotensin II, and AVP. In this regard, it is important to note that loop diuretics block NaCl transport at the macular densa that stimulates the renin–angiotensin system. Angiotensin II is also known to stimulate the sympathetic nervous system. Thus, it is clear that the acute vascular effects that occur with intravenous furosemide are determined, at least in part, by whether the patient has acute (196) versus chronic heart failure (197). With chronic treatment, however, diuretic therapy results in favorable effects on both cardiac preload and afterload, which may result in an improvement in left ventricular function.

Neurohormonal Effects of Diuretics

The acute intravenous administration of furosemide with the resultant diuresis and natriuresis may be associated with activation of the sympathetic nervous system, renin–angiotensin–aldosterone system, and nonosmotic release of AVP in patients with acute heart failure. Likewise, chronic oral diuretic therapy (furosemide, 80 to 240 mg/day for 8 days) has been shown to increase plasma renin, angiotensin II, and aldosterone concentrations in chronic heart failure patients (197). Moreover, Bayliss et al. (198) have demonstrated a similar activation of the renin–angiotensin–aldosterone system during the chronic administration of oral furosemide, 40 mg/day, plus amiloride, 5 mg/day, for 30 days to patients presenting with decompensated heart failure manifest by pulmonary and/or peripheral edema.

In addition to the effect of diuretics to increase renal renin release, the diminished concentrations of natriuretic peptides that occur in association with chronic diuretic administration also may explain the further activation of the renin–angiotensin–aldosterone system, because natriuretic peptides are known to suppress plasma renin and aldosterone synthesis and release. Support for this hypothesis may be found in studies performed in animal models of heart failure. Fett et al. (199) have studied the endocrine and renal effects of intravenous furosemide (1.7 mg/kg) in an animal model of acute low-output heart failure owing to rapid right ventricular pacing at 250 beats/min for 3 hours. In this model, 2 hours after furosemide, there was a fall in plasma ANP, RBF, and GFR as the renin–angiotensin–aldosterone system was activated. The authors then examined the effects of an exogenous infusion of ANP, sufficient to prevent the furosemide-induced fall in the elevated endogenous plasma ANP, in the same experimental model. Maintenance of plasma ANP concentrations was associated with an enhanced natriuretic response to furosemide at 1 hour (182 μEq/min vs. 440 μEq/min, $p < 0.05$) and at 2 hours (72 μEq/min vs. 180 μEq/min, $p < 0.05$), associated with suppression of plasma aldosterone and maintenance of GFR.

Intermittent versus Continuous Intravenous Diuretic Therapy for Decompensated Edematous States

Kaojarern et al. (200) have suggested the time course of delivery of such diuretics as furosemide into the urine as an independent predictor of overall response. This observation led to the concept of a "maximally efficient excretion rate" for furosemide (200). In this regard, it is possible that a continuous infusion of furosemide or similar diuretic at a dose that constantly maintains the most efficient urinary diuretic excretion rate may be superior to intermittent intravenous diuretic administration. Studies in heart failure patients support this hypothesis. Lahav et al. (201) performed a prospective, randomized, crossover trial comparing intermittent intravenous furosemide administration (30 to 40 mg/ 8 hr for 48 hours) with a continuous furosemide infusion following a single loading dose (2.5 to 3.3 mg/hr for 48 hours after a 30- to 40-mg loading dose) in nine patients with advanced heart failure refractory to conventional oral therapy. Total doses of furosemide administered were equivalent in the two groups. The continuous infusion of furosemide produced greater diuresis and natriuresis compared to intermittent furosemide administration in all patients. Similar results have been obtained with furosemide or bumetanide in normal volunteers and patients with advanced renal dysfunction (202). These results suggest that the continuous infusion of a loop diuretic may be the preferred method for intravenous diuretic therapy in patients with decompensated disease or "diuretic resistance" (see the following). Torsemide oral bioavailability may be better and more consistent than other loop diuretics (203).

Side Effects and Complications of Diuretic Therapy

The most common complications of diuretic therapy are volume and potassium depletion (Table 2.4). The thiazide and loop diuretics are most commonly associated with these complications. Volume depletion can be profound and may be associated with symptoms of cerebral or coronary insufficiency, particularly in the elderly. Diminished renal perfusion also may occur, as evidenced by a rise in blood urea nitrogen and serum creatinine concentrations.

A high-potassium diet (e.g., oranges, apricots, and bananas) frequently is sufficient to avoid diuretic-induced hypokalemia. However, potassium chloride supplements or potassium-retaining diuretics may be necessary to avoid this complication in many patients treated with moderate to high doses of loop and/or thiazide-type diuretics and metolazone. It is important to note that potassium supplements and potassium-retaining diuretics only should be administered simultaneously under very close supervision because of the potential danger of fatal hyperkalemia. This also is true for the combination of potassium supplements or potassium-retaining diuretics and ACEIs or ARBs, which inhibit aldosterone and thus promote potassium retention. Spironolactone has been shown to induce or worsen renal tubular acidosis in some cirrhotic patients (204). Even more careful monitoring of serum potassium concentrations is necessary during diuretic therapy for patients receiving cardiac glycosides, because either hypokalemia or hyperkalemia are known to stimulate or exacerbate arrhythmias associated with digoxin excess.

Hyponatremia may result from the impaired water excretion associated with the primary edematous disorder, from the ability of the diuretic to impair urinary diluting capacity, or from a combination thereof. In either case, if diuretic therapy is indicated, any symptomatic hyponatremia associated with edematous states is better treated by water restriction than by cessation of diuretic therapy. If ineffective, the orally active V_2 antagonist, tolvaptan, may be useful. Metabolic acidosis is a complication of the use of carbonic anhydrase inhibition, because these agents block hydrogen ion secretion. The use of thiazide and loop diuretics may be associated with metabolic alkalosis. This is predominantly owing to the excretion of sodium, chloride, and potassium without bicarbonate, which leads to a rise in serum bicarbonate concentration.

The complication of carbohydrate intolerance has been observed with both the thiazide and loop diuretics and may be related to potassium depletion. Hypokalemia is known to blunt the insulin response to a carbohydrate load, and this mechanism accounts at least in part for the carbohydrate intolerance. Patients most affected by this complication are probably those with diabetes mellitus or those predisposed to it.

Hyperuricemia may occur with most diuretics but has been reported most widely with thiazide diuretics or furosemide therapy. The primary cause of the hyperuricemia is a reduced urine clearance, which has been attributed to the enhanced tubular sodium reabsorption associated with volume depletion, because urate reabsorption in the proximal tubule parallels the rate of tubular sodium reabsorption.

TABLE 2.4 COMPLICATIONS OF DIURETIC THERAPY

Metabolic Complications

Volume depletion and azotemia
Hypokalemia and hyperkalemia
Hyponatremia
Acidosis and alkalosis
Carbohydrate intolerance
Hypomagnesemia
Hypocalcemia and hypercalcemia
Hyperuricemia

Hypersensitivity

Rash
Interstitial nephritis
Pancreatitis
Hematologic disorders

Miscellaneous

Deafness
Gastrointestinal symptoms

Hypercalcemia also has been described in conjunction with thiazides given to normal subjects, hyperparathyroid subjects, and hypoparathyroid subjects treated with vitamin D (205). The negative sodium balance and positive calcium balance associated with thiazide treatment seem at least partially responsible for the hypercalcemic effect. An interrelationship between parathyroid hormone and thiazide diuretics also has been demonstrated. Because of their hypocalciuric effect, thiazide diuretics may be used in the treatment of the idiopathic hypercalciuria that afflicts some patients with renal calculi. This may be associated with an effect on Na^+/Cl^- cotransporter to enhance Na^+/Ca_2^+ exchange (206). In contrast, furosemide increases calcium excretion and therefore has been used in conjunction with saline infusions to treat hypercalcemia. Because of this hypocalcemic effect, furosemide may induce symptoms of tetany in patients with borderline hypoparathyroidism (207).

Hypersensitivity reactions causing an interstitial nephritis may occur in association with thiazide diuretics or furosemide. Acute renal failure may occur when nonsteroidal anti-inflammatory drugs (NSAIDs) and triamterene are administered simultaneously (208). Skin rashes and hematologic disorders are other manifestations of hypersensitivity reactions that have been observed with diuretic therapy. A Schönlein–Henoch type of purpuric lesion of the lower extremities has been seen during treatment with ethacrynic acid (209). The diuretic agent should be discontinued in the presence of any signs of hypersensitivity reactions similar to serum sickness. Acute pancreatitis also has been observed in association with thiazide administration. Deafness, which generally is reversible on cessation of the diuretic administration, has been reported both with ethacrynic acid and with furosemide; in occasional cases, however, diuretic-induced deafness has been irreversible. Generally, this has occurred in patients with renal disease receiving acute bolus administration. Thus, the dose of loop diuretics should be given over 20 to 30 minutes when administered intravenously. Gastrointestinal disturbances may occur with any of the diuretic agents.

Causes of Diuretic Resistance

Resistance to diuretic therapy is most often owing to incomplete treatment of the primary disorder, continuation of a high sodium intake, or patient noncompliance. Inadequate diuretic dose or dosing regimen and route of administration also may be implicated in some cases. For example, given the 6-hour duration of action of oral furosemide, once-daily administration of this agent will be inadequate for most patients. As noted, in decompensated patients, continuous intravenous diuretic therapy may be superior to intermittent dosing regimens. Volume depletion is the most common cause of diuretic resistance once these above factors have been excluded. Because the most frequently used diuretics act at sites in the loop of Henle or distal convoluted tubule, their action is dependent on adequate delivery of sodium to these sites. Thus, diuretic-induced volume depletion with attendant decreases in GFR and increases in proximal tubular sodium reabsorption impairs the response to diuretics acting in the distal nephron. Because most diuretic agents exert their diuretic effect from the luminal side of tubular cells (as opposed to the contraluminal or peritubular capillary side), the delivery of the diuretic agent to its site of action in the nephron also may be diminished during volume depletion and decreased RBF. In this regard, it should be noted that triamterene may block the tubular secretion of furosemide, and this combination of diuretics should be avoided.

Diuretic-induced further activation of the sympathetic nervous and renin–angiotensin–aldosterone systems with a concomitant decrease in circulating plasma ANP also may contribute to the development of diuretic resistance, because increased renal nerve activity and angiotensin II may enhance proximal tubular sodium reabsorption, thereby obscuring the beneficial effect of a diuretic that acts in the distal nephron. This mechanism provides the rationale for combination therapy with a diuretic and neurohormonal antagonist, such as an ACEI, in edematous states.

Volume depletion and diuretic-induced renin release also increase aldosterone secretion. The distal tubular effect of aldosterone may blunt the natriuretic and enhance the kaliuretic response to diuretics. Avoidance of diuretic-induced volume depletion can be obtained best by initiating diuretic therapy with one of the diuretic agents of lower potency. Subsequently, the dose may be carefully titrated upward or more potent diuretics added while the patient's weight and orthostatic pulse and blood pressure changes are being monitored. The intermittent use of diuretics may help to avoid intravascular volume depletion. Finally, aldosterone antagonists in combination with more proximally acting diuretics may help to promote a diuresis in patients with "resistance" who do not appear to be profoundly volume depleted.

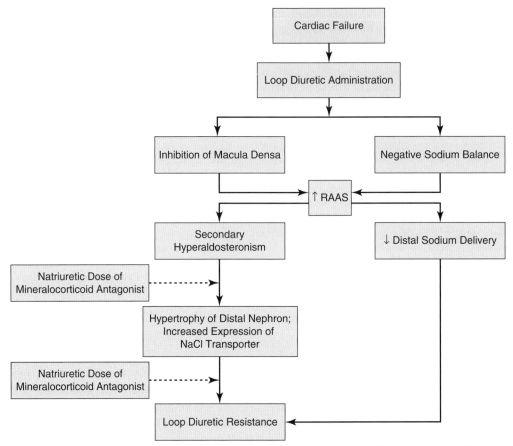

■ **Figure 2.9** Mechanisms of diuretic resistance in heart failure. (With permission from Bansal S, Lindenfeld J, Schrier RW. Sodium retention in heart failure and cirrhosis: potential role of natriuretic doses of mineralocorticoid antagonist? *Circ Heart Fail*. 2009;2:370–376.)

Aldosterone has also been shown to increase the NaCl cotransporter that could contribute to diuretic resistance (210). The role of diminished distal delivery and secondary hyperaldosteronism in diuretic resistance is shown in Figure 2.9.

The loop diuretics and thiazides are effective in the presence of acid–base disturbances. The diuretic effect of carbonic anhydrase inhibitors is blunted by the presence of respiratory or metabolic acidosis, possibly because of the excess of intracellular hydrogen ions even in the presence of carbonic anhydrase inhibition. Finally, the NSAIDs appear capable of attenuating the action of several diuretic agents (206).

USE OF DIURETICS IN SPECIFIC EDEMATOUS STATES

Cardiac Failure

It is the heart and not the kidney that fails in heart failure. The response of the kidney can be viewed as a normal compensatory attempt to restore arterial circulatory integrity. However, the increased renal sodium and water retention with heart failure results in increased venous return, further stretching of the diseased myocardium, pulmonary congestion, increasing renal venous pressure, and ultimately increased capillary filtration of fluid with peripheral and pulmonary edema. One form of therapy in chronic heart failure is to increase the contractile force of the heart with a cardiac glycoside, which has been shown to decrease the frequency of hospitalization but not alter mortality. The chronic use of other inotropic agents, however, has been shown to decrease survival, perhaps secondarily to arrhythmias and sudden death.

In addition to the effect of agents directly influencing the contractile state of the myocardium, it is important to note that the myocardial contractile state also is related to preload (venous return to the heart) and afterload (impedance to left ventricular outflow). Diuretic therapy diminishes preload by reducing venous return. This reduction in preload can reduce left ventricular filling pressure and thus alleviate some of the congestive symptoms of heart failure. Afterload reduction by systemic vasodilator therapy (parenteral nitroprusside or oral hydralazine, ACEIs, ARB, or prazosin) potentially results in improved ventricular function. The combined reduction in both preload and afterload induced by diuretics and vasodilators also may result in a favorable effect on cardiac performance.

In actuality, diuretics alone improve both congestive symptoms and exercise tolerance of patients with chronic heart failure (207–211). These favorable effects may occur at the expense of a reduced cardiac output, however (209). Thus, diuretics should be used cautiously in patients with chronic heart failure. ACEIs alone are often effective in relieving symptoms in mild heart failure without substantial edema. However, this form of therapy may be inadequate, and diuretics and digoxin may be needed in more severe degrees of heart failure. Again, it is important to be aware of diuretic-induced decreases in serum potassium and magnesium concentrations that predispose to digitalis toxicity and cardiac arrhythmias when treating the patient with heart failure.

Specific recommendations after ACE inhibition or ARB for the use of diuretics in heart failure are as follows:

1. Start with a loop or thiazide-type diuretic, depending on the severity of the heart failure. For severe heart failure with substantial volume overload (i.e., overt pulmonary and/or peripheral edema), use a loop diuretic, given the greater potency of this class of agents. Thiazides usually are adequate in patients with mild heart failure.
2. Add a thiazide diuretic or metolazone if a loop diuretic given twice daily in doses equivalent to furosemide, 240 mg/day, is inadequate for diuresis. This combination generally results in a synergistic effect on salt and water excretion. *Note:* This combination also results in a synergistic effect on renal potassium excretion; therefore, anticipate an increase in the requirement for supplemental potassium to avoid hypokalemia.
3. A potassium-retaining diuretic may be added in order to spare potassium or enhance diuresis. However, as mentioned, do not combine triamterene with furosemide, because triamterene blocks the tubular secretion of furosemide, thus inhibiting furosemide effect.
4. The goal of therapy is the resolution of signs and symptoms caused by pulmonary and/or peripheral edema.

In Figure 2.4 are shown the potential mechanisms whereby judicious fluid removal by diuretics or ultrafiltration can improve cardiac function. Nonnatriuretic doses of spironolactone have been shown to improve survival in cardiac failure, presumably via nonrenal effects on vascular and cardiac fibrosis. Natriuretic doses (>50 mg/day) of spironolactone have not been routinely used in heart failure patients, presumably because of the potential for causing hyperkalemia in the presence of ACE inhibition or ARB.

Cirrhosis

Some authors suggested that diuretic therapy is associated with substantial risk of adverse effects for the cirrhotic patient (212). The most feared complication is the induction of azotemia. Often this is the result of overzealous use of diuretics. Shear et al. (213) have demonstrated that the maximum rate of absorption of ascites from the peritoneum is 900 mL/day and is usually much less. A more rapid rate of diuresis (i.e., >1 L/day of negative fluid balance) occurs only at the expense of more easily mobilized peripheral edema fluid or diminished plasma volume. Hence, a profound diuresis may be associated with deterioration in renal function. Fortunately, such diuretic-induced azotemia usually is reversible; however, diuretics have been shown to precipitate hepatorenal syndrome in some cases. Alterations in serum potassium concentration often are encountered during diuretic treatment of the cirrhotic patient with ascites. Because secondary hyperaldosteronism and total body potassium depletion are frequently associated with cirrhosis (214), any diuretic that acts proximally to the distal potassium secretory site may cause profound hypokalemia unless it is accompanied by a potassium-sparing diuretic. Because of the frequently observed temporal relationship between diuretic therapy and induction of hepatic encephalopathy, Gabuzda and Hall (215) have postulated that the enhanced renal ammonia production of hypokalemia may contribute to the encephalopathy. In view of these potential hazards in the use of diuretics for the cirrhotic patient, the following general principles are recommended in the treatment of ascites:

1. Daily body weight and careful clinical and biochemical monitoring is mandatory.
2. Ascertaining that liver and renal functions are stable before instituting diuretic therapy.
3. Mobilizing ascites and edema with an initial period of bed rest and restricting dietary sodium before instituting diuretic therapy, because conservative therapy alone may result in a diuresis in 5% to 15% of cirrhotic patients.
4. Aiming for a daily weight loss of 1 to 2 lb in patients with ascites with peripheral edema and 0.5 to 1 lb in patients with ascites but without peripheral edema.
5. Maintaining the end point of therapy as maximum patient comfort with a minimum of drug-induced complications. Occasionally, this may require slight liberalization of sodium intake at the expense of increased usage of diuretics and maintenance of some residual ascites in selected patients.

The suggested regimen for diuretic therapy of ascites is as follows:

1. Restrict sodium (20 to 40 mEq/day).
2. If there is no diuresis in 3 to 4 days, add spironolactone initially (100 mg/day with increases every 3 to 5 days until natriuresis occurs as assessed by urinary sodium concentration). This approach results in a diuresis in 40% to 60% of patients.
3. If there is no diuresis with 400 mg of spironolactone per day, add hydrochlorothiazide (50 to 200 mg/day) or furosemide (20 to 80 mg/day). Diuretic resistance in cirrhosis has been defined as lack of response to 400 mg/day spironolactone and furosemide 160 mg/day.
4. Increasing doses of furosemide may be used if no diuresis is observed on this regimen after reassessment of dietary intake and hepatic and renal function show no deterioration.

It is of note that using a similar protocol, Gregory et al. (134) have documented that diuretic therapy can safely and efficaciously be given to the cirrhotic patient. Recently, numerous investigators have shown that repeated large-volume paracentesis (4 to 6 L/day) is a fast, effective, and safe therapy for ascites in patients with cirrhosis (216–221). The subsequent administration of diuretics avoids reaccumulation of ascites in the patients responding to these drugs. Of interest, contrary to the traditional concept of the potential danger of rapid and large paracentesis, the mobilization of ascites by paracentesis associated with intravenous albumin (8 g/L of ascites removed) did not alter renal function or systemic hemodynamics, the latter being estimated either directly (by measuring plasma volume, cardiac output, or peripheral resistance) or indirectly (by measuring PRA, plasma norepinephrine, and plasma AVP concentration).

Nephrotic Syndrome

The general approach to the therapy of nephrotic edema is listed in Table 2.5. As pointed out, nephrotic patients may be particularly susceptible to diuretic agents that act in the distal nephron. Distal-acting diuretics of the potassium-sparing variety also prove to be helpful in the management of the hypokalemia that may occur. These patients also respond to mineralocorticoid antagonists.

TABLE 2.5 THERAPY OF NEPHROTIC EDEMA

Treatment of primary disorder

Conservative methods of therapy
    Dietary (protein supplementation, salt restriction, water restriction)
    Physical (recumbency, lower-extremity elevation)

Diuretic therapy
    Pharmacologic agents
    Albumin infusions
    Water immersion
    Miscellaneous (angiotensin-converting enzyme inhibition, increase protein intake)

Acknowledgment

Studies reported in this chapter were supported, in part, by United States Public Health Services Research Grant M01-RR00051 from the General Clinical Research Centers Program of the Division of Research Resources, National Institutes of Health.

REFERENCES

1. Schrier RW. Pathogenesis of sodium and water retention in high-output and low-output cardiac failure, nephrotic syndrome, cirrhosis, and pregnancy. *N Engl J Med.* 1988;319:1065.
2. Schrier RW. Body fluid volume regulation in health and disease: a unifying hypothesis. *Ann Intern Med.* 1990;113:155.
3. Schrier RW. A unifying hypothesis of body fluid volume regulation: the Lilly Lecture 1992. *J R Coll Physicians Lond.* 1992;26:295.
4. Schrier RW. An odyssey into the milieu interieur: pondering the enigmas. *J Am Soc Nephrol.* 1992;2:1549.
5. Schrier RW, Gurevich AK, Cadnapaphornchai MA. Pathogenesis and management of sodium and water retention in cardiac failure and cirrhosis. *Semin Nephrol.* 2001;21:157–172.
6. Abraham W, Schrier RW. Heart disease and the kidney. In: Schrier RW, ed. *Diseases of the Kidney and Urinary Tract.* 8th ed. Philadelphia, PA: Lippincott Williams & Wilkins; 2006:2159–2178.
7. Gines P, Cardenas A, Schrier RW. Liver disease and the kidney. In: Schrier RW, ed. *Diseases of the Kidney and Urinary Tract.* 8th ed. Philadelphia, PA: Lippincott Williams & Wilkins; 2006:2179–2205.
8. Schrier RW, Abraham W. The nephrotic syndrome. In: Schrier RW, ed. *Diseases of the Kidney and Urinary Tract.* 8th ed. Philadelphia, PA: Lippincott Williams & Wilkins; 2006:2206–2213.
9. Verney EB. Croonian lecture: the anti-diuretic hormone and the factors which determine its release. *Proc R Soc Lond (Biol).* 1947;135:25.
10. Starling EH. On the absorption of fluid from the connective tissue spaces. *J Physiol (Lond).* 1896;19:312.
11. Peters JP. The role of sodium in the production of edema. *N Engl J Med.* 1948;239:353.
12. Borst JGG, deVries LA. Three types of "natural" diuresis. *Lancet.* 1950;2:1.
13. Sato F, Kamoi K, Wakiya Y, et al. Relationship between plasma atrial natriuretic peptide levels and atrial pressure in man. *J Endocrinol Metab.* 1986;63:823.
14. de Torrente A, Robertson GL, McDonald KM, et al. Mechanism of diuretic response to increased left atrial pressure in the anesthetized dog. *Kidney Int.* 1975;8:355.
15. Goetz KL, Bond GC, Bloxham DD. Atrial receptors and renal function. *Physiol Rev.* 1975;55:157.
16. Zucker IH, Earle AM, Gilmore JP. The mechanism of adaptation of left atrial stretch receptors in dogs with chronic congestive heart failure. *J Clin Invest.* 1977;60:323.
17. Epstein FH, Post RS, McDowell M. Effects of an arteriovenous fistula on renal hemodynamics and electrolyte excretion. *J Clin Invest.* 1953;32:233.
18. Pearce JW, Sonnenberg H. Effects of spinal section and renal denervation on the renal response to blood volume expansion. *Can J Physiol Pharmacol.* 1965;43:211.
19. Schrier RW, Humphreys MH. Factors involved in the antinatriuretic effects of acute constriction of the thoracic and abdominal inferior vena cava. *Circ Res.* 1971;29:479.
20. Schrier RW, Humphreys MH, Ufferman RC. Role of cardiac output and autonomic nervous system in the antinatriuretic response to acute constricting of the thoracic superior vena cava. *Circ Res.* 1971;29:490.
21. Guyton A, Scanlon CJ, Armstrong GG. Effects of pressoreceptor reflex and Cushing's reflex on urinary output. *Fed Proc.* 1952;11:61.
22. Schrier RW, Berl T, Anderson RJ. Osmotic and non-osmotic control of vasopressin release. *Am J Physiol.* 1979;236:F321–F322.
23. Davis JO. The control of renin release. *Am J Med.* 1973;55:333.
24. Epstein FH, Goodyer AVN, Lawrason FD, et al. Studies of the antidiuresis of quiet standing: the importance of changes in plasma volume and glomerular filtration rate. *J Clin Invest.* 1951;30:63.
25. Gauer OH, Henry JP. Circulating basis of fluid volume control. *Physiol Rev.* 1963;43:423.
26. Smith HW. Salt and water volume receptors: an exercise in physiologic apologetics. *Am J Med.* 1957;23:623.
27. Murdaugh HV Jr, Sieker HO, Manfredi F. Effect of altered intrathoracic pressure on renal hemodynamics, electrolyte excretion and water clearance. *J Clin Invest.* 1959;38:834.
28. Hulet WH, Smith HH. Postural natriuresis and urine osmotic concentration in hydropenic subjects. *Am J Med.* 1961;30:8.
29. Gauer OH, Henry JP, Sieker HO, et al. The effect of negative pressure breathing on urine flow. *J Clin Invest.* 1954;33:287.
30. Reinhardt HW, Kacmarczyk G, Eisele R, et al. Left atrial pressure and sodium balance in conscious dogs on a low sodium intake. *Pflugers Arch.* 1977;370:59.
31. Epstein M, Duncan DC, Fishman LM. Characterization of the natriuresis caused in normal man by immersion in water. *Clin Sci.* 1972;43:275.
32. Henry JP, Gauer OH, Reeves JL. Evidence of the atrial location of receptors influencing urine flow. *Circ Res.* 1956;4:85.
33. Currie MG, Geller DM, Cole BC, et al. Bioactive cardiac substances: potent vasorelaxant activity in mammalian atria. *Science.* 1983;221:71.
34. Atlas SA, Kleinert HD, Camargo MJ, et al. Purification, sequencing, and synthesis of

natriuretic and vasoactive rat atrial peptide. *Nature.* 1984;309:717.

35. Barger AC, Yates FE, Rudolph AM. Renal hemo-dynamics and sodium excretion in dogs with graded valvular damage, and in congestive failure. *Am J Physiol.* 1961;200:601.

36. Zucker IH, Gorman AJ, Cornish KG, et al. Impaired atrial receptor modulation of renal nerve activity in dogs with chronic volume overload. *Cardiovasc Res.* 1985;19:411.

37. Ferguson DW, Abboud FM, Mark AL. Selective impairment of baroreceptor-mediated vasocon-strictor responses in patients with ventricular dysfunction. *Circulation.* 1984;69:451.

38. Sandoval AB, Gilbert EM, Larrabee P, et al. Hemodynamic correlates of increased cardiac adrenergic drive in the intact failing human heart. *J Am Coll Cardiol.* 1989;13:245A.

39. Sklar AH, Schrier RW. Central nervous system mediators of vasopressin release. *Physiol Rev.* 1983;63:1243.

40. Berl T, Henrich WL, Erickson AL, et al. Prostaglandins in the beta adrenergic and baroreceptor-mediated secretion on renin. *Am J Physiol.* 1979;235:F472.

41. Braunwald E, Plauth WH, Morrow AG. A method for detection and quantification of impaired sodium excretion. *Circulation.* 1965;32:223.

42. Schrier RW. Body water homeostasis: clinical disorders of urinary dilution and concentration. *J Am Soc Nephrol.* 2006;17(7):1820–1832.

43. Hope JA. *Treatise on the Diseases of the Heart and Blood Vessels.* London: William Kidd; 1832.

44. Warren JV, Stead EA. Fluid dynamics in chronic congestive heart failure: an interpretation of the mechanisms producing edema, increased plasma volume and elevated venous pressure in certain patients with prolonged congestive heart failure. *Arch Intern Med.* 1944;73:138.

45. Kilcoyne MM, Schmidt DH, Cannon PJ. Intrarenal blood flow in congestive heart failure. *Circulation.* 1973;47:786.

46. Bourdeaux R, Mandin H. Cardiac edema in dogs. II. Distribution of glomerular filtration rate and renal blood flow. *Kidney Int.* 1976;10:578.

47. Meyers BD, Deen WM, Brenner BM. Effects of norepinephrine and angiotensin II on the determinants of glomerular ultrafiltration and proximal tubule fluid reabsorption in the rat. *Circ Res.* 1975;37:101.

48. Ichikawa I, Pfeffer JM, Pfeffer MA, et al. Role of angiotensin II in the altered renal function in congestive heart failure. *Circ Res.* 1984;55:669.

49. Henrich WL, Berl T, MacDonald KM, et al. Angiotensin, renal nerves and prostaglandins in renal hemodynamics during hemorrhage. *Am J Physiol.* 1978;235:F46.

50. Bennett WM, Bagby GC, Antonovic JN, et al. Influence of volume expansion on proximal tubular sodium reabsorption in congestive heart failure. *Am Heart J.* 1973;85:55.

51. Davis D, Baily R, Zelis R. Abnormalities in sys-temic norepinephrine kinetics in human conges-tive heart failure. *Am J Physiol.* 1988;254:E760.

52. Hasking GJ, Esler MD, Jennings GL, et al. Norepinephrine spillover to plasma in patients with congestive heart failure: evidence of increased overall and cardiorenal sympathetic nervous activity. *Circulation.* 1986;73:615.

53. Abraham WT, Hensen J, Schrier RW. Elevated plasma noradrenaline concentrations in patients with low-output cardiac failure: dependence on increased noradrenaline secretion rates. *Clin Sci.* 1990;79:429.

54. Francis GS, Benedict C, Johnstone EE, et al. Comparison of neuroendocrine activation in patients with left ventricular dysfunction with and without congestive heart failure: a substudy of the studies of left ventricular dysfunction (SOLVD). *Circulation.* 1990;82:1724.

55. Leimbach WN, Wallin BG, Victor RG, et al. Direct evidence from intraneural recordings for increased sympathetic outflow in patients with heart failure. *Circulation.* 1986;73:913.

56. Cohn JN, Levine BT, Olivari MT, et al. Plasma norepinephrine as a guide to prognosis in patients with chronic congestive heart failure. *N Engl J Med.* 1984;311:819.

57. DiBona GF, Herman PJ, Sawin LL. Neural control of renal function in edema forming states. *Am J Physiol.* 1988;254:R1017.

58. Bello-Reuss E, Trevino DL, Gottschalk CW. Effect of renal sympathetic nerve stimulation on proxi-mal water and sodium reabsorption. *J Clin Invest.* 1976;57:1104.

59. Lifschitz MD, Schrier RW. Alterations in cardiac output with chronic constriction of thoracic infe-rior vena cava. *Am J Physiol.* 1973;225:1364.

60. Francis GS, Goldsmith SR, Levine TB, et al. The neurohumoral axis in congestive heart failure. *Ann Intern Med.* 1984;101:370.

61. Han HJ, Park SH, Koh HJ, et al. Mechanism of regulation of Na^+ transport by angiotensin II in primary renal cells. *Kidney Int.* 2000;57:2457–2467.

62. Cohn JN, Rector TS. Prognosis of congestive heart failure and predictors of mortality. *Am J Cardiol.* 1988;62(2):25–30.

63. Liu FY, Cogan MG. Angiotensin II: a potent regu-lator of acidification in the rat early proximal convoluted tubule. *J Clin Invest.* 1987;80:272.

64. Abassi ZA, Kelly G, Golomb E, et al. Losartan im-proves the natriuretic response to ANF in rats with high-output heart failure. *J Pharmacol Exp Ther.* 1994;268:224.

65. Watkins L, Burton JA, Haber E, et al. The renin–angiotensin system in congestive failure in conscious dogs. *J Clin Invest.* 1977;57:1606.

66. Cody RJ, Covit AB, Schaer GL, et al. Sodium and water balance in chronic congestive heart failure. *J Clin Invest.* 1986;77:1441.

67. Pierpont GL, Francis GS, Cohn JN. Effect of cap-topril on renal function in patients with conges-tive heart failure. *Br Heart J.* 1981;46:522.

68. Hensen J, Abraham WT, Durr JA, et al. Aldos-terone in congestive heart failure: analysis of de-terminants and role in sodium retention. *Am J Nephrol.* 1991;11:441.

69. Pitt B, Zannad F, Remme WJ, et al. The effect of spironolactone on morbidity and mortality in pa-tients with severe heart failure. Randomized Al-dactone Evaluation Study Investigators. *N Engl J Med.* 1999;341:709–717.

70. van Vliet AA, Donker AJ, Nauta JJ, et al. Spirono-lactone in congestive heart failure refractory to high-dose loop diuretic and low-dose angiotensin-converting enzyme inhibitor. *Am J Cardiol.* 1993;71:21–28.

71. Adams KF Jr, Fonarow GC, Emerman CL, et al. Characteristics and outcomes of patients hospital-ized for heart failure in the United States: ratio-nale, design, and preliminary observations from the first 100,000 cases in the Acute Decompen-sated Heart Failure National Registry (ADHERE). *Am Heart J.* 2005;149:209–216.

72. Juurlink DN, Mamdani MM, Lee DS, et al. Rates of hyperkalemia after publication of the Random-ized Aldactone Evaluation Study. *N Engl J Med.* 2004;351:543–551.

73. Schrier RW. Role of diminished renal function in cardiovascular mortality: marker or pathogenetic factor? *J Am Coll Cardiol.* 2006;47:1–8.

74. Szatalowicz VL, Arnold PA, Chaimovitz C, et al. Radioimmunoassay of plasma arginine vaso-pressin in hyponatremic patients with congestive heart failure. *N Engl J Med.* 1981;305:263.

75. Riegger GA, Niebau G, Kochsiek K. Antidiuretic hormone in congestive heart failure. *Am J Med.* 1982;72:49.

76. Pruszczynski W, Vahanian A, Ardailou R, et al. Role of antidiuretic hormone in impaired water excretion of patients with congestive heart failure. *J Clin Endocrinol Metab.* 1984;58:599.

77. Goldsmith SR, Francis GS, Cowley AW Jr. Argi-nine vasopressin and the renal response to water loading in congestive heart failure. *Am J Cardiol.* 1986;58:295.

78. Ishikawa S, Saito T, Okada T, et al. Effect of vasopressin antagonist on water excretion in inferior vena cava constriction. *Kidney Int.* 1986;30:49.

79. Yamamura Y, Ogawa H, Yamashita H, et al. Characterization of a novel aquaretic agent, OPC-31260, as an orally effective, nonpeptide vasopressin V_2 receptor antagonist. *Br J Pharmacol.* 1992;105:787.

80. Ohnishi A, Orita Y, Okahara R, et al. Potent aquaretic agent: a novel nonpeptide selective vasopressin 2 antagonist (OPC-31260) in men. *J Clin Invest.* 1993;92:2653.

81. Xu D-L, Martin P-Y, Ohara M, et al. Upregulation of aquaporin-2 water channel expression in chronic heart failure rat. *J Clin Invest.* 1997;99:1500–1505.

82. Nielsen S, Terris J, Andersen D, et al. Congestive heart failure in rats is associated with increased expression and targeting of aquaporin-2 water channel in collecting duct. *Proc Natl Acad Sci.* 1997;94:5450–5455.

83. Kim JK, Michel J-B, Soubrier F, et al. Arginine va-sopressin gene expression in congestive heart fail-ure. *Kidney Int.* 1988;33:270.

84. Bichet D, Kortas CK, Mattauer B, et al. Modula-tion of plasma and "platelet fraction" vasopressin by cardiac function in patients with severe con-gestive heart failure. *Kidney Int.* 1986;29:1188.

85. Dunn FL, Brennan TJ, Nelson AE, et al. The role of blood osmolality and volume in regulating vasopressin secretion in the rat. *J Clin Invest.* 1973;52:3212.

86. FDA announcement made May 20, 2009.

87. Schrier RW, Lehman D, Zacherle B, et al. Effect of furosemide on free water excretion in edematous patients with hyponatremia. *Kidney Int.* 1973;3:30.

88. Raine AEG, Erne P, Bürgisser E, et al. Atrial natriuretic peptide and atrial pressure in patients with congestive heart failure. *N Engl J Med.* 1986;315:533.

89. Mukoyama M, Nakao K, Saito Y, et al. Increased human brain natriuretic peptide in congestive heart failure. *N Engl J Med.* 1990;323:757.

90. Molina CR, Fowler MB, McCrory S, et al. Hemo-dynamic, renal, and endocrine effects of atrial natriuretic peptide in severe heart failure. *J Am Coll Cardiol.* 1988;12:175.

91. Hensen J, Abraham WT, Lesnefsky EJ, et al. Atrial natriuretic factor kinetic studies in patients with congestive heart failure. *Kidney Int.* 1992;42:1333.

92. Saito Y, Nakao K, Arai H, et al. Atrial natriuretic polypeptide (ANP) in human ventricle: increased gene expression of ANP in dilated cardiomyopa-thy. *Biochem Biophys Res Commun.* 1987;148:211.

93. Hosoda K, Nakao K, Mukoyama M, et al. Expres-sion of brain natriuretic peptide gene in human heart: production in the ventricle. *Hypertension.* 1991;17:1152.

94. Colucci WS, Elkayam U, Horton DP, et al. Intravenous nesiritide, a natriuretic peptide, in the treatment of decompensated congestive heart failure. Nesiritide Study Group. *N Engl J Med.* 2000;343:246–253.

95. Drexler H, Hirth C, Stasch H-P, et al. Vasodilatory action of endogenous atrial natriuretic factor in a rat model of chronic heart failure as determined by monoclonal ANF antibody. *Circ Res.* 1990;66:1371.

96. Biollaz J, Nussberger J, Porchet M, et al. Four-hour infusion of synthetic atrial natriuretic peptide in normal volunteers. *Hypertension.* 1986;8:II-96.

97. Kim JK, Summer SN, Dürr J, et al. Enzymatic and binding effects of atrial natriuretic factor in glomeruli and nephrons. *Kidney Int.* 1989;35:799.

98. Lee ME, Miller WL, Edwards BS, et al. Role of endogenous atrial natriuretic factor in acute con-gestive heart failure. *J Clin Invest.* 1989;84:1962.

99. Cody RJ, Atlas SA, Laragh JH, et al. Atrial natri-uretic factor in normal subjects and heart failure patients: plasma levels and renal, hormonal, and hemodynamic responses to peptide infusion. *J Clin Invest.* 1986;78:1362.

100. Hoffman A, Grossman E, Keiser HR. Increased plasma levels and blunted effects of brain natriuretic peptide in rats with congestive heart failure. *Am J Hypertens.* 1991;4:597.

101. Sackner-Bernstein J, Skopicki H, Aaronson K. Risk of worsening renal function with nesiritide in patients with acutely decompensated heart failure. *Circulation.* 2005;111:14878–14891.

102. Abraham WT, Hensen J, Kim JD, et al. Atrial natriuretic peptide and urinary cyclic guanosine monophosphate in patients with congestive heart failure. *J Am Soc Nephrol.* 1992;2:697.

103. Abraham WT, Lauwaars ME, Kim JK, et al. Reversal of atrial natriuretic peptide resistance by

increasing distal tubular sodium delivery in patients with decompensated cirrhosis. *Hepatology.* 1995;22:737.

104. Connelly TP, Francis GS, Williams KJ, et al. Interaction of intravenous atrial natriuretic factor with furosemide in patients with heart failure. *Am Heart J.* 1994;127:392.

105. Koepke JP, DiBona GF. Blunted natriuresis to atrial natriuretic peptide in chronic sodium-retaining disorders. *Am J Physiol.* 1987; 252:F865.

106. Dzau VJ, Packer M, Lilly LS, et al. Prostaglandins in severe congestive heart failure: relation to activation of the renin–angiotensin system and hyponatremia. *N Engl J Med.* 1984;310:347.

107. Walshe JJ, Venuto RC. Acute oliguric renal failure induced by indomethacin: possible mechanism. *Ann Intern Med.* 1979;91:47.

108. Riegger GA, Kahles HW, Elsner D, et al. Effects of acetylsalicylic acid on renal function in patients with chronic heart failure. *Am J Med.* 1991; 90:571.

109. Papper S. The role of the kidney in Laennec's cirrhosis of the liver. *Medicine.* 1958;37:299.

110. Lieberman FL, Denison EK, Reynolds TB. The relationship of plasma volume, portal hypertension, ascites, and renal sodium retention in cirrhosis: the overflow theory of ascites formation. *Ann N Y Acad Sci.* 1970;170:202.

111. Schrier RW, Arroyo V, Bernardi M, et al. Peripheral arterial vasodilation hypothesis: a proposal for the initiation of renal sodium and water retention in cirrhosis. *Hepatology.* 1988;8:1151.

112. Rahman SN, Abraham WT, Schrier RW. Peripheral arterial vasodilation hypothesis in cirrhosis. *Gastroenterol Int.* 1992;5:192.

113. Vallance P, Moncada S. Hyperdynamic circulation in cirrhosis: a role for nitric oxide? *Lancet.* 1991; 337:776.

114. Guarner C, Soriano G, Tomas A, et al. Increased serum nitrite and nitrate levels in patients with cirrhosis: relationship to endotoxemia. *Hepatology.* 1993;18:1139.

115. Niederberger M, Ginès P, Tsai P, et al. Increased aortic cyclic guanosine monophosphate concentration in experimental cirrhosis in rats: evidence for a role of nitric oxide in the pathogenesis of arterial vasodilation in cirrhosis. *Hepatology.* 1995; 250:1625.

116. Niederberger M, Martin PY, Ginès P, et al. Normalization of nitric oxide production corrects arterial vasodilation and hyperdynamic circulation in cirrhotic rats. *Gastroenterology.* 1995; 109:1624.

117. Miyase S, Fujiyama S, Chikazawa H, et al. Atrial natriuretic peptide in liver cirrhosis with mild ascites. *Gastroenterol Jpn.* 1990;25:356.

118. Martin P-Y, Ohara M, Gines P, et al. Nitric oxide synthase inhibition for one week improves renal sodium and water excretion in cirrhotic rats with ascites. *J Clin Invest.* 1998; 101:235–242.

119. Albillos A, Rossi I, Cacho G, et al. Enhanced endothelium-derived vasodilation in patients with cirrhosis. *Am J Physiol.* 1995;268:G459.

120. Leehey DJ, Gollapudi P, Deakin A, et al. Naloxone increases water and electrolyte excretion after water loading in patients with cirrhosis and ascites. *J Lab Clin Med.* 1991;118:484.

121. Bichet DG, Groves RM, Schrier RW. Mechanisms of improvement of water and sodium excretion by enhancement of central hemodynamics in decompensated cirrhotic patients. *Kidney Int.* 1983;24:788.

122. Laragh JH, Cannon PJ, Bentzel CJ, et al. Angiotensin II, norepinephrine and renal transport of electrolytes and water in normal man and in cirrhosis with ascites. *J Clin Invest.* 1963;42:1179.

123. Bank N, Aynedijian HS. A micropuncture study of renal salt and water retention in chronic bile duct obstruction. *J Clin Invest.* 1975;55:994.

124. Chaimovitz C, Szylman P, Alroy G, et al. Mechanism of increased renal tubular sodium reabsorption in cirrhosis. *Am J Med.* 1972;52:198.

125. Schubert J, Puschett J, Goldberg M. The renal mechanisms of sodium reabsorption in cirrhosis [abstract]. *Am Soc Nephrol.* 1969;3:58A.

126. Levy M. Sodium retention and ascites formation in dogs with experimental portal cirrhosis. *Am J Physiol.* 1977;233:F575.

127. Lopez-Novoa JM, Rengel MA, Rodicio JL, et al. A micropuncture study of salt and water retention in chronic experimental cirrhosis. *Am J Physiol.* 1977;232:F315.

128. Nicholls KM, Shapiro MD, Van Putten VJ, et al. Elevated plasma norepinephrine concentrations in decompensated cirrhosis. *Circ Res.* 1985; 56:457.

129. Floras JS, Legault L, Morali GA, et al. Increased sympathetic outflow in cirrhosis and ascites: direct evidence from intraneural recordings. *Ann Intern Med.* 1991;114:373.

130. Ring-Larsen H, Hesse B, Henriksen JH, et al. Sympathetic nervous activity and renal and systemic hemodynamics in cirrhosis: plasma norepinephrine concentration, hepatic extraction and renal release. *Hepatology.* 1982;2:304.

131. Bichet DG, Van Putten VJ, Schrier RW. Potential role of increased sympathetic activity in impaired sodium and water excretion in cirrhosis. *N Engl J Med.* 1982;307:1552.

132. Ring-Larsen H, Henriksen JG, Christensen NJ. Increased sympathetic activity in cirrhosis. *N Engl J Med.* 1983;308:1029.

133. Gregory PB, Broekelschen PH, Hill MD, et al. Complications of diuresis in the alcoholic patient with ascites: a controlled trial. *Gastroenterology.* 1977;73:534.

134. Arroyo V, Rodes J, Guiterrez-Lizarrage MA, et al. Prognostic value of spontaneous hyponatremia in cirrhosis with ascites. *Dig Dis.* 1976;21:249.

135. Birchard WH, Prout TE, Williams TF, et al. Diuretic responses to oral and intravenous water-loads in patients with hepatic cirrhosis. *J Lab Clin Med.* 1956;48:26.

136. Vlachecevic ZR, Adham NF, Zick H, et al. Renal effects of acute expansion of plasma volume in cirrhosis. *N Engl J Med.* 1965;272:387.

137. Yamahiro HS, Reynolds TB. Effects of ascitic fluid infusion on sodium excretion blood volume and creatinine clearance in cirrhosis. *Gastroenterology.* 1961;40:497.

138. Bichet D, Szatalowicz VL, Chaimovitz C, et al. Role of vasopressin in abnormal water excretion

in cirrhotic patients. *Ann Intern Med.* 1982; 96:413.

139. Shapiro MD, Nicholls KM, Groves BM, et al. Interrelationship between cardiac output and vascular resistance as determinants of effective arterial blood volume in cirrhotic patients. *Kidney Int.* 1985;28:206.

140. Claria J, Jimenez W, Arroyo V, et al. Blockade of the hydroosmotic effect of vasopressin normalizes water excretion in cirrhotic rats. *Gastroenterology.* 1989;97:1294.

141. Tsuboi Y, Ishikawa SE, Fujisawa G, et al. Therapeutic efficacy of the nonpeptide AVP antagonist OPC-31260 in cirrhotic rats. *Kidney Int.* 1994; 46:237.

142. Fujita N, Ishikawa S, Sasaki S, et al. Role of water channel AQP-CD in water retention in SIADH and cirrhotic rats. *Am J Physiol.* 1995;269:F926.

143. Gerbes AL, Gulberg V, Gines P, et al.; VPA Study Group. Therapy of hyponatremia in cirrhosis with a vasopressin receptor antagonist: a randomized double-blind multicenter trial. *Gastroenterology.* 2003;124(4):933–939.

144. Schrier RW, Gross P, Gheorghiade M, et al. for the SALT Investigators: Tolvaptan, a selective oral vasopressin V_2-receptor antagonist, for hyponatremia. *N Engl J Med.* 2006;355(20):2099–2112.

145. Schrier RW, Better OS. Pathogenesis of ascites formation: mechanism of impaired aldosterone escape in cirrhosis. *Eur J Gastroenterol Hepatol.* 1991;3:721.

146. Skorecki KL, Leung WM, Campbell P, et al. Role of atrial natriuretic peptide in the natriuretic response to central volume expansion induced by head-out water immersion in sodium-retaining cirrhotic subjects. *Am J Med.* 1988;85:375.

147. Koepke JP, Jones S, DiBona GF. Renal nerves mediate blunted natriuresis to atrial natriuretic peptide in cirrhotic rats. *Am J Physiol.* 1987;252: R1019.

148. Zambraski EJ, Dunn MJ. Importance of renal prostaglandins in control of renal function after chronic ligation of the common bile duct in dogs. *J Lab Clin Med.* 1984;103:549.

149. Arroyo V, Planas R, Gaya J, et al. Sympathetic nervous activity, renin–angiotensin system and renal excretion of prostaglandin E2 in cirrhosis: relationship to functional renal failure and sodium and water excretion. *Eur J Clin Invest.* 1983; 13:271.

150. Boyer TD, Zia P, Reynolds TB. Effect of indomethacin and prostaglandin A1 on renal function and plasma renin activity in alcoholic liver disease. *Gastroenterology.* 1979;77:215.

151. Wong F, Massie D, Hsu P, et al. Indomethacin-induced renal dysfunction in patients with well-compensated cirrhosis. *Gastroenterology.* 1993;104:869.

152. Schrier RW, Fassett RG. A critique of the overfill hypothesis of sodium and water retention in the nephrotic syndrome. *Kidney Int.* 1998;53: 1111–1117.

153. Usberti M, Gazzotti RM, Poiesi C, et al. Considerations on the sodium retention in nephrotic syndrome. *Am J Nephrol.* 1995;15:38.

154. Rahman SN, Abraham WT, Van Putten VJ, et al. Increased norepinephrine secretion in patients with the nephrotic syndrome and normal glomerular filtration rates: evidence for primary sympathetic activation. *Am J Nephrol.* 1993; 13:266.

155. Geers AB, Koomans HA, Boer P, et al. Plasma and blood volumes in the nephrotic syndrome. *Nephron.* 1984;38:170.

156. Meltzer JI, Keim HJ, Laragh JH, et al. Nephrotic syndrome: vasoconstriction and hypervolemic types indication by renin–sodium profiling. *Ann Intern Med.* 1979;91:688.

157. Keller H, Noseda G, Morell A, et al. Analbuminemia. *Minerva Med.* 1972;63:1296.

158. Barnett HL, Forman CW, McNamara H, et al. The effect of adrenocorticotrophic hormone on children with the nephrotic syndrome. II. Physiologic observations on discrete kidney functions and plasma volume. *J Clin Invest.* 1951;30:227.

159. Bernard DB, Alexander EA, Couser WG, et al. Renal sodium retention during volume expansion in experimental nephrotic syndrome. *Kidney Int.* 1978;14:478.

160. Kuroda S, Aynedjian HS, Bank NA. A micropuncture study of renal sodium retention in nephrotic syndrome in rats: evidence for increased resistance to tubular fluid flow. *Kidney Int.* 1979; 16:561.

161. Grausz H, Lieberman R, Earley LE. Effect of plasma albumin on sodium reabsorption in patients with nephrotic syndrome. *Kidney Int.* 1972;1:47.

162. Usberti M, Federico S, Cianciaruso B, et al. Relationship between serum albumin concentration and tubular reabsorption of glucose in renal disease. *Kidney Int.* 1979;16:546.

163. Tobian L, Perry S, Mork J. The relationship of the juxtaglomerular apparatus to sodium retention in experimental nephrosis. *Ann Intern Med.* 1962;57:382.

164. Kalant N, Gupta DD, Despointes R, et al. Mechanisms of edema in experimental nephrosis. *Am J Physiol.* 1962;202:91.

165. Ichikawa I, Rennke HG, Hoyer JR, et al. Role for intrarenal mechanisms in the impaired salt excretion of experimental nephrotic syndrome. *J Clin Invest.* 1983;71:91.

166. Brown EA, Markandu ND, Sagnella GA, et al. Evidence that some mechanism other than the renin system causes sodium retention in nephrotic syndrome. *Lancet.* 1982;2:1237.

167. Shapiro MD, Hasbergen J, Cosby R, et al. Role of aldosterone in the Na retention of patients with nephrotic syndrome. *Am J Kidney Dis.* 1986;8:81.

168. Hisanaga S, Yamamoto Y, Kida O, et al. Plasma concentration and renal effect of human atrial natriuretic peptide in nephrotic syndrome. *Jpn J Nephrol.* 1989;31:661.

169. Yokota N, Yamamoto Y, Iemura F, et al. Increased plasma levels and effects of brain natriuretic peptide in experimental nephrosis. *Nephron.* 1993; 65:454.

170. Perico N, Remuzzi G. Renal handling of sodium in the nephrotic syndrome. *Am J Nephrol.* 1993; 13:413.

171. Abassi Z, Shuranyi E, Better OS, et al. Effect of atrial natriuretic factor on renal cGMP

production in rats with adriamycin-induced nephrotic syndrome. *J Am Soc Nephrol.* 1992;2:1538.

172. Kleinknecht C, Broyer M, Gubler MC, et al. Irreversible renal failure after indomethacin in steroid resistant nephrosis. *N Engl J Med.* 1980;302:691.

173. Dorhout-Mees EJ, Roos JC, Boer P, et al. Observations on edema formation in the nephrotic syndrome in adults with minimal lesions. *Am J Med.* 1979;67:378.

174. Pedersen EB, Danielsen H, Madsen M, et al. Defective renal water excretion in nephrotic syndrome: the relationship between renal water excretion and kidney function, arginine-vasopressin, angiotensin II and aldosterone in plasma before and after water loading. *Eur J Clin Invest.* 1985;15:24.

175. Gur A, Adefuin PY, Siegel NJ, et al. A study of the renal handling of water in lipoid nephrosis. *Pediatr Res.* 1976;10:197.

176. Krishna GG, Danovitch GM. Effects of water immersion on renal function in the nephrotic syndrome. *Kidney Int.* 1982;21:395.

177. Berlyne GM, Sutton J, Brown C, et al. Renal salt and water handling in water immersion in the nephrotic syndrome. *Clin Sci.* 1981;61:605.

178. Rascher W, Tulassay T, Seyberth HW, et al. Diuretic and hormonal responses to head-out water immersion in nephrotic syndrome. *J Pediatr.* 1986;109:609.

179. Tulassay T, Rascher W, Lang RE, et al. Atrial natriuretic peptide and other vasoactive hormones in nephrotic syndrome. *Kidney Int.* 1987;31:1391.

180. Usberti M, Federico C, Meccariello S, et al. Role of plasma vasopressin in the impairment of water excretion in nephrotic syndrome. *Kidney Int.* 1984;25:422.

181. Shapiro MD, Nicholls KM, Groves R, et al. Role of glomerular filtration rate in the impaired sodium and water excretion of patients with the nephrotic syndrome. *Am J Kidney Dis.* 1986;8:81.

182. Konstam MA, Dracup K, Baker DW, et al. *Heart Failure: Evaluation and Care of Patients with Left-ventricular Systolic Dysfunction.* Rockville, MD: Agency for Health Care Policy and Research; 1994. Clinical Practice Guideline Number 11.

183. Hooper J Jr, Ryan P, Lee JC, et al. Lipoid nephrosis in 31 adult patients: renal biopsy study by light, electron, and fluorescence microscopy with experience in treatment. *Medicine (Baltimore).* 1970;49:321.

184. Taguma Y, Kitamoto Y, Futaki G, et al. Effect of captopril on heavy proteinuria in azotemic diabetics. *N Engl J Med.* 1985;313:1617.

185. Bjorck S, Nyberg G, Mulec H, et al. Beneficial effects of angiotensin converting enzyme inhibition on renal function in patients with diabetic nephropathy. *Br Med J.* 1986;293:471.

186. Gansevoort RT, De Zeeuw D, De Jong PE. Is the antiproteinuric effect of ACE inhibition mediated by interference in the renin–angiotensin system? *Kidney Int.* 1994;45:861.

187. Morgan T, Berliner RW. A study by continuous microperfusion of water and electrolyte movements in the loop of Henle and distal tubule of the rat. *Nephron.* 1969;6:388.

188. Szatalowicz VL, Miller PD, Lacher J, et al. Comparative effects of diuretics on renal water excretion in hyponatremic edematous disorders. *Clin Sci.* 1982;62:235.

189. Birtch AG, Zakheim RM, Jones LG, et al. Redistribution of renal blood flow produced by furosemide and ethacrynic acid. *Circ Res.* 1967; 21:869.

190. Giebisch G. Renal potassium excretion. In: Rouiller C, Muller AF, eds. *The Kidney: Morphology, Biochemistry, Physiology.* New York: Academic Press; 1971:329.

191. Forrest JN, Cox M, Hong C, et al. Demeclocycline versus lithium for inappropriate secretion of antidiuretic hormone. *N Engl J Med.* 1978;298:173.

192. Miller PD, Linas SL, Schrier RW: Plasma demeclocycline levels and nephrotoxicity. Correlation in hyponatremic cirrhotic patients. *JAMA.* 1980; 243:2513–2515.

193. Schrier RW. The sea within us: disorders of body water homeostasis. *Curr Opin Invest Drugs.* 2007; 8(4):304–311.

194. Dikshit K, Vyden JK, Forrester JS, et al. Renal and extrarenal hemodynamic effects of furosemide in congestive heart failure after acute myocardial infarction. *N Engl J Med.* 1973;288:1087.

195. Johnston GD, Hiatt WR, Nies AS, et al. Factors modifying the early nondiuretic vascular effects of furosemide in man. *Circ Res.* 1983;53:630.

196. Francis GS, Siegel RM, Goldsmith SR, et al. Acute vasoconstrictor response to intravenous furosemide in patients with chronic congestive heart failure. *Ann Intern Med.* 1985;103:1.

197. Ikram H, Chan W, Espiner EA, et al. Haemodynamic and hormone responses to acute and chronic furosemide therapy in congestive heart failure. *Clin Sci.* 1980;59:443.

198. Bayliss J, Norell M, Canepa-Anson R, et al. Untreated heart failure: clinical and neuroendocrine effects of introducing diuretics. *Br Heart J.* 1987;57:17.

199. Fett DL, Cavero PG, Burnett JC. Atrial natriuretic factor modulates the renal and endocrine actions of furosemide in experimental acute congestive heart failure. *J Am Soc Nephrol.* 1993;4:162.

200. Kaojarern S, Day B, Brater DC. The time course of delivery of furosemide into the urine: an independent determinant of overall response. *Kidney Int.* 1982;22:69.

201. Lahav M, Regev A, Ra'anani P, et al. Intermittent administration of furosemide vs continuous infusion preceded by a loading dose for congestive heart failure. *Chest.* 1992;102:725.

202. Van Meyel JJM, Smits P, Russel FGM, et al. Diuretic efficiency of furosemide during continuous administration versus bolus injection in healthy volunteers. *Clin Pharmacol Ther.* 1992; 51:440.

203. Vargo DL, Kramer WG, Black PK, et al. Bioavailability, pharmacokinetics, and pharmacodynamics of torsemide and furosemide in patients with congestive heart failure. *Clin Pharmacol Ther.* 1995; 57(6):601–609.

204. Gabow PA, Moore S, Schrier RW. Spironolactone induced hyperchloremia acidosis in cirrhosis. *Ann Intern Med.* 1979;90:338.

205. Brickman AS, Massry SG, Coburn JW. Changes in serum and urinary calcium during treatment with hydrochlorothiazide: studies on mechanisms. *J Clin Invest.* 1972;51:945.

206. Reilly RF, Ellison DH. Mammalian distal tubule: physiology, pathophysiology, and molecular anatomy. *Physiol Rev.* 2000;80(1):277–313.

207. Gabow PA, Hanson T, Popovtzer M, et al. Furosemide-induced reduction in ionized calcium in hypoparathyroid patients. *Ann Intern Med.* 1977;86:579.

208. Favere L, Glasson P, Reonad A, et al. Interacting diuretics and nonsteroidal antiinflammatory drugs in man. *Clin Sci.* 1983;64:407.

209. Lyons H, Pinn VW, Cortell S, et al. Allergic interstitial nephritis causing reversible renal failure in four patients with idiopathic nephrotic syndrome. *N Engl J Med.* 1973;288:124.

210. Abdallah JG, Schrier RW, Edelstein C, et al. Loop diuretic infusion increases thiazide-sensitive Na(+)/Cl(−)-cotransporter abundance: role of aldosterone. *J Am Soc Nephrol.* 2001;12: 1335–1341.

211. Stampfer M, Epstein SE, Beiser GD, et al. Hemodynamic effects of diuresis at rest and during intense upright exercise in patients with impaired cardiac function. *Circulation.* 1968;37:900.

212. Sherlock S. Ascites formation in cirrhosis and its management. *Scand J Gastroenterol Suppl.* 1970;7:9.

213. Shear L, Ching S, Gauzda GJ. Compartmentalization of ascites and edema in patients with hepatic cirrhosis. *N Engl J Med.* 1970;282:1391.

214. Rosoff L, Zia P, Reynolds T, et al. Studies of renin and aldosterone in cirrhotic patients with ascites. *Gastroenterology.* 1975;69:698.

215. Gabuzda GJ, Hall PW III. Relation of potassium depletion to renal ammonium metabolism and hepatic coma. *Medicine.* 1966;45:481.

216. Ginès P, Arroyo V, Quintero E, et al. Comparison between paracentesis and diuretics in the treatment of cirrhotics with tense ascites. *Gastroenterology.* 1987;93:234.

217. Ginès P, Tito LI, Arroyo V, et al. Randomized comparative study of therapeutic paracentesis with and without intravenous albumin in cirrhosis. *Gastroenterology.* 1988;94:1493.

218. Quintero E, Ginès P, Arroyo V, et al. Paracentesis versus diuretics in the treatment of cirrhotics with tense ascites. *Lancet.* 1985;1:611.

219. Salerno F, Badalamenti S, Incerti P, et al. Repeated paracentesis and i.v. albumin infusion to treat "tense" ascites in cirrhotic patients: a safe alternative therapy. *J Hepatol.* 1987;5:102.

220. Tito L, Ginès P, Arroyo V, et al. Total paracentesis associated with intravenous albumin management of patients with cirrhosis and ascites. *Gastroenterology.* 1990;98:146.

221. Gines P, Schrier RW. Renal failure in cirrhosis. *N Engl J Med.* In press.

CHAPTER 3

Pathogenesis and Management of Metabolic Acidosis and Alkalosis

SHOBHA RATNAM, WILLIAM KAEHNY, AND JOSEPH I. SHAPIRO

A cid–base disorders occur commonly in clinical medicine. Although the degree of acidosis or alkalosis that results is rarely life threatening, the careful evaluation of the acid–base status of the patient often provides insight into the underlying medical problem. Moreover, the pathophysiology and differential diagnosis of these disorders can be approached quite logically with a minimum of laboratory and clinical data. An effective approach to clinical acid–base disorders is accomplished most easily with a stepwise pathophysiologic approach.

Human acid–base homeostasis normally involves the tight regulation of CO_2 tension by respiratory excretion and plasma bicarbonate $[HCO_3^-]$ concentration by renal HCO_3^- reabsorption and elimination of protons (H^+) produced by metabolism. The pH of body fluids (which can be sampled easily) is determined by the CO_2 tension (in arterial blood, Pa_{CO_2}) and the $[HCO_3^-]$. Primary derangements of CO_2 tension are referred to as respiratory disturbances, whereas primary derangements of $[HCO_3^-]$ are called metabolic disturbances (1).

In this chapter, we first review acid–base chemistry and physiology and then present a pathophysiologic approach to the diagnosis and management of metabolic acidosis and alkalosis.

Acid–Base Chemistry and Physiology

The chemistry of acids, bases, and buffers as well as the normal physiology of acid and bicarbonate excretion (2,3) are described in detail in several excellent reviews and are summarized only briefly in this section.

BUFFERING

Clinical acid–base chemistry basically is the chemistry of buffers. For clinical purposes, we may define an acid as a chemical that donates an H^+ and a base as an H^+ acceptor. For any acid (HA), we can define its strength or tendency to donate H^+ by its dissociation constant K according to the relationship:

$$[HA] = K_{eq} \times [H^+][A^-] \tag{3.1}$$

If we rearrange this equation and apply a log transformation, we arrive at the familiar relationship:

$$pH = pK + \log_{10}[A^-]/HA \tag{3.2}$$

Buffering refers to the ability of a solution containing a weak or poorly dissociated acid and its anion (a base) to resist change in pH when a strong acid (i.e., highly dissociated acid) or alkali is added. To illustrate this important point, suppose 1 mL of 0.1 mol/L HCl is added to 9 mL of distilled water, the $[H^+]$ would increase from 10^{-7} to 10^{-2} mol/L. In other words, the pH would fall from 7.0 to 2.0. However, if we added 1 mL of 0.1 mol/L HCl to 9 mL of a 1-mol/L phosphate *buffer* (pK = 6.9) at pH 7.0, most of the dissociated H^+ from HCl would combine with dibasic phosphate (HPO_4^{2-}) and only slightly change the ratio of dibasic to monobasic ($H_2PO_4^-$) phosphate. In fact, the pH would fall by only about 0.1 pH units. The addition of acid has been *buffered* by the phosphate dissolved in water. Another way to think about this is that the pH was stabilized by substances that bound the free H^+ released by the HCl, in this case the phosphate. Such substances are called *buffers* (4).

Biochemical Determinants of pH

The bicarbonate buffer system is the most important buffer in the extracellular space in humans. Proteins and inorganic phosphate are less important buffers. Inorganic phosphate is probably the most important buffer in the intracellular space followed by bicarbonate and intracellular proteins. Although intracellular pH (pHi) is probably more important in predicting physiologic and clinical consequences than extracellular pH (5), it is difficult to measure in vivo without using sophisticated investigational techniques, such as ^{31}P nuclear magnetic resonance (NMR) spectroscopy (6), laser scanning cytometry (7), and fluorescence lifetime imaging (8), which are not available for routine clinical applications. Therefore, our clinical efforts are focused on classifying disease states based on what is measurable, that is, extracellular pH. In particular, our attention focuses on the bicarbonate buffer system (2). We can assume that equilibrium conditions apply because there is abundant carbonic anhydrase in blood. Therefore, we can view the bicarbonate buffer system as the equilibrium reaction:

$$H^+ + HCO_3^- \xrightleftharpoons{K_{eq}} H_2CO_3 \text{ or} \tag{3.3}$$

$$[H^+] = K_{eq} \times [H_2CO_3]/[HCO_3^-] \tag{3.4}$$

H_2CO_3 is defined by the partial pressure of CO_2 and the solubility of CO_2 in physiologic fluids, which is a constant S to all intents and purposes. We can therefore rearrange this equation as

$$[H^+] = K \times (S \times P_{CO_2})/[HCO_3^-] \tag{3.5}$$

which is attributed to Henderson in 1909.

Taking the antilog of both sides gives the following:

$$pH = pK + \log_{10}[HCO_3^-]/(S \times P_{CO_2}) \tag{3.6}$$

which is called the Henderson–Hasselbalch equation and was first described by Hasselbalch in 1916. In blood at 37°C, the pK of the bicarbonate buffer system is 6.1 and the solubility coefficient for CO_2 is 0.03. Therefore, we can simplify our expression to

$$pH = 6.1 + \log_{10}[HCO_3^-]/[0.03 \times Pa_{CO_2}] \tag{3.7}$$

In the above equations, $[HCO_3^-]$ is expressed in mM (or mEq/L) and Pa_{CO_2} is expressed in torr (or mm Hg). Convenient expression allows us to view acid–base disorders as being attributable to the numerator of the ratio (metabolic processes), the denominator (respiratory processes), or both (mixed or complex acid–base disorders) (Fig. 3.1) (1).

Total Body Acid–Base Metabolism

A myriad of enzymatic reactions involve the loss or gain of protons that occurs with ongoing catabolism and anabolism. However, one simply has to examine the initial substrates and final products to understand whether acid or base is produced. To do this, it is helpful to think of acids and bases as "Lewis" acids and bases, in other words, to consider acids as electron acceptors rather than proton donors. In

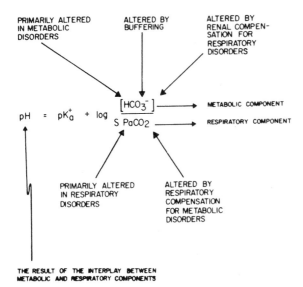

PRIMARILY ALTERED
IN METABOLIC
DISORDERS

ALTERED BY
BUFFERING

ALTERED BY
RENAL COMPEN-
SATION FOR
RESPIRATORY
DISORDERS

METABOLIC COMPONENT

RESPIRATORY COMPONENT

$$pH = pK_a^+ + \log \frac{[HCO_3^-]}{S \; PaCO_2}$$

PRIMARILY ALTERED
IN RESPIRATORY
DISORDERS

ALTERED BY
RESPIRATORY
COMPENSATION
FOR METABOLIC
DISORDERS

THE RESULT OF THE INTERPLAY BETWEEN
METABOLIC AND RESPIRATORY COMPONENTS

■ **Figure 3.1** Modified Henderson–Hasselbalch equation, portraying the interacting effects of the primary acid–base disturbance and the secondary mechanisms on the pH.

concrete terms, acid is generated when a substrate is metabolized to something more anionic (e.g., glucose is metabolized to lactate through the Embden–Meyerhof glycolytic pathway). Conversely, if a substrate is metabolized to something more cationic (e.g., lactate is metabolized to CO_2 and H_2O via the tricarboxylic acid [TCA] cycle), then acid is consumed (9). Because of the importance of the bicarbonate buffer system in overall acid–base homeostasis, we generally consider the addition of a proton as equivalent to the decrease in total body HCO_3^- and loss of a proton as a gain in HCO_3^- (10).

This approach to understanding acid–base metabolism has led to its practical application in treating the acidosis of chronic renal failure with peritoneal dialysis. Although the lactate-based dialysate (generally at about 35 mM) has a pH of only 6.0, virtually all of the lactate is ionized; bicarbonate is generated and the acidosis is corrected via metabolism largely through the TCA cycle to CO_2 and H_2O (11).

Renal Acid Excretion

GENERAL CONSIDERATIONS

In adult men studied at sea level, the kidneys regulate the $[HCO_3^-]$ at approximately 24 mM and the lungs control the $PaCO_2$ at about 38 torr, thus producing an arterial pH of approximately 7.42; for women, the corresponding values for $[HCO_3^-]$, $PaCO_2$, and pH are 24 mM, 37 torr, and 7.43, respectively (12). The kidneys regulate plasma $[HCO_3^-]$ and acid–base balance by reclaiming filtered HCO_3^- and generating new HCO_3^- to replace that lost internally in titrating metabolic acid and externally (e.g., from the gastrointestinal [GI] tract). A normal "Western diet" generates approximately 1 mmol of acid per kilogram of body weight per day. This acid load must be excreted by the kidney to maintain acid–base homeostasis. The easiest way to understand the molecular processes involved in renal acid excretion is to separate renal acid–base handling itself into two functions: bicarbonate reabsorption and net acid excretion (NAE) (13).

RENAL CELLULAR MECHANISMS OF PROTON EXTRUSION

In recent years, our understanding of the renal cellular transport proteins that effect H^+ extrusion has expanded significantly. We know that in addition to the sodium–proton exchanger (Na^+/H^+ exchanger) that exchanges one H^+ for one sodium molecule, the sodium phosphate symporter that transports one sodium with one monobasic phosphate molecule, and the vacuolar H^+ ATPase that directly pumps H^+ into the tubular lumen (14–20), other transport proteins may be of considerable importance. These other transport proteins include the family of chloride–bicarbonate symporters and exchangers, the "colonic" H^+/K^+ ATPase and the Na^+/K^+ ATPase (21–24). These transport proteins are expressed to different degrees in the different nephron segments depending on the function of the cell type within that nephron section.

On a more global basis, there is a tight link between acid secretion and the reclamation of filtered bicarbonate as well as the production of new bicarbonate by the kidney. For example, the reclamation of HCO_3^- filtered from the blood occurs when HCO_3^- formed inside the renal tubular cells by either H^+ secretion or ammonium (NH_4^+) synthesis is transported back into the blood via the basolateral $Na^+(HCO_3^-)_3$ symporter (24) or a Cl^-/HCO_3^- antiporter (14,25). Alternatively, bicarbonate secretion can occur in some nephron segments (26), although the clinical significance of this is uncertain.

RENAL ACID–BASE METABOLISM

Bicarbonate Reabsorption

When plasma is filtered at the glomerulus, HCO_3^- enters the tubule lumen. Mechanistically, each HCO_3^- that is reclaimed requires the epithelial secretion of one H^+. This is accomplished largely by an Na^+/H^+ exchanger on the luminal membrane, although an electrogenic H^+ ATPase also may be involved. On an organ physiology level, HCO_3^- reabsorption can be considered in terms of the *plasma threshold* (PT) for bicarbonate, that is, the plasma HCO_3^- concentration at which HCO_3^- begins to appear in the urine. In terms of the maximal net activity of tubular HCO_3^- reabsorption (also called T_{max}), assuming glomerular filtration rate (GFR) of 100 mL/min and a plasma [HCO_3^-] of 24 mM, the renal tubules must secrete about 2.4 mmol of H^+ per minute to reclaim all of the filtered HCO_3^-. Therefore, HCO_3^- reclamation by the tubules involves a tremendous amount of H^+ secretion. Bicarbonate reclamation is coupled tightly to sodium reabsorption and also is sensitive to a number of other influences. As the T_{max} for HCO_3^- increases, the PT for HCO_3^- increases. Conversely, decreases in T_{max} result in decreases in the PT. In particular, states of extracellular fluid (ECF) expansion and decreases in P_{CO_2} decrease the apparent T_{max} for HCO_3^-, whereas ECF contraction and increases in P_{CO_2} increase the apparent T_{max} for HCO_3^-. Parathyroid hormone inhibits proximal tubule HCO_3^- reabsorption and lowers the apparent T_{max} and PT for HCO_3^-. Most (but not all) of this HCO_3^- reabsorption (about 85% to 90%) occurs in the proximal tubule (3).

Carbonic anhydrase that is present both intracellularly as well as on the tubular surface of the brush border of the proximal tubule allows the secreted H^+ that combines with tubular fluid HCO_3^- to form H_2CO_3. This H_2CO_3 rapidly dissociates to form H_2O and CO_2 that can readily permeate proximal tubule cell membranes. Intracellularly, carbonic anhydrase catalyzes the formation of H_2CO_3 again, which subsequently dissociates into HCO_3^- and H^+. Finally, HCO_3^- leaves the cell via several bicarbonate transport proteins, including the $Na^+(HCO_3^-)_3$ symporter as well as the Cl^-/HCO_3^- exchanger. This process is shown schematically in Figure 3.2 (27).

Net Acid Excretion

NAE is the net amount of H^+ eliminated from the body. If we postulate that an excreted HCO_3^- molecule negates the value of an excreted H^+, then we can consider NAE by the kidney to be the amount of H^+ (both buffered and free) excreted in the urine minus the amount of HCO_3^- excreted in the urine. As discussed, H^+ secretion into the tubule lumen mandates 1:1 stoichiometric HCO_3^- transport across the basolateral segment into the extracellular space; therefore, NAE represents the amount of new HCO_3^- generated by the kidneys and added to the body stores.

NAE is accomplished primarily through elimination of titratable acid (which is mostly phosphate) and nontitratable acid (in the form of NH_4^+) (13). These terms refer to clinical chemistry titration techniques by which known amounts of alkali were added to urine until a color change with a pH indicator (e.g., phenolphthalein) occurred. This color change occurred above the pK for the phosphate buffer system but below the pK for ammonia-ammonium (about 9). It must be stressed that the NAE is relatively insensitive to the urine pH. This concept is illustrated by the observation that addition of

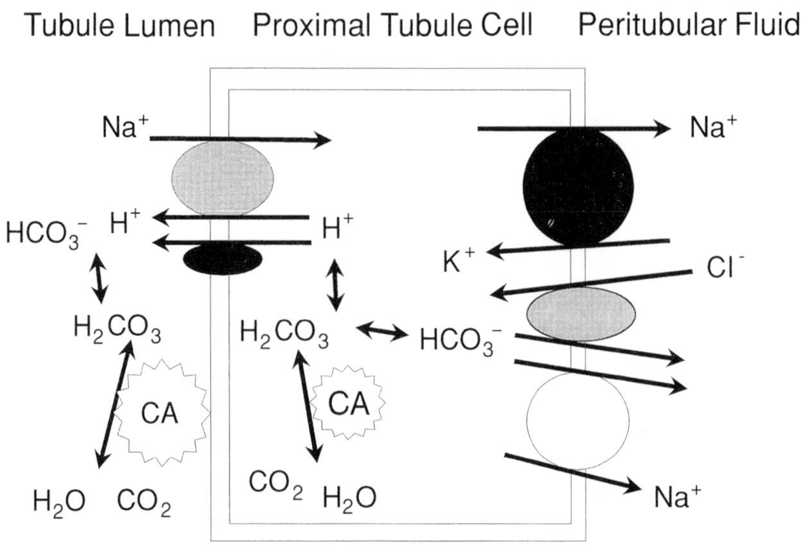

Tubule Lumen   Proximal Tubule Cell   Peritubular Fluid

■ Figure 3.2 Schematic depicting proximal tubule HCO_3^- reclamation process. Two vehicles for apical H^+ secretion: Na^+/H^+ exchanger *(lightly shaded ellipse)* and H^+ ATPase *(filled ellipse on apical side)* are shown. Some basolateral ion pumps and exchangers, including the Na^+/K^+ ATPase *(filled circle)*, $Na^+(HCO_3^-)_3$ symporter *(open circle)*, and HCO_3^-/Cl^- exchanger *(lightly shaded ellipse)*, are also shown. The role of carbonic anhydrase (CA) both in the tubular cell and on the brush border in HCO_3^- reabsorption also is depicted.

1 mmol of HCl to 1 L of distilled water results in a pH of 3 (corresponding to an H^+ concentration of 10^{-3} mol/L). Therefore, in the extreme case (i.e., no buffers in the urine at all), extremely acid urine (i.e., a very low pH) could eliminate very few protons from the body. There are several clinical settings discussed later in which acid urine is elaborated, but NAE is insufficient. NAE requires the adequate function of both the proximal tubule to synthesize NH_4^+ (which generates an HCO_3^- molecule) as well as the distal tubule and collecting tubules where H^+ and NH_4^+ secretion occur (27).

Proton secretion by the distal nephron involves the production of an electrogenic gradient that favors H^+ secretion produced by removal of sodium from the luminal fluid as well as direct pumping of H^+ into the tubular lumen. This is accomplished by Na^+/H^+ exchange as well as the activities of the vacuolar H^+ ATPase and the H^+/K^+ ATPase in intercalated and principal cells, respectively. Notably, chloride exchange with bicarbonate on the basolateral side of these distal tubular cells allows for proton secretion to be translated into bicarbonate addition to the blood. Finally, the epithelial membrane must not allow backleak of H^+ or loss of the electrogenic gradient. Under normal circumstances, humans can elaborate a urine pH as low as 4.4 representing a 1000:1 gradient of H^+ between tubular fluid and cells. However, the excretion of NH_4^+, which is discussed later, is of much greater importance in terms of NAE than is the level of urine pH achieved (28).

NAE is sensitive to a variety of factors, including the plasma K concentration (increases in plasma K decrease NH_4^+ excretion, whereas decreases enhance H^+ secretion by the distal nephron) and the effects of aldosterone. By stimulating the renin–angiotensin–aldosterone system, ECF contraction enhances distal acid secretion (26).

Ammonium Metabolism

The traditional view that NH_4^+ excretion was determined by simple passive trapping of NH_4^+ in the tubular lumen has been revised considerably. Recent seminal studies have identified specific proteins that have led to new insights into mechanisms of renal ammonia transport and metabolism (29). Although many of these proteins are primarily involved in the transport of H^+ or K^+, they also transport NH_4^+ (30). The role of aquaporins and the identification of mammalian Rh glycoproteins are two new exciting areas of research in understanding of ammonia transport in normal acid–base homeostasis (29).

Importantly, proximal tubule cells deaminate glutamine to form alpha ketoglutarate (αKG) and NH_4^+. Proximal tubule cells then secrete NH_4^+ into the lumen, probably via substitution for an H^+ using the luminal Na^+/H^+ antiporter. A key feature is that the further metabolism of αKG generates a new HCO_3^- molecule. Therefore, complete metabolism of each glutamine produces two NH_4^+ and two HCO_3^- ions. Ammonium later is reabsorbed in the thick ascending limb of Henle (via substitution for K^+ using the $Na^+/K^+/2Cl^-$ cotransporter) that ultimately increases medullary interstitial concentrations of NH_4^+. This NH_4^+ is then taken up by distal convoluted tubule and collecting duct cells, substituting for K^+ using the basolateral Na^+/K^+ ATPase, and ultimately is secreted into the tubular lumen and hence into the urine, possibly by substitution for H^+ in the apical Na^+/H^+ antiporter or H^+/K^+ exchanger (29). The net generation of any HCO_3^- from αKG metabolism is ultimately dependent on the excretion of NH_4^+. This is because if this NH_4^+ molecule is not excreted in the urine but rather is returned via the systemic circulation to the liver, it is used to form urea at the expense of generating an H^+. Thus, the HCO_3^- molecule that was generated by the metabolism of the αKG will be neutralized, and no change in acid–base status will occur (29).

Difficulties in the routine clinical measurement of urinary NH_4^+ concentrations have delayed our appreciation of its importance in net acid–base balance during pathophysiologic conditions including chronic metabolic acidosis or acid loads (30). However, recent observations by Batlle et al. suggest that the urinary [NH_4^+] may be inferred fairly accurately by calculations based on urinary electrolyte concentrations as is discussed subsequently (31).

Although the topic under discussion is "renal" acid–base metabolism, the liver may be significantly involved. Hepatic glutamine synthetase expression appears to be regulated by pH as well as protein ingestion (32–34). Perhaps more importantly, administration of amino acids via a parenteral rather than the enteral route often is accompanied by acid retention (35).

Clinical Approach to Acid–Base Disorders

GENERAL APPROACH

We propose a relatively simple six-step method to identify and treat acid–base disturbances. This approach presumes that the clinician has suspected an acid–base disturbance based on history and/or physical examination data or other laboratory data. Once such suspicion exists, a blood gas (which gives pH, O_2, CO_2, and calculated [HCO_3^-] values) and serum chemistry panel (which gives serum Na^+, K^+, Cl^-, and total CO_2 content [TCO_2]) is obtained on which subsequent decisions are based. The TCO_2, which is the sum of the [HCO_3^-] and dissolved CO_2 and usually is determined on a venous serum sample, must be distinguished from the Pco_2, which refers to the partial pressure of CO_2 that is generally measured in arterial blood. The remainder of this chapter and the subsequent chapter contain the information necessary to follow these steps successfully:

1. Examine the pH. Many students get confused by the potential complexity and forget this important and easy first step. Based on a normal sea level pH of 7.42 ± 0.02, significant reduction in pH means that the major process ongoing is an acidosis. Conversely, a significant increase in pH means that the major process ongoing is an alkalosis.
2. Examine the directional changes of Pco_2 and [HCO_3^-] from normal. If the pH is acid and HCO_3^- is low, then metabolic acidosis must be present. Conversely, if the pH is alkalemic and HCO_3^- is high, then a metabolic alkalosis must be present.
3. Assess the degree of compensation. Is this a simple (compensation appropriate) or mixed acid–base disorder? With metabolic acidosis, the Pco_2 (in torr) should decrease; conversely, with metabolic alkalosis, the Pco_2 should increase (Table 3.1). The rules of thumb for adequate compensation are presented in Table 3.2 and displayed graphically in Figure 3.3. Failure of respiratory compensation is equivalent to the presence of a primary respiratory acid–base disturbance. Note that a normal pH is never obtained for a given patient through compensation alone.
4. Calculate the serum anion gap (SAG). The SAG is discussed in detail later in this chapter. This useful calculation helps both in the differential diagnosis of metabolic acidosis as well as in identifying whether metabolic acidosis and alkalosis processes coexist.

TABLE 3.1 SIMPLE ACID–BASE DISORDERS

Type of Disorder	pH	Paco$_2$	[HCO$_3^-$]
Metabolic acidosis	↓	↓^{a}	↓
Metabolic alkalosis	↑	↑^{a}	↑
Respiratory acidosis	↓	↑	↑^{a}
Respiratory alkalosis	↑	↓	↓^{a}

^{a}Change owing to compensation.

TABLE 3.2 RULES OF THUMB FOR BEDSIDE INTERPRETATION OF ACID–BASE DISORDERS

Metabolic acidosis	Paco$_2$ (in torr) should fall by $1-1.5 \times$ the fall in plasma [HCO$_3^-$] (in mmol/L)
Metabolic alkalosis	Paco$_2$ (in torr) should increase by $0.25-1 \times$ the rise in plasma [HCO$_3$] (in mmol/L)
Acute respiratory acidosis	The plasma [HCO$_3$] should rise by $0.1 \times$ the increase in Paco$_3$ (in torr) $\pm$ 3 (in mmol/L)
Chronic respiratory acidosis	The plasma [HCO$_3$] should rise by $0.4 \times$ the increase in Paco$_2$ (in torr) $\pm$ 4 (in mmol/L)
Acute respiratory alkalosis	The plasma [HCO$_3$] (in mmol/L) should fall by $0.1-0.3 \times$ the decrease in Paco$_2$ (in torr) but usually not to <18 mmol/L
Chronic respiratory alkalosis	The plasma [HCO$_3$] (in mmol/L) should fall by $0.2-0.5 \times$ the decrease in Paco$_2$ (in torr) but usually not to <14 mmol/L

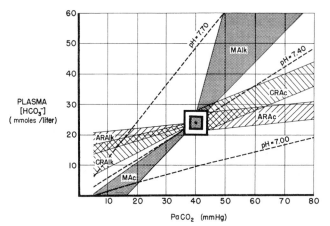

■ **Figure 3.3** Acid–base nomogram derived from Table 3.2 is demonstrated. Regions on nomograms associated with plasma HCO$_3^-$ and Paco$_2$ values seen with primary metabolic alkalosis (MAlk), metabolic acidosis (MAc), chronic respiratory acidosis (CRAc), chronic respiratory alkalosis (CRAlk), acute respiratory acidosis (ARAc), and acute respiratory alkalosis (ARAlk) and appropriate compensation are shown.

5. Determine the underlying cause of the disturbance. Acid–base disorders are merely laboratory signs of an underlying disease of the body fluids. The pathologic cause often is obvious once one has determined what the pathophysiologic nature of the acid–base disturbance is.

6. Determine appropriate therapy. In some situations, the acid–base disturbance must be directly addressed; however, in all situations, treatment of the underlying causes is most advantageous.

Metabolic Acidosis

DEFINITIONS AND CAUSES

Metabolic acidosis is a systemic disorder characterized by a primary decrease in $[HCO_3^-]$. This may occur in three ways: (a) the addition of strong acid that is buffered by (i.e., consumes) HCO_3^-; (b) the loss of HCO_3^- from body fluids, usually through the GI tract or kidneys; and (c) the rapid addition to the ECF of nonbicarbonate solutions (dilutional acidosis). No organic anion is generated when HCO_3^- is lost or diluted. Reciprocal increases in the serum chloride concentration occur to preserve electroneutrality. Thus, these forms of metabolic acidosis generally are referred to as hyperchloremic or nonanion gap metabolic acidosis. When an organic acid consumes HCO_3^-, its organic anion is generated and may be retained in the ECF and serum. The serum chloride concentration does not increase with organic acidosis. An increase in the anion gap marks the existence and concentration of the organic anion (36).

DEFENSE OF SYSTEMIC pH DURING METABOLIC ACIDOSIS

Buffering

The hallmark of metabolic acidosis is a fall in plasma $[HCO_3^-]$. We stress that the fall in $[HCO_3^-]$ always is mitigated by the participation of other buffers in both the ECF and intracellular fluid (ICF). Roughly one half of an administered acid load is buffered by nonbicarbonate buffers (37). Bone is an important buffer pool in states of chronic metabolic acidosis. In fact, the leaching of calcium from bone is one of the major deleterious effects of chronic metabolic acidosis (38–40).

Respiratory Compensation

A fall in $Paco_2$ is a normal compensatory response with simple metabolic acidosis. The failure of this normal adaptive response is indicative of the presence of respiratory acidosis in the setting of a complex or mixed acid–base disturbance. Conversely, an exaggerated fall in $Paco_2$ producing a normal pH indicates the presence of respiratory alkalosis in the setting of a complex or mixed acid–base disturbance (41). The mechanism by which metabolic acidosis induces hypocapnia appears to be mediated in part by peripheral pH receptors in the carotid body, but mostly by central nervous system (CNS) pH receptors. This point is supported by the time course, specifically the temporal delay observed for respiratory compensation seen in experimental metabolic acidosis (42). The degree of chronic compensation varies from person to person; however, based on a large volume of clinical data, we can state with some confidence that the appropriate fall in $Paco_2$ (in torr) should be 1 to 1.5 × the fall in $[HCO_3^-]$ (in mM) (41). Oral acid loading in normal subjects produced a rapid fall in Pco_2 that reached a steady state after 30 minutes that was 0.85 times the fall in HCO_3^-, thus providing direct evidence for the rapid respiratory response to metabolic acidosis in man (43).

Correction

The kidney provides the mechanism for the third line of defense to pH changes. However, this mechanism is rather slow compared to buffering (which begins immediately) and respiratory compensation (which begins within 15 to 30 minutes), since it takes up to 5 days to become maximal. Increases in NAE by the kidney develop in response to either metabolic acidosis (unless the kidney is the cause) or respiratory acidosis. This increase in NAE is largely NH_4^+ excretion because titratable acid excretion is limited by the amount of excreted phosphate, which changes very little. Metabolic acidosis increases the processing of glutamine into NH_4^+, which, in turn, leads to enhanced generation of HCO_3^-, by both transcriptional and translational regulations of key enzymes in this pathway (44). Chronic metabolic acidosis increases renal endothelin-1 activity that activates the NHE3 sodium–hydrogen ion antiporter on the proximal tubule brush border (45). Thus, both the generation of new HCO_3^- via the glutamine system and the enhancement of HCO_3^- reabsorption and titratable acid formation are stimulated. Of interest, the hypocapnia that occurs because of respiratory compensation actually limits renal correction in metabolic acidosis (46). Note that renal correction never corrects the pH to normal until the disorder causing HCO_3^- loss or acid generation is halted.

BIOCHEMICAL AND PHYSIOLOGIC EFFECTS OF METABOLIC ACIDOSIS

Mild degrees of acidemia generally are well tolerated, at least acutely, and even may afford some physiologic advantages, such as favorable oxygen delivery from hemoglobin. However, with marked acidemia, pH <7.10, myocardial contractility is depressed and peripheral resistance falls (47,48). These manifestations may be a result of the effect of acidosis to depress both vascular and myocardial responsiveness to catecholamines as well as innate myocardial contractility. Both myocardial β receptor density as well as physiologic responses to β agonists appear to be decreased by metabolic acidosis (49,50).

Clearly, metabolic acidosis induces an intracellular acidosis in myocytes (45,46). This intracellular acidosis in turn impairs contractile responses to normal or even elevated cytosolic calcium concentrations (51,52). Alterations in troponin I–troponin C interactions mediated by low pH appear to shift the sensitivity of troponin C to calcium (53). Additionally, impairment of actin–myosin cross-bridge cycling caused by increases in the concentration of inorganic phosphate in the monovalent form may be involved in the decreased calcium sensitivity and contractile dysfunction seen with acidosis (54). The increase in monovalent inorganic phosphate results both from the acidic environment, which increases the ratio of monovalent to divalent inorganic phosphate, as well as from an impairment of myocardial energy production, which increases the total intracellular concentration of inorganic phosphate (55,56). Metabolic acidosis and hypoxia appear to additively or synergistically impair myocardial function, a phenomenon consistent with the monovalent inorganic phosphate hypothesis (57). The vasodepressor effect of acidosis likely results from similar molecular mechanisms (58).

CLINICAL FEATURES

Clinically, one can observe an increase in ventilatory effort with even mild degrees of acidosis. With severe metabolic acidosis (e.g., pH <7.20), respirations become extremely deep and rapid (Kussmaul's). Mild degrees of acidosis do not appear to markedly impair hemodynamic stability, at least in subjects with otherwise normal cardiovascular function. However, severe metabolic acidosis may lead to hypotension, pulmonary edema, and ultimately, ventricular standstill (47,59,60). Chronic metabolic acidosis, even if fairly mild, causes hypercalciuria and bone disease as bone buffering of acid leads to marked calcium losses from the bone due to increases in prostaglandin (PGE) (2) production (61). This aspect is extremely important in determining treatment of renal tubular acidosis (RTA) or the acidosis of chronic renal failure.

LABORATORY FINDINGS

Simple metabolic acidosis is characterized by a decrease in blood pH, $[HCO_3^-]$, and P_{CO_2} (through compensation). Note that a failure to lower the P_{CO_2} by 1 to 1.5 × the fall in $[HCO_3^-]$ indicates the coexistence of respiratory acidosis (41). The clinical implications of this are quite profound because this failure of compensation may signify impending severe respiratory failure. Serum electrolytes reveal a fall in $[TCO_2]$. Acidosis tends to shift potassium out of cells in a rather complex manner (62), and renal potassium excretion tends to increase in many states of metabolic acidosis. Normal or increased serum potassium in the face of decreased total body potassium stores occurs commonly in cases of metabolic acidosis (Chapter 5) (62). Some states of metabolic acidosis are characterized by the retention of an organic anion generated in concert with HCO_3^- consumption (organic acidosis), whereas others are not (hyperchloremic). The screening of plasma for such organic anions is not practical on a routine, immediate basis; thus, a calculation performed on the serum electrolytes called the anion gap is employed (63).

Serum Anion Gap

The SAG is a concept used in acid–base pathophysiology to infer whether an organic or mineral acidosis is present. We use the routine venous blood serum electrolytes to calculate the SAG (55):

$$SAG = [Na^+] - [Cl^-] - [TCO_2] \tag{3.8}$$

Here we use TCO_2 as an index of HCO_3^-. We define unmeasured cations (UCs) as cations that are not Na^+ (e.g., K^+, Mg^{2+}, Ca^{2+}) and unmeasured anions (UAs) as anions that are not Cl^- or HCO_3^- (e.g., SO_4^{2-}, $H_2PO_4^-$, HPO_4^{2-}, albumin, organic anions). Thus, electroneutrality demands that

$$[Na^+] + [UC] = [Cl^-] + [TCO_2] + [UA] \tag{3.9}$$

where the UA and UC concentrations are expressed in mEq/L rather than mmol/L. Putting formulas (8) and (9) together, we see that

$$SAG = [UA] - [UC] \tag{3.10}$$

Normally, the SAG is about 9 (6 to 12 mEq/L). Although the SAG is used routinely in the differential diagnosis of metabolic acidosis, we stress that it is a relative rather than absolute indicator of the underlying pathophysiology. Note that the maintenance of stoichiometry (i.e., 1-mEq increase in anion gap for every 1-mmol decrease in HCO_3^-) depends on the clearance mechanisms for the anion as well as the myriad factors that influence HCO_3^- concentration. Therefore, some organic acidoses may manifest trivial or even no increase in the anion gap, whereas some hyperchloremic acidoses may have coincidental increases in the anion gap. This must be kept in mind when evaluating the differential diagnosis of metabolic acidosis. However, a major increase in the anion gap (e.g., SAG >26 mEq/L) always implies the existence of an organic acidosis (64).

Urine Anion Gap

To address a different problem, urinary electrolytes have been used to estimate the quantity of NH_4^+ in the urine, a measurement that has been difficult to develop into a routine clinical test. The concept is quite similar to that described in the preceding for the SAG. In the urine, because of electroneutrality

$$[Na^+] + [K^+] + [UC] = [Cl^-] + [UA] \tag{3.11}$$

When urine pH is <6, UA does not include appreciable amounts of HCO_3^-, but consists primarily of phosphate ($H_2PO_4^-$ more than HPO_4^{2-}), and to a lesser degree, sulfate (SO_4^{2-}) and organic anions. UC is made up mostly of NH_4^+. Therefore, if we define the urinary anion gap (UAG) as

$$UAG = [Na^+] + [K^+] - [Cl^-] \tag{3.12}$$

then, we see that this is determined largely by the amount of NH_4^+ in the urine which holds true in clinical studies of metabolic acidosis (31). In contrast to the SAG, which is useful in many settings of clinical acid–base diagnosis and therapy, the UAG has a very narrow clinical application in the differentiation of renal from nonrenal causes of nonanion gap metabolic acidosis (65).

DIFFERENTIAL DIAGNOSIS OF METABOLIC ACIDOSIS

The differential diagnosis of metabolic acidosis generally is approached clinically by using the SAG. Those acidosis states associated with retention of an organic anion are classified as increased anion gap or simply anion gap metabolic acidosis. Those acidosis states not associated with retention of an organic anion are classified as nonanion gap or hyperchloremic metabolic acidosis (63). These disorders are listed in Table 3.3.

TABLE 3.3 DIFFERENTIAL DIAGNOSIS OF METABOLIC ACIDOSIS

Normal Anion Gap (Hyperchloremic)	Increased Anion Gap (Organic)
Gastrointestinal Loss of HCO₃⁻	**Increased Acid Production**
Diarrhea	Lactic acidosis
Intestinal fistula or drainage	Diabetic ketoacidosis
Anion exchange resins	Starvation
Ingestion of $CaCl_2$ or $MgCl_2$	Alcoholic ketoacidosis
Renal Loss of HCO₃⁻	Inborn errors of metabolism
Renal tubular acidosis	Toxic alcohol ingestion
Carbonic anhydrase inhibitors	Salicylate intoxication
Hypoaldosteronism	Other intoxications
K-sparing diuretics	Failure of acid excretion
Miscellaneous	Acute renal failure
Recovery from ketoacidosis	Chronic renal failure
Dilutional acidosis	
Addition of HCl	
Parenteral alimentation	
Sulfur ingestion	

CAUSES OF HYPOCHLOREMIC METABOLIC ACIDOSIS

Gastrointestinal Loss of HCO₃⁻

Diarrhea

Diarrhea is the most common cause of hyperchloremic metabolic acidosis and always should be considered early in the differential diagnosis. The concentration of HCO_3^- in diarrheal fluid is generally greater than that of plasma. In the extreme case of cholera, patients may lose up to 20 L/day of fluid containing 30 to 50 mEq/L of HCO_3^- (66). However, hypovolemic shock likely will cause lactic acidosis and increase the anion gap in that situation. Ileostomy fluid is also rich in HCO_3^-, especially early after construction (67).

The diagnosis of diarrheal loss of HCO_3^-, however, may be difficult in the very young or very old (68). In the former case, the distinction between diarrhea and an underlying RTA is extremely important. The UAG may be very helpful in this setting. Patients with diarrhea as a cause of metabolic acidosis typically have a very negative UAG (i.e., urinary chloride exceeds the sum of urinary $NA^+ + K^+$ by >10 mEq/L) reflecting the presence of ample urinary NH_4^+ concentrations, whereas patients with all forms of distal RTA have positive UAGs reflecting the inadequate urinary NH_4^+ concentrations present (31).

Gastrointestinal Drainage and Fistulas

The succus entericus and pancreatic and biliary secretions are rich in HCO_3^- and poor in Cl^-. The succus entericus has a daily volume of 600 to 700 mL but may be increased in disease states. Biliary secretions amount to >1 L/day of fluid, with $[HCO_3^-]$ approaching 60 mmol/L. Pancreatic secretion may exceed 2 L/day, with $[HCO_3^-]$ approaching 120 mmol/L. Therefore, it is not surprising that GI drainage or fistulas could cause significant metabolic acidosis (69).

Recently, the technique of simultaneous kidney/pancreas transplant (SPK) has been used for the treatment of type I diabetic patients with end-stage renal disease (70). When urinary drainage of the HCO_3^--rich exocrine secretions of the pancreatic allograft is employed rather than enteric drainage, this addition of pancreatic exocrine fluid causes urinary loss because the bladder cannot absorb the pancreatic secretion. Thus, SPK with urinary drainage is often associated with significant normal anion gap metabolic acidosis (71,72). Many of these patients require sodium bicarbonate supplementation (as high as 100 to 150 mEq/day) on a chronic basis. The incidence of metabolic acidosis can be significantly lowered with enteric drainage compared to urinary drainage because the intestine can absorb the HCO_3^- (73).

Urinary Diversion to Bowel

Patients may require urinary diversion from normal egress through the bladder for a variety of reasons. Approaches to this include the creation of an ileal loop conduit or, less commonly, drainage of the ureters into the sigmoid colon (ureterosigmoidostomy) (74). Although metabolic acidosis can develop with both procedures, it is more severe with ureterosigmoidostomy. The pathophysiology for both situations is the bowel mucosal secretion of HCO_3^- in exchange for Cl^- during water reabsorption, which may lead to significant HCO_3^- losses in the GI tract effluent (69). Newer reconstructive procedures including ileal neobladders, which minimize the time of contact between urine and bowel mucosa, have been successful in limiting HCO_3^- loss (75).

Chloride-containing Anion Exchange Resins

Cholestyramine is a nonabsorbable anion exchange resin used to bind bile acids in the gut for a variety of purposes, including the treatment of obstructive liver disease as well as hypercholesterolemia and the management of acute diarrhea in children (76). However, this resin has some affinity for HCO_3^- and may exchange Cl^- for HCO_3^- across the bowel mucosa. In conditions of renal insufficiency where new HCO_3^- generation is impaired, in volume depletion or patients taking spironolactone, hyperchloremic metabolic acidosis has been reported (77).

Calcium or Magnesium Ingestion

The divalent cations, calcium or magnesium, are absorbed incompletely in the GI tract. If large amounts of these cations are ingested in soluble form (e.g., as the Cl_2 salts), then the unabsorbed Ca^{2+} or Mg^{2+} reacts with HCO_3^-, which has been exchanged across the mucosa for Cl^-, to form an insoluble salt. Thus, plasma HCO_3^- falls to a moderate degree (78).

Renal Loss of HCO_3^-

Renal Tubular Acidosis

RTA refers to a group of functional disorders characterized by impairment of renal HCO_3^- reabsorption and H^+ excretion that is out of proportion to any reduction in GFR. In many cases, the RTAs exist in the presence of a completely normal GFR. Unfortunately, a nomenclature has evolved that confuses many experienced clinicians as well as trainees and students. We provide a pathophysiologic classification of these disorders while referring to this nomenclature. RTAs can be divided into those characterized by disturbed distal nephron function (i.e., impaired NAE) and those caused by impaired proximal HCO_3^- reabsorption (79). Distal RTAs are divided into those associated with hypokalemia (80) and those associated with hyperkalemia, which may be further subdivided into RTA caused by hypoaldosteronism and RTA characterized by a general distal tubular defect (81).

Proximal Renal Tubular Acidosis

Proximal RTA, also called type II RTA, is an uncommon but very interesting disorder (82,83). Basically, the acid–base disturbance is caused by impairment in proximal tubular reabsorption of HCO_3^-, the nephron site where 85% of HCO_3^- usually is reabsorbed. The delivery of HCO_3^--rich fluid to distal nephron sites leads to substantial bicarbonaturia, when plasma levels of HCO_3^- are normal, as well as urinary losses of potassium and sodium. Thus, patients present with hypokalemia and hyperchloremic metabolic acidosis. When the plasma concentration of HCO_3^- is maintained at normal by administration of HCO_3^-, fractional HCO_3^- excretion (i.e., the fraction of filtered HCO_3^- that is excreted in the urine) exceeds 15%.

In physiologic terms, the apparent T_{max} and PT for HCO_3^- are significantly reduced in patients with proximal RTA. However, once a level of plasma HCO_3^- is achieved that is below the patient's PT for HCO_3^-, renal acid handling is normal. In other words, NAE equals dietary and endogenous acid production rates and the subject comes into a steady state of acid–base balance, albeit at a moderately

TABLE 3.4 CAUSES OF RENAL TUBULAR ACIDOSIS

Proximal	Distal (Hypokalemic)	Distal (Hyperkalemic)
Primary	Primary	Hypoaldosteronism
Cystinosis	Hypercalcemia	Obstructive nephropathy
Wilson disease	Nephrocalcinosis	Sickle cell disease/trait
Lead toxicity	Multiple myeloma	Lupus erythematosus
Cadmium toxicity	Lupus erythematosus	Analgesic nephropathy
Mercury toxicity	Amphotericin B	Renal transplant rejection
Amyloidosis	Toluene	Cyclosporine toxicity
Multiple myeloma	Renal transplant rejection	Other interstitial disease
Nephrotic syndrome	Medullary sponge kidney	
Medullary cystic disease		
Outdated tetracycline		
Injury from kidney preservation		

reduced plasma HCO_3^- concentration (and a mild reduction in systemic pH). Because a steady state in acid handling is achieved, patients with proximal RTA have less severe acidosis as well as less nephrocalcinosis (which results from bone calcium mobilization from acidosis) than patients with distal RTAs (see the following).

The problem with proximal HCO_3^- reabsorption may occur independently but more commonly coexists with other defects in proximal nephron function, such as decreased reabsorption of glucose, amino acids, phosphate, and uric acid. The term Fanconi syndrome is employed when general proximal nephron function is disturbed (84). Patients with full-blown Fanconi syndrome may have severe osteomalacia and malnutrition in addition to the mild metabolic acidosis associated with proximal RTA (85). Proximal RTA may occur as a primary disorder and present in infancy or may be acquired in the course of other diseases or as a result of exposure to substances toxic to this nephron segment. A list of causes of proximal RTA is shown in Table 3.4. Treatment of this condition is approached by addressing the underlying cause, but if this is ineffective, administration of large amounts of HCO_3^- (10 to 15 mmol/kg/day) and potassium to compensate for ongoing potassium losses in the urine caused by the bicarbonaturia is necessary. This is necessary to avoid growth retardation in children and osteopenia, which may be produced by even mild degrees of academia (86).

Distal Renal Tubular Acidosis

The distal RTAs are characterized primarily by impaired NAE, which is due, at least in part, to impaired NH_4^+ excretion. The central role of impaired NH_4^+ excretion in this disorder is highlighted by a recent clinical study in which all patients with either hypokalemic distal RTA (also called type I or classic distal RTA) or hyperkalemic distal RTA (previously referred to as type IV RTA), caused by either hypoaldosteronism or a generalized tubular defect, had a positive UAG reflecting decreased NH_4^+ excretion. How NH_4^+ excretion is impaired in this diverse set of clinical disorders is still incompletely understood (81,87).

Hypokalemic distal RTA has long been considered a disorder of the collecting duct in which the quantity of H^+ secretion is inadequate to effect the necessary NAE for the subject to maintain acid–base balance. Clinically, patients with hypokalemic distal RTA present with hyperchloremic metabolic acidosis but are unable to acidify their urine (pH <5.5 is commonly used) in response to an acid challenge. It must be stressed that the failure to acidify the urine does not fully explain the defect in NAE, which is primarily caused by an associated defect in NH_4^+ excretion (88). However, the failure to acidify the urine under conditions of systemic acidosis historically has been considered the clinical hallmark of hypokalemic distal RTA. The physiologic mechanisms for this impaired acidification have been a topic of interest for some time and are summarized with clinical examples in Table 3.5. Basically, four mechanisms have been suggested for impaired acidification by the distal nephron: (a) backleak through a leaky epithelium; (b) pump failure, where the H^+ ATPase cannot pump sufficient amounts of H^+;

TABLE 3.5 EXAMPLES OF PATHOPHYSIOLOGIC MECHANISMS IN CLINICAL DISTAL RENAL TUBULAR ACIDOSIS

Physiologic Defect	Example
Backleak	Amphotericin B
Pump failure	Primary
Voltage defect	Amiloride
Rate defect/NH_4^+ defect	Hypoaldosteronism

(c) voltage defect, where a favorable transepithelial voltage cannot be generated (e.g., decreased sodium delivery to the distal nephron or decreased sodium reabsorption in the distal nephron); or (d) rate defect/NH_4^+ defect, where urinary pH is reduced but NH_4^+ excretion and NAE cannot be increased to normal amounts. Hypokalemic distal RTA appears to be caused by either backleak or pump failure. Patients may have an isolated defect in the H^+/K^+ ATPase or the vacuolar ATPase (89). Hyperkalemic distal RTAs are probably caused by either voltage defect or rate defect/NH_4^+ defect (81).

A number of physiologic maneuvers have been used to examine these mechanisms clinically. The first and simplest test is that of a metered pH (i.e., using a pH meter rather than a dipstick) performed on urine collected under oil. If the subject is already acidemic (e.g., arterial pH <7.35), then there is no need for ammonium chloride loading. In some cases, patients are able to maintain a normal plasma HCO_3^- concentration and systemic pH under most circumstances, but do not respond normally to increases in acid generation by increasing NAE. Recent studies have identified mutations in the vacuolar-ATPase B1 subunit most likely responsible for this defect (90). This is called an incomplete distal RTA. If an incomplete distal RTA is suspected, ammonium chloride is administered to induce a mild case of metabolic acidosis. This test basically screens for backleak, pump failure, or voltage defects. An alternate method, the furosemide–fludrocortisone test, is a better-tolerated test for urine acidification (91). Furosemide increases distal Na^+ delivery, and the mineralocorticoid fludrocortisone increases distal H^+ secretion. Normal subjects all acidify urine to pH <5.3 by 3 or 4 hours, whereas patients with distal RTA fail to do so. Infusion of sodium sulfate or sodium phosphate increases distal sodium delivery. The failure to lower urine pH after these maneuvers suggests pump failure or impaired voltage owing to inadequate distal sodium reabsorption. Another maneuver is to determine the urine to blood P_{CO_2} gradient when the patient has bicarbonaturia (urine $[HCO_3^-]$ >100 mM) induced by HCO_3^- administration. Under conditions where bicarbonaturia is induced, H^+ secreted into the collecting duct lumen will combine with HCO_3^- and form H_2CO_3. Because carbonic anhydrase is absent in the lumen of this segment (as well as the bladder), conversion to CO_2 and water is slow and occurs largely in the urinary collecting system (i.e., renal pelvis, ureters, and urinary bladder), where the surface area for CO_2 absorption is small. This CO_2 essentially is trapped, and, when normalized for the blood P_{CO_2} (i.e., the difference between urine and blood), is a marker for the rate of distal H^+ secretion. Patients with backleak or pump failure generally have a small difference between urine and blood P_{CO_2} (<20 torr).

Hypokalemic distal RTA may be primary or associated with other diseases, most commonly, Sjögren syndrome (92) and toxin exposures. These toxins may vary from wasp sting (93) to toluene inhalation, the latter capable of causing several forms of acidosis (94). A list of causes of hypokalemic distal RTA appears in Table 3.4. Some of the causes also may result in a hyperkalemic distal RTA because of a generalized tubular defect (81). Urinary obstruction and some of the autoimmune disorders are such examples (95). Perhaps the best understood cause of hypokalemic distal RTA is that due to amphotericin toxicity, which results (at least experimentally) in acidification failure owing to backleak of normally secreted H^+. Hypokalemic distal RTA usually occurs in young children in its primary form. The children never achieve a steady state of acid–base balance; therefore, they typically present with extremely severe metabolic acidosis, growth retardation, nephrocalcinosis, and nephrolithiasis (96). Hypokalemia, which usually is present, is actually caused by the associated sodium depletion and stimulation of the renin–angiotensin–aldosterone axis. Therefore, renal potassium losses actually decrease considerably when appropriate therapy with sodium bicarbonate is instituted. This is quite different from patients with proximal RTA, where urinary potassium losses increase considerably during therapy because of the bicarbonaturia-associated urinary K losses. Another contrasting point between proximal RTA and hypokalemic distal RTA is the amount of alkali therapy needed. Once the acute acidosis is corrected, patients with hypokalemic distal RTA only need enough alkali to account for the amount of acid generated from diet and metabolism; therefore, 1 to 3 mmol/kg/day generally is sufficient.

Hyperkalemic distal RTA from hypoaldosteronism occurs in several settings summarized in Table 3.4. Best understood is the case of either selective aldosterone deficiency or complete adrenal insufficiency. Probably the most common form of RTA is the hyporeninemic hypoaldosteronism often seen in patients with diabetic nephropathy. In patients with this form of RTA, urinary acidification as assessed by urine pH appears normal, but the patients are unable to raise NAE to appropriate levels. The defect, at least in some of these individuals, can be traced to impaired NH_4^+ synthesis in the proximal nephron, resulting directly from the hyperkalemia. Treatment of the hyperkalemia in some individuals with this disorder is sufficient to correct the disturbance in NAE. In patients with pure primary aldosterone deficiency, replacement of physiologic amounts of mineralocorticoid results in correction of the disturbance in acid–base metabolism and is both logical and appropriate therapy. However, in patients with the hyporeninemic hypoaldosteronism form, the renal defect requires pharmacologic amounts of mineralocorticoid (i.e., 5 to 10 times the usual physiologic dose) for efficacy. Moreover, the use of mineralocorticoid in this setting may be contraindicated because these patients often have mild renal insufficiency and tend to be total body sodium expanded rather than depleted (as is the case in the pure hypoaldosteronism form). Treatment of the hyperkalemia by increasing renal K excretion (e.g., with loop diuretics) or K excretion through the GI tract with potassium-binding resins (Kayexalate) may be the preferred approach in patients with the hyporeninemic hypoaldosteronism form.

Hyperkalemic distal RTA from a generalized tubular defect is considerably more common than either classic distal or proximal RTA. A list of causes appears in Table 3.4. Urinary obstruction may be the most common and important cause of this form of distal RTA. Other important causes in selected populations include cyclosporine nephrotoxicity and allograft rejection in the renal transplant patient, sickle cell nephropathy in patients homozygous and occasionally heterozygous for the sickle cell gene, and many autoimmune disorders such as lupus nephritis and Sjögren syndrome. Urinary acidification is impaired similarly to the hypokalemic distal RTA patients. Also in contrast to the hypoaldosteronism form, hyperkalemia plays a less significant role in the genesis of impaired NH_4^+ excretion, which is tied directly to the impaired distal nephron function.

Carbonic Anhydrase Inhibitors

Carbonic anhydrase inhibitors such as acetazolamide inhibit both proximal tubular luminal brush border and cellular carbonic anhydrase. The net effect is a pattern of impaired HCO_3^- reabsorption similar to that of proximal RTA. These drugs are commonly used topically to treat glaucoma, but their use may be complicated by systemic effects such as hyperchloremic metabolic acidosis (97). Topiramate is an antiseizure medication widely used in children that causes a mild to moderate proximal RTA by inhibiting carbonic anhydrase (98). The use of this drug has been associated with nephrolithiasis in both adults and children due to the resultant hypocitraturia, hypercalciuria, and elevated urine pH (99).

Hypoaldosteronism

Hypoaldosteronism is associated with a hyperkalemic distal RTA. This may be produced by pharmacologic antagonism of aldosterone action or impaired aldosterone secretion. Impaired aldosterone secretion may be caused by hyporeninemia (e.g., the hyporeninemic hypoaldosteronism associated with diabetes mellitus) or may be part of adrenal insufficiency (e.g., Addison disease). With hyporeninemic hypoaldosteronism, some have suggested that the disorder is, at least in part, an adrenal disorder because plasma potassium concentrations that typically induce aldosterone secretion do not in this disorder. However, permissive amounts of angiotensin II are necessary to allow potassium to be an effective aldosterone secretagogue (100,101).

K-sparing Diuretics

Potassium-sparing diuretics, which either block aldosterone action (e.g., spironolactone, eplerenone) or impair distal nephron sodium reabsorption (e.g., amiloride, triamterene), also may produce a hyperchloremic acidosis in concert with hyperkalemia (102,103). The observation that aldosterone antagonists may ameliorate the progression of congestive heart failure (104) has led to more widespread use, but careful monitoring of plasma potassium is necessary (105).

Miscellaneous Causes of Hyperchloremic Acidosis

Recovery from Ketoacidosis

Although diabetic ketoacidosis (DKA) is one of the best described forms of increased anion gap metabolic acidosis, many patients during recovery from DKA may eliminate the organic anions through renal clearance faster than their acidosis corrects, leaving them with a nonanion gap or hyperchloremic metabolic acidosis (106). This also may occur in patients who drink enough to avoid volume depletion and consequent fall in GFR (107).

Dilutional Acidosis

The rapid expansion of ECF volume with fluids that do not contain HCO_3^- leads to a dilution of HCO_3^- and mild metabolic acidosis. The fall in HCO_3^- produced in this manner is typically quite small (e.g., 10%) and usually is corrected fairly rapidly by renal generation of HCO_3^- (i.e., by renal correction) (108).

Addition of HCl

Administration of HCl or congeners (e.g., ammonium chloride or lysine chloride) rapidly consumes an HCO_3^- molecule without generating an organic anion, thus causing hyperchloremic metabolic acidosis (109).

Parenteral Alimentation

Amino acid infusions without concomitant administration of alkali (or alkali-generating precursors) may produce hyperchloremic metabolic acidosis in a manner similar to addition of HCl. This problem can be avoided by replacing the chloride salt of these amino acids with an acetate salt which is metabolized to HCO_3^- (110).

Sulfur Ingestion

Ingested elemental sulfur or sulfur released during metabolism of sulfur-containing amino acids (e.g., methionine or cysteine) is oxidized to sulfate with accompanying H^+ production. Sulfate is excreted rapidly by the kidneys, usually accompanied by sodium, whereas the excretion of H^+ produced by sulfur metabolism lags, resulting in a hyperchloremic metabolic acidosis. A dietary intake rich in sodium compared to potassium and excessive consumption of sulfur-containing amino acids is a common feature of Western diets. Ingestion of 40 to 50 g/day of flowers of sulfur for several days, a folk remedy for constipation, has also produced profound hyperchloremic metabolic acidosis (111).

CAUSES OF INCREASED ANION GAP (ORGANIC METABOLIC ACIDOSIS)

Organic Acidosis Resulting from Increased Acid Production

Lactic Acidosis

Lactic acidosis is an extensively studied organic acidosis. Causes of lactic acidosis are summarized in Table 3.6. Lactic acid is the final product of mammalian anaerobic metabolism. In general, aerobic tissues metabolize carbohydrates to pyruvate, which then undergoes oxidative metabolism within mitochondria. This oxidative metabolism regenerates NAD^+ consumed at a more proximal site in the glycolytic pathway. When tissues must perform anaerobic glycolysis to regenerate this NAD^+, the net effect is to generate lactic acid from carbohydrates and thus generate H^+. Under normal conditions in

TABLE 3.6 CAUSES OF LACTIC ACIDOSIS

Primary Decrease in Tissue Oxygenation

Septic shock

Cardiogenic shock

Hypovolemic shock

Mesenteric ischemia

Hypoxemia

Excessive Energy Expenditures

Seizures

Extreme exertion

Hyperthermia

Deranged Oxidative Metabolism

Diabetic ketoacidosis

Malignancy

Intoxication (e.g., ethanol, iron, isoniazid, carbon monoxide, strychnine)

Impaired Lactate Clearance

Liver failure

Miscellaneous

D-Lactic acidosis

---

humans, relatively small amounts of lactate, specifically the L-isomer, are formed during normal metabolism and are metabolized by the liver, maintaining relatively low plasma and urine levels of this metabolite. Lactic acidosis may develop under pathologic conditions associated with either local or systemic decreases in oxygen delivery (type A), impairments in oxidative metabolism (type B), or impaired hepatic clearance (112).

The diagnosis of lactic acidosis must be considered in all forms of metabolic acidosis associated with an increased anion gap, particularly those cases occurring in these clinical circumstances. Determination of the serum or plasma lactate level may confirm this diagnosis, although many clinical laboratories may not provide this information on an emergency basis (112). In cases of D-lactic acidosis (e.g., seen with blind intestinal loops colonized with D-lactate-producing organisms), the usual measurement of lactate performed in clinical laboratories using an enzymatic reaction does not detect this D-isomer. Nonroutine measurement techniques such as ^{1}H NMR spectroscopy (which does not distinguish between D and L forms) or specific measurement of the D form with the appropriate enzymatic analysis may be necessary to document elevations of D-lactate in this unusual clinical circumstance (113,114).

Treatment of lactic acidosis must be directed at the underlying pathophysiology. Although the degree of acidemia in this setting may become deleterious in its own right, therapy with $NaHCO_3^-$ to directly address the metabolic acidosis has not been found to be effective clinically (115) and is actually deleterious in several experimental models (47,116–118). This issue remains quite controversial at this time (119).

Diabetic Ketoacidosis

DKA results from insufficient insulin to metabolize glucose and excess glucagon, which generates short-chain fatty ketoacids, specifically, β-hydroxybutyric and acetoacetic acids. These ketoacids are both relatively strong acids that dissociate almost completely at physiologic pH into H^+ and the keto-anions and cause an anion gap metabolic acidosis. Interestingly, the amount of insulin needed for catabolism of short-chain fatty acids is significantly less than that necessary for glucose homeostasis. Thus, DKA is a common presentation in patients with insulin-dependent diabetes mellitus (107). However, DKA also occurs in patients with non–insulin-dependent diabetes mellitus (120). In addition, patients with non–insulin-dependent diabetes mellitus may present with marked increases in serum glucose concentrations without ketosis (121) (e.g., nonketotic hyperglycemic hyperosmolar coma).

Patients with DKA typically present with altered sensorium, deep respirations, and severe anion gap metabolic acidosis with HCO_3^- concentrations as low as 1 to 10 mmol/L and arterial pH values that may be <7.0. Initially, the increase in the anion gap above normal may parallel the decrease in HCO_3^-; however, during therapy, a dissociation of the decrease in anion gap (ΔAG) and the decrease in HCO_3^- concentration ($\Delta[HCO_3^-]$) may develop. This is due to renal elimination of the ketoacidosis as renal perfusion and clearance improve during therapy of the ketoacids; also, it may signify a degree of underlying distal RTA (e.g., hyporeninemic hypoaldosteronism) in some subjects (122).

The diagnosis of DKA is made by finding the combination of anion gap metabolic acidosis, hyperglycemia, and demonstration of serum (or urine) ketoacids. We stress that the presence of serum and urine ketones is not specific for DKA, but also may be present in other conditions such as alcoholic ketoacidosis (AKA) and starvation ketoacidosis (106) as well as some drug intoxications (e.g., salicylate, ketamine) (123,124).

Some patients who present with DKA may be critically ill; however, mortality is quite low with appropriate therapy. Insulin, hydration, and management of electrolyte disturbances are the essentials of therapy. Most patients with DKA present with considerable total body deficits of potassium, magnesium, and phosphorus, even though serum levels (particularly of potassium) may be high on presentation (125). Treatment of DKA with $NaHCO_3$ still has some proponents despite absence of evidence to support its use (126,127). Hazards associated with $NaHCO_3$ in this setting include hyperosmolarity (ampules of $NaHCO_3$ are quite hypertonic), overshoot alkalosis, and paradoxical intracellular acidosis (discussed later in the text), which may further compromise CNS function and hemodynamic stability (126). Thus, we do not recommend $NaHCO_3$ treatment for DKA.

Starvation

Voluntary or involuntary abstinence from caloric intake produces relative insulin deficiency and glucagon excess, which is similar to the hormonal disturbances seen with DKA. Specifically, during starvation, hepatic ketogenesis is accelerated and tissue ketone metabolism is reduced. Thus, an increase in the plasma and urine concentrations of ketoacids occurs. Moreover, with prolonged starvation, decreases in plasma HCO_3^- may also transpire, producing a mild anion gap metabolic acidosis. However, the plasma $[HCO_3^-]$ rarely falls to values <18 mmol/L in this setting. Ketone bodies stimulate pancreatic cells to release insulin, and lipolysis is controlled resulting in much less severe ketoacidosis as compared to patients with frank DKA (128).

Alcoholic Ketoacidosis

AKA is probably the result of the combination of alcohol toxicity and starvation. Serum glucose levels range from very low (i.e., <50 mg/dL) to modestly elevated (e.g., 250 to 275 mg/dL), where confusion with the diagnosis of DKA may occur. Typically, patients present not with simple metabolic acidosis but rather with a complex acid–base disturbance containing features of anion gap metabolic acidosis, metabolic alkalosis produced by vomiting, and respiratory alkalosis owing to hyperventilation. A markedly increased anion gap is a hallmark of this disorder. Rarely devastating complications such as sudden cardiac death occur (129).

At times, this diagnosis may not be easy to make. This is because when the pH is low, the majority of ketoanions circulating in the serum may not be detected by the Acetest assay. Specifically, the Acetest reaction measures acetoacetate but is rather insensitive to β-hydroxybutyrate. When the serum pH is low as might be the case with severe AKA, the proportion of β-hydroxybutyrate increases secondary to an increase in the NADH/NAD$^+$ ratio due to alcohol metabolism. Proton NMR spectroscopy of the urine has been used to identify AKA as well as other causes of anion gap metabolic acidosis (113,130). Treatment of AKA consists of vigorous volume and glucose repletion with additional attention to repletion of potassium, magnesium, phosphorus, and vitamin deficits (131).

Nonketotic Hyperosmolar Coma

Some patients with nonketotic hyperosmolar coma with severe hyperglycemia also may present with anion gap metabolic acidosis. In most cases, the organic anion that accumulates has not been identified but does not appear to be either keto-anions or lactate (132,133).

Inborn Errors of Metabolism

The accumulation of organic acids in body fluids with a resultant metabolic acidosis may be seen in certain inborn errors of metabolism, such as maple syrup urine disease, methylmalonic aciduria, propionic acidemia, and isovaleric acidemia. These disorders generally present shortly after birth (134).

Toxic Alcohol Ingestion

Important causes of anion gap metabolic acidosis are those due to toxic alcohol ingestion, specifically methanol and ethylene glycol. Early diagnosis allows for prompt and usually successful therapy, whereas delay in the diagnosis may be associated with considerable morbidity and mortality. Patients who ingest either methanol or ethylene glycol generally develop profound anion gap metabolic acidosis during the course of their illness, but their acid–base status initially may be normal if they present soon after ingestion. The serum osmolal gap generally is elevated soon after ingestion because of the presence of toxic alcohol in the serum (135–137).

$$\text{Calculated serum osmolality} = 1.86\,[Na^+] + [\text{glucose}]/18 + [\text{urea nitrogen}]/2.8 \qquad (3.13)$$

$$([Na^+] \text{ in mM, the [glucose] and [urea nitrogen] in mg/dL})$$

$$\text{Serum osmolal gap} = \text{measured serum osmolality} - \text{calculated serum osmolality} \qquad (3.14)$$

The osmolal gap tends to collapse further along the course of this disease, whereas anion gap metabolic acidosis worsens. Although useful in suggesting this diagnosis, elevations in the serum osmolar gap are not specific for toxic alcohol ingestion, largely because ethanol is the most common cause of an elevated serum osmolal gap (138,139).

Patients who ingest methanol either as a suicide attempt or accidentally typically present with abdominal pain, vomiting, headache, and visual disturbances. Methanol intoxication characteristically produces severe retinitis, which may lead to blindness, and may be detectable on funduscopic examination. Methanol toxicity generally is believed to result from the metabolism of the methanol by alcohol dehydrogenase, specifically to formic acid. Ingestions of as little as 30 mL of methanol are toxic, and 100 to 250 mL of methanol generally is fatal unless treated (137).

Ethylene glycol is the major osmolyte in most commercial antifreeze formulations. Ingestion may occur as a suicide attempt, but because of its sweet taste, accidental ingestions are quite common. Ethylene glycol intoxication is similar to that of methanol in that both produce CNS disturbances and severe anion gap metabolic acidosis. In contrast to methanol, ethylene glycol does not usually produce retinitis, but can cause acute and chronic renal failure. The major toxicity of ethylene glycol is caused by its metabolism by alcohol dehydrogenase to glycolate, glyoxylate, and oxalate (140). Detection of oxalate crystals in the urine may support the clinical impression of ethylene glycol ingestion. Renal biopsy in this setting is characterized by the deposition of calcium oxalate crystals in the tubular epithelial cells and areas of acute tubular necrosis (141). The lethal dose of ethylene glycol is believed to be as little as 100 mL (135).

Because metabolism of methanol and ethylene glycol directly lead to their major toxicities, immediate prevention of this metabolism plays an important role in the therapy of these intoxications. Fortunately, the affinity of alcohol dehydrogenase for ethanol is considerably greater than for either methanol or ethylene glycol, and infusing ethanol to achieve concentrations >100 mg/dL effectively prevents alcohol dehydrogenase–mediated metabolism of both ethylene glycol and methanol. Hemodialysis is an effective procedure to facilitate clearance of the nontoxic parent compounds. However, during hemodialysis, adjustments in the dosage of ethanol (which also is cleared by hemodialysis) are necessary to maintain sufficient blood concentrations (142). Fomepizole, a specific inhibitor of alcohol dehydrogenase that has been used in veterinary medicine for some time, recently has been approved by the FDA for the treatment of methanol and ethylene glycol intoxications (143).

Salicylate Overdose

Ingestion of large amounts of aspirin, salicylamide, bismuth salicylate, or methyl salicylate may lead to serious and complex acid–base abnormalities. Symptoms correlate quite poorly with blood levels, especially in elderly persons, but almost always accompany extremely elevated blood levels (plasma [salicylate] >50 mg/dL) (123). Salicylates have a CNS effect to stimulate respiration and produce a component of respiratory alkalosis, especially early in the course of toxicity. Most adults with salicylate toxicity present either with respiratory alkalosis or a mixed anion gap metabolic acidosis and respiratory alkalosis. In children, the decreases in plasma [HCO_3^-] and increases in the anion gap develop more rapidly, and presentation with simple anion gap metabolic acidosis is most common. The acids responsible for the metabolic acidosis and increase in the anion gap include salicylate itself as well as endogenous acid anions whose metabolism is affected by the toxic amounts of salicylates. A blood salicylate concentration of 100 mg/dL contributes 7.3 mEq/L to the anion gap. Some component of lactic acidosis generally accompanies severe salicylate toxicity (144).

The diagnosis of salicylate toxicity is suggested by the history of aspirin use, nausea, and tinnitus. This is further supported by the clinical findings of unexplained hyperventilation, anion gap metabolic acidosis, noncardiogenic pulmonary edema, and an elevated prothrombin time. When salicylate toxicity occurs in younger adults, it is generally a result of a suicide attempt and is easily diagnosed; however, the diagnosis may be more elusive in older adults as well as in children. Delayed toxicities have been reported with the use of enteric coated aspirin, salicylate-induced pylorospasm, or the formation of pharmacobezoars. Therefore, it is imperative that salicylate concentrations are monitored every 4 hours until the levels are decreasing and the patient is not symptomatic (145). Advanced age and a delay in the diagnosis of salicylate toxicity are associated with significant mortality.

Treatment of salicylate toxicity generally should include alkalization of the blood and urine with sodium bicarbonate. Despite the potential negatives associated with sodium bicarbonate use in acute anion gap metabolic acidosis, alkalization of the plasma decreases the diffusion of salicylate into CNS sites where it is toxic, and it improves renal excretion as the urine is alkalinized (146). However, hemodynamic compromise and fluid overload must be carefully avoided, especially in older patients or those with underlying heart disease (147). Sustained low-efficiency dialysis has been shown to be quite effective at removing salicylate from the body and should be considered for patients with severely elevated plasma levels (>90 mg/dL), or evidence of severe toxicity, or for patients for whom aggressive alkalization may be hazardous (147).

Other Intoxications

A variety of other agents may produce anion gap metabolic acidosis. These include strychnine, oral iron overdose, isoniazid, papaverine, outdated tetracyclines, hydrogen sulfide, carbon monoxide, and paraldehyde. In general, these produce lactic acidosis (143). Severe lactic acidosis has also been reported with the daily ingestion of mangosteen, a tropical fruit used for weight loss (148). Sedatives used in critical care setting such as propofol and lorazepam can also cause lactic acidosis due to the propylene glycol solvent (149,150).

Other agents that may cause nonlactate anion gap metabolic acidosis include acetaminophen, toluene, and citric acid. Acetaminophen in therapeutic doses may generate pyroglutamic acid (5-oxoproline) in susceptible individuals. Bicarbonate levels as low as 3 mM and anion gaps >35 mEq/L have been seen, and repeated episodes may occur in the same patient (151,152). No metabolic defect has been identified. Toluene, which produces RTA (generally distal, but may include a proximal component), causes an elevation of serum hippurate (a metabolite of the toluene) concentration (153). The hippurate is excreted rapidly if renal function is intact and hyperchloremic metabolic acidosis may ensue. Another exception is citric acid present in toilet bowl cleaner, which increases the anion gap and causes hyperkalemia. Administration of intravenous calcium was necessary to stabilize a reported patient (154).

Failure of Acid Excretion

Acute or Chronic Renal Failure

The failure of the kidney to excrete the usual 1 to 3 mmol/kg of acid produced each day leads to metabolic acidosis. With both acute and chronic renal failure, some retention of anions occurs (including phosphate, sulfate, and some poorly characterized organic anions), which produces some increase in the SAG (155). Metabolic acidosis in the setting of acute and chronic renal failure generally is not severe unless a markedly catabolic state occurs or another acidotic condition supervenes.

With acute renal failure, the sudden loss of renal excretory function is invariably accompanied by a failure of acid excretion. Adaptation has no time to occur in this setting. With chronic renal failure, adaptation in remaining nephrons has time to occur. Specifically, the remaining nephron units markedly increase their NH_4^+ excretion. Metabolic acidosis is caused by a failure of the enhanced ammonia genesis in remaining nephron units to achieve the necessary NAE required for acid–base balance. Phosphate retention, which ultimately decreases urinary phosphate involved in the titratable acid component of NAE, also may contribute to this failure of acid–base balance. In addition, the high concentrations of circulating parathyroid hormone seen in chronic renal failure decrease proximal tubular HCO_3^- reabsorption and participate in the pathogenesis of metabolic acidosis (156). Although therapy of the metabolic acidosis with supplemental sodium bicarbonate may be useful in some cases of chronic renal failure, generally the development of metabolic acidosis is accompanied by other manifestations of chronic renal failure that mandate institution of dialysis or renal transplantation.

TREATMENT OF METABOLIC ACIDOSIS

Although acidosis itself is deleterious to the function of many organs, the treatment of most conditions associated with metabolic acidosis generally is best accomplished by treatment of the underlying disease state. With most of the hyperchloremic states of metabolic acidosis, gradual correction of the acidosis with HCO_3^- administered either as sodium bicarbonate or as a substrate metabolized to HCO_3^- (e.g., citrate) is quite rational, effective, and ultimately beneficial. Oral administration of these agents is preferred. In general, 1 g of sodium bicarbonate delivers about 2 mmol of HCO_3^-. Commercially available sodium or mixed sodium and potassium citrate solutions (e.g., Shohl's solution or Polycitra) contain 1 mmol of HCO_3^- equivalent per milliliter. Although citrate solutions are generally better tolerated than sodium bicarbonate tablets (which cause bloating when they produce CO_2 gas in the stomach), citrate may increase GI absorption of aluminum and should not be administered along with aluminum-based phosphate binders, especially in the setting of chronic renal failure (157).

The acute treatment of metabolic acidosis associated with an increased anion gap with intravenous sodium bicarbonate actually may be deleterious, especially in conditions associated with impaired tissue perfusion. To understand how acute therapy with sodium bicarbonate may be deleterious, one must consider the fate of the administered HCO_3^- molecules. When sodium bicarbonate is given, a change in the serum HCO_3^- concentration results. The magnitude of this change in serum HCO_3^- for a given dose of bicarbonate is determined by the apparent volume of distribution for HCO_3^- ($Vd_{HCO_3^-}$), which we define as

$$Vd_{HCO_3^-} = \text{dose of } HCO_3^-/(\Delta serum[HCO_3^-]) \tag{3.15}$$

This $Vd_{HCO_3^-}$ is not constant, but increases with increasing severity of acidosis. This variation in $Vd_{HCO_3^-}$ probably results both from increased buffering from some extracellular and intracellular proteins as well as from alterations in pHi homeostasis. The addition of HCO_3^- to blood (or an organism) produces CO_2 by mass action. Again, when metabolic acidosis is present, more CO_2 is produced for a given dose of sodium bicarbonate. In fact, recent studies performed in a closed, human blood model demonstrate that the production of CO_2 from administered HCO_3^- is directly dependent on the initial pH. Therefore, when ventilation is normal, this extra CO_2 is rapidly eliminated by the lungs, and a portion of the $Vd_{HCO_3^-}$ can be considered to be extracorporeal. However, when pulmonary ventilation or, more commonly, tissue ventilation is impaired (by poor tissue perfusion), this CO_2 generated by infused HCO_3^- may diffuse into cells (far more rapidly than the original HCO_3^- molecule) and paradoxically decrease the pHi. This is shown schematically in Figure 3.4. Experimentally, administration of sodium bicarbonate in animal models of metabolic acidosis has been associated with a fall in pH in several organs as well as additional hemodynamic compromise. In addition to this paradoxical intracellular acidosis, administration of hypertonic sodium bicarbonate (often given as 50-mL ampules of 1 mol/L $NaHCO_3$) may be associated with development of hypertonicity as well. This hypertonicity itself may have deleterious effects on cardiac function, especially in the setting of cardiac arrest resuscitation (158). In general, we do not advocate the emergency administration of intravenous sodium bicarbonate for acute anion gap metabolic acidosis, although this area remains quite controversial (127). Some small

Extracellular Space

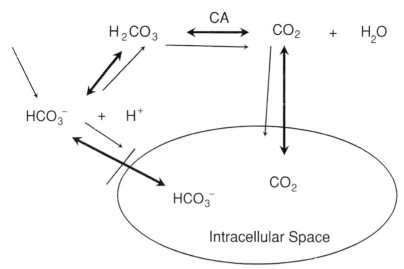

■ **Figure 3.4** Illustration of mechanism underlying paradoxical intracellular acidosis resulting from sodium bicarbonate administration. When additional HCO_3^- is added to the extracellular fluid *(narrow arrow)*, HCO_3^- combines with H^+ and reaction is shifted by mass action to H_2CO_3, which results in increases in extracellular CO_2 tension. Because most cell membranes are more permeable to CO_2 than to HCO_3^-, this transiently causes the cellular CO_2 tension to rise more than the $[HCO_3^-]$, which results in decreases in intracellular pH.

studies suggest that administering large amounts of bicarbonate while providing continuous hemodialysis and ultrafiltration may be a useful approach in this setting (159,160); however, this approach has not been subjected to rigorous study and remains speculative.

To address the concerns for sodium bicarbonate discussed in the preceding, alternatives have been proposed. These alternatives include non–CO_2-generating buffers such as THAM (tris-hydroxymethyl aminomethane) (161) and Carbicarb (a 1:1 mixture of disodium carbonate and sodium bicarbonate) as well as dichloroacetate, an agent which decreases lactate production by stimulating the activity of the pyruvate dehydrogenase complex (162). Although all three of the agents have been studied for some time, none have made it into routine clinical practice.

Metabolic Alkalosis

DEFINITIONS AND CAUSES

Metabolic alkalosis is a systemic disorder caused by a process that leads to an increased pH caused by a primary increase in the plasma $[HCO_3^-]$. This primary elevation of plasma $[HCO_3^-]$ may be caused by three processes (163).

Net Loss of H^+ from the Extracellular Fluid

H^+ can be lost from the ECF externally through the GI tract and kidneys or be shifted (at least theoretically) internally into cells. If H^+ losses exceed the daily H^+ load produced by diet and metabolism, then increases in the plasma $[HCO_3^-]$ will occur. This is because the loss of H^+ at these sites mandates the generation of an HCO_3^- molecule. In the stomach, the gastric parietal cell secretion of H^+ by the luminal H^+ ATPase leaves an HCO_3^- to be reclaimed at the basolateral surface. In the kidney, H^+ secretion via the H^+ ATPase or Na^+/H^+ exchanger also leaves an HCO_3^- molecule for reclamation on the basolateral surface. Shifting of H^+ into cells has been postulated to accompany states of significant potassium depletion, thus increasing ECF $[HCO_3^-]$. Despite the appeal of this concept, evidence of intracellular acidosis developing during experimental potassium depletion has not been observed consistently (164).

Net Addition of Bicarbonate Precursors to the Extracellular Fluid

The administration of HCO_3^- or substances that generate HCO_3^-, such as lactate, citrate, or acetate, at a rate greater than that of metabolic H^+ production also lead to a rise in ECF $[HCO_3^-]$. When renal function is normal, such increases in ECF $[HCO_3^-]$ are offset by marked increases in renal HCO_3^- excretion because the plasma $[HCO_3^-]$ exceeds the PT for HCO_3^- reabsorption.

External Loss of Fluid Containing Chloride in Greater Concentration and Bicarbonate in Lesser Concentration Than the Plasma

Loss of this type of fluid leads to both a contraction of the ECF volume and a rise in $[HCO_3^-]$. In this situation, H^+ is not lost externally, as in vomiting or nasogastric suction, but rather the remaining ECF $[HCO_3^-]$ increases as ECF volume contracts (contraction alkalosis) (108). However, intrarenal mechanisms to generate and reabsorb HCO_3^- also are active in this state.

PATHOPHYSIOLOGY OF METABOLIC ALKALOSIS

The normal kidney has a wonderful protective mechanism against the development of significant increases in ECF $[HCO_3^-]$, namely, a threshold for tubular fluid $[HCO_3^-]$ above which proximal reabsorption falls and HCO_3^- losses in the urine ensue. Therefore, in virtually all cases of metabolic alkalosis, the kidney must participate in the pathophysiology, at least at a passive level, by not excreting the excess HCO_3^-. A useful way to consider the pathogenesis of metabolic alkalosis is to separate factors that initiate or generate the metabolic alkalosis from those that maintain it.

Buffering

When HCO_3^- is added to the ECF, H^+ reacts with the HCO_3^- to produce CO_2, which normally is exhaled in expired gas. Thus, the increase in plasma and ECF $[HCO_3^-]$ is attenuated. Most of the H^+ used in this buffering comes from the ICF and from a small increase in lactic acid production (112).

Respiratory Compensation

The control of ventilation under normal conditions apparently is situated in the brain stem and is most sensitive to interstitial H^+ concentrations. The respiratory compensation to metabolic alkalosis follows the same principles as respiratory compensation to metabolic acidosis. However, the direction of the change of P_{CO_2} is different. Hypercapnia caused by hypoventilation rather than hypocapnia caused by hyperventilation occurs. Constraints regarding oxygenation limit the magnitude of this hypoventilatory response. As a rule of thumb, the Pa_{CO_2} should increase 0.25 to 1.0 $\times$ the increase in plasma $[HCO_3^-]$ during metabolic alkalosis. Failure to demonstrate such compensation in the setting of metabolic alkalosis marks the coexistence of primary respiratory alkalosis (165).

Renal Correction

The response by the kidney to excrete excessive HCO_3^- in the urine, under normal conditions, rapidly corrects metabolic alkalosis. In a manner analogous to tubular reabsorption of glucose, one can consider the maximal amount of tubular bicarbonate reabsorption (T_{max}) as well as the PT above which bicarbonaturia occurs. Bicarbonate excretion in the urine is proportional to the GFR once the PT is exceeded. Therefore, if a patient has normal renal function, it is difficult to produce a sustained increase in plasma $[HCO_3^-]$ without somehow changing the PT and T_{max}.

Biochemical and Physiologic Responses

FACTORS IN THE MAINTENANCE OF METABOLIC ALKALOSIS

Several factors tend to increase the apparent T_{max} for HCO_3^- and thus increase net HCO_3^- reabsorption by the kidney.

Decreases in Effective Arterial Blood Volume

Absolute (e.g., salt losses through vomiting or bleeding) or effective (e.g., heart failure, cirrhosis, nephrotic syndrome) arterial volume depletion increases the T_{max} and PT for HCO_3^-. This is accomplished both proximally (increased proximal tubule reabsorption of Na and water) as well as distally (mineralocorticoid effect) in the nephron (166).

Chloride Depletion

Although chloride depletion occurs as part of the pathophysiology of decreases in ECF volume, detailed physiologic studies show that the chloride anion is independently involved in the process of HCO_3^- reabsorption. Specifically, even in the presence of expansion of the ECF, depletion of chloride leads to increases in the apparent T_{max} and PT for HCO_3^- (167).

Aldosterone

An increase in distal sodium avidity resulting in increased renal HCO_3^- generation may occur in the absence of decreases in effective arterial blood volume if mineralocorticoids are administered or produced locally (168).

Potassium Depletion

Potassium depletion is another factor implicated in increasing the apparent T_{max} and PT for HCO_3^- and maintaining metabolic alkalosis. One explanation is that potassium depletion leads to a relative intracellular acidosis, and this relative intracellular acidosis makes renal H^+ excretion more favorable (169). Evidence against this concept includes the considerable concentration differences involved; that is, it is difficult to evoke the argument of preservation of electroneutrality by an ion that exists in nM concentrations. In addition, investigators have failed to detect a decrease in renal pHi with ^{31}P NMR spectroscopy during potassium depletion (170). Moreover, in human studies, metabolic alkalosis can be corrected almost completely without correction of potassium depletion (171).

Hypercapnia

Increases in Pa_{CO_2} are known to increase the apparent T_{max} and PT for HCO_3^-. This may be mediated through decreases in cellular pHi (which have been documented during acute and chronic hypercapnia). Interestingly, the increases in Pa_{CO_2} that occur during metabolic alkalosis as part of normal respiratory compensation actually tend to impair renal correction through this mechanism (172).

CLINICAL FEATURES

No symptoms or signs are specific for metabolic alkalosis. The disturbance should be suspected, however, in patients who have muscle cramps, weakness, arrhythmias, or seizures, especially if the appropriate clinical scenario (e.g., diuretic use, vomiting) is present. Some of these signs and symptoms may be related to alterations in ionized calcium because increases in pH cause plasma proteins to bind calcium more avidly, thus lowering ionized calcium concentrations. Severe alkalemia (pH >7.6) may be associated with malignant arrhythmias as well as seizures (163).

LABORATORY FINDINGS IN METABOLIC ALKALOSIS

Arterial blood gases reveal the diagnostic pattern, that is, an increased pH, increased $[HCO_3^-]$, and an increased Pa_{CO_2}, with the increase in Pa_{CO_2} being between 0.25 and 1 × the increase in $[HCO_3^-]$. The serum electrolytes demonstrate increased TCO_2 as well as decreased chloride and, usually, diminished potassium concentrations. The hypokalemia results from both shifting of potassium into cells and increased renal losses. Potassium shifts into cells during both respiratory and metabolic alkalosis; however, the magnitude of such changes is difficult to predict. Renal losses are enhanced throughout the course of metabolic alkalosis. The SAG may be increased by up to 9 to 12 mEq/L with severe metabolic alkalosis. This is owing to some small increases in lactate concentrations (112), but mostly to the increased electronegativity of albumin with elevated pH (173).

Urine chemistries represent an important step in the classification of metabolic alkalosis. Specifically, urine electrolytes are used to determine whether decreases in effective arterial blood volume act as a maintenance factor in the pathogenesis of metabolic alkalosis. Although the urine sodium concentration may be inconsistent in this condition especially if bicarbonaturia is present at the time the urine sample is collected, the urine chloride concentration allows one to classify patients into chloride-responsive and chloride-unresponsive categories of metabolic alkalosis. Chloride-responsive metabolic alkalosis corrects when volume expansion or improvement of hemodynamics occurs. Examples include patients who are vomiting or have received diuretics, but have discontinued them. Chloride-unresponsive metabolic alkalosis does not correct with these maneuvers. Examples are patients with primary mineralocorticoid excess or patients who are continuing to take diuretics. In patients with chloride-responsive metabolic alkalosis, the urine chloride concentration is <10 mmol/L, whereas patients with chloride-unresponsive metabolic alkalosis have a urine chloride concentration >20 mmol/L.

DIFFERENTIAL DIAGNOSIS OF METABOLIC ALKALOSIS

The differential diagnosis of metabolic alkalosis generally is approached by separating patients into those who have chloride depletion as a maintenance factor (chloride-responsive), those who do not have chloride depletion as a maintenance factor (chloride-unresponsive), and those who have an unclassified (generally uncommon) form of metabolic alkalosis. As discussed, this generally is accomplished using the urine chloride concentration (Table 3.7).

Chloride-responsive Metabolic Alkalosis

Vomiting

Gastric secretory volume may exceed 1 to 2 L/day in patients with persistent vomiting. The gastric secretions may contain as much as 100 mmol/L of H^+, and because the gastric parietal cells generate an

TABLE 3.7 DIFFERENTIAL DIAGNOSIS OF METABOLIC ALKALOSIS

Chloride-responsive Metabolic Alkalosis
Vomiting
Gastric drainage
Villous adenoma
Chloride diarrhea
Diuretics
Posthypercapnia
Cystic fibrosis
Chloride-resistant Metabolic Alkalosis
Hyperaldosteronism
Cushing syndrome
Bartter syndrome
Licorice
Profound potassium depletion?
Unclassified Metabolic Alkalosis
Alkali administration
Milk–alkali syndrome
Transfusion of blood products
Hypercalcemia
Poststarvation
Large doses of penicillin antibiotics

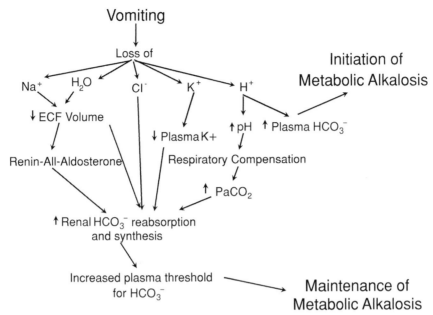

■ **Figure 3.5** Initiation and maintenance factors in the pathogenesis of metabolic alkalosis developing from vomiting are illustrated. Initial loss of H^+ from the stomach is the initiation factor where the concomitant loss of K^+, Na^+, Cl^-, and H_2O along with respiratory compensation set up the maintenance of the alkalosis by increasing renal HCO_3^- reabsorption and synthesis and the plasma threshold for HCO_3^-.

HCO_3^- molecule for each H^+ secreted, as much as 200 mmol of HCO_3^- may be generated in 1 day. Although this represents a significant initiation factor, it must be stressed that the concomitant Na^+ and Cl^- losses (as much as 400 mmol/day), possibly along with the associated K^+ losses (more in the urine than in vomit, which generally has <15 mmol/L potassium), are the maintenance factors that allow metabolic alkalosis to be maintained (174). This is shown schematically in Figure 3.5.

The degree of metabolic alkalosis associated with vomiting generally is mild; however, in conditions where gastric secretions are greatly stimulated, such as Zollinger–Ellison syndrome with gastric outlet obstruction, plasma $[HCO_3^-]$ may exceed 60 mmol/L (69).

Gastric Drainage

The pathophysiology of gastric drainage, usually through a nasogastric tube, is identical to that of vomiting (174).

Villous Adenoma of the Colon

Villous adenoma of the colon may result in profound diarrhea, which is extremely rich in protein, sodium, potassium, and chloride. The losses of sodium, potassium, and chloride and the relatively low $[HCO_3^-]$ concentration in the diarrheal fluid in some patients may lead to metabolic alkalosis (175). However, it must be stressed that this condition more commonly leads to sufficient HCO_3^- losses to produce metabolic acidosis, as discussed earlier (69).

Chloride Diarrhea

Chloride diarrhea is a rare congenital syndrome arising from a defect in small and large bowel chloride absorption that leads to a chronic diarrhea with a stool fluid rich in chloride. Metabolic alkalosis develops through the mechanisms described in the preceding for villous adenoma (69).

Diuretic Therapy

Diuretics that exert their effects either in the thick ascending limb of Henle (loop diuretics such as furosemide, bumetanide, torsemide) or in the distal tubule (thiazide diuretics) may facilitate volume depletion as well as directly stimulate renin secretion (possibly through increases in distal tubular fluid sodium content). Thus, they both initiate metabolic alkalosis through H^+ losses and maintain metabolic alkalosis via volume depletion and ongoing H^+ losses by the kidney (if diuretics are continued). If the urine chloride is obtained while diuretic effects persist, it may be high, whereas if the urine chloride is determined after sufficient time has elapsed to eliminate diuretic effects (generally >24 to 48 hours), it should be low, reflecting volume depletion. Metabolic alkalosis along with hypokalemia is an extremely frequent complication of diuretic use and should suggest the possibility of diuretic use especially in adolescents and adults, even if such drugs are not prescribed. Diuretic abuse is seen commonly in patients suffering from anorexia nervosa (176).

Posthypercapnia

As discussed in Chapter 4, the renal compensation to chronic hypercapnia results in an elevation in plasma $[HCO_3^-]$. When hypercapnia is rapidly corrected (e.g., with intubation and mechanical ventilation), the patient is left with an elevated plasma $[HCO_3^-]$ until renal correction occurs, a process that generally takes at least several hours. This metabolic alkalosis may persist if sufficient chloride is not provided to allow for renal correction (177). Possibly a mild metabolic alkalosis may be seen during waking hours in patients with sleep apnea.

Cystic Fibrosis

Children with cystic fibrosis have been reported in whom metabolic alkalosis developed because of marked loss of chloride in the sweat, which had relatively little HCO_3^-. The resultant volume depletion maintained the metabolic alkalosis in these patients (178).

Chloride-resistant Metabolic Alkalosis

Primary Hyperaldosteronism

Aldosterone directly stimulates distal nephron H^+ secretion by several mechanisms, some of which are tied to sodium reabsorption and potassium secretion, whereas others appear to be independent of sodium or potassium transport. This increased H^+ secretion leads to either reclamation of filtered HCO_3^- destined for excretion or the generation of new HCO_3^- that is ultimately retained in the ECF. Although the increase in ECF $[HCO_3^-]$ produced by such distal effects results in ECF volume expansion and decreases in proximal tubule reabsorptive capacity for HCO_3^-, distal processes are sufficient to maintain an elevated PT for HCO_3^-. Hence, the clinical features of hypokalemic metabolic alkalosis are produced, often in concert with hypertension associated with ECF volume expansion.

Such primary increase in mineralocorticoids may be caused by an adrenal tumor, which selectively makes aldosterone (Conn syndrome) or by hyperplasia (usually bilateral) of the adrenal cortex. The diagnosis of such a primary mineralocorticoid excess state is dependent on the demonstration that volume expansion is present (e.g., nonstimulatable plasma renin activity) and that aldosterone secretion is not suppressible by volume expansion (i.e., demonstration that exogenous mineralocorticoids and high-salt diet or acute volume expansion with saline do not suppress plasma aldosterone levels) (179). In some cases, hyperaldosteronism can be suppressed by the pharmacologic administration of glucocorticoids. Recent studies have demonstrated that this glucocorticoid remediable aldosteronism (GRA) is caused by a gene duplication fusing regulatory sequences of the steroid 11β-hydroxylase gene to the coding sequences of the aldosterone synthase gene (180).

Cushing Syndrome

Adrenocorticotropic hormone (ACTH)-secreting tumors, primary adrenal cortical tumors, or hyperplasia owing to congenital enzyme deficiencies may increase corticosteroid synthesis. Many corticosteroids (specifically cortisol, deoxycorticosterone, and corticosterone) also may have considerable mineralocorticoid effects and produce hypokalemic metabolic alkalosis, sometimes accompanied by hypertension. Detailed metabolic analysis of the plasma and urine as well as imaging studies may be necessary to arrive at the precise diagnosis (168).

Bartter and Gitelman Syndromes

Bartter syndrome is a rare condition usually presenting in children characterized by hyperreninemia, hyperaldosteronemia in the absence of hypertension, or sodium retention. Histologically, hyperplasia of the juxtaglomerular apparatus is noted, a finding not specific for this diagnosis (181,182). Functionally, the disorder is believed to be caused by a failure of chloride reabsorption in the thick ascending limb of Henle, a disturbance that results in a very high delivery of chloride and sodium to the distal nephron, activation of the renin–angiotensin–aldosterone system, and production of hypokalemic metabolic alkalosis. Although the PGE system has been suggested to participate in this disturbance, and sometimes PGE synthesis inhibitors may be beneficial, the increase in renal PGEs in this disorder is secondary. Elegant genetic studies have demonstrated that the molecular basis of Bartter syndrome can be attributed to one of three abnormalities. Specifically, inherited inactivity of the NaKCl$_2$ transporter, ROMK (renal outermedullary potassium) channel, and a chloride channel, transport proteins that are essential to the function of the medullary thick ascending limb of Henle, each can result in Bartter syndrome (183–185). These findings suggest that each of these three components is essential for effective thick ascending limb function. A schematic of how these transporters interact is shown in Figure 3.6. A closely related condition, Gitelman syndrome, now is known to be caused by mutations in the thiazide-sensitive NaCl transporter important in distal tubule function (186). Gitelman syndrome may present in adults and is probably more common than Bartter syndrome.

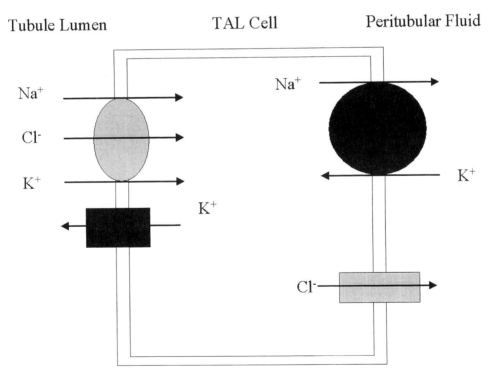

■ **Figure 3.6** Schematic depicting medullary thick ascending limb reabsorption of NaCl from the tubular lumen. Entry of Na$^+$, K$^+$, and Cl$^-$ occurs through the NaKCl$_2$ transporter *(light-colored ellipse)* with 2 Cl$^-$ molecules transported for each Na$^+$ and K$^+$. To allow for a continued supply of K$^+$ in the luminal fluid, K$^+$ must leak out through the ROMK channel *(dark solid rectangle)*. Once Na$^+$ and Cl$^-$ are in the cell, the Cl$^-$ must leave through the basolateral side via a chloride channel *(light gray rectangle)*, whereas the Na$^+$ is pumped out by the Na$^+$/K$^+$ ATPase *(solid dark circle)*.

Because both Bartter and Gitelman syndromes mimic diuretic use so closely on a physiologic basis, it may be difficult to separate them from surreptitious diuretic use unless diuretics are specifically screened for in the urine. The genetic syndromes are uncommon and surreptitious diuretic use is much more common and must be considered foremost in adolescents or adults who present with unexplained hypokalemic metabolic alkalosis (176).

Licorice

A major component of "black" licorice, glycyrrhizic acid, may cause a hypokalemic metabolic alkalosis accompanied by hypertension and thus mimic primary hyperaldosteronism. Recent study demonstrates that glycyrrhizic acid actually inhibits $11\beta\beta$-hydroxysteroid dehydrogenase activity and "uncovers" the mineralocorticoid receptor to be stimulated by glucocorticoids that normally circulate in relatively higher concentrations. Some chewing tobacco also contains this substance and can cause a similar presentation (187).

Profound Potassium Depletion

Several patients with profound hypokalemia (plasma $[K^+]$ <2 mmol/L) have had significant metabolic alkalosis associated with a urine chloride concentration >20 mmol/L without evidence of mineralocorticoid excess. The alkalosis was not corrected during sodium repletion until the potassium deficit also was corrected (169). This suggests that in some cases potassium depletion may convert a chloride-responsive metabolic alkalosis to a chloride-unresponsive metabolic alkalosis. However, correction of metabolic alkalosis without repletion of potassium deficits clearly has been demonstrated in humans (171). Therefore, although potassium supplementation is advisable to correct the potassium deficit and hypokalemia that may contribute to the maintenance of metabolic alkalosis and are problems in their own right, such supplementation does not appear necessary to correct metabolic alkalosis.

Unclassified Metabolic Alkalosis

Alkali Administration

The kidney rapidly excretes alkali, and metabolic alkalosis can be maintained only if a maintenance factor supervenes or the administration of alkali continues. However, in some situations, alkali administration may cause metabolic alkalosis. This alkali load may be in the form of HCO_3^- or organic anions that are metabolized to HCO_3^-, such as citrate or acetate. Specifically, administration of an alkali load may cause sustained metabolic alkalosis in patients with chronic renal failure, where the ability to excrete an HCO_3^- load is impaired because GFR is reduced (188).

Milk–Alkali Syndrome

Milk–alkali syndrome is seen in patients with dyspepsia who consume moderate to large amounts of antacids containing calcium and absorbable alkali (e.g., calcium carbonate). Lack of ECF volume expansion along with hypercalcemia-mediated suppression of PTH secretion contributes to the maintenance of metabolic alkalosis. Hypercalcemia also decreases renal blood flow and glomerular filtration, which can further impair renal correction of metabolic alkalosis. Alkalosis reduces calcium excretion and tends to potentiate associated hypercalcemia. Chronically, nephrocalcinosis may occur, which may ultimately decrease GFR, thus further reducing ability to excrete an alkali load (189).

Transfusion of Blood Products

Infusion of large amounts (>10 units) of blood products containing the anticoagulant citrate can produce moderate metabolic alkalosis. The production of HCO_3^- from citrate is totally responsible for the initiation of metabolic alkalosis. In other situations, some degree of prerenal azotemia (e.g., when packed red blood cells are given to a patient with hemorrhagic shock) may contribute to the maintenance of the metabolic alkalosis. Patients given parenteral hyperalimentation with excessive amounts of acetate or lactate also may develop metabolic alkalosis through an identical mechanism (188).

Hypercalcemia (Nonhyperparathyroid Etiology)

Mild metabolic alkalosis has been associated with hypercalcemia that results from causes other than hyperparathyroidism (e.g., malignancy, sarcoid). This may be caused by a suppression of PTH that then raises the PT for HCO_3^- (190).

Poststarvation (Refeeding Alkalosis)

Patients who break prolonged fasts with meals containing carbohydrates may develop a metabolic alkalosis that can persist for several weeks. The mechanism for the initiation of the metabolic alkalosis is unknown. Increases in renal sodium avidity (resulting from the ECF volume depletion occurring during starvation) appear to be the maintenance factor (128).

Large Doses of Penicillin Antibiotics

Intravenous administration of large doses of some penicillin antibiotics, specifically penicillin and carbenicillin, may result in hypokalemic metabolic alkalosis. The mechanism is believed to be the increase in delivery of poorly reabsorbable anions to the distal nephron with a resultant increase in H^+ and potassium secretion (191).

TREATMENT OF METABOLIC ALKALOSIS

The guiding principle for treating all acid–base disturbances is to address the underlying disease state. However, in some cases, the degree of acid–base abnormality itself becomes life threatening, especially in mixed acid–base disturbances where the respiratory and metabolic components go in the same direction (e.g., respiratory alkalosis + metabolic alkalosis). When an elevated systemic pH becomes life threatening (e.g., pH >7.6 with seizures and ventricular arrhythmias), rapid reduction in systemic pH may be accomplished by control of ventilation. In such situations, airway intubation with sedation and controlled hypoventilation with a mechanical ventilator (sometimes using inspired CO_2 and/or supplemental oxygen to prevent hypoxia) may be lifesaving (192).

Although historically administration of either HCl or its congeners (e.g., arginine chloride or ammonium chloride) had been advocated to correct metabolic alkalosis, we do not advocate this approach alone. Our rationale is that these agents all may have significant potential complications (e.g., hemolysis and tissue necrosis with HCl, ammonia toxicity with ammonium chloride). However, of greater importance, they simply do not work fast enough to prevent or treat life-threatening complications. Therefore, we advocate the control of the $PaCO_2$ as outlined in the preceding for urgent intervention. Once the situation is no longer critical, partial or complete correction of the metabolic alkalosis over 6 to 8 hours with HCl administered as a 0.15-mol/L solution through a central vein may be used. Generally, the "acid deficit" is calculated assuming a bicarbonate distribution space of $0.5 \times$ the body weight in liters, and about one half of this amount of HCl is given with frequent monitoring of blood gases and electrolytes. Hemodialysis well may be faster and safer.

In less urgent settings, therapy of the metabolic alkalosis may be addressed after examining whether it is chloride responsive or not. Chloride-responsive metabolic alkalosis responds quite well to volume repletion and improvement of renal hemodynamics. If hypokalemia is present, it should be corrected as well. Treatment of the chloride-unresponsive metabolic alkalosis conditions generally mandates interference with the mineralocorticoid (or mineralocorticoid-like substance) that is maintaining renal H^+ losses. Sometimes this can be accomplished pharmacologically with spironolactone or other distal K-sparing diuretics, such as amiloride.

In some cases, the proximate cause of the metabolic alkalosis is necessary for the overall well-being of the patient. One example that comes to mind is a patient with severe heart failure who develops hypokalemic metabolic alkalosis as a result of loop diuretics whose continued use is mandated by the patient's congestive symptoms. In such cases, the proximal diuretic acetazolamide, which decreases the PT for HCO_3^- by inhibiting proximal tubule HCO_3^- reabsorption, may be very effective (97). In subjects who are undergoing persistent gastric drainage, administration of either an H_2 blocker or H^+ ATPase inhibitor to decrease gastric H^+ secretion may be advantageous (193). In patients with advanced chronic renal failure in whom metabolic alkalosis has been induced (e.g., with antacid excess), hemodialysis may be necessary for correction.

REFERENCES

1. Filley G. *Acid–Base and Blood Gas Regulation.* Philadelphia: Lea and Febiger; 1971.
2. Stewart P, ed. *How to Understand Acid–Base. A Quantitative Acid–Base Primer for Biology and Medicine.* New York: Elsevier; 1981.
3. Alpern R, Warnock D, Rector F. Renal acidification mechanisms. In: Brenner B, Rector F, eds. *The Kidney.* Philadelphia: WB Saunders; 1986: 206–250.
4. Nelson D, Cox M, eds. *Lehninger Principles of Biochemistry.* 5th ed. New York: W.H. Freeman and Company/Worth Publishers; 2009.
5. Srivastava J, Barber DL, Jacobson MP. Intracellular pH sensors: design principles and functional significance. *Physiology (Bethesda).* 2007;22:30–39.
6. Malhotra D, Shapiro J. Nuclear magnetic resonance measurements of intracellular pH: biomedical implications. *Concepts Magn Reson.* 1993;5:123–150.
7. Koo MK, Oh CH, Holme AL, et al. Simultaneous analysis of steady-state intracellular pH and cell morphology by automated laser scanning cytometry. *Cytometry A.* 2007;71(2):87–93.
8. Hille C, Berg M, Bressel L, et al. Time-domain fluorescence lifetime imaging for intracellular pH sensing in living tissues. *Anal Bioanal Chem.* 2008;391(5):1871–1879.
9. Berg J, Tymoczko J, Stryer L, eds. *Biochemistry.* 6th ed. New York: W.H. Freeman; 2002.
10. Adrogue HE, Adrogue HJ. Acid–base physiology. *Respir Care.* 2001;46(4):328–341.
11. Venkatasen J, Hamilton R, Shapiro J. Dialysis considerations in the patient with chronic renal failure. In: Henrich W, ed. *Hemodialysis: Principles and Practice.* New York: Mosby; 1998.
12. Crapo RO, Jensen RL, Hegewald M, et al. Arterial blood gas reference values for sea level and an altitude of 1,400 meters. *Am J Respir Crit Care Med.* 1999;160(5 pt 1):1525–1531.
13. Vasuvattakul S, Warner LC, Halperin ML. Quantitative role of the intracellular bicarbonate buffer system in response to an acute acid load. *Am J Physiol.* 1992;262(2 pt 2):R305–R309.
14. Watts BA 3rd, George T, Good DW. The basolateral NHE1 Na$^+$/H$^+$ exchanger regulates transepithelial HCO$_3^-$ absorption through actin cytoskeleton remodeling in renal thick ascending limb. *J Biol Chem.* 2005;280(12):11439–11447.
15. Zhang J, Bobulescu IA, Goyal S, et al. Characterization of Na$^+$/H$^+$ exchanger NHE8 in cultured renal epithelial cells. *Am J Physiol Renal Physiol.* 2007;293(3):F761–F766.
16. Vachon V, Delisle MC, Giroux S, et al. Factors affecting the stability of the renal sodium/phosphate symporter during its solubilization and reconstitution. *Int J Biochem Cell Biol.* 1995;27(3):311–318.
17. Paillard M. Na$^+$/H$^+$ exchanger subtypes in the renal tubule: function and regulation in physiology and disease. *Exp Nephrol.* 1997;5(4):277–284.
18. Biemesderfer D, Pizzonia J, Abu-Alfa A, et al. NHE3: a Na$^+$/H$^+$ exchanger isoform of renal brush border. *Am J Physiol.* 1993;265(5 pt 2):F736–F742.
19. Loffing J, Lötscher M, Kaissling B, et al. Renal Na/H exchanger NHE-3 and Na-PO4 cotransporter NaPi-2 protein expression in glucocorticoid excess and deficient states. *J Am Soc Nephrol.* 1998;9(9):1560–1567.
20. Xiao YT, Xiang LX, Shao JZ. Vacuolar H(+)-ATPase. *Int J Biochem Cell Biol.* 2008;40(10):2002–2006.
21. Cougnon M, Bouyer P, Planelles G, et al. Does the colonic H,K-ATPase also act as an Na,K-ATPase? *Proc Natl Acad Sci U S A.* 1998;95(11): 6516–6520.
22. Suzuki Y, Watanabe T, Kaneko K. A novel H+,K(+)-ATPase in the colonic apical membrane? *Jpn J Physiol.* 1993;43(3):291–298.
23. Simpson AM, Schwartz GJ. Distal renal tubular acidosis with severe hypokalaemia, probably caused by colonic H(+)-K(+)-ATPase deficiency. *Arch Dis Child.* 2001;84(6):504–507.
24. Wall SM, Truong AV, DuBose TD Jr. H(+)-K(+)-ATPase mediates net acid secretion in rat terminal inner medullary collecting duct. *Am J Physiol.* 1996;271(5 pt 2):F1037–F1044.
25. Olsnes S, Ludt J, Tønnessen TI, et al. Bicarbonate/chloride antiport in Vero cells: II. Mechanisms for bicarbonate-dependent regulation of intracellular pH. *J Cell Physiol.* 1987;132(2):192–202.
26. Geibel JP. Distal tubule acidification. *J Nephrol.* 2006;19(suppl 9):S18–S26.
27. Halperin ML. How much "new" bicarbonate is formed in the distal nephron in the process of net acid excretion? *Kidney Int.* 1989;35(6):1277–12781.
28. Kamel KS, Briceno LF, Sanchez MI, et al. A new classification for renal defects in net acid excretion. *Am J Kidney Dis.* 1997;29(1):136–146.
29. Weiner ID, Hamm LL. Molecular mechanisms of renal ammonia transport. *Annu Rev Physiol.* 2007;69:317–340.
30. DuBose TD Jr, Good DW, Hamm LL, et al. Ammonium transport in the kidney: new physiological concepts and their clinical implications. *J Am Soc Nephrol.* 1991;1:1193–1203.
31. Batlle DC, Hizon M, Cohen E, et al. The use of the urinary anion gap in the diagnosis of hyperchloremic metabolic acidosis. *N Engl J Med.* 1988;318(10):594–599.
32. Haussinger D. Liver regulation of acid–base balance. *Miner Electrolyte Metab.* 1997;23(3–6):249–252.
33. Lardner AL, O'Donovan DJ. Alterations in renal and hepatic nitrogen metabolism in rats during HCl ingestion. *Metabolism.* 1998;47(2):163–167.

34. Watford M, Chellaraj V, Ismat A, et al. Hepatic glutamine metabolism. *Nutrition.* 2002;18(4):301–303.

35. Parsa MH, Habif DV, Ferrer JM, et al. Intravenous hyperalimentation: indications, technique, and complications. *Bull N Y Acad Med.* 1972;48(7):920–942.

36. Oh MS, Carroll HJ. The anion gap. *N Engl J Med.* 1977;297(15):814–817.

37. Schwartz WB, Orning KJ, Porter R. The internal distribution of hydrogen ions with varying degrees of metabolic acidosis. *J Clin Invest.* 1957;36(3):373–382.

38. Lemann J Jr, Litzow JR, Lennon EJ. The effects of chronic acid loads in normal man: further evidence for the participation of bone mineral in the defense against chronic metabolic acidosis. *J Clin Invest.* 1966;45:1608–1617.

39. Burnell J. Changes in bone sodium and carbonate in metabolic acidosis and alkalosis. *J Clin Invest.* 1971;50:327–335.

40. Cunningham J, Fraher LJ, Clemens TL, et al. Chronic acidosis with metabolic bone disease. Effect of alkali on bone morphology and vitamin D metabolism. *Am J Med.* 1982;73(2):199–204.

41. Elkinton JR. Clinical disorders of acid–base regulation. A survey of seventeen years' diagnostic experience. *Med Clin North Am.* 1966;50(5):1325–1350.

42. Fencl V, Miller TB, Pappenheimer JR. Studies on the respiratory response to disturbances of acid–base balance, with deductions concerning the ionic composition of cerebral interstitial fluid. *Am J Physiol.* 1966;210(3):459–472.

43. Wiederseiner J-M, Muser J, Lutz T, et al. Acute metabolic acidosis: characterization and diagnosis of the disorder and the plasma potassium response. *J Am Soc Nephrol.* 2004;15:1589–1596.

44. Curthoys NP, Gstraunthaler G. Mechanism of increased renal gene expression during metabolic acidosis. *Am J Physiol Renal Physiol.* 2001;281(3):F381–F390.

45. Laghmani K, Preisig PA, Moe OW, et al. Endothelin-1/endothelin-B receptor-mediated increases in NHE3 activity in chronic metabolic acidosis. *J Clin Invest.* 2001;107(12):1563–1569.

46. Madias NE, Schwartz WB, Cohen JJ. The maladaptive renal response to secondary hypocapnia during chronic HCl acidosis in the dog. *J Clin Invest.* 1977;60(6):1393–1401.

47. Shapiro JI, Whalen M, Chan L. Hemodynamic and hepatic pH responses to sodium bicarbonate and Carbicarb during systemic acidosis. *Magn Reson Med.* 1990;16(3):403–410.

48. O'Brodovich HM, Stalcup SA, Pang LM, et al. Hemodynamic and vasoactive mediator response to experimental respiratory failure. *J Appl Physiol.* 1982;52(5):1230–1236.

49. Nimmo AJ, Than N, Orchard CH, et al. The effect of acidosis on beta-adrenergic receptors in ferret cardiac muscle. *Exp Physiol.* 1993;78(1):95–103.

50. Davies AO. Rapid desensitization and uncoupling of human beta-adrenergic receptors in an in vitro model of lactic acidosis. *J Clin Endocrinol Metab.* 1984;59(3):398–405.

51. Orchard C. The effect of acidosis on excitation–contraction coupling in isolated ferret heart muscle. *Mol Cell Biochem.* 1989;89(2):169–173.

52. Allen DG, Orchard CH. The effects of changes of pH on intracellular calcium transients in mammalian cardiac muscle. *J Physiol.* 1983;335:555–567.

53. Endoh M. Acidic pH-induced contractile dysfunction via downstream mechanism: identification of pH-sensitive domain in troponin I. *J Mol Cell Cardiol.* 2001;33(7):1297–1300.

54. Nosek TM, Fender KY, Godt RE. It is diprotonated inorganic phosphate that depresses force in skinned skeletal muscle fibers. *Science.* 1987;236(4798):191–193.

55. Zhou HZ, Malhotra D, Shapiro JI. Contractile dysfunction during metabolic acidosis: role of impaired energy metabolism. *Am J Physiol.* 1991;261(5 pt 2):H1481–H1486.

56. Suleymanlar G, Zhou HZ, McCormack M, et al. Mechanism of impaired energy metabolism during acidosis: role of oxidative metabolism. *Am J Physiol.* 1992;262(6 pt 2):H1818–H1822.

57. Zhou HZ, Malhotra D, Doers J, et al. Hypoxia and metabolic acidosis in the isolated heart: evidence for synergistic injury. *Magn Reson Med.* 1993;29(1):94–98.

58. McGillivray-Anderson KM, Faber JE. Effect of acidosis on contraction of microvascular smooth muscle by alpha 1- and alpha 2-adrenoceptors. Implications for neural and metabolic regulation. *Circ Res.* 1990;66(6):1643–1657.

59. Verdon F. Respiratory response to acute metabolic acidosis in man. *Intensive Care Med.* 1979;5(4):204.

60. Janusek LW. Metabolic acidosis: pathophysiology, signs, and symptoms. *Nursing.* 1990;20(7):52–53.

61. Bushinsky DA, Parker WR, Alexander KM, et al. Metabolic, but not respiratory, acidosis increases bone PGE(2) levels and calcium release. *Am J Physiol Renal Physiol.* 2001;281(6):F1058–F1066.

62. Adrogue HJ, Madias NE. Changes in plasma potassium concentration during acute acid–base disturbances. *Am J Med.* 1981;71(3):456–467.

63. Emmett M, Narins RG. Clinical use of the anion gap. *Medicine (Baltimore).* 1977;56(1):38–54.

64. Gabow PA, Kaehny WD, Fennessey PV, et al. Diagnostic importance of an increased serum anion gap. *N Engl J Med.* 1980;303(15):854–858.

65. Streather CP, Phillips AO, Goodman FR, et al. How often should we measure the urinary anion gap for cases of suspected renal tubular acidosis? *Nephrol Dial Transplant.* 1993;8(6):571.

66. Wang F, Butler T, Rabbani GH, et al. The acidosis of cholera. Contributions of hyperproteinemia, lactic acidemia, and hyperphosphatemia to an increased serum anion gap. *N Engl J Med.* 1986;315(25):1591–1595.

67. Gennari FJ, Weise WJ. Acid–base disturbances in gastrointestinal disease. *Clin J Am Soc Nephrol.* 2008;3:1861–1868.

68. Margolis A, Dziatkowiak H, Bugala I, et al. Urine acidification ability in infants. II. Urinary excretion of hydrogen ions in infants with diarrhea and chronic metabolic acidosis. *Pediatr Pol.* 1972;47(8):979–983.

69. Phillips SF. Water and electrolytes in gastrointestinal disease. In: Maxwell MH,

Kleeman CR, eds. *Clinical Disorders of Fluid and Electrolyte Metabolism.* New York: McGraw-Hill; 1980:1267–1295.

70. Nathan DM, Fogel H, Norman D, et al. Long-term metabolic and quality of life results with pancreatic/renal transplantation in insulin-dependent diabetes mellitus. *Transplantation.* 1991;52(1):85–91.

71. Ketel B, Henry ML, Elkhammas EA, et al. Metabolic complications in combined kidney/pancreas transplantation. *Transplant Proc.* 1992;24(3):774–775.

72. Tom WW, Munda R, First MR, et al. Physiologic consequences of pancreatic allograft exocrine drainage into the urinary tract. *Transplant Proc.* 1987;19(1 pt 3):2339–2342.

73. Monroy-Cuadros M, Salazar A, Yilmaz S, et al. Bladder vs enteric drainage in simultaneous pancreas–kidney transplantation. *Nephrol Dial Transplant.* 2006;21(2):483–487.

74. Mills RD, Studer UE. Metabolic consequences of continent urinary diversion. *J Urol.* 1999;161(5):1057–1066.

75. Hautmann RE, de Petriconi R, Gottfried HW, et al. The ileal neobladder: complications and functional results in 363 patients after 11 years of followup. *J Urol.* 1999;161(2):422–427; discussion 427–428.

76. Thompson WG. Cholestyramine. *Can Med Assoc J.* 1971;104(4):305–309.

77. Scheel PJ Jr, Whelton A, Rossiter K, et al. Cholestyramine-induced hyperchloremic metabolic acidosis. *J Clin Pharmacol.* 1992;32(6):536–538.

78. Haldane JB, Hill R, Luck JM. Calcium chloride acidosis. *J Physiol.* 1923;57(5):301–306.

79. Lash JP, Arruda JA. Laboratory evaluation of renal tubular acidosis. *Clin Lab Med.* 1993;13(1):117–129.

80. Batlle D, Moorthi KM, Schlueter W, et al. Distal renal tubular acidosis and the potassium enigma. *Semin Nephrol.* 2006;26(6):471–478.

81. Karet FE. Mechanisms in hyperkalemic renal tubular acidosis. *J Am Soc Nephrol.* 2009;20(2):251–254.

82. Quigley R. Proximal renal tubular acidosis. *J Nephrol.* 2006;19(suppl 9):S41–S45.

83. Igarashi T, Sekine T, Inatomi J, et al. Unraveling the molecular pathogenesis of isolated proximal renal tubular acidosis. *J Am Soc Nephrol.* 2002;13(8):2171–2177.

84. Izzedine H, Launay-Vacher V, Isnard-Bagnis C, et al. Drug-induced Fanconi's syndrome. *Am J Kidney Dis.* 2003;41(2):292–309.

85. Clarke BL, Wynne AG, Wilson DM, et al. Osteomalacia associated with adult Fanconi's syndrome: clinical and diagnostic features. *Clin Endocrinol (Oxf).* 1995;43(4):479–490.

86. McSherry E. Renal tubular acidosis in childhood. *Kidney Int.* 1981;20(6):799–809.

87. Vasuvattakul S, Nimmannit S, Shayakul C, et al. Should the urine P_{CO_2} or the rate of excretion of ammonium be the gold standard to diagnose distal renal tubular acidosis? *Am J Kidney Dis.* 1992;19(1):72–75.

88. Richardson RM, Halperin ML. The urine pH: a potentially misleading diagnostic test in patients with hyperchloremic metabolic acidosis. *Am J Kidney Dis.* 1987;10(2):140–143.

89. Jefferies KC, Cipriano DJ, Forgac M. Function, structure and regulation of the vacuolar (H+)-ATPases. *Arch Biochem Biophys.* 2008;476(1):33–42.

90. Fuster DG, Zhang J, Xie XS, et al. The vacuolar-ATPase B1 subunit in distal tubular acidosis: novel mutations and mechanisms for dysfunction. *Kidney Int.* 2008;73(10):1151–1158.

91. Walsh SB, Shirley DG, Wrong OM, et al. Urinary acidification assessed by simultaneous furosemide and fludrocortisone treatment: an alternative to ammonium chloride. *Kidney Int.* 2007;71(12):1310–1316.

92. Ren H, Wang WM, Chen XN, et al. Renal involvement and followup of 130 patients with primary Sjogren's syndrome. *J Rheumatol.* 2008;35(2):278–284.

93. D'Cruz S, Chauhan S, Singh R, et al. Wasp sting associated with type 1 renal tubular acidosis. *Nephrol Dial Transplant.* 2008;23(5):1754–1755.

94. Kamijima M, Nakazawa Y, Yamakawa M, et al. Metabolic acidosis and renal tubular injury due to pure toluene inhalation. *Arch Environ Health.* 1994;49(5):410–413.

95. Batlle DC, Arruda JA, Kurtzman NA. Hyperkalemic distal renal tubular acidosis associated with obstructive uropathy. *N Engl J Med.* 1981;304(7):373–380.

96. Sharma AP, Sharma RK, Kapoor R, et al. Incomplete distal renal tubular acidosis affects growth in children. *Nephrol Dial Transplant.* 2007;22(10):2879–2885.

97. DuBose TD Jr. Carbonic anhydrase-dependent bicarbonate transport in the kidney. *Ann N Y Acad Sci.* 1984;429:528–537.

98. Groeper K, McCann ME. Topiramate and metabolic acidosis: a case series and review of the literature. *Paediatr Anaesth.* 2005;15(2):167–170.

99. Welch BJ, Graybeal D, Moe OW, et al. Biochemical and stone-risk profiles with topiramate treatment. *Am J Kidney Dis.* 2006;48(4):555–563.

100. Kurtzman NA, Gonzalez J, DeFronzo R, et al. A patient with hyperkalemia and metabolic acidosis. *Am J Kidney Dis.* 1990;15(4):333–356.

101. DeFronzo RA. Hyperkalemia and hyporeninemic hypoaldosteronism. *Kidney Int.* 1980;17(1):118–134.

102. Allen GG, Barratt LJ. An in vivo study of voltage-dependent renal tubular acidosis induced by amiloride. *Kidney Int.* 1989;35(5):1107–1110.

103. Garty H, Benos DJ. Characteristics and regulatory mechanisms of the amiloride-blockable Na^+ channel. *Physiol Rev.* 1988;68(2):309–373.

104. Effectiveness of spironolactone added to an angiotensin-converting enzyme inhibitor and a loop diuretic for severe chronic congestive heart failure (the Randomized Aldactone Evaluation Study [RALES]). *Am J Cardiol.* 1996;78(8):902–907.

105. Witham MD, Gillespie ND, Struthers AD. Hyperkalemia after the publication of RALES. *N Engl J Med.* 2004;351(23):2448–2450; author reply 2448–2450.

106. Adrogue HJ, Wilson H, Boyd AE 3rd, et al. Plasma acid–base patterns in diabetic ketoacidosis. *N Engl J Med.* 1982;307(26):1603–1610.

107. Gowrishankar M, Carlotti AP, St George-Hyslop C, et al. Uncovering the basis of a severe degree of acidemia in a patient with diabetic ketoacidosis. *QJM.* 2007;100(11):721–735.

108. Garella S, Chang BS, Kahn SI. Dilution acidosis and contraction alkalosis: review of a concept. *Kidney Int.* 1975;8(5):279–283.

109. Relman AS, Shelburne PF, Talman A. Profound acidosis resulting from excessive ammonium chloride in previously healthy subjects. A study of two cases. *N Engl J Med.* 1961;264:848–852.

110. Heird WC, Dell RB, Driscoll JM Jr, et al. Metabolic acidosis resulting from intravenous alimentation mixtures containing synthetic amino acids. *N Engl J Med.* 1972;287(19):943–948.

111. Lemann J Jr, Relman AS. The relation of sulfur metabolism to acid–base balance and electrolyte excretion: the effects of DL-methionine in normal man. *J Clin Invest.* 1959;38:2215–2223.

112. Madias NE. Lactic acidosis. *Kidney Int.* 1986;29(3):752–774.

113. Malhotra D, Shapiro JI, Chan L. Nuclear magnetic resonance spectroscopy in patients with anion-gap acidosis. *J Am Soc Nephrol.* 1991;2(5):1046–1050.

114. Oh MS, Phelps KR, Traube M, et al. D-Lactic acidosis in a man with the short-bowel syndrome. *N Engl J Med.* 1979;301(5):249–252.

115. Cooper DJ, Walley KR, Wiggs BR, et al. Bicarbonate does not improve hemodynamics in critically ill patients who have lactic acidosis. A prospective, controlled clinical study. *Ann Intern Med.* 1990;112(7):492–498.

116. Graf H, Leach W, Arieff AI. Evidence for a detrimental effect of bicarbonate therapy in hypoxic lactic acidosis. *Science.* 1985;227(4688):754–756.

117. Graf H, Leach W, Arieff AI. Metabolic effects of sodium bicarbonate in hypoxic lactic acidosis in dogs. *Am J Physiol.* 1985;249(5 pt 2):F630–F635.

118. Huntley JJ, McCormack M, Jin H, et al. Importance of tonicity of carbicarb on the functional and metabolic responses of the acidotic isolated heart. *J Crit Care.* 1993;8(4):222–227.

119. Adrogue HJ, Madias NE. Management of life-threatening acid–base disorders. First of two parts. *N Engl J Med.* 1998;338(1):26–34.

120. Westphal SA. The occurrence of diabetic ketoacidosis in non-insulin-dependent diabetes and newly diagnosed diabetic adults. *Am J Med.* 1996;101(1):19–24.

121. Filbin MR, Brown DF, Nadel ES. Hyperglycemic hyperosmolar nonketotic coma. *J Emerg Med.* 2001;20(3):285–290.

122. Oh MS, Carroll HJ, Goldstein DA, et al. Hyperchloremic acidosis during the recovery phase of diabetic ketosis. *Ann Intern Med.* 1978;89(6):925–927.

123. Gabow PA, Anderson RJ, Potts DE, et al. Acid–base disturbances in the salicylate-intoxicated adult. *Arch Intern Med.* 1978;138:1481–1484.

124. Lee P, Campbell LV. Diabetic ketoacidosis: the usual villain or a scapegoat? A novel cause of severe metabolic acidosis in type 1 diabetes. *Diabetes Care.* 2008;31(3):e13.

125. Soler NG, Bennett MA, Dixon K, et al. Potassium balance during treatment of diabetic ketoacidosis with special reference to the use of bicarbonate. *Lancet.* 1972;2(7779):665–667.

126. Kaye R. Diabetic ketoacidosis—the bicarbonate controversy. *J Pediatr.* 1975;87(1):156–159.

127. Sabatini S, Kurtzman NA. Bicarbonate therapy in severe metabolic acidosis. *J Am Soc Nephrol.* 2009;20(4):692–695.

128. Stinebaugh BJ, Schloeder FX. Glucose-induced alkalosis in fasting subjects. Relationship to renal bicarbonate reabsorption during fasting and refeeding. *J Clin Invest.* 1972;51(6):1326–1336.

129. Yanagawa Y, Sakamoto T, Okada Y. Six cases of sudden cardiac arrest in alcoholic ketoacidosis. *Intern Med.* 2008;47(2):113–117.

130. Godet C, Hira M, Adoun M, et al. Rapid diagnosis of alcoholic ketoacidosis by proton NMR. *Intensive Care Med.* 2001;27(4):785–786.

131. Halperin ML, Hammeke M, Josse RG, et al. Metabolic acidosis in the alcoholic: a pathophysiologic approach. *Metabolism.* 1983;32(3):308–315.

132. Arieff AI, Carroll HJ. Nonketotic hyperosmolar coma with hyperglycemia: clinical features, pathophysiology, renal function, acid–base balance, plasma–cerebrospinal fluid equilibria and the effects of therapy in 37 cases. *Medicine (Baltimore).* 1972;51(2):73–94.

133. Arieff AI, Carroll HJ. Hyperosmolar nonketotic coma with hyperglycemia: abnormalities of lipid and carbohydrate metabolism. *Metabolism.* 1971;20(6):529–538.

134. Halperin ML. Metabolism and acid–base physiology. *Artif Organs.* 1982;6(4):357–362.

135. Gabow PA. Ethylene glycol intoxication. *Am J Kidney Dis.* 1988;11(3):277–279.

136. Gabow PA, Clay K, Sullivan JB, et al. Organic acids in ethylene glycol intoxication. *Ann Intern Med.* 1986;105(1):16–20.

137. McMartin KE, Ambre JJ, Tephly TR. Methanol poisoning in human subjects. Role for formic acid accumulation in the metabolic acidosis. *Am J Med.* 1980;68(3):414–418.

138. Schelling JR, Howard RL, Winter SD, et al. Increased osmolal gap in alcoholic ketoacidosis and lactic acidosis. *Ann Intern Med.* 1990;113(8):580–582.

139. Sklar AH, Linas SL. The osmolal gap in renal failure. *Ann Intern Med.* 1983;98(4):481–482.

140. Streicher HZ, Gabow PA, Moss AH, et al. Syndromes of toluene sniffing in adults. *Ann Intern Med.* 1981;94(6):758–762.

141. Pomara C, Fiore C, D'Errico S, et al. Calcium oxalate crystals in acute ethylene glycol poisoning: a confocal laser scanning microscope study in a fatal case. *Clin Toxicol (Phila).* 2008;46(4):322–324.

142. Jacobsen D, Hewlett TP, Webb R, et al. Ethylene glycol intoxication: evaluation of kinetics and crystalluria. *Am J Med.* 1988;84(1):145–152.

143. Kraut JA, Kurtz I. Toxic alcohol ingestions: clinical features, diagnosis, and management. *Clin J Am Soc Nephrol.* 2008;3(1):208–225.

144. Hill JB. Salicylate intoxication. *N Engl J Med.* 1973;288(21):1110–1113.

145. Rivera W, Kleinschmidt KC, Velez LI, et al. Delayed salicylate toxicity at 35 hours without early manifestations following a single salicylate ingestion. *Ann Pharmacother.* 2004;38(7/8):1186–1188.

146. Gordon IJ, Bowler CS, Coakley J, et al. Algorithm for modified alkaline diuresis in salicylate poisoning. *Br Med J (Clin Res Ed).* 1984;289(6451):1039–1040.

147. Lund B, Seifert SA, Mayersohn M. Efficacy of sustained low-efficiency dialysis in the treatment of salicylate toxicity. *Nephrol Dial Transplant.* 2005;20(7):1483–1484.

148. Wong LP, Klemmer PJ. Severe lactic acidosis associated with juice of the mangosteen fruit *Garcinia mangostana. Am J Kidney Dis.* 2008;51(5): 829–833.

149. Fodale V, La Monaca E. Propofol infusion syndrome: an overview of a perplexing disease. *Drug Saf.* 2008;31(4):293–303.

150. Zar T, Yusufzai I, Sullivan A, et al. Acute kidney injury, hyperosmolality and metabolic acidosis associated with lorazepam. *Nat Clin Pract Nephrol.* 2007;3(9):515–520.

151. Pitt JJ, Hauser S. Transient 5-oxoprolinuria and high anion gap metabolic acidosis: clinical and biochemical findings in eleven subjects. *Clin Chem.* 1998;44:1497–1503.

152. Tailor P, Raman T, Garganta CL, et al. Recurrent high anion gap metabolic acidosis secondary to 5-oxoproline (pyroglutamic acid). *Am J Kidney Dis.* 2005;46:E4–E10.

153. Batlle DC, Sabatini S, Kurtzman NA. On the mechanism of toluene-induced renal tubular acidosis. *Nephron.* 1988;49(3):210–218.

154. DeMars CS, Hollister K, Tomassoni A, et al. Citric acid ingestion: a life-threatening cause of metabolic acidosis. *Ann Emerg Med.* 2001;38(5):588–591.

155. Widmer B, Gerhardt RE, Harrington JT, et al. Serum electrolyte and acid base composition. The influence of graded degrees of chronic renal failure. *Arch Intern Med.* 1979;139(10):1099–1102.

156. Halperin ML, Ethier JH, Kamel KS. Ammonium excretion in chronic metabolic acidosis: benefits and risks. *Am J Kidney Dis.* 1989;14(4):267–271.

157. Molitoris BA, Froment DH, Mackenzie TA, et al. Citrate: a major factor in the toxicity of orally administered aluminum compounds. *Kidney Int.* 1989;36(6):949–953.

158. Kette F, Weil MH, von Planta M, et al. Buffer agents do not reverse intramyocardial acidosis during cardiac resuscitation. *Circulation.* 1990;81(5):1660–1666.

159. Barenbrock M, Hausberg M, Matzkies F, et al. Effects of bicarbonate- and lactate-buffered replacement fluids on cardiovascular outcome in CVVH patients. *Kidney Int.* 2000;58(4):1751–1757.

160. Gudis SM, Mangi S, Feinroth M, et al. Rapid correction of severe lactic acidosis with massive isotonic bicarbonate infusion and simultaneous ultrafiltration. *Nephron.* 1983;33(1):65–66.

161. Giunti C, Priouzeau F, Allemand D, et al. Effect of tris-hydroxymethyl aminomethane on intracellular pH depends on the extracellular non-bicarbonate buffering capacity. *Transl Res.* 2007;150(6):350–356.

162. Stacpoole PW, Gilbert LR, Neiberger RE, et al. Evaluation of long-term treatment of children with congenital lactic acidosis with dichloroacetate. *Pediatrics.* 2008;121(5):e1223–e1228.

163. Galla JH. Metabolic alkalosis. *J Am Soc Nephrol.* 2000;11(2):369–375.

164. Adam WR, Craik DJ, Kneen M, et al. Effect of magnesium depletion and potassium depletion and chlorothiazide on intracellular pH in the rat, studied by 31P NMR. *Clin Exp Pharmacol Physiol.* 1989;16(1):33–40.

165. Palmer BF. Approach to fluid and electrolyte disorders and acid–base problems. *Prim Care.* 2008;35(2):195–213, v.

166. Shapiro JI, Anderson RJ. Sodium depletion states. In: Brenner BM, Stein J, eds. *Topics in Nephrology.* New York: Churchill Livingstone; 1985:155–192.

167. Kassirer JP, Berkman PM, Lawrenz DR, et al. The critical role of chloride in the correction of hypokalemic alkalosis in man. *Am J Med.* 1965;38:172–189.

168. Melby JC. Assessment of adrenocortical function. *N Engl J Med.* 1971;285(13):735–739.

169. Garella S, Chazan JA, Cohen JJ. Saline-resistant metabolic alkalosis or "chloride-wasting nephropathy". Report of four patients with severe potassium depletion. *Ann Intern Med.* 1970;73(1):31–38.

170. Adam WR, Koretsky AP, Weiner MW. Measurement of renal intracellular pH by ^{31}P NMR. Relationship of pH to ammoniagenesis. *Contrib Nephrol.* 1985;47:15–21.

171. Kassirer JP, Schwartz WB. Correction of metabolic alkalosis in man without repair of potassium deficiency. A re-evaluation of the role of potassium. *Am J Med.* 1966;40(1):19–26.

172. Lucci MS, Tinker JP, Weiner IM, et al. Function of proximal tubule carbonic anhydrase defined by selective inhibition. *Am J Physiol.* 1983;245(4):F443–F449.

173. Madias NE, Ayus JC, Adrogue HJ. Increased anion gap in metabolic alkalosis: the role of plasma-protein equivalency. *N Engl J Med.* 1979;300(25):1421–1423.

174. Kassirer JP, Schwartz WB. The response of normal man to selective depletion of hydrochloric acid. Factors in the genesis of persistent gastric alkalosis. *Am J Med.* 1966;40(1):10–18.

175. Jurgeleit HC. Villous adenoma of the colon with severe fluid and electrolyte depletion: report of a case. *Dis Colon Rectum.* 1976;19(5):445–447.

176. Jamison RL, Ross JC, Kempson RL, et al. Surreptitious diuretic ingestion and pseudo-Bartter's syndrome. *Am J Med.* 1982;73(1):142–147.

177. Brackett NC Jr, Wingo CF, Muren O, et al. Acid–base response to chronic hypercapnia in man. *N Engl J Med.* 1969;280(3):124–130.

178. Fustik S, Pop-Jordanova N, Slaveska N, et al. Metabolic alkalosis with hypoelectrolytemia in infants with cystic fibrosis. *Pediatr Int.* 2002;44(3):289–292.

179. Kassirer JP, London AM, Goldman DM, et al. On the pathogenesis of metabolic alkalosis in hyperaldosteronism. *Am J Med.* 1970;49(3):306–315.

180. Dluhy RG, Lifton RP. Glucocorticoid-remediable aldosteronism. *J Clin Endocrinol Metab.* 1999;84(12):4341–4344.

181. Bartter FC, Pronove P, Gill JR Jr, et al. Hyperplasia of the juxtaglomerular complex with hyperaldosteronism and hypokalemic alkalosis. A new syndrome. *Am J Med.* 1962;33:811–828.

182. Bartter FC. So-called Bartter's syndrome. *N Engl J Med.* 1969;281(26):1483–1484.

183. Simon DB, Karet FE, Hamdan JM, et al. Bartter's syndrome, hypokalaemic alkalosis with hypercalciuria, is caused by mutations in the Na-K-2Cl cotransporter NKCC2. *Nat Genet.* 1996;13(2):183–188.

184. Simon DB, Karet FE, Rodriguez-Soriano J, et al. Genetic heterogeneity of Bartter's syndrome revealed by mutations in the K^+ channel, ROMK. *Nat Genet.* 1996;14(2):152–156.

185. Simon DB, Bindra RS, Mansfield TA, et al. Mutations in the chloride channel gene, CLCNKB, cause Bartter's syndrome type III. *Nat Genet.* 1997;17(2):171–178.

186. Simon DB, Nelson-Williams C, Bia MJ, et al. Gitelman's variant of Bartter's syndrome, inherited hypokalaemic alkalosis, is caused by mutations in the thiazide-sensitive Na-Cl cotransporter. *Nat Genet.* 1996;12(1):24–30.

187. Armanini D, Scali M, Zennaro MC, et al. The pathogenesis of pseudohyperaldosteronism from carbenoxolone. *J Endocrinol Invest.* 1989;12(5):337–341.

188. Rahilly GT, Berl T. Severe metabolic alkalosis caused by administration of plasma protein fraction in end-stage renal failure. *N Engl J Med.* 1979;301(15):824–826.

189. Orwoll ES. The milk–alkali syndrome: current concepts. *Ann Intern Med.* 1982;97(2):242–248.

190. Heinemann HO. Metabolic alkalosis in patients with hypercalcemia. *Metabolism.* 1965;14(11):1137–1152.

191. Lipner HI, Ruzany F, Dasgupta M, et al. The behavior of carbenicillin as a nonreabsorbable anion. *J Lab Clin Med.* 1975;86(2):183–194.

192. Morrison RS. Management of emergencies. 8. Metabolic acidosis and alkalosis. *N Engl J Med.* 1966;274(21):1195–1197.

193. Barton CH, Vaziri ND, Ness RL, et al. Cimetidine in the management of metabolic alkalosis induced by nasogastric drainage. *Arch Surg.* 1979;114(1):70–74.

Pathophysiology and Management of Respiratory and Mixed Acid–Base Disorders

WILLIAM D. KAEHNY

R espiratory acid–base disorders are caused by *primary* changes from normal in excretion of carbon dioxide (CO_2) by the lungs. Primary means that the changes are not secondary to changes in pH caused by metabolic acid–base disorders. Under usual metabolic conditions, the body makes 13,000 to 15,000 mmol of CO_2 per day from the catabolism of carbohydrate, protein, and fat. If the lungs excrete this amount, the quantity of CO_2 in the body remains the same. This is reflected by the amount of CO_2 dissolved in blood and the partial pressure of the CO_2 gas in equilibrium with it (P_{CO_2}). A small amount of the dissolved CO_2 reacts with water to form carbonic acid (H_2CO_3), the acid part of the Henderson–Hasselbalch acid–base equation discussed in Chapter 3 and in detail elsewhere (1). It is simpler to use the P_{CO_2} in arterial blood (Pa_{CO_2}) to represent the respiratory or acid component of this equation:

$$pH \leftarrow \frac{[HCO_3^-]}{Pa_{CO_2}} \tag{4.1}$$

If the lungs fail to excrete the daily production or, conversely, excrete more than the daily production of CO_2, the quantity of CO_2 in the body changes; therefore, the amount dissolved in the blood and the pressure it generates (P_{CO_2}) change in the same direction. This change generates either of the two simple (or primary) respiratory acid–base disorders: hypercapnia, or high CO_2 level, generates respiratory acidosis; hypocapnia, or low CO_2 level, generates respiratory alkalosis.

The whole body responds to this imbalance between CO_2 production (rarely inhalation) and CO_2 excretion via effective ventilation in a programmed fashion. In step 1, the pH change causes rapid chemical *buffering*. Buffers within cells either take up hydrogen ions [H^+], producing a bicarbonate [HCO_3^-] in the blood or give up H^+ to titrate (consume) HCO_3^- in the blood. In step 2, the abnormal blood P_{CO_2} alters the renal tubular cell P_{CO_2}, causing changes in H^+ secretion that result in changes in renal net acid excretion (NAE) that, in turn, raise or lower blood [HCO_3^-]. This process is called by its traditional name of *compensation,* but it is more of an *adaptation* to a new state of CO_2 balance. This process takes days to reach a new steady state. Thus, it occurs only in *chronic* respiratory acid–base disorders. In step 3, the respiratory system *corrects* the problem and restores the whole-body CO_2 content and the arterial P_{CO_2} (Pa_{CO_2}) to previously normal values. Obviously, this can occur only if the causative disorder is cured or corrected. Notably, changes in oxygen (O_2) supply and demand and the Pa_{O_2} do not define respiratory acid–base disorders, but they can cause both respiratory acid–base disorders and metabolic acidosis through their effects on respiratory drive and lactic acid metabolism (2).

Carefully obtained arterial blood for analysis is the unusual way of diagnosing respiratory acid–base disorders. Although a recent study reported the normal values for the acid–base variables at sea level to differ from the standard textbook normals—namely, pH = 7.42 ± 0.02; P_{CO_2} = 38 ± 3 mm Hg; and HCO_3 = 24 mmol/L in men (7.43, 37, and 24, respectively, in women)—the custom remains to use the traditional values of 7.40, 40 mm Hg, and 24 mmol/L to calculate compensation (3).

Respiratory Acidosis

Respiratory acidosis is a disorder caused by processes that increase P_{CO_2}, which thereby leads to a decrease in the pH. The P_{CO_2} increases when the lungs fail to excrete metabolically produced CO_2. A decrease in effective alveolar ventilation is the usual way that the P_{CO_2} is increased. Effective alveolar ventilation can be diminished in two major ways, namely, decreased minute ventilation or ventilation-perfusion inequality (4). If effective ventilation is fixed by a ventilator or respiratory disease, the introduction of nutrition, parenteral or enteral, will increase the generation of CO_2. Using glucose as the source of nonprotein calories increases CO_2 production by 20% compared with glucose–lipid mixtures (5).

With decreased effective alveolar ventilation, CO_2 excretion falls short of production, and the quantity of CO_2 carried per milliliter of blood increases, as reflected in an increased Pa_{CO_2}. When a steady state of hypercapnia is reached, the ventilatory excretion of CO_2 again equals production. This new state occurs because the quantity of CO_2 carried to the pulmonary vascular bed is increased to a degree sufficient to allow the CO_2 excretion to equal the rate of production, despite decreased effective alveolar ventilation. In other words, with stable chronic hypercapnia, the quantity of CO_2 per milliliter of exhaled gas is increased.

When the Pa_{CO_2} rises, the amount of dissolved CO_2 increases and shifts the equilibrium reaction to favor the production of H_2CO_3; thus, $CO_2 + H_2O \rightarrow H_2CO_3$. This increased acid results in a fall in pH or respiratory acidosis. This process can be visualized more simply as a rise in Pa_{CO_2}, which reduces the ratio of the HCO_3^- concentration to the Pa_{CO_2}, thereby causing a fall in pH:

$$\downarrow pH \leftarrow \frac{[HCO_3^-]}{\uparrow Pa_{CO_2}} \tag{4.2}$$

The chemistry of these reactions is discussed in Chapter 3 and in detail in standard physiology and acid–base texts.

PATHOPHYSIOLOGY OF RESPIRATORY ACIDOSIS

Buffering

The immediate response to the low pH generated by the increased Pa_{CO_2} and H_2CO_3 is to buffer (or bind) hydrogen ions with nonbicarbonate buffers. Bicarbonate does not work as an effective buffer in this situation because it reacts with hydrogen ions to form H_2CO_3, which is the original culprit. In the extracellular fluid (ECF) space, proteins constitute the only buffer, while within the cells, hemoglobin, phosphate, proteins, and lactate are the major nonbicarbonate buffers; 97% of the buffering of H_2CO_3 derives from intracellular rather than ECF buffers (6).

Renal Compensation

The definitive compensation for respiratory acidosis resides solely in the kidneys. The kidneys respond to the increased systemic P_{CO_2} by increasing the production and excretion of ammonium (NH_4^+). The cellular mechanisms responsible for the increased ammonium generation are not clear. The renal tubular cells metabolize glutamine to produce two NH_3 molecules and α-ketoglutarate (AKG). The AKG goes to the liver where metabolism produces two HCO_3^-. The kidney excretes the NH_3 as NH_4^+, which marks the addition of the new HCO_3^- to the body stores by the liver. If the kidneys fail to excrete the NH_4^+, it travels to the liver and metabolism generates H^+, which negates the addition of the HCO_3^- to the body. Thus, increased renal excretion of NH_4^+ is a crucial component of the generation of new HCO_3^-. The increased urinary NH_4^+ excretion is balanced by increased Cl^- excretion with a resultant fall in plasma (Cl^-). When a steady state of hypercapnia is reached, chloride excretion returns to normal and equals intake. NH_4^+ excretion also returns to normal, even though H^+ secretion remains increased. The persistently increased H^+ secretion is needed to reclaim the increased filtered HCO_3^- load that results from the increase in plasma concentration (7,8). The increased cortical Na/H antiporter activity is not due to increased mRNA levels (9) but seems to involve

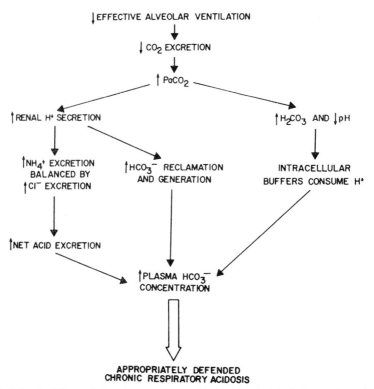

■ Figure 4.1 Pathophysiology of chronic respiratory acidosis. Chemical buffering and renal compensation combine to elevate the plasma [HCO_3^-]. The renal mechanisms involve an adaptive increase in ammonium and chloride excretion until the new steady state is reached.

stimulation by protein kinase C (10). The chemical buffering and renal compensation that occur with chronic respiratory acidosis are diagramed in Figure 4.1.

Correction of Respiratory Acidosis

The third, or corrective, response to respiratory acidosis is the restoration of effective ventilation. Correction or amelioration of an acute neurologic process causing hypoventilation or a ventilatory or gas-exchange defect may be possible. Unfortunately, many processes that result in chronic hypercapnia are caused by irreversible parenchymal lung damage and thus can be corrected only partially at best.

In metabolic acidosis, the corrective agent, the kidney, is sometimes a cause of the disorder, as in uremic acidosis, but at other times is not, as in diabetic ketoacidosis. In respiratory acidosis, however, the respiratory system, which includes neural control—mechanical, circulatory, and membrane exchange components—always is involved as the cause of the disorder and is also the corrective agent.

ACUTE RESPIRATORY ACIDOSIS (ACUTE HYPERCAPNIA)

Acute respiratory acidosis results from acute alveolar hypoventilation with a primary elevation of the Pa_{CO_2}, when only the buffering defense has had time to come into play. Although buffering occurs almost immediately, the renal response does not exert a noticeable influence for 12 to 24 hours (11). This is the period of time in which pure acute respiratory acidosis is observed. An appropriate defense of pH in acute respiratory acidosis is characterized by an elevation of the plasma [HCO_3^-] by about 1 mmol/L (>24) for each 10 mm Hg acute increment in Pa_{CO_2} (>40) (12):

$$\Delta[HCO_3^-] = (\Delta Pa_{CO_2}/10) \pm 3 \qquad (4.3)$$

Clinical Features and Systemic Effects of Acute Respiratory Acidosis

The acute onset of hypercapnia invariably is accompanied by hypoxemia, which usually dominates the clinical picture. Depending on the underlying disorder and the state of consciousness, the patient may present with the signs and symptoms of acute respiratory distress, including marked restlessness, tachypnea, and marked dyspnea. As the process worsens, stupor and eventually coma develop. CO_2 has vasodilating properties, and thus hypercapnia is associated with increased cerebral blood flow (13,14). This increase in blood flow to the brain probably accounts for the headaches and occasional signs of increased intracranial pressure that can occur with both acute and chronic hypercapnia (15,16). Severe acute respiratory acidosis can cause refractory hypotension through two mechanisms (17). First, cardiac contractility is reduced, and cardiac output falls. Second, peripheral arterial smooth muscle relaxes, causing vasodilation and decreased systemic vascular resistance. Modest acute increases in $PaCO_2$ (13–19 mm Hg) actually increase cardiac output as well as pulmonary artery pressure (18).

Laboratory Findings in Acute Respiratory Acidosis

With acute respiratory acidosis, the arterial blood reflects the pathophysiologic state with an elevated PCO_2, a moderately elevated plasma $[HCO_3^-]$ (<30 mmol/L), and a low pH. If the patient is breathing room air, then the PaO_2 is decreased. The venous serum electrolytes reveal a modestly elevated total CO_2 content, with usually normal plasma concentrations of sodium, potassium, and chloride (19).

Causes of Acute Respiratory Acidosis

Some of the causes of acute respiratory failure, which leads to acute CO_2 retention, are listed in Table 4.1.

TABLE 4.1 CAUSES OF ACUTE RESPIRATORY ACIDOSIS

Neuromuscular Abnormalities
Brainstem injury
High cord injury
Guillain–Barré syndrome
Myasthenia gravis
Botulism
Narcotic, sedative, or tranquilizer overdose
Status epilepticus
Postoperative hyponatremia with herniation

Airway Obstruction
Foreign body
Aspiration of vomitus
Laryngeal edema
Severe bronchospasm

Thoracic-Pulmonary Disorders
Flail chest
Pneumothorax
Severe pneumonia
Smoke inhalation
Severe pulmonary edema

Vascular Disease
Massive pulmonary embolism

Respirator-controlled Ventilation
Inadequate frequency, tidal volume settings
Large dead space
Total parenteral nutrition (increased CO_2 production)

Treatment of Acute Respiratory Acidosis

The key to treatment of acute respiratory acidosis is the restoration of effective ventilation. Modest amounts of sodium bicarbonate ($NaHCO_3$) may be given intravenously to mitigate severe acidosis; the latter is only a holding measure to prevent the serious cardiovascular effects of marked acidemia until definitive therapy is established (20). Because equilibration of HCO_3^- across the blood–brain barrier is markedly slower than that of CO_2 with bicarbonate administration, a delay in the correction of the cerebral pH may occur, and cerebrospinal fluid pH falls initially (21).

CHRONIC RESPIRATORY ACIDOSIS (CHRONIC HYPERCAPNIA)

Chronic respiratory acidosis is caused by chronic decreased effective alveolar ventilation with a primary elevation of the Pa_{CO_2}. The duration of the elevation of Pa_{CO_2} must be sufficient to permit adaptation of the renal mechanisms to be maximized. In the dog, a new steady state of blood acid–base values occurs 5 days after the onset of hypercapnia (11). The exact time interval needed to establish "chronic" hypercapnia in humans has not been established. A quantitative relationship has been described between the steady-state Pa_{CO_2} and the H^+ concentration in patients with chronic hypercapnia. This relationship is linear and is described by a slope of about 0.25 nmol of H^+ per 1 mm Hg increase in Pa_{CO_2} (22,23). A clinical guide for bedside use expresses the relationship between Pa_{CO_2} and plasma $[HCO_3^-]$ in chronic hypercapnia as follows: For each increment of 10 mm Hg in Pa_{CO_2}, the plasma $[HCO_3^-]$ rises by 4 mmol/L, with a range of 4 mmol/L in either direction. The following formula summarizes this rule of thumb:

$$\Delta \text{plasma}[HCO_3^-] = 4 \times \frac{\Delta Pa_{CO_2}}{10} \pm 4 \text{ mmol/L} \qquad (4.4)$$

Clinical Features and Systemic Effects of Chronic Respiratory Acidosis

Patients with chronic respiratory acidosis exhibit few if any signs or symptoms related directly to CO_2 retention and acidosis. However, papilledema and other neurologic disturbances have been described in several patients (22,23). These findings are not caused by the hypercapnia per se nor by the pH changes that mediate cerebral vascular reactivity through intracellular calcium. Rather, secondary changes in catecholamines are the likely causes (13). The signs and symptoms of the chronic pulmonary disease, with or without cor pulmonale, usually predominate. Chronic respiratory acidosis causes decreased bone mineralization, although to a lesser degree than does metabolic acidosis (24–26). This effect does not appear to be mediated by altered function of bone osteoclasts or osteoblasts and is not accompanied by hypercalciuria (27,28).

Laboratory Findings in Chronic Respiratory Acidosis

Arterial blood examination reveals a low pH (not <7.25 even with severe chronic CO_2 retention), an elevated Pa_{CO_2}, and an elevated plasma $[HCO_3^-]$. Thus a blood pH <7.25 is a marker of imposed acute hypercapnia or metabolic acidosis. Plasma sodium and potassium concentrations are usually normal. Total plasma CO_2 content is elevated, and plasma chloride concentration is reciprocally decreased. The anion gap usually is normal (22). In the absence of diuretic use or vomiting, these serum electrolyte findings should lead the clinician to check arterial blood gas values. The urine pH is usually acid.

Causes of Chronic Respiratory Acidosis

Chronic respiratory acidosis is seen most commonly in patients with chronic obstructive pulmonary disease (COPD). However, any condition that can lead to chronic retention of CO_2 (27) will cause the same acid–base disturbance. Examples of such conditions are given in Table 4.2.

The epidemic of obesity has led to the need to recognize two acid–base disorders caused by this condition. Obesity-hypoventilation causes chronic day and night hypercapnia and resultant chronic

TABLE 4.2 CAUSES OF CHRONIC RESPIRATORY ACIDOSIS

Neuromuscular Abnormalities
Chronic narcotic or sedative ingestion
Primary hypoventilation
Pickwickian syndrome
Poliomyelitis
Diaphragmatic paralysis
Hypothyroidism
Sleep apnea syndrome

Thoracic-Pulmonary Disorders
Chronic obstructive pulmonary disease
Kyphoscoliosis
End-stage interstitial pulmonary disease

respiratory acidosis (29,30). Sleep apnea causes nocturnal hypercapnia, which can lead to renal generation of bicarbonate. People on low-salt diets (low chloride) are unable to excrete this bicarbonate and thus develop posthypercapnic metabolic alkalosis.

Treatment of Chronic Respiratory Disease

Chronic respiratory acidosis can be corrected effectively only by restoring or improving the ability of the respiratory system to excrete CO_2. Often this is impossible because of an irreversible pathologic condition. However, adequate airway drainage, relief of bronchospasm, and treatment of pulmonary infections and congestive heart failure may lead to significant improvement. Because the arterial pH remains >7.25 even with chronic $Paco_2$ elevations to 110 mm Hg (31), the acidosis per se is not dangerous, although the patient is at more risk for serious acidemia if metabolic acidosis occurs. Attention to the maintenance of adequate oxygen tension (Po_2) is the critical need. Acidemia does cause constriction of venous capacitance vessels, and thus any fluid administration may acutely expand central blood volume and cause cardiac decompensation and pulmonary edema. Therefore, caution should be taken during fluid administration to patients with any form of respiratory acidosis.

People with end-stage renal disease (ESRD) who also have COPD or another cause of chronic hypercapnia are unable to generate the usual amounts of bicarbonate for compensation in chronic respiratory acidosis. Thus they will benefit from dialysis using a higher bicarbonate dialysate.

ACUTE HYPERCAPNIA SUPERIMPOSED ON CHRONIC RESPIRATORY ACIDOSIS

When a patient in a steady state of chronic hypercapnia suffers a new insult to his or her ability to excrete CO_2, the $Paco_2$ rises acutely to a new level. Thus, the plasma [HCO_3^-] and blood pH are lower than predicted for a given chronic level of $Paco_2$. However, the change in pH is not as great as would be expected for a similar acute increment in $Paco_2$ occurring in a previously normal person. That is, the pH is better protected against an acute rise in $Paco_2$ when there is a background of chronic respiratory acidosis than it is with acute respiratory acidosis alone (32,33). The mechanism for this is not entirely clear but has been attributed partially to the physicochemical effect of the preexisting higher [HCO_3^-], which would reduce the fall in pH compared with that seen for a similar increment in $Paco_2$ in a patient with a normal [HCO_3^-]. In addition, the kidney rapidly increases H^+ excretion when an acute rise in Pco_2 is superimposed on chronic respiratory acidosis. This is in contrast to acute respiratory acidosis alone, in which renal acid excretion makes little quantitative contribution to H^+ balance.

Treatment is directed toward correcting the acute disorder and providing supplemental oxygen. In patients with chronic CO_2 retention with acute worsening for whom pressurized mask oxygen administration is not possible, doxapram hydrochloride, given intravenously in doses starting with 2 mg/kg load followed by 1 to 3 mg/min maintenance, may help avoid mechanical ventilation until treatment of the underlying disorder can have effect. This agent works by stimulating both central and peripheral chemoreceptors to enhance respiratory rate and tidal volume. Case reports describe decreases in Pa_{CO_2} of as much as 60 mm Hg (34).

Respiratory Alkalosis

Respiratory alkalosis is caused by a process that leads to a rise in pH owing to a primary decrease in the Pa_{CO_2}. The Pa_{CO_2} can fall only if the excretion of CO_2 by the lungs exceeds the production of CO_2 by metabolic processes. Because the production of CO_2 usually remains relatively constant, a negative CO_2 balance results primarily from increased alveolar ventilation. Hyperventilation can result from two processes: (a) increased neurochemical stimulation of ventilation by central or peripheral neural mechanisms and (b) physically increased ventilation, either artificially with mechanical ventilators or voluntarily with increased conscious effort. Alveolar hyperventilation produces increased CO_2 excretion, which reduces the Pa_{CO_2} and H_2CO_3. This fall in Pa_{CO_2} increases the ratio of the $[HCO_3^-]$ to Pa_{CO_2}, which results in a rise in the pH of the blood, that is, alkalemia.

$$\uparrow pH \leftarrow \frac{[HCO_3^-]}{\downarrow Pa_{CO_2}} \tag{4.5}$$

The buffering response constitutes the *acute* phase of respiratory alkalosis, whereas the renal response to hypocapnia defines the *chronic* stage of respiratory alkalosis.

PATHOPHYSIOLOGY OF RESPIRATORY ALKALOSIS

Buffering

Buffering constitutes the first response in respiratory alkalosis. To return the pH toward normal in the face of the decreased H_2CO_3 or Pa_{CO_2}, the plasma $[HCO_3^-]$ must be decreased. Therefore, H^+ is released from the body buffers, and the plasma $[HCO_3^-]$ is reduced by the following net reaction:

$$H^+ + HCO_3^- \rightarrow CO_2 + H_2O \tag{4.6}$$

Intracellular buffers supply about 99% of the H^+, whereas plasma proteins contribute about 1% to the buffering effort (6). Cellular metabolism contributes by increasing the production of lactic acid and possibly of slight amounts of other organic acids. Lactate concentration increased by 0.5 mmol/L in a study in anesthetized patients; this represents about 10% of the total buffering effort. Buffering is completed within minutes, and the steady state persists for at least 2 hours (35). The alacrity of the response is critical, because the Pa_{CO_2} can decrease abruptly, and without buffering, life-threatening alkalemia would occur. The quantitative change in plasma $[HCO_3^-]$ is not great, however, and the pH therefore may rise markedly. The arterial $[HCO_3^-]$ fell to as low as 18 mmol/L at Pa_{CO_2} levels of 15 to 20 mm Hg in anesthetized patients (35). A rule of thumb for acute respiratory alkalosis is that the $[HCO_3^-]$ should decrease by 1 mmol/L for each 10 mm Hg decrement in Pa_{CO_2}:

$$\Delta[HCO_3^-] = 1 \times (\Delta Pa_{CO_2}/10) \pm 3 \tag{4.7}$$

Renal Compensation

The second adaptive response in respiratory alkalosis is handled by a renal mechanism. The kidney attempts to lower the plasma $[HCO_3^-]$ in either of two ways: by decreasing the reclamation of filtered HCO_3^-, thus leading to bicarbonaturia, or by reducing the generation of new HCO_3^- to replace that consumed in the daily buffering of the dietary metabolic acid load. In animals, the kidney appears to make the second choice, because a decreased NH_4^+ excretion without an increased HCO_3^- excretion occurs during the phase of adaptation to chronic hypocapnia. This reduction in excretion of NH_4^+, a cation, is balanced electrochemically by increased sodium or potassium excretion (36). After a new steady state is reached, excretion of these electrolytes returns to normal. The process of renal adaptation appears to

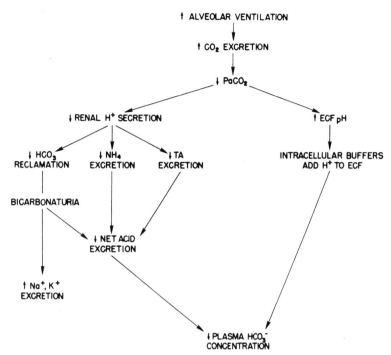

■ **Figure 4.2** Pathophysiology of chronic respiratory alkalosis. Intracellular buffers donate H^+ to the ECF to produce a small decrease in plasma [HCO_3^-] during acute hypocapnia. The net effect on renal function of prolonged hypocapnia is a decrease in H^+ secretion, which results in a fall in net acid excretion below the level necessary to maintain acid balance. Thus, plasma [HCO_3^-] falls. Urinary acid and electrolyte excretion return to normal after steady-state $Paco_2$ and [HCO_3^-] are achieved. ECF, extracellular fluid; TA, titratable acid.

occur rapidly and is probably completed within 24 to 48 hours (36). In humans, the early stage of renal adaptation for prolonged hypocapnia is characterized by bicarbonaturia, natriuresis, and decreased NH_4^+ and titratable acid excretion (37,38). The stimulus for this renal response appears to be independent of systemic pH changes but is a direct effect of the $Paco_2$ level on renal reabsorption of an anion, either HCO_3^- or chloride (39,40). The chemical buffering and proposed renal response in respiratory alkalosis are diagramed in Figure 4.2.

The quantitative contribution of the kidney to pH defense is difficult to judge in humans. Subjects with hypocapnia caused by voluntary hyperventilation or altitude hypoxemia had decreases in plasma [HCO_3^-] of 2.1 to 4.9 mmol/L/10 mm Hg decrease in $Paco_2$ during 1 to 11 days of hypocapnia (37,38,41). Arterial pH remained frankly alkalemic. Climbers adapted to altitude over 60 days had $Paco_2$ levels of 13.3 and [HCO_3^-] of 10.8 mmol/L with resultant pH of 7.53 just below the Everest summit (42). However, some studies of lifelong high-altitude dwellers have shown decreased plasma [HCO_3^-] sufficient to produce pH values of 7.4 with $Paco_2$ levels as low as 28 to 30 mm Hg (43–46). For clinical purposes, a useful rule is to diagnose simple chronic respiratory alkalosis when plasma [HCO_3^-] is decreased 4 mmol/L <24 for each 10 mm Hg chronic decrement <40 in the $Paco_2$.

$$\Delta[HCO_3^-] = 4 \times (\Delta Paco_2/10) \pm 2 \qquad (4.8)$$

Correction of Respiratory Alkalosis

The third, or corrective, response in respiratory alkalosis entails correction of the hyperventilation that maintains the negative CO_2 balance. This, of course, is dependent on removal of the neurohumoral stimulus to the respiratory center or cessation of mechanical or voluntary hyperventilation. The latter is easier to achieve because neural stimulation of ventilation often is caused by pathophysiologic processes that are difficult to correct.

CLINICAL FEATURES AND SYSTEMIC EFFECTS OF RESPIRATORY ALKALOSIS

Hypocapnia may be manifested by symptoms and signs of neuromuscular irritability. Patients may complain of perioral and extremity paresthesias, muscle cramps, and even tinnitus. Hyperreflexia, tetany, and even seizures may occur (47,48). Hypocapnia causes cerebral vasoconstriction with reduced blood flow, which may have deleterious and even fatal effects on the brain, especially in patients with sickle cell disease (49–52). Marked alkalemia may cause serious refractory cardiac arrhythmias and electrocardiographic changes of ischemia (53–57).

LABORATORY FINDINGS WITH RESPIRATORY ALKALOSIS

If arterial blood pH is increased, then a decreased Pa_{CO_2} and plasma $[HCO_3^-]$ are diagnostic of respiratory alkalosis. Venous serum total CO_2 content reflects the decrease in $[HCO_3^-]$, and chloride concentration is slightly increased. Serum potassium is increased by an average of 0.3 mmol/L in acute respiratory alkalosis. This effect appears to be stimulated by the buffering-induced fall in $[HCO_3^-]$, which activates the α-adrenergic system (Chapter 5) (58). Serum phosphorus concentration may decrease only slightly or to seriously low levels (Chapter 6) (59–61). Urine pH is not clinically informative. It may be relatively alkaline (>6.0) during the onset of acute hypocapnia but then fluctuates into the more acidic range, as in the eucapnic state (37).

DIFFERENTIAL DIAGNOSIS OF RESPIRATORY ALKALOSIS

Respiratory alkalosis is the most common acid–base disorder among seriously ill patients (62). The reason for this is apparent from a review of the list of causes of respiratory alkalosis (Table 4.3).

TABLE 4.3 CAUSES OF RESPIRATORY ALKALOSIS

Central Stimulation of Respiration
Anxiety
Head trauma
Brain tumors or vascular accidents
Salicylates
Fever
Pain
Pregnancy

Peripheral Stimulation of Respiration
Pulmonary emboli
Congestive heart failure
Interstitial lung diseases
Pneumonia
"Stiff lungs" without hypoxemia
Altitude
Asthma

Multiple Mechanisms
Hepatic insufficiency
Gram-negative septicemia

Mechanical or Voluntary Hyperventilation

Central stimulation of the medullary respiratory center occurs with anxiety, pain, pregnancy, febrile states, and salicylate intoxication. Mechanical irritation by brain trauma or tumor is another respiratory stimulant.

Stimulation of the peripheral pathways to the medullary respiratory center occurs in pulmonary-thoracic disorders that cause hypoxemia with relatively unimpaired CO_2 transport, altitude hypoxemia, asthma (63), and disorders that decrease lung compliance (stiff lung) without necessarily causing hypoxemia.

Mechanical ventilation may produce respiratory alkalosis if the rate and tidal volume are set so that pulmonary excretion of CO_2 is allowed to exceed CO_2 production. However, increased minute ventilation often is necessary in order to deliver adequate quantities of oxygen to patients with severe pulmonary insufficiency.

Patients with hepatic cirrhosis often have respiratory alkalosis (64,65). The mechanism is probably multifactorial (66), although increased pulmonary shunting (67), hyponatremia (68), and increased blood ammonia levels (69) have been implicated. Respiratory alkalosis is an early manifestation of gram-negative sepsis and other forms of shock; therefore, the clinician should suspect these processes in the appropriate clinical setting (70).

TREATMENT OF RESPIRATORY ALKALOSIS

The only definitive treatment is to correct or ameliorate the basic disorder responsible for the hyperventilation. Correcting significant hypoxemia is more critical for the patient's well-being than is correcting the acid–base disturbance. If alkalemia is causing deleterious neuromuscular or cardiac rhythm problems in a patient on mechanical ventilation, then decreasing the minute ventilation or increasing the dead space may be effective. If this cannot be done without compromising oxygenation, then the use of an inhaled gas mixture containing 3% CO_2 may be helpful for short periods of time (71). Use of morphine to decrease hyperventilation and alleviate anxiety is reasonable if adequate oxygenation is insured. The morphine effect can be reversed rapidly with naloxone.

Mixed Acid–Base Disorders

Mixed acid–base disorders occur when two or even three primary events act independently to alter the acid–base state at the same time. Five double- and two triple-mixed acid–base disorders can occur as listed in Table 4.4. The two primary respiratory acid–base disorders, respiratory acidosis and respiratory alkalosis, cannot coexist.

TABLE 4.4 MIXED ACID–BASE DISORDERS

Disorders	Adaptation	pH
Inadequate Response		
Metabolic acidosis and respiratory acidosis	$Paco_2$ too high and $[HCO_3^-]$ too low for simple disorders	↓↓
Metabolic alkalosis and respiratory alkalosis	$Paco_2$ too low and $[HCO_3^-]$ too high for simple disorders	↑↑
Excessive Response		
Metabolic acidosis and respiratory alkalosis	$Paco_2$ too low and $[HCO_3^-]$ too low for simple disorders	Normal or slightly ↓ or ↑
Metabolic alkalosis and respiratory acidosis	$Paco_2$ too high and $[HCO_3^-]$ too high for simple disorders	Normal or slightly ↑ or ↓
Triple Disorders		
Metabolic alkalosis, metabolic acidosis, and either respiratory acidosis or alkalosis	$Paco_2$ and $[HCO_3^-]$ not appropriate for simple disorders and anion gap >17 mEq/L	Variable

DIAGNOSIS OF MIXED ACID–BASE DISORDERS

A mixed acid–base disorder can be suspected from the clinical setting (e.g., a patient with cor pulmonale on diuretics) and can be diagnosed from arterial blood and venous serum or plasma studies. The key to the diagnosis of a mixed disturbance is the clear understanding of the expected compensation in the primary, uncomplicated acid–base disorders. If the compensation is appropriate, the disorder is simple; if it is out of the expected range for an uncomplicated, primary disorder, a mixed disorder is suspected. To determine whether compensation is appropriate for a given disorder, it is essential to know the expected response. In Table 3.1 are shown the expected directional changes in pH, $Paco_2$, and plasma [HCO_3^-] for each simple disorder. Thumb rules for estimating the expected changes in these values are listed in Table 3.2. A mixed disorder should be suspected if a given set of blood acid–base values does not fall within the range of the expected response for that acid–base disorder (72). This is easy to judge if the bicarbonate and Pco_2 deviate from normal in opposite directions.

Certain of the mixed acid–base disorders may cause dangerous deviations of pH from normal, whereas others may produce pH values within the normal range. The dangerous combinations are those in which the primary disorders block the compensation for each other. For example, the hypercapnia of respiratory acidosis prevents the adaptive hypocapnia of metabolic acidosis, and the hypobicarbonatemia of metabolic acidosis blocks the adaptive rise in plasma [HCO_3^-] expected in respiratory acidosis. The dangerous disorders thus are characterized by *failure of compensation* (Table 4.4).

The "benign" mixed acid–base disorders are those in which the primary disorders provide *excessive compensation* for each other (Table 4.4). For example, salicylate intoxication may produce acidosis, such as plasma [HCO_3^-] of 10 mmol/L or a reduction of 14 mmol/L below normal sea-level values. Application of the rule of thumb for metabolic acidosis (Table 3.2) predicts the maximum fall in $Paco_2$ to be $1.5 \times 14 = 21$ mm Hg. Thus, a $Paco_2$ of <19 mm Hg ($40 - 21$) would not be appropriate for simple metabolic acidosis. Salicylate has a primary stimulating effect on ventilation, however, and may produce sufficient hyperventilation to lower the $Paco_2$ to 14 mm Hg in this example. Thus, the primary hypocapnia would result in excessive compensation for the fall in [HCO_3^-] and pH produced by salicylate intoxication. Reciprocally, the fall in [HCO_3^-] would be greater than that predicted as appropriate for respiratory alkalosis (Table 3.2).

A nomogram for interpreting acid–base variables is displayed in Figure 3.3. A point falling outside the indicated predictive bands suggests the presence of a mixed acid–base disorder. However, a mixed disorder also may result in a set of acid–base variables falling within a band, as discussed in the figure legend; therefore, acid–base variables must be interpreted in light of the entire clinical circumstances and not as an isolated set of numbers.

COMMON MIXED ACID–BASE DISORDERS

Respiratory Acidosis and Metabolic Alkalosis

Patients with chronic lung diseases that produce CO_2 retention and respiratory acidosis often develop congestive heart failure. If diuretics are used to treat the heart failure, then the plasma [HCO_3^-] may rise to levels greater than those appropriate for renal compensation in chronic respiratory acidosis (Table 3.2, Fig. 3.3). The pH may rise to the normal range or even frankly elevated levels. These changes may finally result in a set of acid–base variables appropriate for simple metabolic alkalosis, for example, plasma [HCO_3^-], 48 mmol; $Paco_2$, 60 mm Hg; and pH, 7.52. Clinical information, however, indicated that this particular set of laboratory values resulted from the coexistence of two primary acid–base disorders, chronic respiratory acidosis, with a primary increase in $Paco_2$ and secondary compensatory rise in plasma [HCO_3^-], and metabolic alkalosis, with a primary increase in [HCO_3^-] above the expected level for chronic respiratory acidosis.

Difficulty in interpreting the acid–base variables may arise if clinical information is not available or not clear as to the existence of lung disease with chronic CO_2 retention. In that instance, it is helpful to observe the patient's response to the cessation of diuretics and administration of sodium and potassium chloride. This treatment will correct simple metabolic alkalosis (Chapter 3) but achieve only some improvement in the $Paco_2$ in the mixed disorder. A large alveolar-arterial Po_2 gradient (>15 mm Hg) indicates lung disease and is suggestive of some component of respiratory acidosis.

Although this mixed disorder is one of the excessive compensation variety in which pH does not deviate markedly from normal, it should be treated to maintain the PaO_2 at the best attainable level. The increase in plasma [HCO_3^-] and concomitant rise in pH owing to diuretic-induced metabolic alkalosis are sufficient to suppress ventilation in patients with chronic respiratory acidosis, thus causing a decrease in PaO_2 (73). Treatment of this mixed disorder should be directed at lowering the plasma [HCO_3^-] through sodium chloride and potassium chloride therapy, which best allows the kidney to excrete HCO_3^- retained as a result of diuretic-induced metabolic alkalosis (Chapter 3). Of course, this therapy must be used with caution to avoid exacerbating volume overload. Although the pH will fall to acidemic levels, this is beneficial inasmuch as it stimulates ventilation, thus increasing PaO_2 and decreasing $PaCO_2$. In any event, pH in chronic respiratory acidosis is well defended and does not fall below 7.25, as discussed (30).

Respiratory Acidosis and Metabolic Acidosis

Mixed respiratory and metabolic acidosis may develop in patients with cardiorespiratory arrest, chronic lung disease who are in shock, and metabolic acidosis of any type who develop respiratory failure. This mixed disorder is a failure of compensation (Table 4.4). The respiratory disorder prevents the fall in $PaCO_2$ expected in the defense against metabolic acidosis. The metabolic disorder prevents the buffering and renal mechanisms from raising the plasma [HCO_3^-] as expected in the defense against respiratory acidosis. In the absence of these responses, the pH falls profoundly, even when the changes in plasma [HCO_3^-] and $PaCO_2$ are only moderate.

If the respiratory acidosis is less severe than the metabolic acidosis, then the $PaCO_2$ may be normal or even reduced but not to the level appropriate for the respiratory response expected for the metabolic acidosis. If the respiratory acidosis predominates over the metabolic acidosis, then plasma [HCO_3^-] is normal or even increased but not to the level expected for the degree of CO_2 retention, thus indicating a mixed disturbance. Neither change needs to be major in order to cause a significant academia. This may be a clue to ingestion of agents that cause metabolic acidosis and suppress ventilation, as exemplified by a woman who ingested metformin that caused lactic acidosis and zolpidem that caused respiratory depression: initial pH 7.26, PCO_2 45 mm Hg, and HCO_3^- 19.5 mmol/L. Bicarbonate later fell to 5 (74). This mixed acid–base disorder should be treated with attention to both the respiratory and metabolic acidosis. Mechanical ventilation may be needed to reduce the $PaCO_2$. As respiratory treatment is instituted, $NaHCO_3$ may be administered intravenously to treat the metabolic component of the acidosis while the specific etiology and treatment are sought (20).

Respiratory Alkalosis and Metabolic Acidosis

The combination of respiratory alkalosis and metabolic acidosis is seen often in patients with hepatic failure. Such patients may have respiratory alkalosis due to hyperventilation and metabolic acidosis due to renal failure, renal tubular acidosis, liver failure with lactic acidosis, or any combination. Patients with chronic renal failure and metabolic acidosis are susceptible to bacteremia, which may cause increased ventilation and respiratory alkalosis. Salicylate intoxication may cause mixed metabolic acidosis and respiratory alkalosis (75). This combination is a mixed disorder with excessive compensation (Table 4.4). The respiratory alkalosis lowers the $PaCO_2$ beyond the appropriate range of the respiratory response for metabolic acidosis. The plasma [HCO_3^-] also falls below the level expected in simple respiratory alkalosis. In a sense, the compensation for either disorder alone is enhanced; thus, the pH may be normal or close to normal, with a low $PaCO_2$ and a low plasma [HCO_3^-]. The primary therapeutic approach should be directed at treatment of the underlying disorders. The acid–base problem per se usually does not need treatment because the pH is usually closer to normal than it is in either simple disorder alone.

Respiratory Alkalosis and Metabolic Alkalosis

The combination of respiratory and metabolic alkalosis probably is the most common mixed acid–base disorder. This is a mixed disorder with failure of compensation (Table 4.4). It may be seen in patients with hepatic cirrhosis who hyperventilate, use diuretics, or vomit and in patients with chronic respiratory

TABLE 4.5 EXAMPLE OF A TRIPLE ACID–BASE DISORDER

Clinical Event	Vomiting	→	Hypovolemic Shock	→	Hyperventilation
	↓		↓		↓
Acid–base disorder	Metabolic alkalosis	+	Metabolic acidosis	+	Respiratory alkalosis
pH	7.53		7.35		7.46
Pa_{CO_2} (mm Hg)	44		30		20
[HCO_3^-] (mmol/L)	36		16		14
Anion gap (mEq/L)	12		30		32

acidosis and appropriately elevated plasma [HCO_3^-] who are placed on mechanical ventilators and undergo a rapid fall in Pa_{CO_2} to hypocapnic levels. Each of the two disorders blocks the appropriate compensatory mechanism of the other; therefore, a marked rise in pH may occur. Depending on the severity of each disorder, the Pa_{CO_2} may be normal, reduced, or even increased, whereas the plasma [HCO_3^-] may be normal or elevated. Correction of the metabolic alkalosis by administration of sodium chloride and potassium chloride should be undertaken, and readjustment of the ventilator or treatment of an underlying disorder causing hyperventilation may correct or ameliorate the respiratory disorder.

Metabolic Acidosis and Metabolic Alkalosis

Metabolic acidosis and metabolic alkalosis may coexist in that two separate processes occur sequentially or simultaneously to exert opposing effects on the plasma [HCO_3^-]. This situation should be suspected in cases of metabolic acidosis associated with markedly increased anion gaps when the increments in the anion gap are much greater than the decrements in plasma [HCO_3^-]. Such a picture suggests that the plasma [HCO_3^-] was set at a value above normal at the time the metabolic acidosis developed.

"Triple" Acid–Base Disorders

The occurrence of a primary respiratory disorder in a patient with metabolic acidosis superimposed on metabolic alkalosis results in a "triple" acid–base disorder. That is, three primary processes have acted to alter the acid–base variables. An example is given in Table 4.5. Vomiting raised the plasma [HCO_3^-], which raised the pH, which suppressed ventilation, allowing the Pa_{CO_2} to rise a bit. The patient became hypotensive and began to increase lactic acid production and decrease lactate catabolism, which lowered the [HCO_3^-] from its high level and increased the anion gap well above normal. The hypotension stimulated ventilation beyond that expected for the degree of acidemia, resulting in a further fall in Pa_{CO_2}, which raised the pH to the alkalemic range. Thus, the high pH and low Pa_{CO_2} identify the presence of respiratory alkalosis. The anion gap greater than 27 mEq/L signals the presence of an organic metabolic acidosis. Adding the increase in the anion gap above normal ($32 - 9 = 23$ mEq/L), which marks the replacement of a HCO_3^- by a metabolic acid anion, to the observed [HCO_3^-] ($23 + 14 = 37$ mmol/L) indicates the presence of the metabolic alkalosis that raised the [HCO_3^-] in the first place. The serum anion gap is usually the key to the unraveling of triple acid–base disorders. Treatment should be directed at correcting the underlying diseases and replacing volume and electrolyte deficits.

REFERENCES

1. Bevensee MO, Boron WF. Control of intracellular pH. In: Alpern RJ, Hebert SC, eds. *Seldin and Giebisch's the Kidney: Physiology and Pathophysiology,* 4th ed. Amsterdam: Elsevier; 2008:1429–1480.
2. Sapir DG, Levine DF, Schwartz WB. The effects of chronic hypoxemia on electrolyte and acid-base equilibrium: an examination of normocapneic hypoxemia and of the influence of hypoxemia on the adaptation to chronic hypercapnia. *J Clin Invest.* 1967;46:369–377.
3. Crapo RO, Jensen RL, Hegewald M, et al. Arterial blood gas reference values for sea level and an altitude of 1,400 meters. *Am J Respir Crit Care Med.* 1999;160:1525–1531.
4. Weinberger SE, Schwarzstein RM, Weiss JW. Hypercapnia. *N Engl J Med.* 1989;321:1223–1231.

5. Askanazi J, Nordenstrom J, Rosenbaum SH, et al. Nutrition for the patient with respiratory failure. Glucose vs. fat. *Anesthesiology.* 1981;54:373–377.

6. Giebisch G, Berger L, Pitts RF. The extrarenal responses to acute acid-base disturbances of respiratory origin. *J Clin Invest.* 1955;34:231–245.

7. Krapf R. Mechanisms of adaptation to chronic respiratory acidosis in the rabbit proximal tubule. *J Clin Invest.* 1989;83:890–896.

8. Ruiz OS, Arruda JAL, Talor Z. Na-HCO₃ cotransport and Na-H antiporter in chronic respiratory acidosis and alkalosis. *Am J Physiol.* 1989;256: F414–F420.

9. Krapf R, Pearce D, Xi X-P, et al. Expression of rat renal Na/H antiporter mRNA levels in response to respiratory and metabolic acidosis. *J Clin Invest.* 1991;87:747–751.

10. Pahlavan P, Wang L-J, Sack E, et al. Role of protein kinase C in the adaptive increase in Na-H antiporter in respiratory acidosis. *J Am Soc Nephrol.* 1993;4:1079–1086.

11. Schwartz WB, Brackett NC Jr, Cohen JJ. The response of extracellular hydrogen ion concentration to graded degrees of chronic hypercapnia: the physiologic limitation of the defense of pH. *J Clin Invest.* 1965;44:291–301.

12. Brackett NC Jr, Cohen JJ, Schwartz WB. Carbon dioxide titration curve of normal man: effect of increasing degrees of acute hypercapnia on acid-base equilibrium. *N Engl J Med.* 1965;272:6–12.

13. Brian JE Jr. Carbon dioxide and the cerebral circulation. *Anesthesiology.* 1998;88:1365–1386.

14. Pollock JM, Deibler AR, Whitlow CT, et al. Hypercapnia-induced cerebral hyperperfusion: an underrecognized clinical entity. *AJNR.* 2009;30: 378–385.

15. Dulfano MJ, Ishikawa S. Hypercapnia: mental changes and extrapulmonary complications. An expanded concept of the "CO₂ intoxication" syndrome. *Ann Intern Med.* 1965;63:829–841.

16. Epstein FH. Signs and symptoms of electrolyte disorders. In: Maxwell MH, Kleeman CR, eds. *Clinical Disorders of Fluid and Electrolyte Metabolism,* 3rd ed. New York: McGraw-Hill; 1980:499–516.

17. Potkin RT, Swenson ER. Resuscitation from severe acute hypercapnia: determination of limits of tolerance and survival. *Chest.* 1992;102:1742–1745.

18. Chabot F, Mertes PM, Delorme N, et al. Effect of acute hypercapnia on alpha atrial natriuretic peptide, renin, angiotensin II, aldosterone, and vasopressin plasma levels in patients with COPD. *Chest.* 1995;107:780–786.

19. Natalini G, Seramondi V, Fassini P, et al. Acute respiratory acidosis does not increase plasma potassium in normokalaemic, anesthetized patients. A controlled randomized trial. *Eur J Anaesthesiol.* 2001;18:394–400.

20. Lakshminarayan S, Sahn SA, Petty TL. Bicarbonate therapy in severe acute respiratory acidosis. *Scand J Respir Dis.* 1973;54:128–131.

21. Bulger RJ, Schrier RW, Arend WP, et al. Spinal-fluid acidosis and the diagnosis of pulmonary encephalopathy. *N Engl J Med.* 1966;274: 433–437.

22. Brackett NC Jr, Wingo CF, Muren O, et al. Acid-base response to chronic hypercapnia in man. *N Engl J Med.* 1969;280:124–130.

23. Van Ypersele de Strihou C, Brasseur L, DeConinck J. The "carbon dioxide response curve" for chronic hypercapnia in man. *N Engl J Med.* 1966;275: 117–122.

24. Manfredi F, Merwarth CR, Buckley CE III, et al. Papilledema in chronic respiratory acidosis. *Am J Med.* 1961;30:175–180.

25. Miller A, Bader RA, Bader ME. The neurological syndrome due to marked hypercapnia, with papilledema. *Am J Med.* 1962;33:309–318.

26. Bushinsky DA. The contribution of acidosis to renal osteodystrophy. *Kidney Int.* 1995;47: 1816–1832.

27. Bushinsky DA. Stimulated osteoclastic and suppressed osteoblastic activity in metabolic but not respiratory acidosis. *Am J Physiol.* 1995;268: C80–C88.

28. Bushinsky DA, Parker WR, Alexander KM, et al. Metabolic, but not respiratory, acidosis increases bone PGE2 levels and calcium release. *Am J Physiol Renal Physiol.* 2001;281:F1058–F1066.

29. Strumpf DA, Millman RP, Hill NS. The management of chronic hypoventilation. *Chest.* 1990;98: 474–480.

30. Nowbar S, Burkart KM, Gonzales R, et al. Obesity-associated hypoventilation in hospitalized patients: prevalence, effects, and outcome. *Am J Med.* 2004; 116:1–7.

31. Neff TA, Petty TL. Tolerance and survival in severe chronic hypercapnia. *Arch Intern Med.* 1972; 129:591–596.

32. Goldstein MB, Gennari FJ, Schwartz WB. The influence of graded degrees of chronic hypercapnia on the acute carbon dioxide titration curve. *J Clin Invest.* 1971;50:208–216.

33. Ingram RJ Jr, Miller RB, Tate LA. Acid-base response to acute carbon dioxide changes in chronic obstructive pulmonary disease. *Am Rev Respir Dis.* 1973;108:225–231.

34. Hirshberg AJ, Dupper RL. Use of doxapram hydrochloride injections as an alternative to intubation to treat chronic obstructive pulmonary disease patients with hypercapnia. *Ann Emerg Med.* 1994;24:701–703.

35. Arbus GS, Hebert LA, Levesque PR, et al. Characterization and clinical application of the "significance band" for acute respiratory alkalosis. *N Engl J Med.* 1969;280:117–123.

36. Gennari FJ, Goldstein MB, Schwartz WB. The nature of the renal adaptation to chronic hypocapnia. *J Clin Invest.* 1972;51:1722–1730.

37. Gledhill N, Beirne GJ, Dempsey JA. Renal response to short-term hypocapnia in man. *Kidney Int.* 1975; 8:376–386.

38. Krapf R, Beeler I, Hertner D, et al. Chronic respiratory alkalosis: the effect of sustained hyperventilation on renal regulation of acid-base equilibrium. *N Engl J Med.* 1991;324:1394–1401.

39. Cohen JJ, Madias NE, Wolf CJ, et al. Regulation of acid-base equilibrium in chronic hypocapnia: evidence that the response of the kidney is not geared to the defense of extracellular [H⁺]. *J Clin Invest.* 1976;57:1483–1489.

40. Hilden SA, Johns CA, Madias NE. Adaptation of rabbit renal cortical Na⁺−H⁺ exchange activity in chronic hypocapnia. *Am J Physiol.* 1989;257: F615–F622.

41. Forster HV, Dempsey JA, Chosy LW. Incomplete compensation of CSF [H$^+$] in man during acclimatization to high altitude (4300 m). *J Appl Physiol.* 1975;38:1067–1072.

42. Grocott MPW, Martin DS, Levett DZH, et al. Arterial blood gases and oxygen content in climbers on Mount Everest. *N Engl J Med.* 2009; 360:140–149.

43. Severinghaus JW, Mitchell RA, Richardson BW, et al. Respiratory control at high altitude suggesting active transport regulation of CSF pH. *J Appl Physiol.* 1963;18:1155–1166.

44. Chiodi H. Respiratory adaptations to chronic high altitude hypoxia. *J Appl Physiol.* 1957;10:81–87.

45. Dill DB, Talbott JH, Consolazio WV. Blood as a physiochemical system. XII. Man at high altitudes. *J Biol Chem.* 1937;118:649–666.

46. Lahiri S, Milledge JS. Acid-base in Sherpa altitude residents and lowlanders at 4880 m. *Respir Physiol.* 1967;2:323–334.

47. Edmondson JW, Brashear RE, Li T. Tetany: quantitative interrelationships between calcium and alkalosis. *Am J Physiol.* 1975;228:1082–1086.

48. Kilburn KH. Shock, seizures, and coma with alkalosis during mechanical ventilation. *Ann Intern Med.* 1966;65:977–984.

49. Arnow PM, Panwalker A, Garvin JS, et al. Aspirin, hyperventilation, and cerebellar infarction in sickle cell disease. *Arch Intern Med.* 1978;138:148–149.

50. Ayres SM, Grace WJ. Inappropriate ventilation and hypoxemia as causes of cardiac arrhythmias: the control of arrhythmias without antiarrhythmic drugs. *Am J Med.* 1969;46:495–505.

51. Kety SS, Schmidt CF. The effects of altered arterial tensions of carbon dioxide and oxygen on cerebral blood flow and cerebral oxygen consumption of normal young men. *J Clin Invest.* 1948;27: 484–491.

52. Protass LM. Possible precipitation of cerebral thrombosis in sickle-cell anemia by hyperventilation. *Ann Intern Med.* 1973;79:451.

53. Jacobs WF, Battle WE, Ronan JA Jr. False-positive ST–T-wave changes secondary to hyperventilation and exercise: a cineangiographic correlation. *Ann Intern Med.* 1974;81:479–482.

54. Lawson NW, Butler CH III, Ray CT. Alkalosis and cardiac arrhythmias. *Anesthesiol Analg (Paris).* 1973;52:951–962.

55. Neill WA, Pantley GA, Nakomchai V. Respiratory alkalemia during exercise reduces angina threshold. *Chest.* 1981;80:144–153.

56. Weber S, Cabanes L, Simon J-C, et al. Systemic alkalosis as a provocative test for coronary artery spasm in patients with infrequent resting chest pain. *Am Heart J.* 1988;115:54–59.

57. Yakaitis RW, Cooke JE, Redding JS. Reevaluation of relationships of hyperkalemia and PCO_2 to cardiac arrhythmias during mechanical ventilation. *Anesthesiol Analg (Paris).* 1971;50:368–373.

58. Krapf R, Caduff P, Wagdi P, et al. Plasma potassium response to acute respiratory alkalosis. *Kidney Int.* 1995;47:217–224.

59. Knochel JP. The pathophysiology and clinical characteristics of severe hypophosphatemia. *Arch Intern Med.* 1977;137:203–220.

60. Mostellar ME, Tuttle EP Jr. The effects of alkalosis on plasma concentration and urinary excretion of inorganic phosphate in man. *J Clin Invest.* 1964; 43:138–149.

61. Paleologos M, Stone E, Braude S. Persistent, progressive, hypophosphatemia after voluntary hyperventilation. *Clin Sci.* 2000;98:619–625.

62. Mazzara JT, Ayres SM, Grace WJ. Extreme hypocapnia in the critically ill patient. *Am J Med.* 1974;56:450–456.

63. Mountain RD, Heffner JE, Brackett NC Jr, et al. Acid-base disturbances in acute asthma. *Chest.* 1990;98:651–655.

64. Mulhausen R, Eichenholz A, Blumentals A. Acid-base disturbances in patients with cirrhosis of the liver. *Medicine (Balt).* 1967;46:185–189.

65. Record CO, Iles RA, Cohen RD, et al. Acid-base and metabolic disturbances in fulminant hepatic failure. *Gut.* 1975;16:144–149.

66. Lange PA, Stoller JK. The hepatopulmonary syndrome. *Ann Intern Med.* 1995;122:521–529.

67. Wolfe JD, Tashkin DP, Holly FE, et al. Hypoxemia of cirrhosis: detection of abnormal small pulmonary vascular channels by a quantitative radionuclide method. *Am J Med.* 1977;63:746–754.

68. Wilder CE, Morrison RS, Tyler JM. Relationship between serum sodium and hyperventilation in cirrhosis. *Am Rev Respir Dis.* 1967;96:971–976.

69. Wichser J, Kazemi H. Ammonia and ventilation: site and mechanism of action. *Respir Physiol.* 1974; 20:393–406.

70. Simmons DH, Nicoloff J, Guze LB. Hyperventilation and respiratory alkalosis as signs of gram-negative bacteremia. *JAMA.* 1960;174:2196–2199.

71. Trimble C, Smith DE, Rosenthal MH, et al. Pathophysiologic role of hypocarbia in post-traumatic pulmonary insufficiency. *Am J Surg.* 1971;122: 633–638.

72. Kraut JA, Madias NE. Approach to patients with acid-base disorders. *Respir Care.* 2001;46: 392–403.

73. Bear R, Goldstein M, Phillipson E, et al. Effect of metabolic alkalosis on respiratory function in patients with chronic obstructive lung disease. *Can Med Assoc J.* 1977;117:900–903.

74. Chang L-C, Hung S-C, Yang C. The case. A suicidal woman with delayed high anion gap metabolic acidosis. *Kidney International.* 2009;75:757–758.

75. Yip L, Dart RC, Gabow PA. Concepts and controversies in salicylate toxicity. *Emerg Med Clin North Am.* 1994;12:351–364.

CHAPTER

5

Disorders of Potassium Metabolism

BIFF F. PALMER AND THOMAS D. DUBOSE JR.

Introduction

Potassium plays a key role in maintaining cell function. All cells possess a Na^+/K^+ ATPase, which pumps Na^+ out of the cell and K^+ into the cell. This leads to a K^+ gradient across the cell membrane ($K^+_{in} > K^+_{out}$), which is partially responsible for maintaining the potential difference across the membrane. This potential difference is important to the function of all cells but is especially important in excitable tissues such as nerve and muscle. For these reasons, the body has developed numerous mechanisms for the defense of serum K^+. Total body K^+ is approximately 50 mEq/kg, which in a 70-kg person would be 3,500 mEq. The majority (98%) of this K^+ is within cells with only 2% in the extracellular fluid. The normal concentration of K^+ in the extracellular fluid is 3.5 to 5.3 mEq/L. Large deviations from these values are not compatible with life. The typical U.S. diet includes 50 to 100 mEq/day of K^+. Approximately 90% of the daily K^+ intake is excreted in the urine, while 10% is excreted in the gastrointestinal track. When K^+ intake increases or decreases, both urinary and fecal excretion rates respond directionally.

Potassium Handling: Old and New Concepts

Potassium is freely filtered by the glomerulus. The bulk of filtered K^+ is reabsorbed in the proximal tubule and loop of Henle such that only 10% of the filtered load reaches the distal nephron. In the proximal tubule K^+ absorption is passive and is in rough proportion to Na^+ and water absorption. In the thick ascending limb of Henle's loop K^+ reabsorption occurs via transport on the apical membrane $Na^+/K^+/2Cl^-$ (NKCC2) cotransporter. Secretion of K^+ occurs in the distal nephron, primarily in the initial collecting duct and the cortical collecting duct. Under most physiologic and pathologic conditions, K^+ delivery to the distal nephron remains small and is fairly constant. By contrast, the rate of K^+ secretion by the distal nephron varies significantly and is highly regulated according to physiologic needs. K^+ secretion in the distal nephron is generally responsible for most of urinary K^+ excretion.

The specialized cell that is responsible for K^+ secretion in the initial collecting duct and the cortical collecting duct is the principal cell (Fig. 5.1). This cell possesses a basolateral Na^+/K^+ ATPase, which is responsible for the active transport of K^+ from the blood into the cell. The resultant high intracellular K^+ concentration provides a favorable diffusion gradient for movement of K^+ from the cell into the lumen. In addition to establishing a high intracellular K^+ concentration, activity of this pump lowers intracellular Na^+ concentration, thus maintaining a favorable diffusion gradient for movement of Na^+ from the lumen into the cell. The movement of both Na^+ and K^+ across the apical membrane occurs via well-defined Na^+ and K^+ channels.

The cellular determinants of K^+ secretion include the cell K^+ concentration, luminal K^+ concentration, transepithelial potential difference (voltage) across the luminal membrane, and permeability of the luminal membrane for K^+. Any condition that increases cellular K^+ concentration, decreases luminal K^+ concentration, or renders the lumen more electronegative will increase the rate of K^+ secretion. In addition, any condition that increases the permeability of the luminal membrane for K^+ will increase the

137

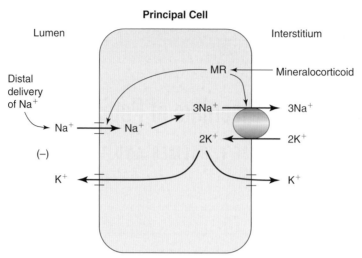

■ **Figure 5.1** Cell model for renal regulation of K^+ secretion by the principal cell in the collecting tubule. The negative sign represents the transepithelial voltage; lumen negative; an important driving force in K secretion.

rate of K^+ secretion. All of the physiologic determinants of renal K^+ secretion are found to affect one or more of the above cellular determinants of collecting tubule K^+ secretion. Two of the most important physiologic determinants are mineralocorticoid activity and distal delivery of Na^+ and water.

The major mineralocorticoid in humans is aldosterone. Aldosterone, secreted by the adrenal gland, interacts with the intracellular mineralocorticoid receptor in the principal cell to stimulate K^+ secretion by affecting several of the cellular determinants discussed above. First, aldosterone stimulates Na^+ reabsorption across the luminal membrane by increasing the open probability of the epithelial sodium channel (ENaC) on the apical membrane, which increases the electronegativity of the lumen, thereby increasing the electrical gradient, favoring K^+ secretion. Second, aldosterone increases intracellular K^+ concentration by stimulating the activity of the Na^+/K^+ ATPase in the basolateral membrane. Third, aldosterone directly increases the permeability of the luminal membrane to K^+. Thus, aldosterone increases the rate of K^+ secretion by increasing cell K^+ concentration, increasing luminal membrane K^+ permeability, and making the luminal potential more negative (Fig. 5.1).

A second important factor that affects K^+ secretion is the rate of distal delivery of Na^+ and water. An increase in the distal delivery of Na^+ stimulates distal Na^+ absorption, which will make the luminal potential more negative and thus increase K^+ secretion. Increased flow rates also increase K^+ secretion. When K^+ is secreted in the collecting duct, the luminal K^+ concentration increases, which decreases the diffusion gradient and slows further K^+ secretion. At higher luminal flow rates, the same amount of K^+ secretion will be diluted by the larger volume such that the increase in luminal K^+ concentration will be less. Thus, increases in the distal delivery of Na^+ and water stimulate K^+ secretion by lowering luminal K^+ concentration and by rendering the luminal potential more negative.

Two populations of K^+ channels have been identified in the cells of the cortical collecting duct (1). The renal outer medullary $\underline{K}^+$ (ROMK) channel is considered the major K^+-secretory pathway. This channel is characterized by having low conductance and a high probability of being open under physiologic conditions. The maxi-K^+ channel is characterized by a large single-channel conductance and is relatively quiescent in the basal state. Where this channel becomes activated is under conditions of increased flow. In addition to increased delivery of Na^+ and dilution of luminal K^+ concentration, recruitment of maxi-K^+ channels plays an important role in mediating flow-dependent increased K^+ secretion (2).

The effect of increased tubular flow to activate maxi-K^+ channels may be mediated by changes in intracellular Ca^{2+} concentration (3). The channel is known to be Ca^{2+} activated, and an acute increase in flow has been shown to increase intracellular Ca^{2+} concentration in the principal cell. It has been suggested that the central cilium (a structure present in principal cells) may play a role in transducing the signal of increased flow to increased intracellular Ca^{2+} concentration. In cultured cells bending of primary cilia results in a transient increase in intracellular Ca^{2+}, an effect blocked by antibodies to polycystin 2 (4).

In addition to stimulating maxi-K^+ channels, increased tubular flow has been shown to stimulate Na^+ absorption through the ENaC in the collecting duct. This increase in absorption is not only due to increased delivery of Na^+ but also appears to be the result of mechanosensitive properties intrinsic to the channel. Increased flow creates a shear stress, leading to an increase in open-channel probability with subsequent activation of the ENaC (5,6).

It has been hypothesized that the biomechanical regulation of renal tubular Na^+ and K^+ transport in the distal nephron may have evolved as a response to defend against sudden increases in extracellular K^+ concentration that would occur in response to ingestion of K^+-rich diets typical of early vertebrates (3). According to this hypothesis an increase in glomerular filtration rate (GFR) following a protein rich meal would lead to an increase in distal flow, activating the ENaC, increasing intracellular Ca^{2+} concentration, and activating maxi-K^+ channels. These events would enhance K^+ secretion, thus providing an important buffer to guard against the development of hyperkalemia.

This interest in the renal response to a high-K^+, low-Na^+ diet characteristic of Paleolithic man has been studied in a rat model (7,8). Wistar rats were fed a diet very low in NaCl and K^+ for several days. A pharmacologic dose of deoxycorticosterone was also given to ensure a constant and nonvariable effect of mineralocorticoids. Following a KCl load administered into the peritoneal cavity, two distinct phases were noted. In the first 2 hours, there was a large increase in the rate of renal K^+ excretion largely accounted for by an increase in the K^+ concentration in the cortical collecting duct. During this early phase, flow through the collecting duct increased only slightly. The authors speculated that insertion of K^+ channels into the lumen of the collecting duct was likely responsible for these early changes. In support, dietary supplementation of K^+ has been shown to increase channel density of both ROMK and maxi-K^+ channels (9).

In the subsequent 4 hours, renal K^+ excretion continued to be high, but during this second phase, the kaliuresis was mostly accounted for by increased flow through the collecting duct. This increased flow was attributed to an inhibitory effect of increased interstitial K^+ concentration on reabsorption of NaCl in the upstream ascending limb of Henle, an effect supported by microperfusion studies published more that 20 years ago (10). Increased interstitial K^+ concentration would have the effect of lowering the negative potential across the basolateral membrane of cells in the thick limb, secondarily decreasing Cl^- exit. The rise in intracellular Cl^- concentration would inhibit apical NaCl reabsorption and thus increase distal delivery.

The timing of the two phases described in this model is presumably important, since the higher flow would be most effective in promoting kaliuresis in the setting of increased channel density. Presumably the inhibitory effect of interstitial K^+ on thick-limb function is short lived and relatively precise so that Na^+ delivered distally is only an amount necessary to maximally stimulate K^+ secretion and nothing more. Excessive delivery of Na^+ would predispose to volume depletion, given the low Na^+ content of the diet.

The ability of dietary K^+ to modulate the density of apical K^+ channels has recently been linked to changes in members of the with-no-lysine [K] (WNK) family of kinases. The name is derived from the atypical placement of the catalytic lysine compared with other types of kinases. There are four mammalian WNK family members, each of which is encoded by a different gene. Mutations in certain members of this family are responsible for the development of Gordon syndrome, which is discussed in more detail in the section dealing with hyperkalemia (11).

WNK1 is ubiquitously expressed throughout the body in multiple spliced forms. For example, a long WNK1 transcript has been identified in all cell lines and tissues examined. By contrast, a shorter WNK1 transcript lacking the N-terminal 1-437 amino acids of the long transcript is highly expressed in the kidney but not in other tissues and is referred to as kidney-specific WNK1 (KS-WNK1). Quantitative analysis shows much greater renal expression of this KS-WNK1 versus long WNK1 (85% vs. 15%) (12).

Changes in the ratio of KS-WNK1 and long WNK1 in response to dietary K^+ play an important role in the physiologic regulation of renal K^+ excretion (13–16). Long WNK1 inhibits ROMK by stimulating its endocytosis, whereas KS-WNK1 functions as a physiologic antagonist to the actions of long WNK1. Under the condition of dietary K^+ restriction, the relative abundance of long WNK1 to KS-WNK1 is increased. These changes lead to decreased abundance of ROMK in the renal cortical collecting duct, which is an adaptive response important for renal K^+ conservation. By contrast, dietary K^+ loading increases the abundance of KS-WNK1 relative to long WNK1 and is accompanied by upregulation of ROMK. In addition to reversing the inhibition of ROMK caused by long WNK1, KS-WNK1 exerts a stimulatory effect on the ENaC, thus increasing the lumen-negative potential. The combined effects of increased ROMK abundance along with a more lumen-negative potential facilitate K^+ secretion in the setting of a high-K^+ diet.

The changes in KS-WNK1 and long WNK1 that occur in response to dietary K^+ intake also have affects on renal Na^+ handling that may be of importance in the observed relationship between dietary K^+ intake and hypertension. Epidemiologic studies have established that K^+ intake is inversely related to the prevalence of hypertension (17). In addition, K^+ supplements and avoidance of hypokalemia lower blood pressure in hypertensive subjects. By contrast, blood pressure increases in hypertensive subjects placed on a low-K^+ diet. This increase in blood pressure is associated with increased renal Na^+ reabsorption (18).

As previously mentioned, K^+ deficiency increases the ratio of long WNK1 to KS-WNK1 and is associated with increased retrieval of ROMK from the plasma membrane. Long WNK1 has also been shown to stimulate ENaC activity through activation of serum and glucocorticoid-regulated kinase (SGK1) (19,20). SGK1 inactivates the ubiquitin–protein ligase Nedd4-2 through phosphorylation, resulting in less retrieval of ENaC from the apical membrane. Increased activity of long WNK1 also releases the inhibitory affect of WNK4 on Na^+ reabsorption mediated by the NaCl cotransporter (NCC). These effects suggest the decrease in K^+ secretion under conditions of K^+ deficiency will occur at the expense of increased Na^+ retention. Such changes could play a role in the genesis of salt-sensitive hypertension in patient populations ingesting a low-K^+, high-Na^+ diet (Fig. 5.2).

Given that WNK1 is ubiquitously expressed, changes in activity may affect blood pressure through effects on the peripheral vasculature. In this regard, WNK1 activates the NKCC2 cotransporter (21). Decreased activity of this cotransporter leads to hypotension and decreased vascular smooth muscle tone. By inference, increased activity of WNK1 might increase blood pressure by increasing vascular resistance. WNK3 is a related member of the WNK kinase family whose function has not been well characterized. Recent data indicated it is expressed throughout the nephron and, like WNK1, is a potent activator of the NKCC2 cotransporter (22). The role of WNK kinases in regulating blood pressure is an unfolding area that deserves further investigation.

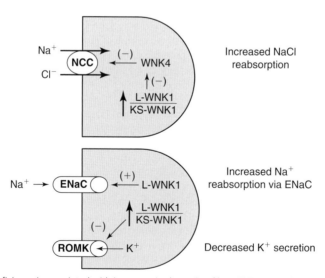

■ **Figure 5.2** K^+ deficiency is associated with increases in the ratio of long WNK1 to KS-WNK1. An increase in this ratio (L-WNK1/KS-WNK1) leads to increased retrieval of ROMK from the apical membrane, thereby minimizing K^+ secretion, which would be an appropriate response to a K^+-deficient diet (*lower cell*). Increased L-WNK1/KS-WNK1 also releases the inhibitory effect of WNK4 on the thiazide-sensitive Na^+/Cl^- cotransporter (*upper cell*). In addition, increased L-WNK1 leads to increased activity of ENaC (*lower cell*). These later two effects lead to salt retention and may explain the genesis of salt-sensitive hypertension in subjects ingesting K^+-deficient diets. KS-WNK1, kidney-specific with-no-lysine [K]; ROMK, renal outer medullary K^+; ENaC, epithelial sodium channel.

Hypokalemia

APPROACH TO THE HYPOKALEMIA PATIENT

Hypokalemia is frequently encountered in clinical practice. Transient causes of hypokalemia are due to cell shift, while sustained hypokalemia is either due to inadequate intake or excessive K^+ loss. Hypokalemia resulting from excessive K^+ loss can be due to renal or extrarenal losses. The clinical history, physical examination with particular emphasis on determination of volume status, and determination of the acid–base status will allow the cause of hypokalemia to be readily determined in most cases.

Assessment of renal K^+ excretion allows one to determine whether hypokalemia is due to renal or extrarenal causes. Renal K^+ handling can be assessed with a 24-hour urine collection or a spot urine, determining the K^+/creatinine ratio. A 24-hour urinary K^+ of <15 mEq or a K^+ (mmol)/creatinine (mmol) ratio <1 suggests an extrarenal cause of hypokalemia.

The main limitation to the use of a spot urine K^+ is the influence of renal water handling on urine K^+ concentration. Two patients with similar renal K^+ excretion would have significantly different urine K^+ concentrations, depending on whether the urine was concentrated or dilute. To overcome this effect the transtubular K^+ gradient (TTKG) has been proposed as a useful tool to assess renal K^+ handling.

$$\text{TTKG} = \frac{[K_{urine}/(U_{osmolality}/S_{osmolality})]}{K_{serum}} \tag{5.1}$$

The K^+ concentration in the final urine will exceed the concentration at the beginning of the collecting duct as a result of water reabsorption along the length of the collecting duct. To account for this effect, the equation divides the urine K^+ concentration by the ratio of the urine osmolality to serum osmolality. In an otherwise normal subject ingesting a typical Western diet, the TTKG ranges from 8 to 9 and will increase to >11 with increased K^+ intake. In a chronically hyperkalemic subject a value <5 would indicate impaired renal K^+ excretion, as a result of either aldosterone deficiency or resistance. In patients with hypokalemia due to extrarenal K^+ losses, the TTKG should fall to values <3.

It is worthwhile considering some of the assumptions made in calculating the TTKG (23). First, the calculation assumes there is no significant solute transport and only water reabsorption as fluid enters the medullary collecting duct. Any Na^+ or urea reabsorption in this segment would tend to lower urine osmolality and cause the TTKG to overestimate the gradient for K^+ secretion in the upstream collecting duct. Second, conditions should be optimal for K^+ secretion at the time the TTKG is measured. In this regard, urine Na^+ should be no less than 25 mEq/L to ensure Na^+ delivery to the collecting duct is not rate limiting in K^+ secretion. In addition, urine osmolality should be equal to and ideally greater than the plasma. A higher urine osmolality reflects increased vasopressin, which is known to exert a stimulatory effect on K^+ secretion in the collecting duct.

While the TTKG is of interest, in most settings a spot urine K^+ concentration and the clinical setting will be sufficient in determining the cause of K^+ disturbances. Calculation of the TTKG may prove useful in those patients in whom the cause of dyskalemia continues to remain in doubt.

ETIOLOGY OF HYPOKALEMIA

Low K^+ Intake

While the kidney can elaborate urine virtually free of Na^+ in response to dietary Na^+ restriction, the kidney can only reduce urinary K^+ to approximately 15 mEq/day in response to a K^+-free diet. As a result extreme dietary restriction of K^+, as might occur with a fad diet or eating disorder, can conceivably lead to hypokalemia over time. An example of such dietary restriction might occur in patients with anorexia nervosa. Hypokalemia is of particular concern, given its association with QT prolongation and ventricular arrhythmias (24). Such changes have been suggested as playing an etiologic role in the increased risk of sudden death reported in these patients.

More commonly, dietary K^+ restriction simply exacerbates the hypokalemia that is due to other causes. In a recent report life-threatening hypokalemia developed in a patient with undiagnosed primary hyperaldosteronism after starting a low-carbohydrate, low-calorie diet (25). In addition to less dietary K^+ intake, worsening hypokalemia can also be the result of increased renal K^+ excretion in this setting. Low-carbohydrate diets are accompanied by a period of increased ketogenesis. The excretion of these acids by the kidney in the form of sodium salts results in increased distal delivery of Na^+ in the setting of increased aldosterone. As a result renal K^+ wasting is exacerbated.

Cellular Redistribution

Total body K^+ content in a typical 70-kg subject is approximately 3,500 mEq. Of the total body K^+, 98% is located in the intracellular space primarily in skeletal muscle, while 2% is found in the extracellular space. The extracellular K^+ concentration is tightly regulated in order to maintain normal cell membrane excitability. The kidney is primarily responsible for maintaining total body K^+ content by matching K^+ intake with K^+ excretion. Since adjustments in renal K^+ excretion can take several hours, changes in extracellular K^+ concentration are initially buffered by movement of K^+ into or out of skeletal muscle. The two most important factors that regulate this movement under normal conditions are insulin and catecholamines. For example, following a meal the postprandial release of insulin not only functions to regulate the serum glucose concentration but also functions to shift dietary K^+ into cells until the kidney excretes the K^+ load reestablishing normal total body K^+ content. During exercise the release of catecholamines through β_2 stimulation limits the increase in extracellular K^+ concentration that would otherwise occur as a result of the normal K^+ release by contracting muscle.

Pathologic stimulation of β_2 receptors can result in symptomatic hypokalemia. For example, hypokalemic paralysis is a potential complication of the hyperadrenergic state that oftentimes accompanies alcohol withdrawal syndromes (26). Clenbuterol is a β_2 adrenergic agonist with a rapid onset and long duration of action approved for limited use in veterinary medicine. The drug has been used illicitly as an alternative to anabolic steroids due to its effects of increasing muscle mass. Hypokalemia as a result of clenbuterol toxicity has now been reported in users of heroin adulterated with clenbuterol (27).

Intracellular K^+ also serves as a reservoir to limit the fall in extracellular K^+ concentration that occurs under pathologic conditions in which there is loss of K^+ from the body. An example of the efficiency of this buffering effect was previously reported in military recruits undergoing training in summer (28). The trainees were found to have K^+ losses of >40 mEq/day in sweat alone. At the end of 11 days, subjects exhibited a total body K^+ deficit of approximately 400 mEq and yet the serum K^+ concentration was maintained near normal.

Recent work has been devoted to better define the role of skeletal muscle in regulating extracellular K^+ concentration (29). In these studies the movement of K^+ into skeletal muscle is indirectly determined by use of a K^+ clamp. With this technique insulin is administered to rats at a constant rate. K^+ is simultaneously infused at a rate designed to prevent any drop in plasma K^+ concentration. Frequent measurements of plasma K^+ values serve as a guide. The amount of K^+ administered is presumed to be equal to the amount of K^+ entering the intracellular compartment.

This model was used to study the effect of total body K^+ depletion on insulin-stimulated K^+ uptake. In rats deprived of K^+ for 10 days, the plasma K^+ concentration decreased from 4.2 to 2.9 mmol/L. Insulin-mediated K^+ disappearance declined by >90% when compared to control values. This decrease in K^+ uptake was accompanied by a >50% reduction in both the activity and the expression of muscle Na^+/K^+ ATPase, suggesting that decreased pump activity might account for the decrease in the effect of insulin. When measured after only 2 days of deprivation, there was also a significant decline in insulin-mediated K^+ uptake despite the fact that plasma K^+ concentration had only decreased slightly (4.2 to 3.8 mmol/L). Interestingly, the expression and activity of the Na^+/K^+ ATPase was still normal, suggesting the initial resistance to insulin-mediated K^+ uptake is due to some other mechanism other than decreased pump activity or expression. This decrease in muscle K^+ uptake under conditions of K^+ depletion may serve to limit an excessive decrease in extracellular K^+ concentration that might otherwise occur under conditions in which insulin is stimulated. These changes would still allow skeletal muscle to buffer any decline in extracellular K^+ concentration by donating some component of its intracellular stores.

Since chronic K^+ depletion decreases skeletal muscle Na^+/K^+ ATPase expression and activity, one would expect that the ability to clear an acute K^+ load under these conditions would be diminished and potentially result in dangerously high levels of plasma K^+. This hypothesis was tested by administering intravenous KCl acutely to rats fed a K^+-free diet for 2 weeks (30,31). In contrast to what was predicted, total

K^+ clearance capacity was actually greater in the K^+-depleted animals when compared with K^+-replete controls. The skeletal muscle Na^+/K^+ ATPase pool size was decreased, but the decrease was found to be specific to the α-2 isoform, which is the major form found in skeletal muscle. There was no change in the less abundant α-1 isoform. By contrast, the cardiac Na^+/K^+ ATPase pool size increased in K^+-deficient animals. Like skeletal muscle there was a decrease in the α-2 isoform but a significant increase in the α-1 isoform, which is the dominant form found in the heart. At baseline the decrease in myocardial K^+ content was considerably less compared with skeletal muscle. Despite a smaller deficit of K^+, the myocardial uptake of K^+ during the intravenous infusion of K^+ was of the same magnitude as skeletal muscle.

These findings indicate significant differences between skeletal and cardiac muscle in the response to K^+ depletion. While skeletal muscle readily relinquishes K^+ to help minimize the drop in plasma K^+ concentration, cardiac tissue K^+ content remains relatively preserved. This difference can be attributed, at least in part, to Na^+/K^+ ATPase isoform differences in the response to K^+ depletion. Cardiac muscle accumulates a considerable amount of K^+ in the setting of an acute load. When expressed on a weight basis, the cardiac capacity for K^+ uptake is comparable to that of skeletal muscle under conditions of K^+ depletion and may actually exceed skeletal muscle under control conditions.

Potassium administration in patients with chronic hypokalemia may result in hyperkalemia. This response may be due to the chronic suppression of aldosterone elaboration by hypokalemia. Therefore, in summary, the rate of potassium replacement in the chronic hypokalemic patient should be relatively slow and monitored closely.

Hypokalemic periodic paralysis is a rare disorder that is characterized by muscle weakness or paralysis due to the sudden movement of K^+ into cells. The attacks are precipitated by rest after exercise, stress, high-carbohydrate meals, and events accompanied by increased release of catecholamines or insulin. This disorder may be familial or acquired.

The acquired form of periodic paralysis typically develops in association with thyrotoxicosis and has been the subject of several recent reviews (32–34). Thyrotoxic periodic paralysis is more commonly seen in Asians but has also been reported with higher frequency in American Indians and Hispanics. While the incidence of thyrotoxicosis is typically more common in women, there is a male to female predominance that ranges from 17:1 to 70:1 in those who develop hypokalemic periodic paralysis. The typical patient is a young adult male aged 20 to 40 who presents with weakness most commonly between 2100 and 0900 hours during the summer months. The attacks are precipitated by conditions characterized by increased release of catecholamines or insulin, such as stress, high-carbohydrate meals, and exercise. With regard to exercise, the timing of attacks is typically in the initial rest period following exertion. Oftentimes the attacks are heralded by muscle cramps and aches, and many patients learn to avoid paralytic episodes by exercising the involved muscle groups. Hypophosphatemia and hypomagnesemia are also common during acute attacks and like K^+ are the result of shifts into the intracellular compartment. There is a single case report of lactic acidosis occurring during an acute attack (35).

Excess thyroid hormone may predispose to paralytic episodes by increasing Na^+/K^+ ATPase activity. The activity of this pump is likely to be increased further by catechols, which are typically increased in this setting. The underlying cause of thyrotoxicosis is most commonly Graves disease but can also be a solitary thyroid adenoma, a thyroid stimulating hormone–secreting pituitary adenoma, or abuse of thyroid hormone. Iodine-induced thyrotoxicosis (Jod–Basedow syndrome) and associated hypokalemic periodic paralysis have been reported following the administration of iodine-containing radiocontrast agents, amiodarone, and kelp supplements (36–38). "Dream Shape" and "Ever Youth" are two herbal medications used for weight reduction, reported to cause iodine-induced thyrotoxicosis without periodic paralysis.

The acute attacks are treated with intravenous KCl and propranolol. It is important to administer KCl in non-dextrose-containing solutions, since glucose will stimulate insulin release, potentially exacerbating the movement of K^+ into cells. In order to minimize the likelihood of rebound hyperkalemia, K^+ should be given at doses <10 mmol/h. Propranolol (a nonspecific β-adrenergic blocker) blocks the effects of catecholamines and inhibits the peripheral conversion of T_4 to T_3. The definitive treatment is to remove the underlying cause of thyrotoxicosis. Periodic paralysis does not recur once the patient is euthyroid.

The familial form of hypokalemic periodic paralysis is inherited as an autosomal dominant disorder and has similar clinical features as the acquired form. Notable differences include a younger age at presentation (usually <20 yr), an equal male–female distribution, and appearance mostly in Caucasians. The familial disorder is most commonly due to mutations in the muscle calcium channel α-1 subunit gene (CACNA1S) on chromosome 1q3132. The α-1 subunit of the calcium channel serves as the pore for movement of calcium into the T tubule and also contains the dihydropyridine binding site. Mutations of this subunit reduce the calcium current into the T tubule. The precise mechanism by which impaired function of the calcium channel dihydropyridine receptor causes the influx of K^+ into muscle cells is not entirely clear. A smaller number of cases have been localized to mutations in the skeletal muscle sodium channel SCN4A and the R83H mutation in the K^+ channel subunit gene KCNE3. Mutations in these genes are not found in patients with thyrotoxic hypokalemic periodic paralysis (39).

The clinical phenotype of patients, together with the pattern of response to therapy, has been shown to differ, depending on the location of the mutation. The carbonic anhydrase inhibitor, acetazolamide, is typically an effective therapy in reducing the number of attacks in patients with the familial disorder. The effectiveness of the drug has been attributed to induction of metabolic acidosis, which would in turn limit the intracellular shift of K^+ into cells. However, recent work in an animal model of periodic paralysis suggests the beneficial effects of the drug are actually due to a direct stimulatory effect on Ca^{2+}-activated K^+ channels and not the induction of metabolic acidosis (40). While generally effective, a small number of patients given acetazolamide may demonstrate an exacerbation of symptoms (41). In this regard, the R83H mutation in the K^+ channel subunit gene KCNE3 reduces single-channel conductance compared to wild-type channels (42). This decrease in conductance is further reduced under conditions of low pH. It has been suggested that this mutation may explain the tendency for paralytic attacks to occur postexercise, since skeletal muscle intracellular pH drops during this period. In addition this sensitivity to acidosis could provide an explanation for why some patients with this disease worsen after acetazolamide therapy.

Another condition that needs to be considered when evaluating a hypokalemic patient with paralysis is distal renal tubular acidosis (dRTA) (43–46). Muscle paralysis in this disorder can begin insidiously with weakness evolving gradually over a 24- to 48-hour time period to complete flaccid quadriplegia. Attacks of flaccid paralysis in dRTA have been referred to as an "RTA crisis" by some authors because this striking clinical manifestation may result in the clinician's overlooking the underlying cause. Most of these cases have occurred in patients with distal renal tubular acidosis that is idiopathic in origin or as a manifestation of Sjögrens syndrome. There is one report of aristolochic acid–induced Fanconi syndrome presenting in this manner (47).

Extrarenal K$^+$ Loss from the Body

Cutaneous loss of K^+ sufficient to cause hypokalemia is uncommon but may occur in the setting of intense exercise in a hot, humid environment. Under these conditions large volumes of sweat can be lost each day. Sweat rates of approximately 2 L/h were found in a study of football players who were members of a National Collegiate Athletic Association Division II team undergoing preseason training (48). The players practiced 4.5 h/day and therefore were losing 9 L of sweat per day. This rate of sweat loss was no different whether practices were conducted in half pads or full pads. Body weight only declined between 1 and 2 kg, depending on the time of day body weight was measured, since the players were allowed free access to water.

A similar sweat volume loss (2.1 L) was found in elite soccer players studied during a single 90-minute preseason training session (49–51). As observed in the football players, body weight declined by a lesser amount (1.2 kg) secondary to fluid intake. Na^+ and K^+ concentration was measured in sweat samples obtained from absorbent sweat pads placed on the chest, forearm, back, and thigh of the soccer players. Sweat Na^+ concentration was 30 mmol/L, and total sweat Na^+ loss was 67 mmol. The respective values for K^+ were 3.58 mmol/L and 8 mmol. There are two points worth emphasizing in these studies. First, sweat losses can be substantial in well-trained athletes during exercise. Despite the free availability of water, these athletes remain mildly dehydrated in the immediate postexercise period. Second, while the K^+ concentration is low in sweat, significant total body K^+ loss can develop when sweat volume is high.

There is an impression by many that cramps that develop in athletes are related to loss of K^+ in sweat. To address this issue sweat Na^+ and K^+ losses were measured in division I collegiate football players undergoing practice sessions twice daily (52). Values obtained were compared between players with a history of heat cramps (C) and teammates with no history of cramping (NC). In a 2.5-hour practice session, sweat loss was similar between the two groups (4.0 l [C] vs. 3.5 l [NC]). Sweat K^+ was also similar in the two groups, but sweat Na^+ was two times higher in players with a history of heat cramps (54 vs. 25 mmol/L). These data suggest it is large, acute Na^+ and fluid loss rather than K^+ loss that is associated with a tendency to develop cramps during exercise.

Gastrointestinal loss is a common cause of hypokalemia and is generally due to diarrhea. Secretory diarrhea is generally believed to be caused by one of two processes that can either occur alone or both together (53,54). First, there can be inhibition of active intestinal NaCl and $NaHCO_3$ reabsorption, and second, there can be stimulation of active chloride secretion, which is then followed by passive secretion of an equal amount of Na^+ so as to maintain electrochemical balance. In both of these instances, the stool electrolyte content is similar to plasma, with high concentration of NaCl and much lower K^+ concentration. The sodium salts in stool cause an isotonic increase in stool water output such that the fecal content of sodium salts roughly parallels the volume of diarrhea. Despite the low K^+ concentration in fecal fluid, significant total body K^+ losses can occur in the setting of large stool volumes.

Severe K^+ depletion due to secretory diarrhea has been the subject of recent case reports. One patient with neurofibromatosis type 1 presented with the syndrome of watery diarrhea, hypokalemia, and achlohydria (WDHA) due to oversecretion of vasoactive intestinal polypeptide (VIP) (55). A neuroendocrine tumor composed of pheochromocytoma and ganglioneuroma was responsible for the VIP production. A second patient presented with hypokalemia complicated by rhabdomyolysis due to oversecretion of pancreatic polypeptide from a pancreatic islet tumor (56). Pancreatic polypeptide (PP) normally exerts an inhibitory effect on gastric emptying and upper gastrointestinal motility but has been reported to cause a watery diarrhea syndrome similar to that as a VIPoma. In this patient severe hypokalemia developed with minimal gastrointestinal complaints. The authors speculated that the inhibitory effect of PP on gut motility may have attenuated the development of watery diarrhea. Hypokalemia and volume depletion can also occur in association with villous adenomas, a symptom complex referred to as the McKittrick–Wheelock syndrome (57). A patient with this syndrome caused by a rectal adenocarcinoma has been reported.

Abnormalities in K^+ transport have not previously been known to be the primary cause of secretory diarrhea. The first such case has recently been described in an elderly woman with colonic pseudo-obstruction (Ogilvie syndrome) (58). One week after undergoing surgical treatment of a hip fracture, a 78-year-old woman developed diarrhea, hypokalemia, and a markedly dilated colon. The work-up excluded identifiable causes of intestinal obstruction and diarrhea. Fecal fluid was collected on multiple occasions, and electrolyte content was measured. In contrast to the high Na^+ concentration (101 to 137 mEq/L) and low K^+ concentration (16 to 51 mEq/L) typically found in various causes of secretory diarrhea, fecal electrolyte concentration in this patient was reversed. Fecal K^+ concentration ranged from 130 to 170 mEq/L, while values for Na^+ concentration varied between 4 to 15 mEq/L. In addition increased stool weight was accompanied by a proportionate increase in fecal K^+ output, while stool Na^+ changed very little. Measurement of the rectosigmoid potential difference in this patient was -13 mV (lumen negative). When the data were interpreted in the context of the Nernst equation, the authors concluded there was evidence of active K^+ secretion along with active Na^+ reabsorption across the colonic mucosa. The patient's pseudo-obstruction spontaneously resolved over a 14-week period.

As in the kidney, K^+ is actively absorbed and secreted in the colon, whereas in the small intestine, K^+ movement is strictly diffusional. Colonic K^+ absorption occurs via an H^+/K^+ ATPase located on the luminal membrane, while K^+ secretion occurs via a luminal channel (59,60). Dietary K^+ restriction increases colonic K^+ absorption, while secretion predominates with high dietary K^+ intake. In patients with end-stage renal disease, increased secretion of K^+ by the colon is an important adaptation to K^+ homeostasis. Recent studies indicate colonic K^+ secretion is mediated by the BK channel (61). This channel is a high-conductance channel that is activated by calcium. It is located exclusively in the colonic crypts and not on surface cells. Increased expression of this channel may mediate the enhanced colonic K^+ secretion in patients with end-stage renal disease.

Bowel-cleansing solutions can occasionally be associated with perturbations in serum electrolyte levels to include hypokalemia, hyperphosphatemia, hypocalcemia, and hypernatremia. Risk factors for these disturbances include advanced age, the presence of bowel obstruction, poor gut motility, and unrecognized renal disease. Use of oral sodium phosphate has recently been linked to the development of acute renal failure characterized histologically by widespread deposition of calcium phosphate crystals (62). A recent study randomly allocated 100 consecutive patients who were to undergo colonoscopy to receive either sodium phosphate or a glycol–electrolyte solution (Golytely, Braintree Laboratories) for bowel cleansing (63). Eleven patients received sodium phosphate despite the presence of factors that would have identified them as being at risk for complications. In six of these high-risk patients, the serum phosphate doubled, and hypokalemia developed in four. In subjects without risk factors, mild hyperphosphatemia developed in 39% and hypocalcemia developed in 5%. In the glycol–electrolyte-solution–treated patients, only mild and clinically insignificant changes in serum electrolyte values occurred. The glycol–electrolyte solution is a nonabsorbable and osmotically balanced solution and has virtually no net effect on electrolyte absorption or secretion.

Severe hypokalemia can result from K^+ binding in the gastrointestinal tract. A serum K^+ concentration of 0.9 mmol/L was found in a 3-year-old girl, following several days of oral and rectal administration of bentonite given as a home remedy for the treatment of constipation (64). Bentonite, also called montmorillonite or fuller's earth, is a type of clay primarily composed of hydrated aluminum silicate. Clay eating (geophagia) can be a manifestation of pica and has been reported to cause hypokalemic paralysis during pregnancy and in the postpartum period (65,66).

Renal Potassium Wasting

The elaboration of aldosterone and distal delivery of Na^+ and water are two important factors in the renal excretion of K^+. Although increased distal delivery of Na^+ and water and increased aldosterone activity can each stimulate renal K^+ secretion, under normal physiologic conditions, these two determinants are inversely related. It is for this reason that K^+ excretion is independent of volume status. For example, under conditions of a contracted extracellular fluid volume, aldosterone levels increase. At the same time, proximal salt and water absorption increase, resulting in decreased distal delivery of Na^+ and water. Renal K^+ excretion remains fairly constant under these conditions, since the stimulatory effect of increased aldosterone is counterbalanced by the decreased delivery of filtrate to the distal nephron. A similar situation occurs in the setting of expansion of the extracellular fluid volume. In this setting, distal delivery of filtrate is increased as a result of decreased proximal tubular fluid reabsorption. Under conditions of volume expansion, circulating aldosterone levels are decreased. The effect of the increased delivery of Na^+ and water to stimulate K^+ excretion is opposed by decreased circulating aldosterone levels such that renal K^+ excretion again remains constant.

Thus, there is a balanced reciprocal relationship between urinary flow rates and circulating aldosterone levels, which serves to maintain K^+ balance during normal volume regulation. It is only under pathophysiologic conditions that distal Na^+ delivery and aldosterone become coupled. In this setting, renal K^+ wasting will occur (Fig. 5.3). When treating patients who are hypokalemic as a result of renal K^+ wasting, it must be determined whether there is a primary increase in mineralocorticoid activity or a primary increase in distal Na^+ delivery.

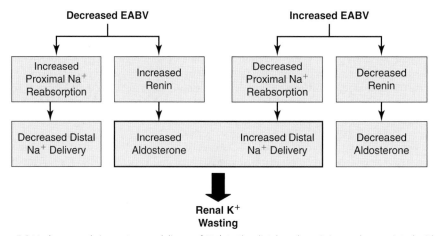

■ **Figure 5.3** Under normal circumstances delivery of Na^+ to the distal nephron is inversely associated with serum aldosterone levels. For this reason, renal K^+ excretion is kept independent of changes in extracellular fluid volume. Hypokalemia due to renal K^+ wasting can be explained by pathophysiologic changes that lead to coupling of increased distal Na^+ delivery and aldosterone or aldosterone-like effects, as shown by events leading to the area within the box.

PRIMARY INCREASE IN MINERALOCORTICOID ACTIVITY

Increases in mineralocorticoid activity can be due to primary increases in renin secretion, primary increases in aldosterone secretion, increases in a nonaldosterone mineralocorticoid, or increases in mineralocorticoid-like effects. In all of these conditions extracellular fluid volume is expanded and hypertension is typically present. The differential diagnosis for the patient with hypertension, hypokalemia, and metabolic alkalosis rests on the renin and aldosterone levels (Fig. 5.4).

Increased Renin, Increased Aldosterone

Renin-secreting tumors are most commonly hemangiopericytomas. These tumors are highly vascular and arise from the pericapillary pericytes of Zimmerman and postcapillary venules. These tumors have also been associated with the development of oncogenic osteomalacia due to overproduction of fibroblast growth factor 23 and the Kasabach–Merritt syndrome. This syndrome describes the presence of a consumptive coagulopathy in which thrombocytopenia is a major feature.

Renal artery stenosis can be associated with activation of the renin–angiotenisn–aldosterone cascade as a result of renal ischemia. Hypokalemia is seen in approximately 15% of cases. When hyponatremia is also present, the term "hyponatremic-hypertensive syndrome" has been applied (67,68).

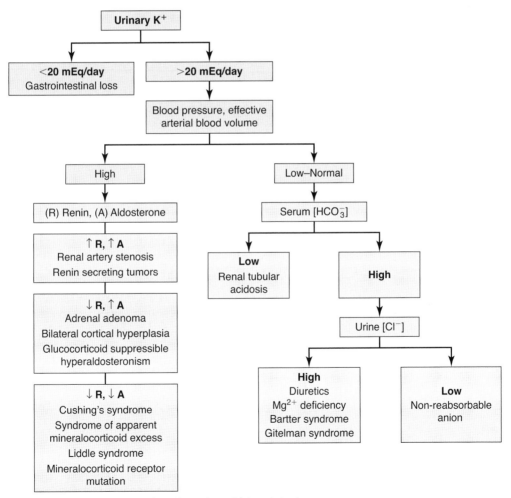

■ **Figure 5.4** Diagnostic approach to the patient with hypokalemia.

Suppressed Renin, Increased Aldosterone

The most common disease in this category is primary aldosteronism due to either an adrenal adenoma or bilateral adrenal hyperplasia. The most common screening test used to detect this entity is measurement of the ratio of plasma aldosterone concentration to plasma renin activity (PAC/PRA). The mean value of this ratio in normals or patients with essential hypertension is 4 to 10. Patients with primary hyperaldosteronism have values of 30 to 50 (69). If this test is positive then confirmatory testing is indicated. Intravenous saline loading, oral sodium loading, or the fludrocortisone suppression test can be used for this purpose (70).

Glucocorticoid-remediable aldosteronism (GRA) is the most common monogenic cause of human hypertension. The disease is inherited in an autosomal dominant fashion and is characterized by adrenocorticotropin hormone (ACTH)-dependent aldosterone secretion. GRA results from the unequal crossover of two genes: the CYP11B1 gene that encodes the enzyme 11β-hydroxylase and the CYP11B2 gene that encodes the enzyme aldosterone synthase (18-hydroxylase). The product of this event creates a chimeric gene in which the ACTH-responsive promoter is fused to the aldosterone-synthase coding sequence. As a result, aldosterone synthase is ectopically expressed in the cortisol-producing zone of the adrenal cortex (zona fasciculata) and is under the control of ACTH. Suppression of aldosterone with exogenous administration of dexamethasone is a useful diagnostic and therapeutic strategy. Measurement of urinary cortisol metabolites can also be useful as a diagnostic tool (71). Increased urinary excretion of 18-hydroxycortisol is typical of this disease.

For unclear reasons, random K^+ levels are frequently normal in patients with GRA. One possibility may be that the stimulatory effect on aldosterone release is only intermittent, since ACTH is secreted centrally in a diurnal fashion with peaks in the early morning and evening. GRA patients have been noted to develop hypokalemia frequently when treated with thiazide or loop diuretics.

Suppressed Renin and Aldosterone

Cushing disease or syndrome is the most common disease within this category. The clinical manifestations of Cushing disease results from the chronic exposure to excess glucocorticoids. Such manifestations include moon facies, abdominal obesity, buffalo hump, and striae. Fluid and electrolyte manifestations include hypertension and hypokalemic alkalosis. High concentrations of cortisol overwhelm the kidneys' ability to convert cortisol to cortisone and result in activation of the mineralocorticoid receptor.

There are monogenic forms of hypertension characterized by suppressed circulating levels of renin and aldosterone (72). An autosomal recessive disorder that prevents the production of cortisol is 11β-hydroxylase deficiency. The lack of feedback control results in high ACTH levels, which in turns drives the synthesis of 11-deoxycortisol and 11-deoxycorticosterone. These compounds have mineralocortiocid-like effects and cause Na^+ retention and renal K^+ wasting. Precursors of cortisol are also driven to increased production of androgens so that such patients have clinical features of virilization.

A rare disorder that also interferes in the synthesis of cortisol is $17\ \alpha$-hydroxylase. As with 11β-hydroxylase deficiency, hypertension and hypokalemia develop due to the accumulation and mineralocorticoid-like effects of 11-deoxycortisol and 11-deoxycorticosterone. This disorder is also accompanied by a reduction in androgen production and estrogen deficiency.

The reabsorption of Na^+ across the apical membrane in the collecting duct occurs through an amiloride-sensitive Na^+ channel formed by the assembly of three subunits: α, β, and γ. Liddle syndrome is an inherited form of hypertension and hypokalemic metabolic alkalosis caused by mutations in this channel. These mutations either delete or alter residues in the C-terminal PY motif of the β and γ subunits. The PY motif of α, β, and γ subunits is the binding site for the WW domain of a cytoplasmic protein called Nedd4–2. The binding of Nedd4–2 to the PY motif on each of the three subunits leads to ubiquination of the epithelial sodium channel, tagging it for eventual endocytosis and degradation. Interference in this binding leads to an inability to retrieve the channel from the membrane and results in increased channel density. The resultant increase in channel density gives rise to the clinical characteristics suggesting constitutive activation of the epithelial sodium channel (73,74).

In addition to increased surface density, there is evidence that Liddle syndrome mutations may also enhance Na^+ transport by increasing the open-state probability of ENaC (75). Under normal conditions

ENaC exists at the cell surface in two distinct pools. In one pool, the extracellular domain of the subunits has been proteolytically cleaved and has a high open-channel probability. A second pool is uncleaved and has a low open-channel probability and/or conductance. Nedd4–2 has the effect of reducing the fraction of cleaved (active) channels at the cell surface. By contrast, Liddle syndrome mutations have the opposite effect. Thus, the increase in Na$^+$ current in Liddle syndrome is the result of a generalized increase in ENaC expression, along with a greater fraction of cleaved channels in the open state.

ENaC activity is also regulated by a negative feedback mechanism sensitive to intracellular Na$^+$. As intracellular Na$^+$ rises there is an inhibitory effect on further Na$^+$ entry via ENaC. Under normal conditions this inhibitory effect is mediated by a reduction in channel density as well as a decrease in open-channel probability. This effect has now been studied in the ENaC harboring a β-subunit mutation associated with Liddle syndrome (76). Compared with wild-type channels, the Liddle syndrome mutants are less sensitive to the inhibitory effect of intracellular Na$^+$. In addition, the reduction in Na$^+$ entry that does occur is solely mediated by a decrease in open-channel probability with no change in channel density.

The syndrome of apparent mineralocorticoid excess is a rare recessive disorder characterized by hypertension, hypokalemia, metabolic alkalosis, and suppressed circulating aldosterone levels. This disease is due to decreased activity of the 11β-hydroxysteroid dehydrogenase enzyme type II. This enzyme is normally found in aldosterone-responsive cells and functions to protect these cells from inappropriate activation of the mineralocorticoid receptor by circulating cortisol.

The mineralocorticoid receptor is capable of binding cortisol and aldosterone with equal affinity. Cortisol circulates in the blood at a concentration >1,000-fold higher than aldosterone. Despite these higher concentrations, cortisol is prevented from binding to the mineralocorticoid receptor because it is rapidly converted to cortisone by 11β-hydroxysteroid dehydrogenase type 2. The enzyme allows aldosterone, rather than cortisol, to gain access to the receptor despite the fact that circulating levels of aldosterone are much lower. A decrease in the activity of this enzyme removes the selectivity for aldosterone and allows cortisol to persistently activate the mineralocorticoid receptor, thus accounting for the development of clinical manifestations. Patients with this disorder can be effectively treated with either spironolactone or a sodium channel blocker such as amiloride or triamterene.

Decreased activity of 11β-hydroxysteroid dehydrogenase type 2 can occur as an acquired disorder due to the chronic ingestion of licorice. The active component in licorice is glycyrrhetinic acid, which has an inhibitory effect on the enzyme. Licorice is used as a flavoring agent in a variety of products such as chewing tobacco. Other agents containing glycyrrhetinic acid reported to cause this syndrome include herbal medications used to treat allergic rhinitis and constipation and the flavoring product "Asam Boi," widely consumed by the Malaysian and Singaporean populations (77,78). Flavonoids found in grapefruit juice have also been shown to have an inhibitory effect on the enzyme (79).

Acquired inhibition of 11β-hydroxysteroid dehydrogenase type 2 may be of importance in the salt retention that occurs in some patients with cirrhosis. Aldosterone is generally believed to play a major role in the renal salt retention observed in cirrhotic patients. However, there are many examples of patients who present with ascites and total body sodium overload who have either normal or suppressed aldosterone levels. Bile acids, which can accumulate in the setting of chronic liver disease, have been shown to inhibit the activity of 11β-hydroxysteroid dehydrogenase type 2 (80–82). Such an effect would allow cortisol-mediated stimulation of the mineralocorticoid receptor and potentially explain aldosterone-independent salt retention in the distal nephron.

Studies in the bile duct ligation and carbon tetrachloride models of chronic liver disease are consistent with a component of cortisol-mediated stimulation of the mineralocorticoid receptor (83,84). In these models there is decreased activity of 11β-hydroxysteroid dehydrogenase type 2 that is temporally related to increased ENaC abundance in the apical membrane of the cortical collecting duct. These changes are most pronounced in the sodium-retaining stage of disease.

An autosomal dominant form of hypertension that results from an activating mutation (S810L) in the mineralocorticoid receptor has been described in a single kindred. The development of hypertension is associated with hypokalemia and suppressed serum aldosterone levels. Hypertension typically develops before the age of 20 in affected family members. In addition there is a marked worsening of hypertension that occurs during pregnancy.

Steroids with a 21-hydroxyl group such as aldosterone and cortisol are capable of activating both the wild-type and the mutant receptor. The crystal structure of the wild-type and mutant receptors has recently been identified (85,86). Under normal conditions steroids that lack the 21-hydroxyl group but contain a 17-keto group are mineralocorticoid receptor antagonists because they bind but do not activate the normal receptor. By contrast, the mutated receptor is activated by these steroids. Progesterone (a 17α-hydroxyl steroid) lacks the 21-hydroxyl group and is capable of activating the mutated receptor, thus explaining the worsening of hypertension that occurs during pregnancy when progesterone levels are increased. Spironolactone (a synthetic steroid with a 17γ-lactone) also activates the mutated receptor and therefore should be avoided in this condition. Cortisone is also capable of activating the mutated receptor and has been implicated in the development of hypertension in young men and nonpregnant women harboring the S810L mutation (87). The sodium channel blockers amiloride or triamterene are treatment options.

Primary Increase in Distal Na$^+$ Delivery

Conditions that give rise to primary increases in distal Na$^+$ delivery are characterized by normal or low extracellular fluid volume. Blood pressure is typically normal. Increases in distal Na$^+$ delivery are most frequently due to diuretics, which act proximal to the cortical collecting duct. Increased delivery can also be the result of nonreabsorbed anions such as bicarbonate as with active vomiting or type II proximal renal tubular acidosis. Ketoanions and the Na$^+$ salts of penicillins are other examples. The inability to reabsorb these anions in the proximal tubule results in increased delivery of Na$^+$ to the distal nephron. Since these anions also escape reabsorption in the distal nephron, a more lumen-negative voltage develops and the driving force for K$^+$ excretion into the tubular fluid is enhanced.

Disorders of hypokalemia due to primary increases in distal Na$^+$ delivery can best be categorized as to the presence of metabolic acidosis or metabolic alkalosis (Fig. 5.4). Falling in the category of metabolic acidosis are disorders that cause renal tubular acidosis. In proximal renal tubular acidosis, the threshold for bicarbonate reabsorption is reduced, resulting in a self-limited bicarbonaturia. The loss of NaHCO$_3$ in the urine leads to volume depletion, which in turns activates the renin–angiotensin–aldosterone system. The coupling of increased aldosterone levels with increased distal Na$^+$ delivery results in renal K$^+$ wasting. In the steady state when virtually all the filtered HCO$_3$ is reabsorbed in the proximal and distal nephron, renal K$^+$ wasting is minimal and the degree of hypokalemia tends to be mild. By contrast, treatment of metabolic acidosis with bicarbonate improves the acidosis but worsens the degree of hypokalemia.

A variety of drugs used in the treatment of human immunodeficiency virus (HIV) have been reported to cause proximal renal tubular acidosis usually in association with the Fanconi syndrome (88). Of all patients, hypokalemia has been particularly prominent in patients receiving tenofovir. Risk factors for tenofovir-associated hypokalemia include prolonged administration, lower body weight, and concomitant rotonavir or didanosine use (89).

The development of hypokalemia in dRTA can be due to several mechanisms. First, systemic acidosis in and of itself can lead to renal K$^+$ wasting. Metabolic acidosis is associated with decreased net proximal Na$^+$ reabsorption. The subsequent increase in distal delivery leads to volume contraction and activation of the renin–angiotensin–aldosterone system. These changes lead to increased renal K$^+$ excretion. Second, dRTA due to a defect in the H$^+$/K$^+$ ATPase will increase renal K$^+$ excretion by directly impairing K$^+$ reabsorption in the distal nephron. Third, K$^+$ wasting can be the result of leakage into the tubular lumen as a result of an ionophoric effect as seen in the gradient type of dRTA due to administration of amphotericin B.

Hypokalemia can be severe and potentially life threatening in dRTA. Recent reports have described profound hypokalemia complicated by paralysis in patients with Sjogren syndrome (90,91). While this disorder typically occurs in middle-aged women, it can also be seen in elderly men (92). A clue to the diagnosis of dRTA can be the discovery of nephrocalcinosis visualized on a normal lung radiograph (93).

Toluene inhalation can give rise to severe and symptomatic hypokalemia in association with hyperchloremic normal-gap metabolic acidosis. These electrolyte derangements are largely due to production of hippuric acid (a metabolite of toluene) and the renal excretion of its sodium salt. Chronic exposure may lead to persistent dRTA due to direct tubular toxicity.

Falling in the category of hypokalemia and metabolic alkalosis is the use of loop diuretics and Bartter syndrome. Bartter syndrome is a hereditary disorder characterized by renal salt wasting and hypokalemic metabolic alkalosis resembling the features of chronic loop diuretic therapy. Hypokalemia can be severe and can result in complications such as rhabdomyolysis and periodic paralysis (94,95). This disease results from gene defects that lead to decreased NaCl reabsorption in the thick ascending limb of Henle (96,97).

The development of hypokalemia in type II Bartter syndrome illustrates the importance of maxi-K^+ channels in renal K^+ excretion, which were discussed earlier (98). These patients have a loss of function mutation in ROMK and present with clinical features of the disease in the perinatal period. ROMK provides the pathway for recycling of K^+ across the apical membrane in the thick ascending limb of Henle. This recycling generates a lumen-positive potential, which drives the paracellular reabsorption of Ca^{2+} and Mg^{2+} and provides luminal K^+ to the NKCC2 cotransporter. Mutations in ROMK decrease NaCl and fluid reabsorption in the thick limb, mimicking a loop diuretic effect, causing volume depletion. Despite the increase in distal Na^+ delivery, one would not predict the development of renal K^+ wasting, since ROMK is also the major K^+-secretory pathway for regulated K^+ excretion in the collecting duct. In fact, in the perinatal period, infants with this form of Bartter syndrome often exhibit a transient hyperkalemia consistent with loss of function of ROMK in the collecting duct. However, over time these patients develop hypokalemia as a result of increased flow-mediated K^+ secretion via maxi-K^+ channels. Studies in an ROMK-deficient mouse model of type II Bartter syndrome are consistent with this mechanism (99). The transient hyperkalemia observed in the prenatal period is likely related to the fact that ROMK channels are functionally expressed sooner than maxi-K^+ channels.

Genetic defects of the NKCC2 cotransporter usually present with evidence of severe salt wasting in the prenatal period. A recent report described two brothers who did not come to clinical attention until they were teenagers (100). The mild phenotype in these subjects was found to be the result of mutations of the SLC12A1 gene that allowed for significant residual activity of the NKCC2 cotransporter. Typically, late onset and mild Bartter syndrome is due to defects in the CLCNKB gene coding for the CLC-Kb chloride channel.

Gitelman syndrome is an inherited disorder with clinical manifestations that mimic the chronic use of a thiazide diuretic. This disease is due to an inactivating mutation in the gene (SLC12A3) for the thiazide sensitive apical NCC in the distal convoluted tubule. Immunohistochemistry performed on renal biopsy material taken from two adults with Gitelman syndrome were devoid of intact NCC immunostaining (101). Although the disease may be relatively benign with either no or minimal symptoms, many patients have difficult hypokalemia and represent a therapeutic challenge. One explanation for difficulty with management with K^+ supplementation, amiloride, and spironolactone is that patients with Gitelman syndrome often manifest salt craving. High dietary salt and fluid intake increase distal Na^+ delivery and drive K^+ secretion by the unaffected CCT principal cell. Although a mouse model exists (NCC $(-/-)$), the serum potassium is normal and hypokalemia develops only with dietary K^+ restriction (102). Paralysis and prolongation of the QT interval with malignant arrhythmias attributed to hypokalemia and hypomagnesemia have been described (103,104) in patients with the features of Gitelman syndrome.

Complications and Treatment of Hypokalemia

Hypokalemia can cause a variety of clinical manifestations due to alterations in the excitability of neuromuscular tissues. Decrease in extracellular K^+ concentration leads to hyperpolarization of the cell membrane, causing the cell to become less sensitive to exciting stimuli. Clinically, this effect accounts for the association of hypokalemia and muscle weakness. Occasionally, muscle weakness can be sufficiently severe to cause paralysis, as occurs in patients with hypokalemic dRTA secondary to Sjögren syndrome (105,106).

Under normal circumstances, exercise is associated with movement of intracellular K^+ into the interstitial space in skeletal muscle. The increase in interstitial K^+ can be as high as 10 to 12 mmol with extreme exertion. This accumulation of K^+ has been implicated as a factor limiting the excitability and contractile force of muscle accounting for the development of fatigue (107,108). In addition, increases in interstitial K^+ are thought to be an important factor in eliciting rapid vasodilation, allowing for blood flow to increase in exercising muscle (109). Hypokalemia is a cause of rhabdomyolysis. Although the mechanism is likely to be multifactorial, total body K^+ depletion may blunt the accumulation of K^+ into the interstitial space, thereby limiting blood flow to skeletal muscle and resulting in muscle breakdown.

Hypokalemic nephropathy or "kaliopenic nephropathy" is a chronic tubulointerstitial disease characterized by polyuria, proteinuria, development of renal cysts, and loss of renal function.

Histologically, there is evidence of tubular atrophy, interstitial infiltration of macrophages, and interstitial fibrosis. Mediators of renal injury in this setting include local ischemia, complement activation due to increased ammoniagenesis, and local effects of angiotensin II and endothelin. Studies in Sprague–Dawley rats fed a low-K^+ diet implicate impaired angiogenesis as an additional mechanism of renal injury in this disorder (110).

Hypokalemia may play a role in the association between new-onset diabetes and use of thiazide diuretics. In a recent review of >50 trials in which thiazides were compared with other drugs or placebo, a significant inverse relationship was found between the decrease in K^+ and the increase in glucose level (111). For every 1 mEq/L decrease in K^+, there was an approximate 10 mg/dL increase in glucose. Further strengthening the argument that hypokalemia plays an important role in the genesis of glucose intolerance is the observation that prevention of hypokalemia with K^+ supplements prevents the development of thiazide-induced glucose intolerance (112). In addition, changes in glucose levels can be normalized following K^+ repletion in patients who are hypokalemic.

The mechanism of thiazide-induced hyperglycemia is thought to be the result of decreased insulin released from the pancreatic β-cell. ATP-sensitive K^+ channels couple β-cell metabolism to electrical activity, thereby playing an essential role in the control of insulin secretion (113). The involvement of K^+ in this process at least raises the possibility that K^+ depletion might alter β-cell insulin release. Impaired insulin release that is reversible with drug discontinuation or K^+ supplements is in contrast to the persistent insulin resistance typical of patients with type II diabetes. This difference in the mechanism of glucose intolerance may help explain the lack of convincing evidence that thiazide-induced diabetes mellitus increases the incidence of morbid or fatal cardiovascular events (114).

In the hypokalemic patient, K^+ can be given orally or intravenously as the KCl salt. Because $KHCO_3$ and potassium citrate are converted to bicarbonate, increase the bicarbonate concentration in plasma, and enhance HCO_3^- excretion, these products may increase K^+ excretion and are therefore not the replacement of choice except for patients with concomitant metabolic acidosis. Oral administration of KCl is safest and most effective. KCl can be given in doses of 100 to 150 mEq/day. Liquid KCl is bitter tasting, and the tablet can be irritating to the gastric mucosa. The microencapsulated or wax-matrix forms of KCl are better tolerated.

Intravenous administration of K^+ may be necessary if the patient cannot take oral medications, or if the K^+ deficit is large and is resulting in cardiac arrhythmias, respiratory paralysis, or rhabdomyolysis. Intravenous KCl should be given at a maximum rate of 20 mEq/h and maximum concentration of 40 mEq/L. Higher concentrations will result in phlebitis. Replacement of KCl in dextrose-containing solutions can result in further lowering of the serum K^+ secondary to insulin release. Thus, saline solutions are preferred.

On rare occasions, higher concentrations of K^+ may have to be given. In a patient with a serum K^+ of 2.6 mmol/L and an implantable cardiac defibrillator, rapid administration of K^+ successfully led to the termination of recurrent unstable ventricular tachycardia (115). This patient was given a rapid bolus of 20 mEq KCl solution through a central access, followed by an additional 80 mEq orally and intravenously during the next 2 hours. A 12-year-old boy with a K^+ of 1.2 mEq/L due to gastrointestinal losses was given 140 mEq of KCl as a bolus after developing pulseless ventricular tachycardia (116). The bolus administration leads to resolution of the arrhythmia. Aggressive K^+ administration requires frequent measurement of serum K^+ and continuous electrocardiographic monitoring to prevent iatrogenic hyperkalemia. In a retrospective survey of 140 hospitalized patients with hypokalemia, 16% of patients developed therapy-induced hyperkalemia. Compared with patients who simply corrected to normal, the amount of K^+ given was greater for patients with iatrogenic hyperkalemia (117).

Hyperkalemia

PSEUDOHYPERKALEMIA

Pseudohyperkalemia is an in vitro phenomenon due to the mechanical release of K^+ from cells during the phlebotomy procedure or specimen processing. This diagnosis is made when the serum K^+ concentration exceeds the plasma K^+ concentration by >0.5 mmol/L. Common causes of pseudohyperkalemia include fist clenching during the phlebotomy procedure, application of tourniquets, and use of small-bore needles. In one instance pseudohyperkalemia was documented to occur when a specimen was sent from the ward to the lab in a pneumatic tube transport system (118,119).

Difficult blood draws are common in pediatric patients, and the avoidance of having to obtain a repeat sample to exclude pseudohyperkalemia would be of great benefit. With this goal in mind, a correction factor has been derived on the basis of idea that measurement of free plasma hemoglobin can be used as an index of in vitro hemolysis (120). Twenty whole-blood samples drawn for healthy individuals were divided into four aliquots: (a) no manipulation, (b) mechanical hemolysis via a 27-gauge needle, (c) addition of potassium acetate to mimic significant hyperkalemia, and (d) addition of potassium acetate plus mechanical hemolysis. On the basis of a linear relationship noted between the free plasma hemoglobin and the change in K^+ going from the nonhemolyzed to hemolyzed specimens, a correction factor of 0.00319 times the free plasma hemoglobin was obtained. As an example, the difference between the serum and plasma K^+ would be 1.6 mEq/L in a specimen with free plasma hemoglobin of 500 mg/dL. The authors concluded that when the lower boundary of the predicted δK^+ falls within the normal reference range, a repeat measurement is not needed.

The presence of a high cell or platelet count is another setting where pseudohyperkalemia is frequently observed. Differences in serum and plasma K^+ concentration were recently compared in patients with increased cellular components of blood of various causes (121,122). Compared with normal controls, the δ serum plasma K^+ concentration was significantly increased in patients with erythrocytosis and thrombocytosis but not in patients with white blood cell disorders. The δ was particularly pronounced in subjects with polycythemia vera with an increase in both red blood cell and platelet counts.

Familial pseudohyperkalemia is a symptomless genetic disorder of red blood cell membrane permeability, in which measurement of K^+ is normal at the time of blood collection but is increased when measured after the sample has been allowed to stand at room temperature for several hours. This temperature-dependent leakage of K^+ out of the cell is inherited in an autosomal dominant fashion and has only been described in several kindreds. In one of these kindreds the disorder maps to the same loci as patients with hereditary stomatocytosis.

EXCESSIVE DIETARY INTAKE

In the presence of normal renal and adrenal function, it is difficult to ingest sufficient K^+ to develop hyperkalemia. Rather, dietary intake as a contributor to hyperkalemia is usually in the setting of impaired kidney function. Dietary sources particularly enriched with K^+ include melons, dried fruits, citrus juice, and salt substitutes. Other hidden sources of K^+ reported to cause life-threatening hyperkalemia include raw coconut juice (K^+ concentration of 44.3 mmol/L) and Noni juice (123,124). While clay ingestion can cause hypokalemia due to binding in the gastrointestinal tract, riverbed clay is K^+ enriched (100 mEq K^+ in 100 g clay) and can cause life-threatening hyperkalemia in chronic kidney disease (CKD) patients (125). Ingestion of burnt match heads (cautopyreiophagia) can also be a hidden source of K^+ (126). This activity was found to add an additional 80 mmol of K^+ to one dialysis patient's daily intake and produced a plasma K^+ concentration of 8 mmol/L.

K^+ supplements need to be used with caution even in patients with renal K^+ wasting disorders, since they may develop loss of kidney function due to unrelated reasons. This scenario was described in a patient with Gitelman syndrome who required 260 mmol of K^+ per day. He developed an episode of acute renal failure due to volume depletion caused by gastroenteritis in the setting of taking a nonsteroidal anti-inflammatory drug (127). After complaining of weakness he was found to have a serum K^+ concentration of 10.4 mmol/L.

Use of dietary K^+ supplements may become more commonplace, given the evidence that diets enriched in K^+ may be associated with clinical benefit. In various animal models K^+ supplementation has been shown to lower blood pressure, prevent stroke, and reduce mortality (128). In a mouse model of hypokalemic alkalosis induced by deoxycorticosterone, correction of hypokalemia with dietary K^+ supplementation prevents the development of cardiac and renal hypertrophy independent of blood pressure that otherwise occurs in untreated animals.

Cardiovascular outcomes were recently examined in elderly Taiwanese veterans living in retirement facilities (129). Five kitchens were randomized to use either NaCl or KCl as the only salt in food preparation. Over a 31-month follow-up, cardiovascular disease–related death was less in the subjects ingesting a K^+-enriched diet compared with the veterans ingesting food prepared with NaCl (age-adjusted hazard ratio, 0.59; 95% confidence interval, 0.37–0.95). Greater consumption of fruit and vegetable juices (foods typically enriched with K^+) has been implicated in delaying the onset of Alzheimer disease (130).

CELLULAR REDISTRIBUTION

Cellular redistribution is more important as a cause of hyperkalemia than as a cause of hypokalemia. Tissue damage is probably the most important cause of hyperkalemia due to redistribution of K^+ out of cells. This can be due to rhabdomyolysis, trauma, hypothermia (during the rewarming phase), burns, massive intravascular coagulation, and tumor lysis (either spontaneous or following treatment) (131).

Drugs may cause hyperkalemia as a result of cellular redistribution. An example of this complication is the use of succinylcholine to induce a paralytic state (132,133). Under normal circumstances acetylcholine receptors are concentrated within the neuromuscular junction. The depolarization of these receptors by succinylcholine leads to efflux of intracellular K^+, but the accumulation of K^+ is confined to the neuromuscular junction such that no change in plasma K^+ concentration occurs. Hyperkalemia can develop when this drug is given under conditions that cause upregulation and widespread distribution of acetylcholine receptors throughout the whole-muscle membrane. In this setting succinylcholine-induced depolarization of receptors causes clinically significant amounts of K^+ to enter the extracellular fluid space. Risk factors for this complication include denervation, prolonged immobilization, chronic infection, and burn injury.

Thalidomide is increasingly being used in the treatment of multiple myeloma and has been implicated in the development of hyperkalemia (134). The mechanism by which this occurs is not known, but cellular shift has been suggested. The reports of this complication have been confined to patients with CKD.

Malignant hyperthermia is a rare clinical syndrome that is manifested by muscle rigidity, tachycardia, increased CO_2 production, skin cyanosis and mottling, rhabdomyolysis, and hyperkalemia. The onset of the disorder is usually within one hour of the administration of general anesthesia, with the most common triggers being halothane and succinylcholine. The syndrome is due to a mutation in the gene that encodes the skeletal muscle ryanodine receptor. This receptor is a calcium channel that when mutated allows excess amounts of calcium to exit the sarcoplasmic reticulum, resulting in tetany and heat production. Mutational analysis is now available to identify individuals who are at risk for this syndrome (135).

Mineral acidosis but not organic acidosis can be a cause of cell shift in K^+. Sevelamer can lead to the development of metabolic acidosis and hyperkalemia due to this mechanism. The drug is a nonabsorbed polymer with covalently linked amino groups, almost half of which consist of amine hydrochloride. Chloride is released in exchange for monovalent phosphate in the gastrointestinal tract so that for each molecule of phosphate bound there is liberation of one molecule of hydrochloric acid. In a study of 20 hemodialysis patients, increasing the dialysate bicarbonate concentration to 40 mEq/L was effective in correcting both acidosis and hyperkalemia over a 24-month period despite the ongoing use of this non-calcium-containing phosphate binder (136).

Hyperkalemic periodic paralysis is most commonly associated with mutations in the sodium channel *SCN4A* gene. In contrast to familial hypokalemic periodic paralysis, patients with the hyperkalemic form are typically younger (<10 vs. 5 to 20 years) and have a greater frequency of attacks that tend to be of shorter duration (<24 vs. >24 hours). The attacks can be precipitated by fasting and K^+ administration.

Decreased Renal Excretion of K^+

Decreased renal excretion of K^+ can be divided into one or more of three abnormalities: a primary decrease in distal delivery of salt and water, abnormal cortical collecting duct function, and a primary decrease in mineralocorticoid levels (Table 5.1).

PRIMARY DECREASE IN DISTAL DELIVERY (RENAL FAILURE)

Acute decreases in GFR, as occurs in acute renal failure, may lead to marked decreases in distal delivery of salt and water, which may secondarily decrease distal K^+ secretion. When acute renal failure is oliguric, distal delivery of NaCl and volume are low and hyperkalemia is a frequent problem. When acute renal failure is nonoliguric, however, distal delivery is usually sufficient and hyperkalemia is unusual.

TABLE 5.1 CAUSES OF HYPERKALEMIA

- Pseudohyperkalemia
- Cellular redistribution
  - Mineral acidosis
  - Cell shrinkage (hypertonicity)
  - Deficiency of insulin
  - β-blockers
  - Hyperkalemic periodic paralysis
  - Cell injury
- Excess intake (very rare)
- Decreased renal excretion
  - Decreased distal delivery of Na^+ (oliguric renal failure)
  - Mineralocorticoid deficiency
  - Defect of cortical collecting tubule

The association of hyperkalemia and CKD is more complicated than with acute renal failure. In addition to decreased GFR and a secondary decrease in distal delivery, there is nephron dropout and a smaller number of collecting ducts to secrete K^+ with CKD. However, this is counterbalanced by an adaptive process in which the remaining nephrons develop an increased ability to excrete K^+. Two other defenses against hyperkalemia include a more rapid shift of K^+ into cells in response to a K^+ load and a markedly increased rate of K^+ excretion in the colon. For all of these reasons hyperkalemia is unusual in CKD patients with a slow decline until the GFR falls to <10 mL/min. The occurrence of hyperkalemia with a GFR of >10 mL/min (unless there has been a sudden decline in GFR, i.e., acute on chronic kidney failure), should raise the question of decreased aldosterone levels or a specific lesion of the cortical collecting duct.

Aldosterone continues to play a role in regulating K^+ even in anephric patients through stimulatory effects on colonic secretion. In this regard, fludrocortisone has been used sporadically to better control the plasma K^+ concentration in hyperkalemic chronic dialysis patients. To test whether the drug is effective in this setting, 37 patients with a midweek predialysis serum K^+ concentration of 5.1 to 5.3 mEq/L were randomized to receive either fludrocortisone at 0.1 mg/day or no treatment for a 3-month period (137). While the drug was safe and well tolerated, no difference was found in serum K^+ concentration between the two groups.

PRIMARY DECREASE IN MINERALOCORTICOID ACTIVITY

Decreased mineralocorticoid activity can result from disturbances that originate at any point along the renin–angiotensin–aldosterone system. Such disturbances can be the result of a disease state or be due to effects of various drugs. Diabetes is perhaps the most common disease state associated with hyporeninemic hypoaldosteronism. A list of drugs and where they interfere in the renin–angiotensin–aldosterone axis is displayed in Table 5.2. Hyperkalemia most commonly develops when one or more of these drugs are administered in a setting where the renin–angiotensin–aldosterone system is already impaired (138).

Hyperkalemia that develops in association with use of ACE inhibitors (ACEIs) and angiotensin receptor blockers is of particular concern, since patients at the highest risk for this complication are oftentimes the same individuals expected to derive the greatest cardiovascular benefit. It is worth emphasizing that in patients with CKD the level of renal function should not be the sole determinant as to whether these drugs should be initiated or continued. In a randomized, double-blind study of 224 patients with a serum creatinine concentration of 3.1 to 5.0 mg/dL, the administration of 20 mg/day of benazepril reduced the composite end point of doubling of the serum creatinine concentration, end-stage renal disease, or death compared to placebo (139). During the 3 years of the study, both groups were treated with conventional antihypertensive drugs so that blood pressure control was no different. Hyperkalemia (defined as a serum K^+ >6.0 mmol/L) developed in 6 patients treated with benazepril and 5 receiving placebo. Of these 11 patients, only 3 had to be withdrawn from the

TABLE 5.2 RISK FACTORS FOR HYPERKALEMIA WHEN USING DRUGS THAT INTERFERE IN THE RENIN–ANGIOTENSIN–ALDOSTERONE SYSTEM

- Chronic kidney disease: Risk is inversely related to glomerular filtration rate and increases substantially at <30 mL/min.
- Diabetes mellitus
- Decompensated congestive heart failure
- Volume depletion
- Elderly
- Concomitant use of drugs that interfere in renal potassium excretion
  - Nonsteroidal anti-inflammatory drugs
  - β-blockers
  - Calcineurin inhibitors: Cyclosporin, Tacrolimus
  - Heparin
  - Ketoconazole
  - Potassium-sparing diuretics: Spironolactone, eplerenone, amiloride, triamterene
  - Trimethoprim
  - Pentamidine
- Potassium supplements including salt substitutes and certain herbs

study. The other 8 patients were successfully treated with dietary modifications, diuretic therapy, and optimized acid–base balance. The study illustrates that withholding these drugs simply on the basis of renal function can potentially deprive many patients the cardiovascular benefit they would have otherwise received, particularly because numerous steps can be taken to minimize the risk of hyperkalemia.

The use of drugs that interfere in the renin–angiotensin system in patients at increased risk for hyperkalemia requires close monitoring. If the patient is to be initiated on an ACEI or an angiotensin receptor blocker, it is best to begin with low doses. The serum K^+ should be checked within one week of starting the drug, and then the drug may be titrated upward if the K^+ remains in the normal range. With each increase in dose the serum K^+ should be remeasured at 1-week intervals. For increases in the serum K^+ concentration up to 5.5 mEq/L, the clinician may reduce the dose, and in some cases, the K^+ concentration will improve, allowing the patient to remain on a lower dose of the renin–angiotensin blocker (Table 5.3).

TABLE 5.3 APPROACH TO PATIENTS AT RISK FOR HYPERKALEMIA WHEN USING DRUGS THAT INTERFERE IN THE RENIN–ANGIOTENSIN–ALDOSTERONE SYSTEM

- Accurately assess level of renal function to better define risk.
- Discontinue drugs that interfere in renal potassium secretion, inquire about herbal preparations, and discontinue nonsteroidal anti-inflammatory drugs to include the selective cyclooxygenase 2 inhibitors.
- Give a low-potassium diet and inquire about potassium-containing salt substitutes.
- Give thiazide or loop diuretics (loop diuretics necessary when estimated glomerular filtration rate <30 mL/min).
- Give sodium bicarbonate to correct metabolic acidosis in chronic kidney disease patients.
- Initiate therapy with low-dose ACE inhibitor or angiotensin receptor blocker.
  - Measure potassium 1 week after initiation of therapy or after increasing dose of drug.
  - For increases in potassium up to 5.5 mEq/L, decrease dose of drug. If taking some combination of ACE inhibitor, angiotensin receptor blocker, and aldosterone receptor blocker, discontinue one and recheck potassium.
  - Ensure the dose of spironolactone does not exceed 25 mg/day when used with an ACE inhibitor or angiotensin receptor blocker. Avoid this combination of drugs with glomerular filtration rate <30 mL/min.
  - For potassium ≥5.6 mEq/L despite the above steps, discontinue drugs.

In a retrospective cohort study conducted in 10 health maintenance organizations, the frequency of serum K^+ and creatinine monitoring was assessed in patients labeled as being treated with ACEIs or angiotensin receptor blockers for at least 1 year (140). More than two-thirds of the 52,906 patients identified received laboratory monitoring. The likelihood of monitoring increased with advancing age, more frequent outpatient visits; recent hospitalizations; concomitant use of drugs such as potassium salts, diuretics, and digoxin; and comorbidities such as diabetes, congestive heart failure, and CKD. Nearly one-third of patients prescribed these drugs had no laboratory monitoring over a 1-year period.

The discovery of hyperkalemia during laboratory testing does not guarantee appropriate follow-up. In a retrospective observational cohort study of a large primary care practice, 109 instances of hyperkalemia (defined as $K^+ > 5.8$ mEq/L) were identified in 86 patients (141). While more than half of the patients were recalled to the clinic for retesting, 25% of the cases had no repeat testing until they were seen on routine follow-up visits or when they came to the clinic for unrelated issues.

The lack of appropriate follow-up is of particular concern, since the electrocardiogram in a hyperkalemic subject can progress from normal to that of ventricular tachycardia and asystole precipitously (142). Most physicians are familiar with the findings of peaked T waves and sine-wave patterns that typify hyperkalemia. Profound bradycardia is a less well-appreciated manifestation of hyperkalemia (143). Particular attention should be given to patients with underlying disturbances of cardiac conduction, since even mild degrees of hyperkalemia may precipitate heart block. This complication can occur whether the conduction disease is intrinsic to the heart or drug induced as with the use of verapamil (144). The electrophysiologic and electrocardiographic changes of hyperkalemia are discussed below.

Distal Tubular Defect

Certain interstitial renal diseases can affect the distal nephron specifically and lead to hyperkalemia in the presence of only mild decreases in GFR and normal aldosterone levels. Amiloride and triamterene inhibit Na^+ absorption by the principal cell in the complex chronic disease (CCD) which makes the luminal potential more positive and secondarily inhibits K^+ secretion. A similar effect occurs with trimethoprim and accounts for the development of hyperkalemia following the administration of the antibiotic trimethoprim-sulfamethoxazole (145). Spironolactone and eplerenone compete with aldosterone and thus block the mineralocorticoid effect.

Pseudohypoaldosteronism type II (Gordon syndrome) is an autosomal dominant form of hypertension in which hyperkalemia and metabolic acidosis are key features. Plasma concentrations of aldosterone are low despite the presence of hyperkalemia, which normally exerts a stimulatory effect on aldosterone release from the adrenal gland. Administration of NaCl worsens the hypertension but Na^+, given with a nonchloride anion such as sulfate or bicarbonate has a beneficial effect. The hypertension and hyperkalemia are particularly responsive to the administration of thiazide diuretics.

The protein kinases WNK4 and WNK1 are responsible for this disease (146). Wild-type WNK4 acts to reduce the surface expression of the thiazide-sensitive Na^+/Cl^- cotransporter likely through a lysosomal-mediated degradative pathway (147). The mutant protein (inactivating mutation of WNK4 loses this capability, resulting in increased cotransporter activity accompanied by marked hyperplasia of the distal convoluted tubule (148). The wild-type protein also stimulates clathrin-dependent endocytosis of the ROMK channel in the renal collecting duct, leading to decreased cell surface expression. The mutant protein enhances this removal, giving rise to decreased K^+ secretion and hyperkalemia. In published pedigrees with the disease, mutations in WNK4 have clustered in a highly conserved acidic motif of the protein (149).

Since the expression of ROMK is decreased in these patients, it is not immediately apparent as to why thiazide diuretics would be effective in correcting the hyperkalemia in this disorder. In a manner analogous to the hypokalemia that occurs in type II Bartter syndrome discussed previously, thiazides likely enhance renal K^+ excretion through flow-stimulated maxi-K^+ channels.

WNK4 has also been shown to affect Cl^- permeability through the paracellular pathway. The mutated WNK4 protein causes an increase in paracellular Cl^- permeability by phosphorylating claudins, which are tight junction proteins involved in regulating paracellular ion transport. This increase in permeability dissipates the lumen-negative charge normally generated by Na^+ reabsorption via the ENaC. The reduction in luminal electronegativity will decrease the driving force for K^+ secretion, thus providing an additional mechanism by which the mutated protein can cause hyperkalemia. This reduction in luminal electronegativity also contributes to the development of metabolic acidosis due to the less favorable electrical gradient for H^+ secretion. In addition, hyperkalemia slows H^+ secretion by limiting buffer availability through its suppressive effect on ammoniagenesis.

Mutations in WNK1 can also give rise to the manifestations of Gordon syndrome (150). Wild-type WNK1 normally exerts an inhibitory effect on WNK4. Mutations in WNK1 that give rise to pseudohypoaldosteronism type II are a gain of function mutations that augment this inhibitory effect on WNK4 activity. As a result, Na^+/Cl^- cotransport activity is increased, and there is increased removal of ROMK from the apical membrane. WNK1 can also cause salt retention by increasing the activity of ENaC through a stimulatory effect on SGK1. In addition, increased activity of WNK1 enhances paracellular Cl^- permeability in a similar manner as disease-causing mutations in WNK4 (151). This increase in Cl^- permeability may be related to WNK1-mediated phosphorylation of claudin-4. The observation that hypertension in patients with the WNK1 mutation is less sensitive to the effects of thiazide diuretics suggest these non-Na^+/Cl^- cotransporter mechanisms of salt retention are quantitatively more important in causing volume expansion in this setting. While less effective in treating hypertension, thiazide diuretics remain effective in correcting hyperkalemia despite the augmented removal of ROMK. As with the inactivating mutations in WNK4, flow-mediated K^+ secretion via maxi-K^+ channels likely accounts for this effect.

One additional difference in the clinical manifestations resulting from mutations in WNK4 and WNK1 relates to urinary calcium excretion. Increased Na^+/Cl^- cotransporter activity is normally associated with hypercalciuria, while inhibition of the cotransporter decreases urinary calcium excretion. This later effect explains the hypocalciuric effect of thiazide diuretics. Patients with the WNK4 mutation are hypercalciuric and show a heightened sensitivity to the hypocalciuric effects of thiazide diuretics compared with normal subjects (152). These findings are consistent with constitutive activation of the Na^+/Cl^- cotransporter as the major cause of salt retention in patients with the WNK4 mutation. By contrast, hypercalciuria is not a feature in patients with the WNK1 mutation, suggesting increased ENaC activity and paracellular Cl^- permeability play a more important role in mediating salt retention in these patients than increased Na^+/Cl^- cotransporter activity.

Pseudohypoaldosteronism type I is a disorder characterized by mineralocorticoid resistance that typically presents in the newborn. Clinical findings include hyperkalemia, metabolic acidosis, and a tendency toward volume depletion due to renal salt wasting. There are two modes of inheritance that give rise to slightly different characteristics. In the autosomal recessive form of the disease, the defect has been localized to homozygous mutations in the three subunits of the epithelial sodium channel. This form of the disease tends to be more severe and requires lifelong therapy with salt to prevent recurrent life-threatening volume depletion. Extrarenal manifestations include frequent respiratory tract infections due to the presence of dysfunctional channels in the lung. Cutaneous lesions can also develop as a result of the chronic irritative effect of high salt concentrations in sweat (153).

The autosomal dominant form of the disease is due to mutations in the mineralocorticoid receptor that result in mineralocorticoid resistance. The clinical manifestations are limited to the kidney and tend to resolve with time such that therapy with potassium-binding resins and salt supplementation can eventually be discontinued. The maintenance of normal-volume homeostasis and electrolyte values occurs at the expense of a persistent increase in circulating aldosterone levels in adults with the disorder (154). Depending on the mutation, several types of disturbances on receptor function have been described. These include a marked decrease in affinity to the total absence of binding of aldosterone to the receptor (155). Other types of mutations lead to a failure of initiating transcription or prevent the receptor from translocating into the nucleus. In unrelated families with the disease, loss of function mutations have been found to cluster within specific codons, suggesting there are mutational hot spots within the mineralocorticoid receptor gene (156).

Clinical Manifestation of Hyperkalemia

All of the clinically important manifestations of hyperkalemia occur in excitable tissue. Neuromuscular manifestations include paresthesias and fasciculations in the arms and legs. As the serum K^+ continues to rise, an ascending paralysis with eventual flaccid quadriplegia supervenes. Classically, trunk, head, and respiratory muscles are spared, but rarely respiratory failure can occur.

The depolarizing effect of hyperkalemia on the heart is manifested by changes observable in the electrocardiogram (ECG). The progressive changes of hyperkalemia are classically listed as peaking of T waves, ST-segment depression, widening of the PR interval, widening of the QRS interval, loss of the P wave, and development of a sine-wave pattern (157). The appearance of a sine-wave pattern is ominous and is a harbinger of impending ventricular fibrillation and asystole (158,159).

Hyperkalemia can also be associated with a number of less common patterns on the ECG. Brugada syndrome is a genetic disease associated with sudden cardiac death due to mutations in a cardiac Na^+ channel. ECG changes are characterized by a right-bundle branch block pattern and right precordial ST-segment elevations. A similar pattern has been reported in patients with hyperkalemia. However, the hyperkalemic Brugada pattern differs from the genetic disorder in that P waves are often absent, abnormal axis deviation is present, and the QRS complex is wider (160).

Hyperkalemia can also give rise to ECG changes typical of cardiac ischemia. The tall, narrow, and symmetrical peaked T waves typical of hyperkalemia can occasionally be confused with the hyperacute T-wave change associated with a ST-segment elevation myocardial infarction (161). However, in this later condition, the T waves tend to be more broad based and asymmetric in shape. A pseudoinfarct pattern has also been described, resembling both an anteroseptal and an inferior wall myocardial infarction (162,163). These changes resolve with treatment of the hyperkalemia and in the absence of increased cardiac enzymes. Double counting of the heart rate by ECG interpretation software can also occur as a result of hyperkalemic ECG changes (164).

The correlation of ECG changes and serum K^+ concentration depends on the rapidity of the hyperkalemia onset. Generally, with acute onset of hyperkalemia, ECG changes appear at a serum K^+ of 6 to 7 mEq/L. However, with chronic hyperkalemia, the ECG may remain normal up to a concentration of 8 to 9 mEq/L. Despite these generalities, clinical studies show a poor correlation between serum K^+ concentration and cardiac manifestations. In a retrospective review, only 16 of 90 cases met strict criteria for ECG changes reflective of hyperkalemia (defined as new peaked and symmetric T waves that resolved on follow-up) (165). In 13 of these cases, the cardiologist read the ECG as showing no T-wave changes. Strict ECG changes were only noted in one of 14 hyperkalemic patients who manifested arrhythmias or cardiac arrest, which calls into question the prognostic use of the ECG in this setting. Given the poor sensitivity and specificity of the ECG, the authors stress that the clinical scenario and serial measurements of K^+ are the preferred tools to guide the management of patients with hyperkalemia.

The treatment of hyperkalemia depends on the degree of the increase in the plasma potassium concentration and whether there are ECG changes or neuromuscular symptoms. A plasma potassium concentration >7.5 mEq/L, severe muscle weakness, and marked ECG changes are potentially life threatening and require immediate and emergent treatment.

Calcium antagonizes the potassium-induced decrease in membrane excitability, restoring membrane excitability toward normal. Hyperkalemia causes sustained subthreshold depolarization, which inactivates sodium channels, rendering the membrane progressively less excitable. The toxicity of hyperkalemia is worsened in patients with coexistent hypocalcemia. Elevation of plasma calcium concentration in hyperkalemic patients normalizes the difference between the resting and threshold potentials and restores sodium channel activity. The protective effect of Ca^{2+} administration is quite rapid and should be used only in patients in whom the P wave is absent or the QRS is widened. The usual dose is 1 ampule (10 mL) of a 10% calcium gluconate solution infused over 2 to 3 minutes under ECG monitoring. This dose can be repeated after 5 minutes if the ECG changes persist.

Insulin lowers the plasma potassium concentration by driving potassium into cells. Insulin is administered as 10 units of regular insulin with 30 to 50 g of glucose to prevent hypoglycemia. This regimen lowers the plasma potassium concentration by 0.5 to 1.5 mEq/L. The effect of insulin is evident within 30 to 60 minutes and may last for 2 to 4 hours. An ongoing glucose infusion after the initial insulin–glucose treatment may be necessary to prevent late hypoglycemia.

Raising the extracellular pH with $NaHCO_3$ drives potassium into the cells. The usual dose is 44 to 50 mEq of $NaHCO_3$ infused over 5 minutes. The effect begins within 30 to 60 minutes and may persist for 2 to 4 hours. As noted, given the concerns of extracellular fluid volume expansion and lack of efficacy of bicarbonate administration in patients with renal insufficiency, bicarbonate administration should not be considered standard treatment for hyperkalemia. Rather, bicarbonate administration should be reserved for hyperkalemic patients with coexisting metabolic acidosis, if needed, after the patient has received calcium, insulin and glucose, and perhaps an adrenergic agent.

Activation of β_2-adrenergic receptors drives potassium into the cells. Albuterol, 10 to 20 mg by neb-ulizer, can lower the plasma potassium concentration by 0.5 to 1.5 mEq/L within 30 to 60 minutes.

The effects of calcium, insulin, $NaHCO_3$, and β_2-agonists are only transient. For the long-term achievement of normokalemia, these acute treatment modalities need to be followed by managements that remove the excess potassium from the body. These treatments include diuretics, cation-exchange resins, and dialysis.

The cation-exchange resin sodium polystyrene sulfonate (Kayexalate) takes up potassium in exchange for sodium in the gut. Each gram of Kayexalate binds 1 mEq of potassium and releases 1 to 2 mEq of sodium. When administered orally, 20 g of resin is given with 100 mL of a 20% sorbitol solution. Lower doses of 5 g once to three times a day can be used to treat chronic hyperkalemia. In patients who cannot take the oral solution, the resin can be given as a retention enema. Caution must be exercised in administering Kayexalate to postoperative patients, because intestinal necrosis has been reported to occur in this setting. However, sorbitol, the vehicle often used when sodium polystyrene sulfonate is administered p.o. or p.r., appears to be the cause of intestinal necrosis and not the resin per se. Kayexelate may be given without sorbitol but causes constipation.

Dialysis is needed to remove the excess potassium load in patients with severe hyperkalemia, especially in the presence of advanced renal failure or when accompanied by a hypercatabolic state or severe tissue necrosis. Acute hemodialysis is more effective than peritoneal dialysis in this setting.

REFERENCES

1. Hebert SC, Desir G, Giebisch G, et al. Molecular diversity and regulation of renal potassium channels. *Physiol Rev.* 2005; 85: 319–371.
2. Wang WH. Regulation of ROMK (Kir1.1) channels: new mechanisms and aspects. *Am J Physiol Renal Physiol.* 2006; 290: F14–F19.
3. Satlin LM, Carattino M, Liu W, et al. Regulation of cation transport in the distal nephron by mechanical forces. *Am J Physiol Renal Physiol.* 2006; 291: F923–F931.
4. Nauli SM, Alenghat FJ, Luo Y, et al. Polycystins 1 and 2 mediate mechanosensation in the primary cilium of kidney cells. *Nat Genet.* 2003; 33: 129–137.
5. Morimoto T, Liu W, Woda C, et al. Mechanism underlying flow stimulation of sodium absorption in the mammalian collecting duct. *Am J Physiol Renal Physiol.* 2006; 291: F663–F669.
6. Carattino MD, Sheng S, Kleyman TR. Mutations in the pore region modify epithelial sodium channel gating by shear stress. *J Biol Chem.* 2005; 280: 4393–4401.
7. Halperin ML, Cheema-Dhadli S, Lin SH, et al. Control of potassium excretion: a Paleolithic perspective. *Curr Opin Nephrol Hypertens.* 2006; 15: 430–436.
8. Cheema-Dhadli S, Lin SH, Keong-Chong C, et al. Requirements for a high rate of potassium excretion in rats consuming a low electrolyte diet. *J Physiol.* 2006; 572: 493–501.
9. Najjar F, Zhou H, Morimoto T, et al. Dietary K^+ regulates apical membrane expression of maxi-K channels in rabbit cortical collecting duct. *Am J Physiol Renal Physiol.* 2005; 289: F922–F932.
10. Stokes JB. Consequences of potassium recycling in the renal medulla. Effects of ion transport by the medullary thick ascending limb of Henle's loop. *J Clin Invest.* 1982; 70: 219–229.
11. Xie J, Craig L, Cobb MH, et al. Role of with-no-lysine [K] kinases in the pathogenesis of Gordon's syndrome. *Pediatr Nephrol.* 2006; 21: 1231–1236.
12. Subramanya AR, Yang CL, McCormick JA, et al. WNK kinases regulate sodium chloride and potassium transport by the aldosterone-sensitive distal nephron. *Kidney Int.* 2006; 70: 630–634.
13. O'Reilly M, Marshall E, MacGillivray T, et al. Dietary electrolyte-driven responses in the renal WNK kinase pathway in vivo. *J Am Soc Nephrol.* 2006; 17: 2402–2413.
14. Wade JB, Fang L, Liu J, et al. WNK1 kinase isoform switch regulates renal potassium excretion. *Proc Natl Acad Sci U S A.* 2006; 103: 8558–8563.
15. Lazrak A, Liu Z, Huang CL. Antagonistic regulation of ROMK by long and kidney-specific WNK1 isoforms. *Proc Natl Acad Sci U S A.* 2006; 103: 1615–1620.
16. Cope G, Murthy M, Golbang AP, et al. WNK1 affects surface expression of the ROMK potassium channel independent of WNK4. *J Am Soc Nephrol.* 2006; 17: 1867–1874.
17. Appel LJ, Brands MW, Daniels SR, et al. Dietary approaches to prevent and treat hypertension: a scientific statement from the American Heart Association. *Hypertension.* 2006; 47: 296–308.
18. Krishna GG, Kapoor SC. Potassium depletion exacerbates essential hypertension. *Ann Intern Med.* 1991; 115: 77–83.
19. Vallon V, Wulff P, Huang DY, et al. Role of Sgk1 in salt and potassium homeostasis. *Am J Physiol Regul Integr Comp Physiol.* 2005; 288: R4–R10.
20. Rozansky DJ. The role of aldosterone in renal sodium transport. *Semin Nephrol.* 2006; 26: 173–181.
21. Anselmo AN, Earnest S, Chen W, et al. WNK1 and OSR1 regulate the Na^+, K^+, $2Cl^-$ cotransporter in

HeLa cells. *Proc Natl Acad Sci U S A*. 2006; 103: 10883–10888.

22. Rinehart J, Kahle KT, de Los Heros P, et al. WNK3 kinase is a positive regulator of NKCC2 and NCC, renal cation-Cl⁻ cotransporters required for normal blood pressure homeostasis. *Proc Natl Acad Sci U S A*. 2005; 102: 16777–16782.

23. Choi M, Ziyadeh F. The utility of the transtubular potassium gradient in the evaluation of hyperkalemia. *J Am Soc Nephrol*. 2008; 19: 424–426.

24. Facchini M, Sala L, Malfatto G, et al. Low-K⁺ dependent QT prolongation and risk for ventricular arrhythmia in anorexia nervosa. *Int J Cardiol*. 2006; 106: 170–176.

25. Advani A, Taylor R. Life-threatening hypokalaemia on a low-carbohydrate diet associated with previously undiagnosed primary hyperaldosteronism [corrected]. *Diabet Med*. 2005; 22: 1605–1607.

26. Chen WH, Yin HL, Lin HS, et al. Delayed hypokalemic paralysis following a convulsion due to alcohol abstinence. *J Clin Neurosci*. 2006; 13: 453–456.

27. CDC. Atypical reactions associated with heroin use—five states, January–April 2005. *MMWR*. 2005; 54: 793–796.

28. Knochel JP, Dotin LN, Hamburger RJ. Pathophysiology of intense physical conditioning in a hot climate. I. Mechanisms of potassium depletion. *J Clin Invest*. 1972; 51: 242–255.

29. McDonough AA, Youn JH. Role of muscle in regulating extracellular [K⁺]. *Semin Nephrol*. 2005; 25: 335–342.

30. Bundgaard H, Kjeldsen K. Potassium depletion increases potassium clearance capacity in skeletal muscles in vivo during acute repletion. *Am J Physiol Cell Physiol*. 2002; 283: C1163–C1170.

31. Bundgaard H. Potassium depletion improves myocardial potassium uptake in vivo. *Am J Physiol Cell Physiol*. 2004; 287: C135–C141.

32. Kung AW. Clinical review: thyrotoxic periodic paralysis: a diagnostic challenge. *J Clin Endocrinol Metab*. 2006; 91: 2490–2495.

33. Diedrich DA, Wedel DJ. Thyrotoxic periodic paralysis and anesthesia report of a case and literature review. *J Clin Anesth*. 2006; 18: 286–292.

34. Pichon B, Lidove O, Delbot T, et al. Thyrotoxic periodic paralysis in Caucasian patients: a diagnostic challenge. *Eur J Intern Med*. 2005; 16: 372–374.

35. Al-Jubouri MA, Inkster GD, Nee PA, et al. Thyrotoxicosis presenting as hypokalaemic paralysis and hyperlactataemia in an oriental man. *Ann Clin Biochem*. 2006; 43: 323–325.

36. Tran HA. Inadvertent iodine excess causing thyrotoxic hypokalemic periodic paralysis. *Arch Intern Med*. 2005; 165: 2536.

37. Kane MP, Busch RS. Drug-induced thyrotoxic periodic paralysis. *Ann Pharmacother*. 2006; 40: 778–781.

38. Ohye H, Fukata S, Kanoh M, et al. Thyrotoxicosis caused by weight-reducing herbal medicines. *Arch Intern Med*. 2005; 165: 831–834.

39. Wang W, Jiang L, Ye L, et al. Mutation screening in Chinese hypokalemic periodic paralysis patients. *Mol Genet Metab*. 2006; 87: 359–363.

40. Tricarico D, Mele A, Camerino DC. Carbonic anhydrase inhibitors ameliorate the symptoms of hypokalaemic periodic paralysis in rats by opening the muscular Ca²⁺-activated-K⁺ channels. *Neuromuscul Disord*. 2006; 16: 39–45.

41. Ikeda K, Iwasaki Y, Kinoshita M, et al. Acetazolamide-induced muscle weakness in hypokalemic periodic paralysis. *Intern Med*. 2002; 41: 743–745.

42. Abbott GW, Butler MH, Goldstein SA. Phosphorylation and protonation of neighboring MiRP2 sites: function and pathophysiology of MiRP2-Kv3.4 potassium channels in periodic paralysis. *FASEB J*. 2006; 20: 293–301.

43. Koul PA, Wahid A, Bhat FA. Primary gradient defect distal renal tubular acidosis presenting as hypokalaemic periodic paralysis. *Emerg Med J*. 2005; 22: 528–530.

44. Kim CJ, Woo YJ, Ma JS, et al. Hypokalemic paralysis and rhabdomyolysis in distal renal tubular acidosis. *Pediatr Int*. 2005; 47: 211–213.

45. Soy M, Pamuk ON, Gerenli M, et al. A primary Sjogren's syndrome patient with distal renal tubular acidosis, who presented with symptoms of hypokalemic periodic paralysis: report of a case study and review of the literature. *Rheumatol Int*. 2005; 26: 86–89.

46. Cheng CJ, Chiu JS, Chen CC, et al. Unusual cause of hypokalemic paralysis in aged men: Sjogren syndrome. *South Med J*. 2005; 98: 1212–1215.

47. Tsai CS, Chen YC, Chen HH, et al. An unusual cause of hypokalemic paralysis: aristolochic acid nephropathy with Fanconi syndrome. *Am J Med Sci*. 2005; 330: 153–155.

48. Godek SF, Godek JJ, Bartolozzi AR. Hydration status in college football players during consecutive days of twice-a-day preseason practices. *Am J Sports Med*. 2005; 33: 843–851.

49. Shirreffs SM, Aragon-Vargas LF, Chamorro M, et al. The sweating response of elite professional soccer players to training in the heat. *Int J Sports Med*. 2005; 26: 90–95.

50. Maughan RJ, Shirreffs SM, Merson SJ, et al. Fluid and electrolyte balance in elite male football (soccer) players training in a cool environment. *J Sports Sci*. 2005; 23: 73–79.

51. Maughan RJ, Merson SJ, Broad NP, et al. Fluid and electrolyte intake and loss in elite soccer players during training. *Int J Sport Nutr Exerc Metab*. 2004; 14: 333–346.

52. Stofan JR, Zachwieja JJ, Horswill CA, et al. Sweat and sodium losses in NCAA football players: a precursor to heat cramps? *Int J Sport Nutr Exerc Metab*. 2005; 15: 641–652.

53. Field M. Intestinal ion transport and the pathophysiology of diarrhea. *J Clin Invest*. 2003; 111: 931–943.

54. Agarwal R, Afzalpurkar R, Fordtran JS. Pathophysiology of potassium absorption and secretion by the human intestine. *Gastroenterology*. 1994; 107: 548–571.

55. Onozawa M, Fukuhara T, Minoguchi M, et al. Hypokalemic rhabdomyolysis due to WDHA syndrome caused by VIP-producing composite pheochromocytoma: a case in

neurofibromatosis type 1. *Jpn J Clin Oncol.* 2005; 35: 559–563.

56. Rossi V, Saibeni S, Sinigaglia L, et al. Hypokalemic rhabdomyolysis without watery diarrhea: an unexpected presentation of a pancreatic neuro-endocrine tumor. *Am J Gastroenterol.* 2006; 101: 669–672.

57. Lepur D, Klinar I, Mise B, et al. McKittrick-Wheelock syndrome: a rare cause of diarrhoea. *Eur J Gastroenterol Hepatol.* 2006; 18: 557–559.

58. van Dinter TG, Fuerst FC, Richardson CT, et al. Stimulated active potassium secretion in a patient with colonic pseudo-obstruction: a new mechanism of secretory diarrhea. *Gastroenterology.* 2005; 129: 1268–1273.

59. Sausbier M, Matos JE, Sausbier U, et al. Distal colonic K($+$) secretion occurs via BK channels. *J Am Soc Nephrol.* 2006;17: 1275–1282.

60. del Castillo JR, Burguillos L. Pathways for K$^+$ efflux in isolated surface and crypt colonic cells. Activation by calcium. *J Membr Biol.* 2005; 205: 37–47.

61. Mathialahan T, Maclennan KA, Sandle LN, et al. Enhanced large intestinal potassium permeability in end-stage renal disease. *J Pathol.* 2005; 206: 46–51.

62. Gonlusen G, Akgun H, Ertan A, et al. Renal failure and nephrocalcinosis associated with oral sodium phosphate bowel cleansing: clinical patterns and renal biopsy findings. *Arch Pathol Lab Med.* 2006; 130: 101–106.

63. Mathus-Vliegen EM, Kemble UM. A prospective randomized blinded comparison of sodium phosphate and polyethylene glycol-electrolyte solution for safe bowel cleansing. *Aliment Pharmacol Ther.* 2006; 23: 543–552.

64. Bennett A, Stryjewski G. Severe hypokalemia caused by oral and rectal administration of bentonite in a pediatric patient. *Pediatr Emerg Care.* 2006; 22: 500–502.

65. Trivedi TH, Daga GL, Yeolekar ME. Geophagia leading to hypokalemic quadriparesis in a postpartum patient. *J Assoc Physicians India.* 2005; 53: 205–207.

66. Ukaonu C, Hill DA, Christensen F. Hypokalemic myopathy in pregnancy caused by clay ingestion. *Obstet Gynecol.* 2003; 102: 1169–1171.

67. Nicholls MG. Unilateral renal ischemia causing the hyponatremic hypertensive syndrome in children—more common than we think? *Pediatr Nephrol.* 2006; 21: 887–890.

68. Seracini D, Pela I, Favilli S, et al. Hyponatraemic-hypertensive syndrome in a 15-month-old child with renal artery stenosis. *Pediatr Nephrol.* 2006; 21: 1027–1030.

69. Mulatero P, Milan A, Fallo F, et al. Comparison of confirmatory tests for the diagnosis of primary aldosteronism. *J Clin Endocrinol Metab.* 2006; 91: 2618–2623.

70. Mattsson C, Young WF Jr. Primary aldosteronism: diagnostic and treatment strategies. *Nat Clin Pract Nephrol.* 2006; 2: 198–208.

71. Reynolds RM, Shakerdi LA, Sandhu K, et al. The utility of three different methods for measuring urinary 18-hydroxycortisol in the differential diagnosis of suspected primary hyperaldosteronism. *Eur J Endocrinol.* 2005; 152: 903–907.

72. New MI, Geller DS, Fallo F, et al. Monogenic low renin hypertension. *Trends Endocrinol Metab.* 2005; 16: 92–97.

73. Snyder PM. Minireview: regulation of epithelial Na$^+$ channel trafficking. *Endocrinology.* 2005;146:5079–5085.

74. Staub O, Verrey F. Impact of Nedd4 proteins and serum and glucocorticoid-induced kinases on epithelial Na$^+$ transport in the distal nephron. *J Am Soc Nephrol.* 2005; 16: 3167–3174.

75. Knight KK, Olson DR, Zhou R, et al. Liddle's syndrome mutations increase Na$^+$ transport through dual effects on epithelial Na$^+$ channel surface expression and proteolytic cleavage. *Proc Natl Acad Sci U S A.* 2006; 103: 2805–2808.

76. Anantharam A, Tian Y, Palmer LG. Open probability of the epithelial sodium channel is regulated by intracellular sodium. *J Physiol.* 2006; 574: 333–347.

77. Hamidon BB, Jeyabalan V. Exogenously-induced apparent hypermineralocorticoidism associated with ingestion of "asam boi". *Singapore Med J.* 2006; 47: 156–158.

78. Iida R, Otsuka Y, Matsumoto K, et al. Pseudoaldosteronism due to the concurrent use of two herbal medicines containing glycyrrhizin: interaction of glycyrrhizin with angiotensin-converting enzyme inhibitor. *Clin Exp Nephrol.* 2006; 10: 131–135.

79. Lee YS, Lorenzo BJ, Koufis T, et al. Grapefruit juice and its flavonoids inhibit 11 beta-hydroxysteroid dehydrogenase. *Clin Pharmacol Ther.* 1996; 59: 62–71.

80. Quattropani C, Vogt B, Odermatt A, et al. Reduced activity of 11 beta-hydroxysteroid dehydrogenase in patients with cholestasis. *J Clin Invest.* 2001; 108: 1299–1305.

81. Ackermann D, Vogt B, Escher G, et al. Inhibition of 11beta-hydroxysteroid dehydrogenase by bile acids in rats with cirrhosis. *Hepatology.* 1999; 30: 623–629.

82. Stauffer AT, Rochat MK, Dick B, et al. Chenodeoxycholic acid and deoxycholic acid inhibit 11 beta-hydroxysteroid dehydrogenase type 2 and cause cortisol-induced transcriptional activation of the mineralocorticoid receptor. *J Biol Chem.* 2002; 277: 26286–26292.

83. Kim SW, Wang W, Sassen MC, et al. Biphasic changes of epithelial sodium channel abundance and trafficking in common bile duct ligation-induced liver cirrhosis. *Kidney Int.* 2006; 69: 89–98.

84. Kim SW, Schou UK, Peters CD, et al. Increased apical targeting of renal epithelial sodium channel subunits and decreased expression of type 2 11beta-hydroxysteroid dehydrogenase in rats with CCl4-induced decompensated liver cirrhosis. *J Am Soc Nephrol.* 2005; 16: 3196–3210.

85. Fagart J, Huyet J, Pinon GM, et al. Crystal structure of a mutant mineralocorticoid receptor responsible for hypertension. *Nat Struct Mol Biol.* 2005; 12: 554–555.

86. Bledsoe RK, Madauss KP, Holt JA, et al. A ligand-mediated hydrogen bond network required for the activation of the mineralocorticoid receptor. *J Biol Chem.* 2005; 280: 31283–31293.

87. Rafestin-Oblin ME, Souque A, Bocchi B, et al. The severe form of hypertension caused by the activating S810L mutation in the mineralocorticoid receptor is cortisone related. *Endocrinology.* 2003; 144: 528–533.

88. Izzedine H, Launay-Vacher V, Deray G. Antiviral drug-induced nephrotoxicity. *Am J Kidney Dis.* 2005; 45: 804–817.

89. Cirino CM, Kan VL. Hypokalemia in HIV patients on tenofovir. *AIDS.* 2006; 20: 1671–1673.

90. Bresolin NL, Grillo E, Fernandes VR, et al. A case report and review of hypokalemic paralysis secondary to renal tubular acidosis. *Pediatr Nephrol.* 2005; 20: 818–820.

91. Harada K, Akai Y, Iwano M, et al. Tubulointerstitial macrophage infiltration in a patient with hypokalemic nephropathy and primary Sjogren's syndrome. *Clin Nephrol.* 2005; 64: 387–390.

92. Cheng CJ, Chiu JS, Chen CC, et al. Unusual cause of hypokalemic paralysis in aged med: Sjogren syndrome. *South Med J.* 2005; 98: 1212–1215.

93. Abad S, Park S, Grimaldi D, et al. Hypokalaemia tetraparesis and rhabdomyolysis: aetiology discovered on a normal lung radiograph. *Nephrol Dial Transplant.* 2005; 20: 2571–2572.

94. Pela I, Materassi M, Seracini D, et al. Hypokalemic rhabdomyolysis in a child with Bartter's syndrome. *Pediatr Nephrol.* 2005; 20: 1189–1191.

95. Duman O, Koyun M, Akman S, et al. Case of Bartter syndrome presenting with hypokalemic periodic paralysis. *J Child Neurol.* 2006; 21: 255–256.

96. Landau D. Potassium-related inherited tubulopathies. *Cell Mol Life Sci.* 2006; 63: 1962–1968.

97. Proesmans W. Threading through the mizmaze of Bartter syndrome. *Pediatr Nephrol.* 2006; 21: 896–902.

98. Pluznick JL, Sansom SC. BK channels in the kidney: role in $K(+)$ secretion and localization of molecular components. *Am J Physiol Renal Physiol.* 2006; 291: F517–F529.

99. Bailey MA, Cantone A, Yan Q, et al. Maxi-K channels contribute to urinary potassium excretion in the ROMK-deficient mouse model of Type II Bartter's syndrome and in adaptation to a high-K diet. *Kidney Int.* 2006; 70: 51–59.

100. Pressler CA, Heinzinger J, Jeck N, et al. Late-onset manifestation of antenatal bartter syndrome as a result of residual function of the mutated renal Na^+-K^+-2Cl-co-transporter. *J Am Soc Nephrol.* 2006; 17: 2136–2142.

101. Jang HR, Lee JW, Oh YK, et al. From bench to bedside: diagnosis of Gitelman's syndrome—defect of sodium-chloride cotransporter in renal tissue. *Kidney Int.* 2006; 70: 813–817.

102. Morris RG, Hoorn EJ, Knepper MA. Hypokalemia in a mouse model of Gitelman's syndrome. *Am J Physiol Renal Physiol.* 2006; 290: F1416–F1420.

103. Pachulski RT, Lopez F, Sharaf R. Gitelman's not-so-benign syndrome. *N Engl J Med.* 2005; 353: 850–851.

104. Morita R, Takeuchi K, Nakamura A, et al. Gitelman's syndrome with mental retardation. *Intern Med.* 2006; 45: 211–213.

105. Comer D, Droogan A, Young I, et al. Hypokalaemic paralysis precipitated by distal renal tubular acidosis secondary to Sjögren's syndrome. *Ann Clin Biochem.* 2008; 45(pt 2): 221–225.

106. Aygen B, Dursun F, Dogukan A, et al. Hypokalemic quadriparesis associated with renal tubular acidosis in a patient with Sjögren's syndrome. *Clin Nephrol.* 2008; 69(4): 306–309.

107. Clausen T, Nielsen O. Potassium, Na^+, K^+-pumps and fatigue in rat muscle. *J Physiol.* 2007; 584: 295–304.

108. McKenna M, Bangsbo J, Renaud J. Muscle K^+, Na^+, and Cl^- disturbances and Na^+-K^+ pump inactivation: implications for fatigue. *J Appl Physiol.* 2008; 104: 288–295.

109. Clifford P. Skeletal muscle vasodilatation at the onset of exercise. *J Physiol.* 2007; 583: 825–833.

110. Reungjui S, Roncal C, Sato W, et al. Hypokalemic nephropathy is associated with impaired angiogenesis. *J Am Soc Nephrol.* 2008; 19: 125–134.

111. Zillich A, Garg J, Basu S, et al. Thiazide diuretics, potassium, and the development of diabetes: a quantitative review. *Hypertension.* 2006; 48(2): 219–224.

112. Alderman M. New onset diabetes during antihypertensive therapy. *Am J Hypertens.* 2008; 21(5): 493–499.

113. Koster J, Remedi M, Masia R, et al. Expression of ATP-insensitive KATP channels in pancreatic beta-cells underlies a spectrum of diabetic phenotyes. *Diabetes.* 2006; 55(11): 2957–2964.

114. Barzilay J, Cutler J, Davis B. Antihypertensive medications and risk of diabetes mellitus. *Curr Opin Nephrol Hypertens.* 2007; 16: 256–260.

115. Philips DA, Bauch TD. Rapid correction of hypokalemia in a patient with an ICD and Recurrent Ventricular Tachycardia. *J Emerg Med.* 2008.

116. Garcis E, Nakhleh N, Simmons D, et al. Profound hypokalemia: unusual presentation and management in a 12-year-old boy. *Pediatr Emerg Care.* 2008; 24(3): 157–160.

117. Crop M, Hoorn E, Lindemans J, et al. Hypokalaemia and subsequent hyperkalaemia in hospitalized patients. *Nephrol Dial Transplant.* 2007; 22: 3471–3477.

118. Kellerman PS, Thornbery JM. Pseudohyperkalemia due to pneumatic tube transport in a leukemic patient. *Am J Kidney Dis.* 2005; 46: 746–748.

119. Colussi G. Pseudohyperkalemia in leukemias. *Am J Kidney Dis.* 2006; 47: 373.

120. Owens H, Siparsky G, Bajaj L, et al. Correction of factitious hyperkalemia in hemolyzed specimens. *Am J Emerg Med.* 2005; 23: 872–875.

121. Sevastos N, Theodossiades G, Savvas SP, et al. Pseudohyperkalemia in patients with increased cellular components of blood. *Am J Med Sci.* 2006; 331: 17–21.

122. Sevastos N, Theodossiades G, Efstathiou S, et al. Pseudohyperkalemia in serum: the phenomenon and its clinical magnitude. *J Lab Clin Med.* 2006; 147: 139–144.

123. Cheng CJ, Chiu JS, Huang WH, et al. Acute hyperkalemic paralysis in a uremic patient. *J Nephrol.* 2005; 18: 630–633.

124. Burrowes JD, Van Houten G. Use of alternative medicine by patients with stage 5 chronic kidney

disease. *Adv Chronic Kidney Dis.* 2005; 12: 312–325.

125. Gelfand MC, Zarate A, Knepshield JH. Geophagia. A cause of life-threatening hyperkalemia in patients with chronic renal failure. *JAMA.* 1975; 234: 738–740.

126. Abu-Hamdan DK, Sondheimer JH, Mahajan SK. Cautopyreiophagia. Cause of life-threatening hyperkalemia in a patient undergoing hemodialysis. *Am J Med.* 1985; 79: 517–519.

127. Phillips DR, Ahmad KI, Waller SJ, et al. A serum potassium level above 10 mmol/l in a patient predisposed to hypokalemia. *Nat Clin Pract Nephrol.* 2006; 2: 340–346.

128. Wang Q, Domenighetti AA, Pedrazzini T, et al. Potassium supplementation reduces cardiac and renal hypertrophy independent of blood pressure in DOCA/salt mice. *Hypertension.* 2005; 46: 547–554.

129. Chang HY, Hu YW, Yue CS, et al. Effect of potassium-enriched salt on cardiovascular mortality and medical expenses of elderly men. *Am J Clin Nutr.* 2006; 83: 1289–1296.

130. Dai Q, Borenstein AR, Wu Y, et al. Fruit and vegetable juices and Alzheimer's disease: the Kame Project. *Am J Med.* 2006; 119: 751–759.

131. Rampello E, Fricia T, Malaguarnera M. The management of tumor lysis syndrome. *Nat Clin Pract Oncol.* 2006; 3: 438–447.

132. Martyn JA, Richtsfeld M. Succinylcholine-induced hyperkalemia in acquired pathologic states: etiologic factors and molecular mechanisms. *Anesthesiology.* 2006; 104: 158–169.

133. Matthews JM. Succinylcholine-induced hyperkalemia. *Anesthesiology.* 2006; 105: 430.

134. Penfield JG. Multiple myeloma in end-stage renal disease. *Semin Dial.* 2006; 19: 329–334.

135. Liman RS, Rosenberg H. Malignant hyperthermia: update on susceptibility testing. *JAMA.* 2005; 293: 2918–2924.

136. Sonikian M, Metaxaki P, Vlassopoulos D, et al. Long-term management of sevelamer hydrochloride-induced metabolic acidosis aggravation and hyperkalemia in hemodialysis patients. *Ren Fail.* 2006; 28: 411–418.

137. Kaisar MO, Wiggins KJ, Sturtevant JM, et al. A randomized controlled trial of fludrocortisone for the treatment of hyperkalemia in hemodialysis patients. *Am J Kidney Dis.* 2006; 47: 809–814.

138. Dharmarajan TS, Nguyen T, Russell RO. Life-threatening, preventable hyperkalemia in a nursing home resident: case report and literature review. *J Am Med Dir Assoc.* 2005; 6: 400–405.

139. Hou FF, Zhang X, Zhang GH, et al. Efficacy and safety of benazepril for advanced chronic renal insufficiency. *N Engl J Med.* 2006; 354: 131–140.

140. Raebel MA, McClure DL, Simon SR, et al. Laboratory monitoring of potassium and creatinine in ambulatory patients receiving angiotensin converting enzyme inhibitors and angiotensin receptor blockers. *Pharmacoepidemiol Drug Saf.* 2007; 16(1): 55–64.

141. Moore CR, Lin JJ, O'Connor N, et al. Follow-up of markedly elevated serum potassium results in the ambulatory setting: implications for patient safety. *Am J Med Qual.* 2006; 21: 115–124.

142. Parham WA, Mehdirad AA, Biermann KM, et al. Hyperkalemia revisited. *Tex Heart Inst J.* 2006; 33: 40–47.

143. Noble K, Isles C. Hyperkalaemia causing profound bradycardia. *Heart.* 2006; 92: 1063.

144. Letavernier E, Couzi L, Delmas Y, et al. Verapamil and mild hyperkalemia in hemodialysis patients: a potentially hazardous association. *Hemodial Int.* 2006; 10: 170–172.

145. Muto S, Tsuruoka S, Miyata Y, et al. Effect of trimethoprim-sulfamethoxazole on Na and K^+ transport properties in the rabbit cortical collecting duct perfused in vitro. *Nephron Physiol.* 2006; 102: 51–60.

146. Xie J, Craig L, Cobb MH, et al. Role of with-no-lysine [K] kinases in the pathogenesis of Gordon's syndrome. *Pediatr Nephrol.* 2006; 21: 1231–1236.

147. Cai H, Cebotaru V, Wang YH, et al. WNK4 kinase regulates surface expression of the human sodium chloride cotransporter in mammalian cells. *Kidney Int.* 2006; 69: 2162–2170.

148. Lalioti MD, Zhang J, Volkman HM, et al. Wnk4 controls blood pressure and potassium homeostasis via regulation of mass and activity of the distal convoluted tubule. *Nat Genet.* 2006; 38: 1124–1132.

149. Golbang AP, Murthy M, Hamad A, et al. A new kindred with pseudohypoaldosteronism type II and a novel mutation (564D>H) in the acidic motif of the WNK4 gene. *Hypertension.* 2005; 46: 295–300.

150. Proctor G, Linas S. Type 2 pseudohypoaldosteronism: new insights into renal potassium, sodium, and chloride handling. *Am J Kidney Dis.* 2006; 48: 674–693.

151. Ohta A, Yang SS, Rai T, et al. Overexpression of human WNK1 increases paracellular chloride permeability and phosphorylation of claudin-4 in MDCKII cells. *Biochem Biophys Res Commun.* 2006; 349: 804–808.

152. Mayan H, Munter G, Shaharabany M, et al. Hypercalciuria in familial hyperkalemia and hypertension accompanies hyperkalemia and precedes hypertension: description of a large family with the Q565E WNK4 mutation. *J Clin Endocrinol Metab.* 2004; 89: 4025–4030.

153. Martin JM, Calduch L, Monteagudo C, et al. Clinico-pathological analysis of the cutaneous lesions of a patient with type I pseudohypoaldosteronism. *J Eur Acad Dermatol Venereol.* 2005; 19: 377–379.

154. Geller DS, Zhang J, Zennaro MC, et al. Autosomal dominant pseudohypoaldosteronism type 1: mechanisms, evidence for neonatal lethality, and phenotypic expression in adults. *J Am Soc Nephrol.* 2006; 17: 1429–1436.

155. Riepe FG, Finkeldei J, de Sanctis L, et al. Elucidating the underlying molecular pathogenesis of NR3C2 mutants causing autosomal dominant pseudohypoaldosteronism type 1. *J Clin Endocrinol Metab.* 2006; 91(11): 4552–4561.

156. Fernandes-Rosa FL, de Castro M, Latronico AC, et al. Recurrence of the R947X mutation in unrelated families with autosomal dominant

pseudohypoaldosteronism type 1: evidence for a mutational hot spot in the mineralocorticoid receptor gene. *J Clin Endocrinol Metab.* 2006; 91: 3671–3675.

157. Petrov D, Petrov M. Widening of the QRS Complex due to severe hyperkalemia as an acute complication of diabetic ketoacidosis. *J Emerg Med.*. 2008; 34(4): 459–461.

158. Scarabeo V, Baccillieri M, Di Marco A, et al. Sine-wave pattern on the electrocardiogram and hyperkalaemia. *J Cardiovasc Med.* 2007; 8: 729–731.

159. Pluijmen M, Hersbach F. Sine-wave pattern arrythmia and sudden paralysis that result from severe hyperkalemia. *Circulation.* 2007; 116: e2–e4.

160. Littmann L, Monroe M, Taylor K, et al. The hyperkalemis Brugada sign. *J Electrocardiol.* 2007;40:53–59.

161. Sovari A, Assadi R, Lakshminarayanana B, et al. Hyperacute T wave, the early sign of myocardial infarction. *Am J Emerg Med.* 2007; 25: 859.el–859.e7.

162. Bellazzini M, Meyer T. Pseudo-myocardial infarction in diabetic ketoacidosis with hyperkalemia. *J Emerg Med.* 2007 September 10. [Epub ahead of print]

163. Tatli E, Buyuklu M, Onal B. Electrocardiographic abnormaility: hyperkalaemia mimicking isolated acute inferior myocardial infarction. *J Cardiovasc Med.* 2008; 9: 210.

164. Tomcsanyi J, Wagner V, Bozsik B. Littman sign in hyperkalemia: double counting of heart rate. *Am J Emerg Med.* 2007; 25: 1077–1080.

165. Montague B, Ouellette J, Buller G. Retrospective review of the frequency of ECG changes in hyperkalemia. *Clin J Am Soc Nephrol.* 2008; 3: 324–330.

CHAPTER 6

Disorders of Calcium, Phosphorus, Vitamin D, and Parathyroid Hormone Activity

MORDECAI M. POPOVTZER

Serum Calcium Concentration

The calcium ion is essential to many physiologic phenomena, including preservation of the integrity of cellular membranes, neuromuscular activity, regulation of endocrine and exocrine secretory activities, blood coagulation, activation of the complement system, and bone metabolism.

Total Serum Calcium Concentration

The normal range for total serum calcium must be established for each laboratory and varies according to the method used. Total serum calcium is divisible into protein-bound and ultrafiltrable (diffusible) calcium (Fig. 6.1).

PROTEIN-BOUND CALCIUM

Approximately 40% of total calcium is bound to serum proteins, and 80% to 90% of this calcium is bound to albumin. Variations in serum protein alter proportionally the concentration of the protein-bound and total serum calcium. An increase in serum albumin concentration of 1 g/dL increases protein-bound calcium by 0.8 mg/dL, whereas an increase of 1 g/dL of globulin increases protein-bound calcium by 0.16 mg/dL. Thus, it is obvious that changes in total serum calcium concentration cannot be used for the assessment of the effect on bound calcium concentration unless the changes in albumin and globulin concentrations also are determined. Marked changes in serum sodium concentration also affect the protein binding of calcium. Hyponatremia increases, whereas hypernatremia decreases protein-bound calcium. Changes in pH also affect protein-bound calcium, and an increase or decrease of 0.1 pH, increases or decreases protein-bound calcium by 0.12 mg/dL. Respectively, in vitro, freezing and thawing serum samples may decrease the binding of calcium as well.

ULTRAFILTRABLE (DIFFUSIBLE) CALCIUM

Serum ultrafiltrable calcium is obtained by applying pressure on serum against a semipermeable membrane. Thus, serum water is forced across the membrane, and the ultrafiltrate is analyzed for calcium concentration and then corrected for total serum solids. The samples must be handled anaerobically, because changes in pH may affect calcium binding. Under normal conditions, ultrafiltrable calcium constitutes 55% to 60% of the total serum calcium.

FREE (IONIZED) CALCIUM

The biologically active component of diffusible calcium is ionized calcium. Flow-through and static ion exchange electrodes, which function similarly to the conventional pH electrodes, are used. Serum

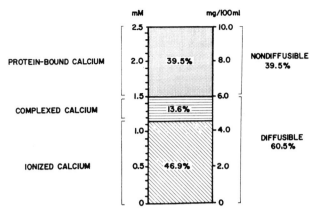

■ **Figure 6.1** Calcium fractions in the serum. (From Moore EW. Ionized calcium in normal serum, ultrafiltrates and whole blood determined by ion-exchange electrode. *J Clin Invest.* 1970; 49: 318, with permission.)

ionized calcium concentration in normal subjects ranges from 4.0 to 4.9 mg/dL, or 47% of total serum calcium. The samples have to be handled anaerobically because changes in pH alter the concentration of ionized calcium. Determinations are best made on freshly separated serum, because heparin creates complexes with calcium, and the presence of fibrin may interfere with the structural integrity of the porous membrane used in the procedure. Storage of serum in oil does not prevent changes in pH, because carbon dioxide dissolves readily in oil. An increase in serum pH of 0.1 unit may cause a decrease in ionized calcium of 0.16 mg/dL (1,2). As with ultrafiltrable calcium, freezing and thawing of serum may alter the level of ionized calcium.

COMPLEXED CALCIUM

The nonionized portion of diffusible or ultrafiltrable calcium is called complexed calcium. The calcium complexes are formed with bicarbonate, phosphate, and acetate. The amount of complexed calcium is measured indirectly by subtracting the ionized calcium (47%) from the ultrafiltrable calcium (60%) and thus equals about 13% of total serum calcium. The complexed calcium has been found to be increased twofold in patients with uremia.

CYTOSOLIC CALCIUM

Cytosolic calcium can be measured by loading the tested cells with fluorescent probe such as indo-1-acetoxymethyl ester and exciting the cells at 350 nM. The ratio of fluorescence emission at 410 nM to that at 490 nM is used an index of free intracellular calcium. The normal concentration of cytosolic calcium is 100 nM/L, which is 10,000-fold lower than the concentration of extracellular calcium. The very steep gradient is maintained by an energy driven calcium pump, known as the plasma membrane Ca^{2+} ATPase (PMCA). In certain type of cells a Na^+/Ca^{2+} exchanger, energized by Na^+-gradient helps drive cytosolic calcium into the extracellular space. Part of cellular calcium is sequestered in intracellular organelles, including endoplasmic reticulum, sarcoplasmic reticulum (SR) in muscle cells and in mitochondria. The calcium-dependent intracellular signaling generally requires 10-fold increase in cytosolic calcium. With each heartbeat the cytosolic calcium concentration in cardiac myocytes is elevated 10-fold, from a resting level of 100 nM to 1000 nM. Likewise, in other signaling events such as T-cell activation, which triggers the transcription of interleukin-2 (IL-2), a 10-fold increase in cytosolic calcium serves as the signal for the response. Elevation of cytosolic calcium is mediated by activation of calcium channels, which allows passive calcium flux down its electrochemical gradient.

Calcium plays an important role in cardiac coupling of excitation and contraction. The lasting phase of cardiac action potential is maintained by L-type calcium channels, whereby extracellular calcium influx into the intracellular space activates calcium-sensitive channels of SR. Relatively small amounts of calcium entering the cell via the L-type channel activate a small number SR calcium channels. This leads to calcium release from SR and marked increase in intracellular calcium concentration, termed "calcium-induced calcium release." Calcium removal from the cytoplasm occurs via active transport back to SR by calcium pump, Ca^{2+} ATPase. A smaller amount, the same that amount that entered the cell through L-type calcium channel, is extruded into the extracellular space via sodium–calcium exchanger (NCX). Glycosides the drugs known for positive inotropic effect act by inhibiting sodium pump (Na^+/K^+ ATPase), increase intracellular sodium load in the myocytes. Subsequent activation of NCX leads to sodium extrusion and calcium into the myocyte cytosol. Glycosides, represented the only effective therapy for congestive heart failure for a long time (3).

Serum Phosphorus Concentration

Serum phosphorus occurs in two forms, organic and inorganic. Organic phosphorus is composed entirely of phospholipids bound to proteins. The inorganic fraction is the principal circulating form of phosphorus and is routinely assayed for clinical uses. About 90% of inorganic phosphorus is ultrafiltrable. About 53% of the ultrafiltrable inorganic phosphorus in serum is dissociated, with a 1:4 ratio of $H_2PO_4^-$ to HPO_4^{2-}; the remainder of ultrafiltrable phosphate is in the form of salts of sodium, calcium, and magnesium. During marked hyperphosphatemia (8 to 10 mg/dL of serum), a significant portion of phosphate forms colloidal complexes with calcium that are rapidly removed from the circulation.

Studies propose that an increase in serum phosphorus leads to a reciprocal fall in serum calcium, so that the product of both ions remains constant. The assumption was that solubility equilibrium exists between the bone and the extracellular fluid (ECF). However, this appears to be an oversimplification of a more complex equilibrium. An inverse relationship between serum calcium and phosphorus is present only under extreme changes of serum phosphorus; for example, a decrease in serum calcium occurs following an acute rise in serum phosphorus. By contrast, this relationship does not hold for acute changes in serum calcium, because a rapid increase in calcium leads to a rise rather than a fall in serum phosphorus before any changes in urinary phosphorus occur (2). This effect may be caused by the release of phosphorus from cells.

Serum phosphorus displays circadian variations. Serum phosphorus levels reach a nadir early in the morning, with an increase to plateau at 4 p.m., followed by a further increase to a peak at 1 to 3 a.m.

Serum phosphorus concentration also is influenced by age. In adults the normal concentration ranges from 2.5 to 4.0 mg/dL, whereas in children it ranges from 4 to 6 mg/dL. The level of alkaline phosphatase in children is higher than in adults. These age differences are probably related to different rates of skeletal growth. Serum phosphorus decreases during hyperventilation and alkalosis and increases during acidosis. Serum phosphorus also varies directly with its content in the diet. Administration of glucose causes a fall in serum phosphate because of the flux of phosphate into cells with the phosphorylation of glucose. The administration of insulin and epinephrine also reduces serum phosphorus concentration. Hypophosphatemia occurring in sepsis and acute myocardial infarction may result from the release of epinephrine into the circulation.

A recent large population study showed that serum phosphorus is only weakly related to dietary phosphorus intake and/or phosphorus rich foods, suggesting that other factors determining serum phosphorus concentration remain to be defined (4). This finding may bear on another earlier population study which showed that higher serum phosphorus levels, even within the normal range, had been associated with increased risk of cardiovascular events in patient with normal kidney function (5). The clinical relevance of these and other population wide studies is uncertain.

Calcium and Phosphorus Balance

Total body calcium ranges from 1.0 to 1.5 kg and that of phosphorus from 0.5 to 0.8 kg. Ninety-nine percent of total calcium and 85% of total phosphorus are stored in the skeleton. Only 1% of both is in the ECF, and the remainder is intracellular.

TABLE 6.1 CALCIUM AND PHOSPHORUS CONTENT IN DIFFERENT FOODS

Food	Calcium (mg/100 g)	Phosphorus (mg/100 g)
Cow's milk	120	100
Hard American cheese	697	771
Cottage cheese	100	110
Eggs	54	205
Meat	13	200

DIETARY CALCIUM AND PHOSPHORUS

Dietary calcium and phosphorus intake varies considerably. In general, balanced diets provide from 800 to 1,200 mg of calcium and from 800 to 1,500 mg of phosphorus per day. The minimum daily requirement of calcium is 400 to 500 mg, and an intake below this amount may cause a negative calcium balance. Dietary calcium can be reduced to about 200 mg by the exclusion of dairy products (6), and boiling of vegetables causes a loss of 25% of their calcium content. It has become common to enrich bread with powdered milk to increase the amount of calcium in the diet. Drinking water is also a source of calcium; "soft" water has 1 to 3 mg/dL of calcium, and "hard" water has 3 to 10 mg/dL. Human diets, almost without exception, contain more phosphorus than calcium, because phosphorus is present in almost all foodstuffs. The amount of calcium and phosphorus in various foods is shown in Table 6.1.

INTESTINAL ABSORPTION OF CALCIUM

Calcium is absorbed along the small intestine, more in the duodenum and proximal jejunum than the ileum (6–8). The absorption of calcium is completed within 4 hours after its oral intake (8,9). Calcium absorption in the gastrointestinal (GI) tract occurs via two transport processes (10–13). Transcellular calcium absorption, which is saturable and physiologically regulated, follows three steps: (a) luminal entry into mucosal cells through apical calcium channels; (b) binding to a protein carrier, calbindin 9k, and transfer to the serosal side; and (c) extrusion from the cell by an active process at the basolateral side by Ca^{2+} ATPase (calcium pump) and also most likely, by NCX. Increasing body demands for calcium activate maximally the transcellular transportation. Paracellular calcium absorption is nonsaturable and is driven by concentration gradients between luminal and serosal spaces. Thus, the rate of absorption primarily depends on calcium concentration in the lumen. This pathway of absorption predominates in distal small bowel. The paracellular absorption route traverses the apical tight junctions of the mucosal cells; therefore, changes in permeability in these sites also may affect the rate of transport. In contrast to the parcellular pathway, the transcellular route represents an actively controlled mechanism of calcium reabsorption. Identification of epithelial calcium channels TRPV6 (also known as ECaC2) to a lesser extent TRPV5 (ECaC1) advanced our understanding of the transcellular calcium reabsorption (14). It appears that ECaC is regulated by vitamin D. ECaC was first cloned from rabbit kidney cortex. In addition to the kidney, ECaC messenger ribonucleic acid (mRNA) is expressed in small intestine as well. Immunohistochemical staining located the channel protein in the apical membrane of renal epithelial cells and the brush-border membrane of duodenal and jejunal villi. ECaC mRNA and protein abundance are decreased in states of vitamin D deficiency and increased with vitamin D repletion. ECaC is the rate-limiting factor in active calcium absorption by regulating the apical entry of calcium into the epithelial cells. The ECaC family consists of two homologous species; ECaC1 refers mainly to the renal channel, whereas ECaC2 is mainly the intestinal channel. Genomic cloning showed that ECaC1 and ECaC2 are products of distinct genes, both are juxtaposed on chromosome 7q35, suggesting evolutionary gene duplication. ECaC2 has been cloned from rat, mouse, and human intestines.

The absorption of calcium becomes more efficient with low calcium intake, thus ensuring that adequate amounts of calcium are delivered to the body. This process of adjustment to low calcium intake, which is not entirely understood, has been termed "adaptation." Younger persons exhibit this phenomenon of adaptation better than older individuals. The absorption of calcium also increases in direct proportion to the requirements; for example, calcium absorption increases during pregnancy and depletion of total body calcium.

Oral calcium may be complexed, chelated, or precipitated in the GI tract by a variety of substances that render it unavailable for absorption. These substances include phytate, oxalate, and citrate. Certain drugs, including colchicine, fluoride, theophylline, and glucocorticoids, also interfere with calcium absorption. Rapid motility or shortening of the length of the GI tract may diminish the absorption of calcium as well. Decreased calcium absorption has been observed with protein depletion both in human subjects and rats. A deficiency of the specific calcium-binding protein in the intestinal mucosal cells has been proposed as the mechanism accounting for this failure of calcium transport.

In the absence of oral intake, calcium continues to be excreted in the feces and a negative calcium balance ensues. Thus, it is apparent that some of the fecal calcium is derived from intestinal secretion. Using an intravenous tracer method, the daily calcium secretion has been estimated to be on the order of 150 mg/day. This amount does not change during an intravenous load of calcium.

Net calcium absorption (dietary calcium minus fecal calcium) can be determined by maintaining the patient on a constant diet and collecting stools. This balance method is time consuming, because it requires an equilibration period of several days followed by a collection period of several days. The results may be expressed in absolute values, where the net calcium absorption is the difference between calcium intake and calcium fecal excretion. Alternatively, the results can be expressed as fractional calcium absorption, as shown in the following formula:

$$\text{Fractional calcium absorption} = \frac{\text{dietary calcium} - \text{fecal calcium}}{\text{dietary calcium} \times 100} \qquad (6.1)$$

INTESTINAL ABSORPTION OF PHOSPHORUS

About 50% to 65% of dietary phosphorus is absorbed, mostly in the jejunum. Evidence from in vitro studies indicates that phosphorus absorption is an active process. The active process is sodium coupled and saturable.

Phosphate is transported across the mucosal brush-border membrane against an electrochemical gradient. This active transport is sodium dependent and is driven by a sodium gradient generated and maintained by the activity of Na^+/K^+ ATPase at the basolateral membrane. A sodium-phosphate (NaPi) cotransporter has been cloned from the mouse small intestine and designated as a type IIb (NaPiIIb) cotransporter in analogy to a type IIa (NaPiIIa) cotransporter cloned from the kidney (15). Type IIb is located in human chromosome 4, whereas type IIa (NaPiIIa) is located in human chromosome 5. NaPiIIb protein was localized in the intestinal brush-border membrane by immunofluorescence and was identified in isolated brush-border membrane vesicles by Western analysis. The type IIb (NaPiIIb) cotransporter was characterized by functional studies in complementary RNA (cRNA)-injected oocytes and shown to have the features of intestinal NaPi transport. Type IIb mediated NaPi cotransport is enhanced by more acidic pH as opposed to the renal type IIa transporter, which is stimulated by more alkaline pH.

It has been shown that $1,25(OH)_2D$ increases phosphorus transport by stimulating NaPiIIb cotransporter. Experimental studies in rodents demonstrated age-dependent response to $1,25(OH)_2D$. In suckling animals vitamin D increased NaPiIIb gene expression and protein abundance. Whereas in adult rodents $1,25(OH)_2D$ increased protein abundance without changes in gene expression of the cotransporters in the small intestine (16). Similarly, low-phosphorus diet stimulated intestinal phosphorus absorption is associated with NaPiIIb protein abundance without changes in gene expression. This response is independent of vitamin D (17). Nicotamide-induced inhibition of intestinal phosphorus absorption is associated with a decrease in NaPiIIb protein abundance in brush-border membrane vesicles.

There, however, is a linear correlation between phosphorus intake and net absorption. This reflects the passive paracellular pathway of transport, which is determined by concentration gradients of phosphorus across the intestinal mucosa. In contrast to findings in animals, high phosphate intake in humans does not seem to cause a decrease in calcium absorption. Rather, the presence of phosphate in the diet is necessary for calcium absorption. Phosphate absorption may be decreased by a high calcium intake or ingestion of aluminum hydroxide antacids, which bind phosphorus in the bowel, thereby inhibiting its absorption. Similarly, sevelamer (Renagel) and lanthanum can reduce intestinal phosphate absorption.

URINARY EXCRETION OF CALCIUM

The urinary excretion of calcium varies considerably in normal subjects, but the oral intake only modestly affects the daily urinary excretion of calcium. The upper normal range of calcium excretion per day has been estimated to be <300 mg for men and <250 mg for women, or 4 mg/kg body weight. Unlike the response to a low-sodium diet, institution of a diet very low in calcium does not lead immediately to a substantial reduction in urinary calcium. However, in clinical states of protracted calcium depletion, such as in patients with intestinal malabsorption and osteomalacia, urinary excretion of calcium may be reduced to 50 mg/day or less.

Only ultrafiltrable calcium crosses the glomerular capillary walls and then is partially reabsorbed by the tubular epithelial cells. In adults, 97% to 99% of filtered calcium is reabsorbed. The tubules reabsorb ionized calcium more easily than complexed calcium, which accounts for the fact that the proportion of ionized calcium in the urine is only 20% of the total, the remainder being complexed calcium. The calcium complexes contain many anions such as citrate, sulfate, phosphate, and gluconate. Citrates in the urine bind calcium most powerfully. Sixty percent of calcium is chelated with citrate at a neutral pH in 1 L of urine containing 100 mg of calcium and 480 mg of citrate; this fraction falls to 40% at a pH of 5.0.

Urinary excretion of calcium is influenced by oral intake and urinary excretion of sodium. Thus, any attempt to assess urinary calcium excretion must take into account the oral intake and excretion of sodium. It has been found also that factors that affect the renal excretion of sodium, such as ECF volume expansion, similarly alter the renal excretion of calcium. Chronic expansion of ECF volume with mineralocorticoid hormone increases the urinary excretion of calcium as well.

It has been estimated that 50% to 70% of filtered calcium is reabsorbed in the proximal nephron, 30% to 40% is reabsorbed between the end of the accessible part of the proximal tubule and the distal tubule, and the remaining 10% is reabsorbed in the distal nephron (13,18). Micropuncture studies have demonstrated that sodium and calcium exhibit very similar reabsorptive characteristics in the proximal tubule. In the thick ascending limb (TAL) of the loop of Henle, the absorption of both ions follows the same direction. Lumen-positive voltage is the driving force for calcium reabsorption in this segment. Furosemide abolishes the transepithelial potential; therefore, it reduces calcium absorption in parallel with reduced sodium reabsorption. Parathyroid hormone (PTH) reduces urinary excretion of calcium but augments urinary excretion of sodium.

Recent studies have provided more detailed insight into the tubular mechanisms underlying calcium transport along various nephron segments. The main fraction of filtered calcium is reabsorbed via paracellular passive flux that is driven by electrochemical gradient in the proximal tubule and in the TAL accounting for 80% to 90% of total filtered calcium. Epithelia permit selective and regulated flux from apical to basolateral surfaces by paracellular flux between cells or transcellular passage through cells. Tight junctions constitute the route for paracellular conductance in TAL for divalent cations, whereas the epithelial calcium channel TRPV5, ECaC1, in the distal convoluted tubule (DCT) and connecting tubule (CNT) constitute the apical entry mechanism of active transcellular calcium transport. Two conditions have to be met in TAL for paracellular reabsorption of divalent cations; the transepithelial voltage must be oriented lumen positive and the paracellular route must allow divalent cation conductance. In this regard, alterations in transepithelial NaCl reabsorption is a determinant of divalent cation reabsorption by means of changes in transepithelial voltage generation. The observations that humoral factors (e.g., PTH) and basolateral concentration changes of divalent ions without changes in transepithelial voltage alter calcium reabsorption suggest a selective effect on paracellular permeability with specificity to divalent cations. In this regard, it is noteworthy that positional cloning has identified a human gene, *Paracellin-1 (PCLN-1)*. Mutation in *PCLN-1* causes renal wasting of calcium and magnesium. This abnormality, known as familial hypomagnesemia with hypercalciuria and nephrocalcinosis (FHHNC), is an autosomal-recessive tubular disorder. PCLN-1 protein is located in tight junctions of TAL and is related to the claudin family of tight junction proteins. *PCLN-1*, therefore, is an essential component of a selective paracellular conductance for divalent cations (19). Recent clinical studies in patients with loss of function mutations of *PCLN-1* (FHHNC) provided results supporting a selective regulatory effect of basolateral divalent cations in TAL. This effect could be mediated by calcium-sensing receptor (CaSR), an important mechanism in determining calcium excretion rate by regulation of paracellular calcium absorption (20–22).

Extracellular CaSR plays a key role in calcium and magnesium reabsorption in TAL. Extracellular calcium and other cations (e.g., Mg^{2+}) activate mechanism(s) that control their paracellular tubular transport by acting on the basolateral CaSR that recognizes those cations as their extracellular ligands. CaSR is a G protein–coupled receptor that leads to a transient rise in intracellular calcium by activation of phospholipase C, hydrolysis of phosphatidylinositol 4,5-biphosphate, and increased formation of inositol triphosphate and diacylglycerol. CaSR is expressed by the cells of the TAL and plays a role in the normal regulation of calcium absorption in this nephron segment. Thus, normal or high calcium concentration is likely to be "sensed" by CaSR activating a signal transduction cascade and leading to reduced paracellular calcium reabsorption. Conversely, low calcium concentration (i.e., hypocalcemia) would fail to activate the signal transduction pathway, thus leading to abnormally avid calcium reabsorption and hypocalciuria. The latter also explains the hypocalciuria observed in patients with familial hypocalciuric hypercalcemia, in whom the gene that encodes the CaSR has undergone an inactivating mutation, leading to a defective receptor (23). Theoretically the CaSR-initiated signaling could regulate calcium absorption by three putative mechanisms: (1) altering the permeability to calcium of the paracellular tight junction pathway, (2) changing the apical electrolyte transport which generates the TAL luminal electropositivity that is the driving force for calcium absorption, or (3) both.

Polymorphism with the R990G allele, which results in gain of function of CaSR, has been reported. This polymorphism has been associated with increased susceptibility to hypercalciuria and renal stone formation (24).

The fine tuning of tubular calcium reabsorption, which is crucial for the maintenance of calcium balance, is regulated by active transcellular calcium transport in distal nephron segments. The calcium channel ECaC1 (TRPV5) plays an important role in this process (14). Immunohistochemical analysis demonstrated the presence of ECaC1 (TRPV5) in the apical membrane of late DCT2 and CNT of the kidney cortex. ECaC1 (TRPV5) is believed to constitute the rate-limiting mechanism, the first step in active calcium reabsorption. Following apical entry into cytosol, calcium is bound to a carrier protein (calbindin D_{28K}) that translocates the cation to the transporters residing in the basolateral cell surface, the NCX and ATP-dependent calcium pump, the PMCA, which extrude the calcium to the extracellular basolateral space. The latter can be inhibited by calcium via the CaSR that resides at the basolateral membrane of DCT.

PTH and 1,25-dihydroxycholecalciferol ($1,25[OH]_2D_3$) are the major regulators of TRPV5 in the distal nephron. Parathyroidectomy in rats leads to fall in TRPV5 expression, as well as diminished calbindin D_{28K} and NCX. PTH supplementation restores the expression of TRPV5. $1,25(OH)_2D_3$ increases the expression of TRPV5, calbindin D_{28K}, PMCA1b and NCX, thus harmonizing enhanced calcium absorption.

Recent observations suggest that Klotho the antiaging hormone upregulates distal calcium reabsorption by two putative mechanisms. The Klotho gene encodes a single-pass transmembrane protein with a sequence similar to β-glucosidase enzyme. The extracellular domain of Klotho, pKlothorotein, is shed and present in the circulation and tubular lumen, potentially functioning as a humoral factor. First, in response to low extracellular calcium level the Klotho binds to Na^+/K^+ ATPase and translocates it to the plasma membrane. The increased sodium gradient generated by Na^+/K^+ ATPase drives the transepithelial transport of calcium by activating the basolateral NCX. Second, the Klotho in the urine increases TRPV5 abundance on the luminal surface by hydrolyzing the N-linked extracellular sugar residues of TRPV5. Both mechanisms augment calcium influx from the lumen (25).

Inhibition of NaCl uptake in DCT by thiazides that bind to NaCl cotransporter leads to hypocalciuria. Studies suggest that suppression of NaCl transport into the DCT cells results in hyperpolarization of the cell that activates the TRPV5 (ECaC1), thus promoting calcium entry into the cytosol. In parallel, the thiazide-induced fall in intracellular sodium concentration facilitates the action of NCX to enhance the exit of calcium from the cytosol to extracellular basolateral compartment. Also amiloride-, triamterene-, and spironolactone-induced inhibition of sodium reabsorption produces hypocalciuria in a similar fashion. Similarly, WNK4 that is a negative regulator of NaCl cotransporter in distal tubule enhances TRPV5-medated calcium transport. Inactivating mutation of WNK4 causes familial hyperkalemic hypertension (PHAII, Gordon syndrome) and leads to reduced calcium reabsorption and hypercalciuria (26).

High extracellular pH stimulates the activity of TRPV5 (ECaC1), whereas low pH suppresses its activity. Consequently, pH-dependent inhibition of ECaC1 in acidosis may contribute to renal calcium wasting in this condition (21).

Changes in the filtered load of calcium also may affect the excretion of this ion. Thus, hypocalcemia is associated with a low urinary calcium excretion, regardless of its cause. A micropuncture study in dogs demonstrated that elevation of plasma calcium from a low to a normal level inhibits calcium reabsorption in the loop of Henle independent of PTH.

The renal capacity to excrete calcium may be severely compromised by a reduction in glomerular filtration rate (GFR) and ECF volume depletion. The reduced absolute and fractional excretion of calcium in early chronic renal failure when the GFR is only moderately reduced is not well understood (27,28). Two factors might contribute to this observation: secondary hyperparathyroidism and abnormalities of vitamin D metabolism with reduced intestinal absorption of calcium (27). In more advanced renal failure, fractional excretion of calcium is enhanced and correlates with the fractional clearance of sodium, suggesting that the renal handling of both ions may be altered by a similar mechanism at this stage of renal insufficiency (27).

Acute and chronic loads of phosphorus may decrease urinary excretion of calcium. It has been proposed that the reduced urinary calcium excretion is owing to an increased deposition of mineral, either in the bone or other tissues. The hypocalciuria following oral phosphates has been used in the treatment of renal calculi.

Phosphate depletion leads to an increased urinary excretion of calcium, although the mechanism for this effect remains to be defined. The possible role of secondary hypoparathyroidism was not supported by studies in animals in which parathyroidectomy did not alter substantially the hypercalciuric response to phosphate depletion. In rats, the hypercalciuric response to phosphate depletion is associated with increased intestinal absorption of calcium. A relevant finding is that phosphate depletion may enhance renal conversion of 25-hydroxy-cholecalciferol or 25-hydroxyvitamin D_3 (25[OH]D_3) into 1,25(OH)$_2D_3$, which stimulates intestinal absorption of calcium. Both metabolic and renal tubular acidosis are associated with an increased urinary excretion of calcium.

URINARY EXCRETION OF PHOSPHORUS

About 85% of serum inorganic phosphorus is filtered, and the ratio of $H_2PO_4^-$ to HPO_4^{2-} depends on the pH. The proximal convoluted and straight tubules are the major sites of phosphorus reabsorption. According to micropuncture studies, when glomerular filtrate reaches the late proximal tubule, 70% of filtered phosphorus is reabsorbed. No phosphate is reabsorbed in the loop of Henle. Evidence was obtained that 10% of filtered load may be absorbed beyond the early distal convoluted tubule. The tubular reabsorption of phosphate is a saturable process and displays a tubular maximum (Tm) reabsorptive capacity.

Phosphorus enters the brush-border membrane of the proximal tubule via the NaPi cotransport against a steep electrochemical gradient. This is energized by the sodium gradient generated by the basolateral sodium pump. Phosphorus moves out of the cell at the basolateral membrane mostly by a sodium-dependent transport (70%) and partly (30%) by a sodium-independent anion exchange system. Only the luminal cotransport is controlled by hormonal and other regulatory factors (e.g., PTH).

Sodium-Phosphate Cotransporters

The structure of a class of NaPi cotransporters in the brush-border membrane of the proximal tubule that facilitates the uptake of both sodium and phosphate in this segment of the nephron has been studied extensively. Many of the changes in the efficiency of phosphate transport are brought about by changes in the amount and activity of the NaPi cotransporters in this segment of the nephron.

Three families of NaPi cotransporters have been identified at the molecular levels, named types I, II, and III NaPi cotransporters. Despite functional similarity, there is very little identity among them. Types I and II were cloned from rat and human renal mRNA by expression cloning strategy, whereas type III cotransporters were first identified on the basis of their function as viral cell surface receptors. PiT-1 cell surface receptor for gibbon ape leukemia virus, *Glvr-1*, and, PiT-2 cell surface receptor for rat amphotropic virus, *RAM-1*. In this regard they are similar to CD_4 that is a surface receptor for HIV. Types I and II cotransporters are expressed predominantly in the kidney and localized to the brush-border membrane of the proximal tubular cells.

Type I cotransporter was the first member to be cloned from rabbit's kidney. Its physiological role, however, has not been well delineated. It is both a NaPi cotransporter and a chloride channel. As opposed to type II, type I produces electrogenic transport only at high concentrations of extracellular phosphorus concentrations. Studies suggest that type I functions as channel permeable not only to phosphorus and chloride but also to organic anions.

Type III is ubiquitously expressed and was initially assigned to fulfill a function of housekeeping NaPi cotransporters with no role as transcellular transporters. They have been assigned the role of supplying the basic cellular metabolic needs for phosphorus and as such were assumed to be located basolaterally in the kidney. The deeply ingrained notion that type III play no role renal transtubular vectorial transport was recently reassessed. New experimental data advanced evidence that PiT-2, a member of type III, which is localized to the brush-border membrane in proximal tubule epithelia, is a novel mediator of phosphorus reabsorption in the proximal tubule and is regulated by dietary phosphorus (29).

Type II cotransporters are the most abundant of the transporters and are also the major target for regulation by metabolic and hormonal factors including PTH, phosphatonins such as fibroblast growth factor 23 (FGF23), vitamin D, and dietary phosphate. Type II is largely responsible for renal phosphate reabsorption, as indicated by knockout experiments. Targeted inactivation of type II (Npt_2) in mice leads to severe phosphate wasting, 70% to 85% reduction in phosphate reabsorption, hypercalciuria, and skeletal abnormalities. It has been generally assumed that NaPiIIc accounts for the remaining 15% to 30% of phosphorus transport capacity. This view has been questioned by recent experiments that suggested that Npt_2c in mice do not play a role in phosphorus transport. Npt_2c knockout mice do not develop phosphaturia or hypophosphatemia. The Npt_2c knockout mice exhibited hypercalcemia, hypercalciuria, elevated plasma $1,25(OH)_2D_3$ and no bone disease (30).

Three isoforms of rat type IIa cotransporter have been described (31,32). They appear to be products of alternative splicing, and are designated NaPiIIaα, NaPiIIβ, and NaPiIIγ. These isoforms are expressed as proteins at the brush-border membrane. None of the three spliced isoforms induced expression of NaPi transporter when injected into oocytes. However, when NaPiIIγ cRNA was coinjected with type IIa transporter into oocytes, it completely abolished the transport function of type IIa cotransporter. Thus, alternative splicing may exert a great impact on phosphate transport in proximal convoluted tubule. The physiological impact of the above-mentioned findings remains to be determined.

Type II cotransporters mediate both electrogenic divalent phosphate transport of $HPO4^-/3Na^+$ by NaPiIIa, and electroneutral divalent phosphate transport $HPO4^-/2Na^+$ by NaPiIIc. Type III mediate monovalent phosphate electrogenic transport $H2PO4^-2Na^+$ by PiT-2. NaPiIIa exhibits the fastest response to dietary phosphorus.

The function of NaPiIIa is closely linked to Na^+/H^+ exchanger regulating factor-1 (NHERF1), a membrane scaffold protein, that plays a crucial role in binding to and anchoring NaPIIIa to apical membrane. Phosphorylation of NHERF1 by PTH leads to reduced binding of NaPiIIa followed by its endocytosis, internalization, and degradation. This results in decreased phosphorus absorption and increased urinary excretion.

By contrast to rodents where NaPiIIa has been the principal player in phosphorus absorption in humans its role is less apparent. There are indications that NaPiIIc may be the dominant phosphorus transporter in humans. Loss-of-function mutation of NaPiIIc gene is associated with excessive urinary wasting of phosphorus in patients with hereditary hypophosphatemic rickets with hypercalciuria, a human phenotype similar to that of NaPiIIa gene knockout rodents. Mutation of NaPiIIa as a cause of hypophosphatemia in humans has not been reported yet. Above observations underscore the importance in species differences in regulation of physiological processes.

The essential role of NaPiIIa in tubular phosphorus in vivo has been challenged when exploring the response to intravenous bolus injection of PTH in parathyroidectomized rats. As expected, the phosphaturic effect of PTH was associated with a striking downregulation of NaPiIIa protein expression in brush-border membrane. However, a complete recovery of tubular phosphorus reabsorption that followed, was not associated with any membrane recovery of the phosphorus transporter, suggesting that other transport mechanisms may fully compensate for the lack of NaPiIIa (33).

Dietary and Metabolic Factors

Urinary excretion of phosphorus depends on oral phosphorus intake to a great extent. Increased dietary phosphorus is associated with increased total and fractional urinary excretion of phosphorus. This may occur even in the absence of detectable changes in the serum level and filtered load of phosphorus. The state of parathyroid activity seems to play an important role in this phosphaturic response to a phosphate load; in fact, this response has been used as a diagnostic test for hyperparathyroidism. Oral intake of 3 g of elemental phosphorus has been reported to increase the excretion of phosphorus to the maximum of 35% of the filtered load in normoparathyroid subjects, but the fractional phosphate excretion exceeds 35% in hyperparathyroid patients. However, although the presence of parathyroid hyperactivity intensifies the phosphaturic response to a phosphate load, the phosphaturic response may be observed in hypoparathyroid patients as well.

Phosphate depletion resulting from phosphate-deficient diets or intestinal phosphate losses is associated with a decrease in urinary excretion of phosphate to negligible amounts. This avid reabsorption of phosphorus is reversed by fasting and acidosis. Animal experiments suggest that increased insulin secretion during phosphorus deprivation contributes to the decreased urinary excretion of phosphorus in the urine.

Animal experiments demonstrated that low phosphate diet increases the apical expression of type II cotransporters. Metabolic acidosis increases urinary phosphate excretion at the level of brush-border membranes and NaPiII abundance is reduced. Animal experiments demonstrated that growth hormone, thyroid hormone, insulin, and insulin-like growth factor increase phosphorus reabsorption and upregulate the NaPiIIa expression.

Acute expansion of ECF volume with intravenous saline increases the urinary excretion of phosphorus; conversely, acute depletion of ECF volume tends to decrease urinary phosphorus (34). However, the effect of chronically increased oral intake of sodium chloride on urinary phosphorus excretion and phosphorus balance is unknown. In this regard, patients with primary hyperaldosteronism showed no changes in urinary phosphorus excretion but exhibited hypercalciuria.

A high oral intake of calcium is associated with a decreased urinary excretion of phosphorus. Two factors may account for this observation. First, calcium may depress intestinal absorption of phosphorus by forming nonabsorbable complexes with phosphorus. Second, large amounts of oral calcium may suppress the secretion of PTH and reduce urinary excretion of phosphorus.

In contrast to its effect when given by the oral route, an intravenous load of calcium produces an acute increase in serum phosphorus concentration and augments excretion of phosphorus in the urine (2). The rise in serum phosphorus has been attributed to a direct effect of hypercalcemia, namely, promotion of the release of intracellular phosphorus into the circulation (2). This transient phosphaturia is followed by a substantial fall in urinary phosphorus excretion owing to suppression of parathyroid activity (7). In addition, hypercalcemia may exert a direct effect on the kidney, enhancing tubular reabsorption of phosphorus independent of parathyroid activity (35). This effect may be mediated by CaSR stimulation in the proximal tubule (36). In contrast to this observation, however, is the finding that restoration of normocalcemia with intravenous calcium in patients with hypoparathyroidism is associated with increased urinary excretion of phosphorus. Likewise, the enhanced excretion of phosphorus that follows the administration of vitamin D to patients with hypoparathyroidism may be at least partly attributable to the restoration of the serum calcium level to normal. Recent study demonstrated that vitamin D downregulates NaPiIIa abundance in patathyroidectomized rats (37).

Acute loads of phosphorus in parathyroidectomized animals produce a net decrease in tubular reabsorption of phosphorus despite markedly increased filtered load. This change has been linked with the attendant fall in serum calcium concentration and indeed may be reversed by maintaining a constant calcium level (38). This and the foregoing observations show the dependence of renal handling of phosphorus on serum levels of calcium and emphasize the complexity of their interrelationship. Rich phosphate diet in experimental animals downregulates the apical tubular expression of the NaPiII protein.

States of rapid catabolism with increased destruction of body tissues and metabolic acidosis are associated with hyperphosphatemia and phosphaturia. Similarly, cytolysis associated with the administration of cytotoxic agents to patients with neoplasms, especially neoplasms of lymphatic origin, is followed by severe hyperphosphatemia, phosphaturia, and hypocalcemia. Conversely, rapid regrowth of lymphatic tumors may lead to hypophosphatemia of marked degree because of incorporation of phosphorus in the tumor (39).

Intravenous administration of glucose has a dual effect on phosphorus metabolism. First, intravenous glucose tends to lower serum phosphorus, probably by incorporating phosphorus into the intracellular pool during the process of glucose phosphorylation. Second, glucose appears to have a direct renal effect in that it suppresses the reabsorption and increases the urinary excretion of phosphate. The competition of glucose and phosphate for transport across the epithelium of the proximal tubule has been demonstrated in studies with isolated renal tubules (40). This competition may be most important in states of massive glucosuria with uncontrolled diabetes mellitus.

Most diuretic agents acutely increase urinary phosphorus excretion. However, with the development of ECF volume depletion, the phosphaturic response of diuretics is blunted and may be restored with replacement of urinary losses of sodium and water. Neither the phosphaturic effect of thiazides nor that of acetazolamide seems to be dependent on the presence of parathyroid glands; however, the phosphaturic effect of these diuretics is linked to their ability to inhibit the enzyme carbonic anhydrase. Acidosis increases and alkalosis reduces urinary excretion of phosphorus.

Denervation of kidneys leads to an increase in urinary excretion of phosphorus because of an increased production of dopamine and decreased α- and β-adrenergic renal receptor activity. This denervation-related phosphaturia may contribute to renal losses of phosphorus after kidney transplantation.

Recent experiments in intact and parathyroidectomized rats demonstrated a rapid phosphaturic response to duodenal load of phosphate. Furthermore protein extracts from homogenates of small intestine that were infused into animals elicited a phosphaturic response. As per suggestions based on the above-mentioned observations, the intestine has luminal "sensors of phosphate" that sense increased luminal phosphate concentration and release a substance into the circulation that inhibits renal phosphate reabsorption. The nature of such substance remains to be defined (41).

Regulation of Serum Calcium and Phosphorus Concentration by Hormonal Factors

VITAMIN D AND ITS METABOLITES

The term "Vitamin D" was first introduced by McCollum in 1922 for the antirachitic factor isolated from cod liver oil (42). There are two naturally occurring sterol precursors of vitamin D, namely, ergosterol, which is present in plants, and 7-dehydrocholesterol, which is found in animals and humans. Under exposure to ultraviolet irradiation, ergosterol is converted into ergocalciferol (calciferol), which is known as vitamin D_2. Vitamin D_1 is not one compound but a mixture of many sterols with antirachitic activity.

The main source of vitamin D in humans is endogenous vitamin D_3, produced by the ultraviolet irradiation of 7-dehydrocholesterol in the skin. Areas of skin in most adults contain 3% to 4% of 7-dehydrocholesterol, which is located beneath the stratum corneum. Therefore, excessive amounts of pigment in the skin may interfere with the production of vitamin D_3. The cutaneous synthesis of vitamin D_3 is quite complex. Previtamin D_3 is formed from its precursor 7-dehydrocholesterol. The preceding conversion depends on the levels of 7-dehydrocholesterol and is mediated by initial exposure to ultraviolet light. However, prolonged exposure to ultraviolate light may inactivate previtamin D_3 and transform it to the inert photoproducts, lumisterol and tachysterol. The levels of 7-dehydrocholesterol decline with age, therefore older age predisposes to vitamin D deficiency. Vitamin D_3, also known as cholecalciferol, is formed from previtamin D_3 by thermal isomerization over 2 to 3 days in the skin and also is rapidly degraded by sunlight. Therefore excessive exposure to sunlight cannot cause vitamin D intoxication because sunlight destroys any excess of vitamin D_3 produced in the skin. Ten to fifteen minutes of exposure to sunlight can provide sufficient amounts of vitamin D_3 for several days' consumption.

The main source of exogenous vitamin D in the United States is milk, which contains about 400 units of vitamin D_2 in each quart. The daily requirement of vitamin D in infants is about 400 units; in older age groups, the requirement is lower, as low as 70 U/day. This modest estimate has been recently challenged because of the high frequency of vitamin D deficiency in the adult and elderly population. Accordingly, higher intake of vitamin D in the range 600 to 800 U/day has been recommended by some investigators (43).

METABOLISM OF VITAMIN D

Cholecalciferol is metabolized in the liver into $25(OH)D_3$, which has a more potent antirachitic activity in vivo than the parent compound. Vitamin D undergoes 25-hydroxylation in the liver by 25(OH)ase. It has been generally accepted that 25(OH)ase is not a tightly regulated enzyme, but its activity is reduced by 50% in animals receiving vitamin D. However, DeLuca's et al. demonstrated inhibition of hepatic production of 25(OH)D$_3$ by 1,25(OH)$_2$D$_3$ in rats, thus suggesting feedback control (44). Decrease in the level of 25(OH)D$_3$ in patients consuming anticonvulsive drugs, such as phenobarbital, phenytoin, primidone, carbamezapine, and rifampin has been attributed to induction of cytochrome P-450 enzymes, which leads to increased turnover of vitamin D, including catabolism resulting in vitamin D deficiency and bone disease (45). After enterohepatic circulation, 25(OH)D$_3$ is further metabolized in the kidney into 1,25(OH)$_2$D$_3$, which is the most active metabolite of vitamin D. On a weight basis, it is 10 times more effective than vitamin D$_3$ in curing rickets and 100 times more potent than 25(OH)D$_3$ in stimulating calcium mobilization from the bone. When plasma calcium and phosphate levels are normal, 25(OH)D-1α(OH) ase activity in the kidney is reduced, and instead 25(OH)D-24(OH)ase activity prevails and metabolizes 25(OH)D$_3$ into 24,25(OH)$_2$D$_3$. Calcitriol is an important negative regulator of itself. It exerts a feedback inhibition of 25(OH)D-1α(OH)ase. Current evidence indicates that this inhibition does not reflect a direct action of 1,25(OH)$_2$D$_3$ on 25(OH)D-1α(OH)ase gene promoter but rather it is an indirect effect. 1,25(OH)$_2$D$_3$ appears to inhibit the known PTH-induced activation of 25(OH)D-1α(OH)ase gene promoter via cyclic-AMP(cAMP). It is the PTH-generated cAMP that induces directly the gene promoter of 25(OH)D-1α(OH)ase resulting in increased production of 1,25(OH)$_2$D$_3$ from 25(OH)D$_3$ (46). In this regard, previous experiments advanced evidence that vitamin D blocks the formation of cAMP by PTH in the kidney, both in vivo and in vitro. The above-mentioned findings shed light on the mechanism by which 1,25(OH)$_2$D$_3$ suppresses the activation of 25(OH)-1α(OH)ase(47).

It has been shown that 25(OH)D$_3$ in complex with its carrier protein, the vitamin D–binding protein, is filtered through the glomerulus and reabsorbed in the proximal tubules by the endocytic receptor megalin. Endocytosis is required to preserve 25(OH)D$_3$ and deliver it to the cells as the precursor for generation of 1,25(OH)$_2$D$_3$. These findings contradict the previously held view that 25(OH)D$_3$ was free, and as such diffused from the circulation across the basolateral surface of proximal tubular cells into the cytosol, to be converted by 25(OH)D-1α(OH) ase to 1,25(OH)$_2$D$_3$. Megalin knockout mice (megalin-1-mice) are unable to retrieve the 25(OH)D$_3$ from the glomerular filtrate and develop vitamin D–deficiency state and bone disease. Such a role of the tubular reabsorption process is suggested by observations in patients with renal tubular defects. Similar to megalin knockout mice, patients who suffer from Fanconi syndrome are unable to reabsorb filtered macromolecules and exhibit vitamin D deficiency and bone disease (rickets and osteomalacia). Furthermore, it has been shown in patients with different degrees of renal failure that the glomerular filtration rate was directly correlated with plasma concentrations of 1,25(OH)$_2$D$_3$, suggesting that glomerular filtration is one of the determinants of 1,25(OH)$_2$D$_3$ synthesis by kidney (48).

PTH seems to act as a tropic hormone in stimulating the production of 1,25(OH)$_2$D$_3$ in the kidney. Thus, with intact parathyroid glands, changes in serum calcium indirectly regulate renal production of 1,25(OH)$_2$D$_3$ by altering the secretion of PTH. Specifically, hypocalcemia stimulates and hypercalcemia inhibits the synthesis of 1,25(OH)$_2$D$_3$. In addition, there is evidence that calcium acts directly to alter the renal synthesis of calcitriol. Low serum phosphorus stimulates and high serum phosphorus suppresses the renal synthesis of 1,25(OH)$_2$D$_3$ independent of PTH. Several other factors control the formation of 1,25(OH)$_2$D$_3$. The novel group of humoral phosphaturic factors, termed "phophatonins," "FGF23" and others, decrease 1,25(OH)$_2$D$_3$ by inhibiting the activity of 25(OH)D-1α(OH)ase. Furthermore, FGF23 synthesis is enhanced by 1,25(OH)$_2$D$_3$. It has been proposed that FGF23 is a negative feedback regulator of 25(OH)D-1α(OH)ase.

Growth hormone via increased synthesis of insulin-like growth factor I stimulates the activity of 25(OH)D-1α(OH)ase. Chronic metabolic acidosis in humans increases serum levels of calcitriol (49). This effect could be mediated by acidosis-induced urinary losses of phosphate leading to cellular phosphate depletion. Once it is formed, 1,25(OH)$_2$D$_3$ is metabolized to several less-active metabolites in target tissues (13,50). These transformations are enhanced by the hormone itself and thus may serve to decrease the biologic activity of the hormone once it has carried out its biologic functions. In addition, 1,25(OH)$_2$D$_3$ is excreted in bile as a monoglucuronide, other polar metabolites, and a 23-carbon acid, calcitroic acid (11,13,51). 1,25(OH)$_2$D$_3$ undergoes enterohepatic circulation in humans and various animal species. Proximal tubular cells are the major site of calcitriol formation. In addition, calcitriol may be produced in decidual cells, keratinocytes, bone cells, endothelial cells, peripheral monocytes, parathyroids, colon, prostate, breast and activated macrophages where it may exert also a local autocrine or paracrine effect. Main aspects of the metabolism of vitamin D are shown in Figure 6.2.

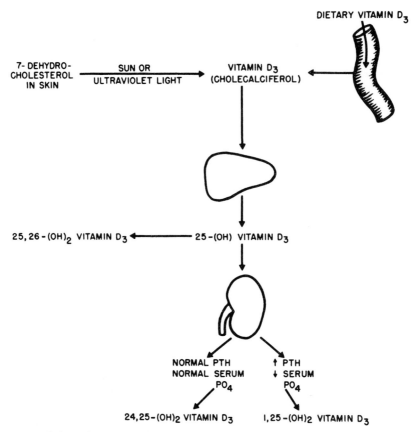

■ **Figure 6.2** Metabolism of vitamin D. The major source of vitamin D_3 is its production in the skin; the other important source is diet. PTH, parathyroid hormone.

Dihydrotachysterol (DHT_3) is an analog of vitamin D used in the treatment of hypoparathyroidism. At high doses it is more effective than vitamin D in mobilizing calcium from the bone, but in low doses it is less effective in curing rickets. DHT_3 undergoes hydroxylation in the liver to $25(OH)DHT_3$, which is the active form of DHT_3. Thus, DHT_3 does not require the presence of the kidneys for the synthesis of its active metabolite. 1α-hydroxycholecalciferol ($1\alpha[OH]D_3$) is a synthetic sterol that undergoes 25-hydroxylation in the liver to $1,25(OH)_2D_3$ and, like DHT_3, does not require the presence of renal tissue for its conversion into the active form of vitamin D_3. Calcitriol stimulates the metabolic clearance of $25(OH)D_3$. Increased calcitriol formation with increased serum concentration leads to a fall in the serum concentration of $25(OH)D_3$ (52).

EFFECT OF VITAMIN D ON INTESTINAL ABSORPTION

Vitamin D_3 stimulates intestinal absorption of calcium and phosphorus. The effect of vitamin D on calcium absorption becomes measurable several hours after its administration and is blocked by actinomycin D. Circulating calcitriol is a major regulator of intestinal calcium absorption. It exerts its effect mainly by a genomic mechanism mediated by binding to cytosolic vitamin D receptors. The calcitriol–vitamin D receptor structure complexes with retinoic X receptor (RXR) in the target cell nucleus, interacts with specific DNA sequences of calcitriol-responsive genes, and modulates transcriptional and posttranscriptional synthetic pathways. $1,25(OH)_2D_3$ complex with its specific cytosolic vitamin D receptor (VDR) promotes mucosal epithelial calcium uptake by induction of the apical calcium channel TRPV6. This is the rate-limiting step in calcium transport. $1,25(OH)_2D_3$ produces a cytosolic calcium-binding protein calbindin D that facilitates transcellular calcium movement, and it upregulates the basolateral PMCA1 that pumps the calcium out of the cell.

The promotion of intestinal calcium absorption by vitamin D, at least partly, may be a rapid nongenomic response; the putative membrane receptors for $1,25(OH)_2D_3$ may mediate this process. The active extrusion of calcium at the basolateral side by plasma membrane-bound Ca^{2+} ATPase operates also in the absence of vitamin D. However, $1,25(OH)D_3$ has been shown conclusively to stimulate the activity and promote the synthesis of the plasma membrane calcium pump. The increased synthesis of calcium-binding protein within the intestinal cell and the synthesis of an increased number of calcium pump units enhance the extrusion of calcium from within the intestinal cell into the ECF space.

Vitamin D Receptors

In addition to intestinal mucosa, calcitriol receptors are present on osteoblasts, monocytes, human breast cancer cells, parathyroid gland, epidermal cells, and cerebellum. Their role will be discussed in other sections (13,50,51).

EFFECT OF VITAMIN D ON BONE METABOLISM

Vitamin D promotes mineralization of the organic bone matrix. This action appears to be at least partly secondary to the effect of vitamin D on enhancing the intestinal absorption of calcium and phosphorus and thus maintaining their normal ECF concentrations. Some evidence supports a direct role of vitamin D in bone accretion (53). However, it has been shown that vitamin D–deficient osteomalacia may be cured with the intravenous administration of calcium and phosphorus despite persistence of a vitamin D deficiency state (54).

Evidence suggests that vitamin D and its metabolites $25(OH)D_3$ and $1,25(OH)_2D_3$ mobilize calcium and phosphorus from bone, an effect that has been demonstrated both in vivo and in vitro (55,56). Therefore, this action of vitamin D may increase serum calcium concentration independently of its enhancement of the intestinal transport of calcium. Studies in animals have shown that vitamin D stimulates both osteocytic and osteoclastic bone resorption, and this action does not require the presence of PTH (55). Calcitriol induces differentiation of monocytic cells into mature osteoclasts, and it increases the number of osteoclasts. $1,25(OH)_2D_3$ interacts with vitamin D receptors in osteoblasts to induce the expression of the receptor activator of nuclear factor kappa B (NF-kB) ligand (RANKL). RANKL binds to RANK on the plasma membrane of preosteoclasts and transforms them into mature osteoclasts. Osteoclasts dissolve the bone and release calcium and phosphorus into the circulation. Calcitriol increases osteoblast size and increases the synthesis of alkaline phosphatase and the blood level of osteocalcin. Interestingly, in vitro studies suggest that $1,25(OH)D_3$, but not other metabolites of vitamin D, may inhibit bone collagen synthesis (56).

The exact role of $24,25(OH)D_3$ in mineral metabolism is unknown and controversial. Many investigators view it as an inactive waste product of vitamin D catabolism. In animals, the hormone is metabolized to $1,24,25(OH)_3D_3$ and becomes active in intestinal absorption of calcium. In normal, hypoparathyroid, and anephric humans, however, $24,25(OH)D_3$ acts directly to increase intestinal absorption of calcium, even when given in relatively low doses (57). This effect of $24,25(OH)D_3$ is associated with positive calcium balance without changes in serum concentration or urinary excretion. In view of this observation and the previously reported effect of $24,25(OH)_2D_3$ to promote the synthesis of protein by chondrocytes, it has been proposed that $24,25(OH)D_3$ may be the metabolite that is directly involved in skeletal metabolism (57). Furthermore, it has been reported that $1\alpha(OH)D_3$ alone does not prevent rickets in chicks, whereas $24,25(OH)D_3$ alone is effective (58). Experimental studies also have demonstrated that $24,25(OH)_2D_3$ may play an important role in the suppression of bone resorption in rats after nephrectomy (59). In vitro studies demonstrated that $24,25(OH)D_3$ antagonizes the osseous calcium mobilizing effect of calcitriol (60).

Recent experiments from our laboratory showed that $1,25(OH)_2D_3$ induced a dose-dependent increase of calcium efflux from cultured bone. This increase was completely obliterated by inhibition of protein kinase C (PKC) with either staurosporine or cephalostin c. In cultured rat calvariae $1,25(OH)_2D_3$ also induced a dose-dependent translocation of PKC from cytosol to membrane. The activation of PKC by $1,25(OH)_2D_3$ occurred following 30 seconds of incubation, peaked at 1 minute, and disappeared by 5 minutes. $1,25(OH)_2D_3$ did not increase cAMP production in similarly cultured calvaria. These results suggest that the action of $1,25(OH)_2D_3$ on calcium flux from bone tissue is mediated by activation of PKC (61).

Similarly, we have shown in the same experimental model that $24,25(OH)_2D_3$ induced a dose-dependent flux of calcium into the bone. This effect was mediated by an inactivation of PKC. Thus, the actions of $1,25(OH)_2D_3$, which mobilizes calcium from bone, and $24,25(OH)_2D_3$, which inhibits bone resorption, are mediated by activation and inhibition of PKC, respectively (62). It is interesting that other investigators demonstrated that $1,25(OH)_2D_3$ activates PKC, rapidly increases intracellular calcium, and stimulates polyphosphoinositide hydrolysis in colonic epithelia (63). Thus, there is mounting evidence demonstrating a role of PKC activation in mediating the nongenomic effects of vitamin D.

EFFECT OF VITAMIN D ON RENAL HANDLING OF PHOSPHORUS AND CALCIUM

The effect of vitamin D on renal handling of phosphorus has been the subject of numerous investigations. The main difficulty encountered in interpreting the changes in urinary excretion of phosphorus has been related to the calcemic actions of vitamin D, which, by suppressing PTH secretion, indirectly alter renal handling of phosphorus. Consequently, the enhanced tubular reabsorption of phosphorus following the administration of vitamin D to patients with osteomalacia and rachitic animals with intact parathyroid glands could be accounted for either by inhibition of PTH secretion or a direct tubular action of vitamin D. The results of studies in animals suggest that both $25(OH)D_3$ and $1,25(OH)_2D_3$ acutely enhance tubular reabsorption of phosphorus (64); in rats, this effect requires the presence of either endogenous or exogenous PTH. The antiphosphaturic effect of minimal doses of $1,25(OH)D_3$ was demonstrated in chronic studies in vitamin D–deficient rats; this effect was reported to be associated with upregulated NaPiII expression. The effects of $1,25(OH)D_3$ are summarized in Figure 6.3.

Recent studies from our laboratory addressed the mechanism(s) underlying the effects of vitamin D on renal handling of phosphate both in acute experiments, using opossum kidney (OK) cell line, and in chronic experiments using metabolic clearances in parathyroidectomized rats infused with $1,25(OH)_2D_3$ without and with PTH via osmotic minipumps over 7 days. The acute studies in OK cells reproduced our previous results in rats (64,65). These experiments demonstrated that pretreatment for 24 hours with $1,25(OH)_2D_3$ antagonized the effect of PTH to inhibit phosphate uptake in OK cells. This action of $1,25(OH)_2D_3$ was associated with suppressed PTH-induced activation of the second messenger

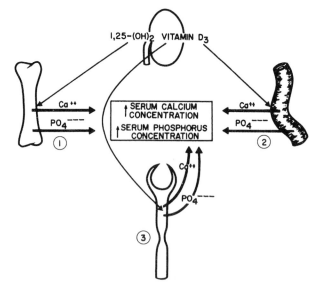

■ **Figure 6.3** Hypercalcemic and hyperphosphatemic effect of $1,25(OH)_2D_3$. Its actions are: (a) mobilization of mineral from bone; (b) enhanced intestinal absorption of calcium and phosphorus; and (c) augmented tubular absorption of phosphorus and calcium. The net physiologic effect is the maintenance of a normal serum calcium and phosphorus product, which allows mineralization of bone.

transduction pathway, the adenylate cyclase/cAMP/PKA system. Interestingly, this response to vitamin D was accompanied by a substantial diminution in the expression of the PTH/PTH-related peptide (PTHrP) receptor. The latter could at least partly account for the inhibition of adenylate cyclase-cAMP activation by PTH. Likewise, it is interesting that the observed PTH triggered rise in intracellular calcium, which presumably resulted from PTH-induced activation of the second signal transduction pathway, namely the activation of PKC, was not altered by $1,25(OH)_2D_3$. By contrast to the acute studies, in chronic experiments $1,25(OH)_2D_3$ enhanced the phosphaturic effect of PTH despite retaining the concomitant reduction in urinary cAMP excretion. We observed that both NaPiII mRNA and NaPiII protein were significantly reduced when $1,25(OH)_2D_3$ was infused alone, when PTH was given alone, and most strikingly when both were given together. Furthermore, the observed vitamin D–induced downregulation of the PTH/PTHrP receptor was reversed in the chronic study when PTH and $1,25(OH)_2D_3$ were given together. The latter could contribute at least partly to the enhancement of PTH-induced phosphaturia by $1,25(OH)_2D_3$. Thus, as opposed to acute conditions where vitamin D blunts the phosphaturic effect of PTH, chronic administration of vitamin D exerts the opposite effect (66). Therefore, it is apparent that the effect of vitamin D on renal handling of phosphate is very complex and depends on many variables.

Large doses of vitamin D cause hypercalciuria, possibly by increasing absorption of calcium from the intestine. In contrast, acute clearance studies in dogs showed an increased renal tubular absorption of calcium after intravenous administration of vitamin D (67,68). Vitamin D, however, does not appear to be essential for the renal conservation of calcium, because urinary calcium excretion may be reduced to extremely low levels in osteomalacia resulting from vitamin D deficiency (54).

In addition to the effect of vitamin D on the intestine, bones, and kidney, vitamin D acts directly on parathyroid tissue to suppress secretion of PTH. Studies in rats in our laboratory demonstrated that physiologic amounts of $1,25(OH)D_3$ inhibit the levels of PTH mRNA, independent of serum calcium levels (69). This action of calcitriol is mediated by the vitamin D receptor. Calcitriol acts on at least two negative regulatory elements upstream in the $5'$ flanking region of the PTH gene to suppress transcription. Furthermore, calcitriol modulates secretion and synthesis of PTH by increasing gene expression of the vitamin D receptor in the parathyroid gland (52).

In view of this information, a feedback loop may be formulated that has the following sequence: PTH stimulates the formation of $1,25(OH)_2D_3$ and $1,25(OH)D_3$ closes the negative feedback loop by suppressing secretion of PTH. Thus, among other functions, $1,25(OH)D_3$ may have a modifying effect on the secretion of PTH (52).

Vitamin D activity in the serum and in other tissues may be measured by both bioassay and radioimmunoassay techniques. The radioreceptor assay can determine the serum levels of the various metabolites. These competitive protein-binding assays have great potential importance in determining the mechanisms underlying clinical disorders secondary to abnormalities in vitamin D metabolism.

Parathyroid Hormone

PTH is a single-chain polypeptide of 84 amino acid residues (mol wt 9,500) with biologic activity in the N-terminal 1 to 34 region of the molecule. The biosynthesis of the hormone starts with prepro-PTH, a 110 amino acid chain polypeptide that is the translation product of PTH mRNA. Pro-PTH is produced after cleavage of 21 amino acids. PTH is produced after additional cleavage and stored in secretory droplets. The amount of stored hormone is sufficient for basal secretion over 5 to 6 hours and 2 hours of augmented secretion. Thus, the synthesis is closely linked to secretory activity.

PTH plays a central role in the physiologic regulation of serum calcium concentration. Serum calcium concentration is maintained within a very narrow range, primarily because of a feedback mechanism in which minimal changes in ionized calcium alter the secretory rate of PTH, which then restores the ionized calcium to its initial normal concentration by its action on bone. Serum concentration of phosphorus is not feedback regulated; therefore, it varies over a relatively wide range. Recent studies, however, suggest that changes in serum phosphate may be involved in the regulation of PTH secretion. There is a direct relationship between serum phosphate level and the secretion rate of PTH. Thus, high–serum phosphate levels increase and low levels decrease the synthesis and secretion of PTH. This appears to be a posttranscriptional effect. This effect appears to be independent of changes in serum calcium and vitamin D (70,71).

It is apparent that serum-ionized calcium is the single most important physiologic factor controlling the secretory rate of PTH. A sensitive inverse relationship has been demonstrated between ionized calcium and serum levels of PTH (8). The parathyroid cells have a cell surface sensing mechanism to extracellular calcium concentration that also recognizes other divalent and polyvalent cations, such as magnesium and neomycin. This mechanism is based on a CaSR. The CaSR is a member of the G protein–coupled receptor family that responds to increased extracellular calcium by triggering the phospholipase C pathway and elevating inositol triphosphate, diacylglycerol, and intracellular calcium concentration. The increased intracellular calcium inhibits PTH secretion from parathyroid cells. The CaSR expressed in the parathyroid, thyroid, and kidney was cloned and characterized (23). Recently, another possible CaSR that is distinct from the G protein–coupled receptor was identified. This receptor (CAS) is a large protein known as gp330 megalin and is a member of the low-density lipoprotein receptor superfamily. It was identified in parathyroid tissue but its role in parathyroid physiology is unknown. In addition, to its acute effect on PTH secretion, chronic changes in serum-ionized calcium concentration, both hypercalcemia and hypocalcemia, reduce or increase the steady-state level of PTH mRNA and synthesis of PTH. In vivo, calcitriol causes a 90% decrease in prepro-PTH mRNA at 48 hours; the effect starts after 2 hours. As opposed to calcium, which exerts both an acute and chronic effect on PTH secretion, calcitriol does not have an acute effect on PTH secretion, but there is a decrease in PTH secretion after 12 to 24 hours (52).

An increase in PTH secretion also has been observed in cows during the administration of epinephrine, raising the possibility that the autonomic nervous system may play a role in controlling PTH secretion (72). The results of an in vitro study with bovine parathyroid cells suggest that the synthesis of PTH is maintained at or very close to maximum capacity at normal serum calcium concentration. Low calcium concentration stimulates secretion and decreases intracellular degradation. High calcium concentration over a short time suppresses secretion and augments degradation.

Peripheral Actions of Parathyroid Hormone and Parathyroid Hormone-Related Peptide

The peripheral actions of PTH and PTHrP on bone and kidney involve binding to cell surface receptors followed by activation of two pathways of signal transduction. Thus, PTH stimulates both the adenylate cAMP–PKA pathway and phospholipase C, which in turn leads to activation of PKC by diacylglycerol and an increase in intracellular calcium by inositol triphosphate. The stimulation of these two signaling pathways is mediated by coupling of the hormone-occupied receptor with two distinct G proteins, which link the receptor to effector pathways (73,74). The gene for the human PTH receptor for bone and kidney has been cloned, sequenced, and expressed in African green monkey kidney (cos) cells. The evaluation of the structure and function relationship of the receptor and PTH is interesting. It has been demonstrated that N-terminal fragment PTH sequence 1 to 34 reproduces all physiologic effects of PTH sequence 1 to 84. It has been shown that the amino acid sequences 10 to 15 and 24 to 34 of PTH are necessary for binding to the receptor. With regard to the biologic effects of PTH, it has shown that the first two N-terminal amino acids 1 and 2 are required for the activation of adenylate cyclase–PKA pathway, whereas the amino acids sequence 28 to 34 are required for the activation of phospholipase C-PKC pathway. Indeed, the fragment PTH sequence 3 to 34 was shown in vitro to suppress phosphate transport without activation of adenylate cyclase–PKA pathway (73–75).

Another PTH receptor (type 2) that binds only PTH and does not bind PTH-related protein has been found in the brain and intestines. The functions of this receptor are unknown.

EFFECT OF PARATHYROID HORMONE ON BONE

PTH plays a major role in bone remodeling. PTH increases bone turnover owing both to increase in osteoclast numbers and resorption and stimulation of bone formation by osteoblast activation. Its receptors are expressed in bone-forming cells, osteoblasts, and proosteoblasts, but not in osteoclasts. Thus, although PTH acts to increase osteoclastic resorption, it appears that this effect is not mediated via receptors on osteoclasts but are indirect, occurring through interaction of PTH with receptors on osteoblasts. PTH–activated osteoblasts may enhance recruitment and stimulation of osteoclasts.

PTH augments release of mineral from bone by stimulating both osteocytic and osteoclastic bone resorption and possibly by enhancing calcium transport from the skeletal ECF into the systemic ECF. There is experimental evidence that the latter is a direct effect. The resulting increase in serum calcium concentration may be preceded by a short period of decreasing concentration because of an initial enhanced entry of calcium into bone cells.

The calcemic effect of PTH on bone requires the presence of vitamin D (76,77). The impaired response to PTH in vitamin D deficiency may be owing either to some permissive action of the vitamin or the mechanical blocking effect of the osteoid that coats the surface of the mineralized bone and thus prevents access of the PTH. Correction of hypocalcemia per se in rats has been shown to restore the responsiveness of the bone to the action of the PTH in states of vitamin D deficiency. This observation is consistent with the possibility that calcium is a cofactor in the skeletal action of PTH. Recently proposals hold that PTH acts on two distinct cellular systems in the bone: (a) the bone remodeling system and (b) the calcium mobilization or calcemic-homeostatic system. The remodeling system consists of osteoclasts that resorb old bone and osteoblasts that form new bone. In this system, bone resorption is balanced by bone formation; therefore, no mineral escapes into the circulation. The homeostatic system is based on the action of surface osteocytes and osteocytes occupying lacunar spaces that regulate the movement of calcium between the bone fluid and ECF. This mineral-releasing system is important in everyday regulation of serum calcium and requires $1,25(OH)_2D_3$ in addition to PTH. Recent in vitro studies suggest that the calcium-mobilizing effect of PTH is mediated by activation of the phospholipase C–PKC signal transduction system (78).

EFFECT OF PARATHYROID HORMONE ON THE KIDNEY

The primary renal effect of PTH is to produce phosphaturia by depressing net phosphate reabsorption in the proximal tubule. This tubular effect involves PTH receptor–mediated intracellular formation of messenger cAMP, inositol triphosphate, diacylglycerol, and free cytosolic calcium and activation of PKA and PKC. These inhibit brush-border transport systems including NaPi cotransport and sodium–proton antiport exchange (73). The results of certain studies suggest additional effects of PTH in more distal parts of the nephron on phosphorus absorption (79). Phosphate depletion produces resistance to the phosphaturic action of PTH in rats; however, this has not been shown yet in humans.

Type II Na/Pi cotransporters are believed to represent the major pathway of renal phosphate reabsorption and are the major target with respect to inhibition of proximal tubular reabsorption by PTH. Both acute and chronic administration of PTH downregulates the NaPiII protein in brush-border membrane of proximal tubular cells, however, only chronic administration downregulates NaPiII mRNA. Experiments in vivo and in vitro showed that PTH causes retrieval of NaPiII cotransporters from the membrane. After internalization, they are routed to the lysosomes where they are degraded.

It had been earlier assumed but never proven that NaPiIIa downregulation by PTH involves phosphorylation of the transporter by cAMP. Recent evidence suggests that PTH induces phosphorylation of the PDZI domain of NHERF1, a scaffold protein that binds to and anchors NaPiIIa to apical membrane. Phosphorylation of the scaffold protein reduces its binding to NaPiIIa and leads to NaPiIIa internalization and degradation in the lysosome (80).

Although the effect of PTH in the proximal tubule is to depress calcium reabsorption, its net effect is to decrease urinary calcium excretion in dogs, rats (81), and humans. The net increase in tubular reabsorption of calcium appears to be primarily caused by a distal action of the hormone, where approximately 10% to 20% of filtered calcium is reabsorbed (18). Thus, it appears that both the renal and skeletal actions of PTH act jointly to increase serum concentrations of calcium. Because PTH may increase bicarbonate, sodium, and amino acid excretion, the hormone does not appear to increase the reabsorption of these substances in the distal nephron.

Parathyroidectomy in rats is associated with downregulation of calcium channel TRPV5, calbindin D_{28K}, and expression of basolateral calcium transporters. The exact molecular mechanism involved in

PTH-induced increase in calcium transport in DCT and CNT has not been elucidated in detail yet. The classic concept that cAMP stimulates calcium reabsorption in this nephron segment has been questioned. Recent studies suggest that PTH stimulates calcium reabsorption in distal nephron, independent of cAMP, via activation of phospholipase C–PKC signal transduction pathway. Activation of PKC increases cell surface abundance of TRPV5 by inhibiting endocytosis. This mechanism of regulation of PKC may contribute to acute stimulation of TRPV5 and calcium absorption by PTH (82).

EFFECT OF PARATHYROID HORMONE ON INTESTINAL ABSORPTION OF CALCIUM

A role for PTH in the intestinal absorption of calcium has been suggested by several studies in both animals and humans. However, at present there is no evidence to support a direct action of PTH on calcium transport in the intestine. The fact that PTH enhances the conversion of $25(OH)D_3$ to $1,25(OH)_2D_3$, which directly acts on the intestinal transport of calcium, may explain the apparent effects of the hormone. Even so, it is obvious that in states of vitamin D deficiency, the elevated levels of circulating PTH fail to maintain normal absorption of calcium. Conversely, vitamin D may affect intestinal absorption in the absence of PTH in patients with hypoparathyroidism. The multiple actions of PTH are summarized in Figure 6.4.

RADIOIMMUNOASSAY OF PARATHYROID HORMONE

Radioimmunoassay for circulating PTH was introduced by Berson and Yalow (83) in 1963. Further studies led to the recognition of the heterogeneity of circulating PTH, which apparently represents various molecular species of the hormone. The glandular hormone (mol wt 9,500) consists of 84 amino acids (1 to 84 sequence) and has two terminals, amino ($-NH_2$) and carboxy ($-COOH$). The circulating PTH consists of the glandular hormone and its fragments. At least two different molecular species of circulating PTH have been detected by different antisera, one with a molecular weight of 4,500 to 5,000 and one with a molecular weight of 7,000 to 7,500. Structurally, there are two major split products that can be characterized by their terminals. The first product has the N-terminal, is the biologically active fragment, and has an amino acid sequence of 1 to 34. The second product has the C-terminal, is the biologically inactive fragment, and has an amino acid sequence of 53 to 84. The level of total circulating immunoreactive

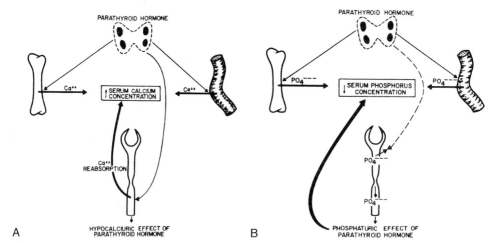

■ **Figure 6.4 A.** The hypercalcemic effect of PTH is a summation of mineral mobilization from bone, calcium absorption from the bowel, and distal tubular reabsorption of calcium in the kidney. The effect on the bowel probably is related to PTH-induced renal production of $1,25(OH)_2D_3$. **B.** The hypophosphatemic effect of PTH is based on its phosphaturic action, which supersedes its effect of mobilizing phosphorus from bone and enhancing phosphate absorption from the intestine. (*Solid lines* represent an enhancement of action; *broken line* represents an inhibition of action.)

PTH that reflects all molecular species appears to represent the chronic state of parathyroid function and is most useful in the diagnosis of parathyroid abnormalities. The level of the glandular (mol wt 9,500) species represents acute changes in parathyroid activity, such as those that occur after calcium infusion. Although it has been suggested that the level of the C-terminal fragment provides the best differentiation between normal persons and patients with hyperparathyroidism, this seems paradoxical in view of the fact that the C-terminal is biologically inactive. It should be emphasized that radioimmunoassays that measure the C-terminal fragments do not provide a reliable estimate of parathyroid function in patients with renal insufficiency. This is because the clearance of C-terminal fragments is delayed in renal failure. Thus, with renal failure, the radioimmunoassay of N-terminal species of PTH or of the intact hormone molecule provides a better indication of parathyroid function. The intact PTH assay employs two antibodies, one binding the N-terminal and the second binding the C-terminal. One antibody is fixed on beads that are then exposed to serum. After incubation with the tested serum, the beads are separated and exposed to radiolabeled antibodies binding the opposite terminal.

Recently, it has been realized that current two-site assays designed to detect, both an N-terminal and C-terminal epitopes of PTH, may not be reliable. PTH molecules that are reactive in these assays are considered intact but some have no bioactivity. For example, a loss of only six amino acids to yield PTH (7–84) eliminates all bioactivity but does not affect the immunoreactivity measured in most of these assays. In fact about 50% of PTH detected in these assays in the serum of patients with chronic renal failure is not only biologically inactive but also exhibits an antagonistic effect on the biological activity of 1-84PTH. The newer immunodetection of PTH by whole PTH two-site assay that recognizes the first 6 amino acids appears to be more reliable in measuring only biologically active PTH.

Calcitonin

The discovery of calcitonin established the presence of a new regulatory system for calcium homeostasis. Calcitonin is a polypeptide with 32 amino acid residues and was isolated from the parafollicular cells of the thyroid gland or ultimobranchial body in a wide variety of species. Hypercalcemia stimulates release of calcitonin, which tends to lower serum calcium concentration (84).

EFFECT OF CALCITONIN ON BONE

The major mechanism by which calcitonin lowers serum calcium and phosphorus concentrations is inhibition of bone resorption. This is associated with decreased osteoclastic activity and decreased urinary hydroxyproline excretion. In organ culture, after prolonged treatment with calcitonin, PTH may overcome the inhibitory effect of calcitonin and induce bone resorption. This phenomenon is termed "escape" and also is observed in vivo in animals with intact parathyroid glands chronically treated with calcitonin. An antagonism exists between calcitonin and glucocorticoid hormones, because glucocorticoids interfere with the hypocalcemic action of calcitonin.

The receptors of calcitonin have been cloned from human giant cell tumors of bone, human ovary, and breast cell lines (74). The calcitonin receptor is expressed by osteoclasts, as opposed to PTH and calcitriol receptors, which are expressed only by osteoblasts. Similar to PTH receptors, calcitonin receptors couple to two signal transduction pathways, adenylate cyclase–PKA and phospholipase C–PKC via linking with G proteins. Calcitonin acts directly to inhibit osteoclast action on the bone and inhibits osteoclast motility in isolated osteoclast preparations.

EFFECT OF CALCITONIN ON THE KIDNEY

Calcitonin increases urinary excretion of phosphorus, sodium, potassium, and calcium. This effect is independent of PTH. In fact, calcitonin acts to reverse the effect of PTH in two organs. It inhibits bone resorption and increases urinary calcium excretion; both actions tend to lower serum calcium. The phosphaturic action of calcitonin has been found to be associated with an increased urinary excretion of cAMP.

Under normocalcemic conditions calcitonin and not PTH has an important role in maintenance serum $1,25(OH)_2D_3$ levels. Calcitonin enhances induction of $25(OH)D-1\alpha(OH)$ase transcription and protein expression. Because plasma calcitonin is increased during pregnancy and lactation, it has been

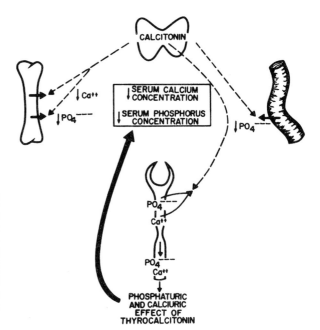

■ **Figure 6.5** The hypocalcemic and hypophosphatemic actions of calcitonin are based on inhibition of mineral mobilization from the bone, decreased tubular reabsorption and increased urinary excretion of calcium and phosphorus, and decreased intestinal absorption of phosphorus. (*Solid lines* represent an enhancing effect of the hormone; *broken lines* represent an inhibitory action.)

proposed that this is the mechanism of increased $1,25(OH)_2D_3$ observed during pregnancy and lactation when calcium requirements are increased (85). Likewise, it is important to remember that experiments conducted in thyroparathyroidectomized animals that are not replaced with calcitonin supplements may invalidate the results.

EFFECT OF CALCITONIN ON INTESTINAL ABSORPTION

The effect of calcitonin on intestinal absorption has not been studied extensively. Preliminary reports indicate, however, that calcitonin has no effect on intestine calcium absorption but may actively decrease the absorption of phosphorus, sodium, potassium, and chloride. The multiple actions of calcitonin are summarized in Figure 6.5.

The development of a sensitive radioimmunoassay for calcitonin has provided the means to study the control of secretion of this hormone. From a clinical standpoint, the radioimmunoassay serves as a valuable aid in the diagnosis of medullary carcinoma of thyroid, which is a calcitonin-secreting tumor.

Disorders of Calcium and Phosphorus Metabolism Associated with Hypocalcemia

VITAMIN D DEFICIENCY

Hypocalcemia is a common feature of vitamin D deficiency; however, this disorder may be present with a normal serum calcium concentration. For example, vitamin D–deficiency rickets in children evolves over three stages. During the first stage, serum calcium concentration is low, serum phosphorus is normal, and immunoreactive PTH in the serum is normal (77,86). There is no satisfactory explanation for the normal PTH in the presence of hypocalcemia. During the second stage, there is a rise in PTH activity, and serum calcium concentration rises to a normal level as serum phosphorus concentration decreases. In the third stage, which is the most severe, both serum calcium and phosphorus concentrations are low (77). It is unknown whether vitamin D–deficiency osteomalacia in adults shows a similar evolution.

TABLE 6.2 COMMON CAUSES OF VITAMIN D DEFICIENCY

Nutritional	Abnormal metabolism of vitamin D
Malabsorption	Vitamin D–dependent rickets
Following gastrectomy	Ingestion of barbiturates and anticonvulsants
Tropical and nontropical sprue	Renal insufficiency
Chronic pancreatitis	Hepatic dysfunction
Biliary cirrhosis	Calcium deprivation
Ingestion of cathartics	Renal losses of vitamin D
Intestinal bypass	Nephrotic syndrome
Anticonvulsant therapy	Fanconi syndrome

The various common etiologies of vitamin D deficiency are listed in Table 6.2. Because vitamin D is a fat-soluble vitamin, nutritional osteomalacia usually is associated with a deficient intake of food products containing fatty substances (77,87). Partial gastrectomy may lead either to a simple dietary deficiency of vitamin D as a result of avoiding fatty foods or malabsorption of vitamin D. Small-bowel disease may produce both malabsorption of vitamin D and mucosal resistance to its action. Bile salt deficiency interferes with vitamin D absorption, and hepatocellular failure may interfere with its metabolism. Factitious diarrhea caused by prolonged ingestion of laxatives also may cause vitamin D deficiency. Likewise, nephrotic syndrome is associated with urinary losses and low levels of circulating $25(OH)D_3$ (88).

In addition to vitamin D deficiency resulting from nutritional and GI causes, a group of disorders has been identified in which the deficiency is caused by an abnormal metabolism of vitamin D. Vitamin D–dependent rickets is an inherited autosomal recessive disorder. It appears during early infancy and responds to pharmacologic doses of vitamin D and physiologic doses of calcitriol. This disorder represents an inherited deficiency in the kidney of the enzyme $25(OH)_2D_3$-$1\alpha(OH)$ase, which converts $25(OH)_2D_3$ into $1,25(OH)_2D_3$ (87).

$25(OH)D$-$1\alpha(OH)$ase is a mitochondrial cytochrome P-450 enzyme that functions in proximal tubular cells. Although it is a key enzyme in vitamin D metabolism, its cloning was difficult because of the low level of gene expression. The recent cloning of the human $25(OH)D$-$1\alpha(OH)$ase deoxyribonucleic acid (DNA) and gene made it possible to screen for mutations. Vitamin D–dependent rickets type I (VDDR-I) occurs at high frequency in French Canadians; the disease locus in this population was mapped to chromosome 12q13–14 by linkage analysis. Renal $1\alpha(OH)$ase activity is regulated by PTH, calcitonin, calcium, phosphate, and $1,25(OH)_2D_3$ itself. By contrast, the recently cloned $1\alpha(OH)$ase in macrophages is not stimulated by PTH or calcitonin; however, 8-Br-CAMP and interferon (IFN)-γ increased the expression of the enzyme (89).

Osteomalacia in patients ingesting phenobarbital is associated with low levels of circulating $25(OH)D_3$. It has been shown that the biologic half-life of vitamin D_3 and $25(OH)D_3$ is shortened in phenobarbital-treated patients and that there is an accumulation of more polar metabolites, some of which are inactive (86). This rapid turnover and the production of inactive forms of vitamin D have been attributed to induction of microsomal enzyme activity in the liver. Phenytoin does not interfere directly with vitamin D metabolism but can induce hypocalcemia through reduced intestinal absorption of calcium and decreased release from bone. Low levels of circulating $25(OH)D_3$ also have been observed in patients with chronic hepatic failure (52,87).

Dietary calcium deprivation per se in rats increases the clearance and inactivation of $25(OH)D_3$ and leads to vitamin D deficiency. It has been suggested that this form of vitamin D deficiency is caused by secondary hyperparathyroidism, which increases the renal production of calcitriol. The latter augments the degradation of $25(OH)D_3$ to inactive metabolites. Hypothetically, this mechanism may account for vitamin D deficiency observed in clinical states of calcium malabsorption, including GI diseases, resection, or bypass; chronic liver disease; anticonvulsant therapy; and morbid obesity (52,90).

The clinical significance of abnormally low serum levels of $25(OH)_2D_3$ in patients with nephrotic syndrome owing to excessive urinary losses of vitamin D–binding globulin has not been fully established yet. However, a study of bone histology in patients with nephrotic syndrome who had normal renal function revealed that the decrease in $25(OH)D_3$ level results in a decrease in ionized calcium, secondary hyperparathyroidism, and enhanced bone resorption as well as defective mineralization (88).

Understanding of the metabolic pathways of vitamin D may facilitate the investigation of various abnormalities. For example, low levels of $1,25(OH)_2D_3$ have been reported in patients with hypoparathyroidism. The lack of PTH and presence of hyperphosphatemia may decrease the conversion of $25(OH)_2D_3$ into $1,25(OH)_2D_3$, which may explain the resistance to vitamin D in some patients with hypoparathyroidism. In support of this possibility is the finding of successful treatment of hypocalcemia with $1,25(OH)_2D_3$ in patients with hypoparathyroidism.

HYPOPARATHYROIDISM

Hypoparathyroidism is a common cause of hypocalcemia. Hypoparathyroidism can cause hypocalcemia with paresthesias, muscle spasms (i.e., tetany), and seizures, especially when it occurs rapidly. Chronic hypoparathyroidism generally causes hypocalcemia so gradually that the only symptoms may be visual impairment from cataracts following years of hypoparathyroidism. Hypoparathyroidism may be secondary or idiopathic.

SECONDARY HYPOPARATHYROIDISM

Hypoparathyroidism may be caused by surgery. This variety of hypoparathyroidism may result from accidental removal of parathyroids or traumatic interruption of their blood supply. Very often the parathyroid deficiency is transient in nature. Hypocalcemia that appears after excision of parathyroid adenoma results from functional suppression and hypofunction of the remaining normal glands. Hypoparathyroidism may be a component of multiple endocrine dysfunction, including adrenal insufficiency owing to an autoimmune disorder. In hypoparathyroidism associated with pernicious anemia, an autoimmune mechanism also has been implicated.

Autoimmune hypoparathyroidism is commonly a part of polyglandular autoimmune syndrome type I (APS-1), which is a familial syndrome. It occurs during childhood and is inherited as an autosomal recessive trait caused by mutations in an autoimmune regulator gene (AIRE). Loss of immunologic tolerance to tissue-restricted antigens due to the absence of AIRE expression in the thymus leads to exit of autoreactive T cells from the thymus that trigger autoimmunity (91). Antibodies against IFN-ω and -α have been recently shown to be a sensitive and specific marker for APS-1. APS-1 is associated with mucocutaneous candidiasis, vitiligo, and adrenal insufficiency. Antibodies against the CaSR in the parathyroid glands were found in many patients with this abnormality. Adrenal insufficiency is a late phenomenon in this syndrome.

Hypoparathyroidism is a recognized complication of thalassemia occurring after multiple transfusions and also has been described in patients with Wilson disease. Deposition of iron and copper, respectively, in the parathyroid glands is the likely mechanism of parathyroid hypofunction in these patients (87). Also, parathyroid granulomas and metastatic cancer can lead to hypoparathyroidism.

Hypocalcemia may occur with magnesium depletion. Hypomagnesemia has been reported to induce skeletal resistance to PTH. It has been proposed that low serum magnesium diminishes the synthesis of PTH. It is interesting that some patients with hypoparathyroidism who exhibit resistance to vitamin D respond after administration of magnesium. Hypocalcemia associated with magnesium depletion responds poorly to intravenous calcium. Profound hypocalcemia may appear after therapeutic use of magnesium sulfate (e.g., in preeclampsia of pregnancy) because of suppression of PTH secretion. Certain drugs such as aminoglycosides and cytotoxic agents may have a direct toxic effect on parathyroid glands, leading to hypocalcemia. Irradiation of neck or administration of radioactive iodine also may affect parathyroid function (87). Symptomatic hypoparathyroidism also has been described in association with HIV infection.

IDIOPATHIC HYPOPARATHYROIDISM

Idiopathic hypoparathyroidism may be sporadic or familial. The familial congenital type is associated with hypocalcemic seizures in infancy. Familial idiopathic hypoparathyroidism is a heterogenous group of disorders. It may result from a mutation of the prepro-PTH gene or mutations of currently unidentified loci that affect the development, structure or function of parathyroid glands (92,93).

The human PTH is encoded by a single gene that was mapped to the short arm of chromosome 11. Mutations in this gene may lead to familial hypoparathyroidism with autosomal dominant transmission. The levels of PTH in serum may be low or undetectable in affected patients (92,93).

The DiGeorge or velocardiofacial syndrome consists of a congenital failure of development of the derivatives of the third and fourth pharyngeal pouches, leading to absence of parathyroid glands and thymus. This syndrome may be inherited as an autosomal dominant disorder. It is associated with deletion of the long arm of chromosome 22 (94).

X-linked recessive hypoparathyroidism, like the DiGeorge syndrome, is associated with parathyroid agenesis and undetectable PTH levels in circulation. The X-linked recessive hypoparathyroidism gene was mapped to the distal long arm of the X chromosome (92,93).

Hypoparathyroidism may be caused by mutations or deletions in transcription factors or regulators of the development of parathyroid glands. Familial hypoparathyroidism due to dysgenesis of parathyroids glands results from mutations in the transcription factors glial cell missing B (GCMB) and glial cell missing 2 (GCM2). The latter GCM2 is the master regulatory gene for parathyroid glands function and transcription factor for parathyroid glands development. Recent study has shown that one of the functions GCM2 is to maintain high levels of CaSR expression in parathyroid glands (95). Mutation in another transcription factor, globin transcription factor (GATA) protein–binding protein 3 (GATA3), which is a critical transcription factor for many developmental processes, causes an autosomal dominant complex disorder that combines hypoparathyroidism, deafness, and renal dysplasia (HDR).

A mutation in the gene coding for tubulin-specific chaperone E (TBCE), a peripheral membrane–associated tubulin-folding cofactor protein that is required for microtubule assembly, causes a rare autosomal recessive complex syndrome which includes hypoparathyroidism. The syndrome consists of hypoparathyroidism, retardation, and dysmorphism (HRD or Sanjat–Sakati syndrome). HRD is characterized by congenital hypoparathyroidism, intrauterine growth retardation, osteosclerosis, calcification of basal ganglia, mental retardation, seizures, and a typical facial dysmorphism featuring prominent forehead, deep-set eyes, and abnormal external ears. Mutation of the same gene was also reported in patients with autosomal recessive Kenny–Caffey syndrome (KCS). KCS resembles HRD phenotype but is characterized by the presence of normal intelligence, late closure of the anterior fontanel, macrocephaly, postnatal growth retardation, and corneal opacity (96). Defects in maternal mitochondrial genes cause the Kearns–Sayre syndrome consisting of hypoparathyroidism, ophthalmoplegia, retinitis pigmentosa, cardiomyopathy with heart block, and diabetes mellitus.

Recently, autosomal dominant hypoparathyroidism was reported in families with activating mutations of the gene that encodes the extracellular CaSR in chromosome 3. In one family, missense mutation was found in the CaSR gene (97). These mutations cause excessive calcium-induced inhibition of PTH secretion. The hypocalcemia is mild and asymptomatic. It should be treated cautiously when mild because raising serum calcium concentrations markedly enhances urinary calcium excretions, with increasing risk of nephrocalcinosis and renal insufficiency.

PSEUDOHYPOPARATHYROIDISM

Pseudohypoparathyroidism is a rare inheritable disorder characterized by mental retardation, moderate obesity, short stature, brachydactyly with short metacarpal and metatarsal bones, exostoses, radius curves, and expressionless face. The biochemical abnormalities are hypocalcemia and hyperphosphatemia (98,99). Some patients only exhibit the biochemical abnormalities. Thus, the disorder may be subdivided into pseudohypoparathyroidism type IA, which is also known as Albright hereditary osteodystrophy and type IB. Pseudohypoparathyroidism type IA is associated with both the somatic and biochemical abnormalities, and type IB, which presents with the biochemical defect without the somatic abnormalities. In patients with pseudohypoparathyroidism, the administration of PTH fails to increase urinary cAMP and is not associated with phosphaturia. It has been shown also that the response to the administration of exogenous dibutyryl cAMP is intact in pseudohypoparathyroidism and causes pronounced phosphaturia. It has been proposed that the skeletal refractoriness to PTH shows a certain degree of selectivity. Accordingly, the bone responds to the remodeling action of the hormone but is resistant to its calcemic-homeostatic effect. Because of the hypocalcemic stimulus, secondary hyperparathyroidism may develop in some patients, leading to osteitis fibrosa cystica. Failure of the kidney to form $1,25(OH)_2D_3$ in response to PTH results in a low circulating level of this metabolite. This deficiency may be responsible, at least partly, for the skeletal refractoriness to the calcemic action of PTH that requires the presence of $1,25(OH)_2D_3$ (98).

Most patients with the type I form of pseudohypoparathyroidism manifest approximately 50% reduction in cellular activity of the α-subunit of the G protein that stimulates adenylate cyclase ($G_s\alpha$) encoded by guanine nucleotide-binding protein alpha-subunit 1 ($GNAS_1$) gene. Patients with type IA show a generalized $G_s\alpha$ deficiency and often manifest resistance to other hormones whose effects are mediated by $G_s\alpha$-coupled receptors (e.g., calcitonin, glucagon, and thyroid-stimulating hormone). Pseudohypoparathyroidism type 1A is caused by an inactivating mutation of the α-subunit of G_s and is inherited as an autosomal dominant trait. At variance with type IA, patients with pseudohypoparathyroidism type IB manifest a selective end-organ resistance to PTH alone (99).

Other mechanisms have been identified in addition to the mechanism of target organ refractoriness. In one patient, the administration of PTH was associated with a normal increase in urinary cAMP but failed to produce phosphaturia (100). The latter is designated as pseudohypoparathyroidism type 2. Production of ineffective PTH, presumably because of a defect in the conversion of parathyroid prohormone into an active form, also was described in one patient (101). The patient had normal to high levels of immunoreactive PTH, which was probably a biologically inactive hormone, because the patient readily responded to exogenous PTH. Recently, a novel mutation of the signal peptide of the prepro-PTH gene has been described. This mutation leads to synthesis of detective PTH molecule and undetectable amounts of PTH in serum. This abnormality is inherited as an autosomal recessive type of isolated familial hypoparathyroidism (102).

Pseudo-pseudohypoparathyroidism occurs in families with pseudohypoparathyroidism type Ia. It presents inactivating mutations of $GNAS_1$ and features of Albright osteodystrophy but without the resistance to PTH and other hormones.

MALIGNANCY ASSOCIATED WITH HYPOCALCEMIA

Medullary carcinoma of the thyroid may present as a familial and autosomal dominant or a sporadic disorder. The tumor is derived from parafollicular cells of ultimobranchial organ, which secrete calcitonin. Patients with this disorder have high levels of circulating calcitonin and exhibit an exaggerated increase of calcitonin in response to calcium infusion. Hypocalcemia has been reported to be present in some subjects. However, it is absent in others, and its absence despite very high levels of calcitonin is not well understood but has been attributed to a secondary increase in PTH. An "escape" from the effect of calcitonin, which has been observed in experimental conditions, is another possible factor. Elevated blood levels of calcitonin also have been reported in tumors other than medullary carcinoma of the thyroid, including carcinoma of the lung.

Hypocalcemia may develop in patients with malignant neoplasms in association with osteoblastic (bone-forming) metastases. These lesions may lead to rapid deposition of mineral in the newly formed matrix, thus causing hypocalcemia (103). Such hypocalcemia has been described in patients with carcinoma of the prostate or carcinoma of the breast with osteoblastic metastases (103). Although most of these patients have shown osteoblastic lesions on radiologic examination, associated osteolytic lesions also have been present (103).

HYPERPHOSPHATEMIA

The various causes of hyperphosphatemia that may lead to hypocalcemia are listed in Table 6.3. The oral or intravenous administration of phosphate lowers serum calcium concentration in normal animals and hypercalcemic human subjects. This observation formed the basis for the clinical use of phosphate administration in states of hypercalcemia. The association of hyperphosphatemia and hypocalcemia has been reported to occur in a variety of circumstances. Hyperphosphatemia has been observed in persons ingesting large quantities of phosphate-containing laxatives or receiving enemas with phosphate. Hyperphosphatemia and hypocalcemia with tetany may develop in babies fed cow's milk, which contains 1,220 mg of calcium and 940 mg of phosphorus per liter (human milk contains 340 mg of calcium and 150 mg of phosphorus per liter).

TABLE 6.3 HYPERPHOSPHATEMIA AS A CAUSE OF HYPOCALCEMIA

Administration of phosphate	Renal disease
Oral phosphate	Acute renal failure
Cow's milk in infants	Chronic renal failure
Laxatives containing phosphate	Neoplasms treated with cytotoxic agents
Potassium phosphate tablets	Lymphomas
Phosphate-containing enemas	Leukemias
Intravenous phosphate	Tumorlysis
	Rhabdomyolysis

The mechanism responsible for lowering serum calcium by the administration of phosphate is not entirely understood. One possibility is that the decrease in serum calcium concentration is caused by deposition of calcium phosphate in the bone, soft tissues, or both. The results of animal studies suggest that the administration of phosphate increases bone formation.

In chronic renal failure, a constant increase in serum phosphorus concentration is observed when GFR is 30 mL/min or less; and hyperphosphatemia is a common accompaniment of acute renal failure. It is important to emphasize, however, that in renal failure causes other than hyperphosphatemia may play an important role in hypocalcemia. An acquired resistance to vitamin D, which might represent a metabolic block in the 1α-hydroxylation of $25(OH)D_3$ to $1,25(OH)_2D_3$, or skeletal resistance to the calcium-mobilizing effect of PTH, or both, is possibly involved (104).

In patients undergoing chemotherapy for neoplastic diseases, particularly of lymphatic origin, large quantities of phosphates may be released into the circulation as a result of the cytolysis. Spontaneous tumor lysis may cause hyperphosphatemia and consequently hypocalcemia. Conversely, rapid regrowth of tumoral masses may lead to profound hypophosphatemia (39).

ACUTE PANCREATITIS

The hypocalcemia associated with acute pancreatitis is not well understood. The precipitation of calcium soaps in the abdominal cavity, which results from the release of lipolytic enzymes and fat necrosis, has been suggested as the mechanism of hypocalcemia. Other studies implicate glucagon-induced hypersecretion of calcitonin as the mechanism of hypocalcemia in acute pancreatitis (87). These latter results have not been confirmed, however.

Even though it has been shown that hypocalcemia and urinary excretion of cAMP respond to pharmacologic doses of PTH, one study suggests a relative peripheral resistance to appropriate levels of endogenous hormone and normal circulating $1,25(OH)_2D_3$. The cause of this refractoriness and its role in the hypocalcemia of acute pancreatitis are not apparent (105).

NEONATAL TETANY

Neonatal tetany with hypocalcemia was first described in 1913. Several mechanisms have been suggested for the pathogenesis of this disorder, namely vitamin D deficiency, parathyroid hypofunction, and hyperphosphatemia owing to a high content of phosphorus in the milk (cow's milk).

Congenital absence of the parathyroid glands, usually in association with other congenital anomalies, has been reported in neonatal tetany. Transient, idiopathic congenital hypoparathyroidism with hypoplasia or dysplasia of the parathyroid glands and with a subsequent compensatory hyperplasia has been described in infants with hypocalcemia (106). In one study, low levels of circulating immunoreactive PTH were detected in a group of babies with hypocalcemia. This finding was attributed to possible immaturity of the parathyroid glands, which was usually transient (107).

Babies born to mothers with osteomalacia caused by vitamin D deficiency have congenital rickets with hypocalcemia and tetany. In one study, serum levels of $25(OH)D_3$ were measured in 15 premature infants with neonatal hypocalcemia and their mothers. In 11 of the 15 cases, plasma $25(OH)D_3$ was low in both mother and infant (108). Babies born to mothers with hyperparathyroidism and hypercalcemia are at risk of hypocalcemia and tetany, probably because of suppression of the babies' own parathyroid glands.

OSTEOPETROSIS (MARBLE BONE DISEASE)

Osteopetrosis is a rare disease, with about 300 cases reported in the literature. The disease is characterized by abnormal bones that fracture easily, increased radiographic bone density, cranial nerve palsies because of compression of the nerves in their foramina, and mandibular osteomyelitis. There are two clinical forms of the disease. The first variant, malignant osteopetrosis, affects infants and usually is fatal. The second, benign osteopetrosis, may be recognized during any stage of adult life (109). The inheritance of the malignant form of the disease is recessive; inheritance of the benign form is autosomal dominant. Hypocalcemia has been found only in a few cases and does not appear to be a constant feature of the disease (109).

The basic abnormality in osteopetrosis is not clear, but indirect evidence suggests that a defect in osteoclast function leading to uncoupling between bone formation and resorption with reduced osteoclastic activity is the underlying mechanism.

The first physiological defect described in human osteopetrosis was an autosomal recessive condition with lack of carbonic anhydrase II activity; 50% to 60% of children with severe osteopetrosis have a mutation in gene proton pump H^+ ATPase. Osteoclasts in patients with proton pump defect are of normal appearance but dysfunctional. Mutations in chloride channel (CLCN7) appear less frequently as a cause of osteopetrosis (110).

Bone marrow transplantation and high doses of $1,25(OH)_2D_3$ with low calcium intake have been used in therapeutic trials. It has been demonstrated that the vitamin D derivative, calcitriol $(1,25(OH)_2D_3)$ may enhance the bone-resorbing activity of osteoclasts that is impaired in osteopetrosis (111). Recent trials of treatment with recombinant human IFN-γ are encouraging (112).

ADMINISTRATION OF PHYTATE, SODIUM ETHYLENEDIAMINETETRAACETATE, CITRATE, AND MITHRAMYCIN

Sodium phytate (sodium–inositol hexaphosphate) binds calcium in the intestine as calcium phytate and thereby inhibits calcium absorption. In normal subjects, the administration of phytate causes only a minimal drop in serum calcium, whereas it may precipitate hypocalcemia in patients with latent hypoparathyroidism. Excessive dietary phytate (cereals) has been implicated as a possible cause of osteomalacia in certain ethnic groups in England (90). Both citrate and sodium ethylenediaminetetraacetate (Na-EDTA), when given intravenously, bind ionized calcium and may induce hypocalcemia with low ionized calcium. Low serum-ionized calcium may be a complication of ethylene glycol (antifreeze) poisoning. This is because calcium binding by oxalic acid, which is the metabolite of the poison, reduces serum-ionized calcium.

Excessive intake of fluoride may induce hypocalcemia. This was reported recently in Alaska in connection with fluorosis that followed excessive addition of fluoride to drinking water (113). Drug-induced hypocalcemia was described in patients with acquired immunodeficiency syndrome. An analog of pyrophosphate foscarnet used to treat cytomegalovirus infection caused hypocalcemia because of chelation of calcium and concomitant hypomagnesemia (114). Ketoconazole and pentamidine have been reported to cause hypocalcemia as well.

The association of low serum-ionized calcium with essential hypertension and secondary hyperparathyroidism has been described and attributed to renal calcium leak (115). This finding may be of clinical significance because a fall in serum-ionized calcium may compromise myocardial performance and worsen the function of a failing heart in patients with hypertension.

Mithramycin is a potent inhibitor of RNA synthesis and has antitumor activity. It produces a decrease in serum calcium and phosphorus levels and in urinary hydroxyproline excretion. Mithramycin has been used to correct the hypercalcemia of various disorders, including malignancy with bone metastases. In experimental studies, mithramycin has been shown to inhibit the rate and magnitude of osteoclastic resorption induced by PTH; however, no demonstrable effect was found on normal bone formation or resorption in growing animals (116,117).

Hypocalcemia has been described recently in critically ill patients admitted to intensive care units. The incidence of hypocalcemia amounted to 88% in these patients. The degree of hypocalcemia correlated with the severity of the disease and was most commonly detected in patients who were septic. The mechanism of this abnormality is unknown. Circulating levels of calcitonin precursors (CTpr) increase up to several thousand-fold in response to microbial infections and this increase correlates with the severity of the infection and mortality. The relationship of elevated CTpr to the emergence of hypocalcemia needs to be investigated (118).

TREATMENT OF HYPOCALCEMIA

Symptomatic hypocalcemia generally responds promptly to the intravenous administration of calcium. The commonly used preparations are 10% calcium gluconate (10-mL ampules containing 90 mg of elemental calcium) and 10% calcium chloride (10-mL ampules containing 360 mg of elemental calcium). The treatment should be instituted immediately, because delay may be associated with further aggravation of tetany and lead to generalized seizures and even cardiac arrest.

Chronic treatment with oral calcium should follow the intravenous therapy in patients with chronic hypocalcemia owing to irreversible causes such as hypoparathyroidism. Oral calcium administration constitutes the best initial therapy in mild cases. The commonly used preparations are in tablet form: calcium lactate, 300 mg (60 mg of elemental calcium); chewable calcium gluconate, 1 g (90 mg of elemental calcium); and calcium carbonate (Os-Cal), 250 mg of elemental calcium. Oral calcium also may be used for patients for whom the diagnosis of irreversible hypoparathyroidism has not been established with absolute certainty. In patients who fail to respond to oral calcium, vitamin D in large doses is the only available treatment. The commonly used preparations are capsules containing 1.25 mg (50,000 units) of vitamin D_2 (ergocalciferol). The average dose ranges between 1.25 and 3.75 mg/day. DHT_3 is three times as potent as vitamin D_2 in raising serum calcium concentration. Each capsule contains 0.125 mg of DHT_3. The average daily dose ranges between 0.25 and 1 mg of DHT_3. Both vitamins are available in liquid oil solutions as well. Both hypoparathyroidism and pseudohypoparathyroidism respond to physiologic doses of $1,25(OH)_2D_3$ and $1\alpha(OH)D_3$ with restoration of serum calcium to normal. Calcitriol is marketed as Rocaltrol and is dispensed in capsules containing 0.25 and 1 μg. Chlorothiazides may enhance the calcemic action of vitamin D and its analogs, whereas furosemide may aggravate the hypocalcemia through its hypercalciuric action.

Patients in whom hypocalcemia is associated with hypomagnesemia respond poorly to intravenous calcium, but serum calcium concentration is restored to normal levels with correction of the hypomagnesemia.

Symptoms rarely develop in patients with chronic renal failure and hypocalcemia. However, very often reduction of elevated serum phosphorus with phosphate-binding antacids cause an increase in serum calcium concentration.

Hypocalcemia associated with osteomalacia resulting from vitamin D deficiency is rarely symptomatic. It usually responds to physiologic doses of vitamin D and increased oral calcium intake.

Disorders of Calcium and Phosphorus Metabolism Associated with Hypercalcemia

Hypercalcemia presents a challenge to every clinician and diagnostician. In some instances, the cause of hypercalcemia is self-evident on the basis of the circumstantial clinical findings, whereas extensive efforts are required to establish the etiology in other situations. The important causes of hypercalcemia are listed in Table 6.4.

HYPERPARATHYROIDISM

Primary hyperparathyroidism is present in 10% to 20% of all patients with hypercalcemia. The annual age-adjusted incidence is approximately 25 cases per 100,000. Making the diagnosis is very important because of this frequency and the amenability to surgical cure. The disease is more common in females

TABLE 6.4 DISORDERS ASSOCIATED WITH HYPERCALCEMIA

Primary hyperparathyroidism	Hypervitaminosis D
Adenoma and carcinoma	Hypervitaminosis A
Hyperplasia	Granulomatous diseases
Multiple endocrine adenomatosis	Sarcoidosis
Extopic secretion of PTH by neoplasms (rare)	Tuberculosis
	Histoplasmosis
Secondary hyperparathyroidism	Coccidioidomycosis
Malabsorption and vitamin D disease	Leprosy
Chronic renal failure	Foreign body granuloma
Following kidney transplantation	Hyperthyroidism
Familial hypocalciuric hypercalcemia	Adrenocortical insufficiency
Hypercalcemia associated with malignancy	Infantile hypercalcemia
Lytic bone metastases	Immobilization
Circulating tumor–secreted factors	Hypophosphatasia
PTHrP	Milk–alkali syndrome
1,25-dihydroxyvitamin D_3–induced hypercalcemia	Parenteral nutrition
Locally acting, noncirculating, tumor-secreted cytokines	Hypercalcemia associated with acute renal failure
IL-1 and -6	Medications
TNF-β	Thiazides
Granulocyte macrophage	Lithium
colony-stimulating factor	Theophylline
TGF-α	Calcium ion exchange resins
Prostaglandins	
Hypercalcemia in patients with hyper-absorptive	
hypercalciuria	

IL, interleukin; PTH, parathyroid hormone; PTHrP, parathyroid hormone–related peptide; TGF, transforming growth factor; TNF, tumor necrosis factor.

than in males; the incidence increases in women after menopause but is less frequent in older men. A single parathyroid adenoma is by far the most common cause of primary hyperparathyroidism. Carcinoma is very infrequent, occurring in <1% of all reported cases. Primary hyperplasia is found in <10% of all cases, but it is the most frequent cause in familial hyperparathyroidism.

The morphologic differentiation between adenomas and hyperplasia sometimes is very difficult. The presence of a capsule and a rim of compressed normal gland tissue around the periphery of an adenoma may be helpful in making a definitive diagnosis. The persistence or recurrence of hypercalcemia after surgery for a purported adenoma warrants a more precise evaluation of the morphologic status of the parathyroid tissue removed. Also, with parathyroid hyperplasia, the quantity of parathyroid tissue to be removed—safely, yet not allowing recurrence of the disease on the other hand—is a very difficult balance to achieve. If more than one gland shows histologic features of hyperplasia, then removal of more than one gland is recommended; generally, approximately 200 mg of parathyroid tissue should remain.

In addition to the uncertainties related to morphologic differences between various forms of hyperparathyroidism, some of its functional characteristics have been questioned also. The widely accepted interpretation of the cause of the hypercalcemia in patients with parathyroid adenomas has been that the normal feedback regulation of PTH secretion is absent. That is, presumably the secreting cells of the adenoma were altered in such a way that their secretory function no longer responded to variations in serum calcium concentration; this state was defined as autonomy. The distinction between parathyroid adenoma and hyperplasia implied that the former is a primary disease rather than an adaptive response and that the latter represents a compensatory adaptation to low serum calcium concentration. The term "tertiary hyperparathyroidism" has been used to describe secondary hyperparathyroidism associated with an enormously enlarged mass of parathyroid tissue. Because of the inordinate number of secreting cells, large amounts of PTH enter the circulation despite the fact that each individual cell may respond normally to an elevation in serum calcium concentration by reducing the secretion of PTH from each cell. This is supported by experimental studies also (119). Some patients with primary hyperparathyroidism have pronounced hypercalciuria despite a very mild degree of hypercalcemia and minimal or no bone disease (120). In patients with primary hyperparathyroidism, a very strong positive correlation was found between $1,25(OH)_2D_3$ in the serum and the urinary calcium excretion. Patients with nephrolithiasis and hypercalciuria had circulating levels of $1,25(OH)_2D_3$ higher than those present in hyperparathyroid patients without renal stones (121). The reason for this difference in the $1,25(OH)_2D_3$ levels is unknown, but it stresses the importance of vitamin D metabolism in the clinical presentation of primary hyperparathyroidism.

New insights regarding additional factors that may predispose to hypercalciuria in patients with primary hyperparathyroidism have emerged recently. Polymorphism of CaSR with the presence of R990G allele brings about gain of function of CaSR and results in increased susceptibility to hypercalciuria with consequent nephrolithiasis. It is likely that increased activation of CaSRs that reside at the basolateral surface of thick ascending loop of Henle triggers mechanisms that inhibit paracellular reabsorption of calcium causing hypercalciuria (9).

The high incidence of parathyroid adenomas in association with various malignant neoplasms is not well understood but warrants consideration in every case in which a malignant tumor is accompanied by hypercalcemia (122).

Molecular biology provides the means to study the role of genomic aberrations as the underlying mechanism of primary hyperparathyroidism. In parathyroid adenomas, changes were reported to occur in the gene that encodes PTH and is located on chromosome 11 (123). Likewise, alterations were identified in the X chromosome. The genomic abnormalities consist of loss of tumor-suppressor genes and/or overexpression of oncogenes on chromosome 11. Likewise, inactivation of tumor-suppressor genes were found in the X chromosome. It is interesting that these genomic changes were found not only in patients with parathyroid adenoma but also in patients with parathyroid hyperplasia, including hyperplasia secondary to chronic renal failure (124).

The familial occurrence of parathyroid adenomas with an autosomal dominant inheritance mandates the biochemical screening of family members of patients with primary hyperparathyroidism. Establishing the diagnosis of familial hyperparathyroidism also may be important to the patient's surgeon, alerting him or her to the high incidence of hyperplasia and multiple adenomas in this group of patients. In some families, primary hyperparathyroidism is associated with other endocrine tumors as well. The syndrome of hyperparathyroidism, medullary carcinoma of the thyroid with amyloid stroma, pheochromocytoma, and multiple neuromas is known as multiple endocrine neoplasia type II (MEN-II) or Sipple syndrome. The syndrome described by Wermer consisted of hyperparathyroidism and tumors of the pituitary and pancreatic islet cells (MEN-I).

MEN-I is an autosomal dominant familial neoplasia syndrome. The gene of MEN-I ("menin") has been cloned. The gene was mapped to the long arm of chromosome 11. MEN-I is a tumor-suppressor gene. Inactivating germ-line mutations of MEN-I gene lead to the growth of multiple endocrine neoplasia. Over 40 different germ-line mutations of MEN-I gene have been identified in MEN-I kindreds, suggesting the absence of founder effect. By contrast, MEN-II is caused by activating mutation of the RET protooncogene and is inherited as an autosomal dominant trait.

The hyperparathyroidism-jaw tumor syndrome consists of hyperparathyroidism cemento-ossifying fibromas of the jaw, renal cysts, Wilms tumor, and renal hamartomas. This syndrome is caused by a mutation of an unknown gene on chromosome 1q24 and is inherited as an autosomal dominant trait.

A small minority of parathyroid adenomas have activating mutation of the cyclin D_1 oncogene $(CCND_1)$. These mutations result in overexpression of the protein cyclin D_1 (125,126). It is interesting in this regard that primary hyperparathyroidism was induced by parathyroid targeted overexpression of cyclin D_1 in transgenic mice.

Primary hyperparathyroidism can best be diagnosed by demonstrating persistent hypercalcemia with elevated serum PTH. Patients presenting with bone, renal, GI, or neuromuscular symptoms are considered symptomatic and usually require surgery. Conversely, in asymptomatic patients, objective manifestations of primary hyperparathyroidism that are indications for surgery include markedly elevated serum calcium concentration, a previous episode of life-threatening hypercalcemia, a reduced creatinine clearance, presence of kidney stones, hypercalciuria, and substantially reduced bone density (127).

Recent progress in the imaging techniques includes the Tc 99m Sestamibi scan. This new technique helps detect and localize parathyroid adenomas with high precision and accuracy. Furthermore, this technique makes it possible to identify the adenoma intraoperatively with use of a portable radioactivity detector probe (Geiger counter) and guide the surgeon directly to the tumor. This advanced technique allows the surgical procedure to be carried out under local anesthesia with reduced morbidity and with more successful outcome. Likewise, progress has been made with use of diagnostic ultrasonography. The close monitoring of PTH levels (PTH has a very short half-life during surgery) may assist in ascertaining the success of parathyroidectomy. A recent clinical study examined the clinical course and development of complications for a period up to 10 years in 121 patients with primary hyperparathyroidism; 101 (83%) of the patients were asymptomatic. During the study, 61 (50%) patients underwent parathyroidectomy and 60 were followed without surgery. Parathyroidectomy resulted in the normalization of biochemical values and increased bone mineral density. Most asymptomatic patients who did not undergo surgery did not have progression of disease; however, approximately one-fourth of them did have some progression. The progression included recurrent kidney stones, decrease of >10% in bone density, rise to >12 mg/dL in serum calcium, and development of hypercalciuria. A recent study showed that in patients with asymptomatic hyperparathyroidism, parathyroidectomy improved the BMD as well as, the quality of life. Parathyroidectomy has been recommended particularly for elderly patients with decreased BMD to prevent later fractures that carry high mortality. These findings raise serious questions regarding the choice of the optimal treatment for so-called "asymptomatic" patients with primary hyperparathyroidism (128).

Vitamin D status is one of the determinants of skeletal complications in patients in patients with primary hyperparathyroidism. Low $25(OH)D_3$ and $1,25(OH)_2D_3$ levels are associated with increased turnover and decreased bone mineral density in patients with primary hyperparathyroidism. This finding suggests that supplementation with vitamin D in deficient patients may be beneficial (129).

Familial hypocalciuric hypercalcemia is an unusual form of parathyroid hyperplasia with autosomal dominant transmission. There is a high incidence of neonatal primary hyperparathyroidism among the offspring of the affected families. The clinical course is relatively benign with an absence of nephrolithiasis and an infrequent occurrence of pancreatitis and chondrocalcinosis. Mild parathyroid hyperplasia with modestly elevated levels of circulating PTH and increased urinary excretion of cAMP have been reported in these patients. The unsatisfactory response to subtotal parathyroidectomy, however, suggests additional underlying abnormalities. The presence of hypocalciuria both before and after subtotal parathyroidectomy provides a strong argument that enhanced tubular reabsorption of calcium plays an important role in maintaining hypercalcemia. Hypermagnesemia, which appears to reflect increased tubular reabsorption of magnesium, is another unique feature of this hypercalcemic disorder. Already in the past, has been proposed that a concurrence of defects in both the parathyroid glands and kidneys in their response to serum calcium concentration is an explanation for this disorder (130).

Inactivating mutations in the human CaSR gene cause both familial hypocalciuric hypercalcemia (FHH) and neonatal severe hyperparathyroidism. The CaSR gene has been mapped to chromosome 3, the same chromosome to which the FHH disease locus was localized in the past. In most families with FHH, linkage to chromosome 3g predominates, although in one family linkage to chromosome 19f was demonstrated. Thus, the disease exhibits genetic heterogeneity. Inheritance of a single copy of mutated gene causes FHH, whereas homozygous patients who inherit two inactive genes develop neonatal severe hyperparathyroidism. The latter is associated with severe hypercalcemia owing to parathyroid hyperplasia that usually requires surgery. These mutations lead to a defective CaSR with a presumable impairment of signal transduction function, possibly resulting from abnormal coupling with G protein. This in turn appears to lead to abnormally reduced parathyroid and renal responsiveness to changes in extracellular calcium, resulting in increased PTH secretion and avid tubular reabsorption of calcium. Thus, the CaSR plays an important role in calcium-regulated secretion of PTH and tubular reabsorption of calcium. The FHH-associated excessive reabsorption of calcium, probably in the thick ascending limb, which persists even after parathyroidectomy, suggests that this abnormality is PTH independent (130,131).

Both familial and acquired forms of hypocalciuric hypercalcemia due to autoantibodies against CaSR have been reported. These autoantibodies inhibit receptor activation. The patient with acquired form of autoimmune hyperparathyroidism presented with systemic autoimmune disease, including psoriasis, rheumatoid arthritis, hypophysitis with diabetes insipidus and hypothyroidism, uveitis and Coombs-positive anemia. The syndrome including hyperparathyroidism responded to immunosuppression with glucocorticoids, featuring a glucocorticoids-responsive hyperparathyroidism (132).

MALIGNANCY ASSOCIATED WITH HYPERCALCEMIA

A malignant neoplasm is the single most common cause of hypercalcemia. Hypercalcemia is most commonly produced by tumors of lung, breast, kidney, and ovary, and by hematologic malignancies. Very often the hypercalcemia is uncontrollable and thus is a harbinger of the patient's demise. Indeed, survival after the appearance of hypercalcemia in association with malignancy is very poor, with a median of 3 months. Two main mechanisms are known to mediate the hypercalcemia of malignancy: local and humoral. The local mechanism is manifested by the presence of osteolytic lesions in the skeleton. The malignant cells may act to destroy the bone directly; however, even local osteolysis is mediated by activated osteoclasts in most instances. Many tumors may produce hypercalcemia by a dual mechanism, that is, both local and humoral. It has become apparent that humoral hypercalcemia of malignancy (HHM) is caused by a circulating factor that is secreted by the neoplasm (133). This circulating substance acts on the bone to induce osteoclastic resorption and on the kidney to reduce phosphate reabsorption, increase calcium reabsorption, and increase nephrogenous cAMP excretion. All of these biochemical effects are characteristic of the actions of native PTH. However, only in four patients, one with small cell carcinoma of lung, the second with ovarian carcinoma, the third with metastatic neuroendocrine tumor of pancreas and the fourth with hepatocellular carcinoma, was ectopic secretion of intact PTH demonstrated (134,135,136). In the vast majority of patients with HHM, the circulating factor is PTH related protein (PTHrP). PTHrP is a 141 amino acid protein that binds to the receptors common to the native PTH, but it is encoded by a distinct gene. Even though PTHrP shares structural homology of N-terminal residues with PTH, immunoradiometric assay of PTH has been able to distinguish completely between patients with HHM and those with primary hyperparathyroidism (137,138). Thus, hypercalcemia with absence of detectable PTH by radioimmunoassay and presence of high urinary cAMP supports the diagnosis of HHM. PTHrP was originally isolated from human malignant tumors associated with HHM. Subsequently, it was detected to be present in a variety of tissues, including parathyroid adenoma, skin, breast, placenta, testis, pancreas, and brain (138). With regard to the presence of PTHrP in parathyroid tissue, it has been suggested that PTH is produced by the chief cells (major component of parathyroid tissue), whereas PTHrP is produced by the oxyphil cells (138). Accordingly, the detection of PTHrP in circulation per se does not rule out parathyroid adenoma. Rather, the absence of PTH and presence of PTHrP by radioimmunoassays in fact rule out parathyroid adenoma and support the diagnosis of HHM.

In vitro PTHrP, similarly to native PTH, has been shown not only to stimulate renal adenylate cyclase and increase the formation of cAMP, but also to activate the $1\alpha(OH)$ase and enhance the formation of $1,25(OH)_2D_3$. In vivo, however, contrary to patients with primary hyperparathyroidism who may have high levels of serum $1,25(OH)_2D_3$, patients with HHM have low serum levels of calcitriol. In this regard, it has been reported that certain solid neoplasms produce substances that may inhibit the activity of $1\alpha(OH)$ase and suppress the formation of $1,25(OH)_2D_3$. This appears to be the most tenable explanation for the low calcitriol levels in patients with HHM (139). The recently documented high circulating levels of FGF23 in malignancy provide a plausible explanation for the above discrepancy. FGF23 is a suppressant of $25(OH)D$-$1\alpha(OH)$ase and inhibits the production of $1,25(OH)_2D_3$ from its precursor $25(OH)D_3$.

Another interesting feature that distinguishes between patients with primary hyperparathyroidism and those with HHM are the findings of bone histomorphometry. Whereas in patients with primary hyperparathyroidism bone resorption is closely matched with bone formation, in patients with HHM bone resorption and formation are uncoupled; specifically in HHM, enhancement of bone resorption and suppression of bone formation occur. The cause of this discrepancy is not readily apparent. Additional studies are necessary to determine whether malignancies produce factors that suppress bone formation (140).

CaSR is expressed in many malignant cells. Pardoxically, activation of CaSR by calcium increases the expression and secretion of PTHrP in cases of humoral hypercalcemia of malignancy, increasing osteolysis. In some cases activation of CaSR promotes growth and spread of the tumor (141).

High PTHrP levels are present in 80% of patients with bone metastases from breast cancer who present with hypercalcemia, whereas PTHrP was present only in 12% of patients with breast cancer and metastases at sites other than bone. These findings are consistent with the notion that PTHrP may promote the development and growth of metastases in the bones by its potent osteolytic activity, which provides the environment for the proliferation of malignant cells (140).

Hypercalcemia is a recognized complication of lymphoma, including both Hodgkin and non-Hodgkin types. Serum levels of $1,25(OH)_2D_3$ are either elevated or inadequately suppressed by the hypercalcemia in many patients with lymphoma-associated hypercalcemia. The elevated $1,25(OH)_2D_3$ levels may play a role in the pathogenesis of hypercalcemia. In some cases, chemotherapy induced normalization of serum calcium and a concomitant fall in $1,25(OH)_2D_3$. Conversely, reappearance of hypercalcemia was associated with recurrent rise above normal of $1,25(OH)_2D_3$ levels. Human T-lymphotrophic virus-transformed lymphocytes are able to produce $1,25(OH)_2D_3$ from $25(OH)D_3$. Thus, there is a possibility that in some cases of lymphoma, the malignant cells may have a similar capacity to produce $1,25(OH)_2D_3$, which may contribute to the development of hypercalcemia. However, it is noteworthy that the levels of PTHrP were elevated and considered to be responsible for the rise in serum calcium in a number of patients with lymphoma-associated hypercalcemia. Obviously, both PTHrP and elevated $1,25(OH)_2D_3$ may act synergistically to cause hypercalcemia (139).

HYPERCALCEMIA OF MALIGNANCY: THE ROLE OF OSTEOCLAST-ACTIVATING CYTOKINES

Tumor cells in bone and tumor-associated macrophages release factors that are known as osteoclast-activating cytokines. These tumor-derived factors, implicated in the development of hypercalcemia of malignancy, are IL-1, IL-6, tumor necrosis factor(TNF)-α (cachectin), TNFβ, lymphotoxin, transforming growth factor-α (TGFα), and arachidonic acid metabolites. In addition, tumor cells may produce mediators (e.g., granulocyte macrophage colony-stimulating factor [M-CSF]) that induce immune cells to produce TNF and IL-1. Cytokines are produced and act locally as osteolytic factors. In most instances, the osteoclast-stimulating activity of the cytokines requires the presence of osteoblastic cells. Intravenous infusion of cytokines causes hypercalcemia in animals; however, these factors are believed to act locally in a paracrine fashion in clinical circumstances (140,142,143).

The role of osteoblastic stromal cell in the tumor-cell induced osteolysis is depicted in Figure 6.6 (144). Tumor cells act indirectly by adapting to the physiologic mechanisms that promote bone resorption. Tumor

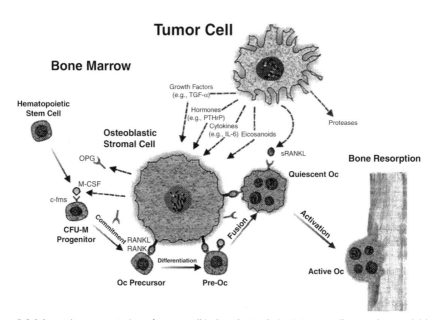

■ **Figure 6.6** Schematic representation of tumor-cell induced osteolysis. A tumor cell may release soluble mediators such as hormones (e.g, PTHrP, eicosanoids, cytokines (e.g., IL-6), or growth factors (e.g., TGFα) that act on an osteoblastic stromal cell. The stromal cell produces RANKL, which binds to its cognate receptor, RANK, expressed on osteoclastic (Oc) precursors. In the presence of M-CSF, which acts on its receptor, c-fms, RANKL can enhance the formation of active osteoclasts that carry out bone resorption. Tumor cells also have been occasionally reported to directly release sRANKL, a soluble form of RANKL. Additionally, proteases can be produced by tumor cells and facilitate their invasion of nonmineralized tissue. (From Goltzman D. Osteolysis and cancer. *J Clin Invest.* 2001;107:1219–1220, with permission.)

cells release hormones (PTHrP), growth factors (TGF$_2$), cytokines (IL-6), and eicosanoids (prostaglandins), which act on osteoblastic cells to enhance the production of osteoclast-activating factors. Most important of these is the cell membrane–associated protein termed "RANKL," a member of TNF family of cytokines. RANKL can then bind to its cognate receptor (RANK) residing on the cell surface membrane on osteoclast precursors and in the presence of M-CSF promote the differentiation and fusion of the preosteoclasts to form active multinucleated osteoclasts. Concomitantly, production of soluble decoy receptors for RANKL termed "oesteoprotegerin" [OPG] by osteoblastic cells inhibit osteoclastic osteolysis. Osteolytic bone matrix releases growth factors, including TGF-β, which accelerate tumor growth in the lysed area. Thus, a cycle is activated where tumor cells and bone matrix interact to promote metastatic expansion. A recent study demonstrated that prostatic tumor cells may produce a soluble RANKL (sRANKL) and thus directly, without the mediating role of osteoblastic cells accelerate the osteoclastogenesis and osteolysis. In the same study, the administration of the decoy receptor for RANK, OPG, prevented the establishment of osseous tumors. These observations bear on possible new therapeutic avenues in preventing spread of prostatic tumor (144).

Hypercalcemia occurs in approximately one-third of patients with myeloma. Osteolytic bone lesions are the most common skeletal radiographic findings. The bone destruction in myeloma is mediated by osteoclasts that accumulate adjacent to the collections of myeloma cells. This association of myeloma cells with osteoclasts in the past was believed to be related to osteoclast-activating effect of cytokines that are locally secreted by the malignant cells. Myeloma cells produce in vitro several osteoclast-activating factors, including TGF-β, IL-1, and IL-6. The increase in bone resorption in most cases is associated with a suppressed osteoblastic bone-forming activity. This explains the depressed skeletal uptake of bone-seeking radiolabeled elements in myeloma, resulting in negative bone scans in the vast majority of the affected patients. Myeloma cells exhibit a unique capability to grow rapidly in the bone. Myeloma cells secrete osteoclast-mobilizing and stimulating cytokines, whereas osteoclasts secrete IL-6, which is a major growth factor of the myeloma cells. This relationship between myeloma cells and osteoclasts explains the rapid destruction of bone in this malignancy (140–143,145,146).

Additional information that accumulated in last years has shed new light on the molecular mechanisms activated by multiple myeloma cells on bone metabolism. Lytic bone destruction is the hallmark of myeloma. The osteolytic bone disease is mediated by osteoclasts. Previous research on the mechanism on myeloma addressed primarily the osteoclasts' role in uncoupling bone remodeling tilting the balance towards resorption. Surprisingly the factor that predisposes certain patients with myeloma to develop osteolytic lesions does not directly act on osteoclasts but rather on osteoblasts. Wnt (wingless/int) gene and its product protein are important factors in bone metabolism. The Wnt signaling pathway is important for the growth, differentiation and maturation of osteoblasts. Interestingly, inactivating mutation of the gene for Wnt coreceptor, the low-density receptor-related protein 5(LRP5), causes an autosomal recessive disorder the osteoporosis–pseudoglioma syndrome with osteopenia and diminished osteoblast proliferation.

Wnt-signaling antagonist Dickkopf 1 (DKK1) levels were found to be elevated in bone marrow plasma cells and peripheral blood from patients with myeloma who have osteolytic lesions. Only myeloma cells obtained from patients who had lytic lesions had detectable DKK1. It was not detected in normal cells, or those in myeloma patients without lytic lesions. It has been proposed that DKK1 could block proliferation and differentiation of osteoblasts by blocking the canonical Wnt signaling. The mechanism by which DKK1 can cause bone lesions in myeloma patients may involve two steps. WNT promotes early proliferation of immature osteoblasts followed by the differentiation into osteoblasts. DKK1 abrogates bone morphometric protein-2 (BMP-2) mediated osteoblast differentiation into mature osteoblasts that build bone. Immature osteoblasts (osteoblast precursors) are rich sources of RANK ligand that plays a dominant role in activation and survival of osteoclast. This leads to bone lytic lesions. On the other hand, reduced number and viability of mature functional osteoblasts downregulates bone formation and prevents filling the lytic lesions with new bone. This explains why the uptake of tracers with affinity to bone formation is absent in myeloma patients (147).

VITAMIN D INTOXICATION AND HYPERCALCEMIA

All patients receiving vitamin D, other than in small doses, for the treatment of hypoparathyroidism may develop hypercalcemia, with the attendant risk of renal failure. The appearance of hypercalcemia in hypoparathyroid patients receiving pharmacologic doses of either ergocalciferol (vitamin D$_2$) or DHT$_3$ is almost unpredictable, because the margin between normocalcemic and hypercalcemic doses of the vitamin is very narrow. Some episodes of hypercalcemia may pass unnoticed and yet may be the underlying cause of reduced renal function in these patients. The administration of thiazide diuretics also may be an aggravating factor in this situation, partly because it reduces the urinary excretion of calcium. The hypercalcemia associated with vitamin D intoxication may be present from 1 to 6 weeks after discontinuation of the treatment, and the normocalcemia may persist for an additional 4 months without any treatment. The toxic effect of vitamin D excess is associated with a high level of circulating $25(OH)D_3$, which is continuously produced by the liver from the adipose tissue stores of vitamin D. The serum level of $1,25(OH)_2D_3$ generally is not elevated and even may be reduced (148). The hypercalcemia associated with $1,25(OH)_2D_3$ administration, however, is much more short-lived (3 to 7 days).

Various factors may alter the response to vitamin D. The inhibitory effect of estrogens on bone resorption may be absent after menopause, which allows more calcium to be released from the bone for any given dose of vitamin D. The administration of corticosteroids may reduce the effect of vitamin D; in fact, corticosteroids may be used to treat vitamin D intoxication. The most important precaution in preventing the complications of vitamin D intoxication is to measure serum calcium concentrations frequently in these patients. Likewise, the presence of excessive hypercalciuria, even in the absence of hypercalcemia, is a risk factor for nephrocalcinosis and renal failure. Thus, monitoring of urinary calcium excretion in these circumstances is recommended as well.

VITAMIN A INTOXICATION AND HYPERCALCEMIA

Hypercalcemia associated with vitamin A intoxication has been much discussed (149–150). This condition has been associated with excessive intake of vitamin A, which is readily available for sale in various pharmaceutic preparations (150). Isotretinoin, a derivative of vitamin A that is effective in the treatment of severe nodulocystic acne, has been reported as a cause of hypercalcemia (151,152). The main symptom of vitamin A intoxication is painful swelling over the extremities. Prolonged hypercalcemia in this condition also has been associated with nephrocalcinosis and impairment of renal function (149). In experimental animals, excessive amounts of vitamin A cause fractures, increased number of osteoclasts, and calcification of soft tissues. In human subjects, periosteal bone deposition constitutes the typical radiographic feature (153).

SARCOIDOSIS AND HYPERCALCEMIA

Hypercalcemia in patients with sarcoidosis is associated with increased intestinal absorption of calcium and increased calcium release from the bone; it is found in about 17% of all patients with sarcoidosis (154). It is more frequent in males than females (125). In a small proportion of patients, very high serum calcium concentration leads to metastatic calcifications and eventual death owing to uremia (155). The hypercalcemia may disappear with the appearance of uremia (156).

Seasonal incidence of hypercalcemia in sarcoidosis is directly related to the amount of sunlight exposure (156). Plasma levels of $1,25(OH)_2D_3$ have been found to be increased in patients with sarcoidosis and hypercalcemia, a finding that accounts for the abnormal calcium metabolism in this disease (157). In most of the patients, hypercalcemia may be corrected with the administration of glucocorticoids, which restores to normal both the elevated calcium and $1,25(OH)_2D_3$ concentrations in the serum (158,159). Serum immunoreactive PTH has been found to be low in patients with sarcoidosis, regardless of the presence or absence of hypercalcemia.

In vitro studies demonstrated production of $1,25(OH)D_3$ by primary cultures of pulmonary alveolar macrophages harvested from patients with active sarcoidosis (160). Thus, the pathogenesis of hypercalcemia in sarcoidosis is extrarenal production of $1,25(OH)_2D_3$ by the macrophage, which is a major constituent of the sarcoid granuloma. A similar mechanism appears to be responsible for the hypercalcemia associated with other granulomatous diseases. Hypercalcemia has been reported in tuberculosis, leprosy, foreign body-induced granuloma, silicone-induced granuloma, disseminated candidiasis and coccidioidomycosis, histoplasmosis, berylliosis, granulomatous lipoid pneumonia, and eosinophilic granuloma (156–159). Whereas $1,25(OH)_2D$ synthesis in renal mitochondria by $25(OH)D\text{-}1\alpha(OH)$ase from $25(OH)D$ is a regulated process, extrarenal synthesis is not well regulated. Recent research results provide evidence that activation of toll-like receptors (TLRs) by microbial LPS results in upregulation of $25(OH)D\text{-}1\alpha(OH)$ase in macrophages. The local production of $1,25(OH)_2D_3$ induces the expression of an antimicrobial peptide cathedicidin, which is considered to be a key factor in the innate immune response. When TLR is activated by infective agent such as mycobacterium tuberculosis it produces the antimicrobial factor. This observation can be used to explain the possible beneficial effect of vitamin D induced by exposure to sunlight at high altitudes in patients with tuberculosis (43).

HYPERTHYROIDISM, HYPOTHYROIDISM, AND HYPERCALCEMIA

The incidence of hypercalcemia in patients with hyperthyroidism varies from 10% to 22% in different reports (161). This hypercalcemia may be reversed by antithyroid therapy. Because the association of hyperthyroidism and hyperparathyroidism has been reported to be common, the therapeutic response of the hypercalcemia to the antithyroid therapy may be of some diagnostic significance (161). The effect of thyroid hormone on calcium metabolism primarily consists of increased bone turnover, increased urinary calcium excretion, and decreased intestinal absorption of calcium, with a resultant negative calcium balance (162). Thus, the action of thyroid hormone on bone is primarily responsible for the hypercalcemia. Thyroid hormone enhances the ability of PTH to increase bone reabsorption and directly enhances bone resorption in vivo in the absence of PTH (163). Serum phosphate may be elevated in hyperthyroidism, possibly because of suppression of parathyroid activity by the hypercalcemia and subsequent enhanced tubular reabsorption of phosphate.

Serum calcium and phosphate levels are normal and alkaline phosphatase is low in the vast majority of patients with hypothyroidism; however, some patients may manifest hypercalcemia. Calcium balance in patients with hypothyroidism tends to be positive as a result of increased intestinal absorption and reduced urinary excretion. Both changes predispose to the development of hypercalcemia. The bone turnover in hypothyroid patients is reduced.

ADRENAL INSUFFICIENCY AND HYPERCALCEMIA

Hypercalcemia is a common abnormality in adrenal insufficiency (164,165). The mechanism of hypercalcemia in this clinical setting is not well understood. One study indicates that the increase in serum calcium concentration is due to an increase in the protein-bound fraction of serum calcium that results from accompanying volume depletion. The volume depletion also may cause an increase in the renal tubular reabsorption of calcium, and vitamin D's enhancement of calcium absorption from the intestine may be greater in the absence of glucocorticoid hormone.

IDIOPATHIC INFANTILE HYPERCALCEMIA

Idiopathic infantile hypercalcemia encompasses a group of disorders characterized by hypercalcemia during infancy, mostly of transient nature. It can be divided into benign and severe types according to the gravity of the clinical manifestation. The benign type is associated with minimal symptomatology and has an excellent prognosis. The severe form is associated with serious somatic sequelae including mental deficiency, "elfin" face with depressed nasal bridge, epicanthal folds, supravalvular aortic stenosis, bladder diverticula, degenerative renal disease, occasionally pulmonic stenosis, ventricular septal defects, and dental abnormalities. These somatic distortions, known as Williams syndrome, was believed to reflect developmental defects resulting from hypercalcemia, probably already present in the fetal stage. The hypercalcemia is of limited duration; however, the somatic abnormalities are permanent. Thus, many patients suffering from Williams syndrome who present with the clinical syndrome fail to show abnormalities in calcium metabolism. The primary genetic abnormality is deletion of one allele of elastin gene. Hemizygosity for this gene was detected in 75% of patients. This defect is probably responsible for the vascular, valvular, and developmental defects.

Idiopathic infantile hypercalcemia has been attributed to hypersensitivity to vitamin D. In support of this possibility is the finding that hypercalcemia in this syndrome may occur with small doses of vitamin D, which are only two to three times larger than the physiologic dose (166). The high incidence of this syndrome in a group of infants in England who were drinking milk fortified with excessive amounts of vitamin D, and its disappearance when vitamin D was eliminated from the diet, supported the possibility that the syndrome was owing to hypersensitivity to vitamin D (167,168).

However, there is no unifying pathogenesis underlying the abnormal calcium metabolism in idiopathic infantile hypercalcemia. Increased serum levels of $1,25(OH)_2D_3$ have been considered to be the mechanism of hypercalcemia by some investigators (166,167). Others have failed to show that abnormality even in the presence of hypercalcemia. Abnormalities in the regulation of calcitonin secretion with reduced stimulation by hypercalcemia were advanced as the possible mechanism by others.

Deletion of approximately 25 to 30 genes spanning about 1.5 megabases in the q11.23 region on chromosome 7 has been identified in some patients with this syndrome. The attention has been recently focused on deletion of so-called Williams syndrome transcription factor (WSTF). The role of WSTF gene deletion in the alleged hypersensitivity to vitamin D is unknown.

It has been proposed that human multiprotein complex (WINAC) that mediates recruitment of unligated VDR to target sites in promoters acts via the WSTF (169,170). Recently evidence has been advanced that WSTF has an intrinsic tyrosine kinase activity that is involved in chromatin remodeling in response to DNA damage. It is possible that the ATP-dependent chromatin complex that incorporates the WSTF potentiates ligand-induced VDR action in both gene transactivation and repression. In the latter case WSTF gene deletion would remove the repression and lead to enhanced response to vitamin D-VDR complex. All above hypotheses are conjectural at this time (171).

Hypercalcemia with fat necrosis is a peculiar variant of the disease. In this syndrome affecting infants, only hypercalcemia occurs, with areas of necrosis of subcutaneous fat tissue (167). In some cases, high levels of $1,25(OH)_2D_3$ were reported. Some investigators maintain that hypercalcemia is not a primary but rather a secondary phenomenon. In the latter instance, it has been proposed that the rise in $1,25(OH)_2D_3$ leading to hypercalcemia is secondary to the granulomatous inflammation of the fat necrosis. Irrespective of the mechanism, idiopathic infantile hypercalcemia is treated by dietary restriction of calcium and vitamin D.

IMMOBILIZATION AND HYPERCALCEMIA

Immobilization may be associated with excessive loss of bone minerals, hypercalcemia, and rapidly developing osteoporosis. The lack of postural mechanical stimuli to the skeleton disturbs the balance between bone formation and reabsorption, thus leading to loss of bone mass and its minerals. Usually, the amount of calcium released from the bone is excreted in the urine and does not increase the serum calcium concentration (172). However, in states of rapid bone turnover, which are present in normal children and adolescents and in patients with bone abnormalities such as Paget disease, immobilization may result in overt hypercalcemia.

HYPOPHOSPHATASIA

Hypophosphatasia is a syndrome characterized by low serum alkaline phosphatase, high serum levels of pyrophosphate, and skeletal abnormalities resembling osteomalacia (173). The disorder may be associated with hypercalcemia, especially in infants.

MILK–ALKALI SYNDROME

Milk–alkali syndrome ranks third, after primary hyperparathyroidism and malignancy as the most common cause of hypercalcemia. It occurs in patients who ingest large amounts of milk and alkali as a therapy to relieve the symptoms of peptic ulcers. Likewise the recommended consumption of calcium carbonate for prevention and treatment of osteoporosis has increased the frequency of this iatrogenic hypercalcemia. The syndrome is characterized by hypercalcemia, hyperphosphatemia, alkalosis, metastatic calcifications, and progressive renal failure. It has been shown that these abnormalities may be reversed by discontinuation of the therapy. Large doses of calcium carbonate seem to be the major factor in the development of this syndrome, because the use of antacids other than calcium carbonate does not lead to hypercalcemia (174). Therefore, it appears that the hypercalcemia of milk–alkali syndrome results from high oral loads of calcium carbonate and causes renal retention of phosphate by suppressing PTH secretion. The resulting serum calcium-phosphorus product leads to metastatic calcification and impairment of renal function. The increased activation by high serum calcium of CaSR at the basolateral surface of loop of Henle cells enhances natriuresis and induces volume depletion that augments proximal reabsorption of calcium. The attendant alkalosis activates the pH sensitive calcium channel, TRPV5, in the distal nephron, thereby contributing to calcium retention and hypercalcemia.

Increased oral intake of calcium carbonate also has been reported to induce hypercalcemia in uremic patients. Similarly, the use of calcium-containing exchange resins for the treatment of hyperkalemia may cause hypercalcemia because of the release of calcium from the resin in the intestinal lumen (175).

Hypercalcemia has been described in patients recovering from acute renal failure. The etiology is not well understood, but in some patients it may result from the combination of secondary hyperparathyroidism and released calcium from traumatized, necrotic muscle (176,177) and to high calcitriol levels produced by the traumatized muscles.

THIAZIDE DIURETICS AND HYPERCALCEMIA

Chronic administration of thiazide diuretics may lead to hypercalcemia in patients treated with large doses of vitamin D (hypoparathyroid patients and patients with osteoporosis) and in patients with hyperparathyroidism. The mechanism of action may involve: (a) reduced urinary excretion of calcium due to a direct tubular effect, or ECF depletion with secondary increase in tubular reabsorption of sodium and calcium, or both; and (b) increased bone responsiveness to the resorptive actions of vitamin D and PTH (177,178). Thiazide-induced inhibition of apical entry of sodium lowers cytosolic sodium concentration. The latter leads to a steeper gradient between intracellular and peritubular sodium concentrations. Increased sodium gradient would favor pumping more calcium out of the cell via NCX, enhancing calcium reabsorption. It has been demonstrated that thiazides may acutely enhance the hypercalcemic skeletal response to PTH in the absence of changes in ECF volume. Recent studies suggest that primary hyperparathyroidism is common in patients who develop hypercalcemia while taking thiazide diuretics. Therefore, it is likely that thiazides "uncover" mild primary hyperparathyroidism in many patients. The above notion is supported by previous studies that demonstrated that the calcemic effect of thiazides is PTH-dependent (179). A recent study demonstrated expression of thiazide-sensitive cotransporters in osteoblasts. In vitro thiazides stimulate osteoblast differentiation and bone formation (169).

LITHIUM AND THEOPHYLLINE

Patients treated chronically with lithium may develop hypercalcemia with elevated PTH levels. In this regard, primary hyperparathyroidism and hypothyroidism have been reported in patients treated with lithium. Theophylline toxicity also may be associated with hypercalcemia, probably because of stimulation of β-receptors in the bone.

TREATMENT OF HYPERCALCEMIA

Lowering of serum calcium concentration can be produced by: (a) inhibiting calcium release from the bone, or increasing its deposition in the bone and other tissues, or both; (b) increasing removal of calcium from the ECF or inhibiting its absorption in the bowel; and (c) decreasing the ionized fraction by complex formation with chelating substances.

Hypercalcemia augments urinary losses of sodium and water, resulting in the contraction of extracellular volume and reduced GFR. The latter leads to diminished urinary excretion of calcium and further aggravation of hypercalcemia. Therefore, the first therapeutic goal is to restore the extracellular volume to normal by intravenous administration of normal saline. This usually requires 3 to 4 L of saline. This therapeutic action per se lowers the serum calcium concentration, partly by the dilutional effect and partly by increased urinary excretion of calcium. There is a risk of extracellular volume overload during a rapid intravenous administration of saline, which is particularly hazardous in elderly patients. Therefore, monitoring of central venous pressure in this situation may be very helpful. Likewise, the addition of loop diuretics as an adjunct therapy not only may minimize the risk of fluid overload but also may substantially increase the urinary excretion of calcium. The effect of loop diuretics as calciuretic agents requires prompt replacement of urinary losses of sodium and water. The use of loop diuretics may be particularly beneficial in patients who develop hypercalcemia as a result of excessive secretion and high serum levels of PTH, PTHrP, or both. Hormone-induced, excessive tubular reabsorption of calcium plays a major role in the development and maintenance of hypercalcemia in these circumstances.

Bisphosphonates

Bisphosphonates (formerly diphosphonates) represent a group of drugs with a high therapeutic potential for the treatment of hypercalcemia in general and that associated with malignancy in particular. Bisphosphonates are related to an endogenous product of bone metabolism, pyrophosphate. The P–O–P bonds of pyrophosphate are cleaved by phosphatase in the process of bone mineralization and osteoclastic bone resorption. In the bisphosphonates, carbon replaces the oxygen moiety, generating a bond P–C–P, which is resistant to hydrolysis by phosphatase. Bisphosphonates have a great affinity for bone and bind tightly to calcified bone matrix, impairing both the mineralization and resorption of bone. In addition, they interfere with the function of osteoclasts. They appear to have several direct effects on the osteoclast function, including prevention of osteoclast attachment to bone matrix and prevention of osteoclast differentiation and recruitment. Bisphosphonates also inhibit the motility of isolated osteoclasts. Thus, they are very potent inhibitors of bone resorption. The first bisphosphonate, ethane-hydroxybisphosphonate (etidronate; Didronel) is now available for clinical use, but its potency as an antihypercalcemic agent is limited, at least when given orally. Probably, this is because its effect to reduce bone resorption is offset by its effect to inhibit bone mineralization. Reduction of serum calcium concentration has been achieved more successfully with the second generation of bisphosphonates, including dichloromethylene bisphosphonate (clodronate) and amino-hydroxypropylidene bisphosphonate (pamidronate; ADP), which causes a reduction in bone resorption with a dose that has a negligible effect on bone mineralization. Pamidronate and etidronate currently are approved for treatment of hypercalcemia of malignancy in the United States. In clinical trials, pamidronate and clodronate have been demonstrated to inhibit hypercalcemia, bone pain, and pathologic fractures in patients with malignancy-associated hypercalcemia. Pamidronate is most effective when given intravenously; a single infusion of 30 mg achieved normocalcemia in 90% of patients in one study. When compared, the effect of 30 mg of pamidronate is equal to 600 mg of clodronate and 1,500 mg of etidronate in controlling hypercalcemia. The third generation of bisphosphonates, including alendronate, risedronate, and tiludronate, in preliminary studies is 500 times more efficient in inhibiting bone resorption than clodronate. Zoledronic acid is a new generation of nitrogen-containing bisphosphonate that in clinical studies was superior to pamidronate. This agent has been approved for clinical use.

The molecular mechanisms underlying the pharmacological anti-osteoclast action differs between the two major classes of bisphosphonate: (1) Non-nitrogen-containing bisphosphonates (etidronate and clodronate) and (2) The more potent, nitrogen-containing bisphosphonates (pamidronate, alendronate, ibandronate, risedronate, and zolendronate). The first class bisphosphonates bind with nonhydrolyzable analogs of ATP that accumulate in osteoclasts and block mitochondrial energy production, leading to osteoclast apoptosis. By contrast the nitrogen-containing class of bisphsphonates inhibit farenesyl pyrophosphate (FPP) synthase, thereby blocking prenylation of small GTPase proteins that are required for normal function and survival osteoclasts.

Glucocorticoids

Glucocorticoids are effective in lowering serum calcium in states of vitamin D intoxication, sarcoidosis, and malignancy. The exact mode of their action is not well understood, but the possible mechanisms are suppression of bone resorption and decreased intestinal absorption. It has been pointed out that glucocorticoids are more effective in hypercalcemia associated with lymphoma, leukemia, and multiple myeloma than with other neoplasms. This effect of glucocorticoids might be related to a tumor lytic effect, interference with the production of osteoclast-activating cytokines, or both. The average effective dose is 3 to 4 mg/kg/day of hydrocortisone given intravenously or orally. The fall in serum calcium concentration occurs 1 to 2 days after starting the therapy.

Calcitonin

Calcitonin lowers serum calcium concentration by inhibiting bone resorption and by increasing urinary calcium excretion. The administration of calcitonin is associated with negligible toxicity; however, its therapeutic action has a limited duration because of the osteoclast escape phenomenon, which is apparent several days after starting therapy. Addition of glucocorticoids may be helpful to maintain efficacy.

Mithramycin (Plicamycin)

Mithramycin is a cytotoxic substance derived from an actinomycete of the genus *Streptomyces* and is used mainly in the treatment of testicular tumors. Mithramycin lowers serum calcium concentration by suppressing bone resorption. The dose, which is lower than the antitumor dose and has fewer side effects, is 25 μg/kg given intravenously. The drug is available commercially as Mithracin. The effect starts 24 to 48 hours after injection and lasts several days. Side effects are suppression of bone marrow activity and hepatocellular and renal toxicity, which usually occur with repeated doses.

Phosphate

Oral and intravenous salts of phosphorus lower serum calcium concentration and reduce urinary excretion of calcium. This effect has been variously attributed to: (a) deposition of mineral in the bone; (b) increased deposition of calcium in soft tissues; and (c) suppression of bone resorption. The major untoward side effects of this therapy are extraskeletal calcifications, including nephrocalcinosis with resulting renal failure. Thus, the use of phosphates to treat hypercalcemia should be discouraged in patients with high serum phosphates and renal insufficiency. Phosphates may be given intravenously at a dose of 20 to 30 mg of elemental phosphorus per kilogram of body weight over 12 to 16 hours. Serum calcium concentration should be determined at close intervals. The commercially available preparation for intravenous use is InPhos; 40 mL of the solution contains 1,000 mg of phosphorus, 65 mEq of sodium, and 8 mEq of potassium.

Other Therapies

Gallium nitrate has been approved by the Food and Drug Administration for therapy of hypercalcemia. It inhibits bone resorption by reducing the solubility of hydroxyapatite crystals. Nephrotoxicity is a major side effect of gallium nitrate. The use of a somatostatin congener (lanreotide) has been reported to successfully inhibit hypercalcemia in a patient with a PTHrP-secreting pancreatic neoplasm. The calcium-lowering effect was associated with suppression of the serum levels of PTHrP (179,180). The hypercalcemia associated with thyrotoxicosis and theophylline toxicity has been successfully treated with intravenous propranolol.

Intestinal absorption of calcium may be reduced by dietary restrictions and binding of calcium in the bowel with cellulose phosphate and sodium phytate to form nonabsorbable complexes. Calcium also may be removed directly from the ECF with hemodialysis or peritoneal dialysis by employing calcium-free dialysate solution. Reduction of serum-ionized calcium may be accomplished with intravenous Na-EDTA, which is a chelating agent. The complexed calcium then is excreted in the urine. The main disadvantage of this therapy is the nephrotoxicity of EDTA.

Metabolic Bone Diseases

RICKETS AND OSTEOMALACIA

Rickets and osteomalacia are metabolic disorders of the bone in which the mineralization process of the epiphyseal cartilage and organic bone matrix is impaired. This abnormality results in a decreased amount of mineralized bone (Fig. 6.7) and an increased amount of osteoid (or cartilage), which cause decreased mechanical strength of the bones. Therefore, the bones become soft, bend easily, and are liable to deformities and pseudofractures (Fig. 6.8). It should be mentioned that such an increase in the width of osteoid seams may be seen in conditions other than osteomalacia. The bone formation is rapid in Paget disease, and there may be a lag between the rate of apposition of bone matrix and its mineralization. Therefore, this sequence leads to an increased width of osteoid seams. Histologically, however, the presence of a calcification front in bones from patients with Paget disease and its absence in osteomalacia allow the distinction between these diseases. The calcification front may be demonstrated by specific histochemical staining techniques or the administration of a tetracycline, which is incorporated specifically in the calcification front. The calcification front reappears during the healing of osteomalacia.

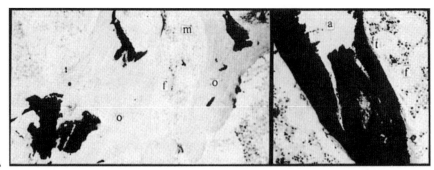

■ **Figure 6.7 A.** Osteomalacia. Bone trabeculae are calcified *(black stain)* only in the center, with a wide rim of osteoid tissue. **B.** Normal bone. All bone trabeculae are calcified *(black stain)*. *a*, artifact; *f*, fat; *m*, marrow; *o*, osteoid; *t*, trabeculae.

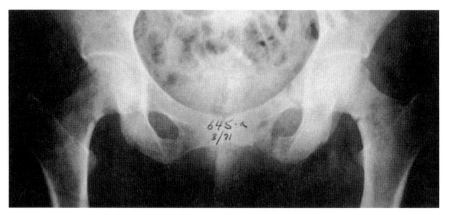

■ **Figure 6.8** Roentgenographic appearance of osteomalacia. The radiolucent lines on the necks of both femurs are pseudofractures.

The major symptoms of osteomalacia are diffuse bone and muscle pains, which cause disability and increasing needs for analgesic medication. The etiologies of osteomalacia (Table 6.5) can be divided into two principal subgroups. The first group, which is the most common, is associated with abnormally low serum concentrations of phosphorus and calcium. In the second group, which is less common, the defect in mineralization is related in some way to abnormalities in the organic matrix and is not associated with a low serum calcium–phosphorus product.

Vitamin D deficiency causes osteomalacia primarily by decreasing the absorption of calcium and phosphorus from the intestine and thereby decreasing the serum concentrations of calcium and phosphorus. As mentioned, osteomalacia caused by vitamin D deficiency may be healed with the intravenous administration of calcium and phosphorus even without repletion of vitamin D (54). It should be emphasized, however, that this finding does not exclude the possibility that vitamin D plays a direct role in the physiologic process of bone accretion. As discussed, vitamin D deficiency may result from poor intake, decreased intestinal absorption, or lack of exposure to ultraviolet light.

Vitamin D-dependent rickets type I (VDDR-I), also designated as pseudo–vitamin D deficiency rickets, is inherited as an autosomal recessive disorder in which 25(OH)D-1α(OH)ase in proximal tubules is deficient due to mutation in its encoding gene. It is manifested by early hypocalcemia, hypophosphatemia, severe secondary hyperparathyroidism, and severe rickets. The serum concentrations of 1,25(OH)$_2$D$_3$ are undetectable or very low, whereas 25(OH)D levels are normal or slightly elevated. The clinical abnormality can be reversed completely by the administration of pharmacologic doses of vitamin D or physiologic doses of 1,25(OH)$_2$D$_3$. Linkage analysis in families with VDDR-I mapped the disease locus to chromosome

TABLE 6.5 CAUSES OF RICKETS AND OSTEOMALACIA

Group I: Low serum calcium–phosphorus product

Vitamin D deficiency

Vitamin D–dependent rickets, type I (1α-hydroxylase deficiency)

Vitamin D–dependent rickets, type II (vitamin D resistance)

Vitamin D–dependent rickets type III

Hypophosphatemic rickets with elevated FGF23:

X-linked hypophosphatemic rickets

Tumor-induced osteomalacia

Autosomal-dominant hypophosphatemic rickets

Autosomal recessive hypophosphatemic rickets

Osteoglophonic dysplasia

McCune–Albright syndrome (polyostotic fibrous dysplasia)

Hypophosphatemic rickets due to abnormal tubular transport

Hereditary hypophosphatemic rickets with hypercalciuria

Lowe oculocerebrorenal syndrome

X-linked recessive hypophosphatemic rickets (Dent disease)

Fanconi syndrome

Other causes of rickets and osteomalacia

Excessive intake of phosphate-binding antacids

Hypophosphatemic norachitic bone disease

Renal tubular acidosis

Group II: Normal or high serum calcium–phosphorus product

Renal (uremic) osteomalacia

Hypophosphatasia

Bisphosphphonates

12q13-14. The synthesis of $1,25(OH)_2D_3$ from its precursor $25(OH)D_3$ is catalyzed by 25(OH)D-$1\alpha(OH)ase(1\alpha[OH]ase)$, a mitochondrial P-450 enzyme in the proximal tubular cells. The cloning of $1\alpha(OH)ase$ was achieved very late because of its very low gene expression and was reported only in 1997, many years after the cloning of 24(OH)ase that catalyzes by an alternative pathway for the metabolism of $25(OH)D_3$ to $24,25(OH)_2D_3$. $1\alpha(OH)ase$ shares high homology with the hepatic vitamin D hydroxylase. Because $1,25(OH)_2D_3$ may alter the hepatic metabolism of $25(OH)D_3$ and the $1,25(OH)_2D_3$-receptor (VDR) is present in the liver, the possibility that $1,25(OH)_2D_3$ acts by binding to its hepatic receptor, to reduce the activity of hepatic vitamin D-25(OH)ase is plausible (44).

The expression of the renal $1\alpha(OH)ase$ has been shown to be inhibited by its product $1,25(OH)_2D_3$ and mice lacking $1,25(OH)_2D_3$-receptor (VDR) develop abnormally high serum levels of $1,25(OH)_2D_3$, suggesting that the expression of $1\alpha(OH)ase$ is regulated by $1,25(OH)_2D_3$ through liganded VDR.

The availability of cDNA and the gene structure that encodes the human $1\alpha(OH)ase$, now makes it possible to analyze for inactivating mutations of $1\alpha(OH)ase$ in patients with VDDR-I. Various mutations were identified in the 12q13–14 locus in patients with VDDR-I, suggesting that there is more than one founder for the $1\alpha(OH)ase$ mutations in these patients (181).

Hypocalcemia and rickets refractory to $1,25(OH)_2D_3$ were described as VDDR-II, also known as hereditary $1,25(OH)_2D_3$-resistant rickets. This familial disorder is inherited by autosomal recessive transmission and is characterized by rickets, impaired intestinal absorption of calcium, hypocalcemia, and alopecia, which may reflect a defect in the physiologic action of $1,25(OH)_2D_3$ in the skin. In contrast to VDDR-I, in type II serum $1,25(OH)_2D_3$ is elevated and the patients either respond to pharmacologic doses of $1,25(OH)_2D_3$ or do not respond at all. In some patients with this disorder, abnormal nuclear uptake, abnormal cytosol receptor binding of $1,25-(OH)_2D_3$, or both are present. These findings suggest that the mechanism of the end-organ resistance is a defect in the receptor. However, this abnormality was not present in other patients, indicating a more distal postreceptor abnormality. In this regard, in one patient with type II vitamin D–dependent rickets with normal receptor function (receptor-positive resistance), failure of $1,25(OH)_2D_3$ to stimulate the enzyme $25(OH)_2D_3$-24(OH)ase was demonstrated (182). In normal people, $1,25(OH)_2D_3$ was shown to stimulate the formation of $24,25(OH)_2D_3$. The event may represent a step in the physiologic action of $1,25(OH)_2D_3$ that is lacking in some patients with type II vitamin D–dependent rickets (182–184). Mutations of VDR genes have been identified in some families with this abnormality. In one family, a nonsense mutation coding for a premature stop codon in exon 7 of the gene-encoding VDR was identified. In other families, the genetic abnormality consisted of a point mutation within the steroid binding domain of the VDR gene (185).

The skeletal lesions in VDR null mutant mice were largely reversed by normalizing ambient calcium and phosphate. This suggested that the skeletal abnormalities resulting from VDR ablation are caused by impaired intestinal absorption of calcium and phosphate. Thus, the absence of vitamin D action does not affect skeletal metabolism so long as mineral homeostasis is restored to normal.

A new type of vitamin resistance has been reported and termed "VDDR type III." The phenotype is identical to VDDR–II, but the resistance to vitamin D results from overexpression of a heterogenous ribonucleoprotein that competes with normally functioning VDR-retinoid X (RXR) receptor dimer for binding to the vitamin D response element of the target gene (186,187).

Hypophosphatemia caused by excessive external losses of phosphorus may cause osteomalacia even in the presence of normal serum calcium concentration. Hereditary and acquired renal losses of phosphorus can be divided into 3 general groups: (1) hypophosphatemia due to excessive phosphaturic action of phosphatonins, mainly due to circulating FGF23, (2) hypophosphatemia due to a defect in NaPi cotransporters, and (3) hypophosphatemia due to enhanced proximal tubular response to PTH.

(1) Phosphatonins include, fibroblast growth factor-23 (FGF23), secreted frizzled-related protein 4 (sFRP4), matrix extracellular phopsphoglycoprotein (MEPE), and, fibroblast growth factor 7 (FGF7).

The presence of a putative circulating phosphaturic substance other than PTH in patients with advanced chronic kidney disease was foreseen 1969. This prediction was based on studies in chronic kidney disease (CKD) patients who underwent total parathyroidectomy for secondary hyperparathyroidism. Fractional excretion of phosphorus that was very elevated before surgery failed to decrease after total removal of parathyroid glands. It was proposed that unidentified circulating factor(s) other than PTH that were present in these patients acted as inhibitors of tubular reabsorption of phosphorus in the absence of PTH (188). Twelve years later, in 1981, a patient was admitted to neurology department with muscular paralysis and generalized bone pains and was found to have serum phosphate of 1.2 mg/dL with high urinary phosphorus, normal serum calcium, and an upper normal concentration of PTH. Bone biopsy showed osteomalacia. A msenchymal giant-cell tumor was resected from his left hip area. The patient recovered after surgery. An extract from the homogenate of the tumor that was infused into parathyroidectomized rats induced a profound phosphaturia. Similar infusion from an unrelated tumor that served as a control did not induce phophaturia. The phosphaturic response was not associated with an increase in urinary cAMP, thus excluding PTH as the phosphaturic factor (189–193).

Phosphaturic humoral factor(s) causing tumor-induced osteomalacia (TIO), called phosphatonins, were extensively studied by the Mayo Clinic group (194,195). It was demonstrated that FGF23 is a causative factor of tumor-induced osteomalacia. This factor was cloned from a tumor tissue following isolation of cDNA clones that were abundantly expressed only in the tumor. Administration of recombinant FGF23 decreased serum phosphate in mice within 12 h. Chinese hamster ovary cells stably expressing FGF23 were subcutaneously implanted into nude mice and hypophosphatemia with increased renal clearance of phosphate was observed.

Conditioned media from such tumors inhibited sodium-dependent phosphate transport in opossum kidney cells. Interestingly, phenotype of TIO is shared by patients with inherited disorders of hypophosphatemic rickets, including autosomal dominant hypophosphatemic rickets (ADHR), X-linked hypophosphatemic rickets (XLH), autosomal recessive hypophosphatemic rickets (ARHR). Sera of all above patient groups tested positive for phosphatonin activity (196).

Further research work identified distinct members of the phosphatonin group from TIO patients, including FGF23, sFRP4, FGF7, and MEPE. FGF23 that was cloned in 2001 attracted most attention and was well characterized by lab animal experiments. Transgenic mice that overexpress FGF23 fully reproduce the abnormalities of patients with TIO and exhibit an important functional feature of FGF23 that is suppression of 25(OH)D-1α(OH)ase with consequent low levels of 1,25(OH)$_2$D$_3$ and hyperparathyroidism. In this regard it has been proposed that FGF-23 may serve as a counterregulatory hormone to 1,25(OH)$_2$D$_3$ to maintain phosphate balance, in face of the effect of 1,25(OH)$_2$D$_3$ to increase phosphate load by increasing intestinal absorption. FGF23 acts primarily as a phosphaturic hormone by inhibiting NaPi cotransporters, NaPiIIa, NaPiIIc, in the kidney, and possibly NaPiIIb in the small bowel. In mice 1,25(OH)$_2$D$_3$ increases FGF23 concentrations and its gene expression. Calcitonin suppresses FGF23 expression (41,196).

Deficiency of FGF23 causes renal phosphorus retention, hyperphosphatemia, increased 1,25(OH)$_2$D$_3$ levels, soft tissue calcification and defective bone mineralization. The latter has been attributed to direct action of 1,25(OH)$_2$D$_3$ on bone (196).

FGF23 binds to and activates FGF23 cognate receptors in cells that express Klotho. Klotho is a transmembrane protein that determines the specificity of tissue targeted by FGF23. In this regard, Klotho binds to FGF23 and converts the canonical FGF receptor to a specific receptor for FGF23. This enables high-affinity binding of FGF23 to all surface receptors in distal convoluted tubule where Klotho is expressed. FGF signaling is mediated by mitogen-activated protein kinase (MAPK) cascade and phospho-ERK1/2 (p-ERK1/2). Klotho is produced in two isoforms by alternating splicing of the 5-exon gene. The first isoform is a single pass transmembrane protein, with extracellular and cytoplasmic domains. Cleavage of the extracellular domain produces a cut segment found in circulation. The second isoform has only extracellular domain without the transcellular portion and is secreted into circulation (196–198).

It is of interest that FGF23-Klotho-receptor signaling is localized in the distal tubule, whereas its physiological effect to reduce phosphorus reabsorption by decreasing NaPiII abundance is in the proximal tubule. The anatomical proximity between proximal and distal tubule perhaps may enable a crosstalk between both of them, thus generating a distal-to-proximal feedback. This perhaps can be mediated by a paracrine factor produced in the distal tubule. FGF23 downregulates renal expression of Klotho resulting in decrease calcium reabsorption by TRPV5 channel in the distal tubule. TRPV5 activity is enhanced by Klotho in the distal tubule independent of FGF23. Klotho directly regulates PTH secretion in the parathyroid glands by recruiting Na$^+$/K$^+$ ATPase to the cell surface in response to low extracellular calcium concentration. It is likely that by reducing cytosolic sodium concentration by sodium-pump, increased sodium gradient enhances NCX. Thus, calcium is pumped out of cell in exchange for sodium that enters the cell down its gradient. In this regard, Klotho signaling may regulate PTH secretion by changing intracellular calcium (196).

Hereditary hypophosphatemic disorders may be divided into three groups—Group I: FGF23-dependent disorders, Group II: Primary disorders of phosphorus transporters, and Group III: Disorders due to hyperresponsiveness to PTH.

Group I: FGF23-Dependent Group of Hereditary Hypophosphatemic Rickets

X-Linked Hypophosphatemic Rickets (XLH)

Hypophosphatemic vitamin D–resistant rickets is a sex-linked dominant disorder also known as XLH, in which renal tubular defects in phosphate reabsorption have been demonstrated (189,190). Serum 1,25(OH)$_2$D$_3$ levels in patients with XLH are in the low-normal or slightly below normal range. Because hypophosphatemia is expected to stimulate 1α(OH)ase activity in the kidney, these relatively low values suggest that, in addition to a defect in tubular phosphate absorption, the response of 1α(OH)ase to low levels of serum phosphate also is impaired in XLH. This hypophosphatemic disorder is associated with mutation of the gene that encodes the phosphate-regulating endopeptidase homolog on the X chromosome (PHEX). PHEX is a type I cell surface zinc metalloprotease that is involved in regulation of FGF23. PHEX cleaves small peptides such as ASARM (acidic serine– and aspartic acid–rich motif) peptide derived from MEPE, but the physiologically relevant peptide for PHEX that regulates FGF23 is unknown. Mutation in PHEX increases transcription of FGF23 in osteocytes. It is assumed that an unidentified substrate of PHEX accumulates and stimulates FGF23 gene promoter activity. Earlier suggestion that PHEX processes FGF23 was not born out. Both the hypophosphatemia and low 1,25(OH)$_2$D$_3$ levels are related to high levels of circulating FGF23.

XLH occasionally respond to treatment with large doses of oral phosphate as well as to pharmacologic doses of vitamin D. The combined administration of oral phosphate supplements with $1,25(OH)_2D_3$ is better than the administration of either alone for the cure of the bone disease in XLH. In hypophosphatemic mice (HYP mice), the animal model of the disease, the administration of phosphate cures the rickets but not the osteomalacia. The combined administration of phosphate supplements and $1,25(OH)_2D_3$ is necessary to achieve improvement of the osteomalacia as well (190,199). It is unknown whether a similar therapeutic response applies to the human disease.

The presence of a tumor may be responsible for excessive urinary loss of phosphate and hypophosphatemic rickets. The tumors that have been identified most frequently consist of mesenchymal and giant cells and often are present in bones. Excision of the tumor has been associated with reversal of the tubular leak of phosphate and cure of the bone disease in many patients (192). Recently, the beneficial effect of the administration of octreotide in a patient with tumor-induced osteomalacia has been reported. It has been proposed that the syndrome is the result of a release of phosphaturic substance by the tumor. Indeed, tumor extracts elicited phosphaturic cAMP-independent effects when injected into animals (193,194). Likewise, in vitro, tumor extracts inhibited NaPi coupled uptake using OK cells (195). FGF23 has been isolated from these tumors.

Hypophosphatemic nonrachitic bone disease is an entity that resembles X-linked hypophosphatemia but is clinically less severe with regard to bone disease and there is no clear evidence of X-linked inheritance.

Autosomal Dominant Hypophosphatemic Rickets (ADHR)

ADHR is a phosphate-wasting disorder that maps to chromosome 12p13 and is characterized by short stature, bone pain, fracture, and lower extremity deformity. It is caused by mutations in the RXXR furin-like cleavage domain of FGF23 that makes it resistant to protelytic inactivation by furin proprotein convertase. Thus patients with ADHR missense mutations produce polypeptides that are less sensitive to protease cleavage than wild FGF23. ADHR mutations protect FGF23 from degradation, thereby elevating circulating concentrations of FGF23 and leading to phosphate wasting in ADHR patients.

Autosomal Recessive Hypophosphatemic Rickets (ARHR)

ARHR, variant of hypophosphatemic rickets, is caused by an inactivating mutation of Dentin matrix protein 1 (DMP_1). DMP_1 is glycophosphoprotein that belongs to the small integrin-binding ligand N-linked glycoprotein family (SIBLING) and is expressed in bones and teeth where it induces mineralization of extracellular matrix. Loss of DMP_1 results in increased transcription of FGF23 in osteocytes. DMP_1 null mice are a model of ARHR and have elevated circulating FGF23.

Osteoglophonic Dysplasia (OGD)

OGD is an autosomal dominant bone dysplastic disorder caused by activating mutation of FGR1 gene that may regulate FGF23 expression in bone, and or increase its phosphaturic effect in the kidney.

Hypophosphatemic Rickets with Hyperparathyroidism

This hypophosphatemic disorder features both rickets and hyperparathyroidism due to parathyroid hyperplasia. The primary abnormality in this hypophosphatemic rickets is elevated levels of Klotho due to Klotho gene translocation. FGF23 levels are elevated in this disorder by yet unknown mechanism . It has been proposed that the elevated levels play a role in parathyroid hyperplasia (197).

Additional Hypophosphatemic Disorders Associated with Elevated FGF23

Other hypophosphatemic disorders in which high levels of FGF23 has been reported to be elevated include McCune–Albright polyostotic fibrous dysplasia with activating mutation of $GNAS_1$. It is unclear if the hypophosphatemia is due to FGF23, which is elevated in 50% of patients, and/or due to activation of the adenylate cyclase/cAMP pathway in the kidney. Epidermal nevus syndrome is caused by activating FGF23 mutations in the affected skin. Some patients with this syndrome have elevated FGF23 levels and hypophosphatemia.

Group II: Primary Disorders of Sodium-Phosphate Cotransporters

Hereditary Hypophosphatemic Rickets with Hypercalciuria (HHRH)

HHRH is an autosomal recessive disorders characterized by hypophosphatemia due renal phosphorus wasting, increased serum levels of $1,25(OH)_2D_3$, increased intestinal absorption of calcium and hypercalciuria, rickets and osteomalacia (200,201). It was originally assumed that this disorder is caused by a mutation in NaPiIIa cotransporter gene, because the human phenotype is similar to that of mice with the deletion of NaPiIIa. Surprisingly, no mutation was identified in the NaPiIIa gene, but a mutation was found in the NaPiIIc cotransporter gene. Thus HHRH is caused by the single-nucleotide deletion in NaPiIIc cotransporter gene (202).

Group III: Hypophosphatemic Disorders Secondary to Hyperresponsiveness to PTH

NHERF1 Mutations and Renal Responsiveness to PTH

NHERF1 is a scaffold protein that links with NaPi cotransporters by interacting with *C*-terminal tail of NaPiIIc and NaPiIIa and anchors them within apical cell membranes. NHERF1 phosphorylation by PTH leads to internalization of Na/Pi cotransporters followed by their degradation in lysosomes. NHERF1 in cultured cells attenuates PTH-induced formation of cAMP. Thus NHERF1 plays an important role in tubular phosphorus transport. Inactivating missense mutations in NHERF1 have been identified in patients with hypercalciuria and nephrolithiasis that exhibited reduced reabsorption of phosphorus below lower limits of normal as well as causing hypophosphatemia. In vitro experiments showed that these mutations potentiated PTH-induced cAMP generation and consequently caused inhibition of phosphorus transport. Patients with this abnormality presented with reduced bone mineralization and elevated $1,25(OH)_2D_3$. Thus inactivating mutations in NHERF1 are a new class of pathogenic factors of hypophosphatemia (203).

Dent Disease or X-Linked Hypercalciuric Nephrolithiasis

Dent disease is characterized by low–molecular weight proteinuria, hyperphosphaturia, and hypercalciuria, which eventually lead to kidney stones, nephrocalcinosis, and renal failure. This hereditary proximal tubulopathy is due to mutation of the chloride channel 5 (CLCN5) gene that encodes the voltage-gated chloride channel and chloride proton antiporter. This mutation results in a defect in proximal tubular endocytosis. This leads to reduced PTH endocytosis with increased tubular PTH concentration available to bind to its PTH1R receptors. This in turn potentiates the tubular effect of PTH causing increased endocytosis of NaPiII cotransporters with reduced phosphorus reabsorption, hyperphosphaturia, and hypophosphatemia (204).

Low oculocerebrorenal syndrome (OCRL1) is caused by mutations of genes that encode phophatidylinositol 4,5-bisphosphonate 5-phosphatase that also produces a defect in endocytosis. OCRL1 patients feature more severe hypophosphatemia, bone disease, and tubular proteinuria than those in patients with Dent's disease.

Jansen Metaphyseal Chondrodysplasia

Jansen chondrodystrophy is characterized by dwarfism with short limbs, bowing of long bones, mild hypercalcemia, nephrolithiasis, hypophosphatemia and low serum PTH level but elevated urinary cAMP excretion. It is caused by activating, gain-of-function mutations of PTH/PTHrP receptor and is inherited as an autosomal dominant trait. It is associated with increased proliferation and delayed maturation of chondrocytes.

OTHER METABOLIC ABNORMALITIES ASSOCIATED WITH RICKETS AND OSTEOMALACIA

Even though calcium deficiency per se has not been recognized as a cause of osteomalacia in humans, several reports suggest that this abnormality may cause rickets in babies and children (205). It is possible that in these circumstances calcium deficiency–induced secondary hyperparathyroidism may lead to vitamin D deficiency. High circulating PTH levels stimulate renal 1α(OH)ase, resulting in high $1,25(OH)_2D_3$ levels. Thus, the proposed mechanism of this abnormality is increased breakdown of $25(OH)_2D_3$ by high levels of $1,25(OH)_2D_3$, causing a state of vitamin D deficiency (90).

Fanconi syndrome is associated with multiple defects in tubular transport. The phosphaturia and renal tubular acidosis associated with this syndrome may be primarily responsible for the occurrence of the hypophosphatemic rickets (206). The exact cause of osteomalacia in patients with renal tubular acidosis is not entirely clear. Another possible mechanism of osteomalacia in Fanconi syndrome is vitamin D deficiency caused by failure to absorb vitamin D bound to a protein carrier in the proximal tubule. Acidosis per se leads to the development of osteoporosis rather than osteomalacia in animals. It has been proposed that hypercalciuria associated with renal tubular acidosis lowers serum calcium and stimulates the secretion of PTH, which in turn causes excessive urinary losses of phosphorus, with hypophosphatemia and osteomalacia. An alternative explanation for the phosphaturia is that acidosis directly increases urinary excretion of phosphorus. Osteomalacia also has been reported in patients with systemic acidosis following ureterosigmoidostomy some years earlier (207). The acidosis occurs as a result of fecal bicarbonate losses in this latter situation. The fact that osteomalacia associated with renal tubular acidosis may be cured in some patients with the correction of the acidosis emphasizes the potential role of acidosis in this disorder (208). Osteomalacia also has been reported in patients with phosphate depletion caused by excessive intake of phosphate-binding antacids and excessive use of laxatives.

All previously discussed disorders causing osteomalacia share one common feature, namely, a reduced serum calcium–phosphorus product that may be responsible for the failure of bone matrix to mineralize. However, osteomalacia in chronic renal failure develops in the presence of a high serum calcium–phosphorus product. In these patients, the mineralization defect may be related to intrinsic abnormalities of the organic matrix, a circulating inhibitor of mineralization, or deficiency of a specific metabolite of vitamin D. Aluminum toxicity causes a mineralization defect in some patients with hemodialysis-associated osteomalacia (209). In osteomalacia associated with hypophosphatasia, the high concentration of pyrophosphates may block bone mineralization despite the presence of normal or high concentrations of serum calcium and phosphorus. Osteomalacia may also develop in association with the administration of bisphosphonates, which share common chemical properties with pyrophosphates.

Osteomalacia may evolve in patients receiving long-term total parenteral nutrition. A normal or slightly elevated serum concentration of calcium and phosphate has been reported in this disorder. In one study, osteomalacia developed during supplementation with vitamin D. Associated abnormalities included hypercalciuria, exceeding the amount of calcium intake, mildly elevated concentrations of serum calcium and serum $25(OH)D_3$, and low serum $1,25(OH)_2D_3$ and serum PTH concentrations. Elimination of vitamin D supplements from the formula of parenteral nutrition reversed the biochemical and hormonal abnormalities and led to recovery from the bone disease (210). This sequence suggests that either vitamin D toxicity or hypersensitivity to vitamin D with consequent loss of mineral in the urine was responsible for osteomalacia. The observed suppression of PTH secretion could play a role in the reduced bone turnover and increased losses of calcium in the urine, which could not be replaced because of the absence of the intestinal supply of calcium. Other studies proposed that either low $1,25(OH)_2D_3$ or aluminum toxicity could be causally related to the observed osteomalacia (211,212). Thus, the total parenteral nutrition–induced osteomalacia remains a poorly understood entity.

OSTEOPOROSIS

Normal bone remodeling is based on matching of bone resorption with bone formation. Each year, 25% of trabecular bone is resorbed and replaced in adults. The turnover rate of cortical bone is substantially slower. Under normal conditions, the bone renewal process proceeds in cycles of resorption followed by formation. During new bone formation the osteoblasts lay down type I collagen in longitudinal layers. The collagen molecules are then interconnected by pyridoline cross-linking to provide strength. Two stages of mineralization then follow. First, hydroxyapatite crystals are deposited between the collagen fibrils. The second stage proceeds over several months as more mineral is added to the bone. The constant bone turnover helps repair microfractures and remodels the bone in response to stress. The quantitative coupling between resorption and formation helps maintain normal bone mass. The hallmark of osteoporosis is loss of bone mass caused by imbalance between bone resorption and formation. Loss of gonadal function and aging are the two most important conditions leading to osteoporosis. The former is known as postmenopausal osteoporosis and the latter as senile osteoporosis.

Peak Bone Mass

Osteoporosis is characterized by low bone mass and disrupted bone architecture, which lead to reduced bone strength and increase the risk of fractures (Table 6.6). Therefore, prevention of low bone mass is of prime importance. One of the means of reaching this goal is to increase the peak bone mass build-up during adolescence. Adolescence is a crucial time for the development of bone mass. Bone mass increases with age throughout childhood, and it reaches its peak by late adolescence and early adulthood. Bone mass accretion during puberty appears to be critical in the development of peak bone mass. Peak bone mass is regarded as a major determinant of osteoporosis in later life (213).

The bone mass remains stable after attainment of peak bone mass under normal conditions. An exception to this rule is the appearance of pregnancy-associated osteoporosis. It consists of four variants: (a) idiopathic osteoporosis of pregnancy, (b) transient osteoporosis of the hip in pregnancy, (c) postpregnancy spinal osteoporosis, and (d) lactation-associated osteoporosis. Whether these are truly independent conditions or they relate specifically to pregnancy remains to be determined. The most important feature of all types of pregnancy-associated osteoporosis is complete recovery without residual damage. Heparin-induced osteoporosis in pregnancy also is reversible after discontinuation of heparin (214).

An annual loss of 0.3% to 0.5% of bone mass may occur starting during the fourth to fifth decade of life. After menopause, the rate of bone loss may increase 10-fold. Loss of bone mass following menopause is characterized by increased bone turnover, featuring both increased bone resorption and increased bone formation. The osteoclastic resorbing activity, however, exceeds the osteoblastic bone-forming activity, resulting in net loss of bone mass. By contrast, the osteoporosis associated with aging, senile osteoporosis, is characterized by low bone turnover (215). The major feature of aging osteoporosis is reduced osteoblastic activity with reduced supply of osteoblasts. Thus, the amount of bone formed during each remodeling cycle is reduced, leading to a net decrease in bone mass. Additional differences between the postmenopausal and senile osteoporosis are that mainly the trabecular bone is affected in the former, whereas cortical and trabecular bones are affected equally in the latter. Estrogen deficiency is the underlying mechanism of postmenopausal osteoporosis. The deficiency of estrogen creates an imbalance in bone metabolism with at least two known abnormalities. First, the resorptive effect of PTH is augmented in the absence of estrogen, with no change in bone formation. Second, estrogen suppresses the production of IL-6 by osteoblastic cells. IL-6 is an osteoclast-activating cytokine (216). Thus, excessive formation of IL-6 leads

TABLE 6.6 CLINICAL FORMS OF OSTEOPOROSIS

Generalized, primary	Generalized, secondary
Type I: Postmenopausal	Corticosteroid
Type II: Senile	Cushing syndrome
Type III: Idiopathic	Hyperthyroidism
Juvenile	Rheumatoid arthritis
Adult	Long-term heparin administration
In pregnancy	Alcoholism
Local	Anorexia nervosa
Transitory migrant osteoporosis	Hypogonadism
Fracture and immobilization	Malabsorption
Neurogenic immobilization	Acidosis
Transient osteoporosis of the hip in pregnancy	Cirrhosis of liver
	Vitamin C deficiency
	Lactation-associated osteoporosis
	Space travel

to excessive bone loss in postmenopausal osteoporosis (217). Serum levels of PTH and calcitriol are low in patients with postmenopausal osteoporosis. PTH levels are increased and calcitriol levels reduced in senile osteoporosis. There is reduced intestinal calcium absorption in both conditions. Estrogen therapy in post-menopausal osteoporosis leads to an increase in plasma calcitriol levels and improves intestinal absorption of calcium (215,216).

Low bone turnover, which is characteristic of senile osteoporosis, also is present in other types of secondary osteoporosis, including steroid-induced osteoporosis, alcohol-induced osteoporosis, osteoporosis associated with malabsorption and chronic liver disease, osteoporosis associated with anorexia nervosa, immobilization-induced osteoporosis, and idiopathic juvenile osteoporosis with and without hypercalciuria. On the other hand, osteoporosis associated with premature menopause, anovulatory cycles, primary hyperparathyroidism, secondary amenorrhea, and male hypogonadism is associated usually with high bone turnover. It is interesting that the two variants of osteoporosis differ also in the abnormalities in microarchitecture. In the high turnover type, the changes consist of thinning and loss of trabecular elements, reduced connectedness, erosions, and penetration of the trabeculas with total disruption of the architecture; in the low bone turnover type, the only change is thinning of the trabecules with loss of horizontal trabecules.

Bone mass is strongly correlated with compressive strength. However, there is a considerable overlap in bone density values between subjects with and without fractures. This emphasizes the importance of factors other than bone mass in the pathogenesis of fractures. These include bone microarchitecture, composition of bone matrix, composition of bone mineral, and factors such as trauma. In this regard, it is of interest that patients with elevated serum levels of homocysteine are at very high risk of osteoporotic fractures. In vivo and in vitro studies suggest that homocysteine interferes with collagen cross-linking in bone, leading to abnormal bone matrix (218).

Even though the vast majority of osteoporotic fractures occur in patients with postmenopausal osteoporosis and elderly persons, it is noteworthy that the association of low bone mass with the occurrence of fractures has been recorded in younger people. It has been shown that athletes with stress fractures had lower bone mineral than did well-matched control athletes. Likewise, there was a good correlation between menstrual irregularity, reduced bone mineral density, and stress fractures. A positive correlation between calcium intake and bone mineral density was demonstrated in young individuals.

Bone Densitometry

Bone densitometry represents a major advance in management osteoporosis. The introduction of advanced technology to assess the bone density has provided clinicians with a valuable tool to assess patients at risk of fractures and monitor response to therapy. These methods include the use of dual energy X-ray absorptiometry (DXA), ultrasonic measurements (SOS), computerized X-ray tomography, and other methods. The indications for bone mineral density measurements recommended by the Scientific Advisory Board of the National Osteoporosis Foundation in the United State are: (a) estrogen deficiency, (b) vertebral deformity and radiographic osteopenia, (c) asymptomatic primary hyperparathyroidism (reduced bone density is an indication for parathyroid surgery), and (d) monitoring of therapy. Optional indications include the presence of several minor risk factors such as genetic factors, alcohol intake, high caffeine intake, smoking, and reduced physical activity.

It is interesting that in recent genetic studies, polymorphism of VDR gene has been linked with bone mineral density in twin studies. It has been shown in postmenopausal women that allelic variants in the gene encoding the VDR can be used to predict differences in bone density. The molecular mechanism by which bone density is regulated by VDR is not certain, although allelic differences in the three untranslated regions may alter mRNA levels. It has been proposed that the use of this genetic marker could allow earlier intervention in those with increased risk of osteoporosis (217). More recent reports have emphasized that the VDR gene acts predominantly to determine peak bone mass, and other genes are likely to be involved in the regulation of bone loss after menopause (219).

TREATMENT OF OSTEOPOROSIS

Undoubtedly, measures aimed at prevention of osteoporosis are most valuable, because in many cases the disease is irreversible and refractory to therapy. Achievement of adequate peak bone mass may be facilitated with adequate intake of calcium and vitamin D, good physical activity, and early detection and treatment of predisposing diseases. Nonsmoking and moderation in alcohol and caffeine intake is recommended.

The therapeutic goals are dual in established osteoporosis: to increase bone formation and decrease bone resorption in order to maintain adequate bone mass and prevent osteoporotic fractures. There is a positive correlation between physical activity and bone density; therefore, gravity exercises and muscle-strengthening exercises should be encouraged.

Estrogen inhibits bone resorption, prevents bone loss, and even may increase bone mass in post-menopausal women. The daily dose of conjugated estrogen is 0.625 mg; it may be given in conjunction with progesterone with good effect. Administration of estrogen not only prevents bone loss but also prevents vertebral and femoral fractures. It is recommended to treat with estrogen for at least 5 years. Reports on the incidence of breast cancer in estrogen-treated women need to be taken into consideration (220).

Bisphosphonates and calcitonin reduce bone turnover and, like estrogens, may potentially lead to increases in bone mass as a result of filling the remodeling space. Estrogens affect equally cortical and cancellous bone, whereas calcitonin and bisphosphonates mainly affect cancellous bone (220–223).

The bisphosphonate, alendronate (Fosamax), gained popularity in the treatment of postmenopausal osteoporosis. Our clinical follow-up experience based on a large population of postmenopausal women shows favorable therapeutic response in 60% to 65% of patients. The drug was discontinued in about 35% to 40% either because of lack of efficacy or because of intolerance due adverse side effects mainly related to upper GI tract. Interestingly, alendronate failed to benefit patients with hypothyroidism receiving hormonal thyroid replacement.

Long-term follow-up studies showed that the therapeutic effects of alendronate on bone density and on bone fractures were sustained over 10 years (224). Concern about the quality of the bone exposed to bisphophonates has been expressed by some investigators. This concern addressed the fact that bisphosphonates are not "bone builders" but "bone hardeners." The bone biopsies from patients treated with bisphosphonates shows that the mineralizing surface which reflects bone formation is markedly reduced and the bone volume does not change significantly. The mineral inside the bone is more densely packed; therefore the bone density on DXA is increased (225). Recent study exploring bone biopsies in patients treated for 3 years with alendronate revealed a peculiar histology showing increased number of giant hypernucleated osteoclasts undergoing protracted apoptosis. This finding is poorly understood (226).

Fluoride increases cancellous bone density. The quality of the bone may be abnormal with fluoride, however, resulting in reduced strength despite increased mass (223,227). Oral calcium supplements, with and without vitamin D (including oral calcitriol), have been reported to be beneficial in certain studies. Obviously the presence of vitamin D deficiency which is common in the elderly needs to be corrected with vitamin D supplements.

All therapeutic interventions addressed to above are based the antiresorptive effects of the therapeutic agents. By contrast, intermittent recombinant PTH (hPTH-[1-34]) administration, has an anabolic effect on bone metabolism as it stimulates bone formation. Older therapeutic trials with alternating calcium and phosphorus infusions that achieved increases in bone volume in fact induced cyclical variations in serum PTH concentrations, similar to intermittent PTH injections (228).

Once-daily injections of injections of hPTH-(1-34) increase the expression of the master osteogenic transcription factor Runx2, which increases osteoblast numbers and thereby enhances bone formation. Intermittent hPTH-(1-34) also increases the decoy protein osteoprotegerin (OPG) expression and reduces osteoclast activity. On the other hand, continuous infusion of PTH as in primary hyperparathyroidism has the opposite effect. It increases the RANK ligand and reduces OPG resulting in increased activity of osteoclasts with increased bone resorption and increase in serum calcium level (229).

A controlled, randomized clinical trial with 1,637 postmenopausal women with osteoporosis demonstrated that once-daily injections of PTH over 21 months increased bone formation and bone mass and decreased the risk of fractures (230).

CHRONIC RENAL DISEASE

Hyperplasia of the parathyroid glands was reported in the early part of this century in autopsies of patients dying of uremia. In 1943, a form of rickets that failed to respond to physiologic doses of vitamin D but responded to pharmacologic doses was reported in children with renal insufficiency (230). These preliminary observations stimulated the evaluation of two major skeletal abnormalities associated with chronic renal disease, osteitis fibrosa cystica and osteomalacia.

Both biochemical studies and measurements of circulating immunoreactive PTH suggest that hyperactivity of parathyroid glands is present in the early stage of chronic renal disease. Assuming that a decrease in serum calcium concentration is the stimulus for secondary hyperparathyroidism in chronic renal failure, several factors may cause the hypocalcemia. Loss of functioning nephrons with a decreased filtered load of phosphorus leads to retention of phosphorus. The resulting increase in serum phosphorus concentration, with a reciprocal decrease in serum calcium concentration, stimulates the secretion of PTH. The increase in parathyroid activity corrects the hyperphosphatemia by decreasing tubular phosphate reabsorption and increasing urinary excretion of phosphorus and returning both serum phosphorus and calcium toward normal, but at the expense ("trade-off") of increasingly rising serum levels of PTH (231). This hypothesis of the pathogenesis of secondary hyperparathyroidism in chronic renal failure is supported by studies in chronically azotemic dogs in which phosphate restriction prevented the development of secondary hyperparathyroidism. However, the major assumptions on which the "trade-off" hypothesis was based were not fulfilled entirely. First, no evidence was presented showing a rise in serum phosphorus in patients with early renal failure. In fact, these patients exhibit a normal or even low serum phosphate, with normal serum calcium. Likewise, sequential sampling of serum phosphate failed to demonstrate transient rises in serum phosphorus or decrements in serum calcium. Second, the patients with early renal failure do not show phosphate retention but rather have an increased ability to excrete phosphorus loads. The fact that phosphate restriction was shown to reverse the rise in PTH cannot be used as favoring the trade-off hypothesis. Phosphate levels per se, independent of serum calcium, have been shown to alter PTH secretion (70,71).

Reduced intestinal absorption of calcium owing to acquired resistance to vitamin D has been proposed as a fundamental abnormality in chronic renal failure (232). This possibility was supported by studies indicating that the conversion of $25(OH)_2D_3$ to $1,25(OH)_2D_3$ takes place in the kidney and that serum levels of $1,25(OH)_2D_3$ are reduced in patients with chronic renal failure. It has been reported that physiologic doses of $1,25(OH)_2D_3$ improve the abnormal GI absorption of calcium in patients with chronic renal failure. These findings, however, apply to advanced renal disease. Intestinal absorption of calcium is normal in early renal failure, whereas serum PTH is already elevated.

Evidence has been advanced demonstrating a direct inhibitory effect of physiologic amounts of $1,25(OH)_2D_3$ on the synthesis of PTH in vivo at the genomic transcriptional level. Thus, reduced $1,25(OH)_2D_3$ levels in chronic renal failure could be responsible for the increased synthesis and secretion of PTH (69). It is noteworthy, however, that in early renal failure serum levels of $1,25(OH)_2D_3$ are variable, normal, low, or even elevated. It has been claimed that the presumably "normal" $1,25(OH)_2D_3$ levels measured in early renal failure may in fact be abnormally low relative to the elevated PTH level. In this regard, it has been demonstrated that the administration of calcitriol or dietary phosphate restriction in early renal disease results in normalization of serum PTH levels. These observations do not necessarily prove conclusively that calcitriol deficiency is the mechanism of secondary hyperparathyroidism.

An additional proposed mechanism of the evolution of secondary hyperparathyroidism is altered number or binding affinity of VDRs for $1,25(OH)_2D_3$, resulting in a blunted response of parathyroid glands to the inhibitory effect of $1,25(OH)_2D_3$ and uninhibited synthesis of PTH. Although reduced density and number of VDRs have been demonstrated in hyperplastic glands removed from uremic patients, this has not yet been demonstrated in patients with early renal failure (233).

Parathyroid glands from uremic patients require higher ambient calcium concentrations than normal glands to suppress the secretion of PTH. Thus, the set point for calcium, that is, the concentration of calcium required to inhibit 50% of maximal PTH secretion, is shifted to the right. This abnormality of response to calcium can be corrected partially by treatment with calcitriol. The possibility that defects in the CaSR might be the mechanism of secondary hyperparathyroidism in early renal failure requires further evaluation. It is of interest that vitamin D deficiency, as defined by low levels $25(OH)D_3$, is more common than assumed in the past. Sustained repletion of vitamin D may reverse secondary hyperparathyroidism. It has been proposed that $25(OH)D$ is indicated before administration of vitamin analogues.

The calcemic response to PTH in chronic renal failure is blunted. This could represent downregulation of PTH receptors in the bone. It has been shown that this abnormality can be reversed after parathyroidectomy, suggesting that high PTH levels may play a role in the blunted calcemic response. The skeletal resistance to PTH has been demonstrated both in early and advanced renal insufficiency (231).

FGF23 is markedly increased in chronic kidney disease (234,235). FGF23 levels show an early rise in chronic kidney disease, perhaps even before the rise in PTH. The rise in FGF23 in early renal failure may explain hypophosphatemia that has been observed in some patients at an early stage of CKD. FGF23 may play an important role in the high fractional excretion of phosphorus that is observed in all stages of CKD and remains elevated after total parathyroidectomy (188). Likewise the reduced levels of $1,25(OH)_2D_3$ in advanced CKD could be partly caused by the inhibitory effect of FGF23 on $25(OH)D-1\alpha(OH)$ase in the kidney and thus contribute to secondary hyperparathyroidism. It has been proposed that FGF23 may also exert a direct effect on bone mineralization independent of serum phosphate. A recent epidemiological study has shown that increased FGF23 levels appear to be independently associated with mortality among patients who are beginning hemodialysis treatment (235).

As renal failure advances, hyperphosphatemia develops and assumes a major role in the aggravation of secondary hyperparathyroidism. Likewise, the serum levels of $1,25(OH)_2D_3$ decrease, and the intestinal absorption of calcium is low. In many patients with advanced renal failure, the hyperplastic parathyroid glands do not respond to physiologic regulation and become refractory to treatment. This sets the stage for the emergence of "tertiary" or "autonomous" hyperparathyroidism, which may require surgical removal of excessive parathyroid tissue. In these circumstances, hypercalcemia may develop as a result of loss of feedback regulation. The combined elevation of serum calcium and phosphorus levels with an increase in their product may lead to metastatic calcifications.

Recent studies have examined the clonality of hyperplastic parathyroid glands from patients with autonomous secondary uremic hyperparathyroidism. Tumor monoclonality was demonstrated in 64% of patients with uremic refractory hyperparathyroidism. Monoclonality implied that somatic mutation of certain genes controlling cell proliferation occurred in a single parathyroid cell, conferring a selective growth advantage to the transformed cell, leading to neoplastic transformation (236).

RENAL BONE DISEASE

Recommendation from the recent conference of Kidney Disease: Improving Global Outcomes (KDIGO)'s Global Mineral and Bone Initiative recommended that (1) the term "renal osteodystrophy" be used exclusively to alterations in bone morphology that are associated with chronic kidney disease and (2) the term "chronic kidney disease-mineral and bone disorder" (CKD-MBD) be used to describe the broader clinical syndrome that develops as a systemic disorder of mineral and bone disorder as a result of chronic kidney disease. The following discussion will focus on some features of renal osteodystrophy.

Secondary hyperparathyroidism causes the development of osteitis fibrosa cystica, which presents radiographically as subperiosteal bone resorption. These lesions are most commonly seen in the middle phalanges of the hands, distal ends of the clavicles, and proximal ends of the tibia. Cystic lesions and brown tumors may be a radiographic feature of hyperparathyroid bone disease.

Osteitis fibrosa cystica is the most common skeletal abnormality both in adults and children with chronic renal failure. This hyperparathyroid osteodystrophy is characterized by rapid bone turnover, featuring both increased osteoclastic resorption and increased osteoblastic bone formation. The rapid bone turnover can be demonstrated by an increased number of double-tetracycline labels. The rapid bone turnover also is associated with marrow fibrosis and increased amounts of woven osteoid. It differs from normal lamellar osteoid in that there is a haphazard arrangement of collagen fibers. Although woven osteoid can be mineralized, the calcium is deposited as amorphous calcium and phosphate instead of hydroxyapatite. The presence of woven bone is characteristic of states of active bone and is visualized with polarizing microscope. Advanced forms of osteitis fibrosa cystica present an abnormal bone architecture in which vast quantities of normal mineralized bone are replaced with fibrous tissue, with multiple cysts, and with woven bone that is mechanically defective. This leads to serious skeletal deformities and fractures.

Another interesting radiographic feature of renal osteodystrophy is osteosclerosis. This entity is associated with increased density of bone, as assessed by X-ray examination, and is most frequently observed in the vertebrae.

In many instances, the secondary hyperparathyroidism seen in advanced renal insufficiency may be reversed with sustained control of serum calcium and phosphorus, which may be accomplished by the use of vitamin D, phosphate-binding antacids, and the administration of calcium carbonate. It has been shown that with continuous control of calcium and phosphorus levels in the serum, the level of circulating PTH

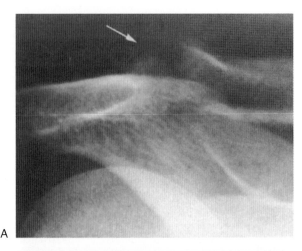

A

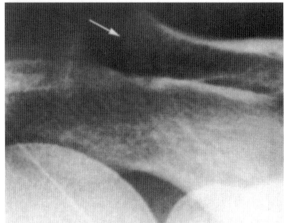

■ Figure 6.9 A. Subperiosteal resorption at the lateral end of the clavicle *(arrow)*, with an irregular appearance and loss of cortical outline. **B.** Healing of bone, with filling of the defect and reappearance of cortical outline after therapy with calcium carbonate and aluminum hydroxide. (*Arrow* indicates distal clavicle.)

B

decreases and radiographically observed bone lesions may resolve (Fig. 6.9) (237). Metastatic calcifications resolve with this regimen as well (238). This therapeutic approach may not be successful in some patients because of extremely severe hyperplasia of the parathyroid glands, and subtotal parathyroidectomy then is the treatment of choice.

Intravenous use of pharmacologic doses of calcitriol, in intermittent doses, has been recommended as a highly efficient way to achieve better suppression of parathyroid hyperactivity in patients with chronic renal failure (239). Indeed, many studies have confirmed the therapeutic efficacy of the intravenous intermittent administration of calcitriol in suppressing PTH levels. The effect of this form of therapy on bone histomorphometry is not entirely clear. In a limited number of studies, intravenous therapy with calcitriol led to marked suppression of bone turnover, with marked reduction in bone formation but with variable effect on osteoclastic resorption (240). It is noteworthy that the initial clinical studies comparing the efficacy of the intermittent intravenous administration of calcitriol with the oral route of administration were uncontrolled. The results of a recent controlled randomized study comparing long-term oral administration of calcitriol with intermittent intravenous administration showed that they were equivalent in the treatment of secondary hyperparathyroidism. Additional observations of that study were that treatment of severe secondary hyperparathyroidism remains difficult regardless of the route of administration. Moreover, the dose of calcitriol was limited by side effects (241).

Additional intravenous preparations of active vitamin D analogs including paracalcitol (Zemplar), and doxecalciferol (Hectorol) are widely used in treatment of secondary hyperparathyroidism in patients undergoing dialysis. These analogs may have an advantage over older intravenous forms of vitamin D by primarily targeting parathyroid glands and exerting minimal effect on intestinal phosphorus absorption (242).

Calcimimetics are allosteric activators of CaSR. Their binding to CaSR stimulates signaling to mobilize and increase intracellular calcium and decrease parathyroid secretion and synthesis. As opposed to vitamin D analogues calcimimetics do not alter directly intestinal absorption of calcium and phosphate, and can lower PTH without increasing circulating phosphorus and calcium. Cinacalcet is the only available calcimimetic drug. Bone histomorphometric studies in dialysis patient showed that treatment with cinacalcet lowered PTH, improved bone histology and reduced bone turnover in most of the studied patients with secondary hyperparathyroidism (243).

A previous trial demonstrated a beneficial effect of oral administration of $24,25(OH)_2D_3$ when combined with $1\alpha(OH)D_3$ on hyperparathyroid bone disease in patients on chronic hemodialysis (244). The potential therapeutic effect of this regimen is uncertain and requires further investigation.

Two additional distinct forms of bone disease in patients with chronic renal disease are osteomalacia and adynamic or aplastic bone disease. A so-called vitamin D–refractory rickets was described in the 1940s in children with advanced renal insufficiency. This form of mineralization defect most likely resulted from deficiency of calcitriol. Osteomalacia may be present in predialysis patients with chronic renal failure also. Most of these patients present with hypocalcemia and normophosphatemia; their kidney disease usually is interstitial and/or obstructive uropathy. Many respond favorably to calcitriol administration.

Aluminum has been recognized as a toxic factor involved in the pathogenesis of uremic osteomalacia. The aluminum-related lesion is characterized by the presence of excessive amounts of inactive osteoid and very low bone turnover. The staining of bone for aluminum is usually strongly positive in states of aluminum overload. Although this type of bone disease has been described mainly in patients undergoing chronic dialysis, it may occur in uremic predialysis patients. Aluminum-associated osteomalacia is a very symptomatic bone disease manifested by severe skeletal pains and fractures (245). Aluminum can be mobilized and removed with the use of the chelating agent deferoxamine mesylate, which binds aluminum. Removal of aluminum leads to recovery. Aluminum-induced bone disease has become less frequent with the restricted use of aluminum-based phosphate binders and the widespread employment of water treatment with reverse osmosis in dialysis units.

Adynamic bone at present is one of the enigmas in the spectrum of renal bone disease. It is characterized by very low bone turnover (low or absent tetracycline uptake) but with no obvious abnormalities in the static parameters of bone histomorphometry. This form of bone pathology has been variously attributed to suppression of parathyroid function by high calcium concentration in dialysate solution or by excessively high levels of circulating calcitriol such as those that follow the intravenous administration of pharmacologic doses of this metabolite of vitamin D (246). It is interesting that patients with the aplastic bone lesion, similarly to those with osteomalacia, frequently develop hypercalcemia following oral or intravenous calcium loads. Thus, both aluminum-associated osteomalacia and adynamic bone are characterized by poor buffering capacity to exogenous calcium. Recent studies indicate that aplastic bone lesion is the prevalent bone abnormality in patients treated with chronic ambulatory peritoneal dialysis (CAPD) and diabetic end-stage renal disease (247). Parathyroid hormone levels are relatively low in both groups. Likewise low turn-over bone lesion has been recently recognized as a common abnormality in patients undergoing chronic hemodialysis.

There are mixed types of renal osteodystrophy, which combine elements characteristic of more than one defined lesion in addition to the discrete forms of bone disease outlined herein. For example, the mixed form of uremic osteodystrophy consists of features typical of osteitis fibrosa; however, in addition, it is characterized by low forming activity with accumulation of excessive quantities of osteoid, as in osteomalacia. Another variant of mixed bone disease is similar to the aforementioned lesion, but the bone-forming parameters are normal. In the latter, the accumulation of osteoid has been attributed to a shortage in the supply of minerals and hence delayed mineralization of organic bone matrix. This lesion responds favorably to vitamin D therapy.

TUMORAL CALCINOSIS

Extraskeletal calcifications with periarticular, vascular, and other soft-tissue calcium deposits are present in patients with chronic renal failure. They usually are associated with advanced secondary hyperparathyroidism featuring hyperphosphatemia with high calcium–phosphate product.

Tumoral calcinosis in nonuremic patients with normal kidney also known hyperphosphatemic familial tumoral calcinosis is a rare autosomal recessive disorder associated large ectopic calcifications in soft tissues. Biochemical abnormalities include hyperphosphatemia secondary to increased tubular reabsorption of phosphorus and inappropriately normal or elevated $1,25(OH)_2D_3$. Recurrence of tumoral calcinosis after kidney transplantation suggests a deficiency of a systemic phosphaturic factor rather than an intrinsic tubular defect as an underlying mechanism (248).

Genetic analyses in patients with tumoral calcinosis identified three mutations that cause decreased bioactive circulating levels of FGF23 or end-organ resistance to FGF23. These mutations involve either genes encoding FGF23, or Klotho, or GalNac transferase 3 ($GALNT_3$). $GALNT_3$ is a Golgi associated enzyme that o-glycolysates the furin-like convertase recognition sequence in FGF23. Mutations in FGF23 gene cause deficiency of FGF23 with renal phosphorus retention. $GALNT_3$ that selectively o-glycosylates the furin-like convertase recognition sequence in FGF23, thereby protecting it from proteolytic processing is missing. This leads to low intact serum of FGF23 and high levels of inactive-terminal FGF23. Mutations in gene-encoding Klotho decreases Klotho expression with decreased level of FGF23–Klotho–FGF receptor complex leading to end-organ resistance to FGF23. No effective treatment other that phosphorus restriction is available for tumoral calcinosis at this time.

CALCIFIC UREMIC ARTERIOLOPATHY (CALCIPHYLAXIS)

Calcific uremic arteriolopathy occurs most often in patients with end-stage renal disease undergoing dialysis or who have recently received a kidney transplant. A similar abnormality has been associated with primary hyperparathyroidism, metastatic breast cancer, alcoholic liver cirrhosis, and Crohn disease. Calcific uremic arteriolopathy is characterized by small vessel calcifications with reduced perfusion and vascular thrombosis leading to acute infarction of subcutaneous fat tissue and cutaneous necrosis. The vascular lesion of small- to medium-size subcutaneous arteries show calcifications of the media. Some arteries are narrowed or occluded by intimal hyperplasia and fibrin thrombi. Interestingly, these changes are restricted to cutaneous arteries only. The reason for this anatomic predilection requires further investigation.

The diagnosis of calciphylaxis is suggested by characteristic features of the skin; painful pruritic skin lesions and subcutaneous nodules. These painful violaceous mottled lesions evolve into necrotic nonhealing ulcerations with gangrene formation. The legs are almost always involved. Severe proximal lesions on the legs and/or trunk are poor prognostic signs. The mortality rate is as high as 80% and principally owing to secondary infection.

In 1962, Selye (249) described an animal model of calciphylaxis in which sensitization of rats with a systemic calcifying factor, such as high phosphate, high calcium diets, and PTH, and then challenge of the animals with trauma, iron salts, or albumin caused an acute local calcinosis followed by inflammation and sclerosis. However, absence of vascular calcifications in experimental calciphylaxis, as opposed to the vascular calcific lesions that are the hallmark of the lesions in uremic patients, led to the term "uremic calcific arteriolopathy" (UCA).

The pathogenesis and risk factors for UCA remain poorly understood. It has been proposed that the vascular smooth muscle cells may assume certain osteoblastic-like features and may play an active role in tissue calcification, including the production of bone matrix protein osteopontin. Indeed, blood vessels from the UCA lesions in patients stained positive for osteopontin and thus expressed an osseous protein (250). However, it is noteworthy that osteopontin, in fact, is an inhibitor of calcification and the role of its presence in UCA vessels requires further evaluation. Whether the vascular calcification is a passive or active process is still a matter of controversy (251). It is of importance that a new noninvasive imaging technology called electron-beam computed tomography has demonstrated that high calcium-phosphate product causes a progressive increase in calcium deposits in coronary arteries and in aortic and mitral valves in patients with advanced renal failure (252). Furthermore, hyperphosphatemia per se is an independent risk factor for high morbidity and mortality.

A recent study evaluating 19 patients with UCA in comparison with 54 patients without UCA with end-stage renal disease, showed that hyperphosphatemia, high alkaline phosphatase level, low serum albumin concentration, and female gender appeared as highly significant risk factors for UCA (253). Other risk factors that were considered in the past included elevated calcium–phosphate product and high PTH. In this regard, parathyroidectomy was deemed as a potential therapeutic modality. In view of the new data, maintenance of normal serum phosphate level by aggressive control of hyperphosphatemia and maintenance of adequate nutritional status are important therapeutic measures.

β_2-MICROGLOBULIN DEPOSITION

Skeletal disease owing to the deposition of β_2-microglobulin is becoming very frequent now that patients are being maintained on hemodialysis for prolonged periods of time. β_2-Microglobulin is part of the major histocompatibility complex-1 and is produced by a large number of cells in the body. It can aggregate to form amyloid, which causes destructive arthropathy of various joints. It may accumulate around intervertebral articular spaces and produce spinal compression syndromes. Likewise, it can produce carpal tunnel syndrome. β_2-Microglobulin induces locally osteoclastic bone resorption. It remains to be established whether it may produce diffuse resorptive bone lesions similar to those present in uremic patients with severe secondary hyperparathyroidism (254).

REFERENCES

1. Moore EW. Ionized calcium in normal serum, ultrafiltrates and whole blood determined by ion-exchange electrode. *J Clin Invest.* 1970;49:318.
2. Chen PS Jr, Neuman WF. Renal excretion of calcium by the dog. *Am J Physiol.* 1955;180:623.
3. Seidler T, Hasenfuss G, Maier LS. Targeting altered calcium physiology in the heart: translational approaches to excitation, contraction, and transcription. *Physiology (Bethesda).* 2007;22:328–334.
4. deBoer IH, Rue TC, Kestenbaum B. Serum phosphorus concentrations in the third National Health and Nutrition Examination Survey (NHANES III). *Am J Kidney Dis.* 2009;53:399–407.
5. Dhingra R, Sullivan LM, Fox CS, et al. Relation of serum phosphate and calcium levels to the incidence of cardiovascular diseasein the community. *Arch Intern Med.* 2007;167:879–885.
6. Fordtran JS, Locklear TW. Ionic constituents and osmolality of gastric and small intestinal fluids after eating. *Am J Dig Dis.* 1966;11:503.
7. Popovtzer MM, Massry SG, Coburn WJ, et al. Calcium infusion test in chronic renal failure. *Nephron.* 1970;7:400.
8. Wills MR. Intestinal absorption of calcium. *Lancet.* 1973;1:820.
9. Wills MR, Zisman E, Worstman J, et al. The measurement of intestinal calcium absorption by external radioisotope counting: application to study of nephrolithiasis. *Clin Sci.* 1970;39:95.
10. Borke JL, Caride A, Verma AK, et al. Cellular and segmental distribution of Ca^{++} pump epitopes in rat intestine. *Pflugers Arch.* 1990;417:120.
11. Borke JL, Penniston JT, Kumar R. Recent advances in calcium transport by the kidney. *Semin Nephrol.* 1990;10:15.
12. Gross MD, Kumar R. The physiology and biochemistry of vitamin D-dependent calcium-binding proteins. *Am J Physiol.* 1990;259:F195.
13. Kumar R. Vitamin D metabolism and mechanisms of calcium transport. *J Am Soc Nephrol.* 1990;3:30.
14. Muller D, Hoenderop JGJ, vanOs CH, et al. The epithelial calcium channel, ECaC1: molecular details of a novel player in renal calcium handling. *Nephrol Dial Transplant.* 2001;16:1329–1335.
15. Hilfiker H, Hattenhauer O, Trtaebert M, et al. Characterization of murine type II sodium phosphate cotransporter expressed in mammalian small intestine. *Proc Natl Acad Sci U S A.* 1998;95:14564–14569.
16. Xu H, Bai L, Collins JF, et al. Age-dependent regulation of rat intestinal type II sodium phosphate cotransporters by 1,25(OH)2D3. *Am J Physiol Cell Physiol.* 2002;282:C487–C493.
17. Capuano P, Rodanovic T, Wagner CA, et al. Intestinal and renal adaptation to phosphate diet of type II NaPi cotransporters in vitamin D receptor- and 1-alpha hydroxylase deficient mice. *Am J Physiol Cell Physiol.* 2005;288:C429–C439.
18. LeGrimellec C, Roinel N, Morel F. Simultaneous Mg, Ca, P, K, Na and Cl analysis in rat tubular fluid: I. During perfusion of either insulin or ferrocyanide. *Pflugers Arch.* 1973;340:181.
19. Simon DB, Lu Y, Choate KA, et al. Paracellin-1, a renal right junction protein required for paracellular MG^{2+} resorption. *Science.* 1999;285(5424):103–106.
20. Blanchard A, Jeunemaitre X, Coudol P, et al. Paracellin-1 is critical for magnesium and calcium reabsorption in the human thick ascending limbs of Henle. *Kidney Int.* 2001;59:2206–2215.
21. Loffing J, Loffing-Cuenl D, Valderrabana V, et al. Distribution of transcellular calcium and sodium transport pathways along mouse distal nephron. *Am J Physiol.* 2001;281:F1021–F1027.
22. Sutton RAL, Wong NLM, Quamme GA, et al. Renal tubular calcium transport: effects of changes in filtered calcium load. *Am J Physiol.* 1983;245:515.
23. Brown EM, Pollak M, Hebert CH. Sensing of extracellular Ca^{2+} by parathyroid and kidney cells: cloning and characterization of extracellular Ca^{2+}-sensing receptor. *Am J Kidney Dis.* 1995;25:506–513.
24. Vezzoli G, Terranegra A, Arcidiacono T, et al. R990G polymorphism of CaSR does produce a gain-of-function and predisposes to hypercalciuria. *Kidney Int.* 2007;71:1155–1162.
25. Neshima Y. Discovery of alpha Klotho and FGF23 unveiled new insights into calcium and

phosphate homeostasis. *Clin Calcium.* 2008;18: 923–934.

26. Tiang Y, Ferguson N, Peng J. WNK4 enhances TRPV5-mediated calcium transport: potential role in hypercalcemia of familial hyperkalemic hypertension cause by gene mutations of WNK4. *Am J Physiol Renal Physiol.* 2007;292:F545–F554.

27. Popovtzer MM, Schainuck LI, Massry SG, et al. Divalent ion excretion in chronic kidney disease: relation to degree of renal insufficiency. *Clin Sci.* 1970;38:297.

28. Popovtzer MM, Massry SG, Coburn JW, et al. The interrelationship between sodium, calcium and magnesium excretion in advanced renal failure. *J Lab Clin Med.* 1969;73:763.

29. Villa-Bellosta R, Ravera S, Sorribas V, et al. The Na^+-Pi cotransporter PiT-2 (SLC20A2) is expressed in the apical membrane of rat renal proximal tubules and is regulated by dietary Pi. *Am J Physiol Renal Physiol.* 2009;296(4): F691–F699.

30. Segawa H, Onitsuka A, Kuwahata M, et al. Type IIc sodium-dependent phosphate cotransporter regulates calcium metabolism. *J Am Soc Nephrol.* 2009;20:1004–1113.

31. Lotz M, Zisman E, Bartter FC. Evidence for a phosphorus depletion syndrome in man. *N Engl J Med.* 1968;278:409.

32. Gamba G. Alternative splicing and diversity of renal transporter. *Am J Physiol.* 2001;281: F781–F794.

33. Friedlaender MM, Wald H, Dranitzki-Elhalel M, et al. Recovery of renal tubule phosphate reabsorption despite reduced levels of sodium-phosphate cotransporter. *Eur J Endocrinol.* 2004;151:797–801.

34. Steele TH. Dual effect of potent diuretics on renal handling of phosphate in man. *Metabolism.* 1971;20:749.

35. Lavender AR, Pullman TN. Changes in inorganic phosphate excretion induced by renal arterial infusion of calcium. *Am J Physiol.* 1963;205:1025.

36. Vezzoli G, Soldatil G, Gambaro G. Role of calcium sensing receptor (CaSR) in renal mineral ion transport. *Curr Pharm Biotechnol.* 2009;10: 302–310.

37. Friedlaender MM, Wald H, Dranitzki-Elhalel M, et al Vitamin D reduces NaPi-2 in PTH-infused rats: complexity of vitamin D action on renal phosphate handling. *Am J Physiol Renal Physiol.* 2001;281:F428–F433.

38. Wong NLM, Quamme GA, Dirks JH, et al. Mechanism of the reduced proximal phosphate reabsorption during phosphate infusion. *Clin Res.* 1978;26:872A.

39. Matzner Y, Prococimer M, Polliack A, et al. Hypophosphatemia in a patient with lymphoma in leukemic phase. *Arch Intern Med.* 1981;141: 805–806.

40. Dennis UW, Brazy PC. Sodium phosphate, glucose, bicarbonate and alanine interactions in the isolated proximal convoluted tubule of the rabbit kidney. *J Clin Invest.* 1978;62:387.

41. Berndt T, Kumar R. Novel mechanisms in the regulation of phosphorus homeostasis. *Physiology.* 2009;24:17–28.

42. McCollum EV. The paths to the discovery of vitamins A and D. *J Nutr.* 1967;91(suppl 1):11.

43. Holick MF. Vitamin D deficiency. *N Engl J Med.* 2007;357:266–281.

44. Reinholz GG, DeLuca HF. Inhibition of $25(OH)D_3$ production by $1,25(OH)2D3$ in rats. *Arch Biochem Biophys.* 1998;355:77–83.

45. Brodie MJ, Boobis AR, Hillyard CJ, et al. Effect of rifampicin and isoniazid on vitamin D metabolism. *Clin Pharmacol Ther.* 1982;32:525.

46. Brenza HE, Kimmel-Jehans C, Jehans F, et al. PTH activation of 25(OH)D-1-alpha hydroxylase gene promoter. *Proc Natl Acad Sci U S A.* 1998;95: 1387–1391.

47. Brezis M, Wald H, Shilo R, et al. Blockade of renal effects of vitamin D by cyclohexemide in the rat. *Pflugers Arch.* 1983;398:247–252.

48. Nykjaer A, Dragun D, Walther D, et al. An endocytic pathway essential for renal uptake and activation of the steroid 25(OH) vitamin D_3. *Cell.* 1999;96:507–515.

49. Krapf R, Vetsch R, Netsch W. Chronic acidosis increases the serum concentration of $1,25(OH)_2$ vitamin D_3 in humans by stimulating its production. *J Clin Invest.* 1992;90:2456–2463.

50. Kumar R, Schnoes HK, DeLuca HF. Rat intestinal 25-hydroxyvitamin D_3 and $1\alpha,25$-dihydroxyvitamin D_3–24-hydroxylase. *J Biol Chem.* 1978;253: 3804.

51. Kumar R. Hepatic and intestinal osteodystrophy and the hepatobiliary metabolism of vitamin D. *Ann Intern Med.* 1983;98:662.

52. Katz BS, Bell NH. The vitamin D endocrine system: current concepts and unanswered questions. *Ital J Miner Electrol Metab.* 1993;7:231–236.

53. Matsumoto T, Igarashi C, Takenchi Y, et al. Stimulation of $1,25(OH)_2$ vitamin D_3 of in vitro mineralization by osteoblast-like (MC3T3-E) cells. *Bone.* 1991;12:27–32.

54. Popovtzer MM, Mathay R, Alfrey AC, et al. Vitamin D deficiency osteomalacia: healing of the bone disease in the absence of vitamin D with intravenous calcium and phosphorus infusion. In: Frame B, Parfitt AM, Duncan H, eds. *Clinical Aspects of Metabolic Bone Disease.* Amsterdam: Excerpta Medica, International Congress Series; 1973:382.

55. Baylink D, Wergedal J, Rich M, et al. Vitamin D-enhanced osteocytic and osteoclastic bone resorption. *Am J Physiol.* 1973;224:1345.

56. Raisz LG. Recent advances in bone cell biology: interactions of vitamin D with other local and systemic factors. *Bone Miner.* 1990;9:191–197.

57. Russell RGG, Kanis JA, Smith R. Physiological and pharmacological aspects of 24,25-dihydroxycholecalciferol in man. In: Massry SG, Ritz E, Rapado A, eds. *Homeostasis of Phosphate and Other Minerals.* New York: Plenum;1978: 487–503.

58. Ornoy A. 24,25-Dihydroxyvitamin D is a metabolite of vitamin D essential for bone formation. *Nature (Lond).* 1978;276:517.

59. Pavlovitch JH, Gournor-Witmer G, Bourdeau S, et al. Suppressive effects of 24,25-dihydroxycholecalciferol or bone resorption induced by acute bilateral nephrectomy in rats. *J Clin Invest.* 1981;68:803.

60. Yamato H, Matsumoto T, Okazaki R, et al. Effect of 24,25(OH)$_2$D$_3$ on the formation and function of osteoclast. In: *Proceedings of the 9th International Workshop of Calcified Tissues. Trends in Calcified Tissue Research.* Jerusalem;1991:11.

61. Dranitzki-Elhalel M, Wald H, Popovtzer M, et al. 1,25(OH)$_2$D$_3$-induced calcium efflux from calvaria is mediated by protein Kinase C. *J Bone Miner Res.* 1999;14:1822–1827.

62. Dranitzki-Elhalel M, Wald H, Sprague SM, et al. The effect of 24,25 (OH)$_2$D$_3$ on calcium efflux in cultured bone: the role of protein Kinase C. *Nephrology.* 1998;4:157–162.

63. Wall RK, Baum CC, Sitrin MD, et al. 1,25(OH)$_2$D$_3$ stimulates membrane phosphoinositide turnover, activates PKC and increases cystolic calcium in rat colonic epithelium. *J Clin Invest.* 1990;85: 1296–1303.

64. Popovtzer MM, Robinette JB, DeLuca HF, et al. Acute effects of 25-hydroxy-cholecalciferol on renal handling of phosphorus: evidence for a parathyroid hormone dependent mechanism. *J Clin Invest.* 1974;53:913.

65. Wald H, Dranitzki-Elhalel M, Backenroth T, et al. Evidence for interference of vitamin D with PTH/PTHrP receptor expression in opossum kidney cells. *Pflugers Arch-Eur J Physiol.* 1998; 436:289–294.

66. Friedlaender MM, Wald H, Dranitzki-Elhalel M, et al. Vitamin D reduces renal NaPi-2 in PTH-infused rats: complexity of vitamin D action on renal handling of phosphate. *Am J Physiol Renal Physiol.* 2001;281:428–433.

67. Brautbar N, Walling MW, Coburn JW. Interactions between vitamin D deficiency and phosphorus depletion in the rat. *J Clin Invest.* 1979;64:335.

68. Puschett JB, Moranz J, Kurnick WS. Evidence for a direct action of cholecalciferol and 25-hydroxycholecalciferol on the renal transport of phosphate, sodium, and calcium. *J Clin Invest.* 1972;51:373.

69. Silver J, Naveh-Many T, Mayer H, et al. Regulation by vitamin D metabolites of parathyroid hormone gene transcription in vivo in the rat. *J Clin Invest.* 1986;78:1296–1301.

70. Lopez-Hilker S, Duso AS, Rapp NS, et al. Phosphorus restriction reverses hyperparathyroidism in uremia independent of changes in calcium and calcitriol. *Am J Physiol.* 1990;28:F432–F437.

71. Aparicio M, Combe C, Lafage MH, et al. In advanced renal failure dietary phosphate restriction reverses hyperparathyroidism independent of changes in the levels of calcitriol. *Nephron.* 1993; 63:122–123.

72. Fischer JA, Blum JW, Biswanger U. Acute parathyroid hormone response to epinephrine in vivo. *J Clin Invest.* 1973;52:2434.

73. Muff R, Fischer JA, Biber J, et al. Parathyroid hormone receptors in control of proximal tubule function. *Annu Rev Physiol.* 1992;54:67–79.

74. Goldring SR, Segre GV. Characterization of structural and functional properties of the cloned calcitonin and parathyroid hormone/parathyroid hormone related peptide receptors. *Ital J Miner Electrol Metab.* 1994;8:1–7.

75. Cole JA, Eber SL, Poelling RE, et al. A dual mechanism for regulation of kidney phosphate transport by parathyroid hormone. *Am J Physiol.* 1987;253:E221–E227.

76. Au WYW, Raisz LG. Restoration of parathyroid responsiveness in vitamin D-deficient rats by parenteral calcium or dietary lactose. *J Clin Invest.* 1967;46:1572.

77. Kruse K. Pathophysiology of calcium metabolism in children with vitamin D deficiency rickets. *J Pediatr.* 1995;126:736–741.

78. Sprague S, Popovtzer MM, Dranitzki-Elhalel M, et al. Parathyroid hormone induced calcium efflux from cultured calvaria is protein kinase C dependent. *Am J Physiol* 1996;271: F1139–F1146.

79. Amiel C, Huntziger H, Richet G. Micropuncture study of handling of phosphate by proximal and distal nephron in normal and parathyroidectomized rats: evidence for distal reabsorption. *Pflugers Arch.* 1970;317:93.

80. Weinman EJ, Biswas RJ, Peng Q, et al. Parathyroid hormone inhibits renal phosphate transport by phosphorylation of serine 77 of sodium hydrogen exchanger regulatory factor-1. *J Clin Invest.* 2007;117:3412–3420.

81. Talmage RV, Kraintz RW, Buchanan GD. Effect of parathyroid extract and phosphate salts on renal calcium and phosphate excretion after parathyroidectomy. *Proc Soc Exp Biol Med.* 1955;88:600.

82. Cha SK, Wu T, Huang CL. Protein Kinase C inhibits caveolae mediated endocytosis of TRPV5. *Am J Physiol Renal Physiol.* 2008;294: F1212–F1221.

83. Berson SA, Yalow RS. Immunochemical heterogeneity of parathyroid hormone in plasma. *J Clin Endocrinol Metab.* 1968;28:1037.

84. Copp DH, Cockeroft DW, Kueh Y. Calcitonin from ultimobranchial glands of dogfish and chickens. *Science.* 1967;158:924.

85. Zhong Y, Armbrecht HJ, Christakos S. Calcitonin a regulator of 25(OH)D-1-alpha hydroxylase gene. *J Biol Chem.* 2009;284:11059–11069.

86. Scriver CR. Rickets and the pathogenesis of impaired tubular transport of phosphate and other solutes. *Am J Med.* 1974;57:43.

87. Guise TA, Mundy GR. Clinical review 69: evaluation of hypocalcemia in children and adults. *J Clin Endocrinol Metab.* 1995;80:1473–1478.

88. Malluche HH, Goldstein DA, Massry SG. Osteomalacia and hyperparathyroid bone disease in patients with nephrotic syndrome. *J Clin Invest.* 1979;63:494.

89. Moncawa T, Yoshida T, Hayashi M, et al. Identification of 25(OH)D$_3$-1α–hydroxylase gene expression in macrophages. *Kidney Int.* 2000;58: 559–568.

90. Smith R. Asian rickets and osteomalacia (editorial). *Q J Med.* 1990;76:899–901.

91. Shikama N, Nusspaumer G, Hollander GA. Clearing the AIRE: on the pathophysiological basis of autoimmune polyendocrinopathy syndrome type I. *Endocrinol Metab Clin North Am.* 2009;38: 273–288.

92. Arnold A, Horst SA, Gardella TJ, et al. Mutation of the signal peptide-encoding region in pre-proparathyroid hormone gene in familial isolated hypoparathyroidism. *J Clin Invest.* 1990;86: 1084–1087.

93. Thakker RV, Davies KE, Whyte MP, et al. Mapping the gene causing X-linked recessive hypoparathyroidism to Xq26-Xq27 linkage studies. *J Clin Invest.* 1990;86:40–45.

94. Cuneo BF. 22q11.2 deletion syndrome: DiGeorge, velocardiofacial and conotruncal anomaly face syndromes. *Curr Opin Pediatr.* 2001;13:465–672.

95. Mizobuchi M, Ritter CS, Krits I, et al. Calcium sensing receptor expression regulator by glial cell missing-2 in human parathyroid cells. *J Bone Miner Res.* 2009;24(7):1173–1179 [Epub]

96. Kortazar D, Fanarroga ML, Cararrza G, et al. role of cofactor B (TBCB) and E (TBCE) in tubulin heterodimer dissociation. *Exp Cell Res.* 2007;313: 425–436.

97. Hirai H, Nakajimas S, Miyauchi A. A novel activating mutation in the calcium-sensing receptor in a Japanese family with autosomal dominant hypocalcemia. *J Hum Genet.* 2001;46:41–44.

98. Breslau NA, Moses AM, Pak CYC. Evidence for bone remodeling but lack of calcium mobilization response in parathyroid hormone in pseudohypoparathyroidism. *J Clin Endocrinol Metab.* 1983; 57:638.

99. Schipani E, Weinstein LS, Bergwitz C, et al. Pseudohypoparathyroidism type lb is not caused by mutations in the coding exons of the human parathyroid hormone (PTH)/PTH-related peptide receptor gene. *J Clin Endocrinol Metab.* 1995;80: 1611–1621.

100. Drezner M, Neelon FA, Lebovitz HE. Pseudohypoparathyroidism type II: a possible defect in the reception of cyclic AMP signal. *N Engl J Med.* 1973;289:1056.

101. Nusynowitz ML, Klein MH. Pseudoidiopathic hypoparathyroidism: hypoparathyroidism with ineffective parathyroid hormone. *Am J Med.* 1973; 55:677.

102. Sunthornthepvarakul T, Churisgaeus T, Ngowngarmratana S. A novel mutation of the signal peptide of the preproparathyroid gene associated with autosomal recessive familial isolated hypoparathyroidism. *J Clin Endocrinol Metab.* 1999;84:3792–3796.

103. Raskin P, McClain CJ, Medsger TA. Hypocalcemia associated with metastatic bone disease. *Arch Intern Med.* 1973;132:539.

104. Massry SG, Coburn JW, Lee DBN, et al. Skeletal resistance to parathyroid hormone in renal failure. Ann Intern Med. 1973;78:357.

105. Hauser CJ, Kamrath RO, Sparks J, et al. Calcium homeostasis in patients with acute pancreatitis. *Surgery.* 1983;94:830.

106. Fanconi G, Prader A. Transient congenital idiopathic hypoparathyroidism. *Helv Paediatr Acta.* 1967;22:342.

107. Fairney A, Jackson D, Clayton BE. Measurement of serum parathyroid hormone with particular reference to some infants with hypocalcemia. *Arch Dis Child.* 1973;48:419.

108. Rosen JF, Roginsky M, Nathenson G, et al. 25-Hydroxyvitamin D: plasma levels in mothers and their premature infants with neonatal hypocalcemia. *Am J Dis Child.* 1974;127:220.

109. Johnston CC, Lavy N, Lord T, et al. Osteopetrosis: a clinical, genetic, metabolic and morphologic study of the dominantly inherited, benign form. *Medicine (Balt).* 1968;47:149.

110. Tolar J, Teitelbaum SL, Orchard PJ. Osteopetrosis. *N Engl J Med.* 2004;351:2839–2840.

111. Key L, Carnes S, Cole S, et al. Treatment of congenital osteopetrosis with high-dose calcitriol. *N Engl J Med.* 1984;310:409.

112. Key LL, Rodriguiz RM, Willi SM, et al. Long-term treatment of osteopetrosis with recombinant human interferon gamma. *N Engl J Med.* 1995; 332:1594–1599.

113. Gessner BD, Beller M, Middaugh JL, et al. Acute fluoride poisoning from public water system. *N Engl J Med.* 1994;330:95–99.

114. Jacobson MA, Gambertoglio JG, Aweeka FT, et al. Foscarnet-induced hypocalcemia and effects of foscarnet on calcium metabolism. *J Clin Endocrinol Metab.* 1991;72:1130–1135.

115. McCarron DA. Low serum concentration of ionized calcium in patients with hypertension. *N Engl J Med.* 1982;307:226.

116. Minkin C. Inhibition of parathyroid hormone stimulated bone resorption in vitro by the antibiotic mithramycin. *Calcif Tissue Res.* 1973;13:249.

117. Robins PR, Jowsey J. Effect of mithramycin on normal and abnormal bone turnover. *J Lab Clin Med.* 1973;82:576.

118. Zivin JR, Gooley T, Zager RA, et al. Hypocalcemia: a pervasive metabolic abnormality in the critically ill. *Am J Kidney Dis.* 2001;37:689–698.

119. Gittes RF, Radde IC. Experimental model for hyperparathyroidism: effect of excessive numbers of transplanted isologous parathyroid glands. *J Urol.* 1966;95:595.

120. Lloyd HM. Primary hyperparathyroidism: an analysis of the role of the parathyroid tumor. *Medicine (Balt).* 1968;47:53.

121. Broadus AG, Horst RL, Lang R, et al. The importance of circulating $1,25(OH)_2$ vitamin D_3 in the pathogenesis of hypercalciuric and renal stone formation in primary hyperparathyroidism. *N Engl J Med.* 1980;302:421.

122. Krementz ET, Yeager R, Hawley W, et al. The first 100 cases of parathyroid tumor from Charity Hospital of Louisiana. *Ann Surg.* 1971;173:872.

123. Arnold A, Kim HG, Gaz RD, et al. Molecular cloning and chromosomal mapping of DNA rearranged within the parathyroid hormone gene in parathyroid adenoma. *J Clin Invest.* 1989;83: 2034–2040.

124. Arnold A, Brown MF, Urena P, et al. Monoclonality of parathyroid tumors in chronic renal failure and in primary parathyroid hyperplasia. *J Clin Invest.* 1995;95:2047–2053.

125. Hory B, Drueke TB. Menin and MEN-I gene: a model of tumor suppressor system. *Nephrol Dial Transplant.* 1998;13:2176–2179.

126. Marx SJ. Hyperparathyroid and hypoparathyroid disorders. *N Engl J Med.* 2000;343:1863–1875.

127. Consensus Development Conference Panel. Diagnosis and management of asymptomatic primary hyperparathyroidism. Consensus Development Conference statement. *Ann Intern Med.* 1991;114: 593–597.

128. Silverberg SJ, Shane E, Jacobs TP, et al. A 10-year prospective study of primary hyperparathyroidism

with or without surgery. *N Engl J Med.* 1999; 341:1249–1255.

129. Moosgaard B, Christensen SE, Vestergaard P, et al. Vitamin metabolism and skeletal consequences of primary hyperparathyroidism. *Clin Endocrinol (Oxf).* 2008;68:707–715.

130. Marx SJ, Spiegel AM, Levine ML, et al. Familial hypocalciuric hypercalcemia. *N Engl J Med.* 1982; 307:416.

131. Janicic N, Pansova Z, Cole DEC, et al. Insertion of ALU sequence in the Ca^{2+}- sensing receptor gene in familial hypocalciuric hypercalcemia and neonatal severe hyperparathyroidism. *Am J Hum Genet.* 1995;56:880–886.

132. Pallais JC, Kifor O, Chen YB, et al Acquired hypocalciuric hypercalcemia due to antibodies against calcium sensing receptor. *N Engl J Med.* 2004;351:362–369.

133. Broadus AE, Mangin M, Ikeda K, et al. Humoral hypercalcemia of cancer: identification of a novel parathyroid hormone-like peptide. *N Engl J Med.* 1988;319:556.

134. Yoshimoto K, Yamasaki R, Sakai H, et al. Ectopic production of parathyroid hormone by small cell lung cancer in a patient with hypercalcemia. *J Clin Endocrinol Metab.* 1989; 68:976–981.

135. Nusbaum SR, Gaz RD, Arnold A. Hypercalcemia and ectopic secretion of parathyroid hormone by an ovarian carcinoma with rearrangement of the gene for parathyroid hormone. *N Engl J Med.* 1990;323:1324–1329.

136. Vanthoven JN. Hypercalcemia of malignancy due to ectopic transactivation of PTH gene. *J Clin Endocrinol Metab.* 2006;91:580–583.

137. Bleizikian JP. Parathyroid hormone–related peptide in sickness and health. *N Engl J Med.* 1990;322:1151–1153.

138. Matsushita H, Hara M, Honda K, et al. Inhibition of parathyroid hormone–related protein release by extracellular calcium in dispersed cells from human parathyroid hyperplasia secondary to chronic renal failure and adenoma. *Am J Pathol.* 1995;146:1521–1528.

139. Cox M, Haddad JG. Lymphoma, hypercalcemia and the sunshine vitamin. *Ann Intern Med.* 1994;21:709–712.

140. Mundy GR. Hypercalcemia of malignancy revisited. *J Clin Invest.* 1988;82:1–6.

141. Chatopadhyay N. Effect of calcium sensing receptor on secretion of PTHrP and its impact on HHM. *Am J Physiol Endocrinol Metab.* 2006;290: E761–E770.

142. Walls J, Bundred N, Howell A. Hypercalcemia and bone resorption in malignancy. *Clin Orthop Relat Res.* 1995;312:51–63.

143. Houston SJ, Rubens RD. The systemic treatment of bone metastases. *Clin Orthop Relat Res.* 1995; 312:95–104.

144. Goltzman D. Osteolysis and cancer. *J Clin Invest.* 2001;107:1219–1220.

145. Mundy GR, Toshiyuki Y. Facilitation and suppression of bone metastasis. *Clin Orthop Relat Res.* 1995;312:34–44.

146. Orr FW, Sanchez-Sweatman OH, Kostenuik P, et al. Tumor-bone interactions in skeletal metastasis. *Clin Orthop Relat Res.* 1995;312:19–33.

147. Heath DJ, Chantry AD, Buckle CH. Antibodies inhibiting Dickkopf (DKK1) remove suppression of bone formation and prevent the development of osteolytic bone disease in multiple myeloma. *J Bone Miner Res.* 2009;24:425–436.

148. Beckman MJ, Johnson JA, Goff JL, et al. The role of dietary calcium in the physiology of vitamin D toxicity: excess dietary vitamin D_3 blunts parathyroid hormone induction of kidney 1-hydroxylase. *Arch Biochem Biophys.* 1995;319: 535–539.

149. Russell RM. The vitamin A spectrum from deficiency to toxicity. *Am J Clin Nutr.* 2000;71: 878–884.

150. Fisher G, Skillern PG. Hypercalcemia due to hypervitaminosis A. *JAMA.* 1974;227:1413.

151. Frame B, Jackson CE, Reynolds WA, et al. Hypercalcemia and skeletal effects in chronic hypervitaminosis A. *Ann Intern Med.* 1974;80:44.

152. Valentic JP, Elias AN, Weinstein GD. Hypercalcemia associated with oral isotretinoin in the treatment of severe acne. *JAMA.* 1983;250:1899.

153. Jowsey J, Riggs BL. Bone changes in a patient with hypervitaminosis A. *J Clin Endocrinol Metab.* 1968;28:1833.

154. Renier M, Sjurdsson G, Nunziata V, et al. Abnormal calcium metabolism in normocalcemic sarcoidosis. *Br Med J.* 1976;2:1473.

155. Myock RL, Bertrand P, Morrison CE, et al. Manifestations of sarcoidosis: analysis of 145 patients with review of nine series selected from literature. *Am J Med.* 1963;35:67.

156. Bell NH, Bartter FC. Transient reversal of hyperabsorption of calcium and of abnormal sensitivity to vitamin D in a patient with sarcoidosis during episode of nephritis. *Ann Intern Med.* 1964;61:702.

157. Anderson J, Dent CE, Harper C, et al. Effect of cortisone on calcium metabolism in sarcoidosis with hypercalcemia: possible antagonistic actions of cortisone and vitamin D. *Lancet.* 1954;2:720.

158. Bell NH, Stern PH, Pantzer E, et al. Evidence that increased circulating $1\alpha,25$-dihydroxyvitamin D is the probable cause for abnormal calcium metabolism in sarcoidosis. *J Clin Invest.* 1979;64:218.

159. Bleizikian JP. Management of acute hypercalcemia. *N Engl J Med.* 1992;326:1196–1203.

160. Adams JS, Sharma OP, Gacad MA, et al. Metabolism of 25-hydroxyvitamin D_3 by cultured pulmonary alveolar macrophages in sarcoidosis. *J Clin Invest.* 1983;72:1856.

161. Occasional survey: calcium metabolism and bone in hyperthyroidism. *Lancet.* 1970;2:1300.

162. Baxter JD, Bondy PK. Hypercalcemia of thyrotoxicosis. *Ann Intern Med.* 1966;65:429.

163. Adams P, Jowsey J. Bone and mineral metabolism in hyperthyroidism: an experimental study. *Endocrinology.* 1967;81:735.

164. Jorgensen H. Hypercalcemia in adrenocortical insufficiency. *Acta Med Scand.* 1973;193:175.

165. Pedersen KO. Hypercalcaemia in Addison's disease: report on 2 cases and review of literature. *Acta Med Scand.* 1967;181:691.

166. Lightwood R. Idiopathic hypercalcemia with failure to thrive. *Proc R Soc Med.* 1952;45:401.

167. O'Brien D. Idiopathic hypercalcaemia of infancy. *Pediatrics.* 1959;23:640.

168. Garabedian M, Jacoz E, Guillozo H, et al. Elevated plasma 1,25(OH)$_2$ vitamin D$_3$ concentration in infants with hypercalcemia and an elfin facies. *N Engl J Med.* 1985;312:948–952.

169. Dvorak MM, De Joussineau C, Carter DH, et al. Thiazide diuretics directly stimulate osteoblast differentiation and mineralized nodules formation. *J Am Soc Nephrol.* 2007;18: 2509–2516.

170. Kitakawa H, Fujiki R, Yoshimura K, et al. The chromatin remodeling complex WINAC targets a nuclear receptor to promoters and is impaired in Williams syndrome. *Cell.* 2003; 113:905–917.

171. Xiao A, Shechter D, Ahn SH, et al. WSTF regulates the H2A.X DNA damage response via novel tyrosine kinaseactivity. *Nature.* 2009;457:57–62.

172. Winters JL, Kleinschmidt AG, Frensili JJ, et al. Hypercalcemia complicating immobilization in treatment of fractures. *J Bone Joint Surg (Br).* 1966;48A:1182.

173. Russell RGG, Bisaz S, Donath A, et al. Inorganic pyrophosphate in plasma in normal persons and in patients with hypophosphatasia, osteogenesis imperfecta, and other disorders of bone. *J Clin Invest.* 1971;50:961.

174. McMillan DE, Freeman RB. The milk alkali syndrome: a study of the acute disorder with comments on the development of the chronic condition. *Medicine (Balt).* 1965;44:485.

175. Sevitt LH, Wrong OM. Hypercalcemia from calcium resin in patients with chronic renal failure. *Lancet.* 1968;2:950.

176. Chertow BS, Plymate SR, Becker FO. Vitamin D resistant idiopathic hypoparathyroidism: acute hypercalcemia during acute renal failure. *Arch Intern Med.* 1974;133:838.

177. deTorrente A, Berl T, Cohn PD, et al. Hypercalcemia of acute renal failure. *Am J Med.* 1976;61:119.

178. Parfitt AM. The interactions of thiazide diuretics with parathyroid hormone and vitamin D: studies in patients with hypoparathyroidism. *J Clin Invest.* 1972;51:1879.

179. Popovtzer MM, Subryan VL, Alfrey AC, et al. The acute effect of chlorothiazide on serum ionized calcium: evidence for a parathyroid hormone dependent mechanism. *J Clin Invest.* 1975;55:1295.

180. Anthony LB, May ME, Oates JA. Case report: lanreotide in the management of hypercalcemia of malignancy. *Am J Med Sci.* 1995;309:312–314.

181. Yoshida T, Monkawa T, Tenenhouse, et al. Two novel 1 alpha-hydroxylase mutations In French-Canadians with vitamin D dependency rickets type II. *Kidney Int.* 1998;54:1437–1443.

182. Griffin JE, Zerwekh JE. Impaired stimulation of 25(OH) vitamin D-24-hydroxylase in fibroblasts from a patient with vitamin D-dependent rickets type II: form of receptor positive resistance of 1,25-dihydroxyvitamin D$_3$. *J Clin Invest.* 1983; 72:1190.

183. Haussler MR, Haussler CA, Jurutka PWL. The vitamin D hormone and its nuclear receptor, molecular action and disease states. *J Endocrinol.* 1997;154(suppl):557–573.

184. Silver J, Popovtzer MM. Hypercalcemia with elevated dihydroxycholecalciferol levels and hypercalciuria. *Arch Intern Med.* 1984;194:162.

185. Malloy PJ, Hochberg Z, Tiosano D, et al. The molecular basis of hereditary 1,25(OH)$_2$ vitamin D3 resistant rickets in seven families. *J Clin Invest.* 1990;86:2071–2079.

186. Coxon FP, Roggers MJ. The role of prenylated small GTPase binding proteins in the regulation of osteoclast function. *Calcif Tissue Int.* 2003;72: 80–84.

187. Chen H, Hewison M, Adams JC. Functional characterization of heterogenous ribonuclear protein C1C2 in vitamin D resistance: a novel response element–binding protein. *J Biol Chem.* 2006;281: 39114–39120.

188. Popovtzer MM, Massry SG, Makoff DL, et al. Renal handling of phosphate in patients with chronic renal failure: the role of variations in serum phosphate and parathyroid activity. *Isr J Med Sci.* 1969;5:1018–1023.

189. Glorieux F, Scriver CR. Loss of parathyroid hormone sensitive component of phosphate transport in X-linked hypophosphatemia. *Science.* 1972;175:997.

190. Short EM, Binder HJ, Rosenberg LE. Familial hypophosphatemic rickets, defective transport of inorganic phosphate by intestinal mucosa. *Science.* 1973;179:700.

191. Marie PJ, Travers R, Glorieux FH. Healing of rickets with phosphate supplementation in the hypophosphatemic male mouse. *J Clin Invest.* 1981; 67:911.

192. Weidner N. Review and update: oncogenic osteomalacia-rickets. *Ultrastruct Pathol.* 1991;15: 317–333.

193. Popovtzer MM. Tumor-induced hypophosphatemic osteomalacia: evidence for a phosphaturic cyclic AMP independent action of tumor extract. *Clin Res.* 1981;29:418A.

194. Wilins GE, Granleese G, Hegele RG, et al. Oncogenic osteomalacia: evidence for a humoral phosphaturic factor. *J Clin Endocrinol Metab.* 1995;80: 1628–1634.

195. Cai Q, Hodgson SF, Kao PC, et al. Brief report: inhibition of renal phosphate transport by a tumor product in a patient with oncogenic osteomalacia. *N Engl J Med.* 1994;330:1645–1649.

196. Quarles LD. Endocrine function of bone in mineral metabolism regulation. *J Clin Invest.* 2008; 118:3820–3828.

197. Brownstein CA, Adler F, Nelson-Williams C, et al. A translocation causing increased alpha-Klotho results in hypophosphatemic rickets and hyperparathyroidism. *Proc Natl Acad Sci U S A.* 2008; 105:3455–3460.

198. Farrow EG, Davis SI, Summers LJ, et al. Initial FGF23-mediated signaling occurs in the distal convoluted tubule. *J Am Soc Nephrol.* 2009;20: 955–960.

199. Holm IA, Nelson AE, Robinson BG, et al. Mutational analysis and genotype-phenotype analysis correlation of the PHEX gene in X-linked hypophosphatemic rickets. *J Clin Endocrinol Metab.* 2001;86:3889–3899.

200. White KE, Carn G, Lorenz-Depiereux, et al. Autosomal-dominant hypophosphatemic rickets

(ADHR) mutations stabilize FGF-23. *Kidney Int.* 2001;60:2079–2086.

201. Tzenova JA, Frappier D, Crumley M, et al. Hereditary hypophosphatemic rickets with hypercalciuria is not caused by mutations in the Na/Pi cotransporter gene. *J Am Soc Nephrol.* 2001;12: 507–514.

202. Bergwitz C, Roslin NM, Tieder M, et al. SLC34A3 mutations in patients with hereditary hypophophatemic rickets with hypercalciuria predict a key role for sodium-phosphate cotransporter NaPi–II c in maintaining phosphate homeostasis *Am J Hum Genet.* 2006; 78:179–192.

203. Karim Z, Gerard B, Barkouh N, et al. NHERF1 mutations and responsiveness of renal parathyroid hormone. *N Engl J Med.* 2008;359: 1128–1135.

204. Jentsch TJ. Chloride transport in the kidney: lessons from human disease and knock out mice. *J Am Soc Nephrol.* 2005;16:1549–1561.

205. Marie PJ, Plettiform JM, Ross P, et al. Histological osteomalacia due to dietary calcium deficiency in children. *N Engl J Med.* 1982;307:584.

206. Fanconi G. Tubular insufficiency and renal dwarfism. *Arch Dis Child.* 1954;29:1.

207. Hossain M. The osteomalacia syndrome after colocystoplasty: a cure with sodium bicarbonate alone. *Br J Urol.* 1970;42:243.

208. Richard P, Chamberlain MJ, Wrong OM. Treatment of osteomalacia of renal tubular acidosis by sodium bicarbonate alone. *Lancet.* 1972;2:994.

209. Ott SM, Maloney NA, Coburn JW, et al. The prevalence of bone aluminum deposition in renal osteodystrophy and its relation to the response to calcitriol therapy. *N Engl J Med.* 1982;307:709.

210. Shike M, Sturtridge WC, Taur CS, et al. A possible role of vitamin D in the genesis of parenteral-nutrition-induced metabolic bone disease. *Ann Intern Med.* 1981;95:560.

211. Klein GL, Horst RL, Norman AW, et al. Reduced serum level of 1-alpha, 25-dihydroxyvitamin D during long-term total parenteral nutrition. *Ann Intern Med.* 1981;94:638.

212. Ott SM, Maloney NA, Klein GL, et al. Aluminum is associated with low bone formation in patients receiving parenteral nutrition. *Ann Intern Med.* 1983;98:910.

213. Chestnut CH. Theoretical overview: bone development, peak bone mass, bone loss and fracture risk. *Am J Med.* 1991;91:25–95.

214. Kohlmeier S, Marcus R. Calcium disorders of pregnancy. *Endocrinol Metab Clin North Am.* 1995; 24:15–39.

215. Manolagas SC, Jilka RL. Bone marrow, cytokines, and bone remodeling: emerging insights into the pathophysiology of osteoporosis. *N Engl J Med.* 1995;332:305–311.

216. Girasole G, Jilka RL, Passeri G, et al. 17β-Estradiol interleukin-6 production by bone marrow–derived stromal cells and osteoblasts in vitro: a potential mechanism for the anti-osteoporotic effect of estrogens. *J Clin Invest.* 1992;89:883–891.

217. Nelson NA, Qi JC, Tokita A, et al. Prediction of bone density from vitamin D receptor alleles. *Nature.* 1994;367:284–287.

218. Van Meurs JBJ, Bhonukshe RAM, Pluijm SMF, et al. Homocysteine levels and the risk of osteoporotic fractures. *N Engl J Med.* 2004;350: 2033–2041.

219. Spector TD, Keen RW, Arden NK, et al. Vitamin D receptor gene alleles and bone density in postmenopausal women: a UK twin study. *J Bone Miner Res.* 1994;9:S143.

220. Belchetz PE. Hormonal treatment of postmenopausal women. *N Engl J Med.* 1994;15: 1062–1071.

221. Rodan GA, Seedor JG, Balena R, et al. Preclinical pharmacology of alendronate. *Osteoporos Int.* 1993;3(suppl 3):S7–S12.

222. Carano A, Teitelbaum SL, Knosek JD, et al. Bisphosphonates directly inhibit the bone resorption activity in isolated avian osteoclasts in vitro. *J Clin Invest.* 1990;85:456–461.

223. Kleerekoper M. Osteoporosis and the primary care physician: time to bone up. *Ann Intern Med.* 1995;123:466–467.

224. Bone HG, Hosking D, Devogelaer J-P, et al. Ten years experience with alendronate for osteoporosis in postmenopausal women. *N Engl J Med.* 2004;350:1189–1199.

225. Ott S. New treatment for brittle bones. *Ann Intern Med.* 2004;141:406–407.

226. Weinstein RS, Robertson P, Manolgas SC. Giant osteoclast formation and long term oral bisphosphonate therapy. *N Engl J Med.* 2009; 360:53–62.

227. Pac CYC, Sakhaee K, Adams-Huet B, et al. Treatment of postmenopausal osteoporosis with slow-release sodium fluoride. *Ann Intern Med.* 1995; 123:401–408.

228. Popovtzer MM, Strejholm M, Huffer WE. Effects of alternating phosphorus and calcium infusions on osteoporosis. *Am J Med.* 1977; 81:478–484.

229. Levine MA. Primary hyperparathyroidism 7000 years in progress. *Cleve Clin J Med.* 2005;72: 1084–1098.

230. Liu SH, Chu HI. Studies of calcium and phosphorus metabolism with special reference to pathogenesis and effects of dihydrotachysterol (AT 10) and iron. *Medicine (Balt).* 1943;22:103.

231. Llach F. Secondary hyperparathyroidism in renal failure: the trade-off hypothesis revisited. *Am J Kidney Dis.* 1995;25:663–679.

232. Stanbury SW, Lumb GA. Metabolic studies on renal osteodystrophy. *Medicine (Balt).* 1962;41:1.

233. Korkor AB. Reduced binding of [^{3}H]-1,25(OH)$_2$D$_3$ in parathyroid glands of patients with renal failure. *N Engl J Med.* 1987;316:1573–1577.

234. Zoccali C. FGF-23 in dialysis patients : ready for prime time? *Nephrol Dial Transplant.* 2009;24: 1078–1081.

235. Gutierrez OM, Mannstadt M, Isakova T, et al. Fibroblast growth factor 23 and mortality among patients undergoing dialysis. *N Engl J Med.* 2008; 359:584–592.

236. Arnold A, Brown MF, Urena P, et al. Monoclonality of parathyroid tumors in chronic renal failure and in primary hyperparathyroid hyperplasia. *J Clin Invest.* 1995;95:2047–2053.

237. Popovtzer MM, Pinggera WF, Robinette JB. Successful conservative management of the

clinical consequences of uremic secondary hyperparathyroidism. *JAMA.* 1975;231:960.

238. Popovtzer MM, Pinggera WF, Hutt MP, et al. Serum parathyroid hormone levels and renal handling of phosphorus in patients with chronic renal disease. *J Clin Endocrinol Metab.* 1972; 35:213.

239. Slatopolsky E, Weerts C, Thielan J, et al. Marked suppression of secondary hyperparathyroidism by intravenous administration of 1,25(OH)$_2$ vitamin D$_3$ in uremic patients. *J Clin Invest.* 1984;74: 2136–2143.

240. Andress DL, Norris KC, Coburn JW, et al. Intravenous calcitriol in the treatment of refractory osteitis fibrosa in chronic renal failure. *N Engl J Med.* 1989;321:274–279.

241. Quarles LD, Yohay DA, Carroll BA, et al. Prospective trial of pulse oral versus intravenous calcitriol treatment of hyperparathyroidism in ESRD. *Kidney Int.* 1994;45:1710–1721.

242. National Kidney Foundation. K-DOQI clinical practice guidelines for bone metabolism and disease in chronic kidney disease. *Am J Kid Dis.* 2003;42(suppl 3):S1–S201.

243. Malluche HH, Mawad H, Moniere-Faugere M-C. Effects of treatment of renal osteodystrophy on bone histology. *Clin J Am Soc Nephrol.* 2008;3: S157–S163.

244. Popovtzer MM, Levi J, Bar-Khayim Y, et al. Assessment of combined 24,25(OH)$_2$D$_3$ and 1α(OH)D$_3$ therapy for bone disease in dialysis patients. *Bone.* 1992;13:369–377.

245. Andress DL, Maloney NA, Endres DB, et al. Aluminum-associated bone disease in chronic renal failure: high prevalence in a long term dialysis population. *J Bone Miner Res.* 1986;1: 391–398.

246. Hercz G, Pei Y, Greenwood C, et al. Aplastic osteodystrophy without aluminum: the role of "suppressed" parathyroid function. *Kidney Int.* 1993;44:860–866.

247. Goodman WG, Ramirez JA, Beilin TR, et al. Development of adynamic bone in patients with secondary hyperparathyroidism after intermittent calcitriol therapy. *Kidney Int.* 1944; 46:1160–1166.

248. Popovtzer MM, Backenroth-Maayan R, Elhalel-Dranitzki M, et al. Recurrence of tumoral calcinosis after kidney transplantation: evidence against an intrinsic defect of tubular phosphate reabsorption (abstract). *J Am Soc Nephrol.* 1995; 6:954.

249. Selye H. *Calciphylaxis.* Chicago: University of Chicago Press;1962.

250. Ahmed S, O'Neill KD, Hood AF, et al. Calciphylaxis is associated with hyperphosphatemia and increased osteopontin expression by vascular smooth muscle cells. *Am J Kidney Dis.* 2001;37: 1267–1276.

251. Schinke T, Karsenty G. Vascular calcification–a passive process in need of inhibitors. *Nephrol Dial Transplant.* 2000;15:1272–1274.

252. Goodman WG, Goldin J, Kuizon BD, et al. Coronary-artery calcification in young adults with end-stage renal disease who are undergoing dialysis. *N Engl J Med.* 2000;342:1478–1483.

253. Mazhar AR, Johnson RJ, Gillen D, et al. Risk factors and mortality associated with calciphylaxis in end-stage renal disease. *Kidney Int.* 2001; 60:324–332.

254. Sprague SM, Popovtzer MM. Is β_2-microglobulin a mediator of bone disease? *Kidney Int.* 1995; 47:1–6.

CHAPTER 7

Normal and Abnormal Magnesium Metabolism

DAVID M. SPIEGEL

M agnesium is the fourth most common cation in the human body, and it plays a critical role in many metabolic processes, including production and use of the energy essential in the maintenance of normal intracellular electrolyte composition. It is predominately an intracellular cation with less than 1% in the extracellular space (1). Owing to this distribution, total body magnesium concentrations are difficult to assess, and currently there is no simple accurate laboratory test to determine total body magnesium.

Magnesium is necessary for a large number of enzymatic actions relating to the basic protein-synthesizing mechanisms. Extracellular magnesium is broadly implicated in neuromuscular transmission and cardiovascular tone. Therefore, cellular and extracellular magnesium concentrations are carefully regulated by the gastrointestinal (GI) tract, kidney, and bone. In general, gastrointestinal losses and renal magnesium wasting constitute the major causes of magnesium deficiency and hypomagnesemia. Hypermagnesemia occurs with excessive magnesium administration, particularly when kidney function is reduced.

Normal Magnesium Metabolism

The average daily diet in North America contains approximately 20 to 30 mEq (240 to 360 mg) of elemental magnesium (2). The requirement for magnesium is considered to be about 18 to 33 mEq/day for young men and 15 to 28 mEq/day for women. This suggests that the average North American diet is only marginally adequate for maintenance of magnesium levels in healthy adults. Moreover, the requirements are higher during the rapid growth of infancy and adolescence as well as pregnancy and lactation. Magnesium is ubiquitous in our diet and is especially abundant in green vegetables rich in chlorophyll (a chelator of magnesium), as well as in seafood, grains, nuts, and meats (2). Under normal circumstances, the GI tract and kidney closely maintain magnesium balance (Fig. 7.1). It has been suggested that the minimum intake of magnesium required to maintain a positive balance in the body is approximately 0.3 mEq/kg/day.

Serum magnesium concentrations can be reported as mEq/L, mmol/L, or mg/dL. One mEq/L = 0.5 mmol/L and is approximately 1.2 mg/dL. Serum magnesium in healthy persons is closely maintained within a normal range that varies between laboratories but is roughly 1.50 to 2.3 mEq/L (0.75 to 1.15 mmol/L). Serum levels <1.5 mEq/L usually indicate magnesium deficiency. When serum magnesium is between 1.5 and 1.7 mEq/L, a magnesium loading test can identify magnesium deficiency (1). Only 20% of the serum magnesium is protein bound, in contrast to calcium, which is 40% bound to serum proteins. Therefore, variations of plasma protein concentration have less effect on serum magnesium than on calcium concentration.

Only about 1% to 2% of the 21 to 28 g (1,750 to 2,400 mEq) of magnesium present in the adult human body is in the extracellular fluid (ECF) compartment (3). The principal cellular stores of magnesium in the body are bone (67%) and muscle (20%) (Fig. 7.1). Normal muscle has 76 mEq of

---

In Memory of Allen Alfrey.

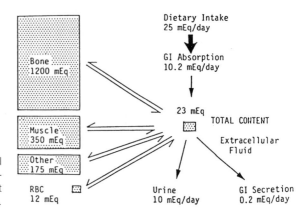

■ Figure 7.1 Schematic display of normal overall body homeostasis of magnesium, including an approximate distribution in different tissues. GI, gastrointestinal; RBC, red blood cells.

magnesium per kilogram of fat-free solids, and much of this is complexed to intracellular organic phosphate and proteins (3). The normal magnesium level in red blood cells is about 4.6 mEq/L, of which 84% is thought to be complexed to adenosine triphosphate (ATP). The magnesium content of erythrocytes appears to be inversely related to the age of the cell, with the reticulocytes containing about two times more magnesium than older red blood cells. As noted, bone is the principal body store of magnesium. The normal calcium to magnesium ratio in bone is 50:1, with the ratio in trabecular bone being consistently higher than that in cortical bone. The major portion of magnesium is complexed with apatite crystal rather than bone matrix. Approximately 30% of bone magnesium is present as a surface-limited ion on the bone crystal and is freely exchangeable (4,5). However, considerable uncertainty exists with regard to the ease of exchangeability of magnesium with its cellular source (4). Intracellular to extracellular distribution of magnesium is dissimilar to that of potassium. Minute changes in extracellular potassium rapidly result in changes in intracellular potassium concentration in muscle. Such shifts do not occur with magnesium because magnesium is bound to intracellular ligands and is not readily available for exchange in muscle. Less than 15% of muscle and erythrocyte magnesium is thought to be exchangeable (6).

In summary, bone and muscle cells are the major intracellular magnesium pools in humans, of which only a small fraction is exchangeable with the ECF.

Gastrointestinal Absorption of Magnesium

About 30% to 40% of the normal dietary intake of magnesium is absorbed by the GI tract. The fraction of magnesium absorbed may increase to as high as 80% when the dietary magnesium intake is restricted to as low as 2 mEq/day and may decrease to 25% at high magnesium intakes of ≥45 mEq/day. Thus, magnesium absorption by the gut is nonlinear and varies inversely with intake. Magnesium absorption in humans and animals occurs primarily in the more distal portion of the small intestine, namely the jejunum and ileum (7). The small intestinal magnesium absorption appears to occur down an electrochemical gradient through a paracellular pathway. In the colon transcellular absorption occurs. Magnesium crosses the brush border of the intestinal cell down an electrochemical gradient via the transient receptor potential melastatin 6 (TRPM6) channel (8). The mechanism for movement across the basolateral membrane has not been identified. The small intestinal paracellular pathway movement of magnesium occurs because of the positive magnesium chemical gradient across the paracellular channels. Magnesium absorption is also affected by paracellular water reabsorption. Bowel water absorption affects magnesium concentration and absorption, and severe prolonged diarrhea results in intestinal secretion of magnesium.

The control of intestinal magnesium absorption is not well understood. Most studies have suggested that vitamin D has little effect on magnesium absorption (9). A study carried out in vitamin D–deficient patients showed that magnesium absorption was only minimally reduced before vitamin D repletion, and even following repletion it was increased only slightly in contrast to the large change in calcium absorption (10). Similarly, Schmulen et al. (11) found that physiologic doses of 1,25-dihydroxyvitamin D_3 (1,25[OH]$_2$$D_3$) normalized the modest defect in jejunal magnesium absorption in uremic patients. This might imply that although vitamin D may have a small effect on proximal absorption of magnesium, it has little effect on the more distal sites for magnesium absorption in the small bowel. Unlike in the kidney, the basic absorptive systems of calcium and magnesium are independent of each other in the intestinal tract; calcium flux is normally twice that of the magnesium flux at similar luminal concentrations. It is probable that only ionized magnesium is available for absorption, and the amount available is affected by progressive precipitation of magnesium as insoluble phosphates, carbonates, and soaps beginning in the ileum, colon, and (ultimately) stool. Alterations of luminal concentrations of calcium and phosphate also indirectly affect magnesium absorption. Conversely, the elevation of intraluminal magnesium concentration may precipitate phosphate and thereby allow for greater calcium absorption. Steatorrhea may potentiate magnesium malabsorption through formation of nonabsorbable magnesium lipid salts (12).

The major portion of magnesium found in the stool is derived from the diet. The magnesium concentration in saliva, gastric secretions, bile, and pancreatic and intestinal secretions ranges from 0.3 to 0.7 mmol and amounts to only about 1% of the daily fecal output. Taken together, overall knowledge of the precise control and regulation of magnesium absorption in the intestinal tract is still lacking.

Renal Excretion of Magnesium

The status of body magnesium balance and particularly ECF magnesium concentration is largely determined by the renal excretion of magnesium. On a normal dietary intake of magnesium, urinary magnesium excretion averages 100 to 150 mg/day or 8 to 12 mEq/day. In patients receiving supplementary oral magnesium-containing antacids, urinary magnesium excretion can increase to 500 to 600 mg/day or more with little change in serum magnesium levels. Similarly, when dietary magnesium restrictions are imposed, 24-hour urinary magnesium excretion decreases in 4 to 6 days to as low as 10 to 12 mg (1 mEq) (13). Thus, the ability of the kidney to conserve magnesium is excellent when it is needed. In chronic kidney disease the fractional excretion of magnesium rises sharply as glomerular filtration rate (GFR) progressively falls, thus protecting against the development of significant hypermagnesemia. Urinary magnesium excretion can approximate the filtered load of magnesium with marked hypermagnesemia secondary to high dietary intake or intravenous magnesium infusion. Studies in several species have shown that there is a threshold value for magnesium excretion, close to the normal magnesium concentration (14). Thus, when serum magnesium concentration falls slightly, urinary magnesium excretion rapidly decreases to very low values. Conversely, when serum magnesium rises slightly above normal, magnesium excretion rapidly increases.

Seventy to eighty percent of plasma magnesium is freely filtered at the glomerulus, and only 20% to 30% of the filtered magnesium is reabsorbed in the proximal tubule. Luminal magnesium concentrations rise along the length of the proximal convoluted tubule to a value as high as 1.5 times greater than that of the ultrafiltrable magnesium in glomerular filtrate (Fig. 7.2) (15). The major influence on proximal magnesium reabsorption is the status of the ECF volume. Absorption is enhanced in states of volume depletion, whereas absorption is decreased in volume-expanded states.

Our knowledge of renal magnesium transport has increased dramatically due to the discovery of the molecules involved in renal magnesium handling from the study of rare human genetic conditions. The early micropuncture studies of Morel et al. (15) indicated that, unlike most cations, the loop of Henle is the major site of magnesium reabsorption. Magnesium concentration in the early distal tubule fluid is only 60% to 70% of the ultrafiltrable magnesium concentration, suggesting that some 50% to 60% of the filtered magnesium is reabsorbed in the loop of Henle, primarily in the thick ascending limb (Fig. 7.2). Magnesium absorption in the loop of Henle is passive via a paracellular pathway and dependent on the transepithelial voltage gradient partly generated by a sodium back-leak into the lumen via the paracellular protein claudin 16 (16) (Fig. 7.3). In hypermagnesemic states, magnesium reabsorption in the loop of Henle approaches zero (17). Conversely, in hypomagnesemic states, the loop of Henle more avidly reabsorbs magnesium, allowing only minimal amounts, <3%, of the filtered load to reach the distal tubules and be excreted in the urine (18).

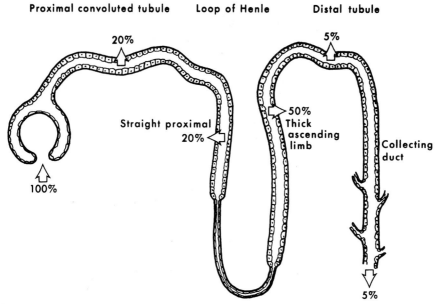

■ Figure 7.2 Normal distribution of magnesium reabsorption as a percentage of the ultrafiltrable magnesium at the glomerulus.

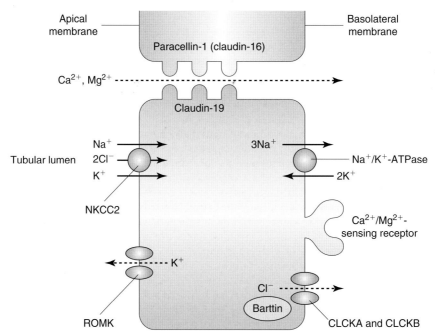

■ Figure 7.3 A model of magnesium transport mechanisms in the TAL. Magnesium absorption is paracellular, driven by the electrochemical gradient partly generated by claudin-16. The Ca/Mg sensing receptor also plays a role in magnesium absorption.

An important interaction between calcium and magnesium has been observed in the thick ascending limb. It is well known that hypercalcemia (17) or hypermagnesemia inhibits both magnesium and calcium reabsorption (19,20). Studies show that this effect is mediated by the calcium-sensing receptor present on the basolateral membrane of the thick ascending limb and distal collecting tubule, which modulates absorption by changes in plasma divalent cation concentrations (21,22).

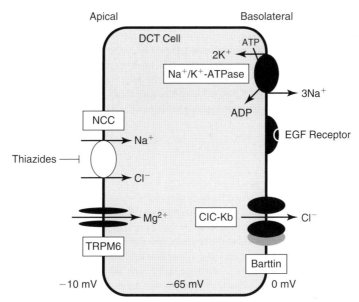

■ **Figure 7.4** A model of magnesium transport mechanisms in the DCT. Magnesium absorption is transcellular via the recently identified magnesium channel TRPM6 in the apical membrane. The link between the defect in the apical thiazide-sensitive NCC seen in Gitleman syndrome or the basolateral Cl⁻ channel (ClC-Kb) defect seen in Bartter syndrome with sensorineural deafness have not been identified. The basolateral EGF receptor that modulates the apical TRPM6 magnesium channel is also depicted. NCC, NaCl cotransporter; DCT, distal convoluted tubule.

In the distal convoluted tubule, fine-tuning of magnesium reabsorption occurs. Magnesium transport in the distal tubule is active and transcellular, with reabsorption occurring via an apical transient receptor potential channel, melastatin subtype 6 (TRPM6) (16,23) (Fig. 7.4). The mechanisms for cytoplasmic diffusion and basolateral transport are not yet known (24). Sex hormones, acid–base status, and peptide hormones such as calcitonin, glucagon, arginine, vasopressin, and parathyroid hormone enhance magnesium uptake in distal convoluted tubule cells (21,24,25) possibly via modulation of TRPM6. Recently, epidermal growth factor (EGF) has been demonstrated to be a magnesiotropic hormone directly stimulating TRPM6 activity (26). This explains the finding that magnesium wasting occurs in patients with colorectal cancer who are treated with cetuximab, an EGF receptor (EGFR)-targeted monoclonal antibody, that prevents receptor stimulation (27). Furthermore, both tacrolimus and cyclosporine A decrease TRPM6 expression, possibly explaining the hypomagnesemia seen in patients treated with these medications (23).

Physiologic and Pharmacologic Effects

Magnesium plays a critical and necessary role in intracellular metabolism. Magnesium is necessary for a wide spectrum of enzymatic reactions, including various phosphokinases and phosphatases (28), which are involved in energy storage and use. Phosphatases are particularly important because magnesium functions primarily to form magnesium ATP, which is a substrate for these enzymes. These ion-sensitive ATPases are situated in the intracellular compartments and membranes to regulate the flow of potential energy from the mitochondria and cytoplasm. Recognized magnesium ATPases include ouabain-sensitive $Mg^{2+}/Na^{+}/K^{+}$ATPase, ouabain-insensitive Mg^{2+}, $HHCO_3$ATPase, and Mg^{2+}/Ca^{2+}ATPase, which are associated with the sodium, proton, and calcium pumps, respectively. They are all essential for ionic control of the cell composition (29). Magnesium also is involved in protein synthesis through its action on nucleic acid polymerization, its role in ribosomal binding to ribonucleic acid (RNA), and in the synthesis and degradation of deoxyribonucleic acid (DNA). In addition to its role in phosphorylation of glucose, magnesium may also control mitochondrial oxidative metabolism (30). Adenylate cyclase, critical in the generation of the intracellular secondary messenger $3',5'$ cyclic adenosine monophosphate (cAMP), also has been shown to be dependent on magnesium (31). Intracellular magnesium has also been shown to have an important regulatory function on both K^+ and Ca^{2+} channels (32).

Intracellular magnesium is found in the free-ion form or complexed to proteins or organophosphates. The free-magnesium concentration determines the effect of concentrations of the high-energy nucleotide complex magnesium ATP. Knowledge of the true ionic concentration of magnesium in the cell is important but difficult to measure. It is thought that only about 5% to 15% of cellular magnesium is truly ionized (33).

Magnesium Deficiency

Because magnesium is an essential element for both plants and animals, it exists almost everywhere in our environment. Thus, it is rare to see spontaneous magnesium depletion from dietary indiscretion unless it is severe. Still, it has been suggested that the normal dietary intake of magnesium is marginal.

The first description of symptoms related to hypomagnesemia was in 1960 when Vallee et al. (34) described five patients with hypomagnesemia and symptoms and signs that are now felt to be classic for magnesium depletion. These patients had carpopedal spasms with positive Chvostek and Trousseau signs, and three of the five subjects also had convulsions. All patients' symptoms and signs abated following magnesium administration. Several investigators have attempted to produce magnesium depletion in humans by placing subjects on a low magnesium intake. In most studies, only minimal magnesium depletion has been induced. Shils (35), however, was able to cause severe magnesium depletion in seven patients who were placed on diets extremely low in magnesium for an extended period of time. Symptoms that appeared to be related to magnesium depletion developed in six of the seven patients; five had a positive Trousseau sign, and two of these patients also had a positive Chvostek sign. All patients became lethargic and showed generalized weakness, anorexia, nausea, and apathy. Biochemical abnormalities included hypomagnesemia, hypocalcemia, hypokalemia, and decreased total body exchangeable potassium. All abnormalities reverted to normal with replacement of magnesium alone.

Clinical Conditions Associated with Magnesium Depletion

DEFECTIVE GASTROINTESTINAL ABSORPTION OF MAGNESIUM

Gastrointestinal causes of magnesium depletion can be divided into four categories: decreased intake, steatorrheic states, severe diarrheal states, and selective magnesium malabsorption (Table 7.1). Caddell and Goddard (36) found serum magnesium to be subnormal in 19 of 28 children with protein calorie malnutrition (kwashiorkor). This was felt to have resulted from the combination of poor intake of magnesium, vomiting, and diarrhea. Similarly, magnesium depletion has been described in hospitalized patients who have been maintained on parenteral nutrition for prolonged periods of time (37,38).

Steatorrheic State

Hypomagnesemia has been described in a number of patients with small-bowel disease. Booth et al. (12) found that 15 of 42 patients with malabsorption syndromes had subnormal serum magnesium levels. They were able to show a rough correlation between serum magnesium levels and the degree of steatorrhea, suggesting that the magnesium malabsorption might be a consequence of the formation of insoluble magnesium soaps. Supporting this possibility is the finding that magnesium absorption was improved when the patients were placed on a low-fat diet. The small-bowel diseases with the highest incidence of hypomagnesemia are idiopathic steatorrhea and disease of the distal ileum.

Diarrheal States

Besides the steatorrheic states, magnesium depletion can occur in any severe diarrheal state (39,40). As with potassium, fecal magnesium excretion is related to the total water content where the stool

TABLE 7.1 CAUSES OF HYPOMAGNESEMIA

Gastrointestinal

Inadequate intake

Steatorrheic states

Severe diarrhea

Hypomagnesemia with secondary hypocalcemia (HSH) (renal defect also exists)

Renal

 Intrinsic

  Inherited disorders

   Familial hypomagnesemia with hypercalciuria and nephrocalcinosis (FHHNC)

   Autosomal-dominant hypomagnesemia with hypocalciuria

   Hypomagnesemia with secondary hypocalcemia (HSH) (main defect may be GI)

   Autosomal-dominant hypocalcemia (ADH)

   Isolated recessive hypocalcemia (IRH)

   Gitelman syndrome

   Bartter syndrome

  Acquired disorders

   Aminoglycosides

   Cis-diaminedichloro platinum

   Cyclosporine/Tacrolimus

   Pentamidine

   Foscarnet

   Amphotericin B

   Cetuximab

 Extrinsic (intrarenal)

  Volume expansion

  Hypercalciuria

  Sodium loads

  Diabetic ketoacidosis

  Diuretics

  Hyperaldosteronism

  Antidiuretic hormone secretion syndrome

Miscellaneous

Alcoholism

Thyrotoxicosis

Burns

Hungry bone syndrome

magnesium concentration is approximately 6 mEq/L (40). Magnesium depletion also has been described in patients following jejunoileal bypass surgery for the treatment of morbid obesity, probably from a combination of factors, including malabsorption, shortened transit time, and diarrhea (41).

Hereditary Magnesium Absorptive Defect

Several patients have been described who have a defect in the GI absorption of magnesium (42–44). In this disorder of hypomagnesemia with secondary hypocalcemia (HSH), profound hypomagnesemia develops in the first few months of life. The absorptive defect can be overcome, however, by high-dose oral intake of magnesium. Most of these patients have severe hypomagnesemia, hypocalcemia, tetany, and seizures. The defect is an autosomal recessive disorder and results in the failure of active transcellular magnesium absorption. It is due to a mutation in the *TRPM6* gene, which encodes for the apical membrane TRPM6 channel in the intestine and the distal convoluted tubule (45,46).

RENAL MAGNESIUM WASTING

Renal magnesium wasting can be of two distinct types. One represents a primary kidney defect, whereas the second represents the kidney's normal response to a variety of systemic and local factors that increase magnesium losses (Table 7.1). Symptomatic hypomagnesemia is much more likely to be seen in the state of primary renal magnesium wasting. The hallmark of both of these states is a disproportionately elevated urinary magnesium excretion in association with hypomagnesemia. Normally, when serum magnesium falls only slightly owing to extrarenal causes, urinary magnesium falls to <1 mEq/day (12 mg/day), whereas if the kidney is responsible for the magnesium losses, urinary magnesium is increased relative to the hypomagnesemic state (>4 mEq/day). Thus, urinary magnesium should be measured before magnesium replacement to determine whether the hypomagnesemic state resulted from renal or extrarenal causes.

Primary Renal Magnesium Wasting

Primary renal magnesium wasting can occur from either inherited or acquired causes. A number of inherited forms of renal magnesium wasting have been described recently. The most severe form of renal magnesium wasting results from an impairment of tubular reabsorption of magnesium and calcium in the thick ascending limb of Henle's loop (47,48). This autosomal recessive disorder known as familial hypomagnesmia with hypercalciuria and nephrocalcinosis (FHHNC) (8) results from mutations in the *CLDN16* gene, which encodes the renal tight junction protein claudin-16 (formally paracellin-1) (Fig. 7.3). This protein is thought to allow selective back-leak of sodium over chloride into the tubule lumen, enhancing the driving force for paracellular magnesium reabsorption (8). Clinical and laboratory features of FHHNC include presentation at a young age with nephrocalcinosis, polyuria, chronic kidney disease, hypomagnesemia, and increased urinary magnesium and calcium excretion. Hypomagnesemia is unresponsive to magnesium replacement, and progression to end-stage renal disease is common.

An autosomal dominate disorder of hypomagnesemia with hypocalcemia has been linked to a heterozygous mutation of FXYD2 on chromosome 11q23. (49). This encodes for a γ subunit of the basolateral Na^+/K^+ ATPase. The mutation results in misrouting of this subunit and defective magnesium reabsorption in the distal convoluted tubule where this subunit is normally expressed in the basolateral membrane (50) (Fig. 7.4).

Isolated recessive hypomagnesemia (IRH) is a rare disorder due to a mutation of the EGF precursor protein. EGF is a magnesiotropic hormone that stimulates TRPM6, an apical magnesium channel in the distal convoluted tubule. The defect in this gene results in decreased TRPM6–mediated apical magnesium uptake in the distal convoluted tubule and magnesium wasting (16,26) (Fig. 7.4).

Activating mutations in the calcium-sensing receptor located in the parathyroid chief cell and basolateral membrane of the thick ascending limb of the loop of Henle and distal convoluted tubule results in autosomal dominate hypocalcemia (ADH). The defect results in decreased kidney calcium and magnesium reabsorption and often hypomagnesemia (51).

Gitelman syndrome is caused by a heterogeneous group of loss-of-function mutations usually in the solute carrier family 12, member 3 gene, *SLC12A3*, which encodes the thiazide-sensitive NaCl cotransporter (NCC) (52) (Fig. 7.3). In a minority of patients the mutation is in the *CLCNKB* gene encoding the chloride channel CID-Kb, the same gene mutation defect found in Bartter syndrome with sensorineural deafness suggesting a highly variable phenotype in patients with *CLCNKB* mutations (52). Gitelman syndrome is an autosomal recessive heritable kidney disease characterized by hypomagnesemia, hypocalciuria, and hypokalemia metabolic alkalosis. This syndrome occurs in an older age group and usually has mild clinical symptoms, although patients may complain of musculoskeletal cramps, muscle weakness, muscle stiffness, arthralgias, nocturia, polydipsia, and thirst (51,52). The mechanism for the moderate renal magnesium wasting in Gitelman syndrome has not been definitively characterized (53) but may relate to reduced abundance of the TRPM6 epithelial magnesium channels in the distal convoluted tubule (54). Bartter syndrome, a defect in the chloride channel of the thick ascending limb cells, also may be associated with mild hypomagnesemia. In contrast to Gitelman syndrome, it occurs at a younger age, has profound clinical symptoms, and is associated with renal calcium wasting (53).

The acquired forms of renal magnesium wasting are largely drug induced. Renal magnesium wasting has been well documented in a number of patients receiving aminoglycosides (55,56). Renal magnesium wasting also has been described in patients receiving *cis*-diaminedichloro platinum (*cis*-DDP) (57). In one series, 23 of 44 patients treated with *cis*-DDP developed hypomagnesemia. Two of these patients required hospitalization because of severe symptomatic magnesium depletion. In an additional report of 50 patients treated with multiple courses of combined chemotherapy with *cis*-DDP, 76% developed hypomagnesemia (58). This defect in renal magnesium handling can persist for months after the *cis*-DDP has been discontinued (57,58). The calcinurin inhibitors, cyclosporine and tacrolimus, are drugs that commonly cause hypomagnesemia (59) possibly by decreasing TRPM6 expression, resulting in renal magnesium wasting (23). In contrast to other hypomagnesemic states, which are usually accompanied by hypokalemia, cyclosporine/tacrolimus-induced hypomagnesemia usually is associated with either normokalemia or hyperkalemia at times (59). The hypomagnesemia rapidly abates on discontinuation of these drugs. Renal magnesium wasting has been described in patients with acquired immunodeficiency syndrome undergoing treatment with pentamidine for *Pneumocystis carinii* pneumonia (60). Symptomatic hypomagnesemia can develop up to 2 weeks after cessation of therapy with this agent. In addition, hypomagnesemia has been reported in patients receiving foscarnet, an antiviral agent used to treat cytomegalovirus disease (61), and amphotericin B treatment of fungi infection (62). Magnesium wasting occurs in patients with colorectal cancer who are treated with cetuximab, an EGFR-targeted monoclonal antibody that prevents receptor stimulation (63). As EGF has been demonstrated to be a magnesiotropic hormone directly stimulating TRPM6 activity, blockade of this receptor simulation results in magnesium wasting (26).

Secondary Forms of Renal Magnesium Wasting

Tubular reabsorption of magnesium is linked to a variety of other cations. Both sodium and calcium infusions can markedly increase urinary magnesium (64). Usually because of the modest nature and short duration of infusions, magnesium depletion does not develop. However, hypomagnesemia may develop when large saline infusions are given in association with diuretics, as are used in the treatment of hypercalcemia. Any chronic hypercalciuric state, such as seen with vitamin D therapy, also can cause magnesium wasting (65,66).

Virtually all diuretics, with the exception of acetazolamide, can increase magnesium excretion but only modestly, and magnesium supplementation usually is not required.

Hypomagnesemia secondary to starvation was first recognized during World War II (67). Jones et al. (68) subsequently showed that patients undergoing total starvation had an average magnesium loss of 10 mEq/day in their urine and suggested that ketoacidosis was responsible for this loss. Similarly, in patients with untreated diabetic ketoacidosis, there is marked renal magnesium wasting in the acidotic period as well as during early treatment (69). Following insulin and fluid therapy, serum magnesium may fall precipitously and tetany may occur (69,70). Phosphate replacement therapy in patients with diabetic ketoacidosis also has been associated with the induction of hypomagnesemia (71). In view of these findings, some (69,70) have suggested that in addition to the other cations commonly given, magnesium replacement should be included in the management of diabetic ketoacidosis. However, the American Diabetic Association recommends magnesium supplementation only in those patients who have documented hypomagnesemia (72).

Increased urinary magnesium excretion also has been reported with primary and secondary hyperaldosteronism (73,74) and inappropriate secretion of antidiuretic hormone (75). The renal magnesium wasting in these settings, however, is usually not severe enough to cause clinically significant magnesium depletion.

MISCELLANEOUS CAUSES OF HYPOMAGNESEMIA

Hypomagnesemia has been a common finding in patients with chronic alcoholism (76). Ethanol has been shown to increase urinary magnesium excretion acutely (77,78); however, this occurs only when the blood alcohol levels are rising. Furthermore, Dunn and Walser (79) showed that alcohol does not increase urinary magnesium excretion in patients maintained on a low-magnesium diet. Thus, it appears that alcohol-induced renal magnesium wasting is probably not the major mechanism responsible for magnesium depletion. A very important cause for the magnesium depletion in alcoholic patients may be the profound reduction in dietary intake of this cation. In view of the frequency with which hypophosphatemia is associated with hypomagnesemia in alcoholic patients, it seems possible that the magnesium depletion is in part a result of phosphate depletion. A number of investigators have reported increased urinary magnesium excretion in rats (80), dogs (81), and humans (82) during phosphorus depletion, although the mechanism of this phenomenon has not been defined.

Hypomagnesemia also has been observed in patients with hyperthyroidism (83,84). This hypomagnesemic state is associated with an increased exchangeable magnesium pool, suggesting that thyroid hormone has a direct stimulatory effect on the transport of magnesium into cells. The degree of hypomagnesemia has been correlated with the severity of the hyperthyroid state, with the lowest values found in apathetic thyrotoxicosis (84).

Hypomagnesemia also has been described in patients with severe burns. This probably results from a combination of factors, including lack of oral intake and losses through the denuded skin (85).

Following parathyroidectomy, especially in patients with severe bone disease, serum magnesium may fall to subnormal levels (86). The most apparent reason for this reduction in the serum magnesium concentration is the rapid deposition of magnesium in the newly formed bone salts.

NEONATAL HYPOMAGNESEMIA

Hypomagnesemia can occur in infants as well. Normally, there is a magnesium gradient between the blood of the mother and fetus, with magnesium being slightly higher in fetal blood. However, this gradient is not great enough to protect the fetus if the mother is magnesium depleted (87). Hypomagnesemia has been described in newborns whose mothers have had malabsorption syndromes, have chronically ingested stool softeners, or have had hyperparathyroidism (88). In a series of 20 children with magnesium depletion, the most common cause was the repeated passage of watery stools regardless of the specific cause (89). A contributory factor was felt to be starvation, which was present in these children. In addition, hypomagnesemia has occurred in association with exchange transfusions, neonatal hepatitis, and polycythemia in infancy (90). Offspring of diabetic mothers also have been reported to have hypomagnesemia (91).

Clinical Consequences of Magnesium Depletion

With the development of atomic absorption spectrophotometry, which made possible the accurate determination of plasma magnesium levels in hospital laboratories, it became apparent that hypomagnesemia is not an uncommon finding, especially in some hospital populations. Patients may have severe hypomagnesemia in the absence of any recognizable symptoms. When symptoms do occur, they are largely confined to the neuromuscular system. These symptoms include weakness, muscle fasciculation, tremors, and positive Chvostek and Trousseau signs. Generalized tetany occasionally may occur (34,35). The mechanism responsible for the development of tetany is poorly understood, but it is clear that tetany can occur in the absence of either hypocalcemia or alkalosis. A decreased concentration of either magnesium or calcium lowers the threshold to stimulation of a nerve, with resulting increased irritability (92,93). However, their effects are antagonistic in muscle. A low concentration of magnesium enhances muscle contraction, whereas a low concentration of calcium inhibits it (94). Studies suggest that the ECF magnesium depletion may increase acetylcholine action at the nerve ending, which then lowers the threshold of the muscle membrane (34).

In addition to the symptoms mentioned, patients with magnesium depletion also may have disturbances of the central nervous system, manifested by marked changes in personality, including excessive anxiety and, at times, delirium and frank psychosis (95).

The clinical importance of reduced tissue stores of magnesium is much less clear, although it is well recognized that hypomagnesemia can be associated with clinical symptomatology. Intracellular magnesium depletion with its effect on intracellular potassium may have an adverse effect on myocardial function and its electrophysiologic response.

Biochemical Consequences of Magnesium Depletion

The earliest biochemical alteration during magnesium depletion is a fall in serum magnesium concentration. In growing animals, serum magnesium falls during the first day the animal is on a magnesium-deficient diet (96). Even humans have been shown to have a significant reduction in serum magnesium concentration within 5 to 7 days after being placed on a diet deficient in magnesium (13).

Erythrocyte magnesium concentration also has been measured during experimentally induced magnesium depletion in humans and has been found to fall but less rapidly than the plasma magnesium concentration. Because factors other than the status of the body magnesium stores, such as erythrocyte age, also influence erythrocyte magnesium concentration, this determination cannot be used as a valid index of the body magnesium content (97).

A more uniform correlation between total body magnesium and bone magnesium concentration has been found. In almost every study in which bone magnesium concentration has been measured during magnesium depletion, it has been found to be decreased (4,5). The surface limited magnesium pool on bone seems to be readily available during magnesium depletion and is rapidly used to replace other body magnesium deficits. In addition, bone magnesium concentration has been shown to strongly correlate with serum magnesium levels in normal, magnesium-deficient, and magnesium-overloaded animals and human subjects (Fig. 7.3) (4,5).

In contrast to bone, there is a poor correlation between plasma magnesium levels and muscle and cardiac magnesium levels (4). However, a reasonably good correlation has been found between mononuclear blood cell magnesium and muscle and heart magnesium (98). Most confusion regarding evaluation of the status of the body magnesium resides around the measurement of muscle magnesium concentrations. Muscle magnesium has been found to be decreased in magnesium-depleted animals (99) but to a lesser extent than bone magnesium. In addition, in a variety of conditions, muscle magnesium has been found to be reduced in association with normal or even increased plasma and bone magnesium levels (4,100,101). There is a close interrelationship between muscle potassium and magnesium levels. During magnesium depletion, in association with the fall in muscle magnesium, there is also a decrease in muscle potassium concentration (4,102).

This change in muscle potassium during magnesium depletion may result from an inability of the muscle to maintain an appropriate gradient for potassium, possibly as a consequence of reduced magnesium-dependent Na^+/K^+ ATPase activity and magnesium's effect on potassium channels (103). A number of investigators have shown that muscle magnesium and potassium concentrations are affected similarly and to a larger extent in primary potassium depletion (4,102) and malnutrition (104), showing that these changes in muscle cation composition are not necessarily characteristic of primary magnesium depletion. It has been found that muscle magnesium falls 0.5 mmol for every 10 mmol fall in muscle potassium during potassium depletion (4). A similar relationship between these two ions exists in the myocardium (105). Because muscle potassium is readily exchangeable and reflects total body potassium, the most likely cause for the reported reduced muscle magnesium levels in patients with a variety of clinical disorders who have normal plasma magnesium levels (100,101) appears to be primary potassium depletion with secondary muscle magnesium depletion.

Therefore, bone and ECF magnesium are the available magnesium pools used to replenish soft-tissue magnesium deficits during magnesium depletion. Furthermore, serum magnesium concentration, not muscle, best reflects bone magnesium content and can be used as an indicator of total body magnesium stores.

Besides the measurement of magnesium concentration in biologic tissues and fluids, the retention of magnesium following an acute intravenous infusion of magnesium also has been used to estimate the status of the body magnesium stores. Normal individuals in magnesium balance excrete the majority of a systemically administered magnesium load in 24 to 48 hours. In contrast, individuals with magnesium deficits retain a significant fraction of the injected magnesium (98,106).

Effect of Magnesium on Calcium Metabolism

Severe magnesium depletion has been found to alter calcium metabolism significantly in animals as well as humans. Studies in cattle (107), sheep (108), pigs (109), dogs (110), monkeys (111), rats (112), and humans (35) have shown that severe magnesium depletion is associated with hypocalcemia in all these species. Subsequently, calcium balance studies in animals, as well as humans, have shown that with the development of hypocalcemia during magnesium depletion, external calcium balances remain unchanged or actually become more positive. Thus, the hypocalcemia results from alterations in internal control mechanisms for calcium. The interrelationship between magnesium and parathyroid hormone (PTH) is quite complex. Acutely, magnesium appears to have a direct effect on PTH secretion (113). Perfusion studies of goat and sheep parathyroid glands have shown that low magnesium concentration acutely stimulates the release of PTH. In vitro studies (114) showed a first-order relationship between PTH release and the combined concentrations of calcium and magnesium. That these divalent cations had an equivalent effect on hormone release was shown by the finding that PTH secretion was unchanged when either cation was decreased in association with a corresponding increase of the other cation.

Parathyroid function appears to be affected in an opposite direction during chronic magnesium depletion. Immunoreactive PTH levels usually have been found to be normal, which is inappropriately low for the hypocalcemic and hypomagnesemic state, or actually low (115–117). Recent studies provide support for an abnormality in PTH release in chronic magnesium depletion. Anast et al. (118) found that PTH levels increased within 5 minutes of administration of magnesium intravenously. Mennes et al. (119) also found that PTH levels rapidly increased in hypomagnesemic patients following intravenous administration of magnesium. Thus, it appears that chronic magnesium depletion is associated with suppression of PTH release from the parathyroid glands rather than a direct effect on decreasing synthesis of this hormone. In further support of this is a recent finding of suppression of PTH secretion by magnesium depletion in a patient with pseudohypoparathyroidism, with subsequent elevated PTH levels noted following magnesium repletion (120). It is interesting that, although chronic magnesium depletion suppresses PTH release, it has little effect on other endocrine glands. Cohan et al. (121) showed normal responsiveness of the adrenal cortex, thyroid, gonads, and liver to their respective trophic hormones in hypomagnesemic patients.

A number of studies have suggested that hypomagnesemia-induced hypocalcemia also results from skeletal resistance to PTH. In vitro techniques (122) revealed that PTH caused less calcium release from fetal rat bone when the medium was low in magnesium. Similarly, bones from magnesium-depleted animals were found to release less calcium and cAMP when exposed to PTH than control bones (123).

Data obtained from in vivo studies have yielded conflicting results. Studies in magnesium-deficient dogs (124), rats (125), and monkeys (111) have shown a normal calcemic response to PTH. In contrast, PTH resistance was found in magnesium-deficient chicks as assessed by the hypercalcemic response (126,127).

Studies in humans also have yielded conflicting results. The earliest studies performed by Estep et al. (128) in hypomagnesemic alcoholic patients, Muldowney et al. (129) in patients with hypomagnesemia secondary to malabsorption syndromes, and Woodard et al. (130) in patients with diarrhea showed an impaired calcemic response from PTH. However, Chase and Slatopolsky (115) found a normal calcemic response from PTH in two hypocalcemic hypomagnesemic adults. A normal calcemic response from PTH has been found in the majority of hypomagnesemic children studied (131).

In human studies (132) as well as some animal studies (133), 1,25(OH)$_2$D$_3$ levels have been found to be low during magnesium-induced hypocalcemia. However, the hypocalcemia does not appear to be related to the low 1,25(OH)$_2$D$_3$ levels, because the hypocalcemia responds to magnesium replacement and the replacement has no effect on vitamin D levels.

Therefore, it can be concluded that several factors may be involved in the pathogenesis of magnesium depletion–induced hypocalcemia. Abnormal PTH release in response to a hypocalcemic stimulus has been well established. There appears to be altered bone solubility as well, possibly as a result of loss of magnesium ions from the crystal surface and hydration shell, with replacement by calcium ions by heteroionic exchange. This could render the bone resistant to PTH as well as other factors that tend to solubilize bone salts. It is possible that PTH secretion is impaired early in the course of magnesium depletion, whereas there is a combination of suppression of PTH release and bone resistance to PTH later in the course of magnesium depletion. This might explain the discrepancies noted in the preceding studies, with the difference in bone response to PTH related to the duration and magnitude of magnesium depletion.

Effect of Magnesium Depletion on Potassium and Other Intracellular Constituents

Whang et al. (134), in studying 106 patients with hypokalemia, found that 42% were also hypomagnesemic. Similarly, Boyd et al. (135) reported a 38% incidence of coexisting hypomagnesemia in hypokalemic patients. However, Watson and O'Kell (136) found a much lower incidence, with only 7.4% of 136 hypokalemic patients also hypomagnesemic. This difference can possibly be explained by the type of patient population studied. The patients studied by Whang et al. (134) were from a University and Veterans Administration hospital, whereas Watson and O'Kell (136) studied patients hospitalized at a tertiary community hospital. From these studies, it would appear that in certain patient populations, such as alcoholic and diabetic patients with ketoacidosis, the combined disturbance of hypokalemia and hypomagnesemia may occur quite commonly.

Whang et al. (137) have suggested that two types of potassium depletion coexist with magnesium depletion. The first represents a combination of intracellular and extracellular potassium and magnesium depletion, whereas the second type represents only intracellular depletion of these two cations. Irrespective of the type of depletion, repletion of potassium frequently cannot be accomplished without the concomitant administration of magnesium. Whang et al. (137) and Rodriguez et al. (138) have used the term "refractory potassium repletion states" to describe this condition. The most common cause has been the use of diuretics to treat edematous disorders. In a review by Whang et al. (137), diuretic therapy was responsible for 63% (46 of 73) of the patients reported who had potassium depletion refractory to only potassium replacement. In the remaining patients, it resulted from a variety of disorders including Bartter syndrome, familial hypokalemic alkalosis, burns, and alcoholism. Whang et al. (137) and Dyckner and Webster (139) have also found that potassium replacement alone may not increase muscle potassium and that a combination of potassium and magnesium replacement is required to normalize muscle potassium and magnesium. Animal studies would add additional support to this contention. Whang and Welt (140) showed that potassium losses from the rat diaphragm maintained in a low-magnesium bath could be prevented by adding more magnesium to the bath. Studies using the isolated rat interventricular septa have shown that increasing extracellular magnesium abruptly decreases ^{42}K efflux (141). Magnesium also has been shown to reduce or prevent the net potassium loss from the heart induced by glycosides (142). This was further supported by showing that a magnesium infusion in animals receiving acetylstrophanthidin prevented potassium loss from the myocardium as determined by measuring arterial and coronary sinus potassium concentrations (143). Findings suggest that this effect of magnesium on intracellular potassium is a result of magnesium enhancing Na^+/K^+ ATPase activity (144). However, this has been criticized by Shine (142), who suggests as an alternative that there might be a direct effect of magnesium on potassium channels in the sarcolemmal membrane or that magnesium's effect might be one of competing with calcium for cellular uptake. An additional factor that may be involved in magnesium-induced potassium depletion is aldosterone. During experimental magnesium depletion–induced kaliuresis, aldosterone levels have been found to be increased, and the kaliuresis can be abolished with spironolactone (145). However, somewhat at variance with this is the finding that magnesium infusion decreases urinary potassium excretion in patients with Bartter syndrome without effecting plasma renin and aldosterone levels (146). This suggests that magnesium repletion may modify kaliuresis by means other than or in addition to its effect on the renin–aldosterone system.

Although most investigators have felt the intracellular alteration in potassium and magnesium to be a result of magnesium depletion, it seems equally as likely, if not more likely under some conditions, that the disturbances are a consequence of primary potassium depletion with secondary magnesium depletion. Studies have shown that potassium can affect the cellular concentration of magnesium. House and Bird (147) showed that goats placed on a high-potassium diet retained more magnesium than goats maintained on a normal potassium intake, given a similar intravenous magnesium load. In addition, as stated earlier, it has been well documented that in primary potassium depletion, intracellular magnesium is also reduced (4,102). This interrelationship between magnesium and potassium could have considerable clinical importance. Under a variety of conditions, it is impossible to replace intracellular deficits of magnesium and potassium without giving both of these cations together, whether the deficiency resulted from either primary potassium or magnesium depletion. In addition, a small number of patients have been reported who have developed tetany following potassium supplementation (148). Although magnesium levels have not been measured in all of these patients, it seems likely in view of their underlying diseases that magnesium deficiency was also present.

Further support for the relationship between these two cations comes from the finding that increased extracellular magnesium causes an abrupt decrease in potassium efflux from the rat intraventricular septa (141). Magnesium also decreased glycoside-induced potassium loss from the myocardium (143). One mechanism by which magnesium may enhance intracellular potassium is by stimulating Na^+/K^+ATPase activity, thus allowing the cell to maintain a potassium gradient (144).

Besides its effect on intracellular potassium, magnesium depletion also causes intracellular phosphorus depletion in muscles. Cronin et al. (149) described rhabdomyolysis in magnesium-depleted dogs and suggested that this resulted from magnesium depletion–induced intracellular phosphate depletion.

Effect of Magnesium on Cardiovascular Function

The effect of magnesium on cardiovascular function has received increasing attention during the last decade. Extracellular and/or intracellular magnesium depletion has been implicated in a variety of cardiovascular disturbances, including ventricular arrhythmias, digitalis intoxication, modulation of vascular tone, and atherogenesis.

Cardiac arrhythmias are an important complication of magnesium depletion, especially in patients on digitalis. Magnesium depletion has been associated with a prolonged QTc interval (150). In addition, magnesium supplementation has been shown to reduce the QTc intervals even in patients with normal serum magnesium levels (151,152). Torsades de pointes is a repetitive polymorphous ventricular tachycardia that occurs in the presence of QT prolongation, which is usually induced by drugs that prolong the QT interval. Because of its effect on prolonging the QT interval, magnesium depletion also has been implicated in the pathogenesis of torsades de pointes, although such a relation has rarely been shown (153). Because of its ability to shorten the QT interval, magnesium supplementation has been used with some success in treating torsades de pointes (154,155).

With regard to cardiac function, there is a close association between magnesium and potassium. Magnesium has been shown to attenuate the electrophysiologic effects of hyperkalemia (156). Furthermore, in view of the relationship between magnesium and intracellular and extracellular potassium depletion, magnesium depletion has been implicated as a potential cause of digitalis intoxication (157). This is supported by the finding that an acute induction of hypomagnesemia in dogs with dialysis facilitates the development of digitalis intoxication and arrhythmias (144). Moreover, ventricular arrhythmias, including those induced by digitalis, are sensitive to magnesium therapy (158). However, it is unclear how much of these cardiovascular alterations are a direct result of magnesium depletion or else a consequence of the associated intracellular potassium depletion.

Therapy of Magnesium Deficiency

Magnesium replacement is indicated in all patients with hypomagnesemia whether symptomatic or not. Symptoms are unusual unless serum magnesium levels are <0.8 mEq/L. Adequate replacement of magnesium deficits usually can be accomplished through dietary sources alone in patients with mild asymptomatic hypomagnesemia. Patients with severe symptomatic hypomagnesemia usually require parenteral replacement of magnesium deficits. Magnesium may be useful, at least as adjuvant therapy, in treating a variety of tachyarrhythmias, including torsades de pointes and some associated with digitalis toxicity. As stated, uncorrected intracellular magnesium deficiency can impair repletion of cellular potassium. At this time, it cannot be recommended that all patients with potassium depletion be given both potassium and magnesium replacement. However, patients with potassium depletion in association with any documented amount of hypomagnesemia should receive combined replacement with both of these cations. In addition, magnesium supplementation should be strongly

TABLE 7.2 MAGNESIUM SALTS USED FOR REPLACEMENT OR PHOSPHORUS BINDER

Compound	Molecular weight	% Mg by weight
$MgCl_2\ 6H_2O^a$	203.23	11.96
$MgSO_4\ 7H_2O^b$	246.50	9.86
$Mg(C_2H_3O_2)_2\ 4H_2O^c$	214.47	11.33
$Mg(OH)_2^d$	58.3	41.68
MgO^e	40	60.30
$MgCO_3^f$	84.32	28.82

[a]Magnesium chloride.
[b]Magnesium sulfate.
[c]Magnesium acetate tetrahydrate.
[d]Magnesium hydroxide.
[e]Magnesium oxide.
[f]Magnesium carbonate.

considered in patients with severe potassium depletion or in those who appear to be resistant to potassium replacement.

Because the kidneys have a marked capability for excretion of magnesium, excessive magnesium treatment usually results in only temporary hypermagnesemia. However, when a patient has compromised kidney function, magnesium should be administered cautiously and with close monitoring of the plasma magnesium levels. The different compounds commonly used for magnesium replacement, including their molecular weights and percent magnesium by weight, are listed in Table 7.2.

The magnesium deficit can be roughly calculated by assuming that the space of distribution is slightly larger than the ECF volume. This assumption seems to be valid because during magnesium depletion, soft-tissue magnesium stores are affected little, if at all, and only the surface limited pool of magnesium on bone would equilibrate during repletion. Therefore, it appears that replacement therapy may be adequate for a number of hypomagnesemic patients if only 30% as much magnesium as recommended by Flink (159) is used. However, in some conditions, the magnesium deficit may be in excess of this amount. It has been estimated that patients with diabetic ketoacidosis may retain 40 to 80 mEq (480 to 960 mg) of magnesium over 2 to 6 days following recovery (70,160). In some alcoholic patients, deficits of up to 1 mEq/kg have been found (161).

Whenever possible, intravenous magnesium replacement should be avoided in small children because of the danger of hypotension. For children weighing 4 to 7 kg, a safe initial dose is 0.5 mL of 50% $MgSO_4$ (2 mEq of magnesium), given intramuscularly. For heavier children, 1.0 mL of 50% $MgSO_4$ may be given intramuscularly (162).

For adults with normal kidney function, suggested magnesium replacement is given in Table 7.3 (159,163). Oral replacement therapy is limited by the amount of magnesium administration that causes

TABLE 7.3 MAGNESIUM REPLACEMENT

Intravenous administration (50% $MgSO_4$):

Symptomatic emergent (seizures) (50% $MgSO_4$)

4 mL (16.3 mEq, 8.2 mmol, or 195 mg of Mg) diluted to 100 mL infused over a 10-min period

Symptomatic nonemergent

Day 1: 12 mL (49 mEq of Mg) in a 1,000-mL solution containing glucose infused over 3 h, followed by 10 mL (40 mEq of Mg) in each of two 1-L solutions administered throughout the day

Days 2–5: 12 mL (49 mEq of Mg) distributed equally in total daily IV fluids

Oral therapy (MgO):

250–500 mg (12.5–25 mEq of Mg) tid to qid

Intramuscular route (50% $MgSO_4$) (painful)

Day 1: 4 mL (16.3 mEq of Mg) q2h for 3 doses and then q4h for 4 doses

Day 2: 2 mL (8.1 mEq of Mg) q4h for 6 doses

Days 3–5: 2 mL (8.1 mEq of Mg) q6h

diarrhea. Oral replacement also can be made with antacids that contain both magnesium and aluminum salts or magnesium calcium salts in patients who develop diarrhea from magnesium oxide replacement. Patients maintained only on intravenous therapy for periods in excess of 5 to 7 days may require some magnesium supplementation to prevent the development of magnesium depletion. This can be accomplished by giving 100 mg (8 mEq) of magnesium daily if there are not excessive losses of this cation through the kidneys and GI tract. For management of arrhythmias, it has been suggested that 8 mmol of magnesium sulfate be administered intravenously over 1 minute or that as much as 1.5 mmol/kg be given over a 10-minute period (155,164,165).

Hypermagnesemia

Most cases of hypermagnesemia are seen in patients with chronic kidney disease but can be seen with shifts or exogenous administration. Normally, plasma magnesium concentration increases in the hibernating animal (166) and during hypothermia (167). Magnesium is commonly given parenterally for the treatment of eclampsia. Blood levels of magnesium usually are increased to 6 to 8 mEq/L but occasionally may be as high as 14 mEq/L (168). This may result in neonatal hypermagnesemia, but in general, blood levels tend to be lower in the infant than in the mother. Other states in which hypermagnesemia has been described with some frequency are in patients with kidney failure (169) and adrenocortical insufficiency (170). The majority of patients with far advanced kidney failure have a modest elevation of serum magnesium levels (171). Severe hypermagnesemia occurs most frequently in patients with marked kidney disease who are given large amounts of oral magnesium salts, usually in the form of magnesium-containing antacids (172,173). Although the normal kidney has a great ability to excrete magnesium, magnesium intoxication can occur in patients with normal kidney function (174,175). This usually results from an individual inadvertently receiving a large oral load of hypertonic magnesium salts. This results in two phenomena that can cause life-threatening hypermagnesemia. First, excessive magnesium is absorbed. Second, and possibly of greater importance, the hypertonic solution pulls fluid from the extracellular space into the GI tract, which causes volume depletion and decreases kidney function, which in turn compromises the excretion of the absorbed magnesium. Hypermagnesemia is being seen with increasing frequency in patients with drug overdoses because of the magnesium-containing laxatives commonly used to treat this condition (176). Another group of patients at risk of developing hypermagnesemia are elderly patients with GI disorders receiving magnesium-containing compounds (177).

Symptoms of Acute Magnesium Intoxication

Acute elevations of the serum magnesium levels depress the central nervous system as well as the peripheral neuromuscular junction. Magnesium in pharmacologic doses has a curare-like action on neuromuscular function. This is probably caused by inhibition of the prejunctional release of acetylcholine owing to displacement of membrane-bound calcium at the neuromuscular junction, which then decreases the depolarizing action of acetylcholine (178). Magnesium also increases the stimulus threshold in nerve fibers, and direct application of magnesium to the central nervous system blocks synaptic transmission. Electrophysiologic studies demonstrate reduced compound muscle action potential amplitudes, decremental amplitude responses to repetitive stimulation at low rates, and a marked amplitude increment following brief exercise (179).

The deep tendon reflexes are depressed when serum magnesium levels exceed 4 mEq/L. A flaccid quadriplegia may develop in the patient at magnesium levels >8 to 10 mEq/L. Deep tendon reflexes are absent at this stage. The patient is typically conscious and reasonably alert. However, because of marked muscle weakness, there is difficulty talking and swallowing, and respiratory paralysis is a real hazard (95). Other symptoms include lethargy, nausea, dilated pupils, and respiratory depression (172,173). There also may be smooth muscle paralysis, resulting in difficulty in micturition and defecation (173). Hypotension and bradycardia are common, and in rare cases, cardiac arrhythmias consisting of complete heart block and cardiac arrest have been observed (173).

Treatment of Acute Magnesium Intoxication

Treatment of hypermagnesemia is primarily directed at reducing the serum magnesium levels. However, calcium acts as a direct antagonist to magnesium, and the injection of as little as 5 to 10 mEq of calcium may readily reverse a potentially lethal respiratory depression or cardiac arrhythmia (95). Thus, intravenous calcium should be used as the initial treatment modality when life-threatening complications of magnesium intoxication are present.

Any parenteral or oral magnesium salt the patient has been taking should be discontinued immediately. Intravenous furosemide should be administered and urine volume replaced with 0.5 N saline if kidney function is adequate. This approach ensures continuing urine output and prevents volume depletion. Calcium gluconate (15 mg of calcium/kg), given over a 4-hour period, also can be used to increase urinary calcium excretion and, in turn, magnesium excretion. In patients with severe impairment of kidney function, dialysis may be required. This should be carried out with a dialysate free of magnesium. The serum magnesium usually can be decreased to a safe level in 4 to 6 hours of dialysis (173).

Chronic Magnesium Excess

Chronic kidney disease is the only state thus far described in which there can be a chronic excess of total body magnesium (169). The body magnesium pools increased during magnesium excess are ECF magnesium and bone magnesium (169). Decreases in the dialysate magnesium concentration since the early days of renal replacement therapy have raised new questions about magnesium balance in dialysis patients. No quantitative bone analyses are available to evaluate the net effect on magnesium balance since these early studies of Alfrey (169). Magnesium has been shown to be an integral part of the soft-tissue calcium phosphate deposits found in uremic patients (180) and in vascular calcification in animal models (181), suggesting that this cation might in part be responsible for this complication. However, in vitro, magnesium impairs hydroxyapitite crystal growth (182,183) and a few observational studies found less vascular and valvular calcification in dialysis patients with higher serum magnesium concentrations (184,185). Futhermore, magnesium has been shown to be an effective phosphate binder (186,187) and has been used in earlier times to decrease aluminum exposure (186) and more recently to decrease net calcium intake (188,189). Additional studies are necessary to determine magnesium balance in dialysis patients and to investigate whether modifications in serum levels or magnesium balance have adverse or favorable consequences with regard to bone disease, vascular calcification, and cardiovascular outcomes.

Summary

In summary, because magnesium determinations have become a routine procedure in most laboratories, it has become apparent that disorders of magnesium metabolism occur with a frequency almost as great as those noted for the other major body elements. Hypomagnesemia is found with some frequency in a variety of conditions, including small-bowel disease, chronic alcoholism, malnutrition, endocrine abnormalities, and certain kidney diseases. At times, the severity of magnesium depletion may be so great that such symptoms as tetany, delirium, psychosis, or even convulsions may occur.

Although acute magnesium intoxication has been repeatedly observed and can lead to death as a result of arrhythmias and respiratory arrest, the consequences of chronic magnesium excess have not been well defined and clearly deserve further study.

REFERENCES

1. Arnaud MJ. Update on the assessment of magnesium status. *Br J Nutr.* 2008;99:S24–S36.
2. Seelig MS. The requirement of magnesium by the normal adult: summary and analysis of published data. *Am J Clin Nutr.* 1964;14:212–218.
3. Walser M. Magnesium metabolism. *Ergeb Physiol.* 1967;59:185–296.
4. Alfrey AC, Miller NL, Butkus D. Evaluation of body magnesium stores. *J Lab Clin Med.* 1974;84:153–162.
5. Alfrey AC, Miller NL, Trow R. Effect of age and magnesium depletion on bone magnesium pools in rats. *J Clin Invest.* 1974;54:1074–1086.

6. Alfrey AC, Miller NL. Bone magnesium pools in uremia. *J Clin Invest*. 1973;52:3019–3027.

7. MacIntyre I, Robinson CG. Magnesium and the gut: experimental and clinical observations. *Ann N Y Acad Sci*. 1970;162:865–873.

8. Alexander RT, Hoenderop JG, Bindels RJ. Molecular determinats of magnesium homeostatis: insights from human disease. *J Am Soc Nephrol*. 2008;19:1451–1458.

9. Miller ER, Ullrey DE, Zutaut CL, et al. Mineral balance studies with the baby pig: effect of dietary vitamin D2 levels upon calcium, phosphorus and magnesium balance. *J Nutr*. 1965;85:255–259.

10. Hodgkinson A, Marshall DH, Nordin BEC. Vitamin D and magnesium absorption in man. *Clin Sci (Lond)*. 1979;57:121–123.

11. Schmulen AC, Lerman M, Pak CYC, et al. Effect of 1,25(OH)$_2$D3 on jejunal absorption of magnesium in patients with chronic renal disease. *Am J Physiol*. 1980;238:G349–G352.

12. Booth CC, Babouris N, Hanna S, et al. Incidence of hypomagnesaemia in intestinal malabsorption. *Br Med J*. 1963;2:141–144.

13. Gitelman HJ, Graham JB, Welt LG. A new familial disorder characterized by hypokalemia and hypomagnesemia. *Trans Assoc Am Physicians*. 1966;79:221–235.

14. Wong NLM, Dirks JH, Quamme GA. Tubular reabsorptive capacity for magnesium in the dog kidney. *Am J Physiol*. 1983;244:F78–F83.

15. Morel F, Roninel N, LeGrimellec C. Electron probe analysis of tubular fluid composition. *Nephron*. 1969;6:350–364.

16. Wagner CA. Disorders of renal magnesium handling explain renal magnesium transport. *J Nephrol*. 2007;20:507–510.

17. Quamme GA, Dirks JH. Effect of intraluminal and contraluminal magnesium on magnesium and calcium transfer in the rat nephron. *Am J Physiol*. 1980;238:187–198.

18. Carney SL, Wong NLM, Quamme GA, et al. Effect of magnesium deficiency on renal magnesium and calcium transport in the rat. *J Clin Invest*. 1980;65:180–188.

19. LeGrimellec C, Roinel N, Morel F. Simultaneous Mg, Ca, P, K, Na and Cl analysis in rat tubular fluid: II. During acute Mg plasma loading. *Pflugers Arch*. 1973;340:197–210.

20. LeGrimellec C, Roinel N, Morel F. Simultaneous Mg, Ca, P, K, Na and Cl analysis in rat tubular fluid: III. During acute Ca plasma loading. *Pflugers Arch*. 1974;346:171–189.

21. Quamme GA. Renal magnesium handling: new insights in understanding old problems. *Kidney Int*. 1997;52:1180–1195.

22. Hebert SC, Brown EM, Harris HW. Role of Ca(2+)-sensing receptor in divalent mineral ion homeostasia. *J Exp Biol*. 1997;200: 295–302.

23. Cao G, Hoenderop JGJ, Bindels RJM. Insights into the molecular regulation of the epithelial magnesium channel. *Curr Opin Nephrol Hypertens*. 2008;17:373–378.

24. Knoers NVAM. Inherited forms of renal hypomagnesemia: an update. *Pediatr Nephrol*. 2008: DOI 10.1007/s00467-008-0968.

25. Dai LJ, Ritchie G, Kerstan D, et al. Magnesium transport in the distal convoluted tubule. *Physiol Rev*. 2001;81:51–84.

26. Groenestege WM, Thebault S, van der Wijst J, et al. Impaired basolateral sorting of pro-EGF causes isolated recessive renal hypomagnesemia. *J Clin Invest*. 2007;117:2260–2267.

27. Tejpar S. Piessevaux H, Claes K, et al. Magnesium wasting associated with epidremal-growth-factor receptor-targeting antibodies in colorectal cancer: a prospective study. *Lancet Oncol*. 2007;8: 387–394.

28. Lehninger AL. *Bioenergetics*. New York: Benjamin; 1965.

29. Kinne-Suffren E, Kinne R. Localization of a calcium-stimulated ATPase in the basolateral plasma membrane of the proximal tubule rat kidney cortex. *J Membr Biol*. 1974;17:264–274.

30. Humes HD, Weinberg JM, Knauss TC. Clinical and pathophysiologic aspects of aminoglycoside nephrotoxicity. *Am J Kidney Dis*. 1982;2:5–29.

31. Bellorin-Font E, Martin KJ. Regulation of PTH receptor-cyclase system of canine kidney: effects of calcium, magnesium and guanine nucleotides. *Am J Physiol*. 1981;241:F364–F373.

32. Kurachi Y, Nakajima T, Sugimoto T. Role of intracellular Mg2+ in the activation of muscarinic K+ channel in cardiac atrial cell membrane. *Pflugers Arch*. 1986;407:572–574.

33. Brinley FJ Jr., Scarpa A, Tiffert T. The concentration of ionized magnesium in barnacle muscle fibers. *J Physiol (Lond)*. 1977;266:545–565.

34. Vallee B, Wacker WE, Ulmer DD. The magnesium deficiency tetany syndrome in man. *N Engl J Med*. 1960;262:155–161.

35. Shils ME. Experimental human magnesium depletion: I. Clinical observations and blood chemistry alterations. *Am J Clin Nutr*. 1964;15: 133–143.

36. Caddell JL, Goddard DR. Studies in protein calorie malnutrition: 1. Chemical evidence for magnesium deficiency. *N Engl J Med*. 1967;276: 533–535.

37. Baron DN. Magnesium deficiency after gastrointestinal surgery and loss of excretions. *Br J Surg*. 1960;48:344–346.

38. Flink EB, Stutzman RL, Anderson AR, et al. Magnesium deficiency after prolonged parenteral fluid administration and after chronic alcoholism, complicated by delirium tremens. *J Lab Clin Med*. 1954;43:169–183.

39. Heaton FW, Fourman P. Magnesium deficiency and hypocalcemia in intestinal malabsorption. *Lancet*. 1965;2:50–52.

40. Thoren L. Magnesium deficiency in gastrointestinal fluid loss. *Acta Chir Scand (Suppl)*. 1963;306: 1–65.

41. Van Gaal L, Delvigne C, Vandewoude M, et al. Evaluation of magnesium before and after jejunoileal versus gastric bypass surgery for morbid obesity. *J Am Coll Nutr*. 1987;6:397–400.

42. Abdulrazzaq YM, Smigura RC, Wettrell G. Primary infantile hypomagnesemia: report of two cases and review of literature. *Eur J Pediatr*. 1989;148:459–461.

43. Suh SM, Tashjian AH, Matsuo N, et al. Pathogenesis of hypocalcemia in primary

hypomagnesemia: normal end organ responsiveness to parathyroid hormone, impaired parathyroid gland function. *J Clin Invest.* 1973;52: 153–160.

44. Milla PJ, Aggett PJ, Wolff OH, et al. Studies in primary hypomagnesaemia: evidence for defective carrier-mediated small intestinal transport of magnesium. *Gut.* 1979;20:1028–1033.

45. Schlingmann KP, Weber S, Peters M, et al. Hypomagnesemia with secondary hypocalcemia is caused by mutations in the TRPM6, a new member of the TRPM gene family. *Nat Genet.* 2002;31: 166–170.

46. Quamme GA. Recent developments in intestinal magnesium absorption. *Curr Opin Gastroenterol.* 2008;24:230–235.

47. Weber S, Schneider L, Misselwitz J, et al. Novel paracellin-1 mutations in 25 families with familial hypomagnesemia with hypercalciuria and nephrocalcinosis. *J Am Soc Nephrol.* 2001;12: 1872–1881.

48. Kuwertz-Broking E, Frund S, Bulla M, et al. Familial hypomagnesemia-hypercalciuria in 2 siblings. *Clin Nephrol.* 2001;56:155–161.

49. Meij IC, Saar K, van den Heuvel LP, et al. Hereditary isolated renal magnesium loss maps to chromosome 11q23. *Am J Hum Genet.* 1999;64: 180–188.

50. Meij IC, Koenderink JB, De Jong JC, et al. Dominant isolated renal magnesium loss is caused by misrouting of the Na^+, K^+-ATPase gamma-subunit. *Ann N Y Acad Sci.* 2003;986:437–443.

51. Naderi ASA, Reilly RF Jr. Hereditary etiologies of hypomagnesemia. *Nat Clin Nephrol.* 2007;4: 80–89.

52. Knoer NV, Levtchenko EN. Gitelman syndrome. Orphanet J Rare Diseases 2008; 3: 22. doi:10.1186/ 1750–1172-3-22.

53. Ellison DH. Divalent cation transport by the distal nephron: insights from Bartter's and Gitelman's syndromes. *Am J Physiol Renal Physiol.* 2000; 279:F616–625.

54. Nijenhuis T, Vallon V, van der Kemp AWCM, et al. Enhanced passive Ca^{2+} reabsorption and reduced Mg^{2+} channel abundance explains thiazide-induced hypocalciuria and hypomagnesemia. *J Clin Invest.* 2005;115:1651–1658.

55. Bar RS, Wilson HE, Mazzaferri EL. Hypo-magnesemia hypocalcemia secondary to renal magnesium wasting. *Ann Intern Med.* 1975;82:646–649.

56. Keating MJ, Sethi MR, Bodey GP, et al. Hypocalcemia with hypoparathyroidism and renal tubular dysfunction associated with aminoglycoside therapy. *Cancer.* 1977;39:1410–1414.

57. Schilsky RL, Anderson T. Hypomagnesemia and renal magnesium wasting in patients receiving cisplatin. *Ann Intern Med.* 1979;90:926–928.

58. Buckley JE, Clark VL, Meyer TJ, et al. Hypomagnesemia after cisplatin combination chemotherapy. *Arch Intern Med.* 1984;144: 2347–2348.

59. Wong NLM, Dirks JH. Cyclosporin-induced hypomagnesaemia and renal magnesium wasting in rats. *Clin Sci (Lond).* 1988;75:505–514.

60. Shah GM, Alvarado P, Kirschenbaum MA. Symptomatic hypocalcemia and hypomagnesemia with renal magnesium wasting associated with

pentamidine therapy in a patient with AIDS. *Am J Med.* 1990;89:380–382.

61. Gearhart ML, Sorg TB. Foscarnet-induced severe hypomagnesemia and other electrolyte disorders. *Ann Pharmacother.* 1993;27:285–289.

62. Narita M, Itakura O, Ishiguro N, et al. Hypomagnesemia-associated tetany due to intravenous administration of amphotericin B. *Eur J Pediatr.* 1997;156:421–422.

64. Wesson LG Jr. Magnesium, calcium and phosphate excretion during osmotic diuresis in the dog. *J Lab Clin Med.* 1962;60:422–432.

65. George WK, George WD, Haan CL, et al. Vitamin D and magnesium. *Lancet.* 1962;1:1300–1301.

66. Richardson JA, Welt LG. The hypomagnesemia of vitamin D administration. *Clin Res.* 1963; 11:250.

67. Mellinghoff K. Magnesium Stoffwechselstorungen bei Inanition. *Deutsche Arch Klin Med.* 1949;95: 475–484.

68. Jones JE, Albrink MJ, Davidson PD, et al. Fasting and refeeding of various suboptimal isocaloric diets. *Am J Clin Nutr* 1966;19:320–328.

69. Butler AM, Talbot NB, Burnett CH, et al. Metabolic studies in diabetic coma. *Trans Assoc Am Physicians.* 1947;60:102–109.

70. Butler AM. Diabetic coma. *N Engl J Med.* 1950; 243:648–659.

71. Winter RJ, Harris CJ, Phillips LS, et al. Diabetic ketoacidosis induction of hypocalcemia and hypomagnesemia by phosphate therapy. *Am J Med.* 1979;67:897–904.

72. White JR, Campbell RK. Magnesium and diabetes: a review. *Ann Pharmacother.* 1993;27: 775–780.

73. Horton R, Biglieri EG. Effect of aldosterone on the metabolism of magnesium. *Clin Endocrinol Metab.* 1962;22:1187–1192.

74. Cohen MI, McNamara H, Finberg L. Serum magnesium in children with cirrhosis. *J Pediatr.* 1970; 76:453–455.

75. Hellman ES, Tschudy DP, Bartter FC. Abnormal electrolyte and water metabolism in acute intermittent porphyria: transient inappropriate secretion of antidiuretic hormone. *Am J Med.* 1962;32: 734–746.

76. Heaton FW, Pyrah LN, Beresford LC, et al. Hypomagnesemia in chronic alcoholism. *Lancet.* 1962; 2:802–805.

77. Kalbfleish JM, Lindeman RD, Ginn HE, et al. Effects of ethanol administration on urinary excretion of magnesium and other electrolytes in alcoholic and normal subjects. *J Clin Invest.* 1963; 42:1471–1475.

78. McCollister RJ, Flink EB, Lewis MD. Urinary excretion of magnesium in man following the ingestion of ethanol. *Am J Clin Nutr.* 1963;12: 415–420.

79. Dunn MJ, Walser M. Magnesium depletion in normal man. *Metabolism.* 1966;15:884–895.

80. Kreusser WJ, Kurokawa K, Aznar E, et al. Effect of phosphate depletion on magnesium homeostasis in rats. *J Clin Invest.* 1978;61: 573–581.

81. Coburn JW, Massry SG. Changes in serum and urinary calcium during phosphate depletion. *J Clin Invest.* 1970;49:1073–1087.

82. Domingues JH, Gray RW, Lemann J Jr. Dietary phosphate deprivation in women and men: effect on mineral and acid balance, parathyroid hormone and metabolism of 25-OH-vitamin D. *J Clin Endocrinol Metab.* 1976;43:1056–1968.

83. Tibbets DM, Aub JC. Magnesium metabolism in health and disease: III. In exophthalmic goiter, basophilic adenoma, Addison's disease and steatorrhea. *J Clin Invest.* 1937;16:511–515.

84. Marks P, Ashraf H. Apathetic hyperthyroidism and hypomagnesaemia and raised alkaline phosphatase concentration. *Br Med J.* 1978;1: 821–822.

85. Broughton A, Anderson IRM, Bowden CH. Magnesium deficiency syndrome in burns. *Lancet.* 1968;2:1156–1158.

86. Heaton FW, Pyrah LN. Magnesium metabolism in patients with parathyroid disorders. *Clin Sci.* 1963; 25:475–485.

87. Dancis J, Springer D, Cohlan SA. Fetal homeostasis in maternal malnutrition: 1. Magnesium deprivation. *Pediatr Res.* 1971;5:131–136.

88. Schindler AM. Isolated neonatal hypomagnesaemia associated with maternal overuse of stool softener. *Lancet.* 1984;2:822.

89. Harris I, Wilkinson AW. Magnesium depletion in children. *Lancet.* 1971;2:735–736.

90. Tsang RC. Neonatal magnesium disturbances. *Am J Dis Child.* 1972;124:282–293.

91. Clark PCN, Carrel IJ. Hypocalcemic, hypomagnesemic convulsions. *J Pediatr.* 1967;70:806–809.

92. Frankenhaeuser B, Meves H. Effect of magnesium and calcium on frog myelinated nerve fiber. *J Physiol.* 1958;142:360–365.

93. Gordon HT, Welsh JH. Role of ions in axon surface reactions to toxic organic compounds. *J Cell Physiol.* 1948;31:395–419.

94. Perry SV. Relation between chemical and contractile function and structure of skeletal muscle cell. *Physiol Rev.* 1956;36:1–76.

95. Welt LG, Gitelman H. Disorders of magnesium metabolism. *DM.* 1965;1:1–32.

96. Chutkow JG. Studies on the metabolism of magnesium in the magnesium deficient rat. *J Lab Clin Med.* 1965;65:912–926.

97. Wallach S, Cahill LN, Rogan FH, et al. Plasma and erythrocyte magnesium in health and disease. *J Lab Clin Med.* 1962;59:195–210.

98. Elin RJ. Assessment of magnesium status. *Clin Chem.* 1987;33:1965–1970.

99. Forbes RM. Effect of magnesium, potassium and sodium nutriture on mineral composition of selected tissues of the albino rat. *J Nutr.* 1966;88: 403–410.

100. Lim P, Jacob E. Magnesium deficiency in liver cirrhosis. *Q J Med.* 1972;41:291–300.

101. Lim P, Jacob E. Tissue magnesium level in chronic diarrhea. *J Lab Clin Med.* 1972;80:313–321.

102. Baldwin D, Robinson PK, Zierler KL, et al. Interrelations of magnesium, potassium, phosphorus and creatinine in skeletal muscle of man. *J Clin Invest.* 1952;31:850–858.

103. Skou JC. The (Na + K)activated enzyme system and its relationship to the transport of sodium and potassium. *Q Rev Biophys.* 1974;7:401–434.

104. Alleyne GA, Millward DJ, Scullard GH. Total body potassium muscle, electrolytes and glycogen in malnourished children. *J Pediatr.* 1970;76: 75–81.

105. Johnson CJ, Peterson DR, Smith EK. Myocardial tissue concentrations of magnesium and potassium in men dying suddenly from ischemic heart disease. *Am J Clin Nutr.* 1979;32:967.

106. Rasmussen HS, McNair P, Goransson L, et al. Magnesium deficiency in patients with ischemic heart disease with and without acute myocardial infarction uncovered by an intravenous loading test. *Arch Intern Med.* 1988;148:329–332.

107. Smith RH. Calcium and magnesium metabolism in calves: 4. Bone composition in magnesium deficiency and the control of plasma magnesium. *Biochem J.* 1959;71:609–615.

108. L'Estrange JL, Axford RFE. A study of magnesium and calcium metabolism in lactating ewes fed a semi-purified diet low in magnesium. *J Agric Sci.* 1964;62:353–368.

109. Miller ER, Ullrey DE, Zutaut CL, et al. Magnesium requirement of the baby pig. *J Nutr.* 1965; 85:13–20.

110. Chiemchaisri H, Phillips PH. Certain factors including fluoride which affect magnesium calcinosis in the dog and rat. *J Nutr.* 1965;86:23–28.

111. Dunn MJ. Magnesium depletion in the rhesus monkey: induction of magnesium-dependent hypocalcemia. *Clin Sci.* 1971;41:333–344.

112. MacManus J, Heaton FW. The effect of magnesium deficiency on calcium homeostasis in the rat. *Clin Sci.* 1969;36:297–306.

113. Buckle RM, Care AD, Cooper CW, et al. The influence of plasma magnesium concentration on parathyroid hormone secretion. *J Endocrinol.* 1968;42:529–534.

114. Targounik JH, Rodman JS, Sherwood LM. Regulation of parathyroid hormone secretion in vitro: quantitative aspects of calcium and magnesium ion control. *Endocrinology.* 1971;88: 1477–1482.

115. Chase LR, Slatopolsky E. Secretion and metabolic efficiency of parathyroid hormone in patients with severe hypo-magnesemia. *J Clin Endocrinol Metab.* 1974;28:363–371.

116. Connor TB, Toskes P, Mahaffey J, et al. Parathyroid function during chronic magnesium deficiency. *Johns Hopkins Med J.* 1972; 131:100–117.

117. Wiegmann T, Kaye M. Hypomagnesemic hypocalcemia: early serum calcium and late parathyroid hormone increase with magnesium therapy. *Arch Intern Med.* 1977;137:953–955.

118. Anast CS, Winnacker LL, Forte LR, et al. Impaired release of parathyroid hormone in magnesium deficiency. *J Clin Endocrinol Metab.* 1976;42:707–713.

119. Mennes P, Rosenbaum R, Martin K, et al. Hypomagnesemia and impaired parathyroid hormone secretion in chronic renal failure. *Ann Intern Med.* 1978;88:206–209.

120. Allen DB, Friedman AL, Greer FR, et al. Hypomagnesemia masking the appearance of elevated parathyroid hormone concentrations in familial pseudohypoparathyroidism. *Am J Med Genet.* 1988;31:153–158.

121. Cohan BW, Singer FR, Rude RK. End-organ response to adrenocorticotropin, thyrotropin,

gonadotropin-releasing hormone and glucagon in hypocalcemic magnesium deficient patients. *J Clin Endocrinol Metab.* 1982;54:975–979.

122. Raisz LF, Niemann I. Effect of phosphate, calcium and magnesium on bone resorption and hormonal responses in tissue culture. *Endocrinology.* 1969;85:446–452.

123. Freitag JJ, Martin KJ, Comrades MB, et al. Evidence for Skeletal-resistance to parathyroid hormone in magnesium deficiency: studies in isolated perfused bone. *J Clin Invest.* 1979;64:1238–1244.

124. Suh SM, Csima A, Fraser D. Pathogenesis of hypocalcemia in magnesium depletion. Normal end-organ responsiveness to parathyroid hormone. *J Clin Invest.* 1971;50:2668–2673.

125. Hahn TJ, Chase LR, Avioli LV. Effect of magnesium depletion on responsiveness to parathyroid hormone in parathyroidectomized rats. *J Clin Invest.* 1972;51:886–891.

126. Breitenbach RP, Gonnerman WA, Erfling WL, et al. Dietary magnesium, calcium homeostasis and parathyroid gland activity of chickens. *Am J Physiol.* 1973;225:12–17.

127. Reddy CR, Coburn JW, Hartenbower DL, et al. Studies on mechanisms of hypocalcemia of magnesium depletion. *J Clin Invest.* 1973;52:3000–3010.

128. Estep H, Shaw WP, Watlington C, et al. Hypocalcemia due to hypomagnesemia and reversible parathyroid hormone unresponsiveness. *J Clin Endocrinol Metab.* 1969;29:942–948.

129. Muldowney FP, McKenna TJ, Kyle LH, et al. Parathormone-like effect of magnesium replenishment in steatorrhea. *N Engl J Med.* 1970;282:61–68.

130. Woodard JC, Webster PD, Carr AA. Primary hypomagnesemia with secondary hypocalcemia, diarrhea and insensitivity to parathyroid hormone. *Am J Dig Dis* 1972;17:612–618.

131. Skyberg D, Stromme JH, Nesbakken HK, et al. Neonatal hypomagnesemia with selective malabsorption of magnesium: a clinical entity. *Scand J Clin Lab Invest.* 1968;21:355–363.

132. Fuss M, Cogan E, Gillet G, et al. Magnesium administration reverses the hypocalcaemia secondary to hypomagnesaemia despite low circulating levels of 25-hydroxyvitamin D and 1,25-dihydroxyvitamin D. *Clin Endocrinol (Oxf).* 1985;22:807–815.

133. Carpenter TO, Carnes DL, Anast CS. Effect of magnesium depletion on metabolism of 25-hydroxyvitamin D in rats. *Am J Physiol.* 1987;252:E106–E113.

134. Whang R, Oei TO, Hamiter T. Frequency of hypomagnesemia associated with hypokalemia in hospitalized patients. *Am J Clin Pathol.* 1979;71:610.

135. Boyd JC, Bruns DE, Wills MR. Occurrence of hypomagnesemia in hypokalemic states. *Clin Chem.* 1983;29:178–179.

136. Watson KR, OiKell RT. Lack of relationship between Mg^{2+} and K^+: concentration in serum. *Clin Chem.* 1980;26:520–521.

137. Whang R, Flink EB, Dyckner T, et al. Magnesium depletion as a cause of refractory potassium repletion. *Arch Intern Med.* 1985;145:1686–1689.

138. Rodriguez M, Solanki DL, Whang R. Refractory potassium repletion due to cisplatin-induced magnesium depletion. *Arch Intern Med.* 1989;149:2592–2594.

139. Dyckner T, Webster PO. Ventricular extrasystoles and intracellular electrolytes before and after potassium and magnesium infusions in patients on diuretic therapy. *Am Heart J.* 1979;97:12–18.

140. Whang R, Welt LG. Observations in experimental magnesium depletion. *J Clin Invest.* 1963;42:305–313.

141. Shine KL, Douglas AM. Magnesium effects on ionic exchange and mechanical function in rat ventricle. *Am J Physiol.* 1974;227:317–324.

142. Shine KL. Myocardial effects of magnesium. *Am J Physiol.* 1979;227:H413–H423.

143. Neff MS, Mendelsohn S, Kim KE, et al. Magnesium sulfate in digitalis toxicity. *Am J Cardiol.* 1971;79:57–68.

144. Seller RH, Cangiano J, Kim KE, et al. Digitalis toxicity and hypomagnesemia. *Am Heart J.* 1970;79:57–68.

145. Francisco LL, Sawin L, Dibona GF. Mechanism of negative potassium balance in the magnesium-deficient rat. *Proc Soc Exp Biol Med.* 1981;168:383–388.

146. Baehler RW, Work J, Kotchen TA, et al. Studies on the pathogenesis of Bartter's syndrome. *Am J Med.* 1980;69:933–939.

147. House WA, Bird RJ. Magnesium tolerance in goats fed two levels of potassium. *J Anim Sci.* 1975;41:1134–1140.

148. Engel FL, Martin SP, Taylor H. On the relation of potassium to the neurological manifestations of hypocalcemic tetany. *Johns Hopkins Med J.* 1949;84:285–301.

149. Cronin RE, Ferbuson ER, Shannon WA, et al. Skeletal muscle injury after magnesium depletion in the dog. *Am J Physiol.* 1982;243:F113–F120.

150. Sellig MS. Electrocardiographic patterns of magnesium depletion appearing in alcoholic heart disease. *Ann N Y Acad Sci.* 1969;162:906–917.

151. Krasner BS, Girdwood R, Smith H. The effect of slow releasing oral magnesium chloride on the QTC interval of the electrocardiogram during open heart surgery. *Can Anaesth Soc J.* 1981;28:329–333.

152. Davis WH, Ziady F. The effect of oral magnesium chloride therapy on the PTC and QUC intervals of the electrocardiogram. *South Afr Med J.* 1978;53:591–593.

153. Topol EJ, Lerman BB. Hypomagnesemic torsades de pointes. *Am J Cardiol.* 1983;52:1367–1368.

154. Tzivoni E, Keren A, Cohen AM, et al. Magnesium therapy for torsades de pointes. *Am J Cardiol.* 1984;53:528–530.

155. Gupta A, Lawrence AT, Krishnan K, et al. Current concepts in the mechanisms and management of drug-induced QT prolongation and trosade de pointes. *Am Heart J.* 2007;153:891–899.

156. Kraft LE, Katholi RE, Woods WT, et al. Attenuation by magnesium of the electrophysiologic effects of hyperkalemia on human and canine heart cells. *Am J Cardiol.* 1980;45:1189–1195.

157. Seller RH. The role of magnesium in digitalis toxicity. *Am Heart J.* 1971;82:551–556.

158. Roden DA. Magnesium treatment of ventricular arrhythmias. *Am J Cardiol*. 1989;63:43G–46G.

159. Flink EB. Therapy of magnesium deficiency. *Ann N Y Acad Sci*. 1969;162:901–905.

160. Nabarro JDN, Spencer AGD, Stowers JM. Metabolic studies in severe diabetic ketosis. *Q J Med*. 1952;21:225–248.

161. Jones JE, Shane SR, Jacobs WH, et al. Magnesium balance studies in chronic alcoholism. *Ann N Y Acad Sci*. 1969;162:934–946.

162. Caddell JL. Magnesium deficiency in extremis. *Nutr Today*. 1967;2:14–20.

163. Parfitt AM, Kleerekiper M. Clinical disorders of calcium, phosphorus and magnesium metabolism. In: Maxwell MH, Kleeman CR, eds. *Clinical Disorders of Fluid and Electrolyte Metabolism*. New York: McGraw-Hill; 1980:1110.

164. Allen BJ, Brodsky MA, Capparelli EV, et al. Magnesium sulfate therapy for sustained monomorphic ventricular tachycardia. *Am J Cardiol*. 1989; 64:1202–1204.

165. Sager PT, Widerhorn J, Petersen R, et al. Prospective evaluation of parenteral magnesium sulfate in the treatment of patients with reentrant AV supraventricular tachycardia. *Am Heart J*. 1990; 119:308–316.

166. Riesdesel ML, Folk GE Jr. Serum magnesium and hibernation. *Nature*. 1956;177:668.

167. Hannon JP, Larson AM, Young DW. Effect of cold acclimatization on plasma electrolyte levels. *J Appl Physiol*. 1958;13:239–240.

168. Pritchard JA. The use of magnesium ion in the management of eclamptogenic toxemias. *Surg Gynecol Obstet*. 1955;100:131–140.

169. Contiguglia SR, Alfrey AC, Miller N, et al. Total body magnesium excess in chronic renal failure. *Lancet*. 1972;1:1300–1302.

170. Wacker WE, Parisi AE. Magnesium metabolism. *N Engl J Med*. 1968;278:658–663,712–717, 772–776.

171. Spencer H, Lesniak M, Gatzo CA, et al. Magnesium absorption and metabolism in patients with chronic renal failure and in patients with normal renal function. *Gastroenterology*. 1980;79:26–34.

172. Randall RE Jr., Chen MD, Spray CC, et al. Hypermagnesemia in renal failure. *Ann Intern Med*. 1949;61:73–88.

173. Alfrey AC, Terman DS, Brettschneider L, et al. Hypermagnesemia after renal homotransplantation. *Ann Intern Med*. 1970;73:367–371.

174. Ditzler JW. Epsom salts poisoning and a review of magnesium-ion physiology. *Anesthesiology*. 1970; 32:378–380.

175. Stevens AR, Wolff HG. Magnesium intoxication: absorption from the intact gastrointestinal tract. *Arch Neurol*. 1950;63:749–759.

176. Weber CA, Santiago RM. Hypermagnesemia, a potential complication during treatment of theophylline intoxication with oral activated charcoal and magnesium containing cathartics. *Chest*. 1989;95:56–59.

177. Clark BA, Brown RS. Unsuspected morbid hypermagnesemia in elderly patients. *Am J Nephrol*. 1992;12:336–343.

178. Ghoneim MM, Long JP. The interaction between magnesium and other neuromuscular blocking agents. *Anesthesiology*. 1970;32:23–27.

179. Swift TR. Weakness from magnesium containing cathartics. *Chest*. 1989;95:56–59.

180. LeGeros RZ, Contiguglia SR, Alfrey AC. Pathological calcification associated with uremia. *Calcif Tissue Res*. 1973;13:173–185.

181. Verberckmoes SC, Persy V, Behets GJ, et al. Uremia-related vascular calcification: more than apatite deposition. *Kidney Int*. 2007; 71: 298–303.

182. Ennever J, Vogel JJ. Magnesium inhibition of apatite nucleation by proteolipid. *J Dent Res*. 1981; 60:838–841.

183. Tomazic B, Tomson M, Nancollas GH. Growth of calcium phosphates on hydroxyapatite cystals: the effect of magnesium. *Arch Oral Biol*. 1975;20: 803–808.

184. Meema HE, Oreopoulos DG, Rapoport A. Serum magnesium level and arterial calcification in end-stage renal disease. *Kidney Int*. 1987;32:388–394.

185. Tzanakis I, Pras A, Kounali D, et al. Mitral annular calcifications in haemodialysis patients: a possible protective role of magnesium. *Nephrol Dial Transplant*. 1997;12:2036–2037.

186. O'Donovan R, Baldwin D, Hammer M, et al. Substitution of aluminum salts by magnesium salts in control of dialysis hyperphosphatemia. *Lancet*. 1986;1:880–882.

187. Parsons V, Baldwin D, Moniz C, et al. Successful control of hyperparathyroidism in patients on continuous ambulatory peritoneal dialysis using magnesium carbonate and calcium carbonate as phosphate binders. *Nephron*. 1993;63:379–383.

188. Delmez JA, Kelber J, Norword KY, et al. Magnesium carbonate as a phosphate binder: a prospective, controlled, crossover study. *Kidney Int*. 1996; 49:163–167.

189. Spiegel DM, Farmer B, Smits G, et al. Magnesium carbonate is an effective phosphate binder for chronic hemodialysis patients: a pilot study. *J Ren Nutr*. 2007;17:416–422.

Disorders of the Renin–Angiotensin–Aldosterone System

MATTHEW K. ABRAMOWITZ, MANISH P. PONDA, AND THOMAS H. HOSTETTER

The renin–angiotensin–aldosterone system (RAAS) has long been known to play a central role in the regulation of bloiod pressure and renal sodium and water excretion. The classic description of the system begins with the conversion of the liver-derived glycoprotein angiotensinogen into the inactive angiotensin (Ang) I by renin, a protease secreted by the juxtaglomerular (JG) cells of the kidney. Ang I is then cleaved by angiotensin-converting enzyme (ACE) into Ang II, which has a diverse range of physiologic effects, including acting as an aldosterone secretagogue in the adrenal cortex. Aldosterone stimulates sodium reabsorption in the distal nephron. The system forms a feedback loop whereby secretion of the main effectors is affected by other members of the RAAS cascade and by other mediators.

The understanding of this system has become increasingly complex over the past two decades with the identification of new Ang receptors, a (pro)renin receptor and additional Ang peptides (Fig. 8.1). Numerous disparate physiologic and pathophysiologic effects have been attributed to the angiotensins and to aldosterone. The notion of the RAAS as an endocrine system has been expanded to include paracrine and autocrine effects with local production of Ang II at the tissue level. This chapter begins with an overview of each component of the RAAS, followed by a discussion of the pathophysiologic importance of each. We then discuss RAAS blockade and its importance in the treatment of individuals with kidney disease.

Angiotensinogen

Angiotensinogen is a 55-to 60-kDa serum glycoprotein that serves as the precursor for all Ang peptides. It is the sole circulating renin substrate; cleavage of a leucine–valine bond produces the decapeptide Ang I. The variability in molecular size of angiotensinogen is attributed to different patterns of glycosylation, as the angiotensinogen gene encodes only a single protein product (1). A high-molecular-weight variant has also been identified that is normally present at low levels. It exists as a greater fraction of total plasma angiotensinogen during the third trimester of pregnancy and is associated with hypertension and preeclampsia in pregnant women (2).

Angiotensinogen is primarily synthesized and released by the liver. Hepatic production may be increased by a number of factors. Angiotensinogen is an acute-phase reactant, and its synthesis is stimulated by stressors such as infection. Glucocorticoids, estrogens, and thyroxine increase angiotensinogen production by the liver (3). Ang II stimulates angiotensinogen synthesis in a positive feedback loop, leading to greater presence of the proximal substrate of the renin–angiotensin system (RAS) at times of increased Ang II production (4).

There is evidence of local angiotensinogen production in multiple organ systems as well. Angiotensinogen mRNA expression has been demonstrated in the kidney, heart, vascular tissues, adrenal gland, central nervous system, fat, and leukocytes (1,5). Within the kidney, angiotensinogen mRNA is most abundant in the cortex, especially in the proximal tubule, but is also present in the glomerulus and medulla (6).

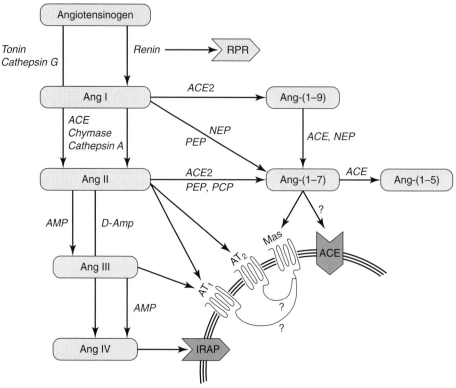

■ **Figure 8.1** Current view of the RAS. ACE, angiotensin-converting enzyme; AMP, aminopeptidase; Ang, angiotensin; AT$_2$, angiotensin II receptors; IRAP, insulin-regulated aminopeptidase; Mas, angiotensin 1-7 receptor; NEP, neutral endopeptidase; PCP, prolyl carboxypeptidase; PEP, prolyl endopeptidase; RAS, renin–angiotensin system; RPR, renin-prorenin receptor. (From Santos RA, Ferreira AJ. Angiotensin-(1-7) and the renin-angiotensin system. *Curr Opin Nephrol Hypertens.* 2007; 16: 122–128, with permission.)

Renin

Renin is a 37- to 40-kDa aspartyl protease with high specificity for angiotensinogen, its only known substrate. Translation of renin mRNA yields the inactive precursor preprorenin, which is converted to prorenin by the removal of a 23–amino acid signal peptide from the carboxyl terminus during insertion into the endoplasmic reticulum (7). Prorenin is a proenzyme that may be rapidly and directly secreted in the intact form or packaged into immature granules and processed into the active renin. Both prorenin and renin are secreted by the JG cells of the kidney. However, prorenin is the major circulating form as the plasma concentration of prorenin is tenfold higher than the concentration of renin (8). Some have speculated that prorenin may be converted to renin in the circulation or locally in tissues, and prorenin-activating enzymes have been found in vascular endothelial cells and neutrophils (9). Renin mRNA has also been demonstrated in multiple organs in addition to the kidney, including the brain, liver, lung, submandibular gland, prostate, testis, ovary, spleen, pituitary, and thymus (10). Nevertheless, renin production outside of the kidney has not been clearly demonstrated, and extrarenal sites that express the renin gene secrete prorenin and not renin (11). Thus the vast majority of circulating renin, if not all, appears to come from the kidney.

A functional renin receptor, called the (pro)renin receptor, has now been described that shows both renin- and prorenin-specific binding. It has been localized to mesangium in glomeruli, smooth muscle cells in renal and coronary arteries, placenta, brain, and liver (12). Binding of renin and prorenin increases the catalytic efficiency of angiotensinogen cleavage and also induces intracellular signaling via activation of the mitogen-activated protein (MAP) kinases ERK1 and ERK2 (12). (Pro)renin receptor binding triggers an increase in the expression of transforming growth factor (TGF)-β1 and other profibrotic molecules such as plasminogen activator inhibitor-1 (PAI-1), fibronectin, and collagen I that is mediated by activation of the MAP kinase pathway (13–15). These results provide evidence of a functional role for prorenin via nonproteolytic activation induced by receptor binding. They demonstrate Ang II-independent, receptor-mediated effects of renin. These findings also suggest that renin itself might be profibrotic and could contribute to the progression of kidney disease.

Regulation of Renin Secretion

As stated earlier, the majority of renin production occurs in the JG cells on the afferent arterioles of the kidney. In normal subjects, sodium intake is the main determinant of renin secretion. Low sodium intake stimulates renin release due to a reduction in extracellular volume. Conversely, high sodium intake causes extracellular volume expansion and inhibits renin secretion. Changes in volume are sensed via several mechanisms that regulate the production and secretion of renin (Table 8.1).

RENAL BARORECEPTORS

The JG cells, of myoepitheliod origin, sense changes in renal perfusion pressure through changes in stretch of the afferent arteriolar wall. JG cells increase renin secretion in response to decreased stretch in the setting of reduced perfusion pressure. Conversely, renin secretion is inhibited in response to increased pressure or stretch within the afferent arteriole. The coupling of perfusion pressure with renin release is thought to be mediated by changes in cytosolic calcium concentration related to JG cell stretch (16).

MACULA DENSA

Renin secretion is also regulated by the macula densa, an area of closely packed specialized tubular cells in the thick ascending limb of the loop of Henle. The composition of tubule fluid delivered to the macula densa regulates renin release via an ion-sensing mechanism that is independent of volume. Infusion of sodium chloride produces a rapid decline in plasma renin activity (PRA) that is not seen with comparable volume expansion with a dextran-containing solution (17). While this effect was initially thought to be sodium dependent, further studies demonstrated the importance of the chloride concentration of tubular fluid. Sodium administered with other anions does not inhibit renin secretion. PRA is not

TABLE 8.1 FACTORS REGULATING RENIN SECRETION

Major Stimuli

Decreased renal perfusion pressure

Decreased NaCl delivery to the macula densa

β-adrenergic stimulation

Other Stimuli

Prostaglandins (PGE$_2$, PGI$_2$)

Dopamine

Glucagon

Nitric oxide

Major Inhibitors

Increased renal perfusion pressure

Increased NaCl delivery to the macula densa

Angiotensin II

Other Inhibitors

Adenosine

Atrial natriuretic peptide

Endothelin

Vasopressin

Calcium

Vitamin D

suppressed by infusion of non-chloride-containing sodium solutions but is suppressed by non-sodium-containing chloride solutions (18). Thus renin inhibition by sodium administration is dependent on the concomitant administration of chloride and is thought to be related to the magnitude of absorptive chloride transport in the macula densa. Isolated perfusion of these structures has shown that lower sodium chloride in the lumen of the macula densa stimulates renin secretion. This depends on salt entry into macula densa cells via the $Na^+/K^+/2Cl^-$ cotransporter (19). As the tubular cells of the macula densa are not in direct contact with the afferent arteriolar JG cells, additional mechanisms have been postulated involving second-messenger signaling and paracrine factors. Adenosine inhibits renin secretion and has been proposed as a mediator of macula densa–regulated renin release (20).

NEURAL MECHANISMS

Neural mechanisms modulate renin release, primarily via the sympathetic nervous system. This appears to be mediated by β-adrenergic receptors, based on several lines of evidence. The JG apparatus (JGA) is densely innervated with sympathetic nerves, and β_1-adrenoreceptors have been localized to the JGA and glomerulus (21–23). β-adrenergic agonists stimulate renin release, while β-adrenergic antagonists reduce renin secretion. Increasing renal sympathetic nerve activity stimulates renin secretion, and β-adrenergic blockade inhibits this effect (20). The mechanism for neural modulation of renin release appears to involve adenylate cyclase activation generating cyclic adenosine monophosphate (cAMP) as a second messenger.

ENDOCRINE AND PARACRINE MECHANISMS

Multiple circulating factors have been shown to regulate renin release. The most important of these is Ang II, which affects renin release in a negative feedback loop independent of volume or tubular transport processes. Higher Ang II levels directly inhibit renin secretion by regulating renin gene expression in the afferent arteriole (24,25). ACE inhibition increases renal renin mRNA expression in animal models (24,26) and increases PRA in humans, at least in part, by interrupting this inhibitory feedback on Ang I (27).

Numerous other hormonal influences affect renin levels via both endocrine and paracrine mechanisms (11). Activators of adenylyl cyclase, by increasing cAMP levels, stimulate renin secretion. These include prostaglandin E_2, prostacyclin, dopamine, and glucagon. Nitric oxide indirectly increases cAMP levels and thus also promotes renin release. Natriuretic hormones, such as atrial natriuretic peptide (ANP), inhibit renin secretion via guanylyl cyclase activation. Calcium has been known to suppress renin release from JG cells. This effect is mediated by calcium-dependent inhibition of adenylyl cyclase (28). Thus, calcium-liberating hormones such as endothelin, vasopressin, and adenosine block renin secretion through the inhibitory effect of calcium. In addition, vitamin D appears to negatively regulate renin expression via a calcium-independent mechanism (29).

Angiotensin-converting Enzyme

ACE is a zinc-containing metalloprotease with a molecular weight of approximately 200 kDa. It cleaves the two C-terminal amino acids (His-Leu) from Ang I to form the octapeptide Ang II. The conversion of Ang I to Ang II occurs rapidly throughout the vasculature. ACE is located on the surface of endothelial cells in many vascular beds, including the kidney. As the main site of synthesis of ACE is in the pulmonary vasculature, a single pass through the lung produces nearly complete conversion of Ang I to Ang II (30).

In contrast to the substrate specificity of renin, multiple small peptides may be hydrolyzed by ACE, including bradykinin, enkephalins, substance P, and luteinizing hormone–releasing hormone (31–35). Thus, in addition to generating the potent vasoconstrictor Ang II, ACE degrades the vasodilator bradykinin into inactive fragments. This underscores the multiple biologic pathways in which ACE may play an important role. The plasma concentration of ACE may be affected by a number of disease states, including hypothyroidism, diabetes mellitus, sarcoidosis, and other granulomatous diseases (36–38). Yet despite significant variation in ACE levels even among healthy subjects, no significant association has been found between levels of the enzyme and the risk of hypertension (39,40).

The human ACE gene has been localized to chromosome 17 (39). There are two catalytic domains that are 68% identical in amino acid sequence. A soluble form of ACE exists in plasma, whose role has yet to be elucidated. A shorter form of ACE with one catalytic domain is present in the testis. In contrast to endothelial ACE, the testicular form is likely regulated by androgens.

Within the kidney, ACE is expressed in the brush border of the proximal tubule and on vascular endothelial cells (41,42). Several functions have been postulated for ACE that is present on the brush border membrane of the proximal tubule epithelium. It may be involved in the cleavage of filtered peptides for subsequent uptake by epithelial cells (42). It may also participate in the local production of Ang II within proximal tubule fluid to facilitate reabsorption.

ACE expression in the vasculature is not limited to the endothelium. Macrophages and other inflammatory cells are significant sources of tissue ACE in human atherosclerotic plaques (43). An insertion/deletion (I/D) polymorphism of a 287-base-pair DNA fragment within the ACE gene has been identified that is associated with clinical outcomes. The deletion polymorphism has been associated with higher ACE levels (40) and with increased risk of microalbuminuria, retinopathy, and left ventricular hypertrophy in hypertensive subjects (44). The D allele has also been associated with the presence of kidney disease in individuals with hypertension (45) and diabetes (46). Patients with diabetic nephropathy homozygous for the D allele compared with the I allele may benefit less from the renoprotective effects of ACE inhibitors (47).

Angiotensins

Ang II is a highly potent vasoconstrictor with multiple actions that regulate vascular tone and renal salt and water excretion. A detailed discussion of its effects appears later. It is formed by ACE via cleavage of the C-terminal dipeptide from Ang I. Alternative pathways for Ang II generation have been demonstrated that do not involve ACE, although their physiologic importance is not yet clear. Tonins, cathepsins, and kallikreins can form Ang I or Ang II directly from angiotensinogen (48). Recent evidence suggests that chymase-dependent pathways may be important for Ang II generation within cardiovascular tissues (49).

The half-life of Ang II in the circulation is very short, approximately 1 to 2 minutes. The major source of degradation is cleavage by aminopeptidases (50). Ang II is hydrolyzed by aminopeptidase A, or glutamyl aminopeptidase, to form Ang III, which is the heptapeptide Ang 2-8. Ang III is a less potent peripheral vasoconstrictor than Ang II (51,52), with a much shorter plasma half-life (53). It has been known since the 1970s to stimulate aldosterone release from the adrenal zona glomerulosa (54). Ang III appears to be an important mediator of the RAS in the central nervous system. Intracerebroventricular injection of Ang II and Ang III produces equivalent pressor and drinking responses (52,55). Ang III may be the main effector of vasopressin release in the brain (56). Further cleavage by aminopeptidases converts Ang III to Ang IV, the hexapeptide Ang 3-8.

Recent data implicate Ang IV in the regulation of cell growth and the vascular inflammatory response. Ang IV stimulates endothelial expression of PAI-1 (57). In vascular smooth muscle cells it activates the nuclear factor kB (NF-kB) pathway, leading to increased expression of monocyte chemoattractant protein-1 (MCP-1), intercellular adhesion molecule-1 (ICAM-1), interleukin-6, and tumor necrosis factor-α (TNF-α) (58). Ang IV may also have a role in memory and cognition (59).

Angiotensins are also subject to hydrolysis by endopeptidases, the most likely of which to be physiologically relevant is neutral endopeptidase (NEP). NEP directly converts Ang I to Ang 1-7 (60). Ang 1-7 can also be formed from Ang II by prolyl endopeptidase and prolyl carboxypeptidase (61), as well as via cleavage by ACE2 (see later). Previously thought to be inactive, Ang 1-7 has been shown to induce renal afferent arteriolar vasodilatation (62) and to stimulate diuresis and natriuresis, possibly via inhibition of the Na^+/K^+ ATPase in the proximal tubule (63). In addition to its vasodilatory properties, Ang 1-7 decreases cardiac hypertrophy and fibrosis and prevents cardiac remodeling (64,65). These actions appear to be mediated via binding to the G protein–coupled receptor Mas (65,66). The ACE2-Ang 1-7-Mas axis has been proposed as a counterregulatory arm within the RAS opposing the actions of Ang II (67).

Angiotensin Receptors

The actions of Ang II are mediated through binding to one of the Ang receptor subtypes. The two most well characterized are the type 1 and type 2 receptors, designated AT_1 and AT_2. Both receptor subtypes are G protein–coupled seven transmembrane receptors. Almost all known Ang II effects, including vasoconstriction, aldosterone secretion, increased sympathetic tone, and cellular growth and proliferation, are mediated by the AT_1 receptor, although the functions of the AT_2 receptor are increasingly being unraveled.

The AT_1 receptor has been localized to multiple organs, including the brain, heart, adrenal gland, kidney, and vasculature (68). It is widely distributed throughout the heart, where Ang II binding causes positive inotropy and chronotropy, but receptor density is greatest within the conducting system (69). Ang II binding to AT_1 receptors stimulates aldosterone secretion from the adrenal zona glomerulosa and catecholamine release from the chromaffin cells of the adrenal medulla. The high levels of the receptor throughout the vasculature on smooth muscle cells mediate changes in vascular tone due to Ang II. Within the kidney, AT_1 receptors have been localized to the afferent arteriole, glomerular mesangial cells, renal medullary interstitial cells, vasa recta, and throughout the tubule (70,71). Ang II stimulates sodium and water reabsorption, regulates the glomerular filtration rate (GFR), and inhibits renin secretion from the macula densa via these receptors. Activation of AT_1 receptors by Ang II stimulates cell growth and proliferation, including activation of the Janus kinases (JAK)/signal transducers and activators of transcription (STAT) pathway (72), expression of growth factors such as TGF-β_1 and basic fibroblast growth factor (bFGF), and vascular smooth muscle cell and cardiac myocyte hypertrophy (73–75).

The AT_2 receptor seems to oppose AT_1 receptor–mediated effects. It is expressed in cardiac fibroblasts (76), the adrenal medulla (68), renal glomeruli, afferent arterioles, proximal tubule, and vasa recta (71,77). Its abundance in kidney mesenchyme during fetal growth suggests an important role in normal development (78). However, AT_2 receptor–knockout mice develop normally but have altered behavior and cardiovascular function, including an increased pressor response to Ang II infusion (79,80). The AT_2 receptor mediates production of vasodilatory substances in the kidney and induces natriuresis via a cascade involving bradykinin and nitric oxide (81). In contrast to the AT_1 receptor, the AT_2 receptor inhibits cell proliferation and promotes differentiation. Thus a generally protective role for AT_2 receptors has been suggested. For example, AT_2 receptor–knockout mice suffer greater kidney injury than do wild-type mice in the partial renal ablation model of chronic kidney disease (CKD) (82).

Additional Ang receptors have been identified that are distinct from the AT_1 and AT_2 receptors. Ang IV binds with high affinity to the AT_4 receptor but has poor affinity for the AT_1 and AT_2 subtypes. The AT_4 receptor has been localized in multiple organs, including the kidney, heart, central nervous system, and adrenal gland (59). Insulin-regulated aminopeptidase (IRAP) has been proposed as a functional receptor for Ang IV (83), although this has been called into question (59). The G protein–coupled receptor Mas has been identified as a functional receptor for Ang 1-7, as described earlier. Mas-knockout mice have impaired cardiac function and altered collagen expression toward a profibrotic state (84).

Angiotensin II

Ang II is the principal effector of the RAS for the regulation of extracellular volume and blood pressure. It acts on multiple organs, including the heart, kidney, vascular system, adrenal gland, central nervous system, and intestine. The effects of Ang II on cardiovascular function include maintenance of systemic blood pressure via direct constriction of vascular smooth muscle cells, leading to increased systemic vascular resistance, and enhanced myocardial contractility. Ang II stimulates catecholamine release from the adrenal medulla and sympathetic nerve endings, increases sympathetic nervous system activity, and may enhance the vasoconstrictor response due to catecholamines (85,86). Ang II acts to preserve extracellular volume via increased salt and water retention by stimulating aldosterone secretion from the adrenal glomerulosa, promoting thirst and water intake, and enhancing renal sodium transport.

In the kidney, Ang II directly affects renal hemodynamics, control of GFR, and tubular transport. The actions of Ang II in the kidney have been nicely reviewed by Ichikawa and Harris (87). It causes arteriolar vasoconstriction, mediated primarily by protein kinase C (PKC) generation (88). Ang II constricts both the afferent and efferent arterioles and the interlobular artery (89–91). Vascular resistance increases more in the efferent than in the afferent arteriole in response to Ang II, partly due to the smaller resting diameter of the efferent arteriole (92). Thus renal blood flow declines, and glomerular capillary hydraulic pressure rises, which preserves GFR in the setting of reduced systemic blood pressure.

The vascular actions of Ang II are modulated by other vasoactive substances produced by endothelial cells, vascular smooth muscle cells, and mesangial cells. Vasodilatory prostaglandins and nitric oxide minimize the increase in vascular resistance, while endothelin-1 (93) and metabolites of the lipoxygenase pathway (94) may mediate Ang II-induced vasoconstriction.

Autoregulatory mechanisms are important for maintaining renal blood flow and GFR in a relatively constant range despite large variations in systemic blood pressure. Two primary mechanisms are recognized to maintain autoregulation. Myogenic stretch receptors in the afferent arteriolar wall respond to changes in perfusion pressure manifested as changes in stretch. Alterations in chloride delivery to the macula densa facilitate a response that returns GFR and tubular flow toward normal. This latter effect is called the tubuloglomerular feedback mechanism (TGF). Ang II might be expected to play a primary role in the maintenance of autoregulation, but this appears not to be the case. Rather, Ang II has a permissive influence on TGF, sensitizing the afferent arteriole or other elements to signals from macula densa cells (95). Other vasopressors do not produce a similar response (96).

Ang II exerts direct effects in the proximal tubule to stimulate the reabsorption of sodium and water, as well as bicarbonate. It increases the activity of the Na^+/H^+ exchanger in the apical membrane of proximal tubule epithelial cells, thereby enhancing Na^+ uptake (97). Ang II stimulates basolateral Na^+/K^+ ATPase activity, further contributing to Na^+ transport (98,99). The Na^+ (HCO_3^-) cotransporter in the basolateral membrane is also activated by Ang II (100). Overall, the effects of Ang II may account for up to 40% to 50% of sodium and water reabsorption in the early (S_1 segment) proximal tubule (101). Ang II also enhances Na^+ reabsorption in the thick ascending limb of the loop of Henle and in the distal tubule (102).

Ang II has effects on cellular growth and proliferation and may contribute to tissue injury in a number of ways (49). It stimulates production of growth factors such as TGF-β and endothelin-1. It appears to have a role in mediating apoptosis. Ang II induces inflammation via mediators such as NF-kB and MCP-1. These proinflammatory and profibrotic actions partly explain the promotion of glomerulosclerosis and tubulointerstitial fibrosis by Ang II (103).

ACE-related Carboxypeptidase

The classical notion of the RAS has been extended by discoveries of the ACE-related carboxypeptidase ACE2 and additional Ang peptides with biologic activity. ACE2 protein expression has been demonstrated in the heart, kidney, and testis (104), as well as in epithelia of the human lung and small intestine (105). Like ACE, ACE2 is both a membrane-associated and membrane-secreted enzyme. It generates its main product, the heptapeptide Ang 1-7, via two pathways. ACE2 cleaves the C-terminal Leu residue from Ang I to generate Ang 1-9, whose function remains unknown. Ang 1-9 is then converted to Ang 1-7 by ACE. Ang 1-7 is also formed by the cleavage of a single residue from Ang II by ACE2. The dual properties of generating the vasodilator Ang 1-7 and degrading Ang II suggest a counterregulatory role for ACE2 in opposing the pressors actions of Ang II (106). Indeed, ACE2-deficient mice show greater pressor sensitivity and higher renal Ang II concentrations during Ang II infusion compared with controls (107). ACE2 may also have an important role in cardiac structure and function (108). In the kidney, ACE2 has been detected in the vascular endothelium, glomerulus, and tubular epithelium (105,109). ACE2-knockout mice develop late glomerulosclerosis that is prevented by Ang II type 1 receptor blockade, suggesting that the glomerular injury is Ang II dependent (110). Early diabetes may be associated with decreased glomerular expression of ACE2, with greater albuminuria induced by ACE2 inhibition (111). However, the association of ACE2 with diabetic nephropathy remains unclear (112–114). An additional unexpected function of ACE2 has been identified, that of a functional receptor for the severe acute respiratory syndrome (SARS) coronavirus (115). SARS infection in ACE2-knockout mice produces more mild disease and reduced viral replication compared with wild-type mice (116).

Local Renin–Angiotensin Systems

It has become clear over the past two decades that the traditional model of the circulating RAS is but one part of the overall picture. There is now abundant evidence of local Ang II synthesis in a variety of sites and the suggestion of complete RASs in several organs. Renin mRNA has been found in multiple tissue sites, although renin secretion has only been demonstrated in the kidney. Ang II production takes place at multiple locations within the kidney, and proximal tubule concentrations of Ang II are 100- to 1000-fold higher than those in plasma. In addition to Ang II generation within JG cells and the tubulointerstitium, it may be formed in the proximal tubule lumen by membrane-bound ACE. Intraluminal Ang II may then stimulate sodium reabsorption in the distal tubule and collecting duct (49). The full spectrum of Ang-mediated effects may need to be viewed as the sum of local and systemic actions of the RAS. In particular, paracrine and autocrine actions have been proposed for the local RAS with effects at the cellular level regulating such diverse processes as cardiac hypertrophy and fibrosis, vascular inflammation and remodeling, temperature regulation, and behavioral control (117).

Aldosterone

Aldosterone is one of the several steroid hormones produced by the adrenal cortex and is the principal steroid regulator of sodium and potassium balance—hence its classification as a mineralocorticoid. Aldosterone's synthesis is localized to the outermost layer of the cortex, the zona glomerulosa. Aldosterone is thought to be secreted by the adrenal as a result of increased synthesis and simple diffusion of the hormone across the adrenal cell membrane, as there have been no specific membrane carriers identified. The circulating aldosterone is about 50% protein bound but nonspecifically so and largely to albumin. The main organ for removal of aldosterone is the liver—one reason that its levels rise with liver disease. It is also inactivated by the kidney through formation of physiologically inert glucuronide conjugates. These and other inactive metabolites are excreted in the urine. In addition to measuring the plasma level of the active hormone, measurement of the excretion of its metabolites in the urine is the usual way of assessing aldosterone secretion (118).

STIMULI TO SECRETION

Several stimuli impinge upon the adrenal to increase aldosterone synthesis and thereby its secretion (Table 8.2). One of the most important of these is Ang II, which is the active peptide produced by the renin–angiotensinogen-converting enzyme cascade described earlier. Ang II acting on its G protein–coupled type 1 receptor on the adrenal cell surface initiates aldosterone synthesis (118). In addition a β arrestin–mediated pathway has also been implicated in transducing Ang II's message in the adrenal (119).

Plasma potassium is the second major signal for aldosterone secretion. Small increases in plasma potassium in the range of 0.1 mEq/L can raise plasma aldosterone by 25% (118). While potassium and Ang II can independently stimulate aldosterone secretion, they appear to have synergistic effects. For example, when Ang II levels are suppressed by pharmacologic inhibition of the converting enzyme, potassium is less potent in stimulating aldosterone than when Ang II levels are at a normal level. However, when Ang II is then administered exogenously, the full potency of potassium is restored. Thus, some tonic action of Ang II seems needed for the full effect of potassium (120). This interaction helps to explain the relative failure of potassium alone to maintain aldosterone secretion in patients receiving drugs that inhibit Ang II production or action.

A large number of other compounds can influence aldosterone secretion. These include adrenocorticotropic hormone (ACTH), atrial natriuretic peptides, endothelin, and dopamine (118).

TABLE 8.2 STIMULI FOR ALDOSTERONE SECRETION

Major Stimuli
Angiotensin II
Potassium
Other Stimuli
ACTH, endothelin, serotonin
Inhibitors
Atrial natriuretic peptides, dopamine, somatostatin

ACTH, adrenocorticotropic hormone.

However, these other factors seem relatively minor in their effects compared with the major controllers, Ang II and potassium.

ACTIONS

Sodium and potassium balance are strongly influenced by aldosterone. Aldosterone enhances sodium reabsorption in the distal nephron through regulation of the epithelial sodium channel (ENaC). Through this and perhaps other tubular effects, aldosterone also augments potassium secretion. Thus, aldosterone acts as a key determinant of extracellular volume and thereby blood pressure as well as plasma potassium levels.

EFFECTS ON SODIUM AND POTASSIUM TRANSPORT

Aldosterone directly and indirectly influences ENaC expression (Fig. 8.2). In the classic model of steroid hormone action, aldosterone binds to a cytoplasmic mineralocorticoid receptor. This complex translocates to the nucleus, which results in increased transcription of target genes such as ENaC subunits (121). Another genomic target of aldosterone is serum- and glucocorticoid-regulated kinase 1 (Sgk1). This enzyme is under transcriptional control by aldosterone (122,123) and is responsible for phosphorylating

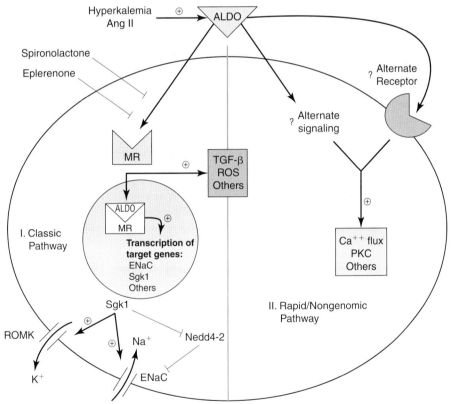

■ **Figure 8.2** Schematic of aldosterone physiology. In renal insufficiency, aldosterone secretion seems to be stimulated principally through the actions of Ang II and hyperkalemia. Other stimuli such as ACTH may be involved. Aldosterone can act through the well-established classic pathway via the mineralocorticoid receptor as well as through a potential rapid, "nongenomic" pathway. Through gene transcription or more direct mechanisms, aldosterone has many downstream effects, as shown. Spironolactone and eplerenone function as competitive antagonists of aldosterone for the mineralocorticoid receptor. *Note:* The "?" signify the uncertain importance or existence of those pathways. ALDO, aldosterone; Ang II, angiotensin II; MR, mineralocorticoid receptor; ROS, reactive oxygen species; TGF-*β*, transforming growth factor beta; PKC, protein kinase C; ENaC, epithelial sodium channel; Nedd 4-2, ubiquitin-protein ligase; Sgk1, serum glucocorticoid kinase 1; ROMK, renal outer medullary potassium channel. (From Ponda MP, Hostetter TH. Aldosterone antagonism in chronic kidney disease. *Clin J Am Soc Nephrol.* 2006;1:668–677 with permission.)

and thereby inhibiting Nedd4-2, a regulatory protein that promotes ENaC degradation (124,125). Thus, aldosterone regulates sodium reabsorption by controlling ENaC trafficking as well.

The mineralocorticoid receptor has an affinity for aldosterone comparable to its affinity for cortisol. Since cortisol is present in much higher concentrations than aldosterone, the presence of the enzyme 11-β hydroxysteroid dehydrogenase is needed to metabolize cortisol at sites of aldosterone action and thereby allow the actions of aldosterone alone unimpeded by ambient cortisol. This effect is thought to be achieved in part by simple degradation of the cortisol and in part through a reduction in the transcriptional activity of the cortisol-mineralocorticoid receptor complex by an associated rise in NADH.

As noted above increases in plasma K^+ increase aldosterone secretion (126). The mineralocorticoid has also been shown to increase expression of the renal outer medullary potassium channel (ROMK), which enhances K^+ secretion (127). This effect is synergistic with sodium reabsorption; the latter allows for an increase in luminal negativity in the renal tubules and thereby facilitates K^+ secretion. Aldosterone also acts through Sgk1 to amplify this effect. Sgk1 appears to work in concert with the Na^+/H^+ Exchange Regulating Factor (NHERF2) to increase ROMK activity (128). This finding is supported by the sgk1-knockout mouse, which has impaired renal K^+ clearance (129).

In addition to renal epithelia, aldosterone exerts control over ENaC expressed in intestinal, salivary, and sweat epithelial tissue, where it also participates in sodium and potassium homeostasis (130).

A number of other non-hemodynamic pathways of aldosterone action have begun to be explored. Some are discussed later. However, several observations give predominance to aldosterone's ability to raise arterial, and probably glomerular, pressure as a major mode of damage to the kidney and the organism as a whole. The requirement for concomitant high salt intake in most animal models of injury and the absence of tissue injury in forms of secondary aldosteronism without hypertension, for example, chronic salt deficiency, both argue for a key role of hypertension (131,132). Also, the appearance of kidney failure in a person with Liddle syndrome in whom aldosterone levels are suppressed suggests that classic salt-dependent hypertension is very important, whatever other aldosterone-dependent pathways may be at work (133).

NONTRANSPORT EFFECTS

Extra-adrenal tissue may synthesize aldosterone. The vasculature, the kidney, and the heart have been reported as synthetic sites (134–136). However, none of these potential sources contributes significantly to plasma levels as the concentration of aldosterone falls to essentially zero with adrenalectomy. Furthermore, recent data have questioned the notion of cardiac synthesis of aldosterone (137,138). However, given the presence of mineralocorticoid receptors in many nonepithelial tissues, including the vasculature and heart, these nontraditional targets may indeed respond to aldosterone whether they produce it or not (139).

Beyond the well-documented effect of aldosterone to expand extracellular volume with the net result of hypertension, direct vascular actions of aldosterone have been proposed. Systemic vascular resistance (SVR) has been reported to change modestly in response to acute aldosterone infusion in normal human subjects (140). Rabbit glomerular afferent and efferent arterioles constrict in response to aldosterone ex vivo (141). In this model, increased calcium flux plays an important role, and calcium channel blockade can inhibit the effect. The direct vascular effects of aldosterone may be complex, involving some interplay with nitric oxide. The homeostatic role of these direct vasoconstrictive actions and their magnitude in vivo are still under investigation.

Beyond raising intravascular pressure, aldosterone may also contribute to injury through stimulation of certain cytokines. TGF-β and PAI-1 are both profibrotic, and the secretion of each is provoked by aldosterone (142,143). In addition to these cytokines, several other inflammatory cytokines are produced in adipocytes under the influence of aldosterone. Finally, production of reactive oxygen species has been observed with aldosterone addition to cells. These findings have given rise to the notion that aldosterone contributes to insulin resistance and the metabolic syndrome through these inflammatory effects and oxidant effects.

NONGENOMIC ACTIONS

Aldosterone can change several markers of cellular signaling within minutes. These effects cannot be explained by its classic genomic actions. Indeed, the effects occur well before any increase in protein expression and are not affected by inhibitors of transcription or protein synthesis (144,145). Therefore, these are so-called "nongenomic" actions. In addition to sodium flux, other rapid or early events such as calcium flux (146), changes in intracellular pH (147), and PKC activity (148) have been demonstrated in response to aldosterone. There are conflicting data as to whether these effects are mediated by the classic mineralocorticoid receptor or an independent pathway, as some studies show inhibition by pharmacologic mineralocorticoid antagonists, for example, spironolactone (see later), whereas others do not (149). Indeed, many of the above-mentioned actions of aldosterone, especially the reported direct vascular actions, are temporally nongenomic or at least partially so. The pleiotropic effects of aldosterone most likely occur through the "classic" mineralocorticoid receptor and gene transcription in parallel with other distinct "rapid" signaling pathways. However, distinct physiologic roles for the nongenomic pathway have yet to be definitively assigned.

The Renin–Angiotensin–Aldosterone System in Hypertension

The major function of the RAAS is to regulate blood pressure and extracellular volume. Changes in either of these parameters lead to either activation or suppression of the system. However, the appropriate coupling of RAAS activity to blood pressure and volume may be altered in a number of pathologic states. In certain conditions, a primary disturbance in the RAAS leads to abnormalities in blood pressure and/or extracellular volume. These disorders can be distinguished by the relationship between PRA and aldosterone secretion (Fig. 8.3).

Individuals with hypertension may be characterized by their PRA profile. In approximately one-third of hypertensive subjects, the PRA is below that of normal subjects (called low-renin hypertension).

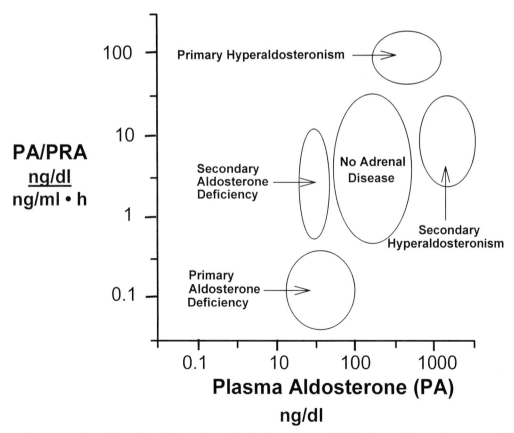

■ **Figure 8.3** The relationship of PA to the ratio of aldosterone to PRA is shown during various states of aldosterone excess or deficiency. PA, plasma aldosterone; PRA, plasma renin activity. (Adapted from McKenna TJ, et al. Diagnosis under random conditions of all disorders. *J Clin Endocrinol Metab* 73:952, 1991.)

Thus, in the remaining two-thirds, renin secretion is normal or supranormal despite the high-pressure state that would be expected to suppress PRA. Some have advocated the use of PRA measurement to guide treatment in essential hypertension, specifically in those with difficult-to-control hypertension (150,151). This is based on the hypothesis that PRA is a marker for the primary pathophysiologic mechanism, that is, low-renin hypertension is a volume excess state best treated with natriuretic agents; in the remainder, hypertension is mediated by renin-dependent vasoconstriction and should be treated with blockers of the RAAS. However, this approach is not routine practice for most clinicians, and its utility has not been rigorously tested.

Primary disorders of the RAAS account for approximately 10% of hypertensive subjects, although prevalence estimates are highly variable depending on the population studied. Mineralocorticoid hypertension is classically accompanied by hypokalemia and metabolic alkalosis. However, this is not universal and should not be considered necessary to raise suspicion for a secondary cause of hypertension. Primary hyperaldosteronism is the most common cause. Disorders of renin secretion and causes of secondary hyperaldosteronism must also be considered (Table 8.3). Unilateral or bilateral vascular lesions of the renal artery stimulate renin release due to decreased renal perfusion pressure. The etiology is most commonly atherosclerotic disease causing renal artery stenosis, especially in older individuals. Fibromuscular dysplasia is the most frequent etiology among younger individuals, presenting most often in women. Renin-secreting tumors are a rare cause of secondary hypertension. Primary hyperaldosteronism may be caused by an adrenal adenoma (Conn syndrome), bilateral adrenal hyperplasia, or, less commonly, an adrenal carcinoma. Glucocorticoid-remediable aldosteronism is an autosomal dominant condition in which a chimeric aldosterone synthase gene results in excess aldosterone secretion under the control of ACTH.

Other syndromes may present similarly to hyperaldosteronism yet be characterized by suppression of aldosterone production. Apparent mineralocorticoid excess (AME) is a rare autosomal recessive disorder marked by inactivity of the enzyme 11-β hydroxysteroid dehydrogenase. The excess cortisol binds the mineralocorticoid receptor, resulting in sodium retention and volume expansion with suppression of renin and aldosterone. An acquired form of AME may result from licorice ingestion due to the actions of glycyrrhizic acid and glycyrrhetinic acid. Liddle syndrome is caused by an inherited gain-of-function mutation in the ENaC, leading to unregulated sodium retention. Ectopic ACTH production and defects in cortisol synthesis may also produce the signs and symptoms of mineralocorticoid excess.

Measurement of the ratio of the plasma aldosterone concentration (measured in ng/dL) to PRA (measured in ng/mL/h) is a useful initial screening test (Fig. 8.4). Values >30, especially with a plasma aldosterone >15 ng/mL, should prompt further testing. Interested readers are referred to several excellent reviews of mineralocorticoid hypertension (152); genetic forms of hypertension, including Liddle syndrome (153); primary aldosteronism (154); and syndromes of aldosterone excess and deficiency (155).

TABLE 8.3 DIFFERENTIAL DIAGNOSIS OF MINERALOCORTICOID HYPERTENSION

Renin

Renovascular hypertension

Renin-secreting tumor

Aldosterone

Adrenal adenoma

Bilateral adrenal hyperplasia

Adrenal carcinoma

Glucocorticoid-remediable aldosteronism

Other

Apparent mineralocorticoid excess

Liddle syndrome

Ectopic ACTH syndrome

Congenital adrenal hyperplasia

ACTH, adrenocorticotropic hormone.

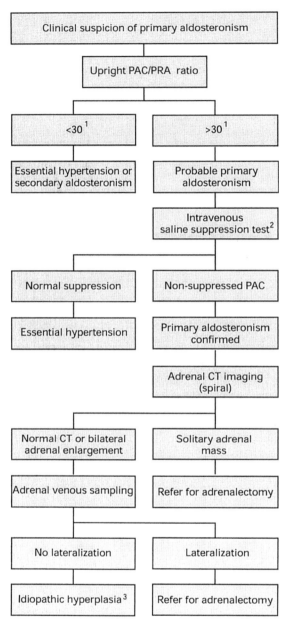

■ **Figure 8.4** Algorithm for diagnosis of primary aldosteronism. [1]PAC, plasma aldosterone concentration; PRA, plasma renin activity. [2]Intravenous saline suppression test: administration of 2L of isotonic saline over 4 hours. PACs should decrease to <6 ng/dL. [3]Consider screening for glucocorticoid remediable aldosteronism if family history is significant for juvenile onset of hypertension. (From Lawrence JE, Dluhy RG. Endocrine hypertension. In: Harris, Bouloux, eds. *Endocrinology in clinical practice,* London: Martin Dunitz, 2002: 390.)

Blockade of the Renin–Angiotensin–Aldosterone System

RENIN INHIBITORS

Aliskiren is the first member of a new class of orally active, nonpeptide, low-molecular-weight renin inhibitors. Its oral bioavailability is quite low (2.6%), but it is highly potent and has a half-life of 40 hours (156). It interferes with the rate-limiting step in Ang II production, the highly substrate-specific cleavage of angiotensinogen by renin. Aliskiren does not undergo hepatic metabolism and is not metabolized by the cytochrome p450 system. It is primariy excreted in the urine, mostly as unchanged drug.

ANGIOTENSIN-CONVERTING ENZYME INHIBITORS

ACE inhibitors inhibit the activity of Ang-converting enzyme. There are three categories based on the ligand that binds to the ACE-zinc moiety: sulfhydryl, carboxyl, and phosphinyl. Despite differences in prodrug, structure, binding affinity, and metabolism, the clinical effects of all ACE inhibitors are quite similar. With the notable exceptions of captopril and cilazopril, the duration of response for most is approximately 24 hours. Drug metabolism varies within the class between liver and kidney, although most are excreted at least partially in the urine. The most common side effect is a dry cough that is reported in up to 20% of patients (157). This is mediated by the accumulation of bradykinins and substance P, which are otherwise degraded by ACE, and by production of prostaglandins. The cough may present immediately after initiation of therapy or may not present until months thereafter. The only established cure is cessation of the drug. The most feared complication of ACE inhibitor therapy is angioedema, which is a potentially life-threatening complication. The mechanism is thought to be related to increased bradykinin levels and inhibition of C1 esterase activity (158).

ANGIOTENSIN II TYPE I RECEPTOR ANTAGONISTS

The AT_1 receptor blockers (ARBs) may provide more complete blockade of the RAS than do ACE inhibitors because ARBs interfere with the system at the point of receptor binding by Ang II. Thus, effects of non-ACE-dependent Ang II formation (due to chymase, cathepsins, etc.; see earlier) are not blocked by ACE inhibitors but are inhibited by ARBs. Like ACE inhibitors, ARBs also increase bradykinin levels. This is due to increased AT_2 receptor activity secondary to lack of Ang II binding to AT_1 receptors.

ARBs also vary in structure, metabolism, potency, and mechanism of receptor inhibition. This class of medication is composed of both peptide and nonpeptide analogs. There are both competitive and noncompetitive antagonists of the AT_1 receptor. Losartan was the first orally active ARB; its derivatives are called biphenyl tetrazoles. Other members of the class are categorized as nonbiphenyl tetrazoles and nonheterocyclic compounds. The duration of response is approximately 24 hours for all. Most ARBs undergo both hepatic and renal metabolism. The incidence of cough in patients with a history of ACE inhibitor–induced cough was no greater than that in controls (159).

ALDOSTERONE RECEPTOR ANTAGONISTS

Spironolactone and eplerenone are steroid analogues with structural similarity to aldosterone and thereby function as competitive antagonists. Compared to spironolactone, eplerenone is equally potent but more specific for the mineralocorticoid receptor by virtue of a 9,11-epoxy moiety that decreases its binding to androgen and progesterone receptors (160). Both drugs are metabolized hepatically, though spironolactone has multiple active metabolites, whereas eplerenone has none (161). This results in a shorter effective half-life and therefore quicker time to peak response for eplerenone.

As described earlier, these molecules are able to antagonize some but not all of aldosterone's actions. This implies that either aldosterone can signal through a mineralocorticoid receptor distinct pathway or differential mineralocorticoid receptor localization somehow favors access to aldosterone but not spironolactone or eplerenone. As an example of the latter, an open-ring water-soluble aldosterone antagonist, RU28318, completely abrogated aldosterone's influence on Na^+/H^+ exchanger activity, whereas spironolactone had no effect in a human vascular preparation ex vivo (162). Hyperkalemia is the most serious side effect. Gynecomastia also occurs and is more frequent with spironolactone.

Progression and the Renin–Angiotensin–Aldosterone System

ACE inhibitors and ARBs are standard drugs for primary hypertension. However, they are each especially effective in slowing the progressive decay of GFR in CKD (163–167). Diabetic nephropathy has been the most studied, and these agents not only lower proteinuria but also slow progressive injury. This general pattern reduction of proteinuria linked to retardation of filtration failure has been observed in the other major classes of renal injury, including hypertensive nephrosclerosis (168). Although these

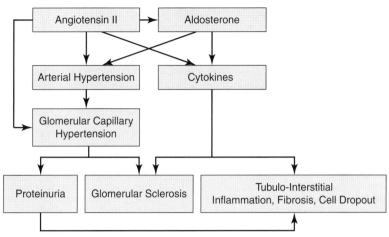

■ **Figure 8.5** RAAS system and renal injury. RAAS, renin–angiotensin–aldosterone system.

drugs reduce proteinuria in autosomal dominant polycystic kidney disease as well, they have not been so clearly proven to mitigate progression in this condition as in other disorders (169). Even in rarer entities such as Alport disease, their use has become routine despite the understandable lack of formal clinical trials in some of these conditions (170).

There are several reasons why ACE inhibitors and ARBs are especially beneficial antihypertensive agents in CKD (Fig. 8.5). They reduce Ang II levels and/or action and thereby also lower aldosterone levels. These actions lower arterial pressure, but intrarenal hemodynamic effects also contribute to their salutary effects. In many animal models of CKD, glomerular capillary pressures are elevated and are thought to be elevated in human CKD. ACE inhibitors and ARBs reduce this capillary hypertension both by reducing arterial perfusion pressure and by relaxation of the efferent arteriole, the dominant site of Ang II action. Relief from this excessive capillary pressure likely prevents mesangial cell proliferation and matrix production as well as podocyte loss (171). The associated reduction in proteinuria may also be a benefit of these drugs, as protein absorption by the proximal tubular cells seems to be toxic (172). Finally, Ang II and aldosterone can cause the release a whole host of profibrotic and inflammatory mediators from even nonimmune cells such as those of the proximal tubule (103,173). Thus, both hemodynamic/antihypertensive actions and antifibrotic and antiinflammatory actions underlie the efficacy of ACE inhibitors and ARBs in CKD.

Since ACE inhibitors and ARBs each slow progression individually, the question has arisen as to whether the combination would provide additional advantage. This issue has not been definitively settled. One early report of the COOPERATE trial claimed that the combination was superior to the individual drugs (174). However, these results and their analysis have been brought into question (175). An analysis of a study designed to examine cardiovascular endpoints in subjects with cardiovascular disease but generally good renal function, the ONTARGET study, found lesser proteinuria with the combination but no benefit in terms of preventing decline in GFR (176). Several trials designed primarily to examine the renal effects of this combination in subjects with CKD are underway (177,178). At present, there is no firm data to support use of the combination.

Aldosterone contributes along with Ang II to the adverse actions of the RAAS in progressive CKD. Recognition of the deleterious effects of aldosterone has led to attempts to selectively block it using the mineralocorticoid receptor blockers (179). A large number of studies in experimental animals have supported this approach. Several trials in human subjects with CKD have shown a reduction in proteinuria when aldosterone blockade was added to an ACE inhibitor or ARB (179). However, there is not yet a large enough trial to assess the effects on decline in GFR. Also, hyperkalemia was more frequent with addition of the mineralocorticoid receptor blocker. Thus, there is not sufficient data to recommend addition of aldosterone blockade to standard therapy in CKD (180).

Inhibition of renin is yet another means of interrupting the RAAS. Addition of a renin inhibitor to an ARB reduced proteinuria in diabetic nephropathy (181). The diminution of proteinuria occurred with little, if any, further reduction in blood pressure, and no additional side effects were noted with the combination. A larger and longer trial is underway to test the value of renin addition to ACE inhibitors or ARBs using cardiovascular and renal endpoints (182).

In summary, blockade of the RAAS with ACE inhibitors or ARBs has proven effective in retarding progression of CKD. Studies are going on to assess the value of interrupting the pathway simultaneously at multiple sites, but such approaches have at this time not been proven more effective than the use of ACE inhibitors or ARBs and have not been adequately assessed for safety.

REFERENCES

1. Lynch KR, Peach MJ. Molecular biology of angiotensinogen. *Hypertension.* 1991;17:263–269.
2. Ward K, Hata A, Jeunemaitre X, et al. A molecular variant of angiotensinogen associated with preeclampsia. *Nat Genet.* 1993;4:59–61.
3. Dzau VJ, Herrmann HC. Hormonal control of angiotensinogen production. *Life Sci.* 1982;30:577–584.
4. Schunkert H, Ingelfinger JR, Jacob H, et al. Reciprocal feedback regulation of kidney angiotensinogen and renin mRNA expressions by angiotensin II. *Am J Physiol.* 1992;263:E863–E869.
5. Campbell DJ, Habener JF. Angiotensinogen gene is expressed and differentially regulated in multiple tissues of the rat. *J Clin Invest.* 1986;78:31–39.
6. Terada Y, Tomita K, Nonoguchi H, et al. PCR localization of angiotensin II receptor and angiotensin mRNAs in rat kidney. *Kidney Int.* 1993;43:1251–1259.
7. Pratt RE, Carleton JE, Richie JP, et al. Human renin biosynthesis and secretion in normal and ischemic kidneys. *Proc Natl Acad Sci U S A.* 1987;84:7837–7840.
8. Danser AH. Prorenin: back into the arena. *Hypertension.* 2006;47:824–826.
9. Dzau VJ, Burt DW, Pratt RE. Molecular biology of the renin-angiotensin system. *Am J Physiol.* 1988;255:F563–F573.
10. Griendling KK, Murphy TJ, Alexander RW. Molecular biology of the renin-angiotensin system. *Circulation.* 1993;87:1816–1828.
11. Krop M, Danser AH. Circulating versus tissue renin-angiotensin system: on the origin of (pro)renin. *Curr Hypertens Rep.* 2008;10:112–118.
12. Nguyen G, Delarue F, Burckle C, et al. Pivotal role of the renin/prorenin receptor in angiotensin II production and cellular responses to renin. *J Clin Invest.* 2002;109:1417–1427.
13. Huang Y, Noble NA, Zhang J, et al. Renin-stimulated TGF-beta1 expression is regulated by a mitogen-activated protein kinase in mesangial cells. *Kidney Int.* 2007;72:45–52.
14. Huang Y, Wongamorntham S, Kasting J, et al. Renin increases mesangial cell transforming growth factor-beta1 and matrix proteins through receptor-mediated, angiotensin II-independent mechanisms. *Kidney Int.* 2006;69:105–113.
15. Nguyen G, Delarue F, Berrou J, et al. Specific receptor binding of renin on human mesangial cells in culture increases plasminogen activator inhibitor-1 antigen. *Kidney Int.* 1996;50:1897–1903.
16. Fray JC, Lush DJ, Park CS. Interrelationship of blood flow, juxtaglomerular cells, and hypertension: role of physical equilibrium and Ca. *Am J Physiol.* 1986;251:R643–R662.
17. Tuck ML, Dluhy RG, Williams GH. A specific role for saline or the sodium ion in the regulation of renin and aldosterone secretion. *J Clin Invest.* 1974;53:988–995.
18. Kirchner KA, Kotchen TA, Galla JH, et al. Importance of chloride for acute inhibition of renin by sodium chloride. *Am J Physiol.* 1978;235:F444–F450.
19. Persson AE, Ollerstam A, Liu R, et al. Mechanisms for macula densa cell release of renin. *Acta Physiol Scand.* 2004;181:471–474.
20. Hackenthal E, Paul M, Ganten D, et al. Morphology, physiology, and molecular biology of renin secretion. *Physiol Rev.* 1990;70:1067–1116.
21. Barajas L. Anatomy of the juxtaglomerular apparatus. *Am J Physiol.* 1979;237:F333–F343.
22. Lew R, Summers RJ. The distribution of beta-adrenoceptors in dog kidney: an autoradiographic analysis. *Eur J Pharmacol.* 1987;140:1–11.
23. McPherson GA, Summers RJ. Evidence from binding studies for beta 1-adrenoceptors associated with glomeruli isolated from rat kidney. *Life Sci.* 1983;33:87–94.
24. Johns DW, Peach MJ, Gomez RA, et al. Angiotensin II regulates renin gene expression. *Am J Physiol.* 1990;259:F882–F887.
25. Lorenz JN, Weihprecht H, He XR, et al. Effects of adenosine and angiotensin on macula densa-stimulated renin secretion. *Am J Physiol.* 1993;265:F187–F194.
26. Sigmund CD, Jones CA, Kane CM, et al. Regulated tissue- and cell-specific expression of the human renin gene in transgenic mice. *Circ Res.* 1992;70:1070–1079.
27. Goldstone R, Horton R, Carlson EJ, et al. Reciprocal changes in active and inactive renin after converting enzyme inhibition in normal man. *J Clin Endocrinol Metab.* 1983;56:264–268.
28. Grunberger C, Obermayer B, Klar J, et al. The calcium paradoxon of renin release: calcium suppresses renin exocytosis by inhibition of calcium-dependent adenylate cyclases AC5 and AC6. *Circ Res.* 2006;99:1197–1206.
29. Li YC, Kong J, Wei M, et al. 1,25-Dihydroxyvitamin D(3) is a negative endocrine regulator of the renin-angiotensin system. *J Clin Invest.* 2002;110:229–238.
30. Ng KK, Vane JR. Conversion of angiotensin I to angiotensin II. *Nature.* 1967;216:762–766.

31. Erdos EG, Johnson AR, Boyden NT. Hydrolysis of enkephalin by cultured human endothelial cells and by purified peptidyl dipeptidase. *Biochem Pharmacol.* 1978;27:843–848.

32. Rieger KJ, Saez-Servent N, Papet MP, et al. Involvement of human plasma angiotensin I-converting enzyme in the degradation of the haemoregulatory peptide N-acetyl-seryl-aspartyl-lysyl-proline. *Biochem J.* 1993;296(pt 2):373–378.

33. Skidgel RA. Characterization of the metabolism of substance P and neurotensin by human angiotensin I converting enzyme and "enkephalinase." *Prog Clin Biol Res.* 1985;192:371–378.

34. Skidgel RA, Erdos EG. Novel activity of human angiotensin I converting enzyme: release of the NH2- and COOH-terminal tripeptides from the luteinizing hormone-releasing hormone. *Proc Natl Acad Sci U S A.* 1985;82:1025–1029.

35. Yang HY, Erdos EG, Levin Y. A dipeptidyl carboxypeptidase that converts angiotensin I and inactivates bradykinin. *Biochim Biophys Acta.* 1970;214:374–376.

36. DeRemee RA, Rohrbach MS. Serum angiotensin-converting enzyme activity in evaluating the clinical course of sarcoidosis. *Ann Intern Med.* 1980;92:361–365.

37. Lieberman J, Sastre A. Serum angiotensin-converting enzyme: elevations in diabetes mellitus. *Ann Intern Med.* 1980;93:825–826.

38. Yotsumoto H, Imai Y, Kuzuya N, et al. Increased levels of serum angiotensin-converting enzyme activity in hyperthyroidism. *Ann Intern Med.* 1982;96:326–328.

39. Jeunemaitre X, Lifton RP, Hunt SC, et al. Absence of linkage between the angiotensin converting enzyme locus and human essential hypertension. *Nat Genet.* 1992;1:72–75.

40. Rigat B, Hubert C, Alhenc-Gelas F, et al. An insertion/deletion polymorphism in the angiotensin I-converting enzyme gene accounting for half the variance of serum enzyme levels. *J Clin Invest.* 1990;86:1343–1346.

41. Metzger R, Bohle RM, Pauls K, et al. Angiotensin-converting enzyme in non-neoplastic kidney diseases. *Kidney Int.* 1999;56:1442–1454.

42. Schulz WW, Hagler HK, Buja LM, et al. Ultrastructural localization of angiotensin I-converting enzyme (EC 3.4.15.1) and neutral metalloendopeptidase (EC 3.4.24.11) in the proximal tubule of the human kidney. *Lab Invest.* 1988;59:789–797.

43. Diet F, Pratt RE, Berry GJ, et al. Increased accumulation of tissue ACE in human atherosclerotic coronary artery disease. *Circulation.* 1996;94:2756–2767.

44. Pontremoli R, Sofia A, Tirotta A, et al. The deletion polymorphism of the angiotensin I-converting enzyme gene is associated with target organ damage in essential hypertension. *J Am Soc Nephrol.* 1996;7:2550–2558.

45. Fabris B, Bortoletto M, Candido R, et al. Genetic polymorphisms of the renin-angiotensin-aldosterone system and renal insufficiency in essential hypertension. *J Hypertens.* 2005;23:309–316.

46. Marre M, Jeunemaitre X, Gallois Y, et al. Contribution of genetic polymorphism in the renin-angiotensin system to the development of renal complications in insulin-dependent diabetes: Genetique de la Nephropathie Diabetique (GENEDIAB) study group. *J Clin Invest.* 1997;99:1585–1595.

47. Parving HH, Jacobsen P, Tarnow L, et al. Effect of deletion polymorphism of angiotensin converting enzyme gene on progression of diabetic nephropathy during inhibition of angiotensin converting enzyme: observational follow up study. *BMJ.* 1996;313:591–594.

48. Belova LA. Angiotensin II-generating enzymes. *Biochemistry (Mosc).* 2000;65:1337–1345.

49. Kobori H, Nangaku M, Navar LG, et al. The intrarenal renin-angiotensin system: from physiology to the pathobiology of hypertension and kidney disease. *Pharmacol Rev.* 2007;59:251–287.

50. Ahmad S, Ward PE. Role of aminopeptidase activity in the regulation of the pressor activity of circulating angiotensins. *J Pharmacol Exp Ther.* 1990;252:643–650.

51. Fink GD, Bruner CA. Hypertension during chronic peripheral and central infusion of angiotensin III. *Am J Physiol.* 1985;249:E201–E208.

52. Wright JW, Morseth SL, Abhold RH, et al. Pressor action and dipsogenicity induced by angiotensin II and III in rats. *Am J Physiol.* 1985;249:R514–R521.

53. Gammelgaard I, Wamberg S, Bie P. Systemic effects of angiotensin III in conscious dogs during acute double blockade of the renin-angiotensin-aldosterone-system. *Acta Physiol (Oxf).* 2006;188:129–138.

54. Goodfriend TL, Peach MJ. Angiotensin III: (DES-aspartic acid-1)-angiotensin II. Evidence and speculation for its role as an important agonist in the renin-angiotensin system. *Circ Res.* 1975;36:38–48.

55. Wright JW, Jensen LL, Roberts KA, et al. Structure-function analyses of brain angiotensin control of pressor action in rats. *Am J Physiol.* 1989;257:R1551–R1557.

56. Zini S, Fournie-Zaluski MC, Chauvel E, et al. Identification of metabolic pathways of brain angiotensin II and III using specific aminopeptidase inhibitors: predominant role of angiotensin III in the control of vasopressin release. *Proc Natl Acad Sci U S A.* 1996;93:11968–11973.

57. Kerins DM, Hao Q, Vaughan DE. Angiotensin induction of PAI-1 expression in endothelial cells is mediated by the hexapeptide angiotensin IV. *J Clin Invest.* 1995;96:2515–2520.

58. Ruiz-Ortega M, Esteban V, Egido J. The regulation of the inflammatory response through nuclear factor-kappab pathway by angiotensin IV extends the role of the renin angiotensin system in cardiovascular diseases. *Trends Cardiovasc Med.* 2007;17:19–25.

59. Wright JW, Yamamoto BJ, Harding JW. Angiotensin receptor subtype mediated physiologies and behaviors: new discoveries and clinical targets. *Prog Neurobiol.* 2008;84:157–181.

60. Yamamoto K, Chappell MC, Brosnihan KB, et al. In vivo metabolism of angiotensin I by neutral endopeptidase (EC 3.4.24.11) in spontaneously hypertensive rats. *Hypertension.* 1992;19:692–696.

61. Welches WR, Santos RA, Chappell MC, et al. Evidence that prolyl endopeptidase participates in

the processing of brain angiotensin. *J Hypertens.* 1991;9:631–638.

62. Ren Y, Garvin JL, Carretero OA. Vasodilator action of angiotensin-(1-7) on isolated rabbit afferent arterioles. *Hypertension.* 2002;39:799–802.

63. Handa RK, Ferrario CM, Strandhoy JW. Renal actions of angiotensin-(1-7): in vivo and in vitro studies. *Am J Physiol.* 1996;270:F141–F147.

64. Grobe JL, Mecca AP, Mao H, et al. Chronic angiotensin-(1-7) prevents cardiac fibrosis in DOCA-salt model of hypertension. *Am J Physiol Heart Circ Physiol.* 2006;290:H2417–H2423.

65. Tallant EA, Ferrario CM, Gallagher PE. Angiotensin-(1-7) inhibits growth of cardiac myocytes through activation of the mas receptor. *Am J Physiol Heart Circ Physiol.* 2005;289:H1560–H1566.

66. Santos RA, Simoes e Silva AC, Maric C, et al. Angiotensin-(1-7) is an endogenous ligand for the G protein-coupled receptor Mas. *Proc Natl Acad Sci U S A.* 2003;100:8258–8263.

67. Santos RA, Ferreira AJ. Angiotensin-(1-7) and the renin-angiotensin system. *Curr Opin Nephrol Hypertens.* 2007;16:122–128.

68. Allen AM, Zhuo J, Mendelsohn FA. Localization of angiotensin AT1 and AT2 receptors. *J Am Soc Nephrol.* 1999;10(suppl 11):S23–S29.

69. Allen AM, Yamada H, Mendelsohn FA. In vitro autoradiographic localization of binding to angiotensin receptors in the rat heart. *Int J Cardiol.* 1990;28:25–33.

70. Zhuo J, Alcorn D, Allen AM, et al. High resolution localization of angiotensin II receptors in rat renal medulla. *Kidney Int.* 1992;42:1372–1380.

71. Miyata N, Park F, Li XF, et al. Distribution of angiotensin AT1 and AT2 receptor subtypes in the rat kidney. *Am J Physiol.* 1999;277:F437–F446.

72. Marrero MB, Schieffer B, Paxton WG, et al. Direct stimulation of Jak/STAT pathway by the angiotensin II AT1 receptor. *Nature.* 1995;375:247–250.

73. Dzau VJ. Cell biology and genetics of angiotensin in cardiovascular disease. *J Hypertens Suppl.* 1994;12:S3–S10.

74. Paradis P, Dali-Youcef N, Paradis FW, et al. Overexpression of angiotensin II type I receptor in cardiomyocytes induces cardiac hypertrophy and remodeling. *Proc Natl Acad Sci U S A.* 2000;97:931–936.

75. Rosendorff C. The renin-angiotensin system and vascular hypertrophy. *J Am Coll Cardiol.* 1996;28:803–812.

76. Tsutsumi Y, Matsubara H, Ohkubo N, et al. Angiotensin II type 2 receptor is upregulated in human heart with interstitial fibrosis, and cardiac fibroblasts are the major cell type for its expression. *Circ Res.* 1998;83:1035–1046.

77. Cao Z, Kelly DJ, Cox A, et al. Angiotensin type 2 receptor is expressed in the adult rat kidney and promotes cellular proliferation and apoptosis. *Kidney Int.* 2000;58:2437–2451.

78. Norwood VF, Craig MR, Harris JM, et al. Differential expression of angiotensin II receptors during early renal morphogenesis. *Am J Physiol.* 1997;272:R662–R668.

79. Hein L, Barsh GS, Pratt RE, et al. Behavioural and cardiovascular effects of disrupting the angiotensin II type-2 receptor in mice. *Nature.* 1995;377:744–747.

80. Ichiki T, Labosky PA, Shiota C, et al. Effects on blood pressure and exploratory behaviour of mice lacking angiotensin II type-2 receptor. *Nature.* 1995;377:748–750.

81. Carey RM, Wang ZQ, Siragy HM. Role of the angiotensin type 2 receptor in the regulation of blood pressure and renal function. *Hypertension.* 2000;35:155–163.

82. Benndorf RA, Krebs C, Hirsch-Hoffmann B, et al. Angiotensin II type 2 receptor deficiency aggravates renal injury and reduces survival in chronic kidney disease in mice. *Kidney Int.* 2009;75:1039–1049.

83. Albiston AL, McDowall SG, Matsacos D, et al. Evidence that the angiotensin IV (AT[4]) receptor is the enzyme insulin-regulated aminopeptidase. *J Biol Chem.* 2001;276:48623–48626.

84. Santos RA, Castro CH, Gava E, et al. Impairment of in vitro and in vivo heart function in angiotensin-(1-7) receptor MAS knockout mice. *Hypertension.* 2006;47:996–1002.

85. Purdy RE, Weber MA. Angiotensin II amplification of alpha-adrenergic vasoconstriction: role of receptor reserve. *Circ Res.* 1988;63:748–757.

86. Zimmerman JB, Robertson D, Jackson EK. Angiotensin II-noradrenergic interactions in renovascular hypertensive rats. *J Clin Invest.* 1987;80:443–457.

87. Ichikawa I, Harris RC. Angiotensin actions in the kidney: renewed insight into the old hormone. *Kidney Int.* 1991;40:583–596.

88. Scholz H, Kurtz A. Role of protein kinase C in renal vasoconstriction caused by angiotensin II. *Am J Physiol.* 1990;259:C421–C426.

89. Heyeraas KJ, Aukland K. Interlobular arterial resistance: influence of renal arterial pressure and angiotensin II. *Kidney Int.* 1987;31:1291–1298.

90. Myers BD, Deen WM, Brenner BM. Effects of norepinephrine and angiotensin II on the determinants of glomerular ultrafiltration and proximal tubule fluid reabsorption in the rat. *Circ Res.* 1975;37:101–110.

91. Yuan BH, Robinette JB, Conger JD. Effect of angiotensin II and norepinephrine on isolated rat afferent and efferent arterioles. *Am J Physiol.* 1990;258:F741–F750.

92. Denton KM, Fennessy PA, Alcorn D, et al. Morphometric analysis of the actions of angiotensin II on renal arterioles and glomeruli. *Am J Physiol.* 1992;262:F367–F372.

93. Herizi A, Jover B, Bouriquet N, et al. Prevention of the cardiovascular and renal effects of angiotensin II by endothelin blockade. *Hypertension.* 1998;31:10–14.

94. Stern N, Golub M, Nozawa K, et al. Selective inhibition of angiotensin II-mediated vasoconstriction by lipoxygenase blockade. *Am J Physiol.* 1989;257:H434–H443.

95. Schnermann J, Briggs JP. Restoration of tubuloglomerular feedback in volume-expanded rats by angiotensin II. *Am J Physiol.* 1990;259:F565–F572.

96. Schnermann J, Briggs JP. Effect of angiotensin and other pressor agents on tubuloglomerular feedback responses. *Kidney Int Suppl.* 1990;30:S77–S80.

97. Wang T, Chan YL. Mechanism of angiotensin II action on proximal tubular transport. *J Pharmacol Exp Ther.* 1990;252:689–695.

98. Garvin JL. Angiotensin stimulates bicarbonate transport and Na+/K+ ATPase in rat proximal straight tubules. *J Am Soc Nephrol.* 1991;1:1146–1152.

99. Yingst DR, Massey KJ, Rossi NF, et al. Angiotensin II directly stimulates activity and alters the phosphorylation of Na-K-ATPase in rat proximal tubule with a rapid time course. *Am J Physiol Renal Physiol.* 2004;287:F713–F721.

100. Ruiz OS, Qiu YY, Wang LJ, et al. Regulation of the renal Na-HCO3 cotransporter: IV. Mechanisms of the stimulatory effect of angiotensin II. *J Am Soc Nephrol.* 1995;6:1202–1208.

101. Cogan MG, Xie MH, Liu FY, et al. Effects of DuP 753 on proximal nephron and renal transport. *Am J Hypertens.* 1991;4:315S–320S.

102. Kwon TH, Nielsen J, Kim YH, et al. Regulation of sodium transporters in the thick ascending limb of rat kidney: response to angiotensin II. *Am J Physiol Renal Physiol.* 2003;285:F152–F165.

103. Ruster C, Wolf G. Renin-angiotensin-aldosterone system and progression of renal disease. *J Am Soc Nephrol.* 2006;17:2985–2991.

104. Donoghue M, Hsieh F, Baronas E, et al. A novel angiotensin-converting enzyme-related carboxypeptidase (ACE2) converts angiotensin I to angiotensin 1-9. *Circ Res.* 2000;87:E1–E9.

105. Hamming I, Timens W, Bulthuis ML, et al. Tissue distribution of ACE2 protein, the functional receptor for SARS coronavirus. A first step in understanding SARS pathogenesis. *J Pathol.* 2004;203:631–637.

106. Burns KD. The emerging role of angiotensin-converting enzyme-2 in the kidney. *Curr Opin Nephrol Hypertens.* 2007;16:116–121.

107. Gurley SB, Allred A, Le TH, et al. Altered blood pressure responses and normal cardiac phenotype in ACE2-null mice. *J Clin Invest.* 2006;116:2218–2225.

108. Crackower MA, Sarao R, Oudit GY, et al. Angiotensin-converting enzyme 2 is an essential regulator of heart function. *Nature.* 2002;417:822–828.

109. Li N, Zimpelmann J, Cheng K, et al. The role of angiotensin converting enzyme 2 in the generation of angiotensin 1-7 by rat proximal tubules. *Am J Physiol Renal Physiol.* 2005;288:F353–F362.

110. Oudit GY, Herzenberg AM, Kassiri Z, et al. Loss of angiotensin-converting enzyme-2 leads to the late development of angiotensin II-dependent glomerulosclerosis. *Am J Pathol.* 2006;168:1808–1820.

111. Ye M, Wysocki J, William J, et al. Glomerular localization and expression of angiotensin-converting enzyme 2 and angiotensin-converting enzyme: implications for albuminuria in diabetes. *J Am Soc Nephrol.* 2006;17:3067–3075.

112. Tikellis C, Johnston CI, Forbes JM, et al. Characterization of renal angiotensin-converting enzyme 2 in diabetic nephropathy. *Hypertension.* 2003;41:392–397.

113. Wysocki J, Ye M, Soler MJ, et al. ACE and ACE2 activity in diabetic mice. *Diabetes.* 2006;55:2132–2139.

114. Ye M, Wysocki J, Naaz P, et al. Increased ACE 2 and decreased ACE protein in renal tubules from diabetic mice: a renoprotective combination? *Hypertension.* 2004;43:1120–1125.

115. Li W, Moore MJ, Vasilieva N, et al. Angiotensin-converting enzyme 2 is a functional receptor for the SARS coronavirus. *Nature.* 2003;426:450–454.

116. Kuba K, Imai Y, Rao S, et al. A crucial role of angiotensin converting enzyme 2 (ACE2) in SARS coronavirus-induced lung injury. *Nat Med.* 2005;11:875–879.

117. Paul M, Poyan Mehr A, Kreutz R. Physiology of local renin-angiotensin systems. *Physiol Rev.* 2006;86:747–803.

118. Williams GH. Aldosterone biosynthesis, regulation, and classical mechanism of action. *Heart Fail Rev.* 2005;10:7–13.

119. Lymperopoulos A, Rengo G, Zincarelli C, et al. An adrenal beta-arrestin 1-mediated signaling pathway underlies angiotensin II-induced aldosterone production in vitro and in vivo. *Proc Natl Acad Sci U S A.* 2009;106:5825–5830.

120. Pratt JH. Role of angiotensin II in potassium-mediated stimulation of aldosterone secretion in the dog. *J Clin Invest.* 1982;70:667–672.

121. Asher C, Wald H, Rossier BC, et al. Aldosterone-induced increase in the abundance of Na+ channel subunits. *Am J Physiol Cell Physiol.* 1996;271:C605–C611.

122. Pearce D. SGK1 regulation of epithelial sodium transport. *Cell Physiol Biochem.* 2003;13:13–20.

123. Naray-Fejes-Toth A, Canessa C, Cleaveland ES, et al. sgk is an aldosterone-induced kinase in the renal collecting duct. Effects on epithelial na+ channels. *J Biol Chem.* 1999;274:16973–16978.

124. Debonneville C, Flores SY, Kamynina E, et al. Phosphorylation of Nedd4-2 by Sgk1 regulates epithelial Na(+) channel cell surface expression. *Embo J.* 2001;20:7052–7059.

125. Flores SY, Loffing-Cueni D, Kamynina E, et al. Aldosterone-induced serum and glucocorticoid-induced kinase 1 expression is accompanied by Nedd4-2 phosphorylation and increased Na+ transport in cortical collecting duct cells. *J Am Soc Nephrol.* 2005;16:2279–2287.

126. Himathongkam T, Dluhy RG, Williams GH. Potassim-aldosterone-renin interrelationships. *J Clin Endocrinol Metab.* 1975;41:153–159.

127. Beesley AH, Hornby D, White SJ. Regulation of distal nephron K+ channels (ROMK) mRNA expression by aldosterone in rat kidney. *J Physiol.* 1998;509(pt 3):629–634.

128. Yun CC, Palmada M, Embark HM, et al. The serum and glucocorticoid-inducible kinase SGK1 and the Na+/H+ exchange regulating factor NHERF2 synergize to stimulate the renal outer medullary K+ channel ROMK1. *J Am Soc Nephrol.* 2002;13:2823–2830.

129. Huang DY, Wulff P, Volkl H, et al. Impaired regulation of renal K+ elimination in the sgk1-knockout mouse. *J Am Soc Nephrol.* 2004;15:885–891.

130. Snyder PM. The epithelial Na+ channel: cell surface insertion and retrieval in Na+ homeostasis and hypertension. *Endocr Rev.* 2002;23:258–275.

131. Funder JW. Aldosterone, salt and cardiac fibrosis. *Clin Exp Hypertens.* 1997;19:885–899.

132. Wang Q, Clement S, Gabbiani G, et al. Chronic hyperaldosteronism in a transgenic mouse model fails to induce cardiac remodeling and fibrosis under a normal-salt diet. *Am J Physiol Renal Physiol.* 2004;286:F1178–F1184.

133. Botero-Velez M, Curtis JJ, Warnock DG. Brief report: Liddle's syndrome revisited—a disorder of sodium reabsorption in the distal tubule. *N Engl J Med.* 1994;330:178–181.

134. Takeda Y. Vascular synthesis of aldosterone: role in hypertension. *Mol Cell Endocrinol.* 2004;217:75–79.

135. Silvestre JS, Robert V, Heymes C, et al. Myocardial production of aldosterone and corticosterone in the rat. Physiological regulation. *J Biol Chem.* 1998;273:4883–4891.

136. Xue C, Siragy HM. Local renal aldosterone system and its regulation by salt, diabetes, and angiotensin II type 1 receptor. *Hypertension.* 2005;46:584–590.

137. Gomez-Sanchez EP, Ahmad N, Romero DG, et al. Origin of aldosterone in the rat heart. *Endocrinology.* 2004;145:4796–4802.

138. Funder JW. Cardiac synthesis of aldosterone: going, going, gone…? *Endocrinology.* 2004;145:4793–4795.

139. Funder JW, Pearce PT, Smith R, et al. Vascular type I aldosterone binding sites are physiological mineralocorticoid receptors. *Endocrinology.* 1989;125:2224–2226.

140. Wehling M, Spes CH, Win N, et al. Rapid cardiovascular action of aldosterone in man. *J Clin Endocrinol Metab.* 1998;83:3517–3522.

141. Arima S, Kohagura K, Xu HL, et al. Nongenomic vascular action of aldosterone in the glomerular microcirculation. *J Am Soc Nephrol.* 2003;14:2255–2263.

142. Brown NJ, Agirbasli MA, Williams GH, et al. Effect of activation and inhibition of the renin-angiotensin system on plasma PAI-1. *Hypertension.* 1998;32:965–971.

143. Brown NJ, Vaughan DE, Fogo AB. The renin-angiotensin-aldosterone system and fibrinolysis in progressive renal disease. *Semin Nephrol.* 2002;22:399–406.

144. Moura AM, Worcel M. Direct action of aldosterone on transmembrane 22Na efflux from arterial smooth muscle. Rapid and delayed effects. *Hypertension.* 1984;6:425–430.

145. Alzamora R, Marusic ET, Gonzalez M, et al. Nongenomic effect of aldosterone on Na+, K+ -adenosine triphosphatase in arterial vessels. *Endocrinology.* 2003;144:1266–1272.

146. Wehling M, Ulsenheimer A, Schneider M, et al. Rapid effects of aldosterone on free intracellular calcium in vascular smooth muscle and endothelial cells: subcellular localization of calcium elevations by single cell imaging. *Biochem Biophys Res Commun.* 1994;204:475–481.

147. Wehling M, Bauer MM, Ulsenheimer A, et al. Nongenomic effects of aldosterone on intracellular pH in vascular smooth muscle cells. *Biochem Biophys Res Commun.* 1996;223:181–186.

148. Christ M, Meyer C, Sippel K, et al. Rapid aldosterone signaling in vascular smooth muscle cells: involvement of phospholipase C, diacylglycerol and protein kinase C alpha. *Biochem Biophys Res Commun.* 1995;213:123–129.

149. Funder JW. The nongenomic actions of aldosterone. *Endocr Rev.* 2005;26:313–321.

150. Blumenfeld JD, Laragh JH. Renin system analysis: a rational method for the diagnosis and treatment of the individual patient with hypertension. *Am J Hypertens.* 1998;11:894–896.

151. Spence JD. Physiologic tailoring of therapy for resistant hypertension: 20 years' experience with stimulated renin profiling. *Am J Hypertens.* 1999;12:1077–1083.

152. Khosla N, Hogan D. Mineralocorticoid hypertension and hypokalemia. *Semin Nephrol.* 2006;26:434–440.

153. Warnock DG. Genetic forms of human hypertension. *Curr Opin Nephrol Hypertens.* 2001;10:493–499.

154. Ganguly A. Primary aldosteronism. *N Engl J Med.* 1998;339:1828–1834.

155. White PC. Disorders of aldosterone biosynthesis and action. *N Engl J Med.* 1994;331:250–258.

156. Nussberger J, Wuerzner G, Jensen C, et al. Angiotensin II suppression in humans by the orally active renin inhibitor Aliskiren (SPP100): comparison with enalapril. *Hypertension.* 2002;39:E1–E8.

157. Dicpinigaitis PV. Angiotensin-converting enzyme inhibitor-induced cough: ACCP evidence-based clinical practice guidelines. *Chest.* 2006;129:169S–173S.

158. Adam A, Cugno M, Molinaro G, et al. Aminopeptidase P in individuals with a history of angio-oedema on ACE inhibitors. *Lancet.* 2002;359:2088–2089.

159. Chan P, Tomlinson B, Huang TY, et al. Double-blind comparison of losartan, lisinopril, and metolazone in elderly hypertensive patients with previous angiotensin-converting enzyme inhibitor-induced cough. *J Clin Pharmacol.* 1997;37:253–257.

160. de Gasparo M, Joss U, Ramjoue H, et al. Three new epoxy-spirolactone derivatives: characterization in vivo and in vitro. *J Pharmacol Exp Ther.* 1987;240:650–656.

161. Sica DA. Pharmacokinetics and pharmacodynamics of mineralocorticoid blocking agents and their effects on potassium homeostasis. *Heart Fail Rev.* 2005;10:23–29.

162. Alzamora R, Michea L, Marusic ET. Role of 11beta-hydroxysteroid dehydrogenase in nongenomic aldosterone effects in human arteries. *Hypertension.* 2000;35:1099–1104.

163. Jafar TH, Schmid CH, Landa M, et al. Angiotensin-converting enzyme inhibitors and progression of nondiabetic renal disease. A meta-analysis of patient-level data. *Ann Intern Med.* 2001;135:73–87.

164. Lewis EJ, Hunsicker LG, Bain RP, et al. The effect of angiotensin-converting-enzyme inhibition on diabetic nephropathy. The Collaborative Study Group. *N Engl J Med.* 1993;329:1456–1462.

165. Lewis EJ, Hunsicker LG, Clarke WR, et al. Renoprotective effect of the angiotensin-receptor antagonist irbesartan in patients with nephropathy due to type 2 diabetes. *N Engl J Med.* 2001;345:851–860.

166. Randomised placebo-controlled trial of effect of ramipril on decline in glomerular filtration rate and risk of terminal renal failure in proteinuric, non-diabetic nephropathy. The GISEN Group (Gruppo Italiano di Studi Epidemiologici in Nefrologia). *Lancet.* 1997;349:1857–1863.

167. Brenner BM, Cooper ME, de Zeeuw D, et al. Effects of losartan on renal and cardiovascular outcomes in patients with type 2 diabetes and nephropathy. *N Engl J Med.* 2001;345:861–869.

168. Agodoa LY, Appel L, Bakris GL, et al. Effect of ramipril vs amlodipine on renal outcomes in hypertensive nephrosclerosis: a randomized controlled trial. *JAMA.* 2001;285:2719–2728.

169. Jafar TH, Stark PC, Schmid CH, et al. The effect of angiotensin-converting-enzyme inhibitors on progression of advanced polycystic kidney disease. *Kidney Int.* 2005;67:265–271.

170. Proesmans W, Van Dyck M. Enalapril in children with Alport syndrome. *Pediatr Nephrol.* 2004;19:271–275.

171. Hostetter TH. Hyperfiltration and glomerulosclerosis. *Semin Nephrol.* 2003;23:194–199.

172. Abbate M, Zoja C, Remuzzi G. How does proteinuria cause progressive renal damage? *J Am Soc Nephrol.* 2006;17:2974–2984.

173. Sowers JR, Whaley-Connell A, Epstein M. Narrative review: the emerging clinical implications of the role of aldosterone in the metabolic syndrome and resistant hypertension. *Ann Intern Med.* 2009;150:776–783.

174. Nakao N, Yoshimura A, Morita H, et al. Combination treatment of angiotensin-II receptor blocker and angiotensin-converting-enzyme inhibitor in non-diabetic renal disease (COOPERATE): a randomised controlled trial. *Lancet.* 2003;361:117–124.

175. Kunz R, Wolbers M, Glass T, et al. The COOPERATE trial: a letter of concern. *Lancet.* 2008;371:1575–1576.

176. Mann JF, Schmieder RE, McQueen M, et al. Renal outcomes with telmisartan, ramipril, or both, in people at high vascular risk (the ONTARGET study): a multicentre, randomised, double-blind, controlled trial. *Lancet.* 2008;372:547–553.

177. Chapman AB. Approaches to testing new treatments in autosomal dominant polycystic kidney disease: insights from the CRISP and HALT-PKD studies. *Clin J Am Soc Nephrol.* 2008;3:1197–1204.

178. Fried LF, Duckworth W, Zhang JH, et al. Design of combination angiotensin receptor blocker and angiotensin-converting enzyme inhibitor for treatment of diabetic nephropathy (VA NEPHRON-D). *Clin J Am Soc Nephrol.* 2009;4:361–368.

179. Ponda MP, Hostetter TH. Aldosterone antagonism in chronic kidney disease. *Clin J Am Soc Nephrol.* 2006;1:668–677.

180. Navaneethan SD, Nigwekar SU, Sehgal AR, et al. Aldosterone antagonists for preventing the progression of chronic kidney disease: a systematic review and meta-analysis. *Clin J Am Soc Nephrol.* 2009;4:542–551.

181. Parving HH, Persson F, Lewis JB, et al. Aliskiren combined with losartan in type 2 diabetes and nephropathy. *N Engl J Med.* 2008;358:2433–2446.

182. Parving HH, Brenner BM, McMurray JJ, et al. Aliskiren Trial in Type 2 Diabetes Using Cardio-Renal Endpoints (ALTITUDE): rationale and study design. *Nephrol Dial Transplant.* 2009;24:1663–1671.

The Kidney in Hypertension

CHARLES R. NOLAN AND ROBERT W. SCHRIER

Global Burden of Hypertension

Cardiovascular disease is the most common cause of death in economically developed countries and is rapidly evolving as a major cause of morbidity and mortality in economically developing nations as well (1). In fact, the World Health Organization projects that ischemic heart disease will soon be the most important, and stroke the fourth most important, contributors to disability-adjusted years of life lost on a worldwide basis. Uncontrolled hypertension also contributes to the progression of chronic kidney disease. Several modifiable risk factors for cardiovascular disease are well established. Certainly, hypertension is among the most important modifiable risk factors. On the basis of currently recommended criteria for diagnosis of hypertension (systolic blood pressure [SBP] ≥140 mm Hg or diastolic blood pressure [DBP] ≥90 mm Hg, or use of antihypertensive medication), the overall prevalence of hypertension in adults in the United States in 1999 to 2000 was 27% in men and 30% in women (2). There is a progressive rise in SBP throughout life, with a difference of 20 to 30 mm Hg between early and late adulthood. Likewise, DBP tends to rise with age up until the fifth decade; in later decades DBP declines. These patterns result in a progressively higher prevalence of hypertension with aging, which consists of predominant elevation of SBP or isolated systolic hypertension. A majority of adults have hypertension by the sixth decade and >70% have it by the seventh and eight decades of life. Among normotensive individuals in their sixth decade, the lifetime risk of developing hypertension approaches 90%. African-American adults have an incidence and prevalence of hypertension that is 50% higher than their white or Mexican-American counterparts. The average level of blood pressure and prevalence of hypertension also increased progressively in children and adolescents between 1988 and 2000. The prevalence of hypertension in many other countries is as high as or higher than that identified in the United States. Estimates suggests that approximately 1 billion adults have hypertension (333 million in economically developed and 639 million in economically developing countries), with the highest prevalence in eastern Europe and the Latin American and Caribbean regions (3). There has also been a progressive increase in the prevalence of age-adjusted hypertension in China. The prevalence of hypertension in economically developing countries appears to be on the rise. Since 80% of the world's population resides in economically developing nations, it is very likely that the worldwide burden of hypertension-related illness will continue to escalate in the coming years. Blood pressure exhibits a dose-dependent relationship with the risk of cardiovascular disease throughout the entire range of blood pressures in the population. The relationship is independent of other cardiovascular risk factors with no evidence of a blood pressure threshold for risk. The blood pressure risk applies to all major manifestations of cardiovascular disease including stroke, sudden cardiac death, coronary heart disease, heart failure, aortic aneurysm, peripheral vascular disease, as well as chronic kidney disease and end-stage renal disease. Although elevations of both SBP and DBP are independently associated with cardiovascular (CV) risk, high SBP is the most potent predictor of risk (4,5). Population-attributable risk estimates indicated that attainment of a population average SBP < 115 mm Hg would reduce the occurrence of ischemic heart disease by 50% and stroke by 60%, thereby preventing about 7 million deaths annually on a worldwide basis (1).

Historical Perspective: The Link Between Hypertension and Renal Dysfunction

The occurrence of hypertension in the setting of renal disease and its impact on the progression of renal insufficiency has long been of interest to clinicians. The concept that hypertension is in some way related to renal dysfunction was first proposed by Bright in 1863 (6). He recognized the association between hypertrophy of the heart and contraction of the kidney and postulated that the cause was increased cardiac work required to force blood through a vascular tree constricted by irritating humoral substances that accumulate in renal failure. The role of fluid retention in the genesis of renal hypertension was first outlined by Traube in 1871 (7), who proposed that with shrinkage of the renal parenchyma, a decreasing amount of fluid is removed from the arterial system by urinary secretion, thereby resulting in hypertension.

Mahomed in 1879 (8) was the first to clearly describe hypertension of unknown cause, without evidence of underlying renal disease (now called essential hypertension). He emphasized that the most frequent complications in individuals with this type of hypertension were cardiovascular and most often occurred in the absence of significant renal dysfunction. However, in 1914 Volhard and Fahr (9) defined a subgroup of patients with essential hypertension who eventually developed severe renal involvement. They distinguished two types of hypertensive nephrosclerosis, benign and malignant. The benign type, characterized by hyaline arteriolosclerosis, was associated with a slowly progressive course with eventual complications caused by heart failure or stroke in the absence of clinically significant renal impairment. In contrast, malignant nephrosclerosis was characterized by arteriolar necrosis and endarteritis that resulted in rapidly progressive renal failure and death. Volhard (10) subsequently introduced the concept of the vicious circle in which renal disease causes hypertension, which in turn exacerbates renal injury.

In recent years, it has been reemphasized that the kidney is both "villain and victim" in hypertension (11). The kidney, even when histologically normal, is felt to play a central role in the pathogenesis of essential hypertension. Elegant molecular genetic studies have now identified mutations in eight genes that cause mendelian forms of hypertension (12). Each of these genetic defects that impart very large effects on blood pressure lead to enhanced renal tubular sodium reabsorption (impaired natriuresis), resulting in salt-sensitive hypertension. In addition, underlying primary renal parenchymal disease or abnormalities of the renal vasculature can cause secondary hypertension. On the other hand, the kidney may also suffer the brunt of hypertension. Essential hypertension that enters a malignant phase can rapidly destroy the kidney. Furthermore, recent evidence suggests that hypertension is a major factor in the progression of chronic kidney disease in the setting of both diabetic nephropathy and nondiabetic of chronic kidney disease.

We address three major questions with regard to the interaction between the kidney and hypertension. What role does the kidney play in the genesis of essential hypertension and the various forms of secondary hypertension? Why does hypertension develop in the setting of primary renal disease? What is the role of treatment of hypertension in slowing the progression of chronic kidney disease?

Circulatory Hemodynamics: Complexity in a Simple Relationship

At face value, the physiology of blood pressure regulation is deceptively simple, behaving according to Ohm's law whereby the mean arterial pressure is defined by the product of the cardiac output times the systemic vascular resistance. Thus, hypertension can only result from an increase in either of these two variables. As such, the kidney is expected to have a major influence on blood pressure given its central role in the regulation of extracellular fluid (ECF) volume (Chapters 1 and 2). An increase in ECF volume caused by renal sodium and water retention should cause increased blood volume, venous return, and filling pressure, which in turn should increase stroke volume and cardiac output via the Frank–Starling mechanism and result in hypertension. Volume expansion, resulting from excess sodium intake or an underlying abnormality in renal sodium excretory mechanisms, has been considered to be an important mechanism for the development of hypertension in animal models as well as in humans with essential hypertension or chronic kidney disease.

The paradox, which we attempt to explain, is that a significant increase in ECF volume or cardiac output is difficult to demonstrate in human essential hypertension as well as animal models, at least in the chronic phase. Chronic essential hypertension is virtually always maintained by an increase in systemic vascular resistance arising primarily at the level of precapillary arterioles throughout the circulatory system (13). This observation has formed the basis for the widely held concept that an increase in systemic vascular resistance is the underlying primary cause of hypertension, and many theories exist regarding the roles of various vasoconstrictor mechanisms (14) or absence of vasodilator substances (15).

However, there are complexities in the seemingly simple equation that relates blood pressure to cardiac output and systemic vascular resistance. The circulatory system is dynamic and a perturbation, such as ECF volume expansion, which initially leads to hypertension via an increase in cardiac output, may result in compensatory hemodynamic responses that ultimately restore sodium balance and thereby normalize ECF volume and cardiac output. This restoration of sodium balance results from a "pressure natriuresis" caused by systemic hypertension that is maintained by a chronic increase in systemic vascular resistance (16–20). The various theories proposed to account for the phenomenon whereby initially volume-dependent hypertension evolves into high systemic vascular resistance hypertension are described in detail in the following sections.

Dietary Salt and Hypertension

Archeological studies of Paleolithic man suggest that the diet of these hunter-gatherers was very low in sodium and relatively high in potassium. Sodium intake averaged 30 mmol/day with a ratio of dietary potassium to sodium of 16:1 (21). Because total body sodium content is the major determinant of ECF volume, a very efficient renal sodium conservation mechanism evolved in the face of this limited availability of sodium. In contrast, the modern urban diet contains 120 to 300 mmol sodium per day (19) and only 65 mmol potassium per day (22). Therefore, the human species today is faced with a much higher daily sodium load than that to which it adapted over roughly 2 million years (21). Because virtually all ingested sodium is absorbed, sodium intake in excess of insensible losses must be excreted by the kidney. Under normal circumstances, even in the face of tremendous dietary sodium excess, humoral and other mechanisms cause an increase in urinary sodium excretion with little increase in ECF volume (23). However, this natriuretic mechanism is aberrant in a segment of the population, so that excessive dietary salt intake results in the development of hypertension (16–20,24).

EPIDEMIOLOGIC STUDIES

Studies throughout the world have suggested a correlation between the mean dietary sodium intake and prevalence of hypertension in the population. In parts of Japan where the mean sodium intake is >400 mmol/day, the prevalence of hypertension approaches 50% (25). In contrast, in certain inland populations where the sodium intake is very low (0.2 to 51 mmol/day), hypertension is virtually nonexistent and there is no tendency for the blood pressure to rise with age (26). The INTERSALT study investigated the relation between dietary sodium intake (defined by 24-hour urine sodium excretion) and blood pressure in 10,000 subjects in 32 countries (27). A significant positive correlation was found between sodium intake and blood pressure even when the data were adjusted for age, gender, body weight, and alcohol consumption. The data suggest that habitually high sodium intake (>150 mmol sodium per day) is a critical environmental factor that contributes to the high prevalence of hypertension in most urban populations, whereas lifelong ingestion of a diet extremely low in sodium (<50 mmol/day) prevents the development of hypertension (25,26). Extremely high sodium intake (>800 mmol sodium per day) has been shown to raise the blood pressure of healthy normotensive individuals (28). On the other hand, diets with <10 mmol sodium per day have been shown to lower the blood pressure of most hypertensive patients (29). Additional support for the importance of dietary sodium in the genesis of hypertension is the finding that, in an adult population, long-term lowering of the sodium intake was associated with a fall in the prevalence of hypertension and a concomitant reduction in cerebrovascular mortality (30).

The effect of dietary composition on blood pressure is a subject of major public health importance. The Dietary Approaches to Stop Hypertension (DASH) diet study demonstrated that a diet that emphasizes on fruits, vegetables, and low-fat dairy foods; includes whole grains, poultry, fish, and nuts;

contains only small amounts of red meat, sweets, and sugar-containing beverages; and has reduced amounts of total and saturated fat and cholesterol substantially lowers blood pressure as compared with the typical diet in the United States (31). In a subsequent report, the effect of different levels of dietary sodium intake, in conjunction with the DASH diet, was studied in subjects with and without hypertension (32). A total of 412 participants were randomly assigned to eat either a control diet typical of intake in the United States or the DASH diet. Within each assigned diet, participants ate foods containing high sodium (150 mmol/day, typical consumption in the United States), intermediate sodium (100 mmol/day, as in the no-added salt diet), and low sodium (50 mmol/day) for 30 consecutive days each, in random order. The DASH diet was associated with significantly lower systolic blood pressure at each sodium intake level. Moreover, the reduction of sodium intake significantly lowered systolic and diastolic blood pressure in a stepwise fashion, with both the control and DASH diets. Reducing dietary sodium intake had approximately twice as great an effect on blood pressure with the control diet as it did with the DASH diet. Reducing the sodium intake from high to intermediate level reduced the systolic blood-pressure by 2.1 mm Hg ($p < 0.001$) during the control diet and by 1.3 mm Hg ($p = 0.03$) during the DASH diet. Reducing intake from intermediate to low level caused additional reductions of 4.6 mm Hg during the control diet ($p < 0.001$) and 1.7 mm Hg during the DASH diet ($p < 0.01$). Dietary sodium restriction resulted in a greater reduction in blood pressure in subjects with hypertension than in normotensive subjects. As compared with the control diet with high sodium intake, the DASH diet with low sodium intake led to a mean systolic blood pressure that was 7.1 mm Hg lower in participants without hypertension and 11.5 mm Hg lower in participants with hypertension. The effects of dietary sodium on blood pressure were observed in participants with and those without hypertension, African-Americans, and those of other races, and in both men and women. On the basis of the levels of dietary sodium intake actually achieved in the study, it appears that blood pressure can be reduced in individuals consuming either a diet that is typical in the United States or the DASH diet by reducing sodium intake from approximately 140 mmol/day (average sodium intake in the United States) to an intermediate level of 100 mmol/day (the currently recommended no-added salt diet), or from this level to a still lower level of 65 mmol/day (equivalent to 1.5 g sodium or 3.8 g sodium chloride). The impact of these findings on public health of course depends on the ability of people to make long-lasting dietary modifications and increased availability of lower sodium foods in the marketplace.

The Genetic Epidemiology Network of Salt-Sensitivity (GenSalt) study recently demonstrated that nondiabetic individuals with metabolic syndrome and underlying insulin resistance have increased sensitivity of blood pressure to changes in dietary sodium intake (33). In GenSalt, 1,906 Chinese participants without diabetes, ages 16 years or more, were selected to receive a low-sodium diet (51.3 mmol/day) for 7 days followed by a high-sodium diet (308.8 mmol/day) for an additional 7 days. Bloodpressure was measured at baseline and on days 2, 5, 6, and 7 of each intervention. Metabolic syndrome was defined as the presence of three or more of the following: abdominal obesity, raised blood pressure, high triglyceride concentration, low high-density lipoprotein (HDL) cholesterol, or high glucose. High salt sensitivity was defined as a decrease in mean arterial pressure (MAP) of >5 mm Hg during low-sodium diet or an increase of >5 mm Hg during the high-sodium diet. Overall 283 (28%) of subjects met criteria for diagnosis of metabolic syndrome. Multivariable-adjusted mean changes in blood pressure in response to changes in dietary sodium intake were significantly different in subjects with and without metabolic syndrome. There was a significant and graded association between number of risk factors for metabolic syndrome and age-adjusted and gender-adjusted proportion of study participants with high salt sensitivity of blood pressure. Compared with those with no risk factors for metabolic syndrome, participants with four or five risk factors had a 3.54-fold increased odds of high salt sensitivity during the low-sodium intervention and a 3.13-fold increased odds of high salt sensitivity after the high-sodium diet. Moreover, compared with participants without metabolic syndrome (less than three risk factors), participants with metabolic syndrome (three or more risk factors) had a 92% increased odds of high salt sensitivity after the low-sodium diet and a 70% increased odds of high salt sensitivity after the high-sodium intervention. The association between metabolic syndrome and salt sensitivity of blood pressure was independent of age, gender, body mass index, physical activity, cigarette smoking, alcohol consumption, and baseline dietary intake of sodium and potassium. Furthermore, the association between metabolic syndrome and salt sensitivity remained significant even if participants with baseline hypertension were excluded. As discussed in more detail later, insulin resistance and concomitant compensatory hyperinsulinemia may lead to renal sodium retention (impaired natriuresis) and thereby explain the blood pressure response to changes in dietary sodium intake in individuals with metabolic syndrome. Data from the GenSalt study suggest that reduction in dietary sodium intake may be an especially important strategy for reducing blood pressure in individual with multiple risk factors for metabolic syndrome.

On balance, it is clear that sodium intake must play a permissive role in the development of hypertension, because a lifelong diet very low in sodium prevents hypertension (26). On the other hand, excessive sodium intake alone is not sufficient to cause hypertension, because the majority of individuals on such a diet fail to develop hypertension. These observations imply that there must be additional predisposing factors that lead to the development of hypertension in certain individuals when the intake of sodium is >60 to 70 mmol/day.

DIETARY SALT AND ANIMAL MODELS OF GENETIC HYPERTENSION

When groups of rats were maintained on a wide range of dietary sodium, the mean blood pressure in each group was directly related to the sodium intake. Dahl noted that at each level of dietary sodium intake, only some rats became hypertensive. By selective inbreeding, he was able to show that the predisposition to develop hypertension was genetically determined, and he produced a salt-sensitive strain that develops hypertension on a high-sodium diet and a salt-resistant strain that remains normotensive (34).

The Role of The Kidney in Essential Hypertension

In *kidney cross-transplantation experiments* between four different strains of genetically hypertensive rats (Dahl salt-sensitive hypertensive rats, Milan hypertensive rats, spontaneously hypertensive rats [SHR], and stroke-prone spontaneously hypertensive rats [SHRSP]), and their respective normotensive control strains, it was found that blood pressure determinants were carried within the kidney (35). Thus, transplantation of a kidney from a hypertensive strain rat into a bilaterally nephrectomized rat from the normotensive strain results in hypertension in the recipient. Conversely, transplantation from a normotensive strain rat into a nephrectomized hypertensive strain rat prevents the development of hypertension. Thus, the blood pressure of the recipient rat is dependent on the source of the donated kidney. On the other hand, it could be argued that the posttransplant hypertension in recipients of kidneys from hypertensive strains is not caused by a primary defect in the donor kidney, but instead results from hypertension-induced changes in the donor kidney and that these acquired secondary structural defects in the kidney lead to hypertension in the recipient. To address this question, the development of hypertension in the SHRSP kidney donors was prevented by chronic antihypertensive drug treatment (35). Despite sustained normalization of blood pressure in the donor rats, the recipients developed posttransplant hypertension. This finding indicates that SHRSP kidneys carry a primary defect that can elicit hypertension. These experiments suggest that the predisposition to genetic hypertension resides in the kidney and is not determined directly by systemic humoral abnormalities or changes in vascular reactivity that have been described in these models. The latter abnormalities must represent either epiphenomena or secondary changes in response to a primary renal abnormality.

These animal models of hypertension bear a remarkable resemblance to human essential hypertension. Indeed, studies of kidney transplant patients also support a primary role for the kidney in the development of essential hypertension. In patients with essential hypertension and renal failure caused by malignant nephrosclerosis, bilateral native nephrectomy in conjunction with a well-functioning renal allograft, from a normotensive cadaver donor, cures essential hypertension (36). In a study of six such patients, before renal transplantation, mean arterial pressure was 168 ± 9 mm Hg despite treatment with a minimum of a four-drug antihypertensive regimen. However, following bilateral native nephrectomy and successful renal transplantation, at a mean follow-up of 4.5 years, mean arterial pressure without antihypertensive treatment was 92 ± 1.9 mm Hg. Another observation that suggests a role for the kidney in the pathogenesis of hypertension is the finding that the incidence of hypertension in recipients of cadaver kidneys correlates with the incidence of essential hypertension in the family of the donor (37). These intriguing reports support the notion that the defect that causes human essential hypertension resides within the kidney.

Pathogenetic Mechanisms of Impaired Natriuresis

If the relationship between sodium intake and hypertension represents cause and effect, then it is important to explain why a high sodium intake leads to hypertension in only some individuals. In this regard, it has been postulated that in the setting of essential hypertension in humans or in salt-sensitive animal models, there is a genetically predetermined impairment in the renal ability to excrete sodium (16–20). This postulated renal abnormality has been termed an "unwillingness to excrete sodium" or "impaired natriuretic capacity." In studies of isolated, perfused kidneys from Dahl salt-sensitive strains, at age 8 weeks, even before the onset of hypertension, there is a defect in natriuresis such that at any given perfusion pressure, less sodium is excreted in comparison to kidneys from salt-resistant strains (38). In humans, the heritability of essential hypertension has been well established in epidemiologic surveys. The prevalence of hypertension among offspring has been reported to be 46% if both parents are hypertensive, 28% if one parent is hypertensive, and only 3% if neither parent is hypertensive (39). The familial aggregation of hypertension is not simply attributable to shared environmental effects because adoption studies show greater concordance of blood pressure among biological siblings than adoptive siblings living in the same household (40). Moreover, twin studies document greater concordance of blood pressure between monozygotic twins than dizygotic twins (41). Analysis of the natriuretic response to slow infusion of saline has revealed that normotensive first-degree relatives of patients with essential hypertension excrete a sodium load less well than control subjects without a family history of hypertension (42). Among blacks and individuals over 40 years old (43)—two groups with an increased incidence of hypertension—studies of normotensive individuals also have demonstrated a slower natriuretic response to saline infusion than in controls, suggesting that a diminished natriuretic capacity may underlie the predisposition to essential hypertension in these groups.

NORMAL RENAL SODIUM HANDLING

On a daily basis, the kidneys filter >170 L of plasma containing 23 mol of sodium. Therefore, in an individual consuming a 2-g sodium diet containing 100 mEq of sodium, maintenance of sodium homeostasis requires that the kidneys reabsorb 99.5% of the filtered sodium load. This efficient process of renal sodium reabsorption is accomplished by a complex integrated array of sodium exchangers, sodium - transporters, and sodium ion channels. Along the entire length of the nephron, the driving force for sodium reabsorption is the Na^+/K^+ ATPase located in the basolateral membrane of tubular cells, which extrudes sodium from the cell into the blood-side of the tubule and maintains low intracellular sodium concentration. The distinct functional properties of various portions of the nephron are determined by differences in the sodium transporters located in the apical membrane (Fig. 9.1). Sixty percent of the filtered sodium is reabsorbed in the proximal tubule (PT), largely by the Na^+/H^+ exchanger (NHE-3) and to a lesser extent by the sodium phosphate cotransporter (NaPi-2). Thirty percent of filtered sodium is reabsorbed in the thick ascending limb (TAL) of Henle by the Na/K/2Cl cotransporter. Seven percent is reclaimed by the thiazide-sensitive Na/Cl cotransporter (NCC) in the distal convoluted tubule (DCT). The remaining 2% to 3% is reabsorbed via the epithelial sodium channel (ENaC) in the cortical collecting tubules (CCTs). Although ENaC accounts for only a small fraction of total renal tubular sodium reabsorption, this is the principal site for regulation of net sodium balance because the activity of this channel is highly regulated by the renin–angiotensin–aldosterone system (RAAS). Decreased perfusion pressure in the afferent arteriole or decreased delivery of sodium to the TAL leads to secretion of renin, an aspartyl protease that acts on angiotensinogen produced in the liver to produce angiotensin I (AI). Through the action of angiotensin-converting enzyme (ACE) in the lung and elsewhere, AI is converted to angiotensin II (AII). A II binds to its specific G protein-coupled receptor in the zona glomerulosa of the adrenal gland, leading to increased secretion of aldosterone, the principal mineralocorticoid steroid hormone. The actions of aldosterone are mediated chiefly by binding to intracellular nuclear hormone mineralocorticoid receptors (MRs) that function as transcription factors when they are in the activated state (44). Aldosterone stimulates sodium retention by the kidney in part through its action to regulate the ENaC, which mediates apical sodium entry across principal cells in the collecting tubules (45). Aldosterone also stimulates sodium reabsorption in the DCT by increasing the abundance of the

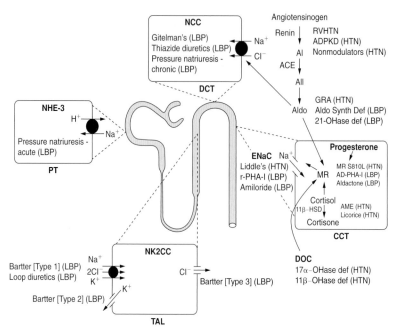

■ **Figure 9.1** Alterations in renal sodium handling that influence systemic blood pressure. This diagram of the nephron illustrates the molecular pathways mediating sodium reabsorption in individual cells in the proximal tubule (PT) (Na^+/H^+ exchanger, NHE-3); the thick ascending limb (TAL) of the loop of Henle (Na/K/2Cl cotransporter, NK2CC); the distal convoluted tubule (DCT) (thiazide-sensitive Na/Cl cotransporter, NCC); and cortical collecting duct (amiloride-sensitive epithelial sodium channel, ENaC, the activity of which is regulated by the mineralocorticoid receptor, MR). Also shown is the pathway of the renin–angiotensin–aldosterone system (RAAS), the major regulator of renal salt reabsorption, sodium balance, and blood pressure. Various inherited diseases, medical disorders, and pharmacologic agents that influence renal sodium handling and blood pressure are listed adjacent to the molecular pathways they involve. Conditions that enhance renal sodium reabsorption and therefore cause hypertension are labeled (*HTN*). Conditions and drugs that impair renal sodium reabsorption and thereby lower blood pressure are labeled (*LBP*). In the PT, downregulation of NHE-3 mediates acute pressure natriuresis. In the TAL, three different variants of Bartter syndrome result from various autosomal recessive loss-of-function mutations that impair sodium reabsorption and lower blood pressure. Type 1 results from mutation in the $Na^+/K^+/2Cl$ cotransporter, which is also the transporter inhibited by loop diuretics. Type 2 results from mutation in the ROMK channel, which is crucial for recycling of potassium from the cell into the lumen to maintain efficiency of the NK2CC. Type 3 results from mutation of the basolateral chloride channel, which is responsible for exit of reabsorbed chloride from the cell. In the DCT, Gitelman syndrome results from autosomal recessive loss-of-function mutation in the NCC, which is also the molecular site of action of thiazide diuretics. Chronic pressure natriuresis is mediated by downregulation of the abundance of the NCC. In the DCT, Liddle syndrome results from gain-of-function mutations in the ENaC leading to enhanced sodium reabsorption and hypertension. ENaC is blocked by the potassium-sparing diuretic amiloride. Loss-of-function mutations in ENaC occur in the autosomal recessive form of pseudohypoaldosteronism type 1 (PHA1). The MR S810L mutation in the MR leads to an autosomal dominant form of hypertension that is markedly exacerbated during pregnancy because the mutant receptor is activated by progesterone. MR is inhibited by spironolactone, another potassium-sparing diuretic. Loss-of-function mutations in the MR cause autosomal dominant PHA 1. In the syndrome of apparent mineralocorticoid excess (AME), loss of function mutations in 11β-hydroxysteroid dehydrogenase (11β-HSD) prevent metabolism of cortisol to cortisone so that cortisol binds and activates the MR leading to enhanced sodium reabsorption and hypertension. Natural licorice causes hypertension by inhibiting 11β-HSD. Cushing syndrome and ectopic secretion of ACTH by certain tumors lead to markedly elevated cortisol levels that overwhelm 11β-HSD, allowing cortisol to bind to MR, leading to enhanced sodium reabsorption and hypertension. Glucocorticoid remediable hyperaldosteronism (GRA) causes hypertension as the result of a chimeric gene that drives constitutive overexpression of aldosterone under the influence of ACTH. Aldosterone synthetase deficiency and 21-hydroxylase deficiency (21-OHase def) result in hypotension because of the inability to produce aldosterone and other 21-hydroxylated mineralocorticoids. The adrenogenital syndromes result from deficiencies of 17α-hydroxylase

(*continued*)

thiazide-sensitive NCC (46). Thus, both NCC and ENaC appear to be primary targets for the regulation of sodium excretion by aldosterone.

MOLECULAR MECHANISMS IMPLICATED IN BLOOD PRESSURE VARIATION IN HUMANS

Landmark molecular genetic studies by Lifton et al. recently have identified a substantial number of genes in which rare mutations impart large effects on blood pressure leading to various mendelian forms of hypertension or hypotension (12). Investigation of the genetic causes of hypertension or hypotension has provided major insights into the pathophysiologic mechanisms that can lead to hypertension. Given the vast array of physiologic systems that can influence blood pressure, it is striking that, in all of the mendelian forms of hypertension and hypotension discussed in detail in the following sections, the fundamental underlying abnormality has been found to involve alternations in renal sodium handling (Fig. 9.1). These findings clearly establish the central role of altered sodium homeostasis in the pathogenesis of hypertension and underscore the pivotal role of the kidney in the long-term regulation of blood pressure. Unfortunately, genetic studies in the general population thus far have been disappointing in that no genetic variants that have a substantial effect on blood pressure have been identified. Nonetheless, the finding that all known inherited and acquired forms of hypertension converge on the same final common pathway leading to impaired natriuresis suggests that the pathophysiologic disorders that lead to essential hypertension in the general population will ultimately be found to result directly or indirectly from abnormalities in renal sodium handling.

BLOOD PRESSURE VARIATIONS CAUSED BY MUTATIONS AFFECTING CIRCULATING MINERALOCORTICOID HORMONE

The major regulator of ENaC activity is the MR and its steroid hormone ligand aldosterone. A number of genetic disorders leading to hypertension or hypotension result from abnormalities in aldosterone secretion or the production of other steroid hormones that activate the MR. *Glucocorticoid remediable aldosteronism* (GRA) is an autosomal-dominant trait with the phenotype of early-onset hypertension with normal or elevated plasma aldosterone despite suppressed plasma renin activity (PRA) (Fig. 9.1) (47). Hypokalemia and metabolic alkalosis are present in some patients. The hallmark of this disease is normalization of blood pressure during treatment with exogenous glucocorticoids, which completely suppresses the overproduction of aldosterone. GRA is caused by a gene duplication arising from an unequal crossover between the gene encoding for steroid 11β-hydroxylase (an enzyme involved in cortisol biosynthesis that contains an adrenocorticotropic hormone [ACTH] response element) and the gene encoding for aldosterone synthetase (the rate-limiting enzyme in aldosterone biosynthesis in the adrenal glomerulosa). The resulting chimeric gene encodes for a protein with aldosterone synthetase enzymatic activity whose expression is regulated by ACTH. The net result is that aldosterone synthetase is ectopically expressed in the adrenal fasciculate under the control of ACTH rather than AII, the normal hormonal regulator. Aldosterone secretion thereby becomes linked to cortisol secretion such that maintenance of normal cortisol levels leads to constitutive aldosterone oversecretion, enhanced ENaC activity with increased distal tubular sodium reabsorption, volume expansion, and hypertension. The expanded plasma volume suppresses PRA but fails to suppress aldosterone production. Exogenous

---

(17α-OHase) or 11β-hydroxylase (11β-OHase), which result in overproduction of the mineralocorticoid hormone deoxycorticosterone (DOC), resulting in enhanced renal sodium reabsorption and hypertension. Increased activity of the renin–angiotensin–aldosterone axis may mediate salt-sensitive hypertension in renovascular hypertension (RVHTN), autosomal dominant polycystic kidney disease (ADPKD), and a subset of patients with essential hypotension who fail to downregulate the RAAS during salt loading (nonmodulators). Additional abbreviations: AI, angiotensin I; ACE, angiotensin-converting enzyme; AII, angiotensin II; HTN, hypertension; LBP, low blood pressure. (From Lifton RP, Gharavi AG, Geller DS. Molecular mechanisms of human hypertension. *Cell.* 2001;104: 545, 2001, with permission of Cell Press.)

administration of glucocorticoid suppresses normal ACTH production and abrogates the ectopic production of aldosterone with normalization of blood pressure.

There are several genetic disorders in which steroids other than aldosterone cause activation of the MR, leading to impaired natriuresis and salt-sensitive hypertension. The *syndrome of apparent mineralocorticoid excess* (AME) is an autosomal recessive disorder that causes early-onset hypertension with hypokalemic metabolic alkalosis (48). The PRA is suppressed and circulating aldosterone is absent. In normal individuals, circulating cortisol levels are 1,000-fold higher than aldosterone levels. In vitro, cortisol is known to bind and activate the MR. However, in vivo, virtually all MR activation is mediated by aldosterone. This paradox is explained by the finding that in the kidney; MR specificity for aldosterone is mediated indirectly by the enzyme 11-β-hydroxysteroid dehydrogenase (11β-HSD). In the ENaC-containing principal cells of the collecting duct, expression of 11β-HSD results in metabolism of cortisol to cortisone, which is not capable of activating the MR. Thus, cortisol does not have a min- eralocorticoid effect in normal individuals. However, in patients with AME, the absence of 11β-HSD allows cortisol to bind and activate the MR, resulting in salt-sensitive hypertension owing to ENaC-mediated enhancement of tubular sodium reabsorption. The development of hypertension following chronic ingestion of large amounts of *natural licorice* shares a similar pathogenesis. A licorice metabolite, glycyrrhetinic acid, is a potent inhibitor of 11β-HSD, resulting in a phenocopy of AME. Likewise, overproduction of cortisol caused by adrenal adenoma, ACTH-producing pituitary adenoma, or ectopic ACTH production, can overwhelm normal 11β-HSD activity so that cortisol is available for binding and activation of the MR, resulting in salt-sensitive hypertension with hypokalemic metabolic alkalosis.

Other genetic disorders are also associated with excess mineralocorticoid activity, resulting in chronic hypertension. In the adrenogenital syndromes, inherited autosomal recessive *11-β-hydroxylase deficiency* (49) and *17α-hydroxylase deficiency* (50) lead to impaired cortisol biosynthesis with compensatory hypersecretion of ACTH, which diverts steroid synthesis into pathways proximal to the enzymatic block. As a result there is overproduction of 21-hydroxylated steroids such as deoxycorticosterone (DOC) and corticosterone, which are potent activators of the MR, leading to ENaC overexpression, enhanced sodium reabsorption in the DCT, and severe salt-sensitive hypertension (Fig. 9.1). The hypertension responds to cortisol replacement in these disorders, which suppresses ACTH and mineralocorticoid overproduction.

In contrast to disorders associated with excess mineralocorticoid that cause salt-sensitive hypertension, genetic disorders that impair aldosterone synthesis, lead to mendelian forms of hypotension. Individuals homozygous for *aldosterone synthase deficiency* (12) have the phenotypic mirror image of GRA, with renal salt wasting and impaired secretion of K^+ and H^+ in the distal nephron (Fig. 9.1). These individuals present with severe hypotension caused by reduced intravascular volume with hyperkalemic metabolic acidosis. Likewise, homozygous *21-hydroxylase deficiency* (51) results in the absence of circulating aldosterone, leading to volume depletion and hypotension (Fig. 9.1).

BLOOD PRESSURE VARIATIONS CAUSED BY MUTATION IN THE MINERALOCORTICOID RECEPTOR

A mutation in the ligand-binding domain of the MR causes an autosomal dominant form of hypertension that develops before the age of 20 years and increases markedly in severity during pregnancy (52). Carriers of this *mineralocorticoid receptor missense mutation (MR S810L)* develop hypertension at a young age. Steroids lacking 21-hydroxyl groups, such as progesterone, normally bind but fail to activate the MR. However, in carriers of the MR S810L mineralocorticoid receptor missense mutation, progesterone binds and functions as a potent activator of MR. Because progesterone levels rise 100-fold during pregnancy, it is not surprising that all pregnancies among women harboring this mutation have been complicated by the development of severe pregnancy-induced hypertension accompanied by complete suppression of the RAAS.

In contrast to gain-of-function mutations of the MR, which cause hypertension, loss-of-function mutations in the MR cause renal salt wasting and hypotension. There are both autosomal-dominant and autosomal-recessive forms of the disease. *Autosomal dominant pseudohypoaldosteronism type I* (PHAI) is characterized by neonatal salt wasting with hypotension despite markedly elevated aldosterone levels in association with hyperkalemic metabolic acidosis (Fig. 9.1). Affected kindred have heterozygous loss of function mutation of the MR due to various premature terminations or frameshift mutations (53). The resulting partial loss of MR function impairs maximal sodium reabsorption, leading to salt wasting and hypotension.

Insufficient ENaC activity causes a diminution in the electrical driving force for H^+ and K^+ secretion resulting in hyperkalemia and metabolic acidosis. In the neonatal period, two normal copies of the MR are apparently required for normal sodium homeostasis because with consumption of a normal salt-rich diet, older affected individuals become normotensive with resolution of the biochemical abnormalities.

BLOOD PRESSURE VARIATIONS CAUSED BY ALTERATIONS IN RENAL SODIUM CHANNELS AND TRANSPORTERS

Mutations leading to a gain-of-function mutation in the ENaC also cause salt-sensitive hypertension. *Liddle syndrome* is characterized by autosomal dominant transmission with early onset of hypertension in association with hypokalemic metabolic alkalosis, suppressed PRA, and low plasma aldosterone levels. This disease is caused by mutations in either the β or γ subunit of the ENaC in which there is deletion of their cytoplasmic carboxy termini (54). These mutations result in enhanced ENaC activity that is attributable to an increase in the number of ENaC inserted into the luminal membrane of principal cells in the DCT. The enhanced number of channels is caused by reduced clearance of ENaC from the cell membrane that substantially prolongs ENaC half-life. The increase in ENaC activity leads to enhanced sodium reabsorption, increase in net renal sodium balance, and salt-sensitive hypertension. The pivotal role of impaired natriuresis in the pathogenesis of hypertension is further illustrated by a case report in which severe hypertension in a patient with Liddle syndrome was cured by successful kidney transplantation from a normotensive donor (55). The most common ENaC variant is the *T594M* mutation, which causes a gain-of-function in the β-subunit, has been found among some individuals with essential hypertension. In a case-control study, 206 hypertensive and 142 normotensive blacks who lived in London were screened for the T594M mutation. It was found that 17 (8.3%) of the hypertensive participants compared with 3 (2.1%) of the normotensive participants possessed the T594M variant (56). These findings suggest that the T594M mutation could be the most common secondary cause of essential hypertension in black people identified to date. Other genes causing mendelian hypertensive syndromes have not yet been systematically studied with regard to their potential roles in the pathogenesis of essential hypertension in the general population (12).

In contrast to gain-of-function mutations in ENaC that cause hypertension, loss-of-function mutations result in hypotension. *Autosomal recessive pseudohypoaldosteronism type I* is caused by loss-of-function mutation in any one of the three ENaC subunits (Fig. 9.1). This disorder causes life-threatening renal salt wasting and hypotension, with hyperkalemic metabolic acidosis despite elevated aldosterone levels (57). Like the autosomal dominant form of PHA1, this disorder begins in the neonatal period; however, it does not resolve on assumption of a salt-rich diet. Affected individuals require lifelong treatment with massive salt supplementation and treatment for hyperkalemia.

To date, hypertension resulting from gain-of-function mutations in the sodium transporters in the PT, TAL, or DCT has not been reported. However, loss-of-function mutations in the Na/K/2Cl cotransporter in the TAL and the thiazide-sensitive NCC in the DCT have been well characterized (12). These autosomal recessive disorders are associated with low–normal blood pressure in association with hypokalemic metabolic alkalosis. In all cases, the disease is caused by mutations that result in renal sodium wasting. Affected individuals can present in the neonatal period with life-threatening hypotension owing to renal sodium wasting or can have disease that is found incidentally. The *Gitelman syndrome* results from homozygous loss-of-function mutations in the thiazide-sensitive NCC (Fig. 9.1) (58). Renal salt wasting leads to blood pressure that is lower than in the general population. Patients present in adolescence with neuromuscular symptoms resulting from hypokalemia. Like thiazide diuretic-treated patients they have hypomagnesemia and hypocalciuria. The salt wasting at the level of DCT leads to compensatory activation of the RAAS. Activation of the MR leads to augmentation of ENaC activity, thereby enhancing sodium reabsorption at the expense of increased H^+ and K^+ secretion leading to hypokalemic metabolic alkalosis. Linkage studies in a large Gitelman kindred indicate that loss-of-function mutations in the NCC indeed lower blood pressure, thereby providing convincing evidence that even a modest enhancement of the natriuretic capacity of the kidney causes a reduction of blood pressure (59). The *Bartter syndrome* occurs in individuals homozygous for various loss-of-function mutations in any of the three genes required for normal function of the Na/K/2Cl cotransporter in the TAL (Fig. 9.1) (12,60). Impaired function of the transporter leads to marked renal salt wasting, reflex activation of the RAAS, and hypokalemic metabolic alkalosis (Fig. 9.1) (12). In type I Bartter syndrome, the mutation may reside in the Na/K/2Cl cotransporter. In type II, the defect resides in the ATP-sensitive K^+ channel ROMK, which is required for potassium recycling and efficient reabsorption of Na^+ and K^+ in the TAL. Type III is caused by homozygous mutation in the chloride channel (CLCNKB), which is required for chloride exit form the cell across the basolateral membrane (12). Individuals with Bartter syndrome often present with premature delivery and life-threatening hypotension caused by salt wasting in the neonatal period. In contrast to Gitelman syndrome, Bartter syndrome is associated with hypercalciuria and normal or only slightly reduced magnesium levels (similar to patients treated with loop diuretics).

Gain-of-function mutations in the sodium–hydrogen ion exchanger (NHE-3) in the PT have been investigated as a possible cause of essential hypertension in the general population; however, linkage analysis studies have failed to demonstrate an association (61).

IMPAIRED NATRIURESIS CAUSED BY HYPERINSULINEMIA

It has been observed that glucose intolerance, hyperlipidemia, and essential hypertension tend to cluster in the same patients. In fact, essential hypertension often occurs many years before the onset of overt diabetes with hyperglycemia. It has been proposed that insulin resistance is central to the pathogenesis of this so-called "Syndrome X," a condition now known as metabolic syndrome (62). Insulin resistance, which may be inherited or acquired (owing to obesity, dietary factors, or sedentary life style), results in compensatory *hyperinsulinemia*. Eventually, the β-cell output of insulin may become inadequate to compensate for insulin resistance, resulting in glucose intolerance or frank type 2 diabetes. The hyperinsulinemia induces abnormalities of lipid metabolism with increased low-density lipoprotein (LDL) and reduced HDL levels. Hyperinsulinemia also may be causally related to the development of hypertension. Insulin has been shown to play an important role in renal sodium handling. In human studies in which euglycemic hyperinsulinemia was generated using an insulin clamp technique, urinary sodium excretion declined significantly within 60 minutes (63). This antinatriuretic effect of insulin was observed in the absence of changes in GFR, renal plasma flow, the filtered load of glucose, or plasma aldosterone concentration. The predominant effect of insulin on tubular sodium reabsorption is in more distal parts of the nephron (TAL of Henle or DCT). Thus, the net effect of insulin resistance and resulting hyperinsulinemia is to induce an impairment in the intrinsic natriuretic capacity of the kidney, which results in the development of salt-sensitive hypertension.

ACQUIRED TUBULOINTERSTITIAL DISEASE IN THE PATHOGENESIS OF SALT-DEPENDENT HYPERTENSION

There is compelling evidence that essential hypertension results from a defect whereby the kidney is unable to maintain sodium homeostasis at a normal blood pressure. However, if the defect that causes impaired natriuresis is genetic, then why does hypertension generally not develop until adulthood? The salt-sensitive hypertension associated with obesity, aging, and black heritage appears to be an acquired disorder. Why does salt sensitivity increase in frequency and magnitude over time? It has been proposed that salt-sensitive hypertension may be the result of acquired tubulointerstitial renal disease (64). The hypothesis is that hypertension consists of two phases. The first phase is characterized by episodic elevations in blood pressure caused by hyperactivity of the sympathetic nervous system (elevated plasma norepinephrine and baroreceptor sensitivity) induced by genetic or environmental factors. Less commonly, the episodic hypertension relates to activation of the renin–angiotensin system (RAAS). Elevations of blood pressure are episodic and renal sodium handling is normal during this initial phase. Transition to the second phase is proposed to occur as a consequence of transient catecholamine or AII-mediated elevations in blood pressure that preferentially damage the juxtamedullary and medullary regions, which do not autoregulate as well as cortical regions in response to sudden changes in renal perfusion pressure. The pressor response may be associated with both an increase in peritubular capillary pressure and a reduction in peritubular capillary flow, resulting in injury to the peritubular capillaries with ischemia of the tubules and interstitium. The resulting tubulointerstitial injury then may trigger local vasoconstrictor mechanisms (AII, adenosine, or renal sympathetic nerves) or inhibit vasodilator mechanisms (nitric oxide [NO], prostaglandins, or dopamine), further augmenting ischemia and resulting in abnormal tubuloglomerular feedback and enhanced tubular sodium reabsorption. Peritubular capillary damage and rarefaction lead to an increase in renovascular resistance, which further blunts the pressure natriuresis mechanism. The predicted consequence of enhanced tubuloglomerular feedback and impaired pressure natriuresis is an acquired functional defect in renal sodium excretion. This resetting of the pressure natriuresis curve to higher pressure is proposed to be the explanation for the development of acquired salt-sensitive hypertension.

Animal models confirm that short-term exposure to catecholamines or AII causes renal injury, which leads to the development of salt-sensitive hypertension that persists even after catecholamine and AII infusions are stopped (65,66). An 8-week infusion of phenylephrine by minipump was found to induce structural and functional changes in the kidneys of rats (65). Glomeruli were spared but focal tubulointerstitial fibrosis was present in association increased expression of transforming growth factor-β (TGF-β), de novo expression of the macrophage adhesive protein osteopontin by injured tubules, macrophage and α-smooth muscle actin-positive myofibroblast accumulation in the interstitium, as well as distortion and rarefaction of the peritubular capillaries. Blood pressure returned to normal in rats maintained on a low-salt diet after discontinuation of catecholamine infusion. However, rats fed on a high-salt diet developed marked hypertension. Short-term (2-week) infusion of AII also caused sustained salt-sensitive hypertension in association with tubulointerstitial damage and fibrosis (66).

This hypothesis may help to explain the development of salt-sensitive hypertension in some high-risk populations. For instance, blacks have enhanced pressor response to exercise or norepinephrine (NE) (67) as well as a relative defect in their renal autoregulatory response to salt loading (68). This could explain their higher frequency of hypertension, increased risk of target organ damage, and salt sensitivity. The prevalence of salt-sensitive hypertension increases progressively with age in the general population. Aging is associated with progressive decline in renal function and the development of glomerulosclerosis and interstitial fibrosis. In rat models, aging is associated with tubulointerstitial fibrosis characterized by tubular injury, myofibroblast proliferation, osteopontin expression, macrophage infiltration, and collagen IV deposition (69). These structural changes could lead to impaired natriuresis with the development of salt-sensitive hypertension. Obesity also is associated with an increased prevalence of hypertension. Obese individuals have been shown to have augmented sympathetic nervous system activity with higher basal NE and plasma renin levels, glomerular hyperfiltration, increased prevalence of interstitial fibrosis and glomerulosclerosis, expanded ECF volume, and salt-dependent hypertension (64). In transplant patients, treatment with cyclosporine A (CsA) to prevent allograft rejection is also associated with interstitial fibrosis, osteopontin and TGF-β expression, and the development of salt-sensitive hypertension in humans (64). Cyclosporine is a vasoconstrictor that can directly inhibit NO production. Rats administered CsA develop interstitial fibrosis identical to that observed in humans with tubulointerstitial injury preferentially involving the juxtaglomerular regions. Interstitial fibrosis develops in association with TGF-β and osteopontin expression and reduction in endothelial NO synthetase. If CsA administration is stopped after the tubulointerstitial lesion develops, placement of the animals on a high-salt diet results in rapid development of hypertension despite the presence of normal GFR (64).

IMPAIRED NATRIURESIS CAUSED BY REDUCED NEPHRON MASS

It has been postulated that the underlying cause of impaired natriuretic capacity in essential (genetic) hypertension may be a congenitally acquired deficit of effective nephron mass (24). In the SHR, the fenestrae of the glomerular capillary endothelium are smaller than in normotensive control rats. In the Milan SHR, there is a decreased glomerular ultrafiltration coefficient and increased proximal sodium reabsorption. Salt-sensitive hypertension in rats is associated with a 15% reduction in nephron number. In humans, major inborn deficits of nephron number such as oligomeganephronia and congenital unilateral renal agenesis are associated with the development of hypertension. Brenner has postulated that the abnormality that predisposes a minority of the population to essential hypertension in the setting of excessive sodium intake is an inherited deficit of nephrons or glomerular filtration surface area leading to a diminished capacity to excrete a sodium load resulting in salt-sensitive hypertension (24). Of course, chronic kidney disease of any etiology could also lead to a state of impaired natriuretic capacity with resulting salt-sensitive hypertension.

IMPAIRED NATRIURESIS CAUSED BY ABNORMAL REGULATION OF THE RENIN–ANGIOTENSIN SYSTEM

Increased circulating levels of AII stimulate increased production of aldosterone with activation of the MR and enhanced sodium reabsorption in the distal nephron as discussed in detail in the preceding section. AII has also been shown to increase renal sodium and water retention independent of its effect to increase aldosterone production (70). In this regard, AII-mediated renal hemodynamic changes lead indirectly to increases in tubular sodium reabsorption. Infusion of AII causes a reduction of renal blood flow with maintenance of near-normal glomerular filtration rate because of an increase in filtration fraction consistent with an increase in efferent arteriolar resistance. The increase in efferent arteriolar resistance caused by AII results in a fall in hydrostatic pressure and an increase in oncotic pressure in the peritubular capillaries of the proximal and distal tubules and collecting ducts, which results in enhanced tubular sodium reabsorption (70). AII also has been shown to directly stimulate sodium reabsorption in the PT (71).

Recent evidence suggests that renal abnormalities involving disordered regulation of the RAAS may be important in the pathogenesis of essential hypertension (72). These fundamental abnormalities, which are present in 45% of patients with essential hypertension, cause impairment in renal sodium handling resulting in sodium-sensitive hypertension. These patients have normal to high PRA and have been termed "nonmodulators" because of their inability to appropriately adjust activity of the RAAS during changes in sodium intake. Renal blood flow changes in parallel to sodium intake in normal individuals or patients with essential hypertension and who are "modulators." Renal blood flow rises with an increase in sodium intake, whereas renal blood flow declines with a decrease in sodium intake. In contrast, the renal blood flow remains fixed in nonmodulators despite changes in sodium intake. This abnormal renal vascular response to changes in sodium intake may account for the limited capacity of the kidney to handle a sodium load. Nonmodulators demonstrate less suppression of renin in response to sodium loading or AII infusion compared with normals or modulators with essential hypertension. Treatment of these nonmodulators with an ACE inhibitor restores the normal natriuretic response to a sodium load and normalizes renin suppression in response to a sodium load or AII infusion. Furthermore, ACE inhibition also results in a decrease in renal vascular resistance and an increase in renal blood flow and natriuresis (72). These findings suggest that enhanced renal vascular responsiveness to AII is present in nonmodulators, even in the absence of increased systemic renin and AII levels, perhaps secondary to in situ AII production by renal-converting enzyme. The resulting decrease in peritubular Starling force and increase in proximal and distal sodium reabsorption may underlie the defect in natriuresis in some cases of essential hypertension. Moreover, restoration of the ability of the kidney to handle a sodium load may explain why treatment with ACE inhibitors leads to a reduction in blood pressure in patients with low-renin essential hypertension.

SYMPATHETIC NERVOUS SYSTEM-MEDIATED IMPAIRMENT IN NATRIURESIS

Neural mechanisms activated in response to perceived changes in blood pressure or intravascular volume act on the kidney to modulate renal sodium excretion. Proximal tubular sodium reabsorption is enhanced by α-adrenergic receptor-mediated sympathetic activation (73). Increased vasoconstrictor responsiveness of the efferent arteriole to α-adrenergic stimuli may cause the intrarenal hemodynamic abnormalities typical of patients with essential hypertension, namely, decreased renal blood flow, increased renal vascular resistance, and increased filtration fraction (74). Akin to the effect of AII, this primary increase in efferent resistance may contribute to the defective natriuresis in essential hypertension by altering peritubular capillary Starling forces. It also should be noted that increased α-adrenergic activity has been shown to directly stimulate sodium reabsorption in the PT (75). Calcium channel blockers (CCBs) decrease renal efferent arteriolar vasoconstriction and improve renal blood flow (74). The natriuretic response to CCBs may be secondary to this phenomenon in addition to their direct effect on tubular sodium transport (76).

The renal nerves contribute to development of hypertension in experimental models, and appear to play a role in the pathogenesis of hypertension in humans (77). In both the SHR and DOC-salt rat models of hypertension, the full development of hypertension is dependent on renal afferent nerve activity, which stimulates renal tubular sodium reabsorption. Denervation of the kidney ameliorates the hypertension in these models (77).

IMPAIRED NATRIURESIS CAUSED BY ABNORMALITIES IN RENAL NITRIC OXIDE

There is increasing evidence that endothelium-derived NO is tonically synthesized within the kidney and that NO plays a crucial role in the regulation of renal hemodynamics and sodium excretion (78). These effects are mediated in part by interactions between NO and the RAAS. Nitric oxide is an important mediator of renal blood flow and the renal microcirculation. Bradykinin and acetylcholine induce renal vasodilation by increasing NO synthesis, which in turn leads to enhancement of diuresis and natriuresis. Blockade of basal NO synthesis, with specific inhibitors of the L-arginine NO pathway (L-NAME or L-NMMA), has been shown to result in an increase in renal vascular resistance with decreases in renal blood flow, urine flow, and sodium excretion. Intrarenal inhibition of NO synthesis leads to reduction of sodium excretory responses to changes in renal perfusion pressure without an effect on renal autoregulation, suggesting that NO exerts a permissive or mediatory role in the tubular responses that regulate the pressure natriuresis mechanism (79,80). Nitric oxide released from the macula densa may modulate tubuloglomerular feedback response by affecting afferent arteriolar constriction. In the collecting duct, an NO-dependent inhibition of solute transport has been suggested. Although most studies indicate that NO synthesis blockade causes reduction in sodium excretion, the exact mechanism is unclear. Reduction in the filtered load of sodium, increased tubular sodium reabsorption, altered medullary blood flow, and decreased renal interstitial hydrostatic pressure may mediate sodium retention during NO blockade. Taken together, these observations suggest that NO-dependent mechanisms have a major impact on renal volume control. Abnormalities in renal NO-mediated sodium excretion have been postulated to cause a state of impaired natriuresis, resulting in salt-sensitive hypertension (78–80). In this regard, impaired NO synthetase activity related to insulin resistance may contribute to the pathogenesis of salt-sensitive hypertension in patients with metabolic syndrome (81).

IMPAIRED NATRIURESIS CAUSED BY ENHANCED PROXIMAL TUBULAR SODIUM REABSORPTION

In some cases, the genetic defect that underlies the development of essential hypertension may be a diminished natriuretic capacity caused by a primary increase in PT sodium reabsorption (82). Lithium clearance often is used as a surrogate marker of proximal tubular sodium reabsorption because lithium reabsorption occurs in parallel to sodium resorption and is limited to the PT. Therefore, a decreased fractional lithium clearance (ratio of lithium clearance to creatinine clearance) implies increased proximal sodium reabsorption. Studies in patients with essential hypertension have revealed a decreased fractional lithium clearance (82). Furthermore, normotensive subjects with a hypertensive first-degree relative had a lower fractional lithium clearance than subjects with no hypertensive relative (82).

IMPAIRED NATRIURESIS: A PREREQUISITE IN HYPERTENSION

Experiments with isolated, perfused kidneys demonstrate that the magnitude of urinary sodium excretion is a direct function of the perfusion pressure (83). The level of perfusion pressure may alter sodium excretion by changing the peritubular hydrostatic pressure. Thus, an increase in perfusion pressure should increase peritubular hydrostatic pressure with a resultant decrease in sodium reabsorption. Micropuncture studies in the rat have shown an inverse relationship between renal perfusion pressure and proximal sodium reabsorption (84).

It has been argued that if this pressure natriuresis mechanism were operating in a normal fashion, then profound volume depletion would occur in the setting of hypertension. The fact that this does not occur suggests that in every hypertensive state, there must be a shift in the pressure natriuresis curve such that a higher perfusion pressure is required to achieve any given level of natriuresis. In this regard, it has been postulated that this shift in the pressure natriuresis curve is actually a reflection of the underlying renal abnormality present in essential hypertension as well as in hypertension caused by chronic kidney disease (17,19,20). If a primary defect in natriuresis does exist in hypertension, then to avert disaster owing to persistent positive sodium balance with inexorable fluid accumulation, compensatory hormonal responses, or other mechanisms must be invoked that restore sodium balance. The theories regarding the pathogenesis of hypertension that follow explain how these compensatory processes restore sodium balance but in the process cause systemic hypertension in association with an elevated systemic vascular resistance.

The Na/K ATPase Inhibitor Hypothesis

There must be an underlying abnormality in the kidney's ability to excrete sodium in both essential hypertension and secondary hypertension caused by renal disease. In individuals with this impairment of natriuretic capacity, if the intake of dietary sodium is >60 mmol/day, then there will be a tendency toward sodium and water retention resulting in ECF volume expansion. Some authors have proposed that in response to this expansion of ECF volume, there is an increase in the plasma concentration of two or more substances, collectively referred to as "natriuretic hormone" (16,17,85,86). The responses induced by this natriuretic hormone include an increase in the natriuretic capacity of the plasma, an increase in the ability of the plasma to inhibit Na/K ATPase, and an increase in vascular responsiveness to vasoconstrictors such as NE, AII, and vasopressin. Atrial natriuretic peptide (ANP), which is released from the atria in response to acute volume expansion, causes a brisk increase in renal sodium and water excretion of rapid onset and short duration. However, ANP does not inhibit Na/K ATPase or increase vascular reactivity, in fact, ANP decreases systemic vascular resistance. It is proposed that another response to the underlying renal impairment in the ability to excrete sodium is an increase in the plasma concentration of a substance, probably of hypothalamic origin, which inhibits Na/K ATPase (87,88). As a result of inhibition of Na/K ATPase, renal tubular sodium reabsorption is reduced and urinary sodium excretion increases, thereby returning sodium balance toward normal. However, this circulating inhibitor also inhibits the sodium pump in other cells, such as erythrocytes and leukocytes and, more importantly, in vascular smooth muscle cells. The increase in cellular sodium is associated with increased Na/Ca exchange and increased cellular calcium concentration. Thus, at the arteriolar level, inhibition of Na/K ATPase theoretically could cause vasoconstriction secondary to increased intracellular calcium with a resultant increase in systemic vascular resistance and a rise in blood pressure (85). As a result of the compensatory release of these natriuretic substances, sodium balance and ECF volume are restored to normal but at the expense of systemic hypertension caused by the increase in systemic vascular resistance (Fig. 9.2). Thus, although the underlying cause of this type of salt-sensitive (volume-dependent) hypertension is a defect in renal natriuretic capacity, this does not result in a

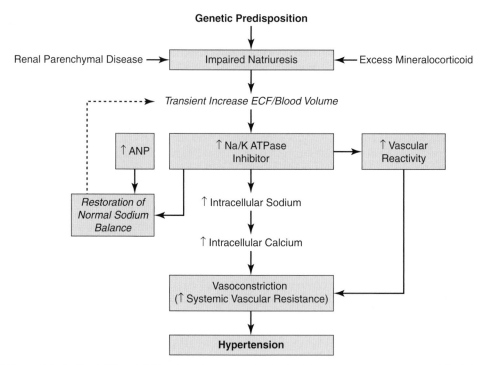

■ **Figure 9.2** The Na/K ATPase inhibitor hypothesis. A defect in the inherent natriuretic capacity of the kidney is thought to be the fundamental abnormality that predisposes to the development of hypertension. The resulting tendency toward extracellular fluid (ECF) volume expansion leads to elaboration of two or more natriuretic hormones. Atrial natriuretic peptide (ANP) and a circulating inhibitor of the Na/K ATPase result in reduced renal tubular sodium reabsorption, thereby compensating for the underlying natriuretic defect and restoring sodium balance and ECF volume to normal. However, Na/K ATPase inhibition in vascular smooth muscle cells causes vasoconstriction because of increased intracellular calcium, resulting in systemic hypertension. Atrial natriuretic peptide causes vasodilation, thereby attenuating the rise in blood pressure.

detectable increase in ECF volume or cardiac output in the steady-state phase. Instead, the hypertension is maintained by the resulting increase in systemic vascular resistance (16,17,85,86).

The Guyton Hypothesis

Guyton's hypothesis is that the most important and fundamental mechanism determining the long-term control of blood pressure is the *renal fluid–volume feedback mechanism*. In simple terms, this is the basic mechanism through which the kidneys regulate arterial pressure by altering renal excretion of sodium and water, thereby controlling circulatory volume and cardiac output. Changes in blood pressure, in turn, directly influence renal excretion of sodium and water, thereby providing a negative feedback mechanism for control of ECF volume, cardiac output, and blood pressure. The hypothesis is that derangements in this renal fluid–volume pressure control mechanism are the fundamental cause of virtually all hypertensive states (17–20,89–91).

RENAL FUNCTION CURVES

Interactions of the renal perfusion pressure–sodium excretion mechanism and modulating neurohormonal factors normally operate very precisely to maintain sodium balance at a normal arterial pressure (89). The physiologic basis of the renal–body fluid feedback mechanism for the regulation of arterial pressure is the direct effect of arterial pressure on output of water and sodium from the kidneys. Studies of the isolated, perfused kidney demonstrate the so-called pressure natriuresis and diuresis whereby an increase in perfusion pressure directly causes the renal output of sodium and water to increase (90,91). Figure 9.3 depicts a *renal function curve* that shows the effect of perfusion pressure on urinary sodium excretion in the isolated perfused kidney. Urinary sodium output falls to zero when the arterial pressure falls to approximately 50 mm Hg. In contrast, the output of sodium increases sixfold to eightfold when the arterial pressure rises from the normal value of 100 mm Hg up to 200 mm Hg (89). This effect of arterial pressure on sodium excretion has been demonstrated in isolated, perfused kidneys and in intact animals. However, for the reasons discussed

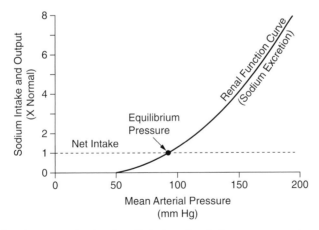

■ **Figure 9.3** Renal function curves showing the effect of renal perfusion pressure on urinary sodium excretion in the isolated, perfused kidney. By using computer modeling, the corresponding sodium intake can be superimposed on the pressure natriuresis curve. An equilibrium pressure point is defined, which represents the unique level at which the arterial pressure will be regulated. It is apparent that a primary increase in systemic vascular resistance alone cannot lead to sustained increase in blood pressure because the pressure-natriuresis mechanism would cause sodium excretion, decreased ECF volume, and cardiac output, thereby returning the blood pressure to the equilibrium point. Likewise, a primary decrease in systemic vascular resistance would not lead to sustained hypotension because reduced natriuresis, sodium retention, increased ECF volume, and cardiac output would once again return blood pressure to the equilibrium point. (From Guyton AC. Renal function curve: a key to understanding the pathogenesis of hypertension. *Hypertension.* 1987; 10: 1, with permission of the American Heart Association, Inc.)

in the following, the upward slope of the renal function curve in the intact animal is much steeper. The horizontal line in Fig. 9.3 represents the level of sodium intake at equilibrium when sodium intake and output are matched. When net intake and output of sodium are matched, the arterial pressure is determined by the point where the two plots intersect, which is known as the *equilibrium pressure point.* Computer model analysis of hypothetical renal function curves in the intact animal suggests that, if the renal function curve and the sodium intake remain unchanged, this is the unique perfusion pressure at which external sodium balance will be maintained (92). If the pressure rises above this level, the sodium output becomes greater than input and negative sodium balance occurs with eventual reduction of ECF volume and cardiac output to a level that returns the blood pressure to the equilibrium point. In contrast, if the blood pressure falls below the equilibrium point, the intake of sodium will be greater than the output and a positive sodium balance will occur until the increase in ECF volume, blood volume, and cardiac output are sufficient to return the pressure to the equilibrium point. Sodium balance can be maintained only at the 100 mm Hg equilibrium pressure point.

If this model is correct, then it is apparent that a primary increase in cardiac output or systemic vascular resistance cannot result in a sustained increase in blood pressure because a normally functioning feedback mechanism would result in natriuresis and diuresis, thereby returning the blood pressure to normal. Thus, a primary increase in systemic vascular resistance would be accompanied by an equal and opposite decrease in cardiac output with return of the blood pressure to normal. This return of the pressure to the equilibrium point illustrates the infinite gain characteristic of the renal fluid–volume feedback mechanism. In this system, a change in the arterial pressure is the critical feedback stimulus that modifies the natriuretic response. In theory, if an initial decrease in blood pressure results from a decrease in cardiac output, for instance in the setting of congestive heart failure, then the compensatory salt and water retention would increase ECF volume but fail to normalize cardiac output and renal perfusion pressure. Thus, renal sodium and water retention would continue unopposed, resulting in massive fluid overload. This mechanism is consistent with the unifying hypothesis recently proposed to explain body fluid volume regulation in disorders characterized by low effective arterial blood volume (23,93). The implication of this renal fluid–volume feedback mechanism is that the finding of sustained hypertension must be a reflection of an underlying abnormality that caused a shift of the renal function curve to the right such that a higher blood pressure is required to maintain sodium balance at any given level of sodium intake (94–96).

ROLE OF THE RENIN–ANGIOTENSIN SYSTEM IN REGULATION OF BLOOD PRESSURE

Unlike the isolated, perfused kidney or computer models, in vivo the position of the renal function curve can be shifted by various neural and endocrine factors. For example, changes in the activity of the RAAS can result in a shift of the curve and thus either magnify or blunt the basic relation between sodium and water excretion and blood pressure (92,94). Different renal function curves can be produced in animals by varying sodium intake in stepwise increments while maintaining AII levels constant at various levels by using combinations of ACE inhibitor and AII infusion (Fig. 9.4) (95). With the AII level maintained above normal, there is a shift in the renal function curve to the right consistent with a blunting of the pressure-induced natriuretic response. In contrast, when AII is totally suppressed by an ACE inhibitor, the curve is shifted to the left, consistent with an exaggerated pressure natriuresis. The vertical line in Figure 9.4 represents a different type of renal function curve called a *salt-loading renal function curve.* It is obtained when sodium intake is varied in a stepwise fashion in animals with an intact RAAS (AII level allowed to vary in response to the sodium intake), which will modulate the intrinsic renal body fluid feedback mechanism. Thus, the renal function curve in the intact animal is much steeper than that seen in the isolated perfused kidney. In this salt-loading curve, blood pressure at equilibrium for each level of sodium intake changes very little. Analysis of the superimposed renal function curves, with AII held constant at different levels, illustrates that the steepness of the curve in the intact animal may be owing to changes in the activity of the RAAS. A high sodium intake suppresses the RAAS and shifts the renal function curve to the left, whereas a low sodium intake activates the RAAS and shifts the curve to the right. This modulation of the renal function curve by the RAAS is thought to result from the effect of AII on renal sodium and water reabsorption. AII directly enhances proximal tubular sodium reabsorption (71). In addition, AII has important renal hemodynamic effects that cause increased tubular sodium reabsorption independent of aldosterone (70). The predominant efferent vasoconstriction produced by

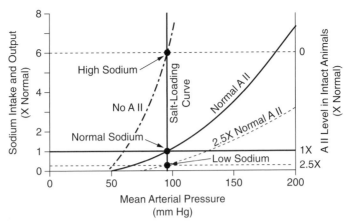

■ **Figure 9.4** Modulation of renal function curves by the renin–angiotensin system. A salt-loading renal function curve is obtained when the sodium intake is varied in stepwise increments in animals with an intact renin–angiotensin system. The curve is extremely steep such that over a wide range of dietary sodium intake, the blood pressure changes very little. Three separate renal function curves were produced by varying the sodium intake in a stepwise fashion in animals, with angiotensin II (AII) levels maintained constant in either the normal range, 2.5 times normal, or with AII absent. The curve obtained when AII production is suppressed by angiotensin converting enzyme inhibitor is shifted to the left, consistent with an enhanced natriuretic response to any given level of perfusion pressure. In contrast, with an AII level at 2.5 times normal, the curve is shifted to the right, reflecting a blunting of the intrinsic renal natriuretic response. Superimposition of these individual renal function curves reveals that the steepness of the salt-loading renal function curve in the intact animal is caused by changes in the natriuretic response to pressure, which are in turn mediated by changes in the activity of the renin–angiotensin system as a function of dietary sodium intake. AII is suppressed with high sodium intake, producing a shift of the renal function curve to the left so the salt load can be excreted at normal blood pressure. In contrast, AII production is enhanced with dietary sodium restriction, leading to a shift of the curve to the right such that the kidney is more avid for sodium such that a normal level of blood pressure is still maintained. (From Guyton AC. Renal function curve: a key to understanding hypertension. *Hypertension*. 1987;10:1, with permission of the American Heart Association, Inc.)

AII causes a drop in peritubular capillary hydrostatic pressure, leading to enhanced tubular reabsorption of sodium and water (70,96). This dynamic interaction between the RAAS and renal fluid–volume feedback mechanism accounts for the observation that tremendous extremes of dietary sodium intake in normal individuals result in relatively little change in the systemic arterial pressure.

AUTOREGULATION LEADS TO INCREASED SYSTEMIC VASCULAR RESISTANCE

The ability to maintain normal blood pressure over a wide range of dietary sodium intake is present only if both the RAA system and the kidney function normally. Aberrations in either the RAA system or the renal fluid–volume mechanism can lead to a significant increase in blood pressure when the sodium intake is increased. Guyton's hypothesis holds that there are two basic ways in which the pressure equilibrium set point can be increased with resulting hypertension. A shift of the renal function curve to the right along the pressure axis owing to either intrinsic renal abnormalities or overactivity of the RAA system can cause hypertension. Alternatively, an increase in the sodium intake without a compensatory leftward shift of the renal function curve also can cause hypertension.

In the setting of an underlying decrease in the inherent natriuretic capacity, the renal fluid–volume feedback mechanism should cause progressive sodium and water retention until the increases in ECF volume, blood volume, and cardiac output are sufficient to raise the blood pressure to the equilibrium pressure point. Sodium and water balance is restored at the equilibrium point; however, this is accomplished at the expense of systemic hypertension (Fig. 9.5). Thus, when the inherent natriuretic capacity is reduced, Guyton's concept holds that an increase in arterial pressure is an essential protective mechanism to restore sodium balance and avert disaster (17–20,91).

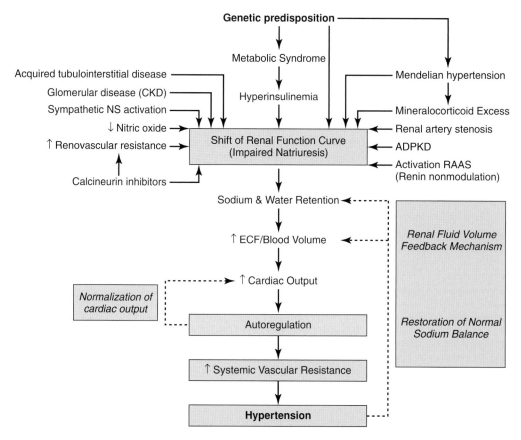

■ **Figure 9.5** The Guyton hypothesis. A defect in the inherent natriuretic capacity of the kidney is thought to be the fundamental abnormality that predisposes to the development of all forms of hypertension. A variety of disorders can lead to a shift in the intrinsic renal function curve with reduced natriuretic capacity. Causes of impaired natriuresis include a genetic predisposition to essential hypertension, primary renal parenchymal disease caused by diabetic nephropathy or other primary glomerular disease with nephron loss, acquired tubulointerstitial disease, inherited or acquired glucose intolerance with hyperinsulinemia, mineralocorticoid excess states, mendelian forms of hypertension that lead to enhanced tubular sodium reabsorption, failure to downregulate the renin–angiotensin in response to volume expansion (renin nonmodulation), renal artery stenosis, activation of sympathetic nervous system (catecholamines or renal nerves), and decreased renal nitric oxide. A rightward shift of the renal function curve with impaired natriuresis is thought to be the fundamental abnormality that underlies all causes of hypertension. Initially, sodium and water retention lead to increases in extracellular fluid (ECF) volume and cardiac output. In the long term, circulatory autoregulation restores cardiac output to normal. However, autoregulation also leads to a sustained increase in systemic vascular resistance and systemic hypertension. Via pressure-induced natriuresis, the renal fluid–volume feedback mechanism, returns sodium balance and ECF volume to normal but at the expense of sustained hypertension. Guyton's hypothesis explains the paradox whereby a primary disorder that involves enhanced renal sodium reabsorption ultimately results in hypertension with elevated systemic vascular resistance in the absence of a detectable increase in ECF volume.

Theoretically, hypertension caused by a rightward shift of the renal function curve should be mediated by an increased cardiac output in response to sodium and water retention. However, in animal models and humans with essential hypertension, even though the initiating mechanism for hypertension is sodium retention with increased ECF volume and cardiac output, ultimately an increase in the peripheral vascular resistance perpetuates the hypertension, whereas the cardiac output and ECF volume return to normal. According to Guyton's hypothesis, this transition from high cardiac output hypertension to the high systemic vascular resistance type of hypertension is explained by the process of autoregulation of blood flow in the systemic circulation (18–20). *Autoregulation* is a local tissue phenomenon that adjusts local blood flow when it becomes too high or low. Acutely, autoregulation may result from local changes in vascular muscle tone; however, structural changes in the resistance vessels develop in the chronic phase (13). In theory, when the cardiac output increases as a result of ECF volume expansion, autoregulatory vasoconstriction in all vascular beds eventually returns the cardiac output to normal. Hypertension persists, however, because the fall in cardiac output is accompanied by an equal and opposite increase in systemic vascular resistance. Given the persistent hypertension, sodium balance can still be maintained by the renal fluid–volume pressure natriuresis mechanism. Figure 9.5 summarizes the pathophysiologic sequence whereby the various disorders that cause an initial defect in natriuretic capacity (shift of renal function curve to the right) eventually lead to sustained hypertension caused by increased systemic vascular resistance in the absence of clinically evident increases in ECF volume, blood volume, or cardiac output.

RENAL FUNCTION CURVES IN SALT-SENSITIVE AND -RESISTANT ESSENTIAL HYPERTENSION

An impairment of the intrinsic natriuretic capacity of the kidney is easy to conceptualize in the setting of the mendelian forms of hypertension, renal artery stenosis, primary renal parenchymal disease, or mineralocorticoid-induced hypertension. However, in the early stages of human essential hypertension, no specific renal histologic abnormality can be identified. At face value, this observation suggests that renal function is entirely normal until damage (nephrosclerosis) secondary to hypertension supervenes. However, if either the Guyton hypothesis or the Na/K ATPase inhibitor hypothesis is correct, it is clear that with sustained hypertension, regardless of etiology, there must be a rightward shift of the renal function curve such that sodium balance is maintained at a hypertensive level.

Salt balance is maintained at a normal blood pressure in the normal individual. Moreover, the slope of the renal function curve is very steep, such that even with dietary salt loading the blood pressure remains near normal (Fig. 9.6). Two subsets of essential hypertension (salt-sensitive and salt-resistant) have been identified based on the response of blood pressure to increases in dietary sodium intake (97,98). Approximately 60% of subjects with essential hypertension have greater than a 10% increase in blood pressure when given a high-sodium diet (>200 mmol/day) and are defined as salt-sensitive, whereas 40% are salt-resistant.

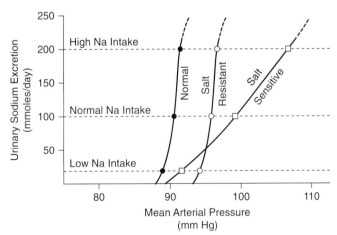

■ **Figure 9.6** Schematic renal function curves in human essential hypertension. In the normal individual, salt balance is maintained at a normal blood pressure. Moreover, the slope of the normal renal function curve is very steep, such that the blood pressure remains near normal even with dietary sodium loading. The salt-loading renal function curve in *salt-resistant hypertension* is shifted to the right, but remains parallel to the curve for normotensive individuals. Thus, salt balance is maintained during normal sodium intake, but at a higher blood pressure set point. However, because the renal function curve is steep, the blood pressure does not increase during dietary salt loading. In contrast, in *salt-sensitive hypertension,* the rightward shift of the curve is accompanied by a depression of the slope. Thus, not only is the blood pressure set point on a normal sodium diet elevated but also the blood pressure increases in response to dietary salt loading. The response to strict dietary sodium intake differs in the two subtypes of essential hypertension as well. Hypertension responds to lowered sodium intake in salt-sensitive hypertension, but not in salt-resistant hypertension.

PRA is low in salt-sensitive patients and usually normal or high in salt-resistant patients. These hypertensive subtypes probably represent differences in the adaptation to a sodium load. The salt-loading renal function curve in *salt-resistant hypertension* is shifted to the right but it remains parallel to the curve for normotensive individuals (Fig. 9.6). Thus, salt balance is maintained on a normal sodium intake, but at a higher blood pressure set point. However, because the renal function curve is steep, the blood pressure does not increase further with dietary salt loading. In contrast with *salt-sensitive hypertension,* the rightward shift of the curve is accompanied by a depression of the slope. Thus, not only is the blood pressure set point on a normal sodium diet elevated, but also the blood pressure increases in response to dietary salt loading (Fig. 9.6). Response to strict dietary sodium restriction also differs in the two subtypes. Hypertension responds to reduced sodium intake in salt-sensitive hypertension but not in salt-resistant hypertension.

Experimental evidence suggests that disorders associated with increased renal vascular resistance, such as one-kidney Goldblatt hypertension, tend to induce salt-resistant hypertension. In contrast, salt-sensitivity with rightward shift of the curve accompanied by a depression in slope occurs in conditions characterized by increased sodium reabsorption by the renal tubules. This phenomenon occurs in DOC-salt hypertension in the rat, in patients with primary hyperaldosteronism, in the various mendelian forms of hypertension with enhanced tubular sodium reabsorption, in the setting of reduced renal mass or chronic kidney disease, and in conditions characterized by blunting of the normal negative feedback of the RAAS. In these instances, as sodium intake increases, an incremental rise in blood pressure is required to overcome excessive sodium reabsorption and maintain normal sodium balance (97).

The precise nature of the defect responsible for the altered pressure natriuresis mechanism in human essential hypertension is unknown. Theoretically, any abnormality that increases renal vascular resistance, reduces renal mass, decreases glomerular basement membrane filtration coefficient, and increases tubular sodium reabsorption (angiotensin, α-adrenergic stimulation, deficient renal NO, aldosterone or other mineralocorticoids, and alterations in net peritubular Starling forces) could impair renal natriuretic capacity and lead to hypertension (18). Changes in renal vascular resistance have been clearly documented in human essential hypertension, especially with advanced nephrosclerosis. On the other hand, the mechanism of increased tubular sodium reabsorption in salt-sensitive patients may relate to abnormalities of the sympathetic nervous system (97). Salt-sensitive patients display an abnormal relation between sodium intake and plasma NE levels. Although plasma NE levels are suppressed by salt loading in normal individuals and salt-resistant patients, they tend to increase in salt-sensitive patients. It has been postulated that increased sympathetic activity and reduced renal sodium excretion in salt-sensitive patients may be related to a defect in sodium-coupled cellular calcium transport. In this regard, CCBs have been shown to have a natriuretic effect and to normalize the derangements in the renal function curve in salt-sensitive essential hypertension in blacks (76,97).

THE DOMINANT ROLE OF PERFUSION RENAL PERFUSION PRESSURE IN MINERALOCORTICOID ESCAPE

To substantiate the role of direct pressure-induced natriuresis in the regulation of sodium balance in mineralocorticoid hypertension, Hall et al. compared the systemic blood pressure and natriuretic effect of aldosterone infusion in a dog model in which the renal perfusion pressure was either allowed to increase or mechanically servocontrolled to maintain perfusion pressure at normal levels (Fig. 9.7) (98). In the intact animal, continuous aldosterone infusion caused a transient period of sodium and water retention with a mild increase in blood pressure. However, the sodium retention lasted only a few days and was followed by an escape from the sodium-retaining effects of aldosterone and restoration of normal sodium balance. In contrast, when the renal perfusion pressure was mechanically servocontrolled at a normal level during aldosterone infusion, there was no escape from aldosterone leading to relentless increase in sodium and water retention accompanied by severe hypertension, edema, ascites, and congestive heart failure. When the servocontrol device was removed and the perfusion pressure was allowed to rise to the systemic level, a prompt natriuresis and diuresis ensued with restoration of sodium balance and a fall in blood pressure. Similar observations have been made in studies of hypertension produced by AII (99) or vasopressin infusion (100). These observations highlight the pivotal role of blood pressure in the regulation of renal sodium and water excretion. It seems that the natriuretic factors proposed in the Na/K ATPase inhibitor hypothesis are not sufficient to offset the antinatriuretic action of mineralocorticoids in the absence of an accompanying increase in renal perfusion pressure.

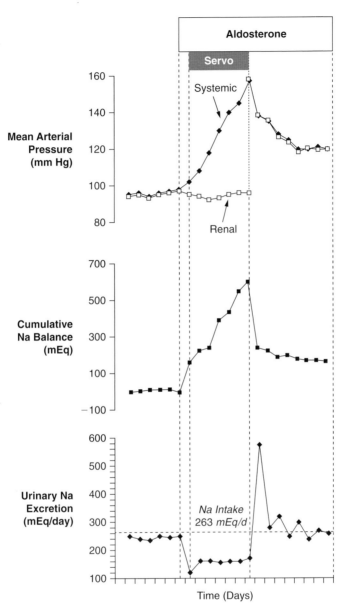

■ **Figure 9.7** The dominant role of renal perfusion pressure in the mineralocorticoid escape phenomenon. In the intact animal, treatment with aldosterone and ingestion of a high-salt diet leads to sodium retention and volume expansion for only a few days, after which a spontaneous natriuresis and diuresis occurs that returns ECF volume toward normal—the so-called mineralocorticoid escape phenomenon. This figure demonstrates the pivotal role of elevated renal perfusion pressure in the escape of the kidney from the sodium retaining effects of aldosterone. Dogs were placed on a 14-day infusion of aldosterone in conjunction with a high-salt diet (263 mEq sodium per day). However, during the first 7 days the renal perfusion pressure was servocontrolled at normal levels by use of a suprarenal aortic clamp. Despite the development of systemic hypertension, when the renal perfusion pressure is normal, urinary sodium excretion remains less than intake and aldosterone escape fails to occur. The net result is inexorable salt and water retention, resulting in pulmonary edema and marked systemic hypertension. However, after day 7, when the clamp is removed such that renal perfusion pressure matches the elevated systemic pressure, there is an immediate natriuresis and diuresis (escape), leading to a return of sodium balance toward normal despite continued aldosterone administration. The systemic blood pressure improves but remains well above the baseline. Servo, servocontrolled renal perfusion pressure to normal level with supraortic cuff. (From Hall JE, Granger JP, Smith MJ, et al. Role of renal hemodynamics and arterial pressure in aldosterone "escape." *Hypertension.* 1984;6(Suppl I):I183, with permission of the American Heart Association, Inc.)

MOLECULAR MECHANISMS OF PRESSURE NATRIURESIS

The phenomenon of pressure natriuresis may be multifactorial and may differ in mechanism depending on whether the increase in arterial pressure is acute (minutes) or chronic (hours to days). In the setting of an acute increase in arterial pressure achieved by cross clamping the infrarenal aorta, pressure natriuresis appears to be the result of inhibition of NaCl absorption in the PT as the result of endocytosis of sodium transporters in the apical (Na^+/H^+ exchanger) and basolateral (Na^+/K^+ ATPase) membranes of the PT (101). In contrast to the findings with acute hypertension, long-term pressure natriuresis is dependent on inhibition of sodium transport in more distal nephron segments. As discussed, in animal models of primary hyperaldosteronism, within a few days the kidneys escape from the sodium-retaining effects of aldosterone via a pressure-mediated natriuresis that acts to return sodium balance and ECF volume to normal. Knepper et al. studied the molecular mechanism of pressure natriuresis in a rat model of primary hyperaldosteronism by using a targeted-proteomics approach (102). They screened rat kidney protein homogenates with rabbit polyclonal antibodies specific for each of the major sodium transporters expressed along the nephron to determine whether escape from aldosterone-mediated sodium retention is associated with decreased abundance of one or more of the transporters. The analysis revealed that the abundance of the thiazide-sensitive NCC was profoundly and selectively decreased during aldosterone escape. The decrease in NCC abundance occurred with a time course of onset that paralleled the increase in renal NaCl excretion associated with the escape process and NCC abundance fell to 17% to 25% of baseline levels. None of the other apical solute-coupled Na transporters (NHE-3, NaPi-2, or the Na/K/2Cl cotransporter) displayed decreased abundance, nor were the total abundance of the three ENaC subunits significantly altered. Immunohistochemical staining confirmed a substantial decrease in NCC labeling in the DCTs of aldosterone-escape rats. Ribonuclease protection assay showed that the decrease in NCC protein abundance was not associated with a significant change in mRNA abundance for NCC, which implies that the decrease in NCC expression in aldosterone escape occurs because of a posttranscriptional mechanism. Thus, downregulation of the thiazide-sensitive NCC of the DCT appears to be the chief molecular target for the regulatory processes responsible for pressure-induced natriuresis in mineralocorticoid escape. Taken together, these observations highlight the pivotal role of blood pressure in the regulation of renal sodium and water excretion. Moreover, the observation that abnormal renal sodium handling is central in the pathogenesis of all forms of hypertension provides sound pathophysiologic rationale for the Seventh Joint National Committee (JNC 7) recommendations regarding thiazide-type diuretics as first-line therapy in most patients with hypertension (2).

Essential Hypertension and Benign Nephrosclerosis

The kidney is usually histologically normal in the early stages of essential hypertension. However, with time there is a gradual loss of nephron mass so that a contracted, granular kidney is found with long-standing benign hypertension. This progressive reduction in renal size is caused by diffuse cortical atrophy and fibrosis owing to hyaline arteriosclerosis, the severity of which is proportional to the duration of the hypertension (103). In benign nephrosclerosis, the afferent arterioles demonstrate hyaline arteriosclerosis with subintimal deposition of a homogenous eosinophilic material (Fig. 9.8A). The interlobular arteries exhibit fibroelastic hyperplasia, which consists of concentric rings of reduplication of the internal elastic lamina (Fig. 9.8B). There is patchy ischemic atrophy of glomeruli, although some glomeruli are normal, others are globally sclerotic. Atrophic tubules filled with eosinophilic material are seen in the areas of glomerular ischemia (Fig. 9.8A).

BENIGN NEPHROSCLEROSIS AS A CAUSE OF END-STAGE RENAL DISEASE

Despite the presence of these renal histologic abnormalities, even with longstanding benign hypertension, the majority of patients with essential hypertension never develop clinically significant renal insufficiency. Benign essential hypertension tends to cause much less damage to the kidney than to other target organs such as the heart and brain. Indeed, the relationship between benign essential hypertension and end-stage renal disease remains circumstantial despite the fact that these syndromes have long been

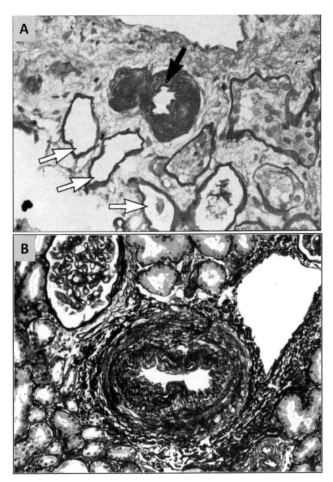

■ **Figure 9.8 (A)** Hyaline arteriolar nephrosclerosis in benign hypertension. In benign arteriolar nephrosclerosis caused by benign hypertension, the characteristic lesion is hyaline arteriolosclerosis with expansion of the intima of afferent arterioles by an eosinophililic amorphous hyaline material which stains a pale pink color on periodic acid–Schiff (PAS) stain (*black arrow*). There is patchy ischemic atrophy of the glomeruli (*not shown*). Some glomeruli are normal, whereas others are completely hyalinized. Atrophic tubules (*white arrows*), sometimes filled with amorphous material, may be seen in the area of sclerotic glomeruli. The severity of tubular atrophy, interstitial fibrosis and glomerulosclerosis are proportional to the extent of vascular involvement with hyaline arteriosclerosis. **(B)** Fibroelastic hyperplasia of interlobular arteries in benign nephrosclerosis. In benign hypertension, the interlobular arteries (cortical radial arteries) are thickened as the result of extensive reduplication of the internal elastic lamina. Reduplicated bands of elastic lamina can be visualized using elastin stain or methenamine silver stain (From Sherry Werner-Abboud, MD; University of Texas Health Sciences Center at San Antonio, with permission). These arterial changes in benign hypertension stand in marked contrast to the proliferation of myointimal fibroblasts typical of malignant nephrosclerosis (see Fig. 9.9).

associated in the medical literature. The widely held notion that benign hypertension with benign nephrosclerosis is a common cause of end-stage renal disease is difficult to support. Recent reviews have suggested that the number of patients reaching end-stage renal disease attributable to benign nephrosclerosis may have been significantly overestimated (104–106). Based on completion of the Health Care Financing Administration (HCFA) 2728 form, practicing nephrologists attribute essential hypertension as the cause of ESRD in 37% of patients initiating Medicare-supported renal replacement therapy (107). Unfortunately, the cause of ESRD more often is based on clinical parameters rather than histologic diagnosis. Two different clinical guidelines have been proposed for the phenotypic identification of hypertensive nephrosclerosis. One guideline suggested that the clinical diagnosis of hypertensive nephrosclerosis include a family history of hypertension, and the presence of left ventricular hypertrophy, proteinuria

<0.5 g/day, and hypertension preceding the onset of renal dysfunction (106). The African American Study of Kidney Disease (AASK) study investigators required a urine protein-to-creatinine ratio <2.0 and no evidence of underlying renal disease for the clinical diagnosis of hypertensive nephrosclerosis (108). Phenotyping of 100 randomly selected patients with a diagnosis hypertensive nephrosclerosis reported on the HCFA 2728 form revealed that only 4% of the patients meet either clinical criterion for diagnosis (107). Analysis of the data for black patients revealed that only 28/91 patients met the AASK criteria for diagnosis of hypertensive nephrosclerosis (107). These data indicate that benign hypertensive nephrosclerosis is a far less common cause of ESRD than commonly assumed and suggest that many patients with presumed hypertensive nephrosclerosis may actually have other undetected causes of chronic kidney disease. Overall, the development of significant renal dysfunction appears to be very rare in uncomplicated essential hypertension. Estimates in white populations have suggested that the relative risk of developing renal failure in essential hypertension is on the order of one in 6,000 cases (108,109). Moreover, serum creatinine levels infrequently increase in patients with longstanding mild to moderate hypertension. An analysis of the data from three recent large clinical trials in patients with essential hypertension revealed that <1% of 10,000 patients developed advanced renal failure during 4 to 6 years of follow-up (110,111). A very low incidence of clinically significant deterioration of renal function was also noted in the Hypertension Detection and Follow-Up Program (HDFP) (112).

Autopsy studies conducted in the preantihypertensive era have documented that benign nephrosclerosis is an uncommon cause of end-stage renal disease. Among 150 hypertensive patients with ESRD, only one was found to have benign nephrosclerosis as the sole underlying etiology (113). Moreover, in a study of renal anatomy and histology of 146 patients with bilateral nephrectomy before initiation of dialysis, approximately half had chronic glomerulonephritis and 20% had reflux nephropathy (114). Only three subjects had hypertension as the primary cause of renal failure: two of these had malignant hypertension and one renal artery stenosis with ischemic nephropathy. Kincaid-Smith maintains that patients with hypertension and renal impairment, in whom renal artery stenosis (ischemic nephropathy) and malignant hypertension have been excluded, most likely have underlying primary renal parenchymal disease rather than benign nephrosclerosis (115).

Patients classified as having hypertensive ESRD typically present with advanced disease, making the processes that initiated the renal disease difficult to discern. It has been proposed that many patients misclassified with ESRD secondary to benign nephrosclerosis actually have primary renal parenchymal disease (such as IgA nephropathy), unrecognized renal artery stenosis with ischemic nephropathy, unrecognized episodes of malignant hypertension, occult renal cholesterol embolic disease, or primary renal microvascular disease (105,106,109).

Hemodynamic studies in essential hypertension demonstrate a near normal GFR despite a significant reduction of renal blood flow, consistent with an increased filtration fraction. Genetic models of essential hypertension in the rat have shown that these alterations in renal hemodynamics arise through an increase in resistance of both the afferent and efferent arterioles, so that glomerular capillary hydraulic pressure is maintained at a normal level (116). In humans with benign essential hypertension there also appears to be a balanced increase in afferent and efferent resistances, thereby shielding the kidney from the high systemic pressure, while enabling the maintenance of near normal glomerular filtration rate. The relative rarity of significant renal impairment in patients with essential hypertension (nonmalignant) is consistent with these hemodynamic observations. In contrast, in animal models of diabetic nephropathy (117) and renal ablation (118), afferent arteriolar vasodilatation occurs such that an increase in arterial pressure is transmitted to the glomeruli. As already discussed, the resulting glomerular capillary hypertension in this setting may be a critical factor in the progression of chronic kidney disease in patients with diabetic nephropathy or another primary renal parenchymal disease.

HYPERTENSION AND END-STAGE RENAL DISEASE IN AFRICAN-AMERICANS

The critical issue, which has yet to be resolved, is why blacks constitute a disproportionate percentage of patients with end-stage renal disease in the United States. The overall rate of ESRD is four times higher in blacks than in whites (119). It has been suggested that the higher incidence of ESRD in blacks compared to whites may be the consequence of a higher risk of progressive hypertensive nephrosclerosis among African-Americans. Epidemiologic studies suggest that essential hypertension occurs more frequently in blacks and is associated with more severe cardiovascular end-organ damage for any given level of blood pressure (120). In angiographic studies of patients with mild to moderate essential hypertension and normal renal function, blacks tended to have more severe angiographic evidence of nephrosclerosis than have whites (121).

There are several plausible explanations for the high frequency with which hypertensive nephrosclerosis is reported as a cause of ESRD in the black population. Because most of the available data are based on clinical diagnoses rather than renal histology, there may be a tendency on the part of physicians to identify hypertension as the cause of ESRD given the known high prevalence of hypertension in blacks (104). In this regard, there appears to be a racial bias with regard to the diagnosis of hypertensive nephrosclerosis. In a recent survey, nephrologists were asked to review identical case histories of patients with end-stage renal disease in which only the race of the patient was randomly assigned as either black or white. It was found that black patients were twice as likely as white patients to be labeled as having end-stage renal disease secondary to hypertensive nephrosclerosis (122). Therefore, in the absences of renal biopsy, it is possible that in many cases ESRD that appears to have resulted from hypertension is in reality the result of an undiagnosed primary renal parenchymal disease.

Another possibility is that recurrent bouts of unrecognized or inadequately treated malignant hypertension are the actual cause of the increase in ESRD, owing to hypertension among blacks. The incidence of malignant hypertension is higher in blacks than in whites. Furthermore, in the epidemiologic studies it is not clear whether the term hypertensive nephrosclerosis refers to benign or malignant nephrosclerosis. In the few available studies detailing the pathologic findings in blacks with end-stage renal disease caused by hypertension, the characteristic findings have been those of malignant nephrosclerosis, namely, musculomucoid intimal hyperplasia of the interlobular arteries and accelerated glomerular obsolescence, rather than benign arteriolar nephrosclerosis (106,114,123). In this regard, a study of 100 patients admitted to an inner-city hospital with a diagnosis of hypertensive emergency showed that two-thirds had malignant hypertension on the basis of funduscopic findings (124). These patients were predominantly young, male, black, or Hispanic individuals of lower socioeconomic status. Over 93% of these patients had been previously diagnosed as hypertensive and most reported to have received prior pharmacologic treatment for hypertension. However, no source of regular health care could be documented in 60% of cases. More than 50% were noted to have stopped their antihypertensive medications more than 30 days before admission and only 24% had taken any medication on the day of admission. If the overrepresentation of young blacks with end-stage renal disease is at least in part owing to undiagnosed or inadequately treated malignant hypertension, this would have tremendous public health implications because malignant hypertension is clearly preventable, and even significant renal dysfunction is potentially reversible with early and aggressive antihypertensive therapy.

Finally, it is entirely possible that blacks with essential hypertension tend to develop more severe benign nephrosclerosis that, unlike benign hypertension in whites, results in progressive renal insufficiency and ESRD. Preliminary results for the AASK trial demonstrate that among nondiabetic hypertensive blacks with mild to moderate renal insufficiency in the absence of marked proteinuria, renal biopsy is overwhelmingly likely to confirm a diagnosis of hypertensive nephrosclerosis (108). The increased prevalence of significant hypertensive nephrosclerosis in blacks could occur because hypertension in blacks tends to be more severe or because their renal vasculature is more susceptible to hypertensive damage (125). Tobian has postulated that the low-potassium diet characteristically consumed by blacks in the United States (30 mmol/day vs. 65 mmol/day in the general population) accelerates the intimal thickening of the renal vasculature that occurs because of hypertensive damage and might contribute to their increased risk of progressive renal disease with benign hypertension. He has proposed that this may account for the increased risk of progressive renal insufficiency among hypertensive blacks (126). Dustan suggested that increased risk of renal injury in essential hypertension in blacks may in part result from the increased expression of growth factors leading to vascular smooth muscle hypertrophy in renal arterioles (127).

A LINK BETWEEN SALT SENSITIVITY AND PROGRESSIVE RENAL DISEASE IN BLACKS WITH ESSENTIAL HYPERTENSION

There is some evidence that essential hypertension may be fundamentally different in blacks and whites. Compared to whites, blacks tend to have a more expanded intravascular volume, lower PRA, reduced natriuretic response to a sodium load, and better antihypertensive responses to diuretics and CCB than

ACE inhibitors or β-blockers. Substantial renal hemodynamic differences between black and white patients with essential hypertension have been described (72,97). For instance, black hypertensive patients have greater reduction in renal blood flow and higher renal vascular resistance than white patients (97). In addition, black hypertensive patients are more likely to be salt-sensitive than are white hypertensives such that an increase in sodium intake leads to an increase in blood pressure (72). In a study of 17 black patients and 9 white patients with essential hypertension, 11 blacks were found to be salt-sensitive, whereas all the whites were salt-resistant (72). Renal hemodynamics were measured during a low-sodium diet (20 mmol/day for 9 days) and a high-salt diet (200 mmol/day for 14 days). During the low-sodium diet period, salt-sensitive and salt-resistant patients had similar mean arterial pressure, GFR, effective renal plasma flow (ERPF), and filtration fraction. During the high-salt diet period, GFR did not change in either group; ERPF increased in salt-resistant patients but decreased in salt-sensitive patients; filtration fraction decreased in salt-resistant patients but increased in salt-sensitive patients; glomerular pressure decreased in salt-resistant patients but increased in salt-sensitive patients. In the salt-sensitive patients, the stable GFR and increased glomerular capillary pressure in the face of reduced ERPF implied that there must be an increase in efferent arteriolar tone leading to an increase in filtration fraction. Given the high prevalence of salt-sensitive hypertension in the blacks, the documented rise in filtration fraction and intraglomerular pressure during high sodium intake suggests that these renal hemodynamic derangements might be partially responsible for the greater propensity to hypertension-induced renal failure in this ethnic group (72). Thus, it is possible that in black patients, essential hypertension may lead to progressive renal injury in the absence of malignant hypertension or underlying primary renal disease.

Experimental evidence in genetic models of hypertension supports this possibility. Renal function deteriorates faster in some strains of rats than others with genetic hypertension. In the spontaneously hypertensive rat, hypertension is accompanied by an increase in renal afferent arteriolar resistance, thus protecting the glomeruli from the adverse effects of hypertension so that progressive renal insufficiency does not occur. In contrast, all salt-sensitive rat models of hypertension share the peculiarity of responding to a rise in blood pressure with a decrease in afferent arteriolar resistance, which leads to an increase in glomerular capillary pressure with progressive renal injury (72).

Malignant Hypertension

Malignant hypertension is a distinct clinical and pathologic entity characterized by a marked elevation of the blood pressure (diastolic pressure often is >120 to 130 mm Hg) and evidence of widespread acute arteriolar injury (128). The clinical sine qua non of malignant hypertension is the funduscopic finding of *hypertensive neuroretinopathy,* which consists of striate (flame-shaped) hemorrhages, cotton wool (soft) exudates, and often papilledema. The development of hypertensive neuroretinopathy heralds the onset of a hypertensive vasculopathy that may cause necrotizing arteriolitis in the central nervous system, kidneys, and other vital organs. If the hypertension is untreated, then there is rapid and relentless progression to renal failure in less than 1 year, often with associated hypertensive encephalopathy, intracerebral hemorrhage, or congestive heart failure. Regardless of the degree of blood pressure elevation, malignant hypertension cannot be diagnosed in the absence of hypertensive neuroretinopathy (128). There has been an unfortunate tendency in recent years to diagnose "malignant hypertension" in any patient with markedly elevated blood pressure. However, given the prognostic and therapeutic implications of true malignant hypertension, it is extremely important to make a clear distinction between benign and malignant hypertension. This is not to say that benign hypertension cannot cause a hypertensive crisis. Benign hypertension that is accompanied by acute end-organ dysfunction such as acute pulmonary edema, dissecting aortic aneurysm, or intracerebral bleeding clearly represents a hypertensive crisis requiring immediate reduction of the blood pressure to avert disaster (128). On the other hand, marked elevation of blood pressure frequently occurs in the absence of hypertensive neuroretinopathy or evidence of acute end-organ dysfunction. This entity, which is called *severe asymptomatic hypertension,* does not represent a true hypertensive crisis, and urgent treatment often is not required (128).

Headache and blurred vision are the most common presenting complaints in malignant hypertension. A striking "asymptomatic" presentation is not uncommon, especially in young black males who deny any prior symptoms when they present in the end stage of malignant hypertension with florid failure of the heart, brain, and kidney. In most patients, the diastolic pressure at presentation is >120 to 130 mm Hg. However, there is no absolute level of pressure above which malignant hypertension develops and there is considerable overlap of blood pressure readings in patients with benign and malignant hypertension (128).

The patient with malignant hypertension (hypertensive neuroretinopathy) may or may not have clinically apparent end-organ involvement at the time of presentation. However, in the absence of adequate treatment, a variety of organ systems eventually will be damaged by the evolving hypertensive vasculopathy. Nervous system manifestations include hypertensive encephalopathy or intracerebral hemorrhage. Congestive heart failure with recurrent bouts of acute pulmonary edema is the most common cardiac complication. Gastrointestinal involvement may cause acute pancreatitis or an acute abdomen because of necrotizing mesenteric vasculitis. Patients with malignant hypertension may present with a spectrum of renal involvement ranging from minimal albuminuria with normal renal function to end-stage renal disease. In the untreated or inadequately treated patient, even if the renal function is initially normal, it is common to observe progressive deterioration to end-stage renal failure over several weeks to months (128).

PATHOLOGY OF MALIGNANT NEPHROSCLEROSIS

Even when terminal renal failure occurs in malignant hypertension, the kidneys may be normal in size. Small, pinpoint petechial hemorrhages on the cortical surface give rise to a peculiar, flea-bitten appearance. Fibrinoid necrosis of the afferent arterioles has traditionally been regarded as the hallmark of malignant nephrosclerosis. There is deposition in the media of a granular material that is pink with hematoxylin and eosin stain and a deep red color with trichrome stain (103). The characteristic finding in the interlobular arteries is severe luminal narrowing owing to intimal thickening (103). This lesion is known as proliferative endarteritis, endarteritis fibrosa, or the onionskin lesion. The arteriolar lumens are severely narrowed because of thickening of the walls or superimposed fibrin thrombi. Focal and segmental fibrinoid necrosis was the predominant glomerular lesion in large autopsy series in the pretreatment era. However, accelerated glomerular obsolescence owing to ischemia is currently the most common finding at renal biopsy. In blacks with malignant hypertension, fibrinoid necrosis of the afferent arterioles is a rare finding. Instead, the afferent arterioles show a marked degree of hyalinization. The most prominent and characteristic finding is musculomucoid intimal hyperplasia of the interlobular arteries and larger arterioles (Fig. 9.9) (123). The intima of interlobular arteries is thickened by hyperplastic smooth muscle cells with variable degrees of fibrosis. The glomeruli show evidence of accelerated

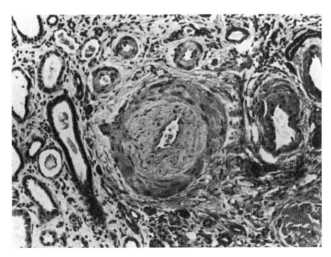

■ **Figure 9.9** Musculomucoid intimal hyperplasia of an interlobular artery in malignant hypertension. The arterial wall is thickened by neointimal proliferation of myofibroblasts (modified smooth muscle cells), resulting in a significant reduction in the caliber of the arterial lumen. A small amount of myxoid material is seen between the smooth muscle cells (hematoxylin and eosin stain). (From Pitcock JA, Johnson JG, Hatch FE, et al. Malignant hypertension in blacks: malignant arterial disease as observed by light and electron microscopy. *Hum Pathol.* 1976;7:333, 1976, with permission.)

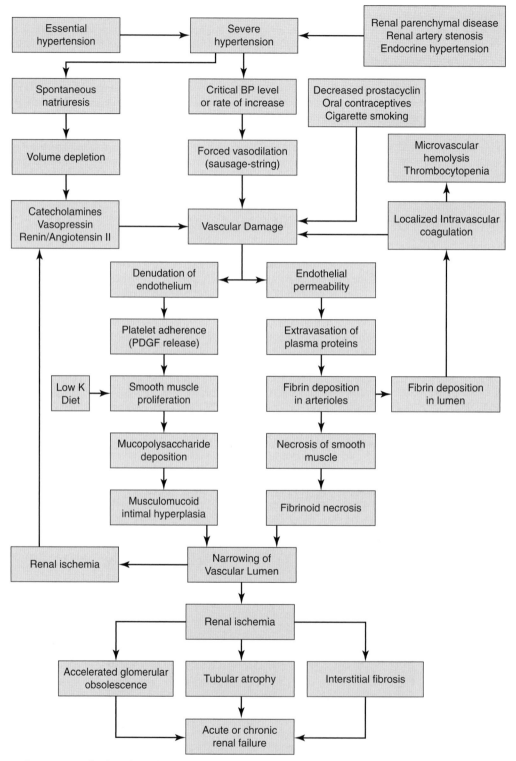

■ **Figure 9.10** Pathophysiology of malignant hypertension. AII, angiotensin II; CHF, congestive heart failure (From Nolan CR, Linas SL. Malignant hypertension and other hypertensive crises. In: RW Schrier, ed. *Diseases of the Kidney and Urinary Tract.* 8th ed. Philadelphia, PA: Lippincott Williams & Wilkins, 2007;1370–1463).

glomerular obsolescence with ischemic wrinkling of the glomerular basement membranes on electron microscopy (128).

PATHOPHYSIOLOGY OF MALIGNANT HYPERTENSION

The mechanism that initiates a transition from benign to malignant hypertension is unknown. Several pathophysiologic mechanisms have been postulated (128). According to the *pressure hypothesis,* the microvascular damage is a direct consequence of the mechanical stress placed on the vessel wall by hypertension. In contrast, the *vasculotoxic theory* holds that AII, vasopressin, and catecholamines not only raise blood pressure but also induce direct vascular injury. Pressure-induced natriuresis with volume depletion and reflex activation of the RAS also may result in an unrelenting vicious cycle of hypertension and ischemic renal injury. The development of localized intravascular coagulation or altered metabolism of glucocorticoids, prostaglandins, or kininogens has been postulated to play a role in acceleration of the vascular injury.

The vicious cycle of malignant hypertension is depicted in Fig. 9.10. In the setting of severe essential hypertension or secondary hypertension, the pressure increases to a critical level or at a rate that overwhelms normal autoregulatory mechanisms and leads to focal areas of overstretched arterioles. The resulting endothelial damage allows extravasation of fibrinogen and other plasma proteins. The deposition of fibrin causes fibrinoid necrosis. Myointimal proliferation occurs, resulting in proliferative endarteritis. In the kidney, there is progressive glomerular injury owing to ischemia. Activation of the RAAS further increases the blood pressure and leads to amplification of the cycle of hypertension and renal ischemia. The end result is renal failure. This widespread hypertensive vasculopathy also results in ischemic damage to other vascular beds. In the retina, ischemia of nerve fiber bundles leads to cotton wool spots and papilledema. Hypertensive neuroretinopathy occurs very early in the course of the disease and is the clinical hallmark of malignant hypertension.

RESPONSE TO TREATMENT IN MALIGNANT HYPERTENSION

In the absence of adequate blood pressure control, malignant hypertension has a grave prognosis. In the preantihypertensive era, the 1-year mortality rate approached 90% and uremia was the most common cause of death. However, it is now clear that adequate treatment of essential hypertension prevents malignant hypertension. Furthermore, early and aggressive treatment of an established malignant phase prevents progressive renal damage. More severe renal dysfunction at presentation correlates with an increased risk of progression to end-stage renal disease. However, there are numerous reports of dramatic recovery of renal function in patients with malignant hypertension, even after months of dialysis-requiring renal failure (128). This recovery of renal function has been attributed to strict blood pressure control with the potent peripheral vasodilator minoxidil used in conjunction with a loop-diuretic and a β-blocker. Presumably, the renal vasculopathy heals and the ischemic glomeruli recover when the inciting stimulus (severe hypertension) is removed.

Renovascular Hypertension

The landmark experimental models of hypertension developed by Goldblatt et al. demonstrated that persistent hypertension could be produced in dogs either by constricting both renal arteries or by removing one kidney and constricting the artery of the remaining kidney (129). Another variant of Goldblatt hypertension is produced by clipping the artery of one kidney and leaving the other kidney untouched. This two kidney/one-clip (2K/1C) hypertension may be analogous to unilateral renal artery stenosis in humans. In this model, constriction of one artery leads to an immediate rise in blood pressure because of increased renin production by the ischemic kidney. The activation of the RAS leads to AII-mediated vasoconstriction, impaired natriuresis in the ischemic as well as contralateral kidney and hypertension. Curiously, after a few days, even though blood pressure continues to rise, the PRA returns to normal. In the early stages of 2K/1C hypertension, removal of the clipped kidney restores blood pressure to normal. In contrast, later in the course, when the PRA is no longer elevated, the blood pressure fails to normalize with angiotensin antagonists, removal of the clipped kidney, or unclipping. Of note, however, is the observation that removal of the contralateral "normal kidney" and unclipping normalizes blood pressure. These findings imply that vascular changes that develop in the normal kidney when it is chronically exposed to elevated pressure may serve to perpetuate hypertension even after the original cause of the renovascular hypertension has been removed. Guyton's hypothesis implies that from the very beginning the contralateral kidney must have an abnormal renal function curve with a blunted natriuretic response to the elevated blood pressure. Early in the course, this shift of the renal function curve may be mediated by functional changes induced by local intrarenal formation of AII. The direct and indirect effects of AII on renal sodium excretion have been discussed in detail in the preceding. The AII-dependent mechanisms that contribute to the development and maintenance of hypertension in the 2K/1C model probably act primarily by attenuating the ability of the animal to exhibit the expected hypertension-induced natriuresis by the contralateral (nonclipped) kidney. In later stages of renovascular hypertension, hypertension-induced structural damage may underlie the reduced natriuretic response to any given level of pressure. These secondary changes in the contralateral kidney may explain the well-known clinical observation that nephrectomy or revascularization for unilateral renal artery stenosis often fails to normalize blood pressure. Preexisting essential hypertension also may explain the failure of revascularization to cure hypertension in many cases.

CAUSES OF RENAL ARTERY STENOSIS

The principal cause of renal artery stenosis is *atheromatous* narrowing of one or both main renal arteries (Fig. 9.11). Atheromatous renal artery stenosis occurs in older individuals, with a peak incidence in the sixth decade. Men are affected twice as often as women. It is most often found in association with diffuse atherosclerotic disease of the aorta, coronary arteries, cerebral arteries, and peripheral vasculature. However, in 15% to 20% of cases renal involvement occurs in the absence of atherosclerotic disease elsewhere (130). The obstructing atheromatous lesion is usually within the proximal 2 cm of the artery. Not uncommonly, a so-called ostial lesion is found with the lesion actually arising in the aorta at the origin of the renal artery.

A second type of arterial lesion, of obscure etiology, which affects the main renal artery is *fibromuscular dysplasia* (hyperplasia) (130). The lesion appears as a multifocal "string-of-beads" beginning in the mid-renal artery and often extending into peripheral branches (Fig. 9.12). This variant is typically seen in young to middle-aged women. The risk of progression to total arterial occlusion is small.

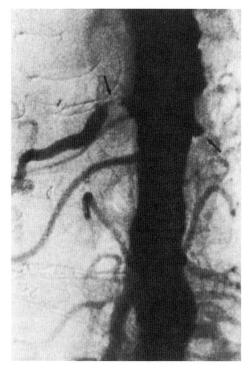

■ **Figure 9.11** Aortogram demonstrating generalized atherosclerosis with bilateral atherosclerotic renal artery stenosis. The left renal artery is totally occluded at its origin. The right renal artery has a high-grade lesion near its origin (ostial lesion). (From Steven D. Brantley, MD, Department of Radiology, Wilford Hall Medical Center, Lackland Air Force Base, Texas, with permission.)

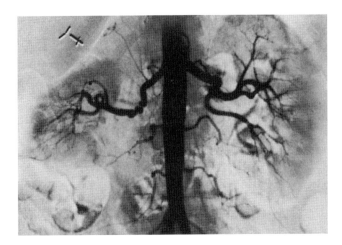

■ **Figure 9.12** Renal angiogram demonstrating right renal artery stenosis owing to medial hyperplasia, the most common variant of fibromuscular dysplasia. The smaller right kidney has a mid-renal artery lesion with the characteristic "string of beads" appearance because of mural aneurysms, caused by thinning of the internal elastica, alternating with areas of narrowing caused by fibrovascular ridges. (From Steven D. Brantley, MD, Department of Radiology, Wilford Hall Medical Center, Lackland Air Force Base, Texas, with permission.)

SCREENING FOR RENOVASCULAR HYPERTENSION

Although renovascular hypertension owing to renal artery stenosis is one of the most common causes of potentially remediable secondary hypertension, available estimates suggest that <0.5% of the hypertensive population has renovascular hypertension (131). Thus, an aggressive approach to screening for this disorder often is not warranted. Several lines of evidence now suggest that an aggressive workup to exclude renovascular hypertension may not be cost-effective because the yield of curable hypertension is low, and the majority of patients can be managed successfully with medical therapy (131–133). The dilemma for the clinician lies in the fact that even the ideal screening test, with high sensitivity and specificity, has a low predictive value when applied indiscriminately to the general hypertensive population where the prevalence of renovascular hypertension is low. In this regard, aggressive screening leads to the generation of many more false-positive results (essential hypertension) than true-positive results (occult renovascular hypertension). This statistical phenomenon undoubtedly accounts for the numerous highly touted screening tests that have come and gone over the years. The rapid sequence intravenous pyelogram (hypertensive IVP) is no longer routinely used as a screening tool because it is not only insensitive but also has a false-positive rate of up to 12% among patients with essential hypertension (131). Isotope renography (renal scan) has proved even less accurate than the hypertensive IVP because of an unacceptable frequency of false-positive results in patients with essential hypertension (131). Casual measurements of PRA are of little value (131). The highly touted "captopril test," which measures the increase in venous PRA in response to captopril, proved to have low specificity (131).

Thus, it is apparent that sound clinical judgment is essential in the selection of patients in whom an aggressive evaluation for renovascular hypertension is indicated. Certain clinical clues suggest the possibility of underlying renovascular hypertension (105). The onset of hypertension before the age of 30 years should suggest secondary hypertension. A truly abrupt onset of hypertension at any age suggests renal vascular disease. However, more often than not, this finding represents newly diagnosed essential hypertension rather than recently developed secondary hypertension. A definite worsening of previously well-controlled hypertension should suggest renovascular hypertension. Clues on physical examination include the finding on funduscopy of striate hemorrhages, cotton wool spots, or papilledema (malignant hypertension) (128), or a continuous systolic and diastolic epigastric bruit.

Even in the presence of diffuse atherosclerotic disease, aggressive evaluation for renovascular hypertension is only indicated if the blood pressure is truly resistant (>150/100 mm Hg) to a rationale triple-drug regimen that includes a diuretic (131). Unexplained deterioration of renal function despite adequate blood pressure control suggests the possibility of ischemic nephropathy and should prompt a search for bilateral renal artery stenosis with ischemic nephropathy (134). Deterioration of renal function on the addition of an ACE inhibitor or angiotensin receptor blocker suggests the possibility of bilateral renal artery stenosis or stenosis of a solitary kidney. This phenomenon probably reflects maintenance of GFR in the ischemic kidneys by AII-mediated vasoconstriction of the efferent arteriole to increase filtration fraction.

In the patient in whom the probability of renovascular hypertension is high, the conventional screening tests are of little value because the predictive value of a negative test is low (132). Computerized tomographic angiography and gadolinium-enhanced three-dimensional magnetic resonance angiography appear to be the best noninvasive tests for detection of anatomic renal artery stenosis (135). Nonetheless, intraarterial contrast angiography remains the gold standard for definitive diagnosis of renal artery stenosis (131). Unfortunately, selective renal angiography carries definite risks including contrast media-associated nephrotoxicity and renal atheroembolic disease (136). Further complicating this issue is the fact that anatomic renal artery stenosis does not always imply functional renovascular hypertension. Incidental renal artery stenosis can clearly occur in essential hypertension. Selective renal vein renin determinations have been used to predict the functional significance of anatomic lesions. A renal vein renin ratio greater than 2:1 (involved to uninvolved) is highly predictive of a beneficial response to intervention. However, a significant number of patients with nonlateralizing ratios ultimately prove to benefit from intervention (137). One study suggests that a change in the Tc 99m-labeled DTPA or MAG_3 renogram after treatment with captopril may help to define the functional significance of a renal artery lesion before intervention with surgery or angioplasty (138).

MEDICAL THERAPY VERSUS ANGIOPLASTY FOR TREATMENT OF RENAL ARTERY STENOSIS

Renal artery stenosis is not an uncommon finding in patients with evidence of atherosclerotic disease elsewhere in the body. In fact, incidental renal angiography in patients undergoing coronary angiography demonstrates renal artery stenosis in 6% to 18% of patients (139,140). Likewise, renal artery stenosis is found in 16% to 40% of patients undergoing aortography for aortic aneurysms or peripheral vascular disease (141,142). However, the clinical utility of renal revascularization via angioplasty and stenting or bypass surgery remains controversial. In this regard, three randomized clinical trials of renal artery angioplasty compared with medical therapy alone showed no convincing benefit of angioplasty with regard to blood pressure control (143–145). A recent review was conducted on the basis of analysis of the MEDLINE database from inception to September 2005 for studies involving adults with atherosclerotic renal artery stenosis that reported morality, renal function, blood pressure, cardiovascular events or adverse events (146). The authors concluded that available evidence does not clearly support renal revascularization over intensive medical therapy for atherosclerotic renal artery stenosis.

Despite the lack of clinical trial evidence demonstrating superiority of renal artery angioplasty compared to intensive medical therapy, there has been an explosive growth in the number of procedures performed in recent years. Murphy et al. recently analyzed claims submitted to Medicare in 1996, 1998, and 2000 and extracted data for renal artery angioplasty, stent placement, or renal artery bypass surgery (147). Between 1996 and 2000, the total volume of renal revascularization (surgical and percutaneous) increased 62% from 13,380 to 21,660 procedures. The annual volume of renal artery surgery decreased 45% in 2000 compared with the volume in 1996. In contrast, annual volumes of renal artery angioplasty and stent placement increased 2.4-fold in 2000 compared with those in 1996. Most of the growth in percutaneous renal artery intervention could be attributed to the added provision of the procedure by cardiologists, who increased their annual volume by 3.9-fold. Moreover, there were large variations across regions. For example, in the Southeast region, the volume of renal artery interventions by cardiologists increased more than 15-fold.

It is apparent that sparse data regarding optimal management of renal artery stenosis limit clinical decision making. Available studies focus on procedural success (reducing the severity of the stenosis) or short-term changes in blood pressure. There remains a paucity of hard clinical outcome data to guide development of clinical practice guidelines for management of renal artery stenosis. To address this important clinical issue the NIH funded the ongoing Cardiovascular Outcomes in Renal Atherosclerosis Lesions (CORAL) trial that will study patients with renal artery stenosis to test the hypothesis that angioplasty and stenting renal artery stenosis in patients with systolic hypertension reduces the number of cardiovascular events. In this multicenter trial, 1,080 patients at 100 sites will be randomized to medical therapy alone versus treatment with angioplasty and non-drug-eluting stents plus intensive medical therapy. Patient will be followed for 3.5 years. Outcome measures include the incidence of myocardial infarction, heart failure, strokes, and renal failure. The CORAL trial results are expected in 2010. Until relevant outcome data become available, management of patients with renal artery stenosis should be individualized. In patients with diffuse atherosclerotic disease, even in the presence of suspected or known renal artery stenosis, medical management may be prudent and entirely appropriate as long as the blood pressure is adequately controlled and the renal function remains stable. At present, the case against an aggressive approach to angioplasty and stenting of atherosclerotic renal artery stenosis is compelling (148). Dworkin and Jamerson cogently argue that published randomized clinical trials provide little support for the notion that angioplasty with stenting significantly improves blood pressure, preserves kidney function, or reduces episodes of congestive heart failure in patients with atherosclerotic RAS. Whether revascularization reduces the incidence of adverse cardiovascular events such as sudden death, myocardial infarction, or stroke is also unknown. In contrast, advances in medical therapy continue to improve outcomes for patients with hypertension and vascular disease. With aggressive medical management of diabetes, chronic kidney disease, antiplatelet therapy, more effective antismoking interventions, and new lower targets for blood pressure and low-density lipoprotein cholesterol, it is quite possible that revascularization, no matter how technically successful, will provide little additional clinical benefit to most patients. They advise that physicians should be conservative in recommending angioplasty and stenting. Ongoing studies including CORAL, Stenting in Renal Dysfunction Caused by Atherosclerotic Renal Artery Stenosis (STAR), and Angioplasty and Stent for Renal Artery Lesions (ASTRAL) are likely to provide insights into the clinical utility of revascularization on the progression of chronic kidney disease due to ischemic nephropathy.

Hypertension Due to Primary Aldosteronism

Primary aldosteronism resulting from an adrenocortical adenoma (aldosteronoma), originally described by Conn, is another of the few potentially curable causes of secondary hypertension (149). *Aldosteronoma* are usually small (<2 cm diameter) benign adrenal nodules, which account for 70% to 80% of cases of primary aldosteronism. *Idiopathic aldosteronism*, which is associated with bilateral micronodular or macronodular adrenal hyperplasia, accounts for 20% to 30% of cases of primary aldosteronism. The prevalence of primary aldosteronism in unselected patients with hypertension is low, on the order of 1% to 2% (149). The clinical features of primary aldosteronism are the result of the effects of aldosterone on renal sodium handling. Aldosterone binds and activates the intracellular MR in principal cells in the DCT resulting in an increase in the number of open ENaCs in the luminal membrane with enhanced sodium reabsorption. The resulting impairment in the natriuretic capacity of the kidney causes salt-sensitive hypertension. Despite the fact that renal sodium handling in the distal tubule is abnormal, patients with primary hyperaldosteronism lack edema or evidence of increased ECF volume. This paradox results from the fact that the kidney escapes from the salt-retaining effects of mineralocorticoid via a pressure natriuresis and diuresis that returns ECF volume to normal. Chronic hypertension in this setting is maintained by an increase in systemic vascular resistance perhaps via a guytonian mechanism. The electronegative potential of the distal tubule lumen favors secretion of potassium and hydrogen ion leading to hypokalemia and metabolic alkalosis in some but not all patients. PRA is suppressed in almost all patients with primary aldosteronism reflecting the state of relative volume expansion. However, PRA is also suppressed in patients with low-renin essential hypertension, so measurement of PRA alone is not a reliable method of screening.

Given the relatively low prevalence of primary hyperaldosteronism in the general hypertensive population, routine screening for this disorder is not recommended. Screening should generally be reserved for hypertensive patients who have spontaneous hypokalemia (not due to diuretics or other secondary causes of hyperaldosteronism) or profound diuretic-induced hypokalemia or patients with severe or resistant hypertension (149). Recent data suggest that determining the ratio of plasma aldosterone concentration (PAC, ng/dL) to PRA (ng/dL/h), in a subject with untreated hypertension is the most acceptable screening method for distinguishing patients with essential hypertension from those with primary aldosteronism (149,150). The timing of the test (morning), the posture of the patient before blood sampling (upright), and the units of measure should be standardized. If the cutoff value of this ratio is kept high enough (e.g., >30 or 50) the test will be sensitive enough to identify most cases of primary aldosteronism while maintaining reasonable specificity. The mean ratio for normal subjects and patients with essential hypertension is 4:10. An elevated PAC/PRA ratio alone does not establish the diagnosis of primary aldosteronism. Further testing is mandatory to establish a definitive biochemical diagnosis based on documentation of nonsuppressible aldosterone secretion during sodium loading and renin hyporesponsiveness to sodium depletion. Aldosterone suppression testing can be performed either with orally administered sodium chloride and measurement of 24-hour urine aldosterone secretion or with intravenous saline loading and measurement of PAC. Before testing, hypokalemia should be corrected because it suppresses aldosterone secretion. If the withdrawal of antihypertensive medications is not feasible, blood pressure should be treated with CCBs, β-blockers or α-blockers that do not affect diagnostic accuracy. ACE inhibitors, angiotensin receptor blockers (ARBs), and spironolactone should be stopped because they interfere with the tests. Oral sodium loading (2 to 3 g sodium chloride/day) is performed by placing the patient on a high-salt diet with supplemental sodium chloride tablets if needed for 3 days. Vigorous replacement of potassium chloride also should be prescribed because sodium loading increases kaliuresis. On the third day of the diet, serum electrolytes are measured and a 24-hour urine is collected for measurement of aldosterone, sodium, and potassium. Adequate sodium loading is present if the 24-hour urine sodium exceeds 200 mEq. Urine aldosterone excretion >14 μg/day is consistent with hyperaldosteronism. Alternatively, aldosterone suppression can be performed by intravenous administration of 2 L of normal saline over 4 hours while the patient is recumbent. The PAC will fall to a level <6 ng/dL in patients with essential hypertension, whereas values >10 ng/dL are consistent with primary aldosteronism. Inability to stimulate renin should then be confirmed by placing the patient on a low-sodium diet (40 mg/day) or treatment with diuretic (furosemide, up to 120 mg/day in divided doses). The PRA should remain below 1 ng/dL/h in patients with primary hyperaldosteronism.

Once the biochemical diagnosis of primary aldosteronism has been confirmed, the approach to therapy depends on whether the disease is caused by aldosteronoma or idiopathic aldosteronism. Computerized tomography (CT) can detect most aldosteronoma >1 cm in size. Unfortunately, CT results can be misleading. A nodule <1 cm in size may be undetected, leading to an erroneous diagnosis of idiopathic aldosteronism. On the other hand, in patients with idiopathic aldosteronism, the adrenal glands are usually either normal in size or bilaterally enlarged. However, the fortuitous presence of an incidental nonfunctional adrenal nodule may lead to an erroneous diagnosis of aldosteronoma. Selective adrenal vein sampling during corticotropin stimulation, with simultaneous measurement of PAC and cortisol is invasive, but represents a much more reliable method to differentiate aldosteronoma from idiopathic aldosteronism (149,150). Measurement of cortisol as well as aldosterone in the adrenal veins and inferior vena cava is critical for evaluating the accuracy and success of adrenal venous sampling. A unilateral excess of aldosterone secretion suggests the presence of aldosteronoma.

Patients with aldosteronoma are best treated with removal of the affected adrenal gland, which dramatically reduces or cures hypertension in the majority patients. The blood pressure response to spironolactone is predictive of the response to surgery in patients with aldosteronoma but not those with idiopathic aldosteronism (149). Spironolactone therapy for 3 to 4 weeks preoperatively is useful to allow for repletion of total body potassium and minimize postoperative hypoaldosteronism. Laparoscopic surgery is now widely employed to resect aldosteronoma and other adrenal tumors. On the other hand, idiopathic aldosteronism is best managed medically, because unilateral or bilateral adrenalectomy fails to normalize blood pressure and patients then need lifelong glucocorticoid and mineralocorticoid replacement in addition to antihypertensive therapy. High-dose spironolactone, an aldosterone antagonist, is the mainstay of therapy that can be used in conjunction with other antihypertensive agents such as CCBs.

GRA (also known as dexamethasone-suppressible hyperaldosteronism or familial hyperaldosteronism type I), is a rare genetic form of hyperaldosteronism caused by an autosomal dominant mutant chimeric gene that drives constitutive aldosterone synthesis under the control of ACTH and independent of volume status and AII (151). The administration of exogenous glucocorticoids that suppress ACTH secretion results in suppression of aldosterone secretion, reversal of the mineralocorticoid state, and resolution of hypertension. Unlike other etiologies of primary aldosteronism, which are usually diagnosed in the third to fifth decades of life, GRA is evident from birth onward. Hypertension associated with GRA is often difficult to control with conventional antihypertensive agents. The diagnosis of GRA should be considered in a patient with hypertension of early onset, especially in childhood or a history of early onset of hypertension in first-degree relatives. Another clue is a prominent family history of hemorrhagic stroke at a young age. There is an increased prevalence of cerebral hemorrhage, which occurs at mean age of 32 years, and is associated with a 60% mortality rate. Some patients with GRA fit the classical description of a mineralocorticoid-excess state, including hypertension, hyporeninemia, and spontaneous hypokalemia. However, analysis of large GRA pedigree has shown that affected patients often are normokalemic except during treatment with potassium-wasting diuretics. Thus, evaluation for spontaneous hypokalemia lacks sensitivity as a screening test for GRA. Patients with GRA have a PAC–PRA ratio >30. The diagnosis of GRA is supported by dexamethasone suppression testing (DST). A fall in PAC to 4 ng/dL after low-dose DST (0.5 mg dexamethasone orally every 6 hours for 2 to 4 days) is sensitive and specific for the diagnosis of GRA. The adrenal cortex in GRA produces large quantities of 18-oxygenated cortisol compounds, 18-oxocortisol (18-oxo-F), and 18-hydroxycortisol (18-OH-F), so-called hybrid steroids because they possess enzymatic features of both zona glomerulosa and zona fasciculata steroids. Significantly elevated levels of these hybrid compounds in a timed 24-hour urine specimen therefore provide a highly sensitive and specific test to diagnose GRA. Genetic testing for the chimeric gene is 100% sensitive and specific to diagnose GRA (151). GRA can be treated with long-term glucocorticoid suppression; however, glucocorticoid therapy has significant long-term complications, especially in children. For this reason, monotherapy with spironolactone (a competitive antagonist of the MR) or amiloride (blocks the aldosterone-regulated ENaC) represents the preferred treatment for GRA. Cerebral hemorrhage in GRA results from intracranial aneurysm; therefore, routine screening of GRA patients with magnetic resonance angiography is recommended, beginning at puberty and every 5 years thereafter (151).

Hypertension Caused by Glucocorticoid Excess in Cushing Syndrome

Glucocorticoid excess may overwhelm the capacity of 11-β HSD to convert cortisol to cortisone in distal tubular cells so that cortisol is available to bind to the MR. The resulting enhancement of renal sodium reabsorption leads to salt-sensitive hypertension. Cushing syndrome most commonly results from overproduction of ACTH either owing to pituitary adenoma or ectopic secretion of the hormone by a nonpituitary tumor. Hypokalemic metabolic alkalosis also may result from activation of the MR. The purpose of the low-dose dexamethasone suppression test is to differentiate patients with Cushing syndrome from those with normal function of the hypothalamic–pituitary axis. Failure of the morning serum cortisol to fall to <140 nmol/L following a single midnight dose of dexamethasone (1 mg), suggests the presence of Cushing syndrome. The high-dose dexamethasone suppression test then is used to differentiate patients with Cushing disease (pituitary hypersecretion of ACTH) from those with ectopic secretion of ACTH.

Hypertension in Chronic Kidney Disease

Virtually all forms of primary renal parenchymal disease can lead to secondary hypertension, especially if renal insufficiency is present (109,115). Glomerulonephritis and vasculitis are more likely to cause hypertension than chronic interstitial nephritis. Hypertension is present in >75% of cases of acute post-streptococcal glomerulonephritis. In a series of patients with biopsy-proven glomerulonephritis, the overall prevalence of hypertension was 60%. Hypertension was found more commonly with IgA nephropathy, membranoproliferative glomerulonephritis, and focal segmental glomerulosclerosis, whereas it was less frequent with membranous nephropathy or minimal change disease. In the setting of lupus nephritis, the frequency of hypertension approaches 50%. In idiopathic rapidly progressive (crescentic) glomerulonephritis, hypertension is uncommon unless overt fluid overload is present. Hypertension is extremely common in diabetic glomerulosclerosis. In fact most patients with type 2 diabetes have longstanding hypertension as part of the metabolic syndrome–insulin resistance syndrome. Autosomal-dominant polycystic kidney disease (ADPKD) is associated with a >50% incidence of hypertension even before the onset of renal insufficiency. Recent studies have found that the incidence of hypertension in ADPKD may be related to the degree of renal cyst enlargement (152).

A variety of disorders of the renal vasculature other than stenosis of the main renal arteries also may produce hypertension. Systemic vasculitis owing to classic polyarteritis nodosa is frequently accompanied by hypertension that may enter a malignant phase. In patients with progressive systemic sclerosis, hypertension plays a central role in the precipitous loss of renal function that occurs with scleroderma renal crisis (153). Thrombotic microangiopathy owing to hemolytic uremic syndrome or thrombotic thrombocytopenic purpura also can cause severe hypertension. Renal cholesterol embolization syndrome following an angiographic procedure in patients with severe aortic atherosclerosis can cause sudden onset of severe hypertension that may enter a malignant phase (154).

The prevalence of hypertension increases with progressive chronic renal insufficiency, regardless of cause, so that at end stage, virtually all patients are hypertensive. Among patients with end-stage renal disease, roughly 70% have hypertension owing to volume overload, and hemodialysis alone normalizes blood pressure. Approximately 30% of patients have dialysis-resistant hypertension, which may be due to hyperactivity of the RAAS or sympathetic nervous system, and thus require long-term antihypertensive therapy (155). Hypertension is also extremely common in the renal transplant recipient and may result from a variety of factors including acute or chronic rejection, stenosis of the transplant renal artery, calcineurin inhibitors (cyclosporine and tacrolimus), high-dose glucocorticoids, or increased renin production by diseased native kidneys (156).

ROLE OF HYPERTENSION IN THE PATHOGENESIS OF DIABETIC NEPHROPATHY

In diabetic patients, hypertension is a major risk factor for large-vessel atherosclerotic disease affecting the coronary, cerebral, and peripheral vascular beds. The incidence of large-vessel disease is dramatically increased in both type 1 and type 2 diabetics and is a major cause of morbidity and premature death. Diabetic patients have a twofold increased risk of coronary artery disease, a twofold to sixfold increased risk of atheroembolic stroke, and a significantly increased risk of peripheral vascular disease (157). Hypertension also hastens the progression of diabetic microangiopathic complications such as nephropathy and retinopathy (157). In non–insulin-dependent (type 2) diabetes mellitus (NIDDM), hypertension is twice as common as in the nondiabetic population. This increased prevalence of hypertension may relate to underlying insulin resistance, one of the sequelae of which is impairment in the intrinsic natriuretic capacity of the kidney. Moreover, control of hypertension, especially in conjunction with the use of ACE inhibitors ARBs, has been shown in clinical trials to slow the progression of diabetic nephropathy (158–160).

The evolution of hypertension in insulin dependent diabetes mellitus (IDDM, type 1) has been well characterized (161). In the early years of type 1 diabetes, hypertension is no more common than in healthy controls. Incipient nephropathy (microalbuminuria) is accompanied by a small but consistent increase in blood pressure compared with controls. With the development of overt diabetic nephropathy (clinically apparent proteinuria), hypertension is the rule, and the severity of the hypertension correlates inversely with the level of renal function. Once the serum creatinine begins to increase, the prevalence of hypertension is >90%. In contrast, in the older patient with NIDDM (type 2) diabetes, the natural history of hypertension is less predictable. Essential hypertension is likely to coexist in a substantial proportion of patients even before the development of nephropathy. As discussed in detail, the presence of hyperinsulinemia, which is present long before overt hyperglycemia develops, may lead to impaired natriuresis with salt-sensitive essential hypertension.

There are a number of experimental and clinical observations that suggest an important role for hypertension in the progression of diabetic nephropathy. Hypertension is thought to accelerate diabetic renal injury by exacerbating the underlying abnormalities in renal hemodynamics and further elevating glomerular capillary flow and pressure. Poor glycemic control may lead to afferent arteriole vasodilation, thereby allowing enhanced transmission of the elevated systemic blood pressure to the glomeruli. Diabetic patients destined to develop nephropathy have a higher prevalence of hypertension and a higher mean blood pressure than diabetic patients not destined to develop nephropathy. Moreover, there is a threefold increase in risk of nephropathy among type 1 diabetics with a parental history of hypertension, suggesting that an inherited predisposition to essential hypertension may increase the risk of nephropathy (162). In a multivariate analysis of patients with overt diabetic nephropathy, more rapid loss of GFR correlated most strongly with higher diastolic blood pressure (163). In contrast, blood sugar control, assessed by hemoglobin A_1C, did not correlate with change in GFR, at least in these patients with overt nephropathy.

In a study of the effect of two-kidney/one-clip Goldblatt hypertension in the streptozotocin-induced diabetic model in rats, severe diabetic nephropathy was observed in the unclipped kidney exposed to the high systemic pressure, whereas in the clipped kidney, protected from the high systemic pressure, nephropathy did not develop (164). This experimental demonstration of the central role of hypertension in the pathogenesis of diabetic nephropathy is further supported by reports of autopsy findings in patients with diabetes and unilateral renal artery stenosis. Glomerular basement thickening and nodu-lar Kimmelstiel–Wilson lesions were found only in the kidney with the patent renal artery and thereby exposed to the high systemic arterial pressure (165).

In rat models, diabetic nephropathy is produced by injection of streptozotocin with maintenance of moderate hyperglycemia with low-dose insulin. Initially there is a substantial increase in whole-kidney GFR akin to the hyperfiltration observed in young juvenile diabetic patients. There is also an increase in single nephron GFR owing to intrarenal vasodilation of both afferent and efferent arterioles, which results in an increase in glomerular capillary pressure and flow. However, after several weeks, progressive proteinuria, hypertension, and glomerulosclerosis develop (117). As in the remnant kidney model, it has been proposed that this increase in glomerular hydraulic pressure is maladaptive and eventually leads to progressive renal injury and nephron loss. In this model, normalization of glomerular capillary pressure with chronic ACE inhibitor therapy prevents the development of proteinuria and glomerulosclerosis, supporting the important pathophysiologic role of glomerular capillary hypertension. In these models of diabetic nephropathy, ACE inhibitors appear to be superior to conventional triple-antihypertensive therapy with a thiazide diuretic, reserpine, and hydralazine. It has been proposed that this is caused by a selective decrease in efferent arteriolar tone with ACE inhibitors, which leads to a direct reduction of glomerular capillary pressure independent of a reduction in systemic pressure (117).

TREATMENT OF HYPERTENSION IN DIABETIC PATIENTS

There is now convincing evidence from clinical trials that ACE inhibitors are beneficial in the treatment of diabetic nephropathy through a mechanism that is independent of their effect on systemic blood pressure. The Collaborative Study Group investigated the effect of ACE inhibitors in type 1 diabetics, 18 to 49 years old, with overt diabetic nephropathy (proteinuria ≥500 mg/day) (158). All subjects had serum creatinine levels ≤2.5 mg/dL. For the 75% of patients who were hypertensive on entering the study, treatment was instituted as required with antihypertensive medications other that ACE inhibitors or CCBs. Subjects (200 each group) were then randomized to receive either captopril (25 mg) or placebo tablets given three times a day for a median of 3 years. The blood pressure goal during the study was <140/90 mm Hg. Over the course of the study, mean arterial pressures were generally slightly lower (<4 mm Hg) in the ACE inhibitor treated group. The primary end point of the study was a doubling of the baseline serum creatinine that was reached in 25 subjects in the captopril group and 43 in the placebo group (*p* = 0.007). Captopril treatment reduced the relative risk of doubling serum creatinine by 48%. Captopril treatment was also associated with a 50% reduction in the relative risk of end-stage renal disease or death. Overall, in the captopril group, the mean rate of increase in serum creatinine was 0.2 ± 0.8 mg/dL per year versus 0.5 ± 0.8 mg/dL per year in the placebo group. Since the inclusion of mean arterial pressure as a time-dependent covariate in the statistical analysis did not alter the risk reduction estimates, it was concluded that there was a specific beneficial effect of ACE inhibitors independent of systemic blood pressure reduction. Recent studies also suggest that ACE inhibitors are useful in normotensive type I diabetic patients with incipient diabetic nephropathy (microalbuminuria), in that they slow the increase in microalbuminuria and reduce the probability of progression to clinical proteinuria (166).

The recent Irbesartan in Diabetic Nephropathy Trial (IDNT) has confirmed a renoprotective effect of ARBs in patients with diabetic nephropathy owing to type 2 diabetes (159). In this trial, 1,715 hypertensive patients with nephropathy caused by type 2 diabetes were randomly assigned to treatment with irbesartan (300 mg/day), the CCB amlodipine (10 mg/day), or placebo. Blood pressure was controlled to a target of 135/85 mm Hg with the addition of antihypertensive agents of classes other than angiotensin-receptor blocker/ACE inhibitor or CCBs if necessary. Treatment with irbesartan was associated with a 20% (compared with placebo) or 23% (compared with amlodipine) reduction in the risk of development of the composite end point of doubling of baseline serum creatinine, development of ESRD, or death from any cause. The risk of doubling of the serum creatinine was 33% lower in the irbesartan group than in the placebo group and 37% lower than in the amlodipine group. The relative risk of ESRD was 23% lower with irbesartan than with either amlodipine or placebo. These differences were not explained by differences in the achieved level of blood pressure control between the groups. It is possible that the dihydropyridine CCBs (e.g., amlodipine or nifedipine) by causing preferential dilatation of the afferent arteriole may allow more aortic pressure to be transmitted to the glomeruli.

Thus, the reduction in systemic blood pressure produced by these CCBs may not be accompanied by a corresponding reduction in intraglomerular pressure. This may well be the pathophysiologic mechanism underling the variable effect of dihydropyridine CCBs on proteinuria and progression of diabetic renal disease.

In the RENAAL trial (Reduction of End points in NIDDM with the Angiotensin II Antagonist Losartan), 1,513 hypertensive type 2 diabetic patients with proteinuria were randomized to losartan 50/mg day to 100/mg day and followed for >3 years (160). The investigators reported a significant reduction in the incidence of end-stage renal disease as well as the end point of doubling of serum creatinine.

Given the diverse effects of the RAS on the kidney, ACE inhibitors, and ARBs may have protective effects in diabetic nephropathy in addition to glomerular hemodynamic effects. Postulated protective mechanisms include improvement in glomerular permselectivity with decreased proteinuria, decreased mesangial matrix expansion, inhibition of glomerular hypertrophy, amelioration of insulin resistance, improvement in serum lipid profiles, changes in AII-mediated renal sodium handling, inhibition of renal procollagen formation, and inhibition of atherogenesis (117). Moreover, there is increasing recognition of the fact that even in primary glomerular diseases such as diabetic nephropathy, the decrement in GFR correlates best with the extent of interstitial disease (tubular atrophy and interstitial fibrosis). The link between glomerular disease and interstitial disease may be explained by the fact that proteinuria leads to increased protein catabolism by tubular epithelial cells, which in turn increases the expression of transforming growth factor-beta (TGF-β). Expression of fibrogenic cytokines therefore might provide a link between proteinuria and the development of interstitial fibrosis. In this regard, therapeutic maneuvers, such as blood pressure reduction or use of ACE inhibitors, which reduce proteinuria might slow progression of renal disease by modulating TGF-β-mediated interstitial damage.

Clinically, it has been shown that effective antihypertensive therapy with a diuretic and a β-blocker can reduce proteinuria and slow the progression of renal disease in patients with established diabetic nephropathy (167). At least in retrospective studies, the correlation between diastolic blood pressure and rate of progression of diabetic nephropathy is valid even at pressures <90 mm Hg (163). This observation suggests that the usual therapeutic target for diastolic blood pressure may be too high and that patients may benefit from reductions of blood pressure into the low–normal range. In this regard, it has recently been demonstrated that aggressive blood pressure control in normotensive type 2 diabetic patients is beneficial (168). In this study, normotensive type 2 diabetic patients were randomized to intensive (10 mm Hg below the baseline diastolic blood pressure) versus moderate diastolic blood pressure control (80 to 89 mm Hg). Patients in the moderate group were given placebo, whereas patients in the intensive group were randomized to treatment with either ACE inhibitor (enalapril) or CCB (nisoldipine). Over the 5-year follow-up period, compared to patients in the moderate group, intensive blood pressure control (average blood pressure 128/75 mm Hg) with either drug slowed the progression to incipient (microalbuminuria) and overt (macroalbuminuria) diabetic nephropathy. Intensive blood pressure control also decreased the progression of diabetic nephropathy and diminished the incidence of stroke.

MECHANISMS OF HYPERTENSION IN CHRONIC KIDNEY DISEASE

In acute nephritic syndrome due to poststreptococcal glomerulonephritis, the hypertension is clearly caused by sodium and water retention with increased ECF volume, plasma volume, and cardiac output with either normal or increased systemic vascular resistance (109,115). In contrast, the cause of hypertension in the setting of chronic renal insufficiency owing to primary renal disease is more controversial. It has been postulated that the hypertension is caused by volume expansion with inappropriately increased renin release. However, in both humans and animal models with hypertension owing to primary renal disease, the ECF volume, plasma volume, and cardiac output are usually normal, whereas the hypertension is maintained by an increased systemic vascular resistance. Nonetheless, sodium intake clearly plays an important role in the genesis of hypertension because blood pressure is much more sodium-sensitive in patients with chronic renal insufficiency than normal subjects (169).

The genesis of hypertension in the setting of primary renal disease can be readily conceptualized on the framework of either the Na/K ATPase inhibitor or Guyton hypotheses. Declining nephron mass is associated with a diminished capacity to excrete a sodium load. A compensatory increase in Na/K ATPase inhibitor may cause an increase in systemic vascular resistance and thus hypertension (Fig. 9.2). On the other hand, Guyton suggests that in the face of this type of primary natriuretic defect, the renal fluid–volume feedback mechanism restores external sodium balance, but does so at the expense of systemic hypertension that is maintained by an increase in peripheral vascular resistance secondary to the autoregulatory response (Fig. 9.5) (18–20,89).

Hypertension caused by intrinsic renal disease also may be related to the activation of renal pressor mechanisms such as the RAAS in ADPKD (152) or diminished production of vasodilator substances (bradykinins, prostaglandins, and NO) (115). The demonstration that ninefold increases in circulating inhibitors of NO synthesis may occur in uremic patients, implies that deficiencies of vasodilatory substances may indeed be an important contributor to the elevated systemic vascular resistance in hypertensive patients with renal failure (170).

ROLE OF HYPERTENSION IN THE PROGRESSION OF CHRONIC KIDNEY DISEASE

In the setting of primary renal parenchymal disease, hypertension clearly has its origin in the kidney. There is now substantial clinical and experimental evidence to support the concept that this secondary hypertension in turn aggravates the underlying disorder and is a major factor in the progression of chronic renal insufficiency (171). Coexistence of hypertension and primary renal disease creates a vicious circle, hastening the progression of renal failure. Systemic hypertension traditionally had been assumed to accelerate primary renal disease by inducing structural damage in the renal microvasculature (hyaline arteriosclerosis) with resultant glomerular hypoperfusion and ischemia (Fig. 9.13). However, it is now widely accepted that the converse may be true, namely, that systemic hypertension induces progressive injury in the already diseased kidneys via hydraulic stress on the glomeruli caused

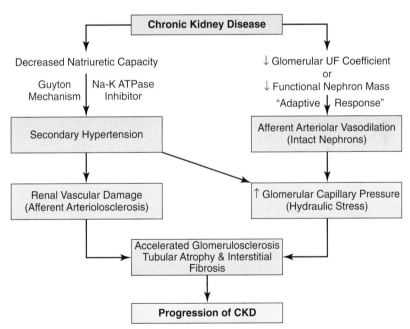

■ **Figure 9.13** Role of hypertension in the progression of chronic kidney disease. Secondary hypertension may contribute to the inexorable progression of primary renal disease by either of two mechanisms. Hypertensive damage to the renal microvasculature may lead to hyaline arteriolosclerosis of the afferent arteriole with further renal injury induced by an ischemic mechanism. Alternatively, following nephron loss caused by the primary disease, compensatory responses in the remaining nephrons cause afferent arteriolar vasodilation. Although this hemodynamic response helps to maintain whole-kidney GFR, in the long term it may be maladaptive. The decrease in afferent arteriolar resistance allows for transmission of the elevated systemic arterial pressure to the glomeruli. The hemodynamic stress caused by elevated glomerular capillary flow and pressure causes accelerated glomerulosclerosis and progression of chronic renal insufficiency. UF, ultrafiltration.

by increased transmission of the elevated systemic pressure to the glomerular capillaries (hyperperfusion theory) (Fig. 9.13) (118,172). The differences in the pathophysiologic mechanism of renal injury between essential hypertension (hypoperfusion/ischemia) and secondary hypertension caused by primary renal disease (hyperperfusion/glomerular hypertension) may be explained by differences in afferent arteriolar resistance in these disorders. Afferent arteriolar resistance determines the fraction of the systemic pressure transmitted to the glomerular capillaries. In benign essential hypertension, the structural changes in the afferent arterioles increase resistance and presumably serve to prevent transmission of the elevated systemic pressure to the glomeruli. In contrast, the glomerular hemodynamic changes in the setting of primary renal disease may be entirely different. The most extensively studied model of hypertension in the setting of a reduced number of normally functioning nephrons is the *remnant kidney* model produced by surgical ablation of renal mass in the rat. Reduction of renal mass below a critical level is associated with the development of proteinuria, systemic hypertension, and progressive renal failure owing to glomerulosclerosis in the remnant kidney (172). The reduction of functioning nephrons leads to a compensatory increase in single nephron glomerular filtration rate in the remaining nephrons. Vasodilatation of both the afferent and efferent arterioles leads to a decrease in renal vascular resistance with a resulting increase in glomerular capillary plasma flow. The glomerular capillary pressure increases because the decrease in efferent resistance is less pronounced than the decrease in afferent resistance. Together the increases in glomerular capillary pressure and perfusion account for the observed compensatory single nephron hyperfiltration. Similar glomerular hemodynamic changes are observed in the DOCA-salt hypertension model and the salt-sensitive model of nephrotoxic serum nephritis (173). Moreover, deterioration of renal function accelerates dramatically when secondary hypertension owing to DOCA-salt administration or renal artery clipping is superimposed on immune complex or nephrotoxic serum nephritis (173). Brenner et al. have suggested that these compensatory increases in glomerular capillary flow and pressure, although sufficient to maintain whole kidney GFR in the short term, are maladaptive in the long term, and that the resulting hydraulic stress is somehow responsible for the eventual development of glomerulosclerosis in the remaining nephrons (118,172). Micropuncture studies have confirmed that in the diseased kidneys autoregulation is lost and afferent arterioles are dilated so that the elevated systemic pressure is transmitted to the glomeruli, resulting in glomerular capillary hypertension, which is thought to induce progressive renal injury (Fig. 9.13).

In the preceding models, treatment of hypertension is associated with a slowing of the progression of renal injury (174). However, in the renal ablation model, although both ACE inhibitor (enalapril) and triple therapy (reserpine, hydralazine, and hydrochlorothiazide) reduced blood pressure equally, only ACE inhibitor treatment ameliorated proteinuria and glomerular scarring (175). The superiority of ACE inhibitor therapy in these models has been attributed to the fact that it leads to a reduction in intrarenal AII-mediated efferent arteriolar tone, thereby directly reducing glomerular capillary pressure in addition to lowering systemic blood pressure. We previously discussed the clinical use of ACE inhibitors and ARBs to slow the progression of renal disease in diabetic nephropathy.

Nonetheless, systemic hypertension and glomerular hypertension do not always coexist. A maladaptive increase in glomerular capillary flow and pressure may be a phenomenon that occurs principally in the setting of reduced functioning renal mass owing either to ablation or intrinsic renal disease. Systemic hypertension occurs without the development of glomerular capillary hypertension in the SHR (176). The glomeruli are protected from the high systemic pressure by afferent arteriolar vasoconstriction, which may explain the absence of progressive renal dysfunction in this model. The critical role that afferent arteriolar tone plays in the protection against hypertensive glomerular injury is illustrated by the fact that reduction of nephron mass by unilateral nephrectomy in the SHR results in a reduction of afferent arteriolar resistance in the remaining kidney. This allows for transmission of the systemic pressure to the glomeruli and, in this model, progressive glomerular injury with glomerulosclerosis does occur (177). The observation may be pertinent to understanding the low risk of progressive loss of renal function in benign essential hypertension in humans. In benign hypertension there is also a relative intrarenal vasoconstriction. It is tempting to speculate that, at least in patients with salt-resistant essential hypertension, there may be an increase in afferent arteriolar resistance that protects the glomeruli from the deleterious effects of systemic hypertension and thus accounts for the infrequent occurrence of progressive renal insufficiency among white patients with essential hypertension.

TREATMENT OF HYPERTENSION TO SLOW DISEASE PROGRESSION IN NONDIABETIC CHRONIC KIDNEY DISEASE

Evidence is accumulating that strict control of blood pressure is also beneficial in slowing the rate of progression of nondiabetic chronic kidney disease. Furthermore, animal and human studies have shown that progression of chronic kidney disease may be exacerbated by secondary hemodynamic factors such as intraglomerular hypertension. Therefore, a vital component of the treatment of hypertension in patients with chronic kidney disease, especially those with proteinuria, is the administration of an ACE inhibitor as part of a multidrug regimen not only to optimally control blood pressure but also with the goal of slowing the progressive loss of renal function. In the Benaepril trial patients already in reasonable blood pressure control were randomized to treatment with benazepril or placebo. Patients on benazepril had a greater reduction in blood pressure and a 25% reduction in protein excretion (178). The risk of progression to a primary end point (doubling of serum creatinine or progression to dialysis) was reduced by 53% in the benazepril-treated patients. The benefits of ACE inhibitor therapy were seen mainly in patients with chronic glomerular diseases or diabetic nephropathy, whereas there was no benefit in patients with polycystic kidney disease or other chronic kidney disease excreting <1 g of protein per day (two settings in which hemodynamically mediated factors may not be as important in disease progression). In the Ramipril Efficacy in Nephropathy (REIN) trial, patients with nondiabetic renal disease were randomized to ramipril or placebo plus other antihypertensive therapy as need to achieve diastolic blood pressure below 90 mm Hg (179). The trial was terminated prematurely among patients excreting >3 g protein per day because of a significant benefit with ACE inhibitor treatment with regard to ameliorating the rate of decline of renal function. The AASK was designed to address the efficacy of different classes of antihypertensive agents (β-blocker, ACE inhibitor, dihydropyridine CCB) in slowing the progressive loss of renal function in blacks with benign hypertensive nephrosclerosis (180). Use of diuretic therapy was allowed as necessary in each treatment groups to achieve target blood pressure goals. The National Institutes of Health (NIH) called a premature halt to the CCB arm of the study when interim analysis by the independent data safety monitoring board revealed that patients with hypertensive nephrosclerosis and proteinuria exceeding 300 mg/day benefited more from treatment with ACE inhibitor (ramapril) than CCB (amlodipine) (181). Results of the AASK trial suggested that ACE inhibitor (ramipril) was more effective in slowing the progression of benign hypertensive nephrosclerosis in blacks that either amlodipine or metoprolol (180). Although the final results of the AASK trial showed no difference among the drug treatment groups in the rate of decline of GFR, the ramipril group had a 22% reduction in risk of the composite end point (reduction in GFR by >50% from baseline, ESRD, or death). In the REIN-2 trial, dihydropyridine channel blocker (CCB) failed to provide renoprotection in patients with nondiabetic renal disease, despite further reduction of blood pressure from that obtained with fixed doses of ACE inhibitors (182). The nondihydropyridine CCBs (diltiazem and verapamil) have antiproteinuric effects; whereas, the dihydropyridines (amlodipine and nifedipine) have been shown to increase proteinuria in some studies. This paradox may be explained by the varied effect of the different classes of CCBs on renal autoregulation. In this regard, dihydropyridines cause preferential afferent arteriolar dilatation that allows more of the systemic pressure to be transmitted to the glomerulus, thereby increasing glomerular pressure and limiting their antiproteinuric effect.

The K/DOQI work group on hypertension and antihypertensive agents in chronic kidney disease recommends that either an ACE inhibitor or an ARB should be used as first-line antihypertensive therapy in proteinuric patients with nondiabetic chronic kidney disease (183). Although the available evidence is strongest for ACE inhibitors, ARBs may be substituted in patients who develop cough during treatment with ACE inhibitors. Although the issue is not as well studied in nondiabetic renal disease, ARBs appear to have similar antiproteinuric activity compared to ACE inhibitors and also significantly slow disease progression in patients with type 2 diabetes and nephropathy. Combination therapy with ACE inhibitor and ARB may also be beneficial given their additive antiproteinuric effect. The optimal goal is to reduce protein excretion to <500 to 1,000 mg/day if possible. A multidrug antihypertensive regimen is usually required to achieve the goal of reduction of blood pressure below 130/80 mm Hg. If this blood pressure goal is not achieved after initial therapy with an ACE inhibitor or an ARB, a diuretic should be added to the regimen. Addition of a diuretic is logical therapy given the central role of impaired natriuresis in the pathogenesis of hypertension in the setting of chronic kidney disease. Thiazide diuretics may be effective in the early stages of chronic kidney disease, whereas loop diuretics may be necessary in patients with more advanced kidney disease or diuretic resistance in the setting of nephrotic syndrome. If the blood pressure goal is not achieved with combination ACE inhibitor and diuretic therapy, additional drugs may be added to the regimen including a β-blocker, or a nondihydropyridine CCB (diltiazem or verapamil). Hydralazine or minoxidil (in combination with appropriate doses of β-blocker to control heart rate and diuretic to prevent fluid retention) may be added to the regimen in patients with resistant hypertension.

Treatment of Hypertension in Dialysis Patients

In the initial era of maintenance hemodialysis therapy in the early 1960s, Scribner et al. convincingly demonstrated that combining long hemodialysis sessions with assiduous attention to dietary sodium restriction resulted in normalization of blood pressure in >90% of hemodialysis patients (184–186). Unfortunately, in recent decades progressive shortening of dialysis sessions, administration of higher sodium dialysate to avoid intradialytic hypotension, and lack of attention to the utility of strict dietary sodium restriction have all collectively resulted in a progressive loss of blood pressure control in dialysis patients (Fig. 9.14) (184). As a result, the vast majority of dialysis patients now require a multidrug regimen to adequately control blood pressure. The key to normalization of blood pressure in dialysis patients without the need for antihypertensive drugs is meticulous attention to the achievement of true dry weight. Charra has defined dialysis dry weight as "the post-dialysis weight at which the patients remains normotensive until the next dialysis session despite modest interdialytic fluid retention and without the need for antihypertensive medications" (184,187). In the absence of residual renal function, there are three basic modalities for control of ECF volume in dialysis patients: dietary sodium restriction, removal of sodium

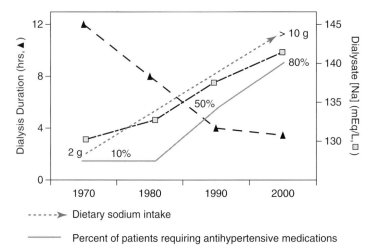

■ **Figure 9.14** Chronological trends in dialysis session time, dialysate sodium concentration, dietary sodium intake and prevalence of hypertension in dialysis patients. In the initial era of maintenance dialysis treatment in the 1960s, prescription of long dialysis session times, moderately low dialysate sodium concentrations and meticulous attention to dietary sodium restriction resulted in normalization of blood pressure in 90% of dialysis patients without the need for antihypertensive medications. Over the ensuing decades, changes in the dialysis prescription, focusing on adequacy of dialysis as defined by urea kinetics, have led to progressively shorter dialysis sessions and increasing use of higher dialysate sodium concentrations and sodium modeling to avoid interdialytic hypotension. Nephrologists have also "forgotten" the importance of restriction of sodium intake as the prime modality for prevention of large intradialytic weight gains; while inappropriately shifting the focus of patient education to "fluid restriction." The net result is that the majority (>80%) of dialysis patients fail to achieve true dry weight and remain hypertensive despite "adequate" dialysis. With current dialysis practice >80% of patients require antihypertensive medication (often a multidrug regimen) to adequately control blood pressure. (Triangles = dialysis session time; squares = dialysate sodium concentration [mmol/L]; dashed line = dietary sodium intake (g/day), triple line = percentage of dialysis patients requiring antihypertensive medications). (From Charra B. Fluid balance, dry weight, and blood pressure in dialysis. *Hemodialysis Int.* 2007;11:21–31, with permission.)

into the dialysate by diffusion (with lower sodium dialysate), and convective losses of sodium by ultrafiltration. Incredibly, most dialysis providers tend to emphasize "fluid restriction" to the patient as the primary means to prevent excessive interdialytic fluid gains, while the value of dietary sodium restriction has been forgotten and is all too often neglected in patient education. In reality, it is excessive dietary sodium intake that is the primary driving force for the typically large interdialytic fluid gains. In this regard, if fluid intake per se were actually the central issue, patients with impressive interdialytic weight gains would present with profound hyponatremia. In fact, even patients with 10-kg weight gains tend to have serum sodium concentrations in the low–normal range. This observation regarding isotonic extracellular volume expansion implies that these patients have actually ingested both salt and water in isotonic proportions. In this regard, a dialysis patient presenting with a 10-kg weight gain and serum sodium of 135 mEq/L has indeed imbibed 10 L of fluid but has also ingested 31 g of sodium. Since the ingested sodium is the factor driving excessive thirst, patient education regarding 'fluid restriction" alone is virtually never effective. In contrast, the interdialytic weight gain can be significantly reduced by moderate sodium restriction (2 g sodium or 5 to 6 g NaCl per day) without emphasis on the need for fluid restriction per se (184). A reasonable dialysate sodium concentration (135 to 138 mmol/L) will also provide for some diffusive loss of sodium during dialysis. Convective removal of sodium by ultrafiltration is the third arm of the triad for achieving true dry weight on dialysis. In this regard long slow dialysis such as that provided by home daily nocturnal dialysis is particularly effective at achieving true dry weight and normalization of blood pressure without the need for antihypertensive medications (188).

Treatment of Essential Hypertension

THIAZIDE DIURETICS IN THE TREATMENT OF ESSENTIAL HYPERTENSION

Because impaired renal handling of sodium plays a central role in the pathogenesis of both essential and secondary forms of hypertension, the use of diuretics is a well-established cornerstone in the treatment of hypertension. Diuretics have been employed for the treatment of hypertension since the discovery of chlorothiazide in 1957. Over the last 40 years, the efficacy of thiazides and related diuretics in preventing complications of essential hypertension has been conclusively demonstrated in long-term controlled clinical trials (189–192). Mild to moderate hypertension often responds to treatment with low-dose thiazide diuretics alone (2). In the setting of severe hypertension, or with concomitant renal insufficiency, diuretics are often an essential element of a stepped-care, multidrug regimen (2). Moreover, the failure to include a diuretic in the antihypertensive regimen is a common cause of "resistant" hypertension that fails to respond to treatment with ACE inhibitors, CCBs, α-adrenergic blockers, β-blockers, or vasodilators used singly or in combination (193).

Thiazide diuretics bind to and inhibit the thiazide-sensitive NCC in the DCT (194). It is interesting to note that the physiologic mechanism that underlies pressure natriuresis also involves downregulation of the NCC (102). The acute effect of diuretic administration is a decrease in ECF and plasma volume with a reduction in cardiac output. However, over a period of days to weeks of chronic thiazide diuretic administration, the negative sodium balance is attenuated such that plasma volume and cardiac output are normalized. Nevertheless, the antihypertensive effect persists, implying a concomitant decrease in systemic vascular resistance. This secondary *decrease in systemic vascular resistance* appears to be the long-term mechanism of the antihypertensive action of thiazides and related diuretics (195–197). The precise mechanism of this reduction in systemic vascular resistance is unknown. However, in the framework of either the Na/K ATPase inhibitor or Guyton hypothesis, a reduction in systemic vascular resistance and blood pressure as an indirect result of the natriuretic action of the diuretics is easy to conceptualize. As discussed, an underlying defect in natriuretic capacity must be present in hypertension, regardless of etiology. Diuretic treatment, by at least partially ameliorating this defect in natriuresis, could result in a decrease in the circulating level of the Na/K ATPase inhibitor, which has been proposed as the cause of the increase in vascular reactivity and systemic vascular resistance in hypertension (Fig. 9.2). In the context of Guyton's hypothesis, restoration of natriuretic capacity toward normal with diuretics means that the renal fluid–volume feedback mechanism no longer necessitates the presence of systemic hypertension (increased systemic vascular resistance) to maintain sodium balance (Fig. 9.5).

SAFETY OF THIAZIDE DIURETICS FOR TREATMENT OF HYPERTENSION

During the past two decades there has been a gradual shift away from diuretics as first-line antihypertensive agents toward the preferential use of newer agents such as converting enzyme inhibitors, CCBs, and selective α-adrenergic blockers. A major cause for concern has been related to the potentially deleterious metabolic effects of diuretics (hypokalemia, hypomagnesemia, hyperuricemia, glucose intolerance, and increased cholesterol). Fortunately, it now appears that use of low-dose thiazide diuretics (12.5 mg/day to 25 mg/day of hydrochlorothiazide, or equivalent) have antihypertensive efficacy similar to high-dose diuretic therapy, while markedly reducing the incidence of metabolic abnormalities. In addition, concern has been expressed that thiazide diuretics may aggravate cardiac arrhythmias and increase the complications of coronary heart disease, including myocardial infarction and sudden death. However, the HDFP study revealed a significant reduction at 8-year follow-up in all-cause mortality in its intensively (high-dose diuretic) treated stepped-care group relative to the referred care control group (190). There was a 16% risk reduction for fatal ischemic heart disease. This difference was noted primarily in the fatal myocardial infarction classification, in which there was a 23% risk reduction. In the European Working Party on High Blood Pressure in the Elderly trial, a double-blind placebo-controlled trial of low-dose hydrochlorothiazide plus triamterene in patients over the age of 60 years, total cardiovascular mortality was reduced 38%, and deaths from myocardial infarction were reduced by 60% (191). In the Systolic Hypertension in the Elderly Program (SHEP) trial, a double-blind placebo-controlled trial of low-dose chlorthalidone in patients over age 60 years with isolated systolic hypertension, the relative risks of stroke, left ventricular failure, nonfatal myocardial infarction or fatal coronary heart disease, and requirement for coronary artery bypass grafting were all significantly reduced in the active treatment group (192).

CHOICE OF DRUGS FOR THE TREATMENT OF HYPERTENSION

Concern over the adverse effects of low-dose thiazide diuretic appears to have been greatly exaggerated (198–200). There is a widespread speculation, fostered to a large extent by the pharmaceutical industry, that the use of antihypertensive drugs without metabolic side effects will inevitably have a more favorable impact on coronary artery disease related morbidity and mortality than thiazide diuretics and β-blockers (200). However, it is currently advisable in clinical practice to follow the latest recommendations of the Joint National Committee on Detection, Evaluation, and Treatment of High Blood Pressure (2), which advocates beginning treatment in uncomplicated essential hypertension with low-dose thiazides or related diuretics. Analysis of the wholesale costs of various antihypertensives demonstrates that thiazide diuretics are clearly the least expensive, with the price for generic hydrochlorothiazide ranging from $1 to $5 for 100 tablets. Thus, it appears that the vast majority of patients with essential hypertension can be treated at low cost without compromising quality of care. That drug costs are often a major impediment to patient compliance provides additional sound rationale for first-line use of diuretics (200). Given existing controversy regarding diuretic-induced hypokalemia and the risk of sudden death, a potassium-sparing diuretic also may be added for patients who require larger doses of diuretic or in patients with evidence of ischemic heart disease (198). Serum potassium levels should be determined before and at periodic intervals after initiation of treatment.

Treatment should be individualized, thiazide diuretics provide a safe, effective, and inexpensive form of treatment in the vast majority of hypertensive patients. However, in some patient groups, drugs other than diuretics may be considered as first-line therapy (2). For instance, given the evidence that ACE inhibitors and ARBs have a beneficial effect in slowing the progression of diabetic nephropathy, they should be considered the initial antihypertensive drug of choice for the treatment of diabetic patients with hypertension. Nonetheless, ACE inhibitor or angiotensin receptor blocker therapy alone may not adequately control blood pressure and the addition of other classes of antihypertensives may be required. In diabetic patients with resistant hypertension or overt diabetic nephropathy with nephrotic syndrome, the use of thiazide or loop diuretics may be imperative. Given their proven benefits with regard to slowing progression of nondiabetic chronic kidney disease, ACE inhibitors also should be included as part of the antihypertensive regimen in patients with chronic renal disease and proteinuria exceeding 1 g/day. Because the risk of progressive renal disease in benign essential hypertension is low, there is currently little rationale for the routine use of ACE inhibitors in patients with essential hypertension that lack evidence of chronic renal insufficiency. ACE inhibitors also should be considered as initial therapy for hypertensive patients with congestive heart failure caused by systolic dysfunction. In hypertensive patients with prior myocardial infarction, β-blockers should be considered first-line therapy because they reduce the risk of reinfarction and sudden death (2). In the setting of hypertension with coexistent renal insufficiency, addition of diuretics is often required to treat refractory hypertension. Substitution of the more potent, loop diuretics may be required in patients failing to respond to thiazide diuretics (i.e., GFR < 25 mL/min). In patients with severe benign hypertension or malignant hypertension, a triple-drug regimen, employing a diuretic and β-blocker in conjunction with the use of a potent peripheral vasodilator such as hydralazine or minoxidil, may be required to achieve adequate blood pressure control (2).

Available data from outcome studies support the conclusion that the achieved level of blood pressure, rather than the class of drug used, is the principal determinant of overall benefit. In this regard, the majority of trials indicate that at the same level of blood pressure control, most antihypertensive drugs provide equivalent cardioprotection. For example, the Captopril Prevention Project (CAPPP) randomized trial (201), the Swedish Trial in Old Patients with Hypertension-2 (STOP-Hypertension-2) study (202), the Nordic Diltiazem (NORDIL) study (203), the Intervention as a Goal in Hypertension Treatment (INSIGHT) study (204), and the Antihypertensive and Lipid-Lowering to Prevent Heart Attach Trial (ALLHAT) (205) each found no significant difference in overall mortality between older classes of drugs (thiazide-like diuretics or β-blockers) and newer antihypertensive drugs (ACE inhibitors or CCBs). The major exception to this generalization regards selective α-blocker therapy, which has been found to be associated with a higher risk of heart failure in high-risk hypertensive patients (206). For this reason, selective α-blockers (prazosin and doxazosin) are not recommended as first-line antihypertensive therapy. The principal finding from ALLHAT is that chlorthalidone (thiazide diuretic), amlodipine (CCB), and lisinopril (ACE inhibitor) provided similar protection from coronary heart disease death and nonfatal myocardial infarction (205). In fact, thiazide diuretic was actually superior to CCB and/or ACE inhibitor in preventing some adverse cardiovascular events. For instance, development of heart failure was significantly less common with chlorthalidone than with either lisinopril or amlodipine. Furthermore, there was a significantly increased risk of stroke and combined cardiovascular disease among black patients given lisinopril compared to those treated with chlorthalidone. A totally unexpected finding was that lisinopril failed to provide an advantage for any outcome measure when compared with chlorthalidone. Indeed, lisinopril-treated patients had higher combined cardiovascular disease outcomes, stroke, and heart failure than chlorthalidone-treated patients. Remarkably, chlorthalidone was even superior to lisinopril among diabetic patients with regard to prevention of new onset heart failure and the combined cardiovascular disease outcome. Thus, results from the ALLHAT strongly suggest that initial therapy with a thiazide diuretic is the appropriate choice for most hypertensive patients. The JNC 7 report recommends initiation of antihypertensive drug therapy with a thiazide diuretic based on the convincing results of ALLHAT and the low cost of generic thiazide diuretics unless there is a compelling reason to use a drug of another class as first-line therapy (2). In fact, results from the ALLHAT trial suggest that low-dose thiazide diuretic therapy in both younger and older patients provides superior cardioprotective effect than either ACE inhibitor or a CCB in a group of patients with at least two risk factors for coronary artery disease including left ventricular hypertrophy, type 2 diabetes, previous myocardial infarction or stroke, current cigarette smoking, hyperlipidemia, or known atherosclerotic cardiovascular disease (205). JNC-7 recommends initiation of therapy with a low dose of a thiazide diuretic, such as 12.5 mg or 25 mg of hydrochlorothiazide or chlorthalidone. This low-dose regimen tends to be associated with a low risk of metabolic complications such as glucose intolerance, hyperlipidemia, hypokalemia, and hyperuricemia (207). If monotherapy with a low-dose thiazide diuretic fails to attain goal blood pressure, then an ACE inhibitor, angiotensin receptor blocker (ARB), β-blocker, or CCB can be added as second- and third-step agents (2).

The recently published Avoiding Cardiovascular Events through Combination Therapy in Patients Living with Systolic Hypertension (ACCOMPLISH) trial was designed to test the hypothesis that treatment with ACE inhibitor combined with amlodipine would result in better cardiovascular outcomes that treatment with the same ACE inhibitor combined with a thiazide diuretic (208). In this randomized double-blind trial, 11,056 patients with hypertension who were at high risk for cardiovascular events were assigned to receive treatment with either benazepril plus amlodipne or benazepril plus hydrdochlorthiazide. The primary end point was the composite of death from cardiovascular causes, nonfatal myocardial infarction, nonfatal stroke, and hospitalization for angina, resuscitation after sudden cardiac arrest, and coronary revascularization. Mean blood pressures where similar in both groups. At 36 months of mean follow-up, there were 552 primary-outcome events in the benazepril–amlodipine group (9.6%) and 679 in the benazepril–hydrochlorothiazide group (11.8%), representing an absolute risk reduction with benazepril–amlodipine therapy of 2.2% and a relative risk reduction of 19.6% (hazard ratio 0.08, 95% confidence interval, 0.72 to 0.90, $p < 0.002$). For the secondary end point of death from cardiovascular causes, nonfatal MI, and nonfatal stroke, the hazard ration was 0.79 (95% CI, 0.67 to 0.92, $p = 0.002$). The authors conclude that the benazepril–amlodipine combination was superior to the benazepril–hydrochlorthiazide combination in reducing cardiovascular events in patients who were at high risk for such events.

Conclusions

It is apparent that the kidney is both the villain and the victim in hypertension. The kidney has a central role in the pathogenesis of both essential hypertension and secondary hypertension caused by primary renal parenchymal disease, renal artery stenosis, and mineralocorticoid excess. Analysis of rare mendelian causes of hypertension has provided convincing evidence that abnormal renal sodium handling plays a central role in the pathogenesis of hypertension. Ongoing genetic linkage analysis studies may provide additional insights into the pathogenesis of essential hypertension and hopefully lead to development of novel treatments to ameliorate the impairment in natriuretic capacity that characterizes both primary and secondary hypertension of all causes (12). At present, there is little hard evidence to support the widely held notion that benign essential hypertension is a common cause of end-stage renal disease. What then, accounts for the tremendous overrepresentation of black patients in the end-stage renal disease population? Is the impact of benign essential hypertension in blacks more pronounced, such that benign nephrosclerosis leads to more rapidly progressive nephron loss? Is there a genetic predisposition to renal injury? Alternatively, does inadequate treatment of hypertension in the black population allow for the development of recurrent episodes of malignant hypertension that culminate in end-stage renal disease? Without question, the critical role of hypertension in accelerating the progression of chronic kidney disease is well established. Rigorous control of blood pressure with a regimen including an ACE inhibitor or angiotensin receptor blocker has been shown to slow the progression of both diabetic and nondiabetic renal disease. Nonetheless, many questions remain even though it has been more than 150 years since Bright's original description of the relationship between hypertrophy of the heart (hypertension) and contraction of the kidney (renal dysfunction). Large outcome trials have produced conflicting results regarding the utility of different classes of antihypertensive agents for reduction of cardiovascular mortality (205,208).

REFERENCES

1. Whelton PK. Epidemiology and prevention of hypertension. *J Clin Hypertens.* 2004; 6: 636–642.
2. Chobanian AV, Bakris GL, Black HR, et al. The seventh report of the Joint National Committee on prevention, detection, evaluation and treatment of high blood pressure. The JNC 7 Report. *JAMA.* 2003; 289: 2560–2572.
3. Kearney PM, Whelton M, Reynolds K, et al. Global burden of hypertension. *Lancet.* 2005; 365: 217–223.
4. Kannel WB. Elevated systolic blood pressure as a cardiovascular risk factor. *Am J Cardiol.* 2000; 85: 251–255.
5. Stamler J, Stamler R, Neaton JD. Blood pressure, systolic and diastolic, and cardiovascular risks: US population data. *Arch Intern Med.* 1993; 153: 598–615.
6. Bright R. Tabular view of the morbid appearances in 100 cases connected with albuminous urine: with observations. *Guy's Hosp Rep.* 1836; 1: 380–402.
7. Traube L. *Ueber den Zusammenhang von Herz-und Nieren Krankheiten. Gesammelte Beitrage zur Pathologie und Physiologie.* Berlin: Hischwald; 1871: 290–350.
8. Mahomed FA. Some of the clinical aspects of chronic Bright's disease. *Guy's Hosp Rep.* 1879; 24(series III): 363–436.
9. Volhard F, Fahr T. *Die Brightische Neirenkrankhert, Klinik Pathologie und Atlas.* Berlin: Julius Springer; 1914.
10. Volhard F. Der arterielle Hochdruck. *Verh Dt Ges Inn Med.* 1923; 35: 134–175.
11. Klahr S. The kidney in hypertension—villain and victim. *N Engl J Med.* 1989; 320: 731–733.

12. Lifton RP, Gharavi AG, Geller DS. Molecular mechanisms of human hypertension. *Cell.* 2001; 104: 545–556.

13. Folkow B. Cardiovascular structural adaptation; its role in the initiation and maintenance of primary hypertension. *Clin Sci Mol Med.* 1978; 55: 3S–22S.

14. Folkow B. Sympathetic nervous control of blood pressure. Role in primary hypertension. *Am J Hypertens.* 1989; 2: 103S–111S.

15. Panza JA, Quyyumi AA, Brush JE Jr., et al. Abnormal endothelium-dependent vascular relaxation in patients with essential hypertension. *N Engl J Med.* 1990; 323: 22–27.

16. de Wardener HE, MacGregor GA. Dahl's hypothesis that a saluretic substance may be responsible for a sustained rise in arterial pressure: its possible role in essential hypertension. *Kidney Int.* 1980; 18: 1–9.

17. de Wardener HE, MacGregor GA. The relation of a circulating sodium transport inhibitor (the natriuretic hormone?) to hypertension. *Medicine.* 1983; 62: 310–326.

18. Guyton AC. Renal function curve—a key to understanding the pathogenesis of hypertension. *Hypertension.* 1987; 10: 1–6.

19. Guyton AC, Cowley AW, Coleman TG, et al. Hypertension: a disease of abnormal circulatory control. *Chest.* 1974; 65: 328–338.

20. Guyton AC, Manning RD, Norman RA, et al. Current concepts and perspectives of renal volume regulation in relationship to hypertension. *J Hypertens.* 1986; 4(Suppl 4): S49–S56.

21. Eaton SB, Konner M. Paleolithic nutrition. A consideration of its nature and current implications. *N Engl J Med.* 1985; 312: 283–289.

22. Tobian L. Potassium and sodium in hypertension. *J Hypertens.* 1988; 6(Suppl 4): S12–S24.

23. Schrier RW. Body fluid volume regulation in health and disease: a unifying hypothesis. *Ann Intern Med.* 1990; 113: 155–159.

24. Brenner BM, Garcia DL, Anderson S. Glomeruli and blood pressure. Less of one, more of the other? *Am J Hypertens.* 1988; 1: 335–347.

25. Sasaki N. The relationship of salt intake to hypertension in the Japanese. *Geriatrics.* 1964; 19: 735–744.

26. Carvalho JJM, Baruzzi RG, Howard PF, et al. Blood pressure in four remote populations in the INTERSALT study. *Hypertension.* 1989; 14: 238–246.

27. Intersalt Cooperative Research Group. Intersalt: an international study of electrolyte excretion and blood pressure. Results for 24 hour urinary sodium and potassium excretion. *Br Med J.* 1988; 297: 319–330.

28. Murray RH, Luft FC, Bloch R, et al. Blood pressure responses to extremes of sodium intake in normal man. *Proc Soc Exp Biol Med.* 1978; 159: 432–436.

29. Watkin DM, Froeb HF, Hatch FT, et al. Effects of diet in essential hypertension II. Results with unmodified Kempner rice diet in fifty hospitalized patients. *Am J Med.* 1950; 9: 441–493.

30. Joossens JV, Geboers J. Salt and hypertension. *Prev Med.* 1983; 12: 53–59.

31. Appel LJ, Moore TJ, Obarzanek E, et al. A clinical trial of the effects of dietary patterns on blood pressure. *N Engl J Med.* 1997; 336: 1117–1124.

32. Sacks FM, Svetkey LP, Vollmer WM, et al. Effects on blood pressure of reduced dietary sodium and the dietary approaches to stop hypertension (DASH) diet. *N Engl J Med.* 2001; 344: 3–10.

33. Chen J, Gu D, Huang J, et al. for the GenSalt Research Group. Metabolic syndrome and salt sensitivity of blood pressure in non-diabetic people in China: a dietary intervention study. *Lancet.* 2009; 373: 829–835.

34. Dahl LK, Schackow E. Effects of chronic excess salt ingestion: experimental hypertension in the rat. *Can Med Assoc J.* 1964; 90: 155–160.

35. Rettig R. Does the kidney play a role in the aetiology of primary hypertension? Evidence from renal transplantation studies in rats and humans (Review). *J Human Hypertens.* 1993; 7: 177–180.

36. Curtis JJ, Luke RG, Dustan HP, et al. Remission of essential hypertension after renal transplantation. *N Engl J Med.* 1983; 309: 1009–1015.

37. Guidi E, Bianchi G, Rivolta E, et al. Hypertension in man with kidney transplant: role of familial versus other factors. *Nephron.* 1985; 41: 14–21.

38. Tobian L, Lange J, Azar S, et al. Reduction of natriuretic capacity and renin release in isolated, blood perfused kidneys of Dahl hypertension-prone rats. *Circ Res* 1978; 43(Suppl I): I92–I98.

39. Ayman D. Heredity in arteriolar (essential) hypertension. A clinical study of the blood pressure of 1,524 members of 277 families. *Arch Intern Med.* 1934; 53: 792–802.

40. Rice T, Vogler GP, Perusse L, et al. Cardiovascular risk factors in a French Canadian population: resolution of genetic and familial environmental effects on blood pressure using twins, adoptees, and extensive information on environmental correlates. *Genet Epidemiol* 1989; 6: 571–588.

41. Feinlab M, Garrison RJ, Fabsitz R, et al. The NHLBI twin study of cardiovascular disease risk factors: methodology and summary of results. *Am J Epidemiol.* 1977; 106: 284–285.

42. Grim CE, Luft FC, Miller JZ, et al. Effects of sodium loading and depletion in normotensive first-degree relatives of essential hypertensives. *J Lab Clin Med.* 1979; 94: 764–771.

43. Luft FC, Grim CE, Fineberg N, et al. Effects of volume expansion and contraction in normotensive whites, blacks, and subjects of different ages. *Circulation.* 1979; 59: 643–650.

44. Bonvalet JP. Regulation of sodium transport by steroid hormones. *Kidney Int.* 1998; 65: S49–S56.

45. Garty H, Palmer LG. Epithelial sodium channels: function, structure, and regulation. *Physiol Rev.* 1997; 77: 359–396.

46. Velasquez H, Bartiss A, Berstein P, et al. Adrenal steroids stimulate thiazide-sensitive NaCl transport by rat renal distal tubules. *Am J Physiol.* 1996; 270: F211–F219.

47. Dluhy RG, Lifton RP. Glucocorticoid-remediable aldosteronism. *J Clin Endocrinol Metab.* 1999; 84: 4341–4344.

48. Mune T, Rogerson FM, Nikkila H, et al. Human hypertension caused by mutations in the kidney isozyme of 11-beta-hydroxysteroid dehydrogenase. *Nat Genet.* 1995; 10: 394–399.

49. White PC. Steroid 11 beta-hydroxylase deficiency and related disorders. *Endocrinol Metab Clin North Am.* 2001; 30: 61–79.

50. Biglieri EG. 17 alpha hydroxylase deficiency. *J Endocrinol Invest.* 1995; 18: 540–544.

51. Amor M, Parker KL, Globerman H, et al. Mutation in the CYP21b gene (ile 172-to-asn) causes steroid 21-hydroxylase deficiency. *Proc Natl Acad Sci U S A* 1988; 85: 1600–1604.

52. Geller DR, Farhi A, Pinkerton N, et al. Activating mineralocorticoid receptor mutation in hypertension exacerbated by pregnancy. *Science.* 2000; 289: 119–123.

53. Geller DS, Rodriguez-Soriano J, Vallo Boado A, et al. Mutations in the mineralocorticoid receptor gene cause autosomal dominant pseudohypoaldosteronism type I. *Nat Genet* 1998; 19: 279–281.

54. Hansson JH, Schild L, Lu Y, et al. A de novo missense mutation of the beta subunit of the epithelial sodium channel causes hypertension and Liddle syndrome, identifying a proline-rich segment critical for regulation of channel activity. *Proc Natl Acad Sci U S A* 1995; 92: 11495–11499.

55. Botero-Velez M, Curtis JJ, Warnock DG. Brief report: Liddle's syndrome revisited—a disorder of sodium reabsorption in the distal tubule. *N Engl J Med.* 1994; 330: 178–181.

56. Baker EH, Dong YB, Sagnella GA, et al. Association of hypertension with T594M mutation in beta subunit of epithelial sodium channels in black people resident in London. *Lancet.* 1998; 351: 1388–1392.

57. Chang SS, Grunder S, Hanukoglu A, et al. Mutations in the subunits of the epithelial sodium channel cause salt wasting with hyperkalemic acidosis, pseudohypoaldosteronism type 1. *Nat Genet.* 1996; 12: 248–253.

58. Simon DB, Nelson-Williams C, Bio MJ, et al. Gitelman's variant of Bartter's syndrome, inherited hypokalemic alkalosis, is caused by mutations in the thiazide-sensitive Na-Cl cotransporter. *Nat Genet.* 1996; 12: 24–30.

59. Cruz DN, Simpn DB, Nelson-Williams C, et al. Mutations in the Na-Cl cotransporter reduce blood pressure in humans. *Hypertension.* 2001; 37: 1458–1464.

60. Simon DB, Karet FE, Hamdan JM, et al. Bartter's syndrome hypokalemic alkalosis with hypercalciuria, is caused by mutations in the Na-K-2Cl cotransporter NKCC2. *Nat Genet.* 1996; 13: 183–188.

61. Lifton RP, Hunt SC, Williams RR, et al. Exclusion of the Na(+)-H(+) antiporter as a candidate gene in human essential hypertension. *Hypertension.* 1991; 17: 8–14.

62. Reaven GM. Role of insulin resistance in human disease: Banting Lecture. *Diabetes.* 1987; 37: 1595–1607.

63. DeFronzo RA. The effect of insulin on renal sodium metabolism. A review of clinical implications. *Diabetologica.* 1981; 21: 165–171.

64. Johnson RJ, Schriener GF. Hypothesis: the role of acquired tubulointerstitial disease in the pathogenesis of salt-dependent hypertension. *Kidney Int.* 1997; 52: 1169–1179.

65. Johnson RJ, Gordon KL, Shinichi S, et al. Renal injury and salt-sensitive hypertension after exposure to catecholamines. *Hypertension.* 1999; 34: 151–159.

66. Lombardi D, Gordon KL, Polinsky P, et al. Salt-sensitive hypertension develops after short-term exposure to angiotensin II. *Hypertension.* 1999; 33: 1013–1019.

67. Dimsdale JE, Graham RM, Ziegler MG, et al. Age, race, diagnosis, and sodium effects on the pressor response to infused norepinephrine. *Hypertension.* 1987; 10: 564–569.

68. Palmer RJ, Stone RA, Cervenka JH. Renal hemodynamics in essential hypertension. Racial differences in response to changes in dietary sodium. *Hypertension.* 1994; 24: 752–757.

69. Thomas SE, Anderson S, Gordon KL, et al. Tubulointerstitial disease in aging: evidence for underlying peritubular capillary damage, a potential role for renal ischemia. *J Am Soc Nephrol.* 1998; 9: 231–242.

70. Hall JE. Intrarenal actions of converting enzyme inhibitors. *Am J Hypertens.* 1989; 2: 875–884.

71. Cogan MG. Angiotensin II: a powerful controller of sodium transport in the early proximal tubule. *Hypertension.* 1990; 15: 451–458.

72. Hollenberg NK, Williams GH. Sodium-sensitive hypertension. Implications of pathogenesis for therapy. *Am J Hypertens.* 1989; 2: 809–815.

73. DiBona GF. Neural control of renal tubular solute and water transport. *Miner Electrolyte Metab.* 1989; 15: 66–73.

74. Frolich ED. Efferent glomerular arteriolar constriction: a possible intrarenal hemodynamic effect in hypertension. *Am J Med Sci.* 1988; 295: 409–413.

75. Bello-Reuss E, Trevino DL, Gottschalk CW. Effect of renal sympathetic nerve stimulation on proximal water and sodium reabsorption. *J Clin Invest.* 1976; 57: 1104–1107.

76. Campese VM, Parise M, Karubian F, et al. Abnormal renal hemodynamics in black salt-sensitive patients with hypertension. *Hypertension.* 1991; 18: 805–812.

77. Wyss JM, Oparil S, Sripairojthikoon W. Neuronal control of the kidney: contribution to hypertension. *Can J Physiol Pharmacol.* 1992; 70: 759–770.

78. Bachmann S, Mundel P. Nitric oxide in the kidney: synthesis, localization, and function. *Am J Kidney Dis.* 1994; 24: 112–129.

79. Majid DSA, Williams A, Navar LG. Inhibition of nitric oxide synthesis attenuated pressure-induced natriuretic responses in anaesthetized dogs. *Am J Physiol.* 1993; 33: F79–F87.

80. Ikenaga H, Suzuki H, Ishii N, et al. Role of NO on pressure natriuresis in Wistar-Kyoto and spontaneously hypertensive rats. *Kidney Int.* 1993; 43: 205–211.

81. Tolin JP, Shultz RJ. Endogenous nitiric oxide synthesis determines sensitivity to pressor effects of salt. *Kidney Int.* 1994; 46: 230–236.

82. Weder AB. Red-cell lithium-sodium countertransport and renal lithium clearance in hypertension. *N Engl J Med.* 1986; 314: 198–201.

83. De Wardener HE. The control of sodium excretion. *Am J Physiol* 1978; 235: F163–F173.

84. Stumpe KO, Lowitz HD, Ochwadt B. Fluid reabsorption in Henle's loop and urinary excretion of sodium and water in normal rats

and rats with chronic hypertension. *J Clin Invest.* 1970; 49: 1200–1212.

85. Blaustein MP. Sodium transport and hypertension. *Hypertension.* 1984; 6: 445–453.

86. Haddy FJ, Overbeck HW. The role of humoral agents in volume expanded hypertension. *Life Sci.* 1976; 19: 935–948.

87. Hamlyn JM, Harris DW, Clark MA, et al. Isolation and characterization of sodium pump inhibitor form human plasma. *Hypertension.* 1989; 13: 681–689.

88. MacGregor GA, Fenton S, Alaghband-Zadeh J, et al. Evidence for a raised concentration of a circulating sodium transport inhibitor in essential hypertension. *BMJ.* 1981; 283: 1355–1357.

89. Guyton AC, Coleman TG, Cowley AW Jr., et al. Arterial pressure regulation. Overriding dominance of the kidneys in long-term regulation and in hypertension. *Am J Med.* 1972; 52: 584–594.

90. Norman RA, Enobakhare JA, DeClue JW, et al. Arterial pressure—urinary output relationship in hypertensive rats. *Am J Physiol.* 1978; 234: R98–R103.

91. Selkurt EE. Effect of pulse pressure and mean arterial pressure modification on renal hemodynamics and electrolyte and water excretion. *Circulation.* 1951; 4: 541–551.

92. Guyton AC, Montani JP, Hall JE, et al. Computer models for designing hypertension experiments and studying concepts. *Am J Med Sci.* 1988; 295: 320–326.

93. Schrier RW. Pathogenesis of sodium and water retention in high-output and low-output cardiac failure, nephrotic syndrome, cirrhosis, and pregnancy (in two parts). *N Engl J Med.* 1988; 319: 1065–1072; 1127–1134.

94. Hall JE, Granger JP, Hester RL, et al. Mechanisms of sodium balance in hypertension: role of pressure natriuresis. *J Hypertens.* 1986; 4(Suppl 4): S57–S65.

95. Hall JE, Guyton AC, Smith MJ, et al. Blood pressure and renal function during chronic changes in sodium intake: role of angiotensin. *Am J Physiol.* 1980; 239: F271–F280.

96. Ichikawa I, Brenner BM. Importance of efferent arteriolar vascular tone in regulation of proximal tubular fluid reabsorption and glomerulotubular balance in the rat. *J Clin Invest.* 1980; 65: 1192–1201.

97. Campese VM. Effects of calcium antagonists on deranged modulation of the renal function curve in salt-sensitive patients with essential hypertension. *Am J Cardiol.* 1988; 62: 85G–91G.

98. Hall JE, Granger JP, Smith MJ, et al. Role of renal hemodynamics and arterial pressure in aldosterone "escape." *Hypertension.* 1984; 6(Suppl I): I183–I192.

99. Hall JE, Granger JP, Hester RL, et al. Mechanisms of escape from sodium retention during angiotensin II hypertension. *Am J Physiol.* 1984; 246: F627–F634.

100. Hall JE, Montani JP, Woods LL, et al. Renal escape from vasopressin. Role of pressure diuresis. *Am J Physiol.* 1986; 250: F907–F916.

101. Zhang Y, Mircheff AH, Hensley CB, et al. Rapid redistribution and inhibition of renal sodium transporters during acute pressure natriuresis. *Am J Physiol.* 1996; 270: F1004–F1014.

102. Wang X-Y, Masilamani S, Nielsen J, et al. The renal thiazide-sensitive Na-Cl cotransporter as mediator of the aldosterone-escape mechanism. *J Clin Invest.* 2001; 108: 215–222.

103. Jennette JC, Olson JL, Schwartz MM. *Heptinstall's Pathology of the Kidney.* 6th ed. Philadelphia, PA: Lippincott Williams & Wilkins; 2006.

104. Whelton PK, Klag MG. Hypertension as a risk factor for renal disease. Review of clinical and epidemiological evidence. *Hypertension.* 1989; 13(Suppl I): I-19–I-27.

105. Freedman BI, Iskandar SS, Appel RG. The link between hypertension and nephrosclerosis. *Am J Kidney Dis.* 1995; 25: 207–221.

106. Schlessinger SD, Tankersley MR, Curtis JJ. Clinical documentation of end-stage renal disease due to hypertension. *Am J Kidney Dis.* 1994; 23: 655–660.

107. Zarif L, Covic A, Iyengar S, et al. Inaccuracy of clinical phenotyping for hypertensive nephrosclerosis. *Nephrol Dial Transplant.* 2000; 15: 1801–1807.

108. Fogo A, Breyer JA, Smith MC, et al. Accuracy of the diagnosis of hypertensive nephrosclerosis in African Americans: a report from the African American Study of Kidney Disease (AASK) Trial. AASK Pilot Study Investigators. *Kidney Int.* 1997; 51: 244–252.

109. Brown MA, Whitworth JA. Hypertension in human renal disease. *J Hypertens.* 1992; 10: 701–712.

110. Bulpitt CJ. Prognosis of treated hypertension 1951–1981. *Br J Clin Pharmacol.* 1982; 13: 73–79.

111. Labeeuw M, Zech P, Pozet N, et al. Renal failure in essential hypertension. *Contrib Nephrol.* 1989; 71: 90–94.

112. Shulman NB, Ford CE, Hall WD, et al. Prognostic value of serum creatinine and effect of treatment of hypertension on renal function. Results from the Hypertension Detection and Follow-up Program. *Hypertension.* 1989; 13(Suppl I): I80.

113. Goldring W, Chasis H. *Hypertension and Hypertensive Disease.* New York: Commonwealth Fund; 1944: 53–95.

114. Kincaid-Smith P. *The Kidney. A Clinicopathological Study.* Oxford: Blackwell; 1975: 212.

115. Kincaid-Smith P, Whitworth, JA. Pathogenesis of hypertension in chronic renal failure. *Semin Nephrol.* 1988; 8: 155–162.

116. Azar S, Johnson MA, Scheinman J, et al. Regulation of glomerular capillary pressure and filtration in young Kyoto hypertensive rats. *Clin Sci (Lond).* 1979; 56: 203–209.

117. Anderson S. Antihypertensive therapy in experimental diabetes. *J Am Soc Nephrol.* 1992; 3: S86–S90.

118. Brenner BM, Meyer TW, Hostetter TH. Dietary protein intake and the progression of kidney disease. The role of hemodynamically mediated glomerular injury in the pathogenesis of progressive glomerulosclerosis in aging, renal ablation, and intrinsic renal disease. *N Engl J Med.* 1982; 307: 652–659.

119. Rostrand SG, Kirk KA, Rutsky EA, et al. Racial differences in the incidence of treatment for

end-stage renal disease. *N Engl J Med.* 1982; 306: 1276–1279.

120. Entwisle G, Apostolides AY, Hebel JR, et al. Target organ damage in black hypertensives. *Circulation.* 1977; 55: 792–796.

121. Levy SB, Talner LB, Coel MN, et al. Renal vasculature in essential hypertension: racial differences. *Ann Intern Med.* 1978; 88: 12–16.

122. Perneger TV, Whelton PK, Klag MJ, et al. Diagnosis of hypertensive end-stage renal disease: effect of patient's race. *Am J Epidemiol.* 1995; 141(1): 10–15.

123. Pitcock JA, Johnson JG, Hatch FE, et al. Malignant hypertension in blacks. Malignant intrarenal arterial disease as observed by light and electron microscopy. *Hum Pathol.* 1976; 7: 333–346.

124. Bennett NM, Shea S. Hypertensive emergency: case criteria, sociodemographic profile, and previous care of 100 cases. *Am J Public Health.* 1988; 78: 636–640.

125. Frolich ED, Messerli FH, Dunn FG, et al. Greater renal vascular involvement in the black patient with essential hypertension. A comparison of systemic and renal hemodynamics in black and white patients. *Miner Electrolyte Metab.* 1984; 10: 173–177.

126. Tobian L. Potassium and sodium in hypertension. *J Hypertens.* 1988; 6(Suppl 4): S12–S24.

127. Dustan HP. Growth factors and racial differences in severity of hypertension and renal diseases. *Lancet* 1992; 339: 1339–1340.

128. Nolan CR, Linas SL. In: Schrier RW, ed. *Diseases of the Kidney and Urinary Tract.* 8th ed. Philadelphia, PA: Lippincott Williams & Wilkins; 2007: 1370–1436.

129. Barger AC. The Goldblatt memorial lecture. Part I: experimental renovascular hypertension. *Hypertension.* 1979; 1: 447–455.

130. Treadway KK, Slater EE. Renovascular hypertension. *Ann Rev Med.* 1984; 35: 665–692.

131. Working Group on Renovascular Hypertension. Detection, evaluation and treatment of renovascular hypertension. Final report. *Arch Intern Med.* 1987; 147: 820–829.

132. Safian RD, Textor SC. Renal artery stenosis. *N Engl J Med.* 2001; 344: 431–442.

133. McNeil BJ, Varady PD, Burrows BA, et al. Measures of clinical efficacy. Cost effectiveness calculations in the diagnosis and treatment of hypertensive renovascular disease. *N Engl J Med.* 1975; 293: 216–221.

134. Mailloux LU, Napolitano B, Bellucci AG, et al. Renal vascular disease causing end-stage renal disease, incidence, clinical correlates, and outcomes: a 20-year experience. *Am J Kidney Dis.* 1994; 24: 622–629.

135. Boudewijn G, Vasbinder C, Nelemans PJ, et al. Diagnostic tests for renal artery stenosis in patients suspected of having renovascular hypertension: a meta-analysis. *Ann Intern Med.* 2001; 135: 401–411.

136. Rudnick MR, Berns JS, Cohen RM, et al. Nephrotoxic risks of renal angiography: contrast media-associated nephrotoxicity and atheroembolism—a critical review. *Am J Kidney Dis.* 1994; 24: 713–727.

137. Marks LS, Maxwell MH. Renal vein renin. Value and limitations in the prediction of operative results. *Urol Clin North Am.* 1975; 2: 311–325.

138. Bourgonie JJ, Rubbert K, Sfakianakis BN. Angiotensin-converting enzyme-inhibited renography for the diagnosis of ischemic kidneys. *Am J Kidney Dis.* 1994; 24: 665–673.

139. Crowley JJ, Santos RM, Peter RH, et al. Progression of renal artery stenosis in patients undergoing cardiac catheterization. *Am Heart J.* 1998; 136: 913–918.

140. Harding MR, Smith LR, Himmelstein SI, et al. Renal artery stenosis: prevalence and associated risk factors in patients undergoing routine cardiac catheterization. *J Am Soc Nephrol.* 1992; 2: 1608–1616.

141. Wachtell K, Ibsen H, Olsen NH, et al. Prevalence of renal artery stenosis in patients with peripheral vascular disease and hypertension. *J Hum Hypertens.* 1996; 10: 83–85.

142. Olin JW, Melia M, Young JR, et al. Prevalence of atherosclerotic renal artery stenosis in patients with atherosclerosis elsewhere. *Am J Med.* 1990; 88: 46N–51N.

143. Webster J, Marshall F, Abdalla M, et al. Randomised comparison of percutaneous angioplasty vs continued medical therapy for hypertensive patients with atheromatous renal artery stenosis: Scottish and Newcastle Renal Artery Stenosis Collaborative Group. *J Hum Hypertens.* 1998; 12: 329–335.

144. Poulin PH, Chatellier G, Darne, B, et al. Blood pressure outcome of angioplasty in atherosclerotic renal artery stenosis: a randomized trial. Essai Multicentrique Medicaments vs Angioplastie (EMMA) Study Group. *Hypertension.* 1998; 31: 823–829.

145. van Jaarsveld BC, Krijnen P, Pieterman H, et al. The effect of balloon angioplasty on hypertension in atherosclerotic renal artery stenosis: Dutch Renal Artery Stenosis Intervention Cooperative Study Group. *N Engl J Med.* 2000; 342: 1007–1014.

146. Balk E, Raman G, Chung M, et al. Effectiveness of management strategies for renal artery stenosis: a systematic review. *Ann Intern Med.* 2006; 145: 901–912.

147. Murphy TP, Soares G, Kim M. Increase in utilization of percutaneous renal artery interventions by Medicare beneficiaries, 1996–2000. *AJR Am J Roentgen* 2004; 183: 561–568.

148. Dworkin LD, Jamerson KA. Case against angioplasty and stenting of atherosclerotic renal artery stenosis. *Circulation.* 2007; 115: 271–276.

149. Ganguly A. Primary aldosteronism. *N Engl J Med.* 1998; 339: 1828–1834.

150. Weinberger MH, Fineberg NS. The diagnosis of primary aldosteronism and separation of two major subtypes. *Arch Intern Med.* 1993; 153: 2125–2129.

151. Dluhy RG, Lifton RP. Glucocorticoids-remdeiable aldosteronism. *J Clin Endocrinol Metab.* 1999; 84: 4341–4344.

152. Chapman AB, Johnson A, Gabow PA, et al. The renin-angiotensin-aldosterone system and autosomal dominant polycystic kidney disease. *N Engl J Med.* 1990; 323: 1091–1096.

153. Cannon PJ, Hassar M, Case DB, et al. The relationship of hypertension and renal failure in scleroderma (progressive systemic sclerosis) to structural and functional abnormalities of the renal cortical circulation. *Medicine (Baltimore)*. 1974; 53: 1–46.

154. Smith MC, Ghose MK, Henry AR. The clinical spectrum of renal cholesterol embolization. *Am J Med*. 1981; 71: 174–180.

155. Zuchhelli P, Santoro A, Zuccala A. Genesis and control of hypertension in hemodialysis patients. *Semin Nephrol*. 1988; 8: 163–168.

156. Curtis JJ. Hypertension after renal transplantation: cyclosporine increases the diagnostic and therapeutic considerations. *Am J Kidney Dis*. 1989; 13(Suppl 1): 28–32.

157. Barnett AH. Diabetes and hypertension. *Br Med Bull*. 1994; 50(No. 2): 397–407.

158. Lewis EJ, Hunsicher LG, Bain RP, et al. The effect of angiotensin-converting-enzyme inhibition on diabetic nephropathy. *N Engl J Med*. 1993; 329: 1456–1462.

159. Lewis EJ, Hunsiker LG, Clark WR, et al. Renoprotective effect of the angiotensin-receptor blocker irbesartan in patients with nephropathy due to type 2 diabetes. *N Engl J Med*. 2001; 345: 910–912.

160. Brenner BM, Cooper ME, de Zeeuw D, et al. The losartan renal protection study–rationale, study design and baseline characteristics of RENALL (Reduction of End points in NIDDM with the Angiotensin II Antagonist Losartan). *J Renin Angiotensin Aldo System*. 2000; 1: 329–335.

161. Mogensen CE, Christensen CK. Blood pressure changes and renal function in incipient and overt diabetic nephropathy. *Hypertension*. 1985; 7(Suppl II): II64–II73.

162. Viberti GC, Earle K. Predisposition to essential hypertension and the development of diabetic nephropathy. *J Am Soc Nephrol*. 1992; 3: S27–S33.

163. Dillon JJ. The quantitative relationship between treated blood pressure and progression of diabetic renal disease. *Am J Kidney Dis*. 1993; 22: 798–802.

164. Mauer SM, Steffes MW, Azar S, et al. The effects of Goldblatt hypertension on the development of the glomerular lesion of diabetes mellitus in the rat. *Diabetes*. 1978; 27: 738–744.

165. Bároniade VC, Lefebvre R, Falardeau P. Unilateral nodular diabetic glomerulosclerosis. Recurrence of an experiment of nature. *Am J Nephrol*. 1987; 7: 55–59.

166. Viberti G, Mogensen CE, Groop LC, et al. Effect of captopril on progression to clinical proteinuria in patients with insulin-dependent diabetes mellitus and microalbuminuria. *JAMA*. 1994; 271: 275–279.

167. Parving H-H, Andersen AR, Smidt UM, et al. Effects of antihypertensive treatment on kidney function in diabetic nephropathy. *BMJ*. 1987; 294: 1443–1447.

168. Schrier RW, Estacio RO, Esler A, et al. Effects of aggressive blood pressure control in normotensive type 2 diabetic patients on albuminuria, retinopathy and strokes, *Kidney Int*. 2002; 61: 1086–1097.

169. Koomans HA, Ross JC, Dorhout Mees EJ, et al. Sodium balance in renal failure. A comparison of patients with normal subjects under extremes of sodium intake. *Hypertension*. 1985; 7: 714–721.

170. Vallance P, Leone A, Calver A, et al. Accumulation of an endogenous inhibitor of nitric oxide synthetase in chronic renal failure. *Lancet*. 1992; 339: 572–575.

171. Dworkin LD, Benstein JA. Impact of antihypertensive therapy on progressive kidney damage. *Am J Hypertens*. 1989; 2: 162S–172S.

172. Hostetter TM, Oslon JL, Rennke HG, et al. Hyperfiltration in remnant nephrons: a potentially adverse response to renal ablation. *Am J Physiol* 1981; 241: F85–F93.

173. Neugarten J, Kaminetsky B, Feiner H, et al. Nephrotoxic serum nephritis with hypertension: amelioration by antihypertensive therapy. *Kidney Int*. 1985; 28: 135–139.

174. Baldwin DS, Neugarten J. Treatment of hypertension in renal disease. *Am J Kidney Dis*. 1985; 5: A57–A70.

175. Anderson S, Meyer TW, Rennke HG, et al. Control of glomerular hypertension limits glomerular injury in rats with reduced nephron mass. *J Clin Invest*. 1985; 76: 612.

176. Arendshorst WJ, Beierwaltes WH. Renal and nephron hemodynamics in spontaneously hypertensive rats. *Am J Physiol*. 1979; 236: F246–F251.

177. Dworkin LD, Feiner HD. Glomerular injury in uninephrectomized spontaneously hypertensive rats. A consequence of glomerular capillary hypertension. *J Clin Invest*. 1986; 77: 797–809.

178. Maschia G, Alberti D, Janin G, et al. Effect of the angiotensin-converting-enzyme inhibitor benazepril on the progression of chronic renal insufficiency. *N Engl J Med*. 1996; 334: 939.

179. The GISEN Group (Gruppo Italiano di Studi Epidemiologici in Nefrologia). Randomised placebo-controlled trial of effect of ramipril on decline in glomerular filtration rate and risk of terminal renal failure in proteinuric, non-diabetic nephropathy. *Lancet*. 1997; 349: 1857.

180. Agadoa LY, Appel L, Bakris GL, et al. Effect of ramipril vs amlodipine on renal outcomes in hypertensive nephrosclerosis: a randomized controlled trial. *JAMA*. 2001; 285: 2719–2728.

181. Sica DA, Douglas JD. The African American Study of Kidney Disease and Hypertension (AASK): new findings. *J Clin Hypertens (Greenwich)*. 2001; 3: 244–251.

182. Ruggenenti P, Perna A, Loriga G, et al. Blood pressure control for renoprotection in patients with non-diabetic renal disease (REIN-2): multicentre, randomized controlled trial. *Lancet*. 2005; 365: 939–946.

183. K/DOQI Clinical Practice Guidelines on hypertension and antihypertensive agents in chronic kidney disease. *Am J Kidney Dis*. 2004; 43: (5 Suppl 1): S1–S290.

184. Charra B. Fluid balance, dry weight, and blood pressure in dialysis. *Hemodialysis Int*. 2007; 11: 21–31.

185. Comty C, Rottka H, Shaldon S. Blood pressure control in patients with end-stage renal failure

treated by intermittent hemodialysis. *Proc Eur Dial Transplant Assoc.* 1964; 1: 209–214.

186. Blumberg A, Nelp WD, Hegstrom RM, et al. Extracellular volume in patients with chronic renal disease treated for hypertension by sodium restriction. *Lancet.* 1967; 2: 69–73.

187. Charra B. Control of blood pressure in long slow haemodialysis. *Blood Purif.* 1994; 12: 252–258.

188. Pierratos A. New approaches to haemodialysis. *Annu Rev Med.* 2004; 55: 179–189.

189. Freis ED. The efficacy and safety of diuretics in treating hypertension. *Ann Intern Med.* 1995; 122: 223–226.

190. Hypertension Detection and Follow-up Program Cooperative Group: persistence of reduction in blood pressure and mortality of participants in the hypertension detection and follow-up program. *JAMA.* 1988; 259: 2113–2122.

191. Amery A, Birkenhäger W, Brixko P, et al. Mortality and morbidity from the European Working Party on High Blood Pressure in the Elderly Trial. *Lancet.* 1985; 1: 1349–1354.

192. SHEP Cooperative Research Group. Prevention of stroke by antihypertensive treatment in older persons with isolated systolic hypertension. Final results of the Systolic Hypertension in the Elderly Program (SHEP). *JAMA.* 1991; 265: 3255–3264.

193. Gifford RW Jr. An algorithm for the management of resistant hypertension. *Hypertension.* 1988; 11(Suppl II): II101–II105.

194. Ellison DH, Velazques H, Wright FS. Thiazide-sensitive sodium chloride cotransport in the early distal tubule. *Am J Physiol.* 1996; 253: F546–F554.

195. Bock HA, Stein JH. Diuretics and the control of extracellular fluid volume. Role of counterregulation. *Semin Nephrol.* 1988; 8: 264–272.

196. Guédon J, Chaignon M, Lucsko M. Diuretics as antihypertensive drugs. *Kidney Int.* 1988; 34(Suppl 25): S177–S180.

197. Shah S, Khatri I, Fries ED. Mechanism of antihypertensive effect of thiazide diuretics. *Am Heart J.* 1978; 95: 611–618.

198. Fries ED. The efficacy and safety of diuretics in treating hypertension. *Ann Intern Med.* 1995; 122: 223–226.

199. Gifford RW Jr., Borazanian RA. Traditional first-line therapy: overview of medical benefits and side effects. *Hypertension.* 1989; 13(Suppl I): I119–I124.

200. Moser M. In defense of traditional antihypertensive therapy. *Hypertension.* 1988; 12: 324–326.

201. Hansson L, Lindholm LH, Miskanen L, et al. Effect of angiotensin-converting enzyme inhibition compared with conventional therapy on cardiovascular morbidity and mortality in hypertension: the Captopril Prevention Project (CAPPP) randomized trial. *Lancet.* 1999; 353: 611–616.

202. Hansson L, Lindholm LH, Ekborn T, et al. Randomized trial of old and new antihypertensive drugs in elderly patients: cardiovascular mortality and morbidity in the Swedish Trial in Old Patients with Hypertension-2 study. *Lancet.* 1999; 354: 1751–1756.

203. Hansson L, Hedner T, Lung-Johansen P, et al. Randomized trial of effects of calcium antagonists compared with diuretics and beta-blockers on cardiovascular morbidity and mortality in hypertension: The Nordic Diltiazem (NORDIL) study. *Lancet.* 2000; 356: 359–365.

204. Brown MJ, Palmer CR, Castaigne A, et al. Morbidity and mortality in patients randomized to double-blind treatment with long-acting calcium-channel blockers or diuretic in the International Nifedipine GITS study: Intervention as a Goal in Hypertension Treatment (INSIGHT). *Lancet.* 2000; 356: 366–372.

205. ALLHAT Collaborative Research Group. Major outcomes in high-risk hypertensive patients randomized to angiotensin-converting enzyme inhibitor or calcium channel blocker vs diuretic: The Antihypertensive and Lipid-Lowering to Prevent Heart Attack Trial (ALLHAT). *JAMA.* 2002; 288: 2981–2997.

206. Anonymous. Major cardiovascular events in hypertensive patients randomized to doxazosin vs chlorthalidone: the Antihypertensive and Lipid-Lowering Treatment to Prevent Heart Attack Trial (ALLHAT). ALLHAT Collaborative Research Group. *JAMA.* 2000; 238: 1967–1975.

207. Carlsen JE, Kober L, Torp-Pedersen C, et al. Relation between dose of bendrofluazide, antihypertensive effect, and adverse biochemical effects. *BMJ.* 1990; 300: 975–978.

208. Jamerson K, Weber MA, Bakris GL, et al. Benazepril plus amlodipine or hydrochlorothiazide for hypertension in high-risk patients. *N Engl J Med.* 2008; 359: 2417–2428.

CHAPTER 10

Acute Kidney Injury: Pathogenesis, Diagnosis, and Management

ROBERT W. SCHRIER AND CHARLES L. EDELSTEIN

A cute kidney injury (AKI) (as defined by an increase of serum creatinine >0.5mg/dL) occurs in 1% of hospital admissions (1), and up to 7% of hospitalized patients develop AKI (1). Twenty five percent of patients in the intensive care unit (ICU) develop AKI as defined by oliguria or a serum creatinine >3.5 mg/dL (1). Five percent of patients in the ICU will need renal replacement therapy (RRT) (1,2). Dialysis is the only Federal Drug Administration (FDA)-approved treatment for AKI (3). Even though both intermittent hemodialysis (IHD) and continuous RRT (CRRT) are widely used, the reported mortality rates of AKI are between 30% and 80% (4,5). In spite of an increase in the degree of comorbidity of patients with AKI, the in-hospital mortality rate has declined over the period 1988 to 2002 (6).

AKI is defined as a sudden decrease in the glomerular filtration rate (GFR) occurring over a period of hours to days. The Acute Dialysis Quality Initiative (ADQI) has developed the RIFLE classification of AKI that divides AKI into the following stages: (a) risk, (b) injury, (c) failure, (d) loss of function, (e) and end-stage kidney disease (Fig. 10.1) (7,8,9). The term "acute kidney injury" replaces the term "acute renal failure" (ARF), and ARF is restricted to patients that have AKI and need RRT. The RIFLE criteria have been validated in multiple studies, that is, as the RIFLE class increases, so does mortality (7,8,9).

When AKI is not the result of primary vascular, glomerular, or interstitial disorders, it is referred to as acute tubular necrosis (ATN). In fact, in the clinical setting, the terms "acute renal failure" and "acute tubular necrosis" have become synonymous (10). However, ATN is a renal histologic finding and may not be consistently detectable in patients with AKI, despite profound kidney dysfunction (11–14). Thus in the strictest sense, the terms AKI and ATN should not be used interchangeably (15). ATN has recently been defined as a syndrome of physiologic and pathologic dissociation (15).

Causes of AKI

INTRARENAL OR INTRINSIC AKI

After prerenal and postrenal azotemia have been excluded, the diagnosis of intrarenal or intrinsic AKI can be entertained. These problems may be renal vascular (large or small vessel), tubular, interstitial, or glomerular (Table 10.1). The Madrid AKI Study Group reported that the commonest cause of AKI was ATN accounting for 38% of hospitalized patients with AKI and 76% of ICU patients with AKI (4). The second and third leading causes of AKI were prerenal azotemia and urinary tract obstruction. Sepsis was the leading cause of AKI and more common than ischemic causes in the ICU (4,16–18). The diseases may be primary renal or part of a systemic disease. The diseases of vessels and glomeruli will be dealt with in Chapter 15. This chapter therefore will focus primarily on the ischemic and nephrotoxic causes of AKI and acute interstitial nephritis (AIN).

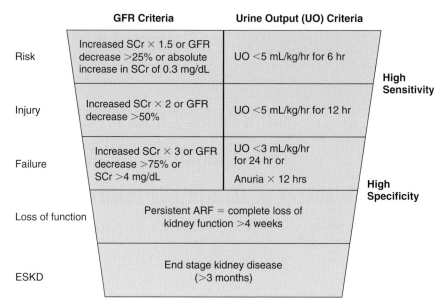

	GFR Criteria	Urine Output (UO) Criteria	
Risk	Increased SCr × 1.5 or GFR decrease >25% or absolute increase in SCr of 0.3 mg/dL	UO <5 mL/kg/hr for 6 hr	High Sensitivity
Injury	Increased SCr × 2 or GFR decrease >50%	UO <5 mL/kg/hr for 12 hr	
Failure	Increased SCr × 3 or GFR decrease >75% or SCr >4 mg/dL	UO <3 mL/kg/hr for 24 hr or Anuria × 12 hrs	High Specificity
Loss of function	Persistent ARF = complete loss of kidney function >4 weeks		
ESKD	End stage kidney disease (>3 months)		

■ **Figure 10.1** RIFLE criteria for the classification of AKI. RIFLE includes three grades of severity of AKI (risk, injury, and failure) and two oucome variables (loss of function and end-stage kidney disease). The RIFLE criteria attempt to convey the notion that kidney injury occurs before kidney failure. Studies have demonstrated that as the RIFLE class goes up, so does mortality. RIFLE, risk, injury, failure, loss of function, and end-stage kidney disease; SCr, serum creatinine; AKI, acute kidney injury.

**TABLE 10.1 CONDITONS THAT CAUSE "INTRINSIC"
OR PARENCYMAL AKI**

Vascular—Large Vessels
Bilateral renal artery stenosis
Bilateral renal vein thrombosis
Operative arterial cross clamping

Vascular—Small Vessels
Vasculitis
Atheroembolic disease
Thrombotic microangiopathies
   Hemolytic uremic syndrome
   Thrombotic thrombocytopenic purpura
   Scleroderma renal crisis
   Malignant hypertension
Hemolysis, elevated liver enzymes, and low platelets (HELLP) syndrome of pregnancy

Glomerular
In AKI, in the setting of glomerulonephritis, a rapidly progressive glomerulonephritis (RPGN) should be excluded. Extracapillary proliferation in the glomerulus forms crescents that can rapidly destroy the glomeruli.

Diseases with Linear Immune Complex Deposition
Goodpasture's syndrome

Diseases with Granular Immune Complex Deposition
Acute postinfectious glomerulonephritis
Lupus nephritis
Infective endocarditis
Immunoglobulin A (IgA) glomerulonephritis
Henoch–Schonlein purpura
Membranoproliferative glomerulonephritis
Cryoglobulinemia

TABLE 10.1 (continued)

Diseases with Few Immune Deposits ("Pauci-Immune")
Wegener granulomatosis
Polyarteritis nodosa
Idiopathic crescentic glomerulonephritis
Churg–Strauss syndrome

Interstitium
Acute allergic interstitial nephritis
Antibiotics
   β-lactam antibiotics (penicillins, methicillin, cephalosporins, rifampicin)
   sulphonamides
   erythromycin
   ciprofloxacin
Diuretics (furosemide, thiazides, chlorthalidone)
Nonsteroidal antiinflammatory drugs (NSAIDs)
Anticonvulsant drugs (phenytoin, carbamazepine)
Allopurinol
Interstitial nephritis associated with infection, granuloma, crystals
Streptococcal
Staphylococcal
Diphtheria
Leptospirosis
Brucellosis
Legionnaire's disease
Toxoplasmosis
Infectious mononucleosis
Salmonella typhi
Tuberculosis
Sarcoidosis
Acute uric acid nephropathy, e.g., tumor lysis syndrome
Hypercalcemia
Melamine toxicity

Acute Tubular Necrosis
Renal ischemia (50% of cases)
  Shock
  Complications of surgery
  Hemorrhage
  Trauma
  Gram-negative bacteremia
  Pancreatitis
  Pregnancy (postpartum hemorrhage, abruptio placenta, septic abortion)
Nephrotoxic drugs (35% of cases)
  Antibiotics (aminoglycosides, amphotericin, pentamidine, foscarnet, acyclovir)
  Antineoplastics (cisplatin, methotrexate)
  Iodine-containing X-ray contrast
  Organic solvents (carbon tetrachloride)
  Ethylene glycol (antifreeze)
  Anesthetics (enflurane)
  Acute phosphate nephropathy
Endogenous toxins
  Myoglobin due to rhabdomyolysis
  Hemoglobin (incompatible blood transfusion, acute falciparum malaria)
  Uric acid (acute uric acid nephropathy)
AKI, acute kidney injury

Pathogenesis of AKI

THE NATURE OF PROXIMAL TUBULAR INJURY

The nature of proximal tubular injury in ischemic AKI (19,20) includes reversible sublethal dysfunction (loss of polarity, swelling, loss of the apical brush border) and lethal injury (necrosis and apoptosis) (12,19). In rat models of ischemic AKI and in posttransplant AKI in humans, there is reversible sublethal injury during the first 6 hours of reperfusion followed by necrosis at 24 hours of reperfusion (21–23). Proximal tubular cell death due to ischemic AKI in vivo in rodents and hypoxia in vitro results predominantly in necrosis, hence the term "acute tubular necrosis," or ATN (24). Apoptotic cell death in ischemic renal injury in vivo has been demonstrated (25,26). When apoptosis has been demonstrated in early ischemic AKI, it is often present in the distal tubules (27–29). The significance of apoptosis in distal tubules is uncertain. Apoptosis in proximal tubules may play a role in tubular regeneration and was demonstrated to occur later at 3 days after ischemic injury in regenerating proximal tubules (30).

Dissociation of spectrin and other basolateral cytoskeletal proteins plays a major role in the well-documented sublethal injury and loss of polarity, which leads to proximal tubule dysfunction during renal ischemia (21,31,32). Spectrin is the major component of the membrane-associated cytoskeleton and is also important in the maintenance of cell membrane structural integrity. In the cytoskeleton of the proximal tubule, Na^+/K^+ ATPase is linked to the cytoskeleton/membrane complex by a variety of cytoskeletal proteins including spectrin (31,33). ATP depletion and renal ischemia cause dissociation of the basolateral cytoskeleton in rat kidneys (32,34) and in human transplanted kidneys (21). Na^+/K^+ ATPase and spectrin dissociate from the cytoskeleton during ischemic AKI (21).

A complete redistribution of Na^+/K^+ ATPase from the basolateral to the apical membrane, that is, total loss of polarity, is not necessary to decrease sodium reabsorption. It has been demonstrated that (a) translocation of Na^+/K^+ ATPase to the cytoplasm results in depolarization confined to the proximal tubule; (b) fractional excretion of lithium, a surrogate measure for the fraction of filtered sodium that is delivered to the macula densa, the site of tubuloglomerular feedback, is massively increased; and (c) these abnormalities persist for the duration of the maintenance phase of postischemic AKI (21,22). These results provide evidence for decreased proximal reabsorption of sodium, resultant increased sodium delivery to macula densa, tubuloglomerular feedback ("tubular communication with the glomerulus"), and resultant filtration failure that accompanies ischemic AKI.

The loss of polarity is also associated with redistribution of integrins. Tubular cells detach from their matrix, which results in increased cast formation and provides an experimental mechanism for the back-leak of glomerular filtrate. The consequences of loss of polarity, that is, tubuloglomerular feedback, cast formation with tubular obstruction, and back-leak of glomerular filtrate are major factors in the pathogenesis of experimental ischemic AKI (25).

Potential mediators/mechanisms of AKI cause tubular injury, inflammation, or vascular injury (Table 10.2). These mediators of tubular injury, inflammation, or vascular injury will now be discussed in more detail.

Tubular Injury

Ca^{2+} ACCUMULATION AND CELL INJURY

Ca^{2+} overload is characteristic of tissues with lethally injured cells, since the breakdown of the plasma membrane barrier to Ca^{2+} causes a large increase in cytosolic Ca^{2+}, which is sequestered in part by the mitochondria. Specifically, building on the hypothesis that homeostatic mechanisms controlling cellular Ca^{2+} are disturbed in AKI, it has been shown that radiocontrast-induced AKI (35,36) and cadaveric kidney transplant dysfunction (37,38), for example, can be attenuated by administration of chemically dissimilar Ca^{2+} channel blockers. These are two clinical conditions in which intense renal vasoconstriction is demonstrable,

TABLE 10.2 MEDIATORS/MECHANISMS OF ISCHEMIC AKI

Tubular Injury
Ca^{2+} influx (proximal tubules and afferent arterioles)
Disruption of actin cytoskeleton
Loss of polarity
Ca^{2+}-dependent PLA_2
Ca^{2+}-independent PLA_2
Calpain
Caspase-1
Caspase-3
Interleukin-18
Nitric oxide (generated by iNOS)
Metalloproteases
Defective heat shock response
Apoptosis
Altered gene expression
HIF-1 α

Tubular Obstruction
Increased tubular pressure
Tamm-horsfall protein
RGD peptides

Vascular Injury
Prostaglandins
Natriuretic peptides
Fractalkine
Abnormal vascular function
　Increased sensitivity to vasoconstrictors
　Increased sensitivity to renal nerve stimuli
　Impaired autoregulation

Inflammation
Neutrophils
CD4 (+) T cells
Macrophages
NK cells
Uric acid
Oxygen radicals
Endotoxin
Cytokines
Chemokines
Adhesion molecules

PLA_2, Phospholipase A_2; HIF, hypoxia-inducible factor; NOS, inducible nitric oxide synthase; RGD, arginine–glycine–aspartic acid.

a situation where delivery of oxygen and nutrients to renal tubules is compromised. The administration of Ca^{2+} channel blockers reduces the intensity of renal vasoconstriction and provides better delivery of nutrients to renal tissues. With ischemia, the poor nutrient flow to renal tubules also results in tubule Ca^{2+} overload, which can be lessened by the Ca^{2+} channel blockers. Although Ca^{2+} channel blockers have been shown to be efficacious in these two aforementioned clinical conditions, a full understanding of the mechanisms by which cytosolic or tissue Ca^{2+} increases in underperfused situations and how this increase may contribute to organ injury is the focus of much recent research. It is important, therefore, to understand the normal cellular Ca^{2+} regulation before discussing the newer insights that have been gained using experimental approaches to further improve our understanding of the pathogenesis of AKI.

Normal Regulation of Cell Ca^{2+}

Three major cellular Ca^{2+} pools exist: (a) a pool bound to plasma membranes, (b) a pool bound to or sequestered within intracellular organelles, and (c) a pool both free and bound within the cytoplasm (39).

Although 60% to 70% of all Ca^{2+} in renal epithelial cells is located in the mitochondria, cytosolic free ionized Ca^{2+} is the most critical with regard to regulation of intracellular events. Cytosolic free Ca^{2+} is normally kept at about 100 nM, which is 1/10,000 of the extracellular level (40). Ca^{2+} efflux is mediated on basolateral membranes by both Ca^{2+} ATPase, which is adenosine triphosphate (ATP) dependent, and a Na^{+}/Ca^{2+} exchanger on the basolateral membrane, which is ATP independent (41). Normally, the cell membrane is impermeable to Ca^{2+} and maintains a steep Ca^{2+} gradient between the cytosol and the extracellular space. However, when cytosolic Ca^{2+} increases in response to increased cellular membrane permeability or decreased Ca^{2+} efflux or both, the mitochondria and endoplasmic reticulum actively increase their Ca^{2+} uptake. Mitochondrial uptake and retention of Ca^{2+} become substantial only when cytosolic levels exceed 400 to 500 nM, as occurs with cell injury (40). Mitochondrial uptake is regulated by a Ca^{2+} uniporter in the mitochondrial inner membrane. During cell injury, active mitochondrial sequestration appears to be quantitatively the most important process for buffering elevations in cytosolic Ca^{2+}.

Tubular Effects of Ca^{2+} Accumulation

In vivo studies of intact kidney cannot discriminate between protective effects at the vascular sites compared to tubular sites or a combination thereof. As the proximal tubule is the main site of injury in ischemia-reperfusion models in vivo and the human allograft with AKI (42), the study of isolated proximal tubules during conditions of oxygen deprivation either in suspension or in primary culture has provided insight into the pathophysiology of proximal tubular injury. Numerous studies in both freshly isolated rabbit and rat proximal tubules as well as various models of proximal and distal tubules in culture have demonstrated an increase in cytosolic Ca^{2+} in these renal epithelial cells during chemical anoxia, hypoxia, and Ca^{2+} ionophore treatment (43–51). When exposed to anoxia in vitro, proximal and distal tubules in culture rapidly exhibit cell death after reoxygenation (52). However, if Ca^{2+} is removed from the bathing medium during the first 2 hours of reoxygenation and then replaced, cell viability is greatly enhanced (52). Ca^{2+} channel blockers have also been shown to delay the onset of anoxic cell death in primary cultures of rabbit proximal tubules and cortical collecting tubules, suggesting that Ca^{2+}-mediated hypoxic cell death is not limited to the proximal tubules (53).

Ca^{2+} channel blockers have no effects on the rate of Ca^{2+} influx into normoxic proximal tubules. However, during hypoxia or anoxia in vitro, Ca^{2+} influx rate into tubules is increased above normal levels, and Ca^{2+} channel blockers reduce this rate to or toward normal (54). This is an important observation because cytosolic free Ca^{2+} could increase as the result of normal influx rates in the presence of reduced efflux rates secondary to decreased ATP-dependent Ca^{2+} ATPase or decreased Na^{+}/Ca^{2+} antiporter activity. The efficacy of Ca^{2+} channel blockers to prevent the increased Ca^{2+} influx rate during hypoxia and not during normoxia suggests a hypoxia-induced alteration in membrane permeability to Ca^{2+} that is sensitive to Ca^{2+} channel blockers. This permeability pathway appears to be sensitive, in part, to the decrease in ATP that occurs during hypoxia. For example, reduced ATP levels in rat proximal tubules with a phosphate-free incubation medium result in increased Ca^{2+} influx rate (55). This ATP-dependent change in Ca^{2+} permeability has not been examined in detail; however, acidosis prevents the increased Ca^{2+} influx rate in tubules and delays the onset of cell injury, as assessed by lactate dehydrogenase (LDH) release even though ATP remains at low levels (56). Cellular protection is also observed with an acidotic perfusate in the isolated perfused kidney (57). Intracellular acidosis is more likely to develop in complete anoxia than in hypoxia, and this may explain the only very short-lived increase in Ca^{2+} influx rate (54) as well as the absence of appreciable tissue Ca^{2+} overload during anoxia, as assessed by atomic absorption spectroscopy (58).

On the basis of these observations, the role of Ca^{2+} influx rate in mediating proximal tubule hypoxic injury was examined. By employing a combination of ethylene glycol tetraacetic acid (EGTA) and various Ca^{2+} concentrations in the tubule bathing medium (Ca^{2+}-modified Krebs buffer), a delay in the onset of cell injury during hypoxia was seen when extracellular Ca^{2+} concentration was $<10^{-5}$ M (48).

Thus, Ca^{2+} ions enter renal proximal tubules at a faster rate than normal during oxygen deprivation. The removal of extracellular Ca^{2+} ions or administration of Ca^{2+} channel buffers reduces the injury associated with this increased influx rate of Ca^{2+}. Acidosis also reduces Ca^{2+} influx rate (56) and exerts cytoprotective effects (55–58). Finally, if Ca^{2+} ions do enter hypoxic or anoxic cells, their deleterious effects can be mitigated by calmodulin inhibitors (53). Together, these data strongly suggest that it is the increased cytosolic or intracellular burden of Ca^{2+} that initiates the development of cell injury.

The level of the free cytosolic Ca^{2+} increase during ATP depletion in proximal tubules has been studied. Previously it was difficult to determine peak cytosolic Ca^{2+} levels using the high-affinity Ca^{2+} fluorophore Fura-2. The cytosolic free Ca^{2+} increases to $>100\ \mu$M in ATP-depleted proximal tubules using the low-affinity Ca^{2+} fluorophore Mag-Fura-2 (59). Experiments were done in the presence of 2 mM glycine, which approximates the physiologic concentration in vivo. Ninety-one percent of the tubules studied in an individual experiment had a free cytosolic Ca^{2+} that exceeded 10 μM. Thirty-five percent had levels $>500\ \mu$M with no cell membrane damage. In this study, proximal tubules had a remarkable resistance to the deleterious effects of increased Ca^{2+} during ATP depletion in the presence of glycine. In the isolated perfused rat kidney, intracellular Ca^{2+} increases have also been measured using 19^F NMR and 5^F BAPTA. In these studies, there was a partially reversible increase from 256 nM to 660 nM of Ca^{2+} (60,61).

The level of oxygen deprivation that is required to increase cytosolic Ca^{2+} has also been studied. A rise in cytosolic Ca^{2+} in anoxic but not hypoxic tubules was demonstrated (62). In hypoxic perfusion oxygen tension measured with a very sensitive electrode was 5 to 6 mm Hg. Complete anoxia was achieved with oxyrase in a nonperfused system. Ca^{2+} did not increase during hypoxia, but there was an increase in Ca^{2+} during anoxia. This increase paralleled the collapse in mitochondrial membrane potential as measured by rhodamine fluorescence. Because cell membrane damage occurred during both anoxia and hypoxia, it was concluded that an increase in cell Ca^{2+} is not always necessary for cell injury.

However, despite these studies, a crucial question remained to implicate Ca^{2+} as the primary factor in cell injury. Does the increase in cytosolic Ca^{2+} precede the injury, or is it a postlethal event? To answer this question, a videoimaging system was designed in which the rise in cytosolic Ca^{2+} as well as cell membrane injury could be simultaneously measured in freshly isolated proximal tubules (63). Cytosolic free Ca^{2+} $(Ca^{2+})i$ in freshly isolated proximal tubules, as assessed with Fura-2, increased significantly after 2 minutes of hypoxia and continued to increase progressively with continued hypoxia (51). This increase in $(Ca^{2+})i$ precedes the uptake by nuclei of the membrane-impermeable dye propidium iodide (PI) (51). PI staining is reduced when hypoxic rat proximal tubules are incubated either in a Ca^{2+}-free medium or with the intracellular Ca^{2+} chelator BAPTA (51). This study strongly supports the hypothesis that a cause-and-effect relationship exists between the elevation in $(Ca^{2+})i$ and the development of hypoxic membrane damage. Furthermore, this early rise in $(Ca^{2+})i$ after 5 to 10 minutes of hypoxia is reversible, since return to a well-oxygenated medium results in a prompt (1 minute) return of $(Ca^{2+})i$ to baseline level. If membrane injury had been the cause of the increase in $(Ca^{2+})i$, a return to basal levels would not have occurred with reoxygenation.

In support of a pathogenic role of Ca^{2+} in cell injury, it has been demonstrated that voltage-dependent Ca^{2+} channels are involved in cellular and mitochondrial accumulation of Ca^{2+} that follows ATP depletion and that voltage-dependent Ca^{2+} channels play an important role in regulating mitochondrial permeability transition, cytochrome c release, caspase activation, and apoptosis (64). In this study, in a rat renal proximal tubular cell line treated with antimycin A, ATP depletion–induced apoptosis was preceded by increased $[Ca^{2+}]i$ and mitochondrial Ca^{2+} before activation of mitochondrial signaling. Antagonizing L-type Ca^{2+} channels with azelnidipine administration ameliorated cellular and mitochondrial Ca^{2+} accumulation, mitochondrial permeability transition, cytochrome c release, caspase-9 activation, and resultant apoptosis.

MECHANISMS OF Ca^{2+}-INDUCED PROXIMAL TUBULAR INJURY

There is now compelling evidence that hypoxia-induced rise in cytosolic free Ca^{2+} activates Ca^{2+}-dependent intracellular events that mediate membrane injury. These potential Ca^{2+}-dependent mechanisms include changes in the actin cytoskeleton of proximal tubule microvilli, activation of PLA2, and activation of the calcium-dependent cysteine protease, calpain.

Ca^{2+}-Dependent Changes in the Actin Cytoskeleton

In the presence of ATP depletion, both Ca^{2+}-independent as well as Ca^{2+}-mediated processes can disrupt the actin cytoskeleton during acute hypoxic proximal tubule cell injury (65,66). To better define the role of Ca^{2+} in pathophysiologic alterations of the proximal tubule microvillus actin cytoskeleton, freshly isolated tubules were studied. The intracellular free Ca^{2+} was equilibrated with highly buffered, precisely defined medium Ca^{2+} levels using a combination of the metabolic inhibitor, antimycin, and the ionophore, ionomycin, in the presence of glycine, to prevent lethal membrane damage (67). Increases of Ca^{2+} to $>= 10$ micromolar were sufficient to initiate concurrent actin depolymerization, fragmentation of F-actin into forms requiring high-speed centrifugation for recovery, redistribution of villin to sedimentable fractions, and structural microvillar damage consisting of severe swelling and fragmentation of actin cores. These observations implicate Ca^{2+}-dependent, villin-mediated actin cytoskeletal disruption in hypoxic tubule cell microvillar damage.

Ca^{2+}-Dependent Activation of Phospholipase A$_2$

Phospholipase A$_2$ (PLA$_2$) hydrolyzes the acyl bond at the sn-2 position of phospholipids to generate free fatty acids and lysophospholipids. Free fatty acid release has been well documented in rat proximal tubules (68). This release is thought to be mediated to a large extent by activation of intracellular PLA$_2$ during hypoxia (69). It has been shown that both the messenger RNA (mRNA) for PLA$_2$ and the PLA$_2$ enzyme activity are increased in hypoxic rabbit tubules (70).

The mechanism of PLA$_2$-induced cell membrane damage is controversial. In proximal tubules hypoxia has been shown to cause an increase in free fatty acids, which was initially believed to contribute to cell injury (68). However, a recent study has shown that unsaturated free fatty acids protect against hypoxic injury in proximal tubules and that this protection may be mediated by negative feedback inhibition of PLA$_2$ activity (71).

There are various isoforms of PLA$_2$, and most isoforms of PLA$_2$ require Ca^{2+} for catalytic activity (72). The cytosolic form, cPLA$_2$, preferentially releases arachidonic acid from phospholipids and is regulated by changes in intracellular Ca^{2+} concentration (72).

PLA$_2$ enzymatic activity was measured in cell-free extracts prepared from rat renal proximal tubules (69). Both soluble and membrane-associated PLA$_2$ activity was detected. All PLA$_2$ activity detected during normoxia was Ca^{2+} dependent. Fractionation of cytosolic extracts by gel filtration revealed three peaks of PLA$_2$ activity. Exposure of tubules to hypoxia resulted in stable activation of soluble PLA$_2$ activity, which correlated with disappearance of the highest molecular mass form (>100 kDa) and appearance of a low-molecular-mass form (approximately 15 kDa) of PLA$_2$. Hypoxia also resulted in release of a low-molecular-mass form of PLA$_2$ into the extracellular medium. This study provides direct evidence for Ca^{2+}-dependent PLA$_2$ activation during hypoxia. However, Ca^{2+}-independent forms of PLA$_2$ have also been found to play a role in hypoxic proximal tubular injury (73).

cPLA$_2$-deficient mice have been developed. The cPLA$_2$ knockout mice have smaller infarcts and develop less brain edema and fewer neurologic deficits after transient middle cerebral artery ischemia (74,75).

There is evidence of an increased macula densa cell calcium concentration with a reduction in fluid load to the macula densa (76). An increase in macula densa cell calcium activates PLA$_2$ to release arachidonic acid, the rate-limiting step in the formation of prostaglandins like PGE$_2$. Adenosine also has an important function in the juxtaglomerular apparatus. It stimulates calcium release in afferent arteriolar smooth muscle cells, leading to contraction of the afferent arteriole as part of the tubuloglomerular feedback mechanism.

CYSTEINE PROTEASES

The cysteine proteases are a group of intracellular proteases that have a cysteine residue at their active site. The cysteine proteases consist of three major groups: cathepsins, calpains, and caspases. The cathepsins are non-Ca^{2+}-dependent lysosomal proteases that do not appear to play a role in the initiation of lethal cell injury (77–79). Calpain is a cytosolic Ca^{2+}-activated neutral protease. The caspases are a family of intracellular cysteine proteases. The term "caspase" embodies two properties of these proteases in which "c" refers to "cysteine" and "aspase" refers to their specific ability to cleave substrates after an aspartate residue. Caspases play a crucial role in inflammation and apoptotic cell death.

Calpain

Calpain is a cytosolic neutral cysteine protease that has an absolute dependence on Ca^{2+} for its activation (80). There are two major ubiquitous or conventional isoforms of calpain, the low Ca^{2+}-sensitive μ-calpain and the high Ca^{2+}-sensitive m-calpain (81,82). The isoenzymes have the same substrate specificity but differ in affinity for Ca^{2+}. Procalpain exists in the cytoplasm as an inactive proenzyme and becomes active proteolytically at the cell membrane only after it has become autolysed (83,84). The autolysed calpain is released either into the cytoplasm, where it hydrolyses substrate proteins, or it remains associated with the cell membrane and degrades cytoskeletal proteins involved in the interaction between the cell cytoskeleton and the plasma membrane. Activity of the autolyzed calpain is subject to a final regulation by a specific endogenous inhibitor called calpastatin (83,84). Calpain plays a role in platelet activation and aggregation (85), cytoskeleton and cell membrane organization (86,87), regulation of cell growth, differentiation and development (88–90), and pathologic states, including Alzheimer disease, aging, cataract, muscular dystrophy, sepsis, Wiskott–Aldrich syndrome, Chediak–Higashi syndrome, inflammation, arthritis, and malaria (91). Calpain 10 is a recently discovered mitochondrial calpain that plays a role in calcium-induced mitochondrial dysfunction (92).

The Ca^{2+}-dependent calpains have been shown to be mediators of hypoxic/ischemic injury to brain, liver, and heart (93–96). Calpain plays a role in hypoxic injury to rat renal proximal tubules (97–99). This role of calpain in proximal tubule injury has been confirmed in subsequent studies (100,101). The calpain inhibitors PD150606 and E-64 ameliorate the functional and histologic parameters in a rat model of ischemic AKI (102). Injection of a fragment of calpastatin, which inhibits calpain, protects against the functional and histologic changes in the kidney in a mouse model of AKI (103). In recent studies, it has been demonstrated that calpains increase epithelial cell mobility and play a critical role in tubule repair. In vitro, exposure of human tubular epithelial cells (HK-2 cells) to m-calpain reduced adhesion of HK-2 cells to extracellular matrix and increased their mobility. In a murine model of ischemic AKI, injection of a fragment of calpastatin, which specifically blocked calpain activity, delayed tubule repair and increased the worsening of kidney function and histologic lesions after 24 and 48 hours of reperfusion.

Caspases

Caspases are Ca^{2+}-independent cysteine proteases. There are now 14 members of the caspase family, caspases 1–14. Caspase-14 has recently been characterized and found to be present in embryonic tissues but absent from adult tissues (104). Caspases share a predilection for cleavage of their substrates after an aspartate residue at P1 (105,106). The members of the caspase family can be divided into three subfamilies on the basis of substrate specificity and function (107). The peptide preferences and function within each group are remarkably similar (107). Members of group 1 (of which caspase-1 is the most important) prefer the tetrapeptide sequences WEHD and YVAD. This specificity is similar to the activation sequence of caspase-1, suggesting that caspase-1 may employ an autocatalytic mechanism of activation. Caspase-1 (previously known as interleukin-1 [IL-1] converting enzyme, or ICE) plays a major role in the activation of proinflammatory cytokines. Caspase-1 is remarkably specific for the precursors of IL-1 and IL-18 (interferon-γ-inducing factor), making a single initial cut in each procytokine that activates them and allows exit from the cytosol (108,109). Group III "initiator" caspase-8 and caspase-9 prefer the sequence (L/V)EXD. This recognition motif resembles activation sites within the "executioner" caspase proenzymes, implicating this group as upstream components in the proteolytic cascade that serve to amplify the death signal. These "initiator" caspases pronounce the death sentence. They are activated in response to signals indicating that the cell has been stressed or damaged or has received an order to die. They clip and activate another family of caspases, the "executioners." The optimal peptide sequence motif for group II, or "executioner caspases" (of which caspase-3 is the most important), is DEXD (107,110,111). This optimal recognition motif is identical to proteins that are cleaved during cell death.

There are two major pathways of caspase-mediated apoptosis (112). In the mitochondrial or "intrinsic" pathway, stress-induced signals affect the balance between pro- and antiapoptotic Bcl-2 family proteins to cause cytochrome c release from mitochondria. Caspase-2 is a recently discovered caspase that is a crucial initiator of the mitochondrial apoptosis pathway (113). Activation and increased activity of caspase-2 is required for the permeabilization of mitochondria and release of cytochrome c (113). Cytochrome c binds to the cytosolic protein, apoptosis protease-activating factor-1 (APAF-1), which recruits and activates caspase-9. Active caspase-9 in turn recruits and activates the "executioners" procaspase-3 and procaspase-7. In the "extrinsic" pathway, the binding of a ligand to its death receptor recruits an adaptor protein that in turn recruits and activates procaspase-8. For example, Fas ligand (FasL) binds to its death receptor Fas that recruits an adaptor protein called Fas-associated death domain (FADD). FADD in turn recruits and activates procaspase-8.

The caspase pathways that are centrally important in cell death involve the "initiator" caspase-8 and caspase-9 and the "executioner" caspase-3 (114). The central role of these caspases is supported by caspase-8, caspase-9, and caspase-3 ($-/-$) mice that have strong phenotypes based on cell death defects, developmental defects, and usually fetal/perinatal mortality. The critical role of "initiator" caspases is illustrated in caspase-9 ($-/-$) mice that demonstrate the absence of downstream caspase-3 activation (115). Activation of caspase-1, caspase-8, caspase-9, and caspase-3 has been widely described in hypoxic renal epithelial cells and cerebral ischemia (27,116,117). Caspase-1 may also cause cell injury by activation of the proinflammatory cytokines IL-1 and IL-18 (109). To establish a direct pathogenic role of specific caspases in this well-established cascade, knockout mice have been used. Caspase-1 ($-/-$) mice are protected against cerebral ischemia (118). Caspase-3 ($-/-$) mice are protected against Fas-mediated fulminant hepatitis (119).

For many years it was not known how caspase-1 was activated. It has recently been discovered that procaspase-1 is activated in a complex called the inflammasome (120,121). The inflammasome is a protein scaffold that contains pyrin domain-containing protein (NALP) proteins, an adaptor protein apoptosis-associated speck-like protein containing a caspase-recruiting domain (CARD) (ASC), procaspase-1, and caspase-5. The interaction of the CARD of procaspase-1 is mediated by the CARD of ASC and the CARD present in the C-terminus of NALP-1. Active caspase-1 in the inflammasome is a regulator of the "unconventional" protein secretion of "leaderless" proteins like IL-33, IL-1α, and fibroblast growth factor (FGF)-2 (122). IL-33 is an IL-1-like cytokine that signals via the IL-1 receptor-related protein ST2 and induces T helper type-2 associated cytokines like IL-4, IL-5, and IL-13 that can lead to pathologic changes in mucosal organs (123). IL-1α is increased in the kidney in mice in endotoxemic AKI (124) and cisplatin-induced AKI (125).

Caspases participate in two distinct signaling pathways, (a) activation of proinflammatory cytokines and (b) promotion of apoptotic cell death (105,111,126,127). While caspases play a crucial and extensively studied role in apoptosis, there is now considerable evidence that the caspase pathway may also be involved in necrotic cell death (128). Caspases and calpain are independent mediators of cisplatin-induced endothelial cell necrosis (129). Caspase inhibition has been demonstrated to reduce ischemic and excitotoxic neuronal damage (118,130,131). Moreover, mice deficient in caspase-1 demonstrate reduced ischemic brain injury produced by occlusion of the middle cerebral artery (117;118;132). Inhibition of caspases also protects against necrotic cell death induced by the mitochondrial inhibitor antimycin A in PC12 cells, Hep G2 cells, and renal tubules in culture (133,134). Caspases are also involved in hypoxic and reperfusion injury in cultured endothelial cells (135). Rat kidneys subjected to ischemia demonstrate an increase in both caspase-1 and caspase-3 mRNA and protein expression (24).

An assay for caspases in freshly isolated rat proximal tubules using the fluorescent substrate Ac-Tyr-Val-Ala-Asp-7-amido-4-methyl coumarin (Ac-YVAD-AMC) was developed (136). Freshly isolated proximal tubules were preincubated with the caspase inhibitor z-Asp-2, 6-dichlorobenzoyloxymethylketone (Z-D-DCB) for 10 minutes before being exposed to hypoxia. Tubular caspase activity was increased after 15-minute hypoxia in association with increased cell membrane damage as assessed by LDH release. Z-D-DCB attenuated the increase in caspase activity during 15-minute hypoxia and markedly decreased LDH release in a dose-dependent fashion. The fluorescent substrate Ac-DEVD-AMC, which is cleaved by caspase-3, was also used. Caspase activity was measured in normoxic and hypoxic tubules with both caspase-1 and caspase-3 substrates. Significant fluorescent activity was detected with Ac-YVAD-AMC (caspase-1 substrate) compared with Ac-DEVD-AMC (caspase-3 substrate), suggesting that caspases-1 is predominantly involved in hypoxic injury. In another study, the deleterious effect of caspase-1 on proximal tubules in vitro in the absence of inflammatory cells and vascular effects was demonstrated (137).

Caspase-1-Mediated Production of Interleukin-18

To establish a pathogenic role of caspase-1 in cell injury, caspase-1-deficient $(-/-)$ mice have been used. These caspase-1 $(-/-)$ mice have a defect in production of mature IL-1β and IL-18 and are protected against lethal endotoxemia (132,138). The fact that IL-1β $(-/-)$ mice are not protected against endotoxemia (139) suggests a potential role of IL-18 in the lethal outcome during sepsis. Moreover, in ischemic AKI, IL-1 receptor knockout mice or mice treated with IL-1 receptor antagonist (IL-1Ra) are not protected against ischemic AKI (140). Taken together, therefore, these previous studies suggest that IL-18 may be a potential mediator of ischemic AKI.

Since caspase-1 activates IL-18, lack of mature IL-18 might protect these caspase-1 $(-/-)$ mice from AKI. Thus it was determined whether mice deficient in the proinflammatory caspase-1, which cleaves precursors of IL-1 beta and IL-18, were protected against ischemic AKI (141). Caspase-1 $(-/-)$ mice developed less ischemic AKI as judged by renal function and renal histology. These animals had significantly reduced blood urea nitrogen (BUN) and serum creatinine levels and a lower morphologic tubular necrosis score than did wild-type mice with ischemic AKI. In wild-type animals with ischemic AKI, kidney IL-18 levels more than double and there is a conversion of the IL-18 precursor to the mature form. This conversion was not observed in caspase-1 $(-/-)$ AKI mice or sham-operated controls. Wild-type mice were then injected with IL-18-neutralizing antiserum before the ischemic insult, and there was a similar degree of protection from AKI as seen in caspase-1 $(-/-)$ mice. In addition, there was a fivefold increase in myeloperoxidase activity, as an index of leukocyte infiltration, in control mice with AKI but no such increase in caspase-1 $(-/-)$ or IL-18 antiserum-treated mice. Caspase-1 $(-/-)$ mice also show decreased neutrophil infiltration, suggesting that the deleterious role of IL-18 in ischemic AKI may be due to increased neutrophil infiltration.

IL-18 function is neutralized in IL-18-binding protein transgenic (IL-18BP Tg) mice. It was determined whether IL-18BP Tg mice are protected against ischemic acute kidney injury (AKI) (142). IL-18BP Tg mice were functionally and histologically protected against ischemic AKI, as determined by the BUN, serum creatinine, and ATN score. The number of macrophages was significantly reduced in IL-18BP Tg compared with wild-type kidneys. Multiple chemokines/cytokines were measured using flow cytometry–based assays. Only CXCL1 (also known as KC or IL-8) was significantly increased in AKI versus sham kidneys and significantly reduced in IL-18BP Tg AKI versus wild-type AKI kidneys. This study demonstrates that protection against ischemic AKI in IL-18BP Tg mice is associated with less macrophage infiltration and less production of CXCL1 in the kidney.

It was determined whether macrophages are a source of injurious IL-18 in ischemic AKI in mice (143). On immunofluorescence staining of the outer strip of the outer medulla, the number of macrophages staining for IL-18 was significantly increased in AKI and significantly decreased by macrophage depletion using tail vein injection of liposomal-encapsulated clodronate (LEC). Adoptive transfer of RAW 264.7 cells, a mouse macrophage line that constitutively expresses IL-18 mRNA, or mouse peritoneal macrophages deficient in IL-18 reversed the functional protection against AKI in LEC-treated mice. In summary, adoptive transfer of RAW cells, that constitutively express IL-18, reverses the functional protection in macrophage-depleted wild-type mice with AKI. In addition, adoptive transfer of peritoneal macrophages in which IL-18 function was inhibited also reverses the functional protection in macrophage-depleted mice, suggesting that IL-18 from adoptive transfer of macrophages is not sufficient to cause ischemic AKI. Possible sources of injurious IL-18 in AKI include the proximal tubule and lymphocytes. In this regard, freshly isolated proximal tubules from mice release IL-18 into the medium when exposed to hypoxia, and proximal tubukles from caspase-1-deficient mice are protected against hypoxic injury (137).

Caspase-1-deficient $(-/-)$ mice are protected against sepsis-induced hypotension and mortality. The role of caspase-1 and its associated cytokines was investigated in a nonhypotensive model of endotoxemic AKI. In mice with endotoxemic AKI, the GFR was significantly higher in caspase-1 $(-/-)$ versus wild-type mice at 16 and 36 hours. IL-1β and IL-18 protein were significantly increased in the kidneys of mice with endotoxemic AKI versus vehicle-treated mice. However, inhibition of IL-1β with IL-1 receptor antagonist (IL-1Ra), or inhibition of IL-18 with IL-18-neutralizing antiserum-treated or combination therapy with IL-1Ra plus IL-18-neutralizing antiserum did not improve the GFR in mice with endotoxemic AKI, suggesting that neither IL-1β nor IL-18 is the mediator on endotoxemic AKI (124).

Interaction Between Calpain and Caspases in Hypoxic/Ischemic Proximal Tubular Injury

Studies suggest that both calpain and caspases play a role in hypoxia-induced cell membrane damage in proximal tubules (24,97,99,133,136). A prelethal increase in cytosolic Ca^{2+} is a cardinal feature of the hypoxic proximal tubule model (51). How are the non-Ca^{2+}-dependent caspases activated during hypoxia? There are two possibilities. Caspase activation may be downstream of Ca^{2+}-mediated activation of calpain, or caspases may be activated in a separate pathway independent of Ca^{2+}. Since an interaction between caspases and calpains during cell injury has been suggested (132), the effect of the specific calpain inhibitor (2)-3-(4-iodophenyl)-2-mercapto-2-propenoic acid (PD150606) on the hypoxia-induced increase in caspase activity in proximal tubules was studied (136). PD150606 inhibited calpain activity and protects against hypoxic injury in rat proximal tubules (98). PD150606 also attenuated the hypoxia-induced increase in caspase activity. However, PD150606 did not inhibit the activity of purified caspase-1 in vitro, suggesting that calpain may be upstream of caspases during hypoxic proximal tubular injury. Next the effect of caspase inhibition on calpain activity was determined (136). The specific caspase inhibitor Z-D-DCB attenuated the hypoxia-induced increase in calpain activity in proximal tubules. However, Z-D-DCB did not inhibit the activity of purified calpain in vitro.

In summary, these data suggest that both caspase-mediated activation of calpain and calpain-mediated activation of caspases occur during hypoxic proximal tubular injury. These data are supported by other studies that demonstrate simultaneous activation of both calpain and caspases during cell death (144). Thus, it is possible that during hypoxic proximal tubule injury, there are different proteolytic pathways involving different caspases and calpains.

The interaction between calpain and caspases during ischemic AKI in vivo was investigated (145). An increase in the activity of calpain, as determined by (a) the appearance of calpain-mediated spectrin breakdown products and (b) the conversion of procalpain to active calpain, was demonstrated. Since intracellular calpain activity is regulated by its endogenous inhibitor, calpastatin, the effect of ischemia on calpastatin was determined. On immunoblot of renal cortex, there was a decrease of a low-molecular-weight (LMW) form of calpastatin during ischemic AKI compared to sham-operated controls. Calpastatin activity was also significantly decreased compared to sham-operated rats, indicating that the decreased protein expression had functional significance. In rats treated with the caspase inhibitor Z-D-DCB, the decrease in both calpastatin activity and protein expression was normalized, suggesting that caspases may be proteolyzing calpastatin. Caspase-3 activity increased significantly after ischemia-reperfusion compared to sham-operated rats and was attenuated in ischemic kidneys from rats treated with the caspase inhibitor. In summary, during ischemic AKI there is (a) calpain activation associated with downregulation of calpastatin protein and decreased calpastatin activity and (b) activation of caspase-3. In addition, in vivo caspase inhibition reverses the decrease in calpastatin activity. The proposed relationship between calpain and caspases in hypoxic/ischemic injury is shown in Figure 10.2 (136,141,146).

ROLE OF NITRIC OXIDE IN HYPOXIA/ISCHEMIA-INDUCED PROXIMAL TUBULE INJURY

Nitric oxide (NO) is a messenger molecule mediating diverse functions, including vasodilatation, neurotransmission, and antimicrobial and antitumor activities (147). A variety of cells produce NO via oxidation of L-arginine by the enzyme nitric oxide synthase (NOS) (148). Thus far, four distinct NOS isoforms have been isolated, purified, and cloned: neuronal, endothelial, macrophage, and vascular smooth muscle cell (VSMC)/hepatocyte (149,150). Identification of the specific isoform of NOS is important because the four isoforms vary in subcellular location, amino acid sequence, regulation, and hence functional roles. Neuronal and endothelial NOS (eNOS) are continuously present and thus are termed constitutive NOS (cNOS) (150). NO is produced by these enzymes when Ca^{2+}/calmodulin interaction permits electron transfer from NADPH via flavin groups within the enzyme to a hemecontaining active site (151). This activation is very short lived. In contrast, VSMC/hepatocyte and macrophage

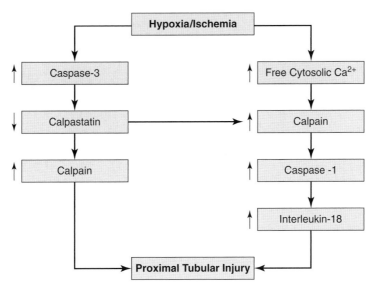

■ **Figure 10.2** Hypoxic/ischemic proximal tubular necrosis results in activation of cysteine protease pathways involving calpains and both caspase-1 and caspase-3 (146). There is increased activity of calpain (97–99) and caspase-1 (136) in hypoxic proximal tubular injury. During ischemic AKI there is early calpain activation associated with downregulation of calpastatin protein, decreased calpastatin activity and activation of caspase-3 (145). Also impaired IL-18 processing protects caspase-1 deficient mice from ischemic AKI (141).

isoforms are only expressed when the cells have been induced by certain cytokines, microbes, and microbial products and are therefore called inducible NOS (iNOS) (152). iNOS expression results in sustained production of NO. Unlike cNOS, iNOS activity is believed to be insensitive to changes in intracellular Ca^{2+}, since calmodulin is tightly bound to the molecule. Once synthesized, iNOS remains tonically activated, producing NO continuously for the life of the enzyme (153).

Both cNOS and iNOS isoforms have been identified in the kidney, specifically in macula densa cells (cNOS), inner medullary collecting ducts (cNOS and iNOS), and proximal tubules (cNOS and iNOS) (150,154). In the kidney, physiologic amounts of NO play an important role in hemodynamic regulation and salt and water excretion (155).

It has been demonstrated that NOS activity is increased during hypoxia in freshly isolated rat proximal tubules. In this study, membrane damage, as assessed by LDH release into the medium, was prevented by both a nonselective NOS inhibitor (L-NAME) and a NO scavenger (hemoglobin) (156). In a separate study, hypoxia stimulated prompt and sustained NO release in the proximal tubule suspension as assessed by a NO-selective sensing electrode (157). NO concentration remained unmeasurable during normoxia. L-NAME completely inhibited hypoxia-induced NO release in parallel with marked cytoprotection. Further studies in freshly isolated proximal tubules from knockout mice have also been revealing about the role of NO in hypoxic/ischemic tubular injury. Hypoxia-induced proximal tubule damage, as assessed by LDH release, was no different between wild-type mice in which eNOS and nNOS were "knocked out." However, proximal tubules from the iNOS knockout mice demonstrated resistance to the same degree of hypoxia (158).

In vivo, targeting of iNOS with oligodeoxynucleotides protects the rat kidney against ischemic AKI (159). This study provided direct evidence for the cytotoxic effects of NO produced via iNOS in the course of ischemic AKI. Augmented expression of iNOS and the prevalence of nitrotyrosine residues in kidneys have been demonstrated in osteopontin-deficient mice versus wild-type counterparts (160). Animals with the disrupted osteopontin gene exhibited ischemia-induced renal dysfunction and structural damage, which was twice as pronounced as that observed in mice with the intact osteopontin response to stress, also suggesting a role of iNOS in ischemic AKI. iNOS-deficient mice also have less renal failure and better survival than the wild-type mice after renal artery clamping (161). An induction of heat shock protein (HSP) was also observed in the iNOS knockout mice as a potential contributor to the protection.

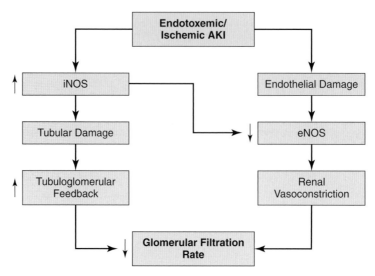

■ **Figure 10.3** Proposed imbalance of NO production in ischemic/septic AKI. In ischemic AKI, increased NO derived from iNOS is damaging to proximal tubules (158,159,161). In ischemic AKI, renal endothelial damage results in decreased NO derived from eNOS (25). In endotoxemic AKI, increased iNOS activity decreases eNOS activity possibly via NO autoinhibition (346) The nonselective NOS inhibitor, L-NAME, worsens ischemic and endotoxemic AKI due to an overriding blocking effect on eNOS.

In a renal artery clamp model in mice in which alpha melanocyte-stimulating hormone (α MSH) was shown to block the induction of iNOS, there was decreased neutrophil infiltration and functional and histologic protection (162). A subsequent study examined the relative importance of α MSH on the neutrophil pathway by examining the effects of α MSH in ICAM-1 knockout mice and the neutrophil-independent isolated perfused kidneys (163,164). In this study it was found that α MSH decreases renal injury when neutrophil effects are minimal or absent, indicating that α MSH inhibits neutrophil-independent pathways of renal injury.

Interestingly, however, L-NAME administration to the rat kidney clamp model actually worsens ischemic and endotoxemic AKI (159). This result was interpreted as an overriding blocking effect of eNOS activity with the nonspecific effects of L-NAME (25). This would worsen the renal vasoconstriction and resultant injury, thus obscuring any salutary effect at the level of the proximal tubule (165). Thus, opposing abnormalities in NO production within the endothelial and tubular compartments of the kidney may contribute to renal injury (25) (Fig. 10.3). Reduced eNOS-derived NO production causes vasoconstriction and worsens ischemia; increased iNOS-derived NO production by tubular cells adds to the injurious effects of ischemia on these cells. Therapeutic interventions to modulate NO production in ischemic AKI may require selective modulation of different NOS isoforms in the tubular and vascular compartments of the kidney (166).

MATRIX METALLOPROTEINASES

Matrix metalloproteinases (MMP) play a crucial role in remodeling of the extracellular matrix, which is an important physiologic feature of normal growth and development. In the kidney, interstitial sclerosis and glomerulosclerosis have been associated with an imbalance of extracellular matrix synthesis and degradation (167). Alterations in renal tubular basement membrane matrix proteins, laminin and fibronectin, occur after renal ischemia-reperfusion injury (168).

Meprin A is a zinc-dependent metalloendopeptidase that is present in the brush border membrane of renal proximal tubular epithelial cells. The redistribution of this metalloendopeptidase to the basolateral membrane domain during AKI results in degradation of the extracellular matrix and damage to adjacent peritubular structures. The effect of meprin A, the major matrix-degrading metalloproteinase in rat kidney, on the laminin–nidogen complex was examined. Following ischemic injury, meprin A undergoes redistribution and/or adherence to the tubular basement membrane. Nidogen-1 (entactin), which acts as a bridge between the extracellular matrix molecules, laminin-1 and type IV collagen breakdown products, is produced as the result of partial degradation of tubular basement membrane by meprin A following renal tubular ischemia-reperfusion injury (169).

Inbred strains of mice with normal and low meprin A activity have been studied (170). The strains of mice with normal meprin A developed more severe renal functional and structural injury following renal ischemia or the injection of hypertonic glycerol compared with the two low-meprin A strains. These findings suggest that meprin A plays a role in the pathophysiology of AKI following ischemic and nephrotoxic AKI (170).

The disruption of cadherin/catenin complexes in AKI may be associated with the transtubular back-leak of glomerular filtrate. In endothelial cells isolated from ischemic kidneys, the proteolytic activity of proMMP-2, proMMP-9, and MMP-9 was increased. Occludin, an in vivo MMP-9 substrate, was partly degraded in the endothelial fractions during ischemia, suggesting that the upregulation of MMP-9 was functional. These data suggest that AKI leads to the degradation of the vascular basement membrane and to increased permeability related to the increase of MMP-9 (171). In renal cells, in vitro cleavage of cadherins in normal rat kidney (NRK) cells requires active membrane-type (MT)1-MMP (MT1-MMP), also known as MMP-14 (172). In contrast to the potential injurious role of some MMPs, MMP9 protects the S3 segment of the proximal tubule and the intercalated cells of the collecting duct from apoptosis in AKI, most likely by releasing soluble stem cell factor (sSCF), an MMP9 substrate (173).

HEAT SHOCK PROTEINS

HSPs protect cells from environmental stress damage by binding to partially denatured proteins and dissociating protein aggregates to regulate the correct folding and to cooperate in transporting newly synthesized polypeptides to the target organelles (174). Stresses that trigger the heat shock response include hyperthermia, hypothermia, generation of oxygen radicals, hypoxia/ischemia, and toxins (175).

HSPs are identified by their molecular weight. The most important families include proteins of 90, 70, 60, and 27 kDa (175). The HSP 70 family includes proteins that are both constitutively expressed and induced by stress. They are the most highly induced proteins by stress and function as chaperones binding to unfolded or misfolded proteins.

Renal ischemia results in both a profound fall in cellular ATP and a rapid induction of HSP-70 (176,177). It has been demonstrated that a 50% reduction in cellular ATP in the renal cortex during ischemia must occur before the stress response is detectable. Reduction of ATP below 25% control levels produces a more vigorous response. Reperfusion is not required for initiation of a heat shock response in the kidney (178).

In vitro studies have demonstrated that HSP induction protects cultured renal epithelial cells from injury. It has been determined that prior heat stress protects cultured opossum kidney (OK) cells from injury mediated by ATP depletion (179). Also HSP 70 overexpression is sufficient to protect LLC- PK1 proximal tubular cells from hyperthermia but is not sufficient for protection from hypoxia (180).

The effect of HSP induction by hyperthermia on ischemic AKI has been studied. One study found that prior heat shock protected kidneys against warm ischemia (181). In another study, prior induction of HSP by hyperthermia was not protective against the functional and morphologic parameters of ischemic AKI in ischemia reflow in intact rats or medullary hypoxic injury (182). These variable results may be explained by the complexity of the intact animal compared with cultured cells; the degree, duration, and timing of the hyperthermic stimulus; and the differential response of mature and immature kidneys (183,184).

The mechanism of HSP protection against ischemic AKI is evolving. It has been demonstrated that HSPs participate in the postischemic restructuring of the cytoskeleton of proximal tubules (185). HSP 72 complexes with aggregated cellular proteins in an ATP- dependent manner, suggesting that enhancing HSP 72 function after ischemic renal injury assists refolding and stabilization of Na^+/K^+ ATPase or aggregated elements of the cytoskeleton, allowing reassembly into a more organized state (186). Another study suggested that there are specific interactions between HSP 25 and actin during the early postischemic reorganization of the cytoskeleton (187).

Another potential mechanism of HSP protection against proximal tubular injury is the inhibition of apoptosis. OK proximal tubule cells exposed to ATP depletion develop apoptosis, and prior heat stress reduced the number of apoptotic cells and improved cell survival compared with controls (188).

APOPTOSIS

Apoptosis is a physiologic form of cell death that occurs in a programmed pattern and can be triggered by external stimuli (189). The triggers of apoptosis include (a) cell injury, for example, ischemia, hypoxia, oxidant injury, NO, and cisplatinum; (b) loss of survival factors, for example, deficiency of renal growth factors, impaired cell-to-cell or cell-to-matrix adhesion; and (c) receptor-mediated apoptosis, for example, Fas (CD 95) and TGF-beta (190).

Apoptosis has been demonstrated in cultured proximal and distal tubules exposed to hypoxia and chemical ATP depletion (188,191–193,116). A feature of these in vitro studies is that severe or prolonged ATP depletion leads to necrosis, while milder and shorter ATP depletion leads to apoptotic cell death (116). Apoptosis has been demonstrated in distal and proximal tubules during both the early phases and the recovery phase of ischemic AKI in rats and mice (27–29,194–204). The role that apoptosis of proximal and distal tubular cells plays in the loss of renal function and the recovery phase of ischemic AKI, as well as the relationship between apoptosis and necrosis in ischemic AKI, still needs to be elucidated (190,205,206).

Cisplatin is a commonly used chemotherapeutic agent that causes apoptosis or necrosis of renal tubular epithelial cells in vitro. After cisplatin injection in mice, renal apoptosis peaks on day 2, which precedes the peak in serum creatinine, ATN scores, and neutrophil counts, which peak on day 3. Renal dysfunction, apoptosis, ATN scores, and neutrophil infiltration were all reduced in the caspase-1 $(-/-)$ mice treated with cisplatin. Active caspase-3 was also reduced in caspase-1 $(-/-)$ mice (207). This study confirms the injurious role of caspases and apoptosis in cisplatin-induced AKI.

Erythropoietin (EPO) is upregulated by hypoxia. EPO receptors are expressed in many tissues, including renal tubules. Multiple animal studies have shown that EPO is protective against AKI, and the protective effect may be related to inhibition of caspases and apoptosis (Table 10.3). In a cisplatin-induced AKI model in the rat, functional recovery was significantly improved in animals that received

TABLE 10.3 ERYTHROPOEITIN PROTECTS AGAINST AKI

Model	Mechanism	Reference
Cisplatin-induced AKI in rats	Increased tubular regeneration	(208)
Ischemic AKI in rats	Functional protection Less apoptosis	(209)
Ischemic AKI in rats	Decreased apoptosis Increased tubular cell regeneration	(210)
Rat AKI	Functional protection Decreased caspase-3, caspase-8, and caspase-9 Less apoptosis	(215)
Proximal tubules exposed to oxidative stress	Decreased caspase-3 and cell death	(215)
Tubular cells exposed to iohexol	Decreased activation of caspase-3 and caspase-8 Less apoptosis	(213)
Hemorrhagic shock in rats	Less AKI Less liver injury Decreased caspase-3, caspase-8, and caspase-9	(216)
Ishemic AKI in rats	Prevented downregulation of renal sodium transporters and aquaporins	(214)
Cyclosporin nephrotoxicty in rats	Less inflammation Less interststial fibrosis	(211)
Contrast nephropathy in rats	Less AKI	(212)
Endotoxemic AKI in mice	Decreased superoxide dismutase Less renal dysfunction	(217)

AKI, acute kidney injury.

EPO compared with controls, and the enhanced recovery was secondary to increased regeneration of tubules, as shown by increased uptake of radioactive thymidine (208). In another study, rats that were pretreated with EPO before induction of ischemic AKI had a lower serum creatinine and decreased apoptosis compared with controls (209). In both in vivo and in vitro models of tubular injury, EPO provided protection from ischemia-reperfusion injury by inhibiting apoptosis and increasing tubular cell regeneration (210). EPO was shown to be protective against interstitial fibrosis and inflammation in a rat model of cyclosporine nephrotoxicity (211). EPO prevents the decrease in the GFR in a rat model of contrast nephropathy (212). Kolyada et al. demonstrated that EPO decreased iohexol-induced activation of caspase-3 and caspase-8 and subsequent apoptosis in renal tubular epithelial cells (213). EPO and/or α-MSH treatment significantly prevented urinary-concentrating defects and downregulation of renal AQPs and sodium transporters in ischemic AKI in rats (214). EPO (300 U/kg) reduced tubular injury, prevented caspase-3, caspase-8, and caspase-9 activation, and reduced apoptotic cell death in vivo in mice (215). In human proximal tubule epithelial cells in vitro, EPO reduced DNA fragmentation, prevented caspase-3 activation, and attenuated cell death in response to oxidative stress (215). In a rat model of hemorrhagic shock, administration of EPO before resuscitation reduced the increase in the activities of caspase-3, caspase-8, and caspase-9 and prevented renal dysfunction and liver injury (216). In a model of endotoxemia-induced AKI in mice, EPO significantly decreased renal superoxide dismutase and attenuated the renal dysfunction as assessed by insulin-GFR (217).

ALTERED GENE EXPRESSION

Immediate early genes and protooncogenes are induced during the early reperfusion period after renal ischemia (218). There is c-fos and c-jun activation as well as an increase in DNA synthesis (219). There is accumulation of early growth response factor-1 (Egr-1) and c-fos mRNAs in the mouse kidney after occlusion of the renal artery and reperfusion (220,221). Transient expression of the genes c-fos and Egr-1 may code for DNA-binding transcription factors and initiate the transcription of other genes necessary for cell division (222). JE and KC, growth-factor-responsive genes with cytokine-like properties that play a role in inflammation, are also expressed during early renal ischemia (223). These genes may code for proteins with chemotactic effects that can attract monocytes and neutrophils into areas of injury (221). Studies demonstrate that c-fos and c-jun are expressed following renal ischemia as a typical immediate early gene response, but they are expressed in cells that do not enter the cell cycle (224,225). The failure of the cells to enter the cell cycle may depend on the coexpression of other genes.

The pathways that lead to the early gene response are interesting. At least two quite different pathways lead to the activation of c-jun (226–228). Growth factors activate c-jun via the mitogen-activated protein kinases (MAPKs), which include extracellular regulated kinases (ERKs) 1 and 2. This pathway is proliferative in nature. In contrast, the stress-activated protein kinase (SAPK) pathway is separate from the MAPK pathway. These kinases include c-Jun N-terminal kinase (JNK) 1 and 2. Activation and the effect on cell fate of the SAPK pathway are very different from the MAPK pathway. The SAPK pathway is essentially antiproliferative and can lead to either cell survival or cell death. During renal ischemia, SAPKs are activated, and inhibition of SAPKs after ischemia protects against renal failure (229,230). Thus, it is possible that manipulation of this pathway could lead to therapies that may ameliorate AKI. Also, exploration of the early gene response in renal ischemia using DNA microarrays and other genome-scale technologies should extend our knowledge of gene function and molecular biology (231).

Microarray analysis of kidney has given clues to the pathogenesis of AKI (231,232). There was an increase in genes involved in cell structure, extracellular matrix, intracellular calcium binding, and cell division/differentiation in kidneys from mice with AKI (233). In another study in mice with AKI, transcription factors, growth factors, signal transduction molecules, and apoptotic factors demonstrated consistent patterns of altered gene expression in the first 24 hours of postischemic reperfusion (234). In rats with AKI, microarray analysis demonstrated that nine genes were upregulated in the early phase (ADAM2, HO-1, UCP-2, and thymosin β4) and established phase (clusterin, vanin1, fibronectin, heat-responsive protein 12, and FK506) (235). Nine genes were downregulated in the early phase (glutamine synthetase, cytochrome p450 IId6, and cyp 2d9) and established phase (cyp 4a14, Xist gene, PPARγ, α-albumin, uromodulin, and ADH B2) Laser capture microdissection of immunofluorescently defined cells (IF-LCM) can isolate pure populations of targeted cells from the kidney for microarray analysis (236). This technique has been used to label and isolate thick ascending limb cells in the kidney for mRNA analysis (236).

HYPOXIA-INDUCIBLE FACTOR-1 α

Hypoxia-inducible factor-1 (HIF-1) α is an important molecule for the adaptation of cells to low oxygen or hypoxia. Systemic hypoxia, anemia, renal ischemia, or cobalt chloride results in an increase in HIF-1 α in renal tubules (237). HIF-1 α activation with carbon monoxide protects against ischemic (238) and cisplatin-induced (239) AKI. HIF-1 α heterozygous deficient mice have worse AKI compared with control mice (240). Treatment of mice with l-mimosine and dimethyloxalylglycine (DMOG), agents that activate HIF-1 α by inhibiting HIF hydroxylases, protects against ischemic AKI in mice (240). Pharmacologic agents that induce HIF-1 α may in the future be a potential therapy for AKI.

TUBULAR OBSTRUCTION IN RENAL CELL INJURY

Increased excretion of tubular epithelial casts is a hallmark of recovery from AKI (183). The presence of tubular casts on renal biopsy as well as urinary casts has provided morphologic support for a role of tubular obstruction due to intraluminal cast formation in the pathogenesis of ischemic AKI (241). Finn and Gottschalk using micropuncture techniques during saline loading demonstrated clear evidence of increased tubular pressures in postischemic compared with normal kidneys (242). Renal vasodilation to restore renal blood flow also demonstrated increased tubular pressures in ischemic AKI in the rat. Tanner et al. (243) found that perfusing the proximal tubule with artificial tubular fluid at a rate that did not increase tubule pressure in normal animals increased tubule pressures in animals after a renal ischemic insult. Moreover, venting those obstructed tubules led to improved nephron filtration rates. Burke et al. also demonstrated that prevention of ischemic AKI in dogs with mannitol led to a decrease in intratubular pressures, suggesting that the induced-solute diuresis led to relief of cast-mediated tubular obstruction (244).

While it is clear that brush border membranes, necrotic cells, viable cells, and perhaps apoptotic tubular epithelial cells enter tubular fluid after an acute renal ischemic insult, the actual process and predominant location of the cast formation is, however, less clear. In AKI, distal tubules are obstructed by casts formed by tubular debris, cells, and Tamm–Horsfall protein (THP) (241). Since there are arginine–glycine–aspartic acid (RGD) adhesive sequences in human THP, there may be direct integrin-mediated binding of tubular cells to THP. Alternatively, polymerization of THP may result in entrapment of the cells in its gel. Adhesion of LLC-PK(1) cells to THP-coated wells was directly measured, and THP concentrate was dissolved in solutions of high electrolyte concentration that mimic urine from AKI and collecting ducts (245). LLC-PK(1) cells did not directly adhere to THP, a finding against integrin-mediated binding as a mechanism for in vivo tubular cell/THP cast formation. The high electrolyte concentration of AKI solutions was associated with THP gel formation. Thus, with renal ischemia and proximal tubule cell shedding, AKI and collecting duct fluid composition enhance THP gel formation and thus favor tubular cast formation and obstruction.

Integrins also play a role in cast formation. They recognize the most common universal tripeptide sequence, RGD, which is present in a variety of matrix proteins (246). These integrins can mediate cell-to-cell adhesion via an RGD-inhibitable mechanism (247). Experimental results support a role for adhesion molecules in the formation of casts. It has been shown that a translocation of integrins to the apical membrane of tubular epithelial cells may occur with ischemia (247–249). Possible mechanisms for the loss of the polarized distribution of integrins include cytoskeletal disruption, state of phosphorylation, activation of proteases, and production of NO (250,251). These integrins are known to recognize RGD tripeptide sequences (252,253). Thus, viable intraluminal cells could adhere to other luminal or paraluminal cells. There is experimental evidence for this cell-to-cell adhesion process as a contributor to tubule obstruction in ischemic AKI. Synthetic cyclical RGD peptides were infused before the renal ischemic insult in order to block cell-to-cell adhesion as a component of tubule obstruction (254–258). Using micropuncture techniques the cyclic RGD tripeptides blocked the rise in tubular pressure postischemic insult (252). In vivo study of RGD peptides (cyclic RGDDFLG and RGDDFV) in ischemic AKI in rats demonstrated attenuation of renal injury and accelerated recovery of renal function (254). Systemic administration of fluorescent derivatives of two different cyclic RGD peptides, a cyclic Bt-RGD peptide and a linear RhoG-RGD peptide, infused after the release of renal artery clamp–ameliorated ischemic AKI in rats (254,257). The staining of these peptides suggests that cyclic RGD peptides inhibited tubular obstruction by predominantly preventing cell-to-cell adhesion rather than cell-to-matrix adhesion (253).

ROLE OF ABNORMAL VASCULAR FUNCTION IN AKI

In organ ischemia, the restoration of perfusion may add to the problem of organ injury. Organ dysfunction attributable to reperfusion has been demonstrated in the heart, lung, brain, intestine, liver, and other organs. The importance of these findings is in their probable contribution to clinical features of myocardial infarction, AKI, and stroke. The implications of reperfusion injury are important in the clinical settings of flow diversion in surgical bypass and for function of transplanted heart, lung, kidney, and other organs.

Injury induced by ischemia-reperfusion leads to organ dysfunction, in part by direct injury of parenchymal cells. Vascular dysfunction is an early and prominent aspect of ischemia-reperfusion injury, with consequent impairment of blood flow and its regulation. For instance, there may be a progressive loss of regional organ blood flow following ischemia-reperfusion. There also may be an exaggerated constriction to neurohumoral agonists, failure to respond to physiologic and pharmacologic vasodilators, and paradoxical vasoconstrictor responses to changes in arterial pressure and blood flow following a period of transient organ ischemia and reperfusion. Evidence suggests that disordered vascular function subsequent to ischemia-reperfusion injury may itself have a substantial impact on organ recovery, since normalization of blood flow influences the rate of parenchymal cell restoration.

Normal Vascular Tone and Reactivity

Basal vascular tone is essential for perfusion of complex and distinct vascular beds and is dictated in large part by metabolic requirements of individual organs. It is clear that both transmural pressure and shear stress from blood flow contribute to basal arterial vascular tone. The predominant effect of vessel wall pressure is to increase tone; that of flow is to reduce tone. The mechanisms mediating the tonal response to these physical forces are only partially understood. Ca^{2+} entry, at least in part, through unique stretch-operated channels is important in pressure-induced vasoconstriction. VSMC transmembrane Na^+ concentrations are a factor in flow-related vasodilation. In addition, endothelial factors (NO, prostaglandins) are involved in flow-related vasodilation. Apart from its role in mediating shear-induced vasodilation, evidence indicates that endothelial-generated NO independently contributes to normal vascular tone. Other neurohumoral factors that contribute to changes in arterial tone dictated by metabolic demand are adenosine, oxygen, and carbon dioxide (259). Factors that modify vascular tone are listed in Table 10.4.

Vascular Dysfunction due to Ischemia-Reperfusion Injury

The kidney model that exemplifies ischemia-reperfusion injury is ischemia-induced AKI. A severe form of this disorder in which the renal artery is clamped for 40 to 70 minutes followed by immediate reflow (260,261) and a less severe form in which high-dose norepinephrine (NE) is infused into the renal artery for 90 minutes with slow spontaneous return of blood flow (260,262) have been studied extensively in rats. In the clamp model, there is a brief postocclusion hyperemia, then a sustained small

---

TABLE 10.4 FACTORS THAT MODIFY VASCULAR TONE

Endocrine or Neural

Renal nerves
Catecholamines
Angiotensin II
Natriuretic peptides

Paracrine

Endothelial derived, e.g., nitric oxide, endothelin-1
Angiotensin II
Arachidonic acid metabolites, e.g., thromboxane A2, prostaglandins, leukotrienes
Purinoreceptors and vasoactive purine agonists, e.g., P1 receptors and adenosine
Dopamine and serotonin

reduction in renal blood flow, and an attenuated response to endothelium-dependent dilators (262). In the first few hours after reflow, in the NE model there is a modest reduction in renal blood flow compared with the preischemia level without hyperemia, a decreased response to endothelium-dependent vasodilators, and a small but significant reduction in the constrictor response to the NOS inhibitor L-NAME (259). There is partial endothelial cell detachment without ultrastructural changes in individual endothelial cells at 6 hours in both the renal artery clamp and NE AKI models. By 48 hours of reperfusion, the basal renal blood flow remains 20% reduced in the renal artery clamp model, and there is a reduced vasoreactive response to changes in renal perfusion pressure to constrictor agonists and to endothelium-dependent and endothelium-independent dilators (259). The predominant histologic finding at this time in the small resistance arteries and arterioles is VSMC necrosis, present in 55% to 60% of the vessels (263,264). It is assumed that the lack of response to vasoactive stimuli is due to the diffuse VSMC injury related to both the relative severity of ischemia and the rapidity of reperfusion. In the NE AKI model, at 48 hours, the basal renal blood flow also is approximately 20% less than normal (259,260). However, vascular reactivity is strikingly different from that in the renal artery clamp AKI model. The difference likely is due to less severe ischemia and a slower rate of reperfusion. There is an exaggerated renal vasoconstrictor response to angiotensin II and endothelin-1 (ET-1) both in vivo and in arterioles isolated from these kidneys (259,265). Response to endothelium-dependent vasodilators is reduced, but the constrictor response to L-NAME is actually increased (259). cNOS can be identified as at least as strongly reactive or more reactive than normal, as determined with cNOS monoclonal antibody in the resistance arterial vessels (266). While there is a dilator response to cyclic adenosine monophosphate–dependent PGI2 in the 48-hour postischemic renal vasculature, there is no increase in renal blood flow to the NO donor sodium nitroprusside. Taken together, these data indicate that at 48 hours after ischemia in NE AKI in the rat kidney, vascular cNOS activity is not diminished but rather is maximal such that it cannot be stimulated further by endothelium-dependent vasodilators. The available NO under basal conditions has fully activated VSMC-soluble cyclic guanosine monophosphate such that there is no additional response to an exogenous NO donor.

In examining the mechanism for the constrictor hypersensitivity in the 48-hour postischemic vasculature in NE AKI, measurements of VSMC cytosolic Ca^{2+} have been made in the isolated arterioles from these kidneys perfused at physiologic pressures (265). Compared to similar vessels from sham AKI kidneys, there is a significantly higher baseline and an earlier and greater increase in VSMC Ca^{2+} in response to a normal half-maximal constricting concentration (EC50) of angiotensin II, which correlates with the initially lower and more intense reduction in lumen diameter in the postischemic AKI vessels.

Another novel observation regarding VSMC Ca^{2+} in 48-hour postischemic renal arterioles in vitro is a paradoxical change in VSMC cell Ca^{2+} in response to changes in lumen pressure. In normal afferent and efferent arterioles, increasing lumen pressure (stretch) within an autoregulatory range for these vessels results in an increase in VSMC Ca^{2+}. Conversely, decreasing lumen pressure is associated with a decrease in VSMC Ca^{2+}. In the NE AKI vessels, the reverse relationships are observed. There are also corresponding paradoxical changes in lumen diameter, representing, at least, a loss of the myogenic response and, at most, a "reverse" myogenic response. This abnormal VSMC Ca^{2+} and myogenic response to pressure is suggested to be the basis of the markedly abnormal in vivo autoregulatory response between 48 hours and 1 week after AKI induction that is likely the most significant and clinically relevant ischemia-reperfusion disorder of vasoreactivity in the kidney.

It was at first thought that Ca^{2+} channel blockers might be exerting their protective effects entirely at the vascular level by promoting the enhancement of renal blood flow. There are unquestioned renal vascular effects of Ca^{2+} channel blockers, with renal blood flow improving more rapidly after ischemia with Ca^{2+} channel blocker treatment (267). Renal blood flow and glomerular filtration will not decrease as severely during radiocontrast administration in dogs when Ca^{2+} channel blockers are coadministered (268). Ischemic AKI is characterized by a loss of autoregulatory ability, an enhanced sensitivity of renal blood flow to renal nerve stimulation, and injury to the endothelial lining of renal vessels (267). Much of this injury may be related to Ca^{2+} overload in VSMCs and/or endothelial cells, since verapamil and diltiazem partially obviate the loss of autoregulatory capacity and hypersensitivity to renal nerve stimulation (267).

Warm and cold ischemia during transplantation surgery may also contribute to vascular injury, and Ca^{2+} channel blockers are protective in experimental models of these clinical entities (269,270). However, other renal vasodilators such as prostacyclin do not restore autoregulatory integrity or reverse the increased sensitivity to renal nerve stimulation (267). Thus, it also seems that a unique effect of Ca^{2+} channel blockers is exerted at the vascular level.

At 1 week after ischemic injury, the endothelium appears normal, smooth muscle necrosis is less evident, but perivascular fibrosis is marked in the mid- to small-sized arterial vessels (260). Functionally, the response to endothelium-dependent dilators is reduced, L-NAME constrictor response is increased, and immunologically detectable NOS is present (266). There is a decreased dilator response to sodium nitroprusside but a measurable, albeit slightly reduced, dilator response to PGI2 (266). These findings suggest maximal endothelial cNOS activity similar to that at 48 hours. Unlike 48-hour vessels, the vasoconstrictor response to angiotensin II was markedly attenuated both in vivo and in vitro at 1 week (259,271). On the other hand, as previously alluded, a paradoxical vasoconstriction to a reduction in perfusion pressure in the autoregulatory range could be demonstrated in vivo. It is difficult to suggest a single mechanism that explains this series of functional aberrations at 1 week. It is likely that more than one pathophysiologic process is operating to produce these complex responses.

Intravital two-photon microscopy has been used to study the microvascular events within the functioning kidney in vivo (272–275). Intravital two-photon microscopy enables investigators to follow functional and structural alterations with subcellular resolution within the same field of view over a short period of time. Endothelial cell dysfunction within the microvasculature was observed and quantified using the infusion of variously sized, differently colored dextrans or proteins. Movement of these molecules out of the microvasculature and accumulation within the interstitial compartment are readily observed during AKI. The FVB-TIE2/GFP mouse, in which the endothelium is fluorescent, has been used to study morphologic changes in the renal microvascular endothelium during ischemia-reperfusion injury in the kidney (276). Alterations in the cytoskeleton of renal microvascular endothelial cells correlated with a permeability defect in the renal microvasculature as identified using fluorescent dextrans and two-photon intravital imaging. This study demonstrates that renal vascular endothelial injury occurs in ischemic AKI and may play an important role in the pathophysiology of ischemic AKI.

In patients with AKI, it has been demonstrated that diminished NO generation by injured endothelium and loss of macula densa neuronal NOS may impair the vasodilatory ability of the renal vasculature and contribute to the reduction in the GFR (277). Fifty patients that had a cadaveric renal transplant were studied: urinary nitrite and nitrate levels were determined, and intraoperative allograft biopsies were performed. In patients with sustained AKI, urinary nitrite and nitrate excretion was lower than in patients without AKI. In the kidney biopsies, endothelial NOS expression diminished from the peritubular capillaries of 6 of 7 subjects in the sustained AKI group but from only 6 of 16 subjects in the recovery group.

In summary, ischemia-reperfusion injury is accompanied by dramatic changes in basal and reactive vascular function of the organ involved. Endothelial injury also occurs in ischemic AKI in mice. There are similarities in altered organ vascular function, particularly in the early reperfusion period of 24 to 48 hours, including changes in permeability, decreased basal organ blood flow, hypersensitivity to vasoconstrictor stimuli, and attenuated response to vasodilators. The reduced responsiveness to endothelium-dependent vasodilators may be due to an actual reduction in endothelial NOS activity or to an actual spontaneous maximal NOS/NO activity that cannot be stimulated further by endothelium-dependent agents.

ROLE OF VASODILATORY SUBSTANCES

Endogenous vasodilators are involved in the hemodynamic changes that both initiate and maintain AKI. In this section, the roles of endogenously generated vasodilators in the pathophysiology of ischemic, septic, and nephrotoxic AKI will be considered, as well as the therapeutic use of vasorelaxing substances in animal models and in clinical AKI.

Prostaglandins

When renal perfusion pressure is reduced, preglomerular arterial resistance decreases and efferent arteriolar resistance increases to maintain glomerular capillary hydraulic pressure (PGC) and single-nephron GFR relatively constant. The efferent arteriolar constriction is mediated, in large part, through the local renin–angiotensin system (RAS) (278). Activation of the RAS stimulates synthesis of cyclooxygenase products, including the vasodilator prostaglandins PGI2 and PGE2 (279). PGI2 and

PGE2 oppose the constrictor effects of angiotensin II, thereby attenuating the reduction in renal blood flow as renal perfusion pressure declines. The modulating vasodilator effect of prostaglandins in the setting of reduced renal perfusion appears to be greater in afferent than efferent arterioles. When PGI2 and PGE2 were administered exogenously during reduced renal perfusion, filtration fraction increased, with better preservation of the GFR than renal blood flow (280,281), suggesting that vasodilator prostaglandins preferentially caused preglomerular vasorelaxation under these conditions.

Prostaglandin synthesis was found to be increased in animal models of ischemic AKI (280,282), aminoglycoside nephrotoxicity (283), sepsis, and endotoxic shock (284,285). The indication that an increase in prostaglandin activity was renoprotective by maintaining glomerular hemodynamics showed that cyclooxygenase inhibitors in these disorders augmented the reduction in renal blood flow and the GFR (286,287).

Other evidence of protection in AKI was the finding that infusion of biologic prostaglandins and their analogs in ischemic (280,281), mercuric chloride— (288), and glycerol-induced AKI (289) results in protection against AKI. The prostaglandin E1 analog, misoprostol, was found to provide significant protection against ischemia-induced renal dysfunction in rats subjected to renal artery occlusion (290). Misoprostol-treated rats had GFRs almost threefold greater than control animals, although renal blood flow and renal vascular resistance were not significantly different. Misoprostol also protected against renal dysfunction in a model of toxic renal injury produced by mercuric chloride. In an in vitro model employing primary cultures of proximal tubule epithelial cells subjected to hypoxia and reoxygenation, misoprostol, prostaglandin E2, and prostacyclin limited cell death. This study demonstrated that prostaglandins protect renal tubule epithelial cells from hypoxic injury at the cellular level independent of hemodynamic factors. Another study demonstrated that inhibitors of cyclooxygenase and lipoxygenase pathways exert a direct protective effect against the hypoxia-reoxygenation-induced cell injury in renal tubules, a model independent of vascular and inflammatory factors (291).

The PGE1 study group has performed a pilot study with intravenous PGE1 administered before radiocontrast media in patients with renal impairment (292). Results from this pilot study suggest that intravenous PGE1 may be used efficaciously and safely to prevent radiocontrast medium (RCM) induced renal dysfunction in patients with preexisting impaired renal function.

Natriuretic Peptides

In 1981 the natriuretic effects of an extract of mammalian atrial myocytes was first reported (293). Subsequently, this substance has been characterized as a polypeptide. The primary stimulus to atrial natriuretic peptide (ANP) synthesis and release is distention of the atria, where storage granules have been identified. Infusion of normal saline into human volunteers increases plasma ANP (294), and plasma ANP levels were elevated in edematous states that involved increased intravascular volume and atrial enlargement such as congestive heart failure.

Natural and synthetic ANPs cause dose-dependent reductions in systemic arterial pressure. The mechanism involves both peripheral vasorelaxation and a reduction in cardiac output (295,296). The magnitude of arterial pressure reduction is dependent on the state of basal vascular tone. ANP has been shown to inhibit both secretion and activity of the renin–angiotensin–aldosterone (297) and adrenergic nervous systems (298), as well as that of vasopressin (299) and ET-1 (300).

ANP has an important effect on the kidney. In vivo infusion of ANPs, both synthetic and naturally occurring from a variety of species, markedly increased the GFR while having a proportionately smaller effect on renal blood flow (301). Studies suggest that ANP-induced renal vasorelaxation was specific for the preglomerular arterioles (302,303). Other studies examining the rat renal microvasculature in vitro indicated that ANP not only directly vasodilated the afferent arteriole but also constricted the efferent arteriole (304,305). The tubular natriuretic effects of ANP involve inhibition of sodium and water transport in the loop of Henle, connecting tubules, and collecting ducts. Among other possible mechanisms, ANP has been shown to interfere with vasopressin effect and alter adenylate cyclase activity.

Other natriuretic peptides have been discovered. Another class of natriuretic peptides is referred to as brain natriuretic peptide (BNP). It has been isolated from both brain and heart (306,307). BNP, which contains 32 amino acids, has diuretic and natriuretic effects similar to ANP, while the hypotensive effect is not as potent. BNP is now FDA approved for clinical use in congestive heart failure (308).

Numerous animal studies have demonstrated a protective effect of ANPs on ischemic and nephrotoxic in models of AKI (304,309–312). ANP is effective in AKI models even when given after the initiating insult.

On the basis of the encouraging animal experimental results and the unique combination of pharmacologic properties, clinical studies were performed. A multicenter, randomized, double-blind, placebo-controlled clinical trial of ANP in 504 critically ill patients with AKI was performed. The patients received a 24-hour intravenous infusion of either ANP or placebo. The primary end point was dialysis-free survival for 21 days after treatment. The administration of ANP did not improve the overall rate of dialysis-free survival in critically ill patients with acute tubular necrosis. However, ANP decreased the need for dialysis in patients with oliguria (313). In a subsequent study, 222 patients with oliguric AKI were enrolled into a multicenter, randomized, double-blind, placebo-controlled trial. There was no statistically significant beneficial effect of ANP in dialysis-free survival or reduction in dialysis in these subjects with oliguric AKI (314). Mortality rates through day 60 were 60% versus 56% in the ANP and placebo groups, respectively. However, 95% of the ANP-treated patients versus 55% of the placebo-treated patients had systolic blood pressures <90 mm Hg during the study-drug infusion (P < 0.001). The hypotensive effect of ANP in these recent trials no doubt obscured any intrarenal beneficial effect of the compound.

Calcium Channel Blockers

Calcium channel blockers (CCBs), which inhibit voltage-gated Ca^{2+} entry, have been shown to protect against ischemic and nephrotoxic (cisplatinum, gentamicin) AKI in various animal models (315–321). The protective effect involves less renal vasoconstriction and improved renal blood flow. At a tubular level, there is less AKI and improved mitochondrial function. More recently, it has been demonstrated that the CCB benidipine can ameliorate the ischemic AKI in rats and that the renoprotective effect was associated with the reduction of apoptosis in tubular epithelial cells (322). Diltiazem also improves renal function in endotoxin-induced AKI in the rat (323).

CCBs have also been examined in clinical studies. Gallopamil resulted in more rapid recovery of renal function in five patients with malaria- or leptospirosis-related AKI (324). Other human experience with CCBs has largely been in the setting of renal transplantation. Verapamil improved early graft function when administered to donors before harvesting the kidneys (38). Diltiazem administered to transplant patients immediately after graft placement resulted in better graft function and a lower incidence of posttransplant AKI (325). More recently, it was demonstrated that isradipine results in a better renal function after kidney transplantation (326). However, the protective effect was independent of delayed graft function or acute rejection.

Fractalkine

Proinflammatory cytokines increase expression of the CX_3C chemokine, fractalkine, on injured endothelial cells. The fractalkine receptor (CX_3CR1) is expressed on natural killer (NK) cells, monocytes, and some CD8+ T cells (327). Fractalkine has a mucinlike stalk that extends the chemokine domain away from the endothelial cell surface, enabling presentation of the CX_3C-chemokine domain to leukocytes. Expression of fractalkine enables bypassing of the first two steps of the adhesion cascade (i.e., rolling and triggering) and mediates cell adhesion between circulating leukocytes and endothelial cells as well as extravasation of these cells. Thus, fractalkine serves the dual function of an adhesion molecule and a chemoattractant (327). Fractalkine is a major chemoattractant for NK cells and monocytes but not neutrophils (328). Fractalkine expression is increased in patients with renal tubulointerstitial inflammation, with the strongest expression localized to vascular sites near to macrophage inflammation (329). Fractalkine is a strong candidate for directing mononuclear cell infiltration induced by vascular injury (329). Fractalkine expression is increased in the endothelium of large blood vessels, capillaries, and glomeruli in ischemic AKI (330). Fractalikine receptor inhibition is protective against ischemic AKI (330). Fractalkine expression is also increased in the blood vessels in mouse kidneys exposed to cisplatin (331). However, fractalkine inhibition did not protect against the functional and histologic abnormalities in cisplatin-induced AKI in mice (331).

Clinical Relevance of Ischemia-Reperfusion Vascular Injury

The course of human ischemia-induced AKI is highly variable. An important and relevant observation regarding the variable duration and, in particular, the prolonged course in AKI patients was made by Solez et al. (13). In individuals with AKI duration of longer than 3 weeks, a prominent finding in biopsy or autopsy specimens was fresh tubular renal ischemic lesions that could not be related to the remote initial ischemic insult. A possible explanation for the fresh ischemic lesions was altered reactivity of the renal vasculature. Abnormal vascular reactivity in established ischemic AKI animal models includes loss of renal blood flow autoregulation. A number of investigators (263,271,332) have found an attenuated autoregulatory response from 2 to 7 days after AKI induction in the renal artery clamp model in rats.

On the background of these postischemic vascular perturbations is the observation that a decrease in renal perfusion pressure is not associated with autoregulation of either the GFR or renal blood flow (259,266,267,271,333,334). In fact, rather than renal vasodilation, renal vasoconstriction occurs with a fall in renal perfusion pressure in the postischemic kidney. Thus, a degree of hypotension, which is of no clinical significance in the normal kidney, may cause renal damage in the kidney during the recovery phase of AKI. The same increased sensitivity in the postischemic kidney has also been shown to occur with nephrotoxic agents such as aminoglycosides.

These data have important clinical implications, as a modest arterial pressure reduction during the course of this disease, such as frequently occurs with hemodialysis treatment, can actually result in recurrent ischemic injury and prolongation of AKI (335).

VASOACTIVE RESPONSE TO SEPSIS

Sepsis is the most frequent cause of AKI in ICUs (4,16). AKI occurs in approximately 19% of patients with moderate sepsis, 23% of patients with severe sepsis, and 51% of patients with septic shock (18). The combination of AKI and sepsis is associated with a >80% mortality (4).

Complex vasoactive responses occur in septic AKI. Over the past 3 decades, sepsis has been studied in various species, including rats, dogs, pigs, primates, and humans. Recently a mouse model of septic AKI has been developed; this model allows the use of newer molecular techniques, including knockout and transgenic mice, to study the pathogenesis of AKI associated with sepsis.

The initial effects of sepsis in causing AKI primarily involve renal vasoconstriction (336). This renal vasoconstriction can be demonstrated in the absence of sepsis-mediated hypotension (336) as well as in the absence of later events, including apoptosis, leukocyte infiltration, and morphologic evidence of coagulation (e.g., glomerular fibrin) (337–340).

There is evidence that several vasoconstrictor and vasodilator pathways are activated during sepsis in various experimental models. During sepsis the cytokine-mediated induction of NO results in a hyperdynamic state in which systemic vasodilation is associated with a secondary increase in cardiac output (18). The rise in cardiac output, however, may not be maximal for the degree of afterload reduction because of the myocardial depressant effect of cytokines such as tumor necrosis factor alpha (TNFα). The arterial underfilling associated with systemic arterial vasodilation is known to activate the RAS and the sympathetic nervous system (SNS) (341–344). While these events attenuate or abolish any systemic hypotension, they also lead to renal vasoconstriction. The vasoactive events of sepsis are, however, more complex than those initiated by arterial underfilling. The endotoxin-mediated increase in TNFα is associated with an increase in iNOS (337,345). There is evidence in the endotoxemic rat that the increased NO that results from the upregulation of iNOS exerts a negative feedback on the eNOS in the kidney (Fig. 10.3) (346). Moreover, the secondary messenger of NO, cyclic guanosine 5'-monophosphate (GMP) has been shown to increase in the renal cortex during the initial 16 hours of sepsis but then at 24 hours to be downregulated in spite of continued high plasma levels of NO (347). Both of these events, namely, NO-mediated decreased eNOS and downregulation of cyclic GMP, would impair the normal counterregulatory vasodilator pathways that attenuate the renal vasoconstriction associated with activation of the RAS and SNS. ET-1 has been shown to be increased during endotoxemia in several species (348–352). The capillary leak that leads to interstitial edema and decreased plasma volume during endotoxemia has been reversed with ET receptor blockade in the rat, albeit with a decrease in blood pressure (348).

INFLAMMATION

The inflammatory response may play a major role in the pathogenesis of ischemic ARF (353,354). The role of neutrophils, lymphocytes, macrophages, and NK cells has been studied in AKI and will be discussed in the next section.

Neutrophils

The role of neutrophils in AKI has been addressed in many studies and remains controversial (355). There is evidence that leukocytes, particularly neutrophils, mediate tubular injury in AKI derived from studies that show an accumulation of neutrophils in ischemic AKI and studies demonstrating a beneficial role of anti-ICAM-1 therapy in AKI (356). Rats depleted of peripheral neutrophils by antineutrophil serum were not protected against ischemic AKI (357). In another study, mice depleted of peripheral neutrophils by antineutrophil serum were protected against ischemic AKI (356).

The adherence of neutrophils to the vascular endothelium is an essential step in the extravasation of these cells into ischemic tissue (358). After adherence and chemotaxis, infiltrating leukocytes release reactive oxygen species and enzymes that damage the cells (358). Activated neutrophils have been shown to enhance the decrease in the GFR in response to renal ischemia, at least in part due to release of oxygen radicals (359–362). In contrast, infusion of oxygen radical–deficient neutrophils from patients with chronic granulomatous disease did not worsen the course of ischemic injury (361). The mechanism by which adherent leukocytes cause ischemic injury is unclear but likely involves both the release of potent vasoconstrictors including prostaglandins, leukotrienes, and thromboxanes (363) as well as direct endothelial injury via release of endothelin and a decrease in NO (25,364).

Increased systemic levels of the cytokines, TNF-α and IL-1 may upregulate ICAM-1 after ischemia and reperfusion in the kidney (356). The administration of a monoclonal antibody against ICAM-1 protected against ischemic AKI in rats (361,365). ICAM-1-deficient mice are protected against renal ischemia (356). Thus, ICAM-1 is a mediator of ischemic AKI probably by potentiating neutrophil–endothelial interactions. There is also evidence that upregulation of adhesion molecules may contribute to this impaired medullary blood flow postischemic injury (366–368).

P-selectin is another important molecule involved in adherence of circulating leukocytes to tissue in inflammatory states. Renal ischemia has also been shown to be associated with upregulation of endothelial P-selectin with enhanced adhesion of neutrophils (369). A soluble P-selectin glycoprotein ligand prevents infiltration of leukocytes and protects functionally against ischemic AKI (251).

The role of neutrophils in AKI has been explored in many studies and remains controversial (355,370). There is evidence that neutrophils mediate renal tubular injury in AKI. This evidence is derived from studies that show an accumulation of neutrophils in ischemic AKI and studies demonstrating a beneficial role of anti-ICAM-1 therapy in AKI (356). In another study, mice depleted of peripheral neutrophils by antineutrophil serum were protected against ischemic AKI (356). However, rats depleted of peripheral neutrophils by antineutrophil serum were not protected against ischemic AKI (357).

Mice with ischemic AKI were treated with the pan-caspase inhibitor Quinoline-val-asp(Ome)-CH$_2$-OPH (OPH-001) (371). OPH-001 induced a marked (100%) reduction in BUN and serum creatinine and a highly significant reduction in the ATN score compared to vehicle-treated mice. OPH-001 significantly reduced the increase in caspase-1 activity and IL-18 and prevented neutrophil infiltration in the kidney during ischemic AKI. To further investigate whether the lack of neutrophil infiltration was contributing to the protection against ischemic AKI, a model of neutrophil depletion was developed. Mice were injected with 0.1 mg of the rat IgG2b monoclonal antibody RB6-8C5 intraperitoneally 24 hours before renal pedicle clamp (372). This resulted in depletion of neutrophils in the peripheral blood and in the kidney during ischemic AKI. Neutrophil-depleted mice had a small (18%) reduction in serum creatinine during ischemic AKI but no reduction in the ATN score despite a lack of neutrophil infiltration in the kidney. Remarkably, caspase-1 activity and IL-18 were still significantly increased in the kidney in neutrophil-depleted mice with AKI. Thus, to investigate the role of IL-18 in the absence of neutrophils, neutrophil-depleted mice with ischemic AKI were treated with IL-18-neutralizing antiserum. IL-18-antiserum-treated neutrophil-depleted mice with ischemic AKI had a significant (75%) reduction in serum creatinine and a significant reduction in the ATN score compared with vehicle-treated neutrophil-depleted mice. These results suggested a novel neutrophil-independent mechanism of IL-18-mediated ischemic AKI (371).

Lymphocytes

The role of other leukocytes, for example, lymphocytes has recently been reported. Mice with genetically engineered deficiency of both CD4+ and CD8+ T cells demonstrate a marked improvement in renal function and less neutrophil infiltration in the ischemic kidney compared with control mice. Also mice deficient in CD4 T cells, not CD8 T cells, are significantly protected from AKI (373). Direct evidence for a pathophysiologic role of the CD4 T cell was obtained when reconstitution of CD4-deficient mice with wild-type CD4 T cells restored postischemic injury.

However, there is also a study that CD4 T cell depletion is not sufficient to protect against ischemic AKI (374). Mice were injected with 10 mg/kg of the rat IgG monoclonal antibody GK1.5 IP or vehicle. Complete CD4+ T cell depletion with GK1.5 was confirmed by flow cytometry of lymph nodes before induction of AKI and at 24 hours of postischemic reperfusion. Serum creatinine and the ATN score were not different in vehicle-treated and CD4 T cell–depleted mice with ischemic AKI. These results suggest that CD4+ T cells are not required for the development of ischemic AKI. Therefore, the hypothesis was tested that more than one subset of lymphocyte may need to be depleted for protection against ischemic AKI. T cell receptor α chain (TCRα) $-/-$ mice lack conventional $\alpha\beta$ T cells and are deficient in both CD4+ and CD8+ T cells. TCRα $-/-$ mice were not protected against ischemic AKI.

Macrophages

Both monocyte/macrophages and NK cells are well-known sources and targets of injurious cytokines and chemokines (375–378). In a model of macrophage depletion using liposomal clodronate, it was demonstrated that macrophages contribute to tissue damage during acute renal allograft rejection (379) and ischemic AKI (380,381,330). Gene therapy in rats expressing an amino-terminal truncated monocyte chemoattractant protein-1 (MCP-1) reduced macrophage infiltration and ATN (382).

It was determined whether macrophages are a source of IL-18 in ischemic AKI in mice (143). On immunofluorescence staining of the outer stripe of the outer medulla, the number of macrophages double-stained for CD11b and IL-18 was significantly increased in AKI and significantly decreased by macrophage depletion using clodronate. Adoptive transfer of RAW 264.7 cells, a mouse macrophage line that constitutively expresses IL-18 mRNA, reversed the functional protection against AKI in both macrophage-depleted wild-type and caspase-1 $(-/-)$ mice. To test whether IL-18 in macrophages is necessary to cause AKI, macrophages in which IL-18 was inhibited were adoptively transferred. Peritoneal macrophages isolated from wild-type mice, IL-18 binding protein transgenic (IL-18 BP Tg) mice, and IL-18 $-/-$ mice were used. IL-18 BP Tg mice overexpress human IL-18 BP and exhibit decreased biologic activity of IL-18. Adoptive transfer of peritoneal macrophages from wild-type as well as IL-18 BP Tg and IL-18 $-/-$ mice reversed the functional protection against AKI in LEC-treated mice. In summary, adoptive transfer of peritoneal macrophages in which IL-18 function was inhibited reverses the functional protection in macrophage-depleted mice, suggesting that IL-18 from adoptive transfer of macrophages is not sufficient to cause ischemic AKI.

NK Cells

NK cells are a type of lymphocyte that mediate innate immunity against pathogens and tumors via their ability to secrete cytokines (383). NK cells are unique in their constitutive expression of receptors for cytokines, for example, IL-18, that are produced by activated macrophages (384). NK cells are activated by IL-18 independently of IL-12 (385). NK cells in mice express mostly the same receptors as humans, including NK 1.1. A model of NK cell activation in injured tissues has been proposed (386). In this model, it is hypothesized that NK cells are recruited to sites of injury from the bloodstream. Once in the tissue, NK cells become activated and release cytokines like IL-18 (386). In support of this hypothesis, it is known that NK cells play a role in numerous disease processes (387).

NK cell depletion in wild-type C57BL/6 mice is protective against ischemic AKI (388). Adoptive transfer of NK cells worsened injury in NK, T, and B cell-null Rag2$(-/-)$ γ(c)$(-/-)$ mice with ischemic AKI. NK cell–mediated kidney injury was perforin (PFN) dependent as PFN$(-/-)$ NK cells had minimal capacity to kill tubular epithelial cells in vitro compared with NK cells from wild-type mice.

Uric Acid

The hypothesis has been presented that uric acid, at levels that do not cause tubular obstruction, may contribute to AKI (389). There are a number of mechanisms by which uric acid may contribute to AKI. Uric acid induces inflammation. Uric acid increases production of the chemotactic factor MCP-1 in VSMCs and

C reactive protein (CRP) synthesis in human vascular endothelial and smooth muscle cells (390). Hyperuricemic rats have a significant increase in macrophage infiltration in their kidneys independent of crystal deposition (391). Renal vasoconstriction also occurs in rats with experimentally induced hyperuricemia. The vasoconstriction is caused by an increase in resistance of the afferent (and, to a lesser extent, efferent) arterioles and a reduction in the single-nephron GFR, which can be attenuated by lowering the uric acid with allopurinol (392). The vasoconstriction is reversed by l-arginine, suggesting that a loss of nitric oxide in endothelial cells may be the cause of the vasoconstriction (393). In summary uric acid may have vasoconstrictive, proinflammatory and pro-oxidative, properties that could promote the development of AKI.

Adenosine

Extracellular adenosine is derived mainly *via* phosphohydrolysis of adenosine 5′-monophosphate (AMP) by ecto-5′-nucleotidase (CD73). Extracellular adenosine plays an anti-inflammatory role, especially during conditions of limited oxygen availability. The four known adenosine receptor (AR) subtypes (A_1, A_{2a}, A_{2b}, A_3) are expressed in the kidney (394). CD73-dependent adenosine production plays a crucial role in the regulation of the tubuloglomerular feedback (395). It has been demonstrated that protection from ischemic AKI in mice by adenosine A2A agonists or endogenous adenosine requires activation of receptors expressed on bone marrow–derived cells (396). In addition, adenosine A2A agonists mediate protection against ischemic AKI by an action on CD4 T cells (397). Activation of the adenosine A1A receptor plays a protective role in ischemic AKI. Adenosine A1 receptor knockout mice demonstrate increased ischemic AKI (394), and adenosine A1 receptor activation inhibits inflammation, necrosis, and apoptosis in ischemic AKI in mice (398). The adenosine A2B receptor antagonist PSB1115 blocks renal protection induced by ischemic preconditioning, whereas treatment with the selective adenosine A2B receptor agonist BAY 60-6583 dramatically improves renal function and histology following ischemia alone (399). Adenosine A2B receptors were exclusively expressed in the renal vasculature (399). Studies using A2BAR bone marrow chimera conferred kidney protection selectively to renal A2BARs. These results identify the A2BAR as a novel therapeutic target for providing potent protection from renal ischemia. Pharmacologic or gene-targeted inhibition of CD 73 abolishes renal protection induced by ischemic preconditioning, and treatment of mice with soluble 5′-nucleotidase restores the renal protection induced by ischemic preconditioning (400). In summary, adenosine receptors are novel therapeutic targets in ischemic AKI.

THERAPEUTIC ROLE OF GROWTH FACTORS

The growth factors insulin-like growth factor (IGF—1), epidermal growth factor (EGF), and hepatocyte growth factor (HGF) are known to bind specific receptors in the proximal tubule and regulate metabolic, transport, and proliferative responses in these cells (401). Studies in this area have fallen into two broad categories: (a) those that have examined the renal expression of genes encoding growth factors or transcriptional factors associated with the growth response that is induced after AKI and (b) those that have examined the efficacy of exogenously administered growth factors in accelerating recovery of renal function in experimental models of AKI (402). EGF, HGF, and IGF-1 accelerate the recovery of renal function and regeneration of damaged proximal tubular epithelium and improve the mortality in postischemic rat tubular injury (403–405). IGF-1 attenuates delayed graft function in a canine renal autotransplantation model (406). A relationship between expression of antiapoptotic Bcl-2 genes and growth factors in ischemic AKI in the rat has recently been described (204). It has been demonstrated that antiapoptotic Bcl-2 genes as well as both EGF and IGF-1 are upregulated in the surviving distal tubules and are detected in the surviving proximal tubules, where these growth factors are not usually synthesized (204,407).

A clinical study has been performed. The study was designed as a randomized, double-blind, placebo-controlled trial in ICUs in 20 teaching hospitals (408). Seventy-two patients with AKI were randomized to receive recombinant IGF-1 (rhIGF-I) (35 patients) or placebo (37 patients). In this study, rhIGF-I did not accelerate the recovery of renal function in severely ill AKI patients.

THERAPEUTIC ROLE OF MESENCHYMAL STEM CELLS

Mesenchymal stem cells (MSCs) have a well-known role in regeneration and immunomodulation. A search of clinicaltrials.gov revealed 40 clinical trials of MSCs in patients with Crohn disease, multiple sclerosis, graft versus host disease, ischemic stroke, organ rejection, cartilage repair, lupus nephritis, and heart disease. Administration of MSCs protects against ischemic AKI in rats (409). In this study, the expression of IL-1β, TNF-α, IFN-γ, and iNOS was significantly reduced by intravenous administration of MSCs. In addition, the beneficial effects of MSCs were found to be mediated by paracrine actions and not by their differentiation into target cells. Human MSCs improve renal function and survival in mice with cisplatin-induced AKI (410). Treatment of mice with autologous and allogeneic MSCs after AKI was safe and reduced renal fibrosis in mice that survived AKI (411). A phase 1 study of MSCs in patients at risk for AKI after cardiac surgery is underway.

Diagnosis of AKI

PRERENAL AZOTEMIA

The conditions causing prerenal azotemia are listed in Table 10.5. There are four clinical criteria required for a diagnosis of prerenal azotemia: (a) an acute rise in BUN and/or serum creatinine, (b) renal hypoperfusion, (c) a bland urine sediment (absence of cells and cellular casts), and (d) the return of renal function to normal within 24 to 48 hours of correction of the hypoperfused state.

The azotemic state can be corrected if the renal hypoperfusion causing the renal ischemia is reversed. Such an improvement in renal function may involve increasing extracellular fluid (ECF) volume, enhancing cardiac output, or correcting the cause of systemic arterial vasodilation, such as bacteremia or excessive use of antihypertensive drugs. Correction or improvement of an insult, such as anesthesia,

TABLE 10.5 CONDITIONS CAUSING PRERENAL AZOTEMIA

Hypovolemia
Hemorrhage
Gastrointestinal losses
Third space
   Burns
   Peritonitis
   Muscle trauma
Renal fluid losses
   Overdiuresis

Impaired Cardiac Function
Congestive heart failure
Cardiogenic shock
   Acute myocardial infarction
Pericardial tamponade
Massive pulmonary embolism

Systemic vasodilatation
Gram-negative bacteremia
Antihypertensive medications
Anaphylaxis
Cirrhosis

Increased renal vascular resistance
Anesthesia
Surgery
Hepatorenal syndrome
Prostaglandin inhibitors
   NSAIDs
Renal vasoconstricting drugs
   Cyclosporin

NSAID, nonsteroidal anti-inflammatory drug.

surgical trauma, liver disease, or bilateral renal vascular occlusion, may also reverse a state of prerenal azotemia. A careful search by history and physical examination for causes of prerenal azotemia, therefore, must constitute the initial undertaking in the evaluation of patients with the potential diagnosis of AKI.

POSTRENAL AZOTEMIA

Obstruction of urine flow in both ureters, the bladder, or urethra may cause postrenal AKI. The common causes of postrenal AKI are listed in Table 10.6. The common denominator of acute azotemia in this setting is obstruction to the flow of urine. The patient most at risk for acute postrenal azotemia is the elderly man in whom prostatic hypertrophy or prostatic cancer may lead to complete or partial obstruction to urine flow. In addition to anatomic causes, functional disturbances of bladder emptying also must be considered. Autonomic insufficiency, spinal cord lesions, and anticholinergic agents may cause functional bladder-neck obstruction and thus postrenal azotemia. Young boys with congenital urethral valves may also have acute obstruction. In women, complete urinary tract obstruction is relatively uncommon in the absence of pelvic surgery, pelvic malignancy, or previous pelvic irradiation. A pelvic examination is mandatory in the evaluation of postrenal azotemia because patients with cervical or endometrial carcinoma or endometriosis may present with azotemia secondary to bilateral ureteral obstruction. A history of analgesic nephropathy, sickle cell anemia, diabetes mellitus, or acute pyelonephritis may suggest obstruction secondary to papillary necrosis.

In the absence of a single kidney or previously impaired renal function, postrenal azotemia occurs only with bilateral obstruction of the urinary tract at these sites. Renal ultrasonography will detect pelvicalyceal dilatation secondary to obstruction in >90% of patients. Staghorn calculi and small shrunken kidneys, however, decrease this sensitivity, and extrarenal pelvices may produce a false-positive diagnosis. Pelvicalyceal dilatation may not occur in some cases of retroperitoneal fibrosis. With the recognition and increased evidence of radiocontrast-induced AKI, it is most appropriate to use ultrasonography to exclude urinary tract obstruction. In some cases, retrograde pyelography may be necessary to exclude urinary tract obstruction definitively. The rapidity of the recovery of renal function depends on the duration and completeness of the obstruction.

TABLE 10.6 CONDITIONS CAUSING POSTRENAL AZOTEMIA

Urethral Obstruction
Valves
Stricture

Bladder Neck Obstruction
Prostatic hypertrophy
Bladder carcinoma
Bladder infection
Functional
   Autonomic neuropathy
   Alpha adrenergic blockers

Obstruction of Ureters, Bilateral
Unilateral Obstruction in Solitary Kidney
   Intraureteral
   Sulphonamide, uric acid, acyclovir, antiretroviral agent crystals
   Blood clots
   Stones
   Necrotizing papillitis
  Extraureteral
   Tumor of cervix, prostate, bladder
   Endometriosis
   Periureteral fibrosis
   Accidental ureteral ligation
   Pelvic abscess or hematoma

INTRARENAL OR INTRINSIC AKI

After prerenal and postrenal azotemia have been excluded, the diagnosis of intrarenal or intrinsic AKI can be entertained (Table 10.1). Clinically it can be diagnosed by one of the following:

1. An increase in BUN only (prerenal AKI).
2. An increase in BUN and serum creatinine. Normal BUN is 8 to 18 mg/dL, and normal serum creatinine is 0.6 to 1.2 mg/dL. Serum creatinine should be interpreted in relationship to the muscle mass of the patient.
3. Oliguria. Oliguria is defined as a urine output <400 mL/day—the minimum amount of urine that a person in a normal metabolic state needs to excrete to get rid of his or her daily solute production. However, in as many as half the cases of AKI, the daily urine volume may exceed this amount and actually be as high as 1.5 to 2.0 L/day (412). This form of AKI has been termed nonoliguric AKI. It is frequently associated with nephrotoxin-induced disease and tends to carry a lower morbidity and mortality than oliguric failure. In nonoliguric renal failure, urinary sodium concentration, fractional excretion of sodium, and the urine to plasma creatinine ratio are lower at the time of diagnosis than in oliguric AKI (413). The exact mechanism for the higher urine flow in this variety of AKI is not known. However, the finding of a higher creatinine clearance in nonoliguric patients suggests that the GFR may be better preserved. Despite liberal daily urine volumes, progressive azotemia with nonoliguric AKI may occur in the following manner. Since the abolition of the renal concentration capacity is a characteristic of AKI, approximately 300 mOsm of solute can be excreted in each liter of isotonic urine. The catabolic rate of patients with AKI is often markedly increased. In these individuals, there may be an exogenous plus endogenous solute load as great as 900 mOsm/day. The daily excretion of 2 L of isotonic urine thus will eliminate only 600 mOsm of the 900-mOsm solute load. Therefore, despite a daily urine output of 2 L, progressive azotemia will result because of the 300-mOsm daily positive solute balance. Such is the sequence of events that occurs in nonoliguric renal failure.
4. Anuria. Anuria has been defined in the past as a 24-hour urine volume <75 mL and has been suggested to be more compatible with urinary tract obstruction or renal vascular occlusion than with AKI. Such a definition of anuria, however, is probably not appropriate. During the first few days of oliguric AKI, urine volumes may frequently be <75 mL/day when assessed by bladder catheterization. It has been documented that such severe oliguria can occur with AKI in the absence of renal vascular or urinary tract obstruction (414). Anuria, therefore, is best defined as the excretion of no urine as documented by bladder catheterization. Anuria by this definition may suggest bilateral renal artery occlusion and thus the need for emergency renal arteriography, particularly in the appropriate clinical setting, such as atrial fibrillation with arterial emboli, abdominal trauma, or a dissecting aortic aneurysm. Because of the slower progression of irreversible functional loss with urinary tract obstruction, some minimal delay (a few days) in establishing this diagnosis may be acceptable, depending on the clinical status of the patient.
5. Biomarkers of AKI. Serum creatinine is the most widely used parameter to assess renal function. There are many renal and nonrenal factors that influence serum creatinine independent of kidney function. For example, creatinine generation is proportional to muscle mass and is affected by age, gender, body weight, and diet (415). In addition, alterations in serum creatinine may lag several days behind actual changes in the GFR in AKI (416,417). A biomarker that is released into the blood or urine soon after AKI may be an earlier marker of AKI than serum creatinine. Early diagnosis of AKI may result in more optimal dosing of antibiotics, avoidance of nephrotoxic agents, and earlier nephrology consultation. Ideally, early diagnosis of AKI may result in the initiation of specific therapies, for example, EPO (Table 10.3). Biomarkers of AKI that have been widely studied include IL-18, neutrophil gelatinase–associated lipocalin (NGAL), kidney injury molecule-1 (KIM-1), tubular enzymes, and cystatin C. In addition to being a mediator of AKI, IL-18 is also a biomarker of AKI. IL-18 is increased in the urine in mice with AKI (141,371). IL-18 is increased in the urine in patients with AKI compared to other kidney diseases and in renal transplant patients with delayed graft function (418,419). Urine IL-18 increases 48 hours before a 50% increase in serum creatinine in critically ill adults with acute respiratory distress syndrome (ARDS) (420), children with AKI in the ICU (421), children that develop AKI postcardiopulmonary bypass (CPB) (422), and adults with contrast nephropathy (423).

NGAL is a small protein of the lipocalin superfamily and is expressed by renal tubular cells (424). NGAL protein increases in the kidney and in the urine in early ischemic AKI in rats and mice (425) and in the early stage of cisplatin-induced nephrotoxicity (426). NGAL increases in the urine before serum creatinine in children and adults with AKI post-CPB (427,428), children with AKI in the ICU (429,430), and adults and children with contrast nephropathy (431,432). In addition to being a biomarker of AKI, NGAL also plays a role in the pathophysiology of AKI. Administration of NGAL to mice protects against ischemic AKI (424,433).

KIM-1 is an epithelial cell adhesion molecule that is expressed at a low level in normal kidney. KIM-1 is increased in the kidney in ischemic AKI in rats and mice (434,435). Urinary KIM-1 is increased in patients with ATN (436) and is a predictor of graft loss in kidney transplant patients (437).

Tubular enzymes are released from damaged proximal and/or distal tubular cells. Tubular enzymuria may be very sensitive to tubular injury from multiple causes. For example, in kidney transplant patients, alkaline phosphatase (AP), γ-glutamyl transferase (GGT), leucine aminopeptidase (LAP), and dipeptidyl peptidase IV (DPP) were increased with both acute rejection and ATN (438).

Cystatin C is a protein produced by all nucleated cells compared to creatinine that is mainly produced by muscle. It is freely filtered by the glomerulus (439). Some serum cystatin C is an earlier marker of AKI than serum creatinine in patients with AKI and adults post-CPB (440,441). Serum cystatin C is a more accurate marker of the GFR than serum creatinine in contrast nephropathy (442), liver cirrhosis (443,444), and critically ill adults and children (445,446).

In patients who are not acutely ill, an increased BUN and serum creatinine may be caused by acute or chronic renal failure. Features suggesting chronic renal failure are:

1. Symptoms for longer than 3 months, for example, malaise and nocturia.
2. An increased BUN or serum creatinine documented months earlier.
3. A normocytic normochromic anemia. However, patients with AKI and a microangiopathic hemolytic anemia, for example, hemolytic uremic syndrome, may have a normocytic anemia.
4. Small kidneys (<10 cm) on renal ultrasound. However, some patients with chronic renal failure, for example, diabetic nephropathy, amyloidosis, autosomal dominant polycystic kidney disease, rapidly progressive glomerulonephritis, or malignant hypertension, may have normal-sized or enlarged kidneys.

EVALUATION OF THE PATIENT WITH AKI

A comprehensive history, thorough physical examination, and urinalysis (sediment and chemistry) will suggest the diagnosis in the majority of patients.

History and Physical Examination

Careful tabulation and recording of data are the first steps in diagnosis and treatment. Vital signs, daily weights, records of intake and output, past and current laboratory data, and the fluid and medication list should be recorded on a flow sheet and included in the patient's chart. When the patient has been hospitalized for weeks or months with a complicated course before developing AKI, a carefully prepared flow sheet may often be the only way to detect causes of AKI, such as administration of nonsteroidal anti-inflammatory drugs (NSAIDS) or prophylactic antibiotics.

It is helpful to determine whether the AKI developed outside the hospital, inside the hospital, or in the ICU. The causes and management of AKI may differ in these circumstances. Common causes of AKI developing outside the hospital are acute systemic illness, for example, viral influenza; gastroenteritis that may lead to AKI through a variety of mechanisms, for example, volume depletion; and rhabdomyolysis with myoglobinuria. Trauma as the cause of acute azotemia is usually apparent at the time of admission to the hospital, but the unconscious or comatose patient may harbor internal injuries, extensive muscle damage, or acute urinary retention that is not discovered on the initial examination. Male patients with acute azotemia should be screened carefully for symptoms of prostatism. Aspirin, NSAIDs, antibiotics, and diuretics are the main causes of AIN. They are often prescribed outside the hospital. Accidental or intentional intoxication with heavy metal compounds, solvents, ethylene glycol, salicylates, or sedatives, especially in a patient presenting with disordered mentation, may explain an otherwise unexpected episode of AKI.

TABLE 10.7 URINE FINDINGS IN PRERENAL AZOTEMIA AND "INTRINSIC" OR PARENCHYMAL AKI

Laboratory test	Prerenal azotemia	ATN
Urine sodium (U_{Na}), mEq/L	<20	>40
Urine osmolality, mOsm/kg H_2O	>500	<400
Urine to plasma urea nitrogen	>8	<3
Urine to plasma creatinine	>40	<20
Fractional excretion of filtered sodium	<1	>1
Urinary sediment	Bland	"Muddy" brown granular casts, cellular debris, tubular epithelial cells

AKI, acute kidney injury; ATN, acute tubular necrosis.

When azotemia develops in the hospital setting, but not in the ICU, the list of possible causes narrows. Most of the patients have either ATN (38%) or prerenal azotemia (28%). Predisposing factors to AKI in this setting include fluid and electrolyte depletion, for example, excessive diuresis, nasogastric suction, surgical drains, and diarrhea in a patient who is too ill to control his or her own solute and water intake. Both surgery and anesthesia cause a vasoconstriction of the renal arteries and release of antidiuretic hormone; both of these effects may persist for 12 to 24 hours into the postoperative period. Nephrotoxic drugs and diagnostic agents, for example, radiocontrast media, represent a major and serious cause of acute azotemia (Table 10.7).

The majority of patients who develop AKI in the ICU have ATN (76%), and most of the rest have prerenal azotemia (18%). The mortality rate of these patients is >70%, which is much higher than the mortality of AKI developing in other areas of the hospital. Patients with respiratory failure secondary to ARDS requiring mechanical ventilation that subsequently develop AKI in the ICU requiring dialysis have a very high mortality >90% (447). In the ICU, AKI is often part of the multiorgan dysfunction syndrome (MODS).

Urinalysis

Assessment of the urinary sediment also is crucial in the diagnosis of AKI. An active sediment with renal tubular epithelial cells, cellular debris, and "muddy-brown" broad tubular cell casts supports the diagnosis of ATN. Large amounts of urinary protein (>3.0 g/day) and numerous red blood cell casts are indicative of AKI secondary to acute glomerulonephritis or vasculitis. The absence of cellular elements and protein in the urine is most compatible with prerenal and postrenal azotemia. An abundance of crystals in the urine, such as uric acid or oxalate crystals, secondary to ethylene glycol or methoxyflurane toxicity or crystalluria in an acquired immunodeficiency syndrome (AIDS) patient being treated with acyclovir or Indinavir also may provide a clue to the specific cause of the AKI.

Considerable information may be obtained from the assessment of the urinary composition (413,448). A study by Miller et al. (413) evaluated the differences in urinary composition between prerenal azotemia and both oliguric and nonoliguric AKI. Those differences are summarized in Table 10.6. Since tubular function is preserved in prerenal azotemia and the tubules are able to reabsorb sodium, the urinary sodium concentration decreases in response to the renal ischemia. In prerenal azotemia, the renal concentrating mechanism also is activated so that the urine osmolality exceeds plasma osmolality. With the intact tubular function in prerenal azotemia and tubular fluid resorption, the urine to plasma (U/P) creatinine ratio >40:1 with prerenal azotemia. This ratio is generally <20:1 in intrinsic or parencymal AKI. If mannitol or a diuretic has been administered within a few hours of obtaining the urine for examination, the interpretation of the urinary composition is difficult because with prerenal azotemia the administration of either of these substances may raise the urinary sodium concentration and impair renal concentrating capacity. Thus, the urinary composition of such a patient with prerenal azotemia who has received a diuretic may mimic that of a patient with AKI. There are a few other limitations to interpreting the urinary composition in differentiating AKI from prerenal azotemia. The urine of older patients and patients with chronic renal disease may not be concentrated despite the presence of prerenal azotemia. Fractional excretion of sodium (Fe_{Na}) is increased in ATN but may be low in association with AKI caused by nonoliguric ATN, radiocontrast, hepatorenal syndrome (HRS), rhabdomyolysis, acute glomerulonephritis, vasculitis, and early obstructive uropathy (449).

In a recent study, urine NGAL performed best at detecting AKI in patients entering the emergency room (450). In this study, patients with prerenal azotemia or chronic kidney disease did not have increased urine NGAL. Fe_{Na}—but not urinary NGAL concentration—distinguished prerenal azotemia from chronic kidney disease in this group of patients.

Finally, since urea clearances are flow dependent, the decreased urine flow and intact tubular function with prerenal azotemia or acute urinary tract obstruction are associated with reduced urea clearances. The rise in BUN, therefore, may be more rapid than the increase in serum creatinine concentration, since creatinine clearances are not flow dependent. In this regard, a ratio of BUN to serum creatinine concentration considerably >10 to 15:1 suggests prerenal azotemia or acute postrenal failure. With uncomplicated AKI, this ratio usually does not exceed 10 to 15:1. However, increased protein intake, blood in the gastrointestinal tract, or enhanced endogenous catabolic rate (e.g., fever, steroids, or trauma) may also increase the ratio of BUN to plasma creatinine. Alternatively, a low-protein diet or liver disease could lower the ratio of BUN to serum creatinine with prerenal or postrenal azotemia, or an increased catabolic rate could increase the ratio to >10 to 15:1 with AKI. Thus, as with evaluation of the composition of the urine, the interpretation of the ratio of BUN to plasma creatinine must be made with caution.

THE PATHOPHYSIOLOGY AND CLINICAL FEATURES OF THE COMMON CAUSES OF AKI

Nephrotoxins are an important cause of AKI. Some important nephrotoxins are aminoglycoside antibiotics, x-ray contrast media, NSAIDs, cisplatin, and amphotericin B.

Aminoglycoside Nephrotoxicity

Aminoglycosides are major antibiotics in the treatment of serious gram-negative infections. Their increased use and potential nephrotoxic risk have made them a frequent cause of AKI. AKI occurs in 10% to 25% of patients on aminoglcosides even with careful dosing and therapeutic plasma levels. The nephrotoxicity of the aminoglycosides probably is related to their binding to the renal cortical tissue (451,452). Specifically, the binding at the apical surface of proximal tubule cells is now known to involve megalin. Once endocytosed, aminoglycosides inhibit endosomal fusion. They may also be directly trafficked to the Golgi apparatus (453). The tissue half-life of the aminoglycosides is much longer than that in serum; specifically, in the rat the half-life in serum of gentamicin has been shown to be 30 minutes, while in renal tissue it is 109 hours (454). The long tissue half-life explains why renal failure secondary to aminoglycosides can occur even after cessation of the antibiotics. A large body of in vitro and in vivo evidence indicates that reduced oxygen metabolites are important mediators of gentamicin nephrotoxicity (455). Gentamicin has been shown to enhance the generation of superoxide anion and hydrogen peroxide by renal cortical mitochondria. The interaction between superoxide anion and hydrogen peroxide in the presence of metal catalyst can lead to the generation of hydroxyl radical. Gentamicin has been shown to release iron from renal cortical mitochondria and to enhance generation of hydroxyl radical. These in vitro observations have been supported by in vivo studies in which scavengers of reactive oxygen metabolites and iron chelators have shown to be protective in gentamicin-induced AKI.

Several factors may predispose to aminoglycoside nephrotoxicity. These include advancing age, underlying renal disease, volume depletion, hypertension, and recent exposure to aminoglycosides or other nephrotoxic drugs. The clinical course of aminoglycoside nephrotoxicity is usually gradual in onset and is related to the dose and duration of drug exposure. Frequently, mild proteinuria, lysozymuria, a defect in concentrating ability, and polyuria precede a decline in glomerular filtration. Early findings are isothenuria secondary to nephrogenic diabetes insipidus, magnesium, and potassium wasting. Later findings include azotemia. The AKI of aminoglycoside toxicity is characteristically nonoliguric and reversible with a low mortality. Frank azotemia secondary to aminoglycosides may

TABLE 10.8 CLINICAL DIFFERENCES BETWEEN CONTRACT-INDUCED NEPHROPTHY AND AMINIOGLYCOSIDE NEPHROTOXICITY

Aminoglycoside Nephrotoxicity	CIN
Nonoliguric	Oliguric more than nonoliguric
Slow onset (days to weeks)	Fast onset (24 h)
Slow recovery	Faster recovery
Normal or high Fe_{Na}	Low Fe_{Na}

CIN, contract-induced nephropthy; Fe_{Na}, fractional excretion of sodium.

develop for the first time after the drug has been discontinued; conversely, recovery of renal function following discontinuation of the nephrotoxic aminoglycoside is often delayed and may require weeks to months to be complete. The clinical differences between aminoglycoside nephrotoxicity and contrast-induced nephropathy (CIN) are shown in Table 10.8.

Contrast Induced Nephropathy

Radiocontrast media-induced AKI has clinically different features compared to aminoglycoside toxicity. The essential clinical differences between CIN and aminoglycoside nephrotoxicity are shown in Table 10.8.

CIN has been recognized to be a cause of renal failure with increasing frequency in the past few years. The incidence of CIN is about 11.3% using the definition of a 25% increase in serum creatinione or an absolute increase in serum creatinine of 0.5 mg/dL (456). Radiocontrast agents cause AKI by causing renal vasoconstriction. Hypoxic tubular injury is important in the pathophysiology of radiocontrast nephropathy. Radiologic contrast agents markedly aggravate outer medullary physiologic hypoxia (457). Endothelins have been implicated in the pathophysiology of radiocontrast nephropathy (458). However, in a recent clinical study of 158 patients with chronic renal failure undergoing cardiac angiography, administration of a mixed endothelin A and B receptor antagonist with intravenous hydration resulted in an exacerbation of radiocontrast nephrotoxicity compared with hydration alone (459).

Predisposing factors include age (>55 years), prior renal insufficiency, diabetes mellitus with neurovascular complications, proteinuria, volume depletion, acute liver failure, and recent nephrotoxic drug exposure (460). Renal failure has been reported following a variety of arteriographic procedures as well as intravenous urography, computed tomography (CT) scan with contrast medium, cholangiography, and oral cholecystography (460). The onset of renal failure usually is abrupt within 24 hours after exposure to contrast media and is characterized by oliguria, but it may be nonoliguric (461). Recovery of renal function generally occurs. However, patients with advanced renal failure, particularly diabetic patients with nephropathy, may never recover function following x-ray contrast-induced AKI and may require chronic hemodialysis (CHD) therapy. Newer nonionic agents may be less nephrotoxic in high-risk patients (462).

It can be minimized by hydration with saline before and after the contrast load (463). Diuretics should be avoided if possible. The hemodynamic effect of radiocontrast may to be mediated by Ca^{2+}, since Ca^{2+} channel blockers attenuate the AKI. Recovery from radiocontrast related AKI tends to begin within 2 to 3 days. Prophylactic oral administration of the antioxidant acetylcysteine, along with hydration, attenuates the reduction in renal function induced by contrast agents in patients with chronic renal insufficiency (464). However, in this study, a reduction in renal function was defined by a small increase in serum creatinine of at least 0.5 mg/dL, which did not result in morbidity or mortality. Also the acetylcysteine-treated group actually had a decrease in serum creatinine compared with the baseline.

Trials that compare intravenous sodium chloride to intravenous sodium bicarbonate for the prophylaxis of CIN have demonstrated conflicting results (465). Two recent meta-analyses have attempted to provide a more definitive answer to whether intravenous sodium chloride is better than intravenous sodium bicarbonate in preventing CIN (456,466). Both meta-analyses demonstrated that intravenous sodium bicarbonate is better in preventing CIN as defined by an increase in serum creatinione of 25% or an absolute increase in serum creatinine of 0.5 mg/dL. Intravenous sodium chloride was no different to intravenous sodium bicarbonate in preventing the need for RRT or death (456,466). The clinical trials of intravenous sodium chloride versus intravenous sodium bicarbonate performed to date in CIN have major limitations (465). Adequately powered, well-designed clinical trials of interventions to prevent or treat CIN are urgently needed.

NSAIDs

NSAIDs, which are used in the management of pain and rheumatic disorders, are increasingly recognized as etiologic factors in AKI. These substances, which include a large group of newer nonsteroidal agents, COX-2 inhibitors, as well as aspirin and its derivatives, have in common the inhibition of prostaglandin synthesis (464). They have been incriminated in several renal abnormalities, including ischemic AKI (467), AIN (468), hyporeninemic hypoaldosteronism (469), papillary necrosis (470), and nephrotic syndrome (471).

Studies indicate that NSAID-induced AKI is due to the diminished renal vasodilatory effect of prostaglandins. In individuals receiving a 50-mEq sodium diet daily, indomethacin doses of 150 mg caused decrements in the GFR of <10 percent but no change in renal blood flow (472). However, chronic renal failure patients treated with the same indomethacin dose and diet regimen had more profound decrements in both the GFR and renal blood flow. Similar effects of diminished renal function and blood flow associated with the use of indomethacin and other NSAIDs have been reported in patients with lupus nephritis (473), nephrotic syndrome (474), cirrhosis with ascites (475), and severe congestive heart failure (476). Common to all of the edematous disorders is reduced effective arterial circulating volume (decreased cardiac output or arterial vasodilatation) and renal vasoconstriction mediated by stimulation of sympathetic tone and the RAS. This renal vasoconstriction is normally attenuated by the vasodilatory effect of prostaglandins. Blocking prostaglandin synthesis with NSAIDs disrupts this balance, thus causing severe renal vasoconstriction and a reduced GFR. Other predisposing factors to NSAID-induced ischemic renal dysfunction include diuretic use, elderly age, atherosclerotic cardiovascular disease, renovascular disease, diabetes, and acute gouty arthritis (476). Patients with chronic renal insufficiency are also at risk of acute vasomotor decline in renal function with NSAIDs. Typical clinical features include the presence of risk factors, modest salt and water retention, decreased urinary output, a benign urine sediment, low FE_{Na} (<1%), and prompt improvement in renal function on discontinuation of NSAIDs (467,469). Several of the NSAIDs have been associated with an acute allergic interstitial nephritis that is highlighted by renal failure, heavy proteinuria, and interstitial nephritis with foot process fusion (minimal change) on renal biopsy. This renal failure with NSAIDs is also generally reversible but in a slower fashion.

Cyclooxygenase metabolizes arachidonic acid into prostaglandin H2. There are two isoforms of cyclooxygenase, designated COX1 and COX2. In the kidney, COX1 predominates in vascular smooth muscle and collecting ducts, whereas COX2 predominates in the macula densa and nearby cells in the cortical thick ascending limb. COX2 is also highly expressed in medullary interstitial cells (477). COX1 is constitutively expressed, while COX2 expression is typically low (478). COX2 expression is subject to regulation by salt intake, water intake, medullary tonicity, growth factors, cytokines, and adrenal steroids. Recently, COX2-selective NSAIDs have become widely available. Many of the adverse renal effects of nonselective NSAIDs appear to be mediated by the inhibition of COX2 rather than COX1. While COX2-selective NSAIDs spare the gastrointestinal tract, they appear to have the same adverse effects on the kidney as the nonselective NSAIDs. Clinical and experimental studies have shown that renal effects of COX-2 inhibitors are similar to those of nonselective NSAIDs (479). These adverse effects include sodium, potassium, and water retention and decreases in renal function, as well as mild to modest increases in blood pressure and aggravation of edema. These adverse effects are potentiated in patients with volume and/or sodium depletion. Also, experimental studies showed increased renal COX-2 expression in models of renal injury, including the remnant kidney, renovascular hypertension, diabetes, as well as during the progression of renal failure (478). This suggests that COX-2 inhibitors may confer a renoprotective effect in diverse renal disorders.

Cisplatin

Cisplatin is a very effective chemotherapeutic agent used in a number of tumor types. Despite routine use of hydration and mannitol, there is still a significant incidence of renal failure. Cisplatin nephrotoxicity is cumulative and dose dependent (480). A significant and transient increase in BUN and serum creatinine is observed in most patients after a single dose of 40 to 100 mg/m^2. At a high dose of 100 mg/m^2 given over 1 week, there is a prolonged renal failure that can last up to 2 years (481). Cisplatin causes tubular necrosis predominantly of S3 segments of proximal tubules (482). The decrease in renal plasma flow by cisplatin precedes the decrease in the GFR, suggesting that the primary effect of the drug in causing tubular necrosis may be due to decreased circulation in the vasa recta, causing damage to the adjacent S3 segments (483). In this regard, caspases and calpain are independent mediators of cisplatin-induced endothelial cell necrosis (129). Also the circulating von Willebrand factor (vWF), a measure of systemic endothelial injury, is increased in mice with cispatin-induced AKI (331). However, cisplatin causes tubular cell death by apoptosis in cultured tubules, an in vitro system independent of renal vasculature (484,485). This suggests that cisplatin can also cause tubular injury directly. Cisplatin nephrotoxicity is also associated with urinary losses of magnesium, sodium, potassium, and Ca^{2+}, as well as hypomagnesemia and hypokalemia.

The pathogenesis of cisplatin-induced AKI has been widely studied in rodents. The antioxidant N-acetylcysteine (486) and the reducing agent glutathione (487) protect against cisplatin-induced AKI in rat models. Caspase-1-deficient mice are protected against cisplatin-induced ATN and tubular cell apoptosis (207). Cisplatin-induced ARF is associated with an increase in the cytokines IL-1β, IL-18, and IL-6 and neutrophil infiltration in the kidney.(125). However, inhibition of IL-1β, IL-18, and IL-6 or neutrophil infiltration in the kidney is not sufficient to prevent cisplatin-induced ARF. Cisplatin-induced AKI in mice is associated with an increase in CD11b-positive macrophages in the kidney and increased expression of fractalkine (CX3CL1), a potent macrophage chemoattractant that is expressed on activated endothelial cells (331). However, macrophage depletion or fractalkine receptor (CX3CR1) inhibition is not sufficient to protect against the histologic and functional changes in cisplatin-induced AKI. The role of other proinflammatory cytokines and inflammatory cells, for example, T cells, merits study in cisplatin-induced AKI.

Angiotensin Converting Enzyme Inhibitors

Angiotensin converting enzyme (ACE) inhibitors are cells widely used for the treatment of hypertension, congestive heart failure, and diabetic nephropathy. AKI may occur in conditions where angiotensin plays a crucial role in maintaining the GFR, such as volume depletion, bilateral renal artery stenosis, autosomal dominant polycystic kidney disease, cardiac failure, cirrhosis, and diabetic nephropathy. Diuretic-induced sodium depletion and underlying chronic renal insufficiency are major predisposing factors. Renal insufficiency is usually asymptomatic, nonoliguric, and associated with hyperkalemia. AKI is reversible in most cases after discontinuation of the ACE inhibitor.

Hepatorenal Syndrome

In cirrhosis of the liver, according to the systemic arterial vasodilation hypothesis, relative underfilling of the arterial tree triggers a neurohumoral response (activation of the renin–angiotensin–aldosterone system, SNS, nonosmotic release of vasopressin) aimed at restoring circulatory integrity by promoting renal sodium and water retention. Evidence has accumulated for a major role of increased vascular production of NO as the primary cause of arterial vasodilation in cirrhosis (342,488).

HRS should be considered in patients with decompensated cirrhosis with ascites presenting with AKI. This condition is typical of prerenal azotemia, as the urine sediment is bland and the kidney functions normally if transplanted into a person with a normal liver. It is a diagnosis of exclusion as other causes of AKI like ATN, hypovolemia, AIN, acute glomerulonephritis, and urinary obstruction need to be excluded. It has a 95% mortality rate but can be reversed by liver transplantation. Recent studies have shown that a V1 vasopressin antagonist, terlipressin, with albumin for 7 to 10 days can reverse type 1 HRS (high risk for mortality within weeks) in approximately 50% of patients.

Recently, new diagnostic criteria for HRS have been proposed (489). The diagnosis of HRS is based on the exclusion of other causes of renal failure. The revised diagnostic criteria for HRS differ from the previously established criteria in that (a) renal failure in the setting of ongoing sepsis, but not septic shock, is considered as HRS; (b) plasma volume expansion should be performed with albumin rather than saline; and (c) minor diagnostic criteria like urine volume <500 mL/day, urine sodium <10 mEq/l, urine osmolality greater than plasma osmolality, and serum sodium concentration <130 mEq/L have been excluded. Major criteria that should be present to make a diagnosis of HRS are (a) cirrhosis with ascites, (b) serum creatinine >1.5 mg/dL, (c) absence of shock and no current or recent treatment with nephrotoxic drugs, (d) no sustained improvement of serum creatinine to a level <1.5 mg/dL following at least 2 days of diuretic withdrawal and volume expansion with albumin (1 g/kg/day up to a maximum of 100 g/day), and (e) absence of intrinsic kidney disease as indicated by proteinuria >500 mg/day, hematuria (>50 red blood cells [RBCs] per high-power field), or abnormal renal ultrasound.

Atheroembolic Disease

Atheroembolic disease, sometimes separately designated as cholesterol crystal embolism, is an increasing and still underdiagnosed cause of renal dysfunction antemortem in elderly patients (490,491). A history of AKI occurring after cardiovascular surgery, angiography-induced aortic intimal trauma, or intravenous administration of streptokinase for myocardial infarction should raise a suspicion of atheroembolic disease as the cause of AKI. Occasionally it occurs spontaneously or in patients on coumadin. There are showers of cholesterol crystals or microemboli from the surface of ulcerated plaques that travel distally to occlude small arterioles. Small emboli to the gut and pancreas may cause abdominal pain. Clinical examination may reveal peripheral vascular insufficiency, a "blue" toe, or livido reticularis. Laboratory investigation may reveal an increased erythrocyte sedimentation rate (ESR), eosinophilia, and hypocomplementemia. The presentation and clinical findings can be confused with those of polyarteritis nodosa, allergic vasculitis, subacute bacterial endocarditis, or left atrial myxoma. The confirmatory diagnosis can be made by means of biopsy of the target organs, including kidneys, skin, and the gastrointestinal system. The renal outcome may be variable; some patients deteriorate or remain on dialysis, some improve, and some remain with chronic renal impairment. Prevention of the disease involves avoiding unnecessary invasive procedures, for example, a renal arteriogram—manipulation of the aorta during surgery in patients with clinical evidence of widespread atherosclerosis. An aggressive therapeutic approach, for example, surgical bypass of infrarenal lesions with patient-tailored supportive measures, may be associated with a favorable clinical outcome (492).

Thrombotic Microangiopathies

Thrombotic microangiopathies are characterized by microangiopathic hemolytic anemia, thrombocytopenia, and variable renal and neurologic manifestations. This condition should be suspected in patients with AKI, thrombocytopenia, and neurologic signs like confusion and seizures. The causes of thrombotic microangiopathy and AKI are listed in Table 10.1. A peripheral blood smear will always show increased RBC fragmentation. The clotting profile, for example, international normalized ratio (INR) and partial thromboplastin time (PTT), is usually normal.

All of these disorders most likely begin with endothelial injury followed by secondary platelet thrombi formation in renal arterioles. Recent advances in the pathophysiology of thrombotic thrombocytopenic purpura (TTP) and hemolytic uremic syndrome (HUS) are the newly discovered vWF, multimer-cleaving protease, endothelial cell apoptosis induced by serum from patients with TTP, and atypical HUS and the activation of the complement system (493). Renal cortical necrosis may result from the arterial lesions. When acute azotemia develops in association with these disorders, it often represents only one of many serious complications of an underlying disease. Moreover, the primary site of injury is the glomerulus or the vascular supply of the glomerulus, with the proximal tubule and the interstitial areas relatively uninvolved. Recovery of renal function following HUS in children is expected. Plamapheresis is the treatment of choice in TTP.

Acute Uric Acid Nephropathy

Acute uric acid nephropathy causes AKI due to intratubular deposition of uric acid crystals. There is a very high serum uric acid concentration. It typically occurs during induction chemotherapy for malignancies with high cell turnover, for example, leukemias and lymphoproliferative malignancies. Acute uric acid nephropathy and AKI occur in the tumor lysis syndrome. Clinical features of acute uric acid nephropathy are hyperuricemia, hyperkalemia, hyperphosphatemia, and a urine urate:creatinine ratio >2. Preventive measures include vigorous hydration and alkaline diuresis. Allopurinol should be started several days before the chemotherapy.

Acute Phosphate Nephropathy

AKI has been reported after the administration of oral sodium phosphate solution as bowel preparation for colonoscopy (494). A common bowel-cleaning regimen is 45 mL of oral sodium phosphate solution containing 21.6 g of monobasic sodium phosphate and 8.1 g of dibasic sodium phosphate, which is equal to 5.8 g of elemental phosphorus. Five criteria have been proposed to make a diagnosis of acute phosphate nephropathy (494): (a) AKI, (b) recent exposure to oral phosphate, (c) renal biopsy findings of acute and chronic tubular injury with abundant calcium phosphate deposits (usually involving >40 tubular lumina in a single biopsy), (d) no evidence of hypercalcemia, and (e) no other significant pattern of renal injury on renal biopsy. Risk factors for the development of acute phosphate nephropathy include preexisting chronic kidney disease, inadequate hydration, older age, hypertension treated with ACE inhibitors, ARBs or loop diuretics, female gender, and NSAIDs. Oral phosphate solution is contraindicated in patients with chronic kidney disease, congestive heart failure, gastrointestinal obstruction, and preexisting electrolyte disorders like hypercalcemia. In animal studies, it remains controversial whether acute phosphate administration alone can cause AKI in the absence of kidney injury from other causes, for example, hypotension and NSAIDs. Female rats fed purified diets containing either 0.4% or 0.6% (wt/wt) phosphorus for 28 days develop nephrocalcinosis and renal impairment (495). However in another study, rats fed oral phosphate did not get renal failure or nephrocalcinosis (496).

Melamine Toxicity

Melamine is an organic nitrogenous compound used commercially in the production of various products like plastics. Recently, in China, melamine was added to milk to falsely elevate protein assay results (497). This resulted in melamine toxicity mostly in children, causing kidney stones due to melamine/cyanuric acid crystals, chronic inflammation in the kidneys, and AKI. An outbreak of AKI in dogs and cats was related to melamine in pet foods (498).

Acute Interstitial Nephritis

AIN is a disorder characterized by acute renal insufficiency usually due to infection or drug exposure. In the kidney, the pathologic changes include an acute interstitial inflammatory exudate and edema. The pathology as seen on renal biopsy is similar regardless of the etiology. There is interstitial edema with variable numbers of polymorphonuclear leukocytes, eosinophils, mononuclear cells, and plasma cells. The glomeruli appear normal, and the tubules show abnormalities that include necrosis, degeneration, or atrophy. The distribution of the tubular changes is patchy.

The earliest cases of this disease were detected in association with diphtheria, syphilis, and streptococcal and other bacterial infections (499). More recently, AIN has been diagnosed in leptospirosis (500), Legionnaires disease, infectious mononucleosis, and falciparum malaria (501). Other protozoan, fungal, and rickettsial agents have also been causally incriminated in AIN. Infection-related AIN usually presents as renal failure complicating the underlying disease.

There are arguments to suggest that drug-induced AIN is secondary to an immune reaction in humans (502). It only occurs in a small proportion of people taking the drug. It is not dose dependent. It is sometimes associated with extrarenal manifestations of hypersensitivity and it recurs after reexposure to the drug or a closely related drug.

Endogenous renal antigens can induce AIN. In a rat model, antisera to Tamm–Horsfall protein caused in situ granular immune complexes in the ascending limb of the loop of Henle (503). In another animal model, Brown–Norway rats have been found to develop antitubular basement membrane antibodies and tubulointerstitial nephritis when injected with homologous tubular basement membrane (504). Renal mononuclear cell infiltration has also been shown in rats injected with homologous or heterologous kidney preparations, suggesting a cell-mediated inflammatory response to autologous antigens (505). Other studies in rats (506) identified activated and immunologically suppressible T cells in inflammatory kidney infiltrates, which also suggests a cell-mediated immunologic response in interstitial nephritis. Human counterparts of these animal studies have been suggested by a number of investigators. Tubular immune complexes have been demonstrated in 50% of lupus nephritis patients (507). Interstitial inflammatory infiltrates are frequently found in association with tubular deposits. Antitubular basement membrane antibodies have been detected in patients with antiglomerular basement membrane–mediated disorders such as Goodpasture syndrome (507). Antitubular basement membrane antibodies have also been found in renal allografts and poststreptococcal glomerulonephritis (507). In antiglomerular basement membrane disease (507), evidence exists that cell-mediated immunity develops against renal antigens. Interstitial lymphocyte infiltrates are frequently seen in this disorder.

Experimental AIN can also be induced by promoting immune reactions against extrarenal proteins that become trapped in the kidney ("planted" antigens) (502). AIN can be induced by injecting rabbits with bovine serum albumin or by injecting aggregated bovine gamma globulins into the kidney of presensitized animals (508).

In animal models of AIN there is either cell-mediated or antibody-mediated immunity (509). However, in humans, AIN probably involves cell-mediated immunity, as immune deposits are not usually seen on renal biopsy. Also, interstitial infiltrates consist of T cells.

Experimental studies show that macrophages, lymphocytes, and activated tubular cells in vitro can produce cytokines that result in proliferation of fibroblasts and/or increase in extracellular matrix (510). The agents produced by these inflammatory cells include TGF-β, IL-1, IL-4, IGF-1, ET-1, and lipid peroxidation products. Accumulation of extracellular matrix may lead to permanent impairment of renal function and the anti-inflammatory TGF-β may induce interstitial fibrosis.

Most drug-related reports of AIN have been with the use of penicillin and, in particular, its synthetic analogs such as methicillin. The antibiotic-induced acute allergic interstitial nephritis may have the clinical findings of a hypersensitivity reaction, with fever, rash, joint pain, and eosinophilia. The urinary sediment is not diagnostic, showing mild proteinuria (<1.5 g/day), pyuria, hematuria, and granular casts. Urine cultures are usually negative. Other urinary findings include impaired concentrating ability, urinary acidification, as well as decreasing potassium excretion. Renal failure is variable. Drug-related AIN also may have a paucity of clinical findings. There may be raised IgE levels in the serum of patients with drug-induced interstitial nephritis.

Recently, there has been considerable interest in the role of NSAIDs in acute allergic interstitial nephritis. The interstitial disorder associated with NSAIDs can occur separately from the ischemic injury and often presents with nephrotic range proteinuria in the absence of clinical findings of a hypersensitivity reaction. However, acute deterioration of renal function may be the only manifestation. The clinical features of the two major forms of acute allergic interstitial nephritis are listed in Table 10.9.

TABLE 10.9 TWO MAJOR FORMS OF ACUTE ALLERGIC INTERSTITIAL NEPHRITIS

	β-Lactam Antibiotics	NSAIDs
Age	Any age	Older than 60
Duration of therapy	Days	Months
Fever, rash, eosinophilia/uria	80%	20%
Proteinuria	<1 g/day	Nephrotic
Requirement for dialysis	20%	40%
Commonest agent	Methicillin	Fenoprofen
Other common agents	β-lactam antibiotics	Aspirin
	Ciprofloxacin	Ibuprofen
	Sulphonamides	Indomethacin
	Erythromycin	Naproxen
	Rifampicin	Phenylbutazone
	Phenytoin	Piroxicam
	Furosemide	Tolemetin
	Allopurinol	Zomepirac
	Cimetadine	Any NSAID
	Omeprazole	

NSAID, nonsteroidal antiinflammatory drug.

In general, recovery occurs with treatment of the underlying disease or removal of the offending drug. However, there have been reports of permanent impairment of renal function or death (501). There is some indication that heavy proteinuria in the nephrotic range and renal granulomas on biopsy are associated with a poor outcome. The use of steroid therapy is controversial, since there is no large randomized prospective controlled study indicating a beneficial effect of steroids (502). However, a brief course of corticosteroids can hasten the recovery of renal function (502). Despite the lack of scientific evidence, a short course of prednisone in a patient whose renal function fails to improve within 1 week of stopping the inciting drug is recommended, provided the diagnosis of AIN is confirmed by renal biopsy (502).

AKI in Patients with Acquired Immunodeficiency Syndrome

The approach to the causes of AKI in AIDS patients is the same as that for other patients, that is, prerenal, intrinsic renal, and postrenal causes. Causes of AKI that are especially associated with human immunodeficiency virus (HIV) infection are given in Table 10.8. AKI may develop in 6% to 20% of hospitalized patients with AIDS and is in most cases multifactorial (511). In a study of 449 patients admitted to a hospital in New York City, the causes of AKI were hypovolemia (38%), drug toxicity (37%), ATN from shock or sepsis (8%), and radiocontrast nephropathy 4% (512). AKI secondary to tenofovir nephrotoxicity has recently been described (513). A distinct form of AIN secondary to diffuse infiltrative lymphocytosis syndrome (DILS) has also been reported in AIDS patients (513) (Table 10.10).

New antiviral agents for the treatment of AIDS have led to increased survival and improved quality of life. Protease inhibitors are important drugs in patients with AIDS. AKI is a rare but important complication of Indinavir treatment (514). The renal function of patients receiving indinavir should be closely monitored. Benign and asymptomatic crystalluria occurs in 4% to 13% of AIDS patients receiving indinavir. Interstitial nephritis has also been reported. A hydration protocol consisting of 1 to 2 L of fluid should be initiated 3 hours after each indinavir dose. If AKI persists, temporary indinavir withdrawal or switching to another protease inhibitor should be considered.

Importantly it should be realized that ATN in AIDS patients may be avoidable in some cases when preventative measures are used, for example, maintaining adequate hydration before use of radiocontrast agents and during use of antibiotics and antiretroviral therapy that precipitates crystalluria (515).

TABLE 10.10 AKI IN AIDS PATIENTS

Prerenal
Hypovolemia (diarrhea)
Hypotension (sepsis, bleeding)
Vasoconstriction (radiocontrast agents)

Renal
ATN (shock, bacteremia, aminoglycosides, amphotericin, tenofovir)
Rhabdomyolysis (pentamidine, zidvudine, didanosine)
Acute allergic interstitial nephritis (penicillins, sulphonamides)
Postinfectious glomerulonephritis
Hemolytic uremic syndrome and thrombotic thrombocytopenic purpura
Diffuse infiltrative lymphocytosis syndrome (DILS)

Postrenal
Tubular obstruction due to crystalluria (intravenous acyclovir, sulphadiazine, indinavir, saquinavir, ritonavir)
Extrinsic ureteral compression (lymph nodes, tumors)
Intrinsic ureteral obstruction (fungus balls)
Bladder obstruction (tumors, fungus balls)

AKI, acute kidney injury; AIDS, acquired immunodeficiency virus; ATN, acute tubular necrosis.

Management of AKI

FLUID AND ELECTROLYTES

The use of dialysis therapy for oliguric AKI may permit fluid intakes of 1.5 to 2.0 L/day, depending on the volume status of the patient. If dialysis is not immediately available, fluid balance usually can be maintained by replacing insensible losses (400 to 600 mL/day) with 10% dextrose in water and measured losses (e.g., urine, gastric drainage, diarrhea) liter for liter with 0.45% saline. The best way to monitor the adequacy of fluid therapy is a clinical examination of ECF volume status, urine output, and daily weights. A serum sodium determination is useful in deciding whether water intake is appropriate to solute intake. Hyponatremia generally indicates excessive water intake, and hypernatremia indicates too little water intake. Since hypokalemia is rarely a problem in patients with oliguric AKI, and because of the dangers of hyperkalemia, potassium chloride is not added to intravenous fluids.

In general, fluid management in nonoliguric AKI tends to be easier. These patients ordinarily should receive a volume of fluid per day that equals their urine output plus insensible losses. The salt content of their diets should be approximately equal to what is excreted in the urine and lost in other measurable bodily fluids.

DIURETICS

The use of diuretic agents in the treatment of AKI has several theoretical benefits. As tubular obstruction by casts is thought to contribute to the pathophysiology of AKI, prevention of cast formation might be protective. Osmotic diuretics in addition to increasing mean arterial pressure could serve to augment tubular flow and "flush out" obstructed tubules. Loop diuretics could similarly increase flow and, by inhibiting the NaK$_2$Cl transporter in the thick ascending limb of the loop of Henle, decrease medullary oxygen demand (516). Additionally, it has been observed that nonoliguric patients fare better than oliguric patients (412). While conversion of oliguria to nonoliguria has not been shown to decrease mortality, it may facilitate fluid and electrolyte management in patients with AKI.

In the setting of prevention of myoglobinuric-related AKI, mannitol is widely used. Prospective randomized controlled data, however, are lacking. There have been reports of patients with rhabdomyolysis treated with mannitol (517,518) with the suggestion that when aggressive hydration is begun early following muscle injury, AKI can be prevented (519). Mannitol coupled with bicarbonate diuresis is commonly prescribed in rhabdomyolysis (520).

While loop diuretics have been used to facilitate fluid management in AKI, they do not attenuate the course of illness or improve mortality (474,521–523). Also, in these studies, deafness as a complication of high-dose loop diuretics has been reported. In a study of 552 patients with AKI in the ICU setting, the use of diuretics was associated with an increased risk of death and nonrecovery of renal function (524). It was concluded that it is unlikely that diuretics confer benefit in AKI patients in the ICU.

NUTRITIONAL SUPPORT

AKI in the setting of multiorgan failure is a state of metabolic stress (525). Catabolism of protein stores to support gluconeogenesis can result in marked muscle and visceral protein wasting and is associated with excess morbidity and mortality.

While the benefits of nutritional support of critically ill patients with AKI are unproven, enteral compared with parenteral feeding may be of benefit. In a study of 75 patients with abdominal trauma undergoing laparotomy, enteral nutrition was associated with improved nutritional markers and decreased infectious complications and sepsis compared with parenteral nutrition (526).

However, in the setting of AKI, parenteral nutrition has not been proven to be of benefit. With multiorgan dysfunction, uremia is known to accelerate catabolism due to a variety of factors, including acidosis, altered counterregulatory hormonal status, increase in plasma protease activity, and insulin resistance. A prospective double-blind study randomizing 30 patients with AKI to three isocaloric regimens—glucose alone, glucose plus essential amino acids, and glucose plus essential and nonessential amino acids—has been performed (527). All patients remained in negative nitrogen balance throughout the study, and no difference in recovery of renal function or of survival between treatment groups was noted. In patients on CRRT, despite an intake of 2.5 g/kg/day of protein, these patients remained in negative nitrogen balance (528).

In recent reviews of the topic, the following recommendations were made (529,530): (a) protein and nonprotein calories should be provided to meet calculated energy expenditures and at a rate not to exceed 1.5 g/kg/day protein intake, (b) nutritional recommendations should not be different from that of critically ill patients as a whole, (c) total parenteral nutrition (TPN) should be administered only to patients who are severely malnourished or patients expected to be unable to eat for >14 days, and (d) enteral feeding is the preferred means of nutritional supplementation.

Specific Therapies for AKI

Although the mortality in patients with AKI has declined between 1988 and 2002 (6), the mortality of AKI in the ICU remains high (1). Most interventional therapeutic trials in AKI, for example, furosemide (523), dopamine and furosemide (531), anaratide (313,314), IGF-1 (408), and fenoldopam (532) have failed in humans. A possible reason for the failure of interventional trials in AKI is the dependence on serum creatinine to diagnose AKI. Alterations in serum creatinine may lag 24 to 48 hours behind actual changes in the GFR (416,417). Ideally, in the future, early diagnosis of AKI using urine or plasma biomarkers may allow early initiation of specific therapies, for example, EPO to treat or prevent worsening of AKI.

DIALYSIS

The various complications of AKI are listed in Table 10.11. The presence of severe hyponatremia may mimic or accentuate symptoms of uremia, and hyperkalemia may lead to severe cardiac disturbances. Symptomatic hypermagnesemia probably occurs only when patients with AKI are treated with magnesium-containing antacids. Hyperuricemia of moderate degree (10 to 14 mg/dL) is a frequent accompaniment of AKI, but the occurrence of gouty arthritis is very rare. In severely catabolic states associated with muscle breakdown, for example, rhabdomyolysis, the level of hyperuricemia may be substantially greater. Fluid overload is generally primarily responsible for the occurrence of hypertension and cardiac failure in AKI, and removal of fluid by dialysis is the most appropriate treatment. Gastrointestinal and neurologic symptoms and hemorrhagic disorders of the uremic patient with AKI should be immediately treated with dialysis. The anemia of AKI may occur more rapidly than expected from bone marrow suppression of erythropoiesis, and thus, in contrast to chronic renal failure, hemolysis may have a predominant role. However, the anemia generally does not necessitate treatment with transfusions unless simultaneous blood loss occurs. Infections remain the main cause of death in patients with AKI despite the vigorous use of dialysis. Thus, meticulous aseptic care of intravenous catheters and wounds and avoidance of the use of an indwelling urinary catheter are important in the management of such patients. Fluid overload, which leads to hypoxia, and mechanical ventilation increase mortality and, if possible, should be avoided.

The main considerations when starting a patient with AKI on dialysis are the following: (a) initiation of dialysis, (b) dose of dialysis, (c) modality of dialysis, and (d) type of dialysis membrane.

Initiation of Dialysis

The indications for starting dialysis in AKI are not specific and may differ in individual patients. Guidelines are given in Table 10.12 (533). The medical records of 100 adult trauma patients treated with CRRT for posttraumatic ARF were retrospectively reviewed (534). Patients were characterized as "early" or "late" starters, on the basis of BUN < or >60 mg/dL, before CRRT initiation. Survival was 39% in early starters compared with 20% in late starters ($p = 0.041$). In a study of 106 critically ill patients with oliguric ARF, survival at 28 days and recovery of renal function were not improved by early (within 12 hours of a creatinine clearance <20 mL/min) initiation of CVVH. In 243 patients from the Program

TABLE 10.11 COMPLICATIONS OF AKI

Metabolic
Hyponatremia
Hyperkalemia
Hypocalcemia, hyperphosphatemia
Hypermagnesemia
Hyperuricemia

Cardiovascular
Pulmonary edema
Arrhythmias
Hypertension
Pericarditis

Neurologic
Asterixis
Neuromuscular irritability
Myoclonus
Somnoloence
Seizures
Coma

Hematologic
Anemia
Bleeding

Gastrointestinal
Nausea
Vomitting
Bleeding

Infectious
Pneumonia
Bacteremia, e.g., secondary to dialysis-catheter infection
Wound infection

AKI, acute kidney injury.

TABLE 10.12 GUIDELINES FOR INITIATION OF DIALYSIS IN AKI(533)

1. Oliguria (<400 mL/day)
2. Anuria
3. Serum creatinine >6−7 mg/dL
4. Plasma urea >80−100 mg/dL
5. Pulmonary edema unresponsive to conservative therapy
6. Hyperkalemia (serum potassium >6.5 mEq/dL)
7. Symptomatic uremia, i.e., encephalopathy, pericarditis
8. Metabolic acidosis

Note: One criterion = grounds to start dialysis.
More than one criterion = mandatory to start dialysis.
AKI, acute kidney injury.

to Improve Care in Acute Renal Disease (PICARD) study, the risk of death was determined in patients with BUN > or <76 mg/dL at the initiation of dialysis. After adjustment for age, hepatic failure, sepsis, thrombocytopenia, and serum creatinine and stratified by site and initial dialysis modality, the relative risk for death was 1.85 (95% confidence interval [CI] 1.16 to 2.96) for the patients with BUN >76 mg/dL (535). This study provides the rationale for prospective trials of the early initiation of renal replacement therapy in AKI patients.

Dose of Dialysis

There have been studies evaluating the dose of dialysis in AKI. In a small prospective study of Vietnam soldiers with ATN due to trauma, patients were assigned to intensive dialysis to keep predialysis serum creatinine <5 mg/dL and BUN <70 mg/dL or conventional dialysis to keep serum creatinine <10 mg/dL and BUN <150 mg/dL (536). Mortality was reduced with intensive versus conventional therapy, 3 of 8 patients dying (36%) versus 8 of 10 patients dying (80%). In a prospective paired study in 34 civilian patients with AKI, patients were assigned to intensive dialysis (predialysis BUN <60mg/dL and serum creatinine <5 mg/dL) or conventional dialysis (BUN <100 mg/dL and creatinine <9 mg/dL). Intensive dialysis resulted in a decrease in hemorrhagic events, and the mortality was 58.8% in the intensive group and 47.1% in the conventional group, which was not statistically significant (537). In a more recent study, an inverse relationship was found between the delivered dose of dialysis and patient survival (538).

The KT/V is a dimensionless index that takes into account the urea clearance rate, K, the time on dialysis, T, and the size of the urea pool, V, and is calculated for an individual hemodialysis therapy (539). The measurement of the delivered dose of dialysis with KT/V, which was designed for use in chronic renal failure, has recently been tested in AKI in a study of 46 dialysis treatments in 28 consecutive patients (540). Blood-based kinetics used to estimate the dose of dialysis in AKI patients on IHD provided internally consistent results. However, when compared with dialysate-side kinetics, blood-based kinetics substantially overestimated the amount of solute (urea) removal. In another study in AKI, nearly 70% of the treatments delivered a KT/V <1.2, the minimally acceptable dose defined in the Dialysis Outcomes Quality Initiative (DOQI) guidelines for CHD patients (541).

In recent trials employing biocompatible membranes in CRRT, there has been a suggestion that an increased dialysis dose was beneficial. The effect of the delivered dose of dialysis on mortality among different strata of a novel scoring system for critical ill AKI patients was examined (542). Among the patients with the lowest and the highest scores, the delivered dose of dialysis had no effect on mortality. Among patients at intermediate risk for death, a higher dose of dialysis (e.g., >58% urea reduction ratio) was associated with improved survival. As the delivered KT/V in these studies was observed and was not assigned by random allocation, the significance of these findings remains in question. For example, the patients who achieved a higher KT/V may have been able to tolerate hemodialysis better than the other patients, thereby introducing bias into the analysis. Thus, the optimal KT/V in AKI is not known (543).

Three recent single-center studies have demonstrated that an increased dose of dialysis is associated with lower mortality. A prospective randomized study of the impact of different ultrafiltration doses in CRRT on survival has recently been performed (544) on 425 patients, with a mean age of 61 years, in intensive care, who had AKI. The patients were randomly assigned ultrafiltration at 20 mL h(−1) kg(−1) (group 1, $n = 146$), 35 mL h(−1) kg(−1) (group 2, $n = 139$), or 45 mL h(−1) kg(−1) (group 3, $n = 140$). The primary endpoint was survival at 15 days after stopping hemofiltration. Survivors in all groups had lower concentrations of BUN before continuous hemofiltration was started than nonsurvivors. The frequency of complications was similarly low in all groups. Mortality among these critically ill patients was high, but patients receiving the higher dose of ultrafiltration (groups 2 and 3) had significantly improved survival. In another study, 160 patients with ARF were assigned to receive daily or alternate-day IHD. The mortality rate, according to the intention-to-treat analysis, was 28% for daily dialysis and 46% for alternate-day dialysis ($p = 0.01$) (545). The hypothesis that an increase in dialysis dose obtained by using continuous venovenous hemodiafiltration (CVVHDF) is associated with better survival than continuous venovenous hemofiltration (CVVH) was tested in 206 patients (546). Twenty-eight-day and three-month survival was significantly higher in the CVVHDF group that received an increased dose of dialysis. In view of the promising single-center studies, a large multicenter study, the ATN study, was performed by the Veterans Administration/National Institutes of Health ARF Trial network (547). In 1,124 critically ill patients with AKI, intensive renal support did not decrease mortality, improve recovery of kidney function, or reduce the rate of nonrenal organ failure compared with less-intensive therapy. The Randomized Evaluation of Normal vs. Augmented Level of Replacement Therapy (RENAL) study in over 1,500 patients plans to be the largest interventional trial in AKI patients and will determine whether an

TABLE 10.13 DOSE OF DIALYSIS IN AKI

Study	Results	Ref
425 patients; single center; dose of CVVH	Ultrafiltration at 35 or 45 mL/h/kg better patient survival than 20 mL/h/kg	(544)
160 patients; single center; daily or alternate day hemodialysis	Daily hemodialysis, better patient survival than alternate-day hemodialysis	(545)
206 patients; single center; increase in dialysis dose by adding CVVHDF to CVVH	CVVH + CVVHDF better patient survival than CVVH alone	(546)
ATN study; 1,124 patients; multicenter; intensive vs. conventional dose of dialysis	Patient survival the same, intensive dialysis vs. conventional dialysis	(547)
RENAL study; 1,500 patients; effect of increased dialysis dose on survival	Study in progress	(548)

AKI, acute kidney injury; CVVH, continuous veno-venous hemofiltration; CVVHDF, continuous veno-venous hemodiafiltration; ATN,acute tubular necrosis; RENAL, Randomized Evaluation of Normal versus Augmented Level Replacement Therapy.

increased dose of dialysis improves mortality (548). The studies examining the dose of dialysis in AKI are listed in Table 10.13.

Modality of Dialysis

In critically ill patients with AKI in the ICU, either a continuous or intermittent modality of dialysis is chosen. In IHD, the patient is connected to a dialysis machine for 2 to 5 hours at a time daily or every second day. Rapid removal of solutes and fluids leads to peaks and troughs in BUN and serum creatinine and hemodynamic instability. Daily treatment for 4 hours, with a blood urea clearance of 200 mL/min, can achieve a weekly urea clearance of 350 L (549). In CRRT, the patient undergoes continuous dialysis for 24 hours a day. There is a slow, continuous, and more gradual removal of solutes and fluid. This may allow massive fluid removal and remove some proinflammatory cytokines. Disequilibrium and hemodynamic instability caused by rapid solute and fluid removal are avoided. Minimization of hypotension theoretically avoids the perpetuation of renal injury. The technique, however, requires immobilization and continuous anticoagulation. The most widely used CRRTs are CVVH and continuous venovenous hemodialysis (CVVHD). CVVHD can achieve a weekly urea clearance of 340 L by use of any combination of ultrafiltration rate and dialysate flow rate that add up to 2 L/h (549).

Several retrospective and prospective studies have attempted to compare outcomes for continuous versus intermittent modalities. In a retrospective study of 349 patients, the mortality rate was higher for continuous versus intermittent dialysis (68% vs. 41%, $p < 0.001$) (550). However when multivariate cox analysis was employed to adjust for reasons for patient assignment to continuous treatment (e.g., systolic blood pressure <90 mm Hg, liver failure, etc.), there was no increase in risk of death with continuous treatment. In another prospective study, 225 patients in the ICU were divided into three groups: group I (control group), 156 patients with AKI who did not receive dialysis; group II, 21 patients who received IHD or peritoneal dialysis (PD); and group III, 43 patients who received continuous hemodiafiltration. The mortality was higher in patients with renal failure who required dialysis. There was no difference in mortality between patients who required IHD versus CRRT (551).

A multicenter, randomized, controlled trial was conducted comparing IHD and continuous hemodiafiltration in the ICU (552). One hundred sixty-six patients were randomized. Principal outcome measures were ICU and hospital mortality, length of stay, and recovery of renal function. Despite randomization, there were significant differences between the groups in several covariates independently associated with mortality, including gender, hepatic failure, APACHE II and III scores, and the number of failed organ systems, in each instance biased in favor of the intermittent dialysis group. Using logistic regression to adjust for the imbalances in group assignment, the odds of death associated with continuous therapy was 1.3 (95% CI, 0.6 to 2.7, $p = $ NS vs. IHD). In the most recent study of intermittent versus continuous dialysis in 316 critically ill patients, the modality of RRT had no effect on the outcome (553). In a meta-analysis of 1,635 patients from nine randomized control trials, it was concluded that CRRT does not confer a survival advantage over IHD (554).

A new hybrid technique named sustained low-efficiency dialysis (SLED), in which standard IHD equipment is used with reduced dialysate and blood flow rates, has recently been described in a single-center study (555). Twelve-hour treatments were performed nocturnally, allowing unrestricted access to the patient for daytime procedures and tests. One hundred forty-five SLED treatments were performed in 37 critically ill patients in whom IHD had failed or been withheld. The study concluded that SLED is a viable alternative to traditional CRRTs for critically ill patients in whom IHD has failed due to hypotension or been withheld (555).

The difficulties in designing trials comparing intermittent with continuous modalities and also in AKI in general were recently reviewed (417). Prospective randomized studies are difficult to do, since hemodynamically unstable patients or patients who cannot tolerate IHD will almost always be started on CRRT. In patients with liver and renal failure, CRRT is the treatment of choice (556). Alternately it may be unethical to confine a mobile patient to bed to receive CVVHD. Thus randomization may be biased. CRRT therefore may be considered the modality of choice in very ill patients, while IHD is used in less ill patients. At present, IHD and CRRT are regarded as equivalent methods for the treatment of AKI (417). The choice of IHD or CRRT should be made in consultation with a nephrologist and tailored for the individual patient. The decision may also depend on facility-specific issues like experience, nursing resources, and technical proficiency. The decision with respect to the mode of dialysis must be an individual one. For example, a severely catabolic patient with trauma, fever, or rhabdomyolysis or following an operation will present initially with high BUN. Aggressive and even daily treatment with hemodialysis therefore is indicated for this group of patients.

TYPE OF DIALYSIS MEMBRANE

Interaction between blood and artificial membranes may cause adverse effects. Adverse effects of bioincompatible membranes, for example, cellulose, cuprophane, hemophane, and cellulose acetate, include activation of complement and hypotension. Biocompatible membranes are made of synthetic polymers and include polyamides, polycarbonate, and polysulfone. Synthetic membranes are regarded as being more "biocompatible" in that they incite less of an immune response than cellulose-based membranes.

The first three randomized prospective studies performed comparing bioincompatible versus biocompatible dialysis membranes demonstrated statistically significant decreases in mortality in patients dialyzed with biocompatible dialysis membranes (557–559). However, subsequent studies did not confirm these promising initial studies. In a prospective study of 57 patients with AKI, alternately assigned to a cuprophane bioincompatible versus polyamide bioincompatible membranes, the survival rate was no different—72% and 64%, respectively (560). In another study of 133 consecutive ventilated patients with AKI, randomized to CRRT, with high-flux polyacrylonitrile versus polysulfone (low protein adsorption, low kinin generation), the mortality was 70% in both groups and there was no difference in renal recovery (561). In the largest trial to date on the subject, 180 patients with AKI were randomized to cuprophane bioincompatible versus polymethacrylate biocompatible dialysis membranes (562). High rates of hypotension were seen in both groups, and there was no difference in survival between groups: 42% with cuprophane and 40% with polymethacrylate. A prospective single-center study randomizing 159 patients with AKI to one of three dialyzer membranes—low-flux polysulfone, high-flux polysulfone, and a less biocompatible meltspun cellulose diacetate membrane—was recently reported (563). There was no significant difference between the three treatment groups for survival, time to renal recovery, and number of required dialysis treatments.

Conclusion

This chapter has reviewed the causes, pathophysiology, diagnosis, and management of AKI. Animal studies have greatly expanded our knowledge of the potential mediators of vascular and tubular cell injury in AKI. Several new clinical studies have been performed in humans. In Table 10.14 (564), the emerging new therapies for AKI are correlated with the pathophysiology.

TABLE 10.14 EMERGING THERAPIES FOR AKI CORRELATED WITH THE PATHOPHYSIOLOGY(564)

Epithelial Cell Injury
Cysteine protease inhibitors
Selective NOS inhibition
Oxgen radical scavengers
NGAL
EPO
EPO receptor antagonist

Tubular Obstruction
Synthetic RGD peptides
Mannitol

Epithelial Repair
Growth factors
Mesenchymal stem cells (MSCs)

Leukocyte-Endothelial Interactions
Anti-ICAM, E-selectin antibodies
IL-18 binding protein
α-MSH
CRRT with increased ultrafiltration
Biocompatible dialysis membranes
Lymphocyte or macrophage depletion
Fractalkine receptor (CX3CR1) inhibition
Adenosine A1A, A2A, A2B receptor agonists

Renal Vasodilatation
Atrial natriuretic peptide
Ca^{2+} channel blockers
Endothelin antagonists
Nitric oxide
MSCs

AKI, acute kidney injury; NOS, nitric oxide synthase; NGAL, neutrophil gelatinase associated lipocalin; EPO, erythropoietin; RGD, arginine–glycine–aspartic acid; CRRT, continuous renal replacement therapy; IL,interleukin.

Acknowledgment

This work was supported by NIH grant RO1 DK56851 (to Charles L. Edelstein).

REFERENCES

1. Lameire N, Van Biesen W, Vanholder R. The changing epidemiology of acute renal failure. *Nat Clin Pract Nephrol.* 2006; 2: 364–377.
2. Waikar SS, Liu KD, Chertow GM. The incidence and prognostic significance of acute kidney injury. *Curr Opin Nephrol Hypertens.* 2007; 16: 227–236.
3. Esson ML, Schrier RW. Update on diagnosis and treatment of acute tubular necrosis. *Ann Intern Med.* 2002; 137(9): 744–752.
4. Liano F, Junco E, Pascual J, et al. The spectrum of acute renal failure in the intensive care unit compared with that seen in other settings. The Madrid Acute Renal Failure Study Group. *Kidney Int Suppl.* 1998; 66: S16–S24.
5. Liano F, Pascual J. Epidemiology of acute renal failure: a prospective, multicenter, community-based study. The Madrid Acute Renal Failure Study Group. *Kidney Int.* 1996; 50: 811–818.
6. Waikar SS, Curhan GC, Wald R, et al. Declining mortality in patients with acute renal failure, 1988 to 2002. *J Am Soc Nephrol.* 2006; 17(4): 1143–1150.
7. Lassnigg A, Schmidlin D, Mouhieddine M, et al. Minimal changes of serum creatinine predict prognosis in patients after cardiothoracic surgery: a prospective cohort study. *J Am Soc Nephrol.* 2004; 15: 1597–1605.
8. Van Biesen W, Vanholder R, Lameire N. Defining acute renal failure: RIFLE and beyond. *Clin J Am Soc Nephrol: CJASN.* 2006; 1(6): 1314–1319.
9. Bellomo R, Kellum JA, Ronco C. Defining and classifying acute renal failure: from advocacy to consensus and validation of the RIFLE criteria. *Intensive Care Med.* 2007; 33(3): 409–413.
10. Edelstein CL, Schrier RW. Pathophysiology of ischemic acute renal injury. In: Schrier RW, ed. *Diseases of the Kidney and Urinary Tract.* Vol 2.

8th ed. Philadelphia: Lippincott, Williams and Wilkins; 2007: 930–961.

11. Olsen TS, Olsen HS, Hansen HE. Tubular ultrastructure in acute renal failure in man: epithelial necrosis and regeneration. *Virchows Arch A Pathol Anat Histpathol*. 1985; 406: 75–89.

12. Racusen LC. Renal histopathology and urine cytology and cytopathology in acute renal failure. In: Goligorsky MS, Stein JH, eds. *Acute Renal Failure. New Concepts and Therapeutic Strategies*. New York: Churchill Livingstone; 1995: 194.

13. Solez K, Marel-Maroger L, Sraer J. The morphology of acute tubular necrosis in man. Analysis of 57 renal biopsies and comparison with glycerol model. *Medicine (Baltimore)*. 1979; 58: 362–376.

14. Solez K, Racusen LC, Olsen S. New approaches to renal biopsy assessment in acute renal failure: extrapolation from renal transplantation. *Kidney Int Suppl*. 1994; 44: S65–S69.

15. Rosen S, Stillman IE. Acute tubular necrosis is a syndrome of physiologic and pathologic dissociation. *J Am Soc Nephrol*. 2008; 19: 871–875.

16. Brivet FG, Kleinknecht DJ, Loirat P, et al. Acute renal failure in intensive care units—causes, outcome, and prognostic factors of hospital mortality; a prospective, multicenter study. French Study Group on Acute Renal Failure. *Crit Care Med*. 1996; 24: 192–198.

17. Schrier RW, Wang W, Poole B, et al. Acute renal failure: definitions, diagnosis, pathogenesis, and therapy [erratum appears in *J Clin Invest*. 2004; 114(4): 598] [review] [94 refs]. *J Clin Invest*. 2004; 114: 5–14.

18. Schrier RW, Wang W. Acute renal failure and sepsis. *N Engl J Med*. 2004; 351: 159–169.

19. Edelstein CL, Ling H, Schrier RW. The nature of renal cell injury. *Kidney Int*. 1997; 51: 1341–1351.

20. Kribben A, Edelstein CL, Schrier RW. Pathophysiology of acute renal failure. *J Nephrol*. 1999; 12(suppl 2): S142–S151.

21. Alejandro VSJ, Nelson WJ, Huie P, et al. Postischemic injury, delayed function and NaK-ATPase distribution in the transplanted kidney. *Kidney Int*. 1995; 48: 1308–1315.

22. Kwon O, Corrigan G, Myers BD, et al. Sodium reabsoption and distribution of NaK-ATPase during postischemic injury to the renal allograft. *Kidney Int*. 1999; 55: 963–975.

23. Van Why SK, Mann AS, Ardito T, et al. Expression and molecular regulation of NaK-ATPase after renal ischemia. *Am J Physiol*. 1994; 267: F75–F85.

24. Kaushal GP, Singh AB, Shah SV. Identification of gene family of caspases in rat kidney and altered expression in ischemia reperfusion injury. *Am J Physiol*. 1998; 274: F587–F595.

25. Lieberthal W. Biology of acute renal failure: therapeutic implications. *Kidney Int*. 1997; 52: 1102–1115.

26. Iwata M, Myerson D, Torok-Storb B, et al. An evaluation of renal tubular DNA laddering in response to oxygen deprivation and oxidant injury. *J Am Soc Nephrol*. 1994; 5: 1307–1313.

27. Daemen MARC, Van t'Veer C, Denecker G, et al. Inhibition of apoptosis induced by ischemia-reperfusion prevents inflammation. *J Clin Invest*. 1999; 104: 541–549.

28. Nogae S, Miyazaki M, Kobayashi N, et al. Induction of apoptosis in ischemia-reperfusion model of mouse kidney: possible involvement of Fas. *J Am Soc Nephrol*. 1998; 9: 620–631.

29. Schumer M, Colombel MC, Sawczuk IS, et al. Morphologic, biochemical and molecular evidence of apoptosis during the reperfusion phase after brief periods of renal ischemia. *Am J Pathol*. 1992; 140: 831–838.

30. Basile DP, Liapis H, Hammerman MR. Expression of bcl-2 and bax in regenerating rat tubules following ischemic injury. *Am J Physiol*. 1997; 272: 640–647.

31. Molitoris BA. Ischemia-induced loss of epithelial polarity: potential role of the cytoskeleton. *Am J Physiol*. 1991; 260: F769–F778.

32. Molitoris BA, Dahl R, Geerdes AE. Cytoskeleton disruption and apical redistribution of proximal tubule Na^+K^+ATPase during ischemia. *Am J Physiol*. 1992; 263: F488–F495.

33. Molitoris BA. New insights into the cell biology of ischemic acute renal failure. *J Am Soc Nephrol*. 1991; 1: 1263–1270.

34. Molitoris BA, Geerdes A, McIntosh JR. Dissociation and redistribution of Na^+, K^+ -ATPase from its surface membrane cytoskeletal complex during cellular ATP depletion. *J Clin Invest*. 1991; 88: 462–469.

35. Neumayer HH, Kunzendorf U, Schreiber M. Protective effect of calcium antagonists in human renal transplantation. *Kidney Int*. 1992; 41: 87–93.

36. Russo D, Testa A, Della VL, et al. Randomised prospective study on renal effects of two different contrast media in humans: protective role of a calcium channel blocker. *Nephron*. 1990; 55: 254–257.

37. Neumayer HH, Wagner K. Prevention of delayed graft function in cadaver kidney transplants by diltiazem: outcome of two prospective, randomized clinical trials. *J Cardiovasc Pharmacol*. 1987; 10: S170–S177.

38. Duggan KA, MacDonald GJ, Charlesworth JA. Verapamil prevents post-transplant oliguric renal failure. *Clin Nephrol*. 1985; 24: 289–291.

39. Humes HD. Role of calcium in pathogenesis of acute renal failure. *Am J Physiol*. 1986; 250: F579–F589.

40. Weinberg JM. The cell biology of ischemic renal injury. *Kidney Int*. 1991; 39: 476–500.

41. Schrier RW, Arnold PE, Van Putten VJ, et al. Cellular calcium in ischemic acute renal failure: role of calcium entry blockers. *Kidney Int*. 1987; 32: 313–321.

42. Lieberthal W, Nigam SK. Acute renal failure. Relative importance of proximal vs. distal tubular injury. *Am J Physiol*. 1998; 275: F623–F632.

43. Mandel LJ, Murphy E. Regulation of cytosolic free calcium in rabbit proximal tubules. *J Biol Chem*. 1984; 259: 11188–11196.

44. Tamura S, Lynch KR, Larner J, et al. Molecular cloning of rat type 2C (IA) protein phosphatase mRNA. *Proc Natl Acad Sci U S A*. 1989; 86: 1796–1800.

45. McCoy CE, Selvaggio AM, Alexander EA, et al. Adenosine triphosphate depletion induces a rise in cytosolic free calcium in canine renal epithelial cells. *J Clin Invest.* 1988; 82: 1326–1332.

46. Phelps PC, Smith MW, Trump BF. Cytosolic ionized calcium and bleb formation after acute cell injury of cultured rabbit renal tubule cells. *Lab Invest.* 1989; 60: 630–642.

47. Jacobs WR, Sgambati M, Gomez G, et al. Role of cytosolic Ca in renal tubule damage induced by hypoxia. *Am J Physiol.* 1991; 260: C545–C554.

48. Wetzels JFM, Yu L, Wang X, et al. Calcium modulation and cell injury in isolated rat proximal tubules. *J Pharmacol Exp Ther.* 1993; 267: 176–180.

49. Li H, Long D, Quamme GA. Effect of chemical hypoxia on intracellular ATP and cytosolic Mg levels. *J Lab Clin Med.* 1993; 122: 260–272.

50. Greene EL, Paller MS. Calcium and free radicals in hypoxia/reoxygenation injury of renal epithelial cells. *Am J Physiol.* 1994; 266: F13–F20.

51. Kribben A, Wieder ED, Wetzels JFM, et al. Evidence for role of cytosolic free calcium in hypoxia-induced proximal tubule injury. *J Clin Invest.* 1994; 93: 1922–1929.

52. Wilson PD, Schrier RW. Nephron segment and calcium as determinants of anoxic cell death in primary renal cell cultures. *Kidney Int.* 1986; 29: 1172–1179.

53. Schwertschlag U, Schrier RW, Wilson P. Beneficial effects of calcium channel blockers and calmodulin binding drugs on in vitro renal cell anoxia. *J Pharmacol Exp Ther.* 1986; 238: 119–124.

54. Almeida AR, Bunnachak D, Burnier M, et al. Time-dependent protective effects of calcium channel blockers on anoxia and hypoxia-induced proximal tubule injury. *J Pharmacol Exp Ther.* 1992; 260: 526–532.

55. Almeida AR, Wetzels JFM, Bunnachak D, et al. Acute phosphate depletion and in vitro rat proximal tubule injury: protection by glycine and acidosis. *Kidney Int.* 1992; 41: 1494–1500.

56. Burnier M, Van Putten VJ, Schieppati A, et al. Effect of extracellular acidosis on 45Ca uptake in isolated hypoxic proximal tubules. *Am J Physiol.* 1988; 254: C839–C846.

57. Shanley PF, Johnson GC. Calcium and acidosis in renal hypoxia. *Lab Invest.* 1991; 65: 298–305.

58. Weinberg JM. Oxygen deprivation-induced injury to isolated rabbit kidney tubules. *J Clin Invest.* 1985; 76: 1193–1208.

59. Weinberg JM, Davis JA, Venkatachalam MA. Cytosolic-free calcium increases to greater than 100 micromolar in ATP-depleted proximal tubules. *J Clin Invest.* 1997; 100: 713–722.

60. Dowd TL, Gupta RK. Multinuclear NMR studies of intracellular cations in perfused hypertensive rat kidney. *J Biol Chem.* 1992; 267: 3637–3643.

61. Gupta RK, Dowd TL, Spitzer A, et al. 23Na, 19F, 35Cl and 31P multinuclear nuclear magnetic resonance studies of perfused rat kidney. *Ren Physiol Biochem.* 1989; 12: 144–160.

62. Peters SMA, Tijsen MJ, Bindels RJ, et al. Rise in cytosolic calcium and collapse of mitochondrial potential in anoxic, but not hypoxic, rat proximal tubules. *J Am Soc Nephrol.* 1998; 7: 2348–2356.

63. Kribben A, Wetzels JFM, Wieder ED, et al. New technique to assess hypoxia-induced cell injury in individual isolated renal tubules. *Kidney Int.* 1993; 43: 464–469.

64. Tanaka T, Nangaku M, Miyata T, et al. Blockade of calcium influx through L-type calcium channels attenuates mitochondrial injury and apoptosis in hypoxic renal tubular cells. *J Am Soc Nephrol.* 2004; 15: 2320–2333.

65. Nurko S, Sogabe K, Bloomfield A, et al. Relationships of glycine and reduced pH cytoprotection to Ca—induced alterations of the proximal tubule actin cytoskeleton (abstract). *J Am Soc Nephrol.* 1993; 4: 742.

66. Nurko S, Sogabe K, Davis JA, et al. Contribution of actin cytoskeletal alterations to ATP depletion and calcium-induced proximal tubule cell injury. *Am J Physiol.* 1996; 270: F39–F52.

67. Sogabe K, Roeser NF, Davis JA, et al. Calcium dependence of integrity of actin cytoskeleton of proximal tubule microvilli. *Am J Physiol.* 1996; 271: F292–F303.

68. Wetzels JFM, Wang X, Gengaro PE, et al. Glycine protection against hypoxic but not phospholipase A2- induced injury in rat proximal tubules. *Am J Physiol.* 1993; 264: F94–F99.

69. Choi KH, Edelstein CL, Gengaro PE, et al. Hypoxia induces changes in phospholipase A2 in rat proximal tubules: evidence for multiple forms. *Am J Physiol.* 1995; 269: F846–F853.

70. Portilla D, Mandel LJ, Bar-Sagi D, et al. Anoxia induces phospholipase A2 activation in rabbit renal proximal tubules. *Am J Physiol.* 1992; 262: F354–F360.

71. Alkhunaizi AM, Yaqoob MM, Edelstein CL, et al. Arachidonic acid protects against hypoxic injury in rat proximal tubules. *Kidney Int.* 1996; 49: 620–625.

72. Bonventre JV. Calcium in renal cells. Modulation of calcium-dependent activation of phospholipase A2. *Environ Health Perspect.* 1990; 84: 155–162.

73. Portilla D, Shah SV, Lehman PA, et al. Role of cytosolic calcium-independent plasmalogen-selective phospholipase A2 in hypoxic injury to rabbit proximal tubules. *J Clin Invest.* 1994; 93: 1609–1615.

74. Bonventre JV, Huang Z, Taheri MR, et al. Reduced fertility and postischaemic brain injury in mice deficient in cytosolic phospholipase A2. *Nature.* 1997; 390: 622–625.

75. Bonventre JV. The 85-kD cytosolic phospholipase A2 knockout mouse: a new tool for physiology and cell biology. *J Am Soc Nephrol.* 1999; 10: 404–412.

76. Persson AE, Ollerstam A, Liu R, et al. Mechanisms for macula densa cell release of renin. *Acta Physiol Scand.* 2004; 181(4): 471–474.

77. Bronk SF, Gores GJ. pH dependent non-lysosomal proteolysis contributes to lethal anoxic injury of rat hepatocytes. *Am J Physiol.* 1993; 264: G744–G751.

78. Plomp PJAM, Gordon PD, Meijen AJ, et al. Energy dependence of different steps in the autophagic-lysosomal pathway. *J Biol Chem.* 1989; 264: 6699–6704.

79. Hawkins HK, Ericsson JLE, Biberfield P, et al. Lysosomal and phagosome stability in lethal cell injury. *Am J Pathol.* 1972; 68: 255–288.

80. Suzuki K. Calcium activated neutral protease: domain structure and activity regulation. *Trends Biochem Sci.* 1987; 12: 103–105.

81. Barrett MJ, Goll DE, Thompson VF. Effect of substrate on Ca2(+)-concentration required for activity of the Ca2(+)-dependent proteinases, mu- and m-calpain. *Life Sci.* 1991; 48: 1659–1669.

82. Yoshimura N, Hatanaka M, Kitahara A, et al. Intracellular localization of two distinct Ca^{2+} proteases (calpain I and II) as demonstrated using discriminative antibodies. *J Biol Chem.* 1984; 259: 9847–9852.

83. Suzuki K, Saido TC, Hirai S. Modulation of cellular signals by calpain. *Ann N Y Acad Sci.* 1992; 674: 218–227.

84. Mellgren RL. Calcium dependent proteases: an enzyme system active at cellular membranes? *FASEB J.* 1987; 1: 110–115.

85. Saido TC, Suzuki H, Yamazaki H, et al. In situ capture of calpain activation in platelets. *J Biol Chem.* 1993; 268: 7422–7426.

86. Kumamoto T, Ueyama H, Watanabe S, et al. Immunohistochemical study of calpain and its endogenous inhibitor in the skeletal muscle of muscular dystrophy. *Acta Neuropathol.* 1995; 89: 399–403.

87. Komatsu K, Inazuki K, Hosoya J, et al. Beneficial effect of new thiol protease inhibitors, epoxide derivatives, on dystrophic mice. *Exp Neurol.* 1986; 91: 23–29.

88. Nakamura M, Mori M, Nakazawa S, et al. Replacement of m-calpain byu-calpain during maturation of megakaryocytes and possible involvement in platelet formation. *Thromb Res.* 1992; 66: 757–764.

89. Giancotti FG, Stepp MA, Suzuki S, et al. Proteolytic processing of endogenous and recombinant B4 integrin. *J Cell Biol.* 1992; 118: 951–959.

90. Covault J, Liu QY, Eil Deeb S. Calcium activated proteolysis of intracellular domains of cell adhesion molecules NCAM and N-adherin. *Brain Res Mol Brain Res.* 1991; 11: 11–16.

91. Saido TC, Sorimachi H, Suzuki K. Calpain: new perspectives in molecular diversity and physiological-pathological involvement. *FASEB J.* 1994; 8: 814–822.

92. Arrington DD, Van Vleet TR, Schnellmann RG. Calpain 10: a mitochondrial calpain and its role in calcium-induced mitochondrial dysfunction. *Am J Physiol Cell Physiol.* 2006; 291(6): C1159–C1171.

93. Seubert P, Lee KS, Lynch G. Ischemia triggers NMDA receptor linked cytoskeletal proteolysis in hippocampus. *Brain Res.* 1989; 492: 366–370.

94. Lee KS, Frank S, Vanderklish P, et al. Inhibition of proteolysis protects hippocampal neurons from ischemia. *Proc Natl Acad Sci U S A.* 1991; 88: 7233–7237.

95. Lizuka K, Kawaguchi H, Yasuda H. Calpain is activated during hypoxic myocardial cell injury. *Biochem Med Metab Biol.* 1991; 46: 427–431.

96. Tolnadi S, Korecky B. Calcium dependent proteolysis and its inhibition in ischemic rat myocardium. *Can J Cardiol.* 1986; 2: 442–447.

97. Edelstein CL, Wieder ED, Yaqoob MM, et al. The role of cysteine proteases in hypoxia-induced renal proximal tubular injury. *Proc Natl Acad Sci U S A.* 1995; 92: 7662–7666.

98. Edelstein CL, Yaqoob MM, Alkhunaizi A, et al. Modulation of hypoxia-induced calpain activity in rat renal proximal tubules. *Kidney Int.* 1996; 50: 1150–1157.

99. Edelstein CL, Ling H, Gengaro PE, et al. Effect of glycine on prelethal and postlethal increases in calpain activity in rat renal proximal tubules. *Kidney Int.* 1997; 52: 1271–1278.

100. Yang X, Schnellmann RG. Proteinases in renal cell death. *J Toxicol Environ Health.* 1996; 48: 319–332.

101. Tijsen MJH, Peters SMA, Bindels RJM, et al. Glycine protection against hypoxic injury in isolated rat proximal tubules: the role of proteases. *Nephrol Dial Transplant.* 1997; 12: 2549–2556.

102. Chatterjee PK, Todorovic Z, Sivarajah A, et al. Inhibitors of calpain activation (PD150606 and E-64) and renal ischemia-reperfusion injury. *Biochem Pharmacol.* 2005; 69(7): 1121–1131.

103. Frangie C, Zhang W, Perez J, et al. Extracellular calpains increase tubular epithelial cell mobility. Implications for kidney repair after ischemia. *J Biol Chem.* 2006; 281(36): 26624–26632.

104. Hu S, Snipas SJ, Vincenz C, et al. Caspase-14 is a novel developmentally regulated protease. *J Biol Chem.* 1998; 273: 29648–29653.

105. Fraser A, Evan G. A license to kill. *Cell.* 1996; 85: 781–784.

106. Barinaga M. Death by dozens of cuts. *Science.* 1998; 280: 32–34.

107. Thornberry NA, Rano TA, Peterson EP, et al. A combinatorial approach defines specificities of members of the caspase family and granzyme B. Functional relationships established for key mediators of apoptosis. *J Biol Chem.* 1997; 272: 17907–17911.

108. Dinarello CA. Biologic basis for interleukin-1 in disease. *Blood.* 1996; 87: 2095–2147.

109. Fantuzzi G, Puren AJ, Harding MW, et al. Interleukin-18 regulation of interferon gamma production and cell proliferation as shown in interleukin-1 beta-converting enzyme (caspase-1)-deficient mice. *Blood.* 1998; 91: 2118–2125.

110. Talanian RV, Quinlan C, Trautz S, et al. Substrate specifities of caspase family proteases. *J Biol Chem.* 1998; 272: 9677–9682.

111. Salvesen GS, Dixit VM. Caspases: intracellular signaling by proteolysis. *Cell.* 1997; 91: 443–446.

112. Green DR. Apoptotic pathways: paper wraps stone blunts scissors. *Cell.* 2000; 102: 1–4.

113. Lassus P, Opitz-Araya X, Lazebnik Y. Requirement for caspase-2 in stress-induced apoptosis before mitochondrial permeabilization. *Science.* 2002; 297: 1352–1354.

114. Green DR. Apoptotic pathways: the roads to ruin. *Cell.* 1998; 94: 695–698.

115. Kuida K, Haydar TF, Kuan CY, et al. Reduced apoptosis and cytochrome c — mediated caspase

activation in mice lacking caspase 9. *Cell*. 1998; 94: 325–337.

116. Feldenberg LR, Thevananther S, del Rio M, et al. Partial ATP depletion induces Fas- and caspase-mediated apoptosis in MDCK cells. *Am J Physiol*. 1999; 276: F837–F846.

117. Krajewski S, Krajewska M, Ellerby LM, et al. Release of caspase-9 from mitochondria during neuronal apoptosis and cerebral ischemia. *Proc Natl Acad Sci U S A*. 1999; 96: 5752–5757.

118. Schielke GP, Yang GY, Shivers BD, et al. Reduced ischemic brain injury in interleukin-1 beta converting enzyme-deficient mice. *J Cereb Blood Flow Metab*. 1998; 18: 180–185.

119. Woo M, Hakem A, Elia AJ, et al. In vivo evidence that caspase-3 is required for Fas-mediated apoptosis of hepatocytes. *J Immunol*. 1999; 163: 4909–4916.

120. Srinivasula SM, Poyet JL, Razmara M, et al. The PYRIN-CARD protein ASC is an activating adaptor for caspase-1. *J Biol Chem*. 2002; 277(24): 21119–21122.

121. Martinon F, Burns K, Tschopp J. The inflamma-some: a molecular platform triggering activation of inflammatory caspases and processing of proIL-beta. *Mol Cell*. 2002; 10(2): 417–426.

122. Keller M, Ruegg A, Werner S, et al. Active caspase-1 is a regulator of unconventional protein secretion. *Cell*. 2008; 132(5): 818–831.

123. Schmitz J, Owyang A, Oldham E, et al. IL-33, an interleukin-1-like cytokine that signals via the IL-1 receptor-related protein ST2 and induces T helper type 2-associated cytokines. *Immunity*. 2005; 23(5): 479–490.

124. Wang W, Faubel SG, Ljubanovic D, et al. Endotoxemic acute renal failure is attenuated in caspase-1 deficient mice. *Am J Physiol Renal Physiol*. 2005; 288: F997–F1004.

125. Faubel S, Lewis EC, Reznikov L, et al. Cisplatin-induced ARF is associated with an increase in the cytokines IL-1β, IL-18, IL-6 and neutrophil infiltration in the kidney. *J Pharmacol Exp Ther*. 2007; 322: 8–15.

126. Barinaga M. Cell suicide: by ICE, not fire. *Science*. 1994; 263: 754–756.

127. Nicholson DW, Ali A, Thornberry NA, et al. Identification and inhibition of the ICE/CED-3 protease neccessary for mammalian apoptosis. *Nature*. 1995; 376: 37–43.

128. Suzuki A. Amyloid B-protein induces necrotic cell death mediated by ICE cascade in PC12 cells. *Exp Cell Res*. 1997; 234: 507–511.

129. Dursun B, He Z, Somerset H, et al. Caspases and calpain are independent mediators of cisplatin-induced endothelial cell necrosis. *Am J Physiol Renal Physiol*. 2006; 291: F578–F587.

130. Hara H, Friedlander RM, Gagliardini V, et al. Inhibition of interleukin 1beta converting enzyme family proteases reduces ischemic and excitotoxic neuronal damage. *Proc Natl Acad Sci. U S A*. 1997; 94: 2007–2012.

131. Loddick SA, MacKenzie A, Rothwell NJ. An ICE inhibitor, z-VAD-DCB attenuates ischaemic brain damage in the rat. *Neuroreport*. 1996; 7: 1465–1468.

132. Kuida K, Lippke JA, Ku G, et al. Altered cytokine export and apoptosis in mice deficient in interleukin-1B converting enzyme. *Science*. 1995; 267: 2000–2002.

133. Kaushal GP, Ueda N, Shah SV. Role of caspases (ICE/CED 3 proteases) in DNA damage and cell death in response to a mitochondrial inhibitor, antimycin A. *Kidney Int*. 1997; 52: 438–445.

134. Shimizu S, Eguchi Y, Kamiike W, et al. Retardation of chemical hypoxia-induced necrotic cell death by Bcl-2 and ICE inhibitors: possible involvement of common mediators in apoptotic and necrotic signal transductions. *Oncogene*. 1996; 12: 2045–2050.

135. Harrison-Shostak DC, Lemasters JJ, Edgell CJ, et al. Role of ICE-like proteases in endothelial cell hypoxic and reperfusion injury. *Biochem Biophys Res Commun*. 1997; 231(3): 844–847.

136. Edelstein CL, Shi Y, Schrier RW. Role of caspases in hypoxia-induced necrosis of rat renal proximal tubules. *J Am Soc Nephrol*. 1999; 10: 1940–1949.

137. Edelstein CL, Hoke TS, Somerset H, et al. Proximal tubules from caspase-1 deficient mice are protected against hypoxia-induced membrane injury. *Nephrol Dial Transplant*. 2007; 22: 1052–1061.

138. Li P, Allen H, Banerjee S, et al. Mice deficient in IL-1 beta-converting enzyme are defective in production of mature IL-1 beta and resistant to endotoxic shock. *Cell*. 1995; 80: 401–411.

139. Fantuzzi G, Zheng H, Faggioni R, et al. Effect of endotoxin in IL-1 beta-deficient mice. *J Immunol*. 1996; 157: 291–296.

140. Haq M, Norman J, Saba SR, et al. Role of IL-1 in renal ischemic reperfusion injury. *J Am Soc Nephrol*. 1998; 9: 614–619.

141. Melnikov VY, Ecder T, Fantuzzi G, et al. Impaired IL-18 processing protects caspase-1-deficient mice from ischemic acute renal failure. *J Clin Invest*. 2001; 107: 1145–1152.

142. He Z, Altmann C, Hoke TS, et al. Interleukin-18 (IL-18) binding protein transgenic mice are protected against ischemic AKI. *Am J Physiol Renal Physiol*. 2008; 295: F1414–F1421.

143. He Z, Dursun B, Oh DJ, et al. Macrophages are not the source of injurious interleukin-18 in ischemic acute kidney injury in mice. *Am J Physiol Renal Physiol*. 2009; 296(3): F535–F542.

144. Wang KKW, Posmantur R, Nadimpalli R, et al. Caspase mediated fragmentation of calpain inhibitor protein calpastatin during apoptosis. *Arch Biochem Biophys*. 1998; 356: 187–196.

145. Shi Y, Melnikov VY, Schrier RW, et al. Downregulation of the calpain inhibitor protein calpastatin by caspases during renal ischemia-reperfusion. *Am J Physiol Renal Physiol*. 2000; 279: F509–F517.

146. Edelstein CL. Editorial comment: calcium-mediated proximal tubular injury-what is the role of cysteine proteases? *Nephrol Dial Transplant*. 2000; 15: 141–144.

147. Moncada S, Palmer RMJ, Higgs EA. Nitric oxide: physiology, pathophysiology, and pharmacology. *Pharmacol Rev*. 1991; 43: 109–142.

148. Ignarro LJ. Biosynthesis and metabolism of endothelium derived relaxing factor. *Annu Rev Pharmacol Toxicol*. 1990; 30: 535–560.

149. Knowles RG, Moncada S. Nitric oxide synthases in mammals. *Biochem J*. 1994; 298: 249–258.

150. Mohaupt MG, Elzie JL, Ahn KY, et al. Differential expression and induction of mRNAs encoding two inducible nitric oxide synthases in rat kidney. *Kidney Int*. 1994; 46: 653–665.

151. Abu-Soud HM, Stuehr DJ. Nitric oxide synthases reveal a role for calmodulin in controlling electron transfer. *Proc Natl Acad Sci U S A*. 1993; 90: 10769–10772.

152. Nussler AK, Biliar TR. Inflammation, immunoregulation, and inducible nitric oxide synthase. *J Leukoc Biol*. 1993; 54: 171–178.

153. Morris SM, Billiar TR. New insights into the regulation of inducible nitric oxide synthase. *Am J Physiol*. 1994; 266: E829–E839.

154. Terada Y, Tomito K, Nonoguchi H, et al. Polymerase chain reaction localization of constitutive nitric oxide synthase and soluble guanylate cyclase messenger RNAs in microdissected rat nephron segments. *J Clin Invest*. 1992; 90: 659–665.

155. Romero JC, Lahera V, Salom MG, et al. Role of endothelium dependent relaxing factor nitric oxide on renal function. *J Am Soc Nephrol*. 1992; 2: 1371–1387.

156. Yu L, Gengaro PE, Niederberger M, et al. Nitric oxide: a mediator in rat tubular hypoxia/reoxygenation injury. *Proc Natl Acad Sci U S A*. 1994; 91: 1691–1695.

157. Yaqoob MM, Edelstein CL, Wieder ED, et al. Nitric oxide kinetics during hypoxia in proximal tubules: effects of acidosis and glycine. *Kidney Int*. 1996; 49: 1314–1319.

158. Ling H, Edelstein CL, Gengaro PE, et al. Effect of hypoxia on tubules isolated from nitric oxide synthase knockout mice. *Kidney Int*. 1998; 53: 1642–1646.

159. Noiri E, Peresleni T, Miller F, et al. In vivo targeting of inducible NO synthase with oligodeoxynucleotides protects rat kidney against ischemia. *J Clin Invest*. 1996; 97: 2377–2383.

160. Noiri E, Dickman K, Miller F, et al. Reduced tolerance to acute renal ischemia in mice with a targeted disruption of the osteopontin gene. *Kidney Int*. 1999; 56: 74–82.

161. Ling H, Edelstein CL, Gengaro P, et al. Attenuation of renal ischemia-reperfusion injury in inducible nitric oxide synthase knockout mice. *Am J Physiol*. 1999; 277: F383–F390.

162. Chiao H, Kohda Y, McLeroy P, et al. Alphamelanocyte-stimulating hormone protects against renal injury after ischemia in mice and rats. *J Clin Invest*. 1997; 99: 1165–1172.

163. Chiao H, Kohda Y, McLeroy P, et al. Alphamelanocyte-stimulating hormone inhibits renal injury in the absence of neutrophils. *Kidney Int*. 1998; 54: 765–774.

164. Kohda Y, Chiao H, Star RA. Alphamelanocyte-stimulating hormone and acute renal failure. *Curr Opin Nephrol Hypertens*. 1998; 7: 413–417.

165. Gabbai FB, Blantz RC. Role of nitric oxide in renal hemodynamics. *Semin Nephrol*. 1999; 19: 242–250.

166. Goligorsky MS, Noiri E. Duality of nitric oxide in acute renal injury. *Semin Nephrol*. 1999; 19: 263–271.

167. Lenz O, Elliot SJ, Stetler-Stevenson WG. Matrix metalloproteinases in renal development and disease. *J Am Soc Nephrol*. 2000; 11: 574–581.

168. Walker PD. Alterations in renal tubular extracellular matrix components after ischemia-reperfusion injury to the kidney. *Lab Invest*. 1994; 70: 339–345.

169. Walker PD, Kaushal GP, Shah SV. Meprin A, the major matrix degrading enzyme in renal tubules, produces a novel nidogen fragment in vitro and in vivo. *Kidney Int*. 1998; 53: 1673–1680.

170. Trachtman H, Valderrama E, Dietrich JM, et al. The role of meprin A in the pathogenesis of acute renal failure. *Biochem Biophys Res Commun*. 1995; 208: 498–505.

171. Caron A, Desrosiers RR, Beliveau R. Ischemia injury alters endothelial cell properties of kidney cortex: stimulation of MMP-9. *Exp Cell Res*. 2005; 310(1): 105–116.

172. Covington MD, Burghardt RC, Parrish AR. Ischemia-induced cleavage of cadherins in NRK cells requires MT1-MMP (MMP-14). *Am J Physiol Renal Physiol*. 2006; 290(1): F43–F51.

173. Bengatta S, Arnould C, Letavernier E, et al. MMP9 and SCF protect from apoptosis in acute kidney injury. *J Am Soc Nephrol*. 2009; 20(4): 787–797.

174. Craig EA, Weissman JS, Horwich AL. Heat shock proteins and molecular chaperones: mediators of protein conformation and turnover in the cell. *Cell*. 1994; 78: 365–372.

175. Kashgarian M. Stress proteins induced by injury to epithelial cells. In: Goligorsky MS, Stein JH, eds. *Acute Renal Failure; New Concepts and Therapeutic Strategies*. 1st ed. New York: Churchill Livingstone; 1995: 75–95.

176. Van Why SK, Hildebrandt F, Ardiro T, et al. Induction and intracellular localization of HSP-72 after renal ischemia. *Am J Physiol*. 1992; 263: F769–F775.

177. Emami A, Schwartz JH, Borkan SC. Transient ischemia or heat stress induces a cytoprotectant protein in rat kidney. *Am J Physiol*. 1991; 260: F479–F485.

178. Van Why SK, Mann AS, Thulin G, et al. Activation of heat-shock transcription factor by graded reductions in renal ATP, in vivo, in the rat. *J Clin Invest*. 1994; 94: 1518–1523.

179. Wang YH, Borkan SC. Prior heat stress enhances survival of renal epithelial cells after ATP depletion. *Am J Physiol*. 1996; 270: F1057–F1065.

180. Turman MA, Rosenfeld SL. Heat shock protein 70 overexpression protects LLC-PK1 tubular cells from heat shock but not hypoxia. *Kidney Int*. 1999; 55: 189–197.

181. Chatson G, Perdrizet G, Anderson C, et al. Heat shock protects kidneys against warm ischemic injury. *Curr Surg*. 1990; 47: 420–423.

182. Joannidis M, Cantley LG, Spokes K, et al. Induction of heat-shock proteins does not prevent renal tubular injury following ischemia. *Kidney Int*. 1995; 47: 1752–1759.

183. Kelly KJ, Molitoris BA. Acute renal failure in the new millennium: time to consider combination therapy. *Semin Nephrol*. 2000; 20: 4–19.

184. Gaudio KM, Thulin G, Mann A, et al. Role of heat stress response in the tolerance of immature renal tubules to anoxia. *Am J Physiol.* 1998; 274: F1029–F1036.

185. Schober A, Burger-Kentischer A, Muller E, et al. Effect of ischemia on localization of heat shock protein 25 in kidney. *Kidney Int Suppl.* 1998; 67: S174–S176.

186. Aufricht C, Lu E, Thulin G, et al. ATP releases HSP-72 from protein aggregates after renal ischemia. *Am J Physiol.* 1998; 274: F268–F274.

187. Aufricht C, Ardito T, Thulin G, et al. Heat-shock protein 25 induction and redistribution during actin reorganization after renal ischemia. *Am J Physiol.* 1998; 274: F215–F222.

188. Wang Y, Knowlton AA, Christensen TG, et al. Prior heat stress inhibits apoptosis in adenosine triphosphate-depleted renal tubular cells. *Kidney Int.* 1999; 55: 2224–2235.

189. Savill J. Apoptosis and the kidney [editorial]. *J Am Soc Nephrol.* 1994; 5: 12–21.

190. Lieberthal W, Koh JS, Levine JS. Necrosis and apoptosis in acute renal failure. *Semin Nephrol.* 1998; 18: 505–518.

191. Allen J, Winterford C, Axelsen RA, et al. Effects of hypoxia on morphological and biochemical characteristics of renal epithelial cell and tubule cultures. *Ren Fail.* 1992; 14: 453–460.

192. Lieberthal W, Menza SA, Levine JS. Graded ATP depletion can cause necrosis or apoptosis of cultured mouse proximal tubular cells. *Am J Physiol.* 1998; 274: F315–F327.

193. Wiegele G, Brandis M, Zimmerhackl LB. Apoptosis and necrosis during ischaemia in renal tubular cells (LLC-PK1 and MDCK). *Nephrol Dial Transplant.* 1998; 13: 1158–1167.

194. Shimizu A, Yamanaka N. Apoptosis and cell desquamation in repair process of ischemic tubular necrosis. *Virchows Arch.B Cell Pathol Incl Mol Pathol.* 1993; 64: 171–180.

195. Nakajima T, Miyaji T, Kato A, et al. Uninephrectomy reduces apoptotic cell death and enhances renal tubular cell regeneration in ischemic ARF in rats. *Am J Physiol.* 1996; 271: F846–F853.

196. Raafat AM, Murray MT, McGuire T, et al. Calcium blockade reduces renal apoptosis during ischemia reperfusion. *Shock.* 1997; 8: 186–192.

197. Burns AT, Davies DR, McLaren AJ, et al. Apoptosis in ischemia/reperfusion injury of human renal allografts. *Transplantation.* 1998; 66: 872–876.

198. Vukicevic S, Basic V, Rogic D, et al. Osteogenic protein-1 (bone morphogenetic protein-7) reduces severity of injury after ischemic acute renal failure in rat. *J Clin Invest.* 1998; 102: 202–214.

199. Padanilam BJ, Lewington AJ, Hammerman MR. Expression of CD27 and ischemia/reperfusion-induced expression of its ligand Siva in rat kidneys. *Kidney Int.* 1998; 54: 1967–1975.

200. Oberbauer R, Rohrmoser M, Regele H, et al. Apoptosis of tubular epithelial cells in donor kidney biopsies predicts early renal allograft function. *J Am Soc Nephrol.* 1999; 10: 2006–2013.

201. Toronyi E, Hamar J, Perner F, et al. Prevention of apoptosis reperfusion renal injury by calcium channel blockers. *Exp Toxicol Pathol.* 1999; 51: 209–212.

202. Cuevas P, Martinez-Coso V, Fu X, et al. Fibroblast growth factor protects the kidney against ischemia- reperfusion injury. *Eur J Med Res.* 1999; 4: 403–410.

203. Forbes JM, Leaker B, Hewitson TD, et al. Macrophage and myofibroblast involvement in ischemic acute renal failure is attenuated by endothelin receptor antagonists. *Kidney Int.* 1999; 55: 198–208.

204. Gobe G, Zhang XJ, Willgoss DA, et al. Relationship between expression of Bcl-2 genes and growth factors in ischemic acute renal failure in the rat. *J Am Soc Nephrol.* 2000; 11: 454–467.

205. Hammerman MR. Renal programmed cell death and the treatment of renal disease [editorial]. *Curr Opin Nephrol Hypertens.* 1998; 7: 1–3.

206. Ueda N, Kaushal GP, Shah SV. Apoptotic mechanisms in acute renal failure. *Am J Med.* 2000; 108: 403–415.

207. Faubel SG, Ljubanovic D, Reznikov LL, et al. Caspase-1-deficient mice are protected against cisplatin-induced apoptosis and acute tubular necrosis. *Kidney Int.* 2004; 66: 2202–2213.

208. Vaziri ND, Zhou XJ, Liao SY. Erythropoietin enhances recovery from cisplatin-induced acute renal failure. *Am J Physiol.* 1994; 266: F360–F366.

209. Yang CW, Li C, Jung JY, et al. Preconditioning with erythropoietin protects against subsequent ischemia-reperfusion injury in rat kidney. *FASEB J.* 2003; 17: 1754–1755.

210. Vesey DA, Cheung C, Pat B, et al. Erythropoietin protects against ischaemic acute renal injury. *Nephrol Dial Transplant.* 2004; 19: 348–355.

211. Lee SH, Li C, Lim SW, et al. Attenuation of interstitial inflammation and fibrosis by recombinant human erythropoietin in chronic cyclosporine nephropathy. *Am J Nephrol.* 2005; 25: 64–76.

212. Goldfarb M, Rosenberger C, Ahuva S, et al. A role for erythropoietin in the attenuation of radiocontrast-induced acute renal failure in rats. *Ren Fail.* 2006; 28: 345–350.

213. Kolyada AY, Liangos O, Madias NE, et al. Protective effect of erythropoietin against radiocontrast-induced renal tubular epithelial cell injury. *Am J Nephrol.* 2008; 28: 203–209.

214. Gong H, Wang W, Kwon TH, et al. EPO and alpha-MSH prevent ischemia/reperfusion-induced down-regulation of AQPs and sodium transporters in rat kidney. *Kidney Int.* 2004; 66: 683–695.

215. Sharples EJ, Patel N, Brown P, et al. Erythropoietin protects the kidney against the injury and dysfunction caused by ischemia-reperfusion [see comment]. *J Am Soc Nephrol.* 2004; 15: 2115–2124.

216. Abdelrahman M, Sharples EJ, McDonald MC, et al. Erythropoietin attenuates the tissue injury associated with hemorrhagic shock and myocardial ischemia. *Shock.* 2004; 22: 63–69.

217. Mitra A, Bansal S, Wang W, et al. Erythropoietin ameliorates renal dysfunction during endotoxaemia. *Nephrol Dial Transplant.* 2007; 22(8): 2349–2353.

218. Bonventre JV. Pathogenetic and regenerative mechanisms in acute tubular necrosis. *Kidney Blood Press Res*. 1998; 21: 226–229.

219. Megyesi J, Di Mari J, Udvarhelyi N, et al. DNA synthesis is dissociated from the immediate-early gene response in the post-ischemic kidney. *Kidney Int*. 1995; 48: 1451–1458.

220. Ouellette AJ, Malt RA, Sukhatme VP, et al. Expression of two "immediate early" genes, Egr-1 and c-fos, in response to renal ischemia and during compensatory renal hypertrophy in mice. *J Clin Invest*. 1990; 85: 766–771.

221. Safirstein R. Renal stress response and acute renal failure. *Adv Ren Replace Ther*. 1997; 4: 38–42.

222. Witzgall R, Brown D, Schwarz C, et al. Localization of proliferating cell nuclear antigen, vimentin, c-Fos, and clusterin in the postischemic kidney. Evidence for a heterogenous genetic response among nephron segments, and a large pool of mitotically active and dedifferentiated cells. *J Clin Invest*. 1994; 93: 2175–2188.

223. Safirstein R, Megyesi J, Saggi SJ, et al. Expression of cytokine-like genes JE and KC is increased during renal ischemia. *Am J Physiol*. 1991; 261: F1095–F1101.

224. Safirstein R. Gene expression in nephrotoxic and ischemic acute renal failure [editorial]. *J Am Soc Nephrol*. 1994; 4: 1387–1395.

225. Safirstein R, Price PM, Saggi SJ, et al. Changes in gene expression after temporary renal ischemia. *Kidney Int*. 1990; 37: 1515–1521.

226. Ip YT, Davis RJ. Signal transduction by the c-Jun N-terminal kinase (JNK)—from inflammation to development. *Curr Opin Cell Biol*. 1998; 10: 205–219.

227. Kyriakis JM, Banerjee P, Nikolakaki E, et al. The stress-activated protein kinase subfamily of c-Jun kinases. *Nature*. 1994; 369: 156–160.

228. Force T, Bonventre JV. Growth factors and mitogen-activated protein kinases. *Hypertension*. 1998; 31: 152–161.

229. Bonventre JV, Force T. Mitogen-activated protein kinases and transcriptional responses in renal injury and repair. *Curr Opin Nephrol Hypertens*. 1998; 7: 425–433.

230. Pombo CM, Bonventre JV, Avruch J, et al. The stress-activated protein kinases are major c-Jun amino-terminal kinases activated by ischemia and reperfusion. *J Biol Chem*. 1994; 269: 26546–26551.

231. Brown PO, Botstein D. Exploring the new world of the genome with DNA microarrays. *Nat Genet*. 1999; 21: 33–37.

232. Devarajan P, Mishra J, Supavekin S, et al. Gene expression in early ischemic renal injury: clues towards pathogenesis, biomarker discovery, and novel therapeutics. *Mol Genet Metab*. 2003; 80: 365–376.

233. Yoshida T, Tang SS, Hsiao LL, et al. Global analysis of gene expression in renal ischemia-reperfusion in the mouse. *Biochem Biophys Res Commun*. 2002; 291: 787–794.

234. Supavekin S, Zhang W, Kucherlapati R, et al. Differential gene expression following early renal ischemia/reperfusion. *Kidney Int*. 2003; 63: 1714–1724.

235. Yoshida T, Kurella M, Beato F, et al. Monitoring changes in gene expression in renal ischemia-reperfusion in the rat. *Kidney Int*. 2002; 61: 1646–1654.

236. Murakami H, Liotta L, Star RA. IF-LCM: laser capture microdissection of immunofluorescently defined cells for mRNA analysis rapid communication. *Kidney Int*. 2000; 58: 1346–1353.

237. Rosenberger C, Mandriota S, Jurgensen JS, et al. Expression of hypoxia-inducible factor-1alpha and -2alpha in hypoxic and ischemic rat kidneys. *J Am Soc Nephrol*. 2002; 13(7): 1721–1732.

238. Bernhardt WM, Campean V, Kany S, et al. Preconditional activation of hypoxia-inducible factors ameliorates ischemic acute renal failure. *J Am Soc Nephrol*. 2006; 17(7): 1970–1978.

239. Weidemann A, Bernhardt WM, Klanke B, et al. HIF activation protects from acute kidney injury. *J Am Soc Nephrol*. 2008; 19(3): 486–494.

240. Hill P, Shukla D, Tran MG, et al. Inhibition of hypoxia inducible factor hydroxylases protects against renal ischemia-reperfusion injury. *J Am Soc Nephrol*. 2008; 19: 39–46.

241. Kumar S. Tubular cast formation and Tamm-Horsfall glycoprotein, In: Goligorsky MS, Stein JS, eds. *Acute Renal Failure. New Concepts and Therapeutic Strategies*. New York, Churchill Livingstone; 1995: 274.

242. Arendhorst WJ, Finn WF, Gottschalk C, et al. Micropuncture study of acute renal failure following temporary renal ischemia in the rat. *Kidney Int*. 1976; 10(suppl 6): S100–S105.

243. Tanner GA, Steinhausen M. Kidney pressure after temporary artery occlusion in the rat. *Am J Physiol*. 1976; 230: 1173–1181.

244. Burke TJ, Cronin RE, Duchin KL, et al. Ischemia and tubule obstruction during acute renal failure in dogs: mannitol in protection. *Am J Physiol*. 1980; 238: F305–F314.

245. Wangsiripaisan A, Gengaro PE, Edelstein CL, et al. Role of polymeric Tamm-Horsfall protein in cast formation: oligosaccharide and tubular fluid ions. *Kidney Int*. 2001; 59: 932–940.

246. Ruoslahti E. RGD and other recognition sequences for integrins. *Annu Rev Cell Dev Biol*. 1996; 12: 697–715.

247. Gailit J, Colflesh D, Rabiner I, et al. Redistribution and dysfunction of integrins in cultured renal epithelial cells exposed to oxidative stress. *Am J Physiol*. 1993; 33: F149–F157.

248. Goligorsky MS, Lieberthal W, Racusen LC, et al. Integrin receptors in renal tubular epithelium: new insights into pathophysiology of acute renal failure [editorial]. *Am J Physiol*. 1993; 264: F1–F8.

249. Goligorsky MS. Abnormalities of integrin receptors. In: Goligorsky MS, Stein J, eds. *Acute Renal Failure. New Concepts and Therapeutic Strategies*. New York: Churchill Livingstone; 1995: 255.

250. Wangsiripaisan A, Gengaro P, Nemenoff R, et al. Effect of nitric oxide donors on renal tubular epithelial cell-matrix adhesion. *Kidney Int*. 1999; 55: 2281–2288.

251. Manns M, Sigler MH, Teehan BP. Intradialytic renal haemodynamics—potential consequences for the management of the patient with acute renal failure [editorial]. *Nephrol Dial Transplant.* 1997; 12: 870–872.

252. Goligorsky MS, DiBona GF. Pathogenic role of Arg-Gly-Asp recognizing integrins in acute renal failure. *Proc Natl Acad Sci U S A.* 1993; 90: 5700–5704.

253. Goligorsky MS, Kessler H, Romanov VI. Molecular mimicry of integrin ligation: therapeutic potential of arginine-glycine-aspartic acid (RGD) peptides. *Nephrol Dial Transplant.* 1998; 13: 254–263.

254. Noiri E, Gailit J, Sheth D, et al. Cyclic RGD peptides ameliorate ischemic acute renal failure in rats. *Kidney Int.* 1994; 46: 1050–1058.

255. Noiri E, Forest T, Miller F, et al. Effects of RGD peptides on the course of acute renal failure. In: Stein J, Goligorsky MS, eds. *Acute Renal Failure. New Concepts and Therapeutic Statgies.* New York: Churchill Livingstone; 1995: 379.

256. Noiri E, Romanov V, Forest T, et al. Pathophysiology of renal tubular obstruction. Therapeutic role of synthetic RGD peptides in ARF. *Kidney Int.* 1995; 48: 1375–1385.

257. Goligorsky MS, Noiri E, Kessler H, et al. Therapeutic effect of arginine-glycine-aspartic acid peptides in ARF. *Clin Exp Pharmacol Physiol.* 1998; 25: 276–279.

258. Goligorsky MS, Noiri E, Kessler H, et al. Therapeutic potential of RGD peptides in acute renal injury. *Kidney Int.* 1997; 51: 1487–1492.

259. Conger JD, Weil JU. Abnormal vascular function following ischemia-reperfusion injury. *J Invest Med.* 1995; 43: 431–442.

260. Conger JD, Robinette JB, Hammond WS. Differences in vascular reactivity in models of ischemic acute renal failure. *Kidney Int.* 1991; 39: 1087–1097.

261. Conger JD, Schultz MF, Miller F, et al. Responses to hemorrhagic arterial pressure reduction in different ischemic renal failure models. *Kidney Int.* 1994; 46: 318–323.

262. Lieberthal W, Wolf EF, Rennke HG, et al. Renal ischemia and reperfusion impair endothelium-dependent vascular relaxation. *Am J Physiol.* 1989; 256: F894–F900.

263. Matthys E, Patton MK, Osgood RW, et al. Alterations in vascular function and morphology in acute ischemic renal failure. *Kidney Int.* 1983; 23: 717–724.

264. Ueda M, Becker AE, Tsukada T, et al. Fibrocellular tissue response after percutaneous transluminal coronary angioplasty. An immunocytochemical analysis of the cellular composition. *Circulation.* 1991; 83: 1327–1332.

265. Conger JD, Falk SA, Robinette JB. Angiotensin II-induced changes in smooth muscle calcium in rat renal arterioles. *J Am Soc Nephrol.* 1993; 3: 1792–1803.

266. Conger JD, Robinette J, Villar A, et al. Increased nitric oxide synthase activity despite lack of response to endothelium-dependent vasodilators in postischemic acute renal failure in rats. *J Clin Invest.* 1995; 96: 631–638.

267. Conger JD, Robinette JB, Schrier RW. Smooth muscle calcium and endothelium-derived relaxing factor in the abnormal vascular responses of acute renal failure. *J Clin Invest.* 1988; 82: 532–537.

268. Bakris GL, Burnett JC. A role for calcium in radiocontrast-induced reduction in renal hemodynamics. *Kidney Int.* 1985; 27: 465.

269. Shapiro JI, Cheung C, Itabashi A, et al. The effect of verapamil on renal function after warm and cold ischemia in the isolated perfused rat kidney. *Transplantation.* 1985; 40: 596–600.

270. Mills S, Chan L, Schwertschlag U, et al. The protective effect of ($-$) Emopamil on renal function following warm and cold ischemia. *Transplantation.* 1987; 43: 928–930.

271. Kelleher SP, Robinette JB, Conger JD. Sympathetic nervous system in the loss of autoregulation in acute renal failure. *Am J Physiol.* 1984; 15: F379–F386.

272. Molitoris BA, Sandoval RM. Intravital multiphoton microscopy of dynamic renal processes. *Am J Physiol Renal Physiol.* 2005; 288: F1084–F1089.

273. Dagher PC, Herget-Rosenthal S, Ruehm SG, et al. Newly developed techniques to study and diagnose acute renal failure. *J Am Soc Nephrol.* 2003; 14: 2188–2198.

274. Dunn KW, Sandoval RM, Molitoris BA. Intravital imaging of the kidney using multiparameter multiphoton microscopy. *Nephron Exp Nephrol.* 2003; 94: e7–e11.

275. Dunn KW, Sandoval RM, Kelly KJ, et al. Functional studies of the kidney of living animals using multicolor two-photon microscopy. *Am J Physiol Cell Physiol.* 2002; 283: C905–C916.

276. Sutton TA, Mang HE, Campos SB, et al. Injury of the renal microvascular endothelium alters barrier function after ischemia. *Am J Physiol Renal Fluid Electrolyte Physiol.* 2003; 285: F191–F198.

277. Kwon O, Hong SM, Ramesh G. Diminished NO generation by injured endothelium and loss of macula densa nNOS may contribute to sustained acute kidney injury after ischemia-reperfusion. *Am J Physiol Renal Physiol.* 2009; 296(1): F25–F33.

278. Myers BD, Deen WM, Brenner BM. Effects of norepinephrine and angiotensin II on the determinants of glomerular ultrafiltration and proximal tubule fluid reabsorption in the rat. *Circ Res.* 1975; 37: 101–110.

279. Stahl RA, Paravicini M, Schollmeyer P. Angiotensin II stimulation of prostaglandin E2 and 6-keto-F1 alpha formation by isolated human glomeruli. *Kidney Int.* 1984; 26: 30–34.

280. Torsello G, Schror K, Szabo A. Effects of prostaglandin E1 (PGE1) on experimental renal ischemia. *Eur J Vasc Surg.* 1989; 3: 5–10.

281. Klausner JM, Paterson IS, Kobzik L, et al. Vasodilating prostaglandins attenuate ischemic renal injury only if thromboxane is inhibited. *Ann Surg.* 1989; 209: 219–224.

282. Oliver JA, Sciacca RR, Pinto J, et al. Participation of the prostaglandins in the control of renal blood flow during acute reduction of cardiac output in the dog. *J Clin Invest.* 1981; 67: 229–237.

283. Assael BM, Chiabrando C, Gagliardi L, et al. Prostaglandins and aminoglycoside nephrotoxicity. *Toxicol Appl Pharmacol.* 1985; 78: 386–394.

284. Badr KF, Kelley VE, Rennke HG, et al. Roles for thromboxane A2 and leukotrienes in endotoxin-induced acute renal failure. *Kidney Int.* 1986; 30: 474–480.

285. Freund HR, Barcelli UO, Muggia-Sullam M, et al. Renal prostaglandin production is increased during abdominal sepsis in the rat and unaffected by the infusion of different amino acid formulations. *J Surg Res.* 1988; 44: 99–103.

286. Walshe JJ, Venuto RC. Acute oliguric renal failure induced by indomethacin: possible mechanism. *Ann Intern Med.* 1979; 91: 47–49.

287. Fink MP, MacVittie TJ, Casey LC. Effects of nonsteroidal anti-inflammatory drugs on renal function in septic dogs. *J Surg Res.* 1984; 36: 516–525.

288. Papanikolaou N, Darlametsos J, Hatziantoniou C, et al. Partial protection against acute renal failure by Efamol. *Prog Clin Biol Res.* 1989; 301: 271–277.

289. Werb R, Clark WF, Lindsay RM, et al. Protective effect of prostaglandin [PGE2] and in glycerol-induced acute renal failure in rats. *Clin Sci Mol Med.* 1978; 55: 505–507.

290. Paller MS, Manivel JC. Prostaglandins protect kidneys against ischemic and toxic injury by a cellular effect. *Kidney Int.* 1992; 42: 1345–1354.

291. Kim YK, Hwang MY, Woo JS, et al. Effect of arachidonic acid metabolic inhibitors on hypoxia/reoxygenation-induced renal cell injury. *Ren Fail.* 2000; 22: 143–157.

292. Koch JA, Plum J, Grabensee B, et al. Prostaglandin E1: a new agent for the prevention of renal dysfunction in high risk patients caused by radiocontrast media? PGE1 Study Group. *Nephrol Dial Transplant.* 2000; 15: 43–49.

293. DeBold AJ, Borenstein HB, Veress AT, et al. A potent and rapid natriuretic response to intravenous injection of atrial myocardial extract in rats. *Life Sci.* 1981; 28: 89–94.

294. Yamaji T, Ishibashi M, Takaku F. Atrial natriuretic factor in human blood. *J Clin Invest.* 1985; 76: 1705–1709.

295. Bussien JP, Biollaz J, Waeber B, et al. Dose-dependent effect of atrial natriuretic peptide on blood pressure, heart rate, and skin blood flow of normal volunteers. *J Cardiovasc Pharmacol.* 1986; 8: 216–220.

296. Lappe RW, Smits JF, Todt JA, et al. Failure of atriopeptin II to cause arterial vasodilation in the conscious rat. *Circ Res.* 1985; 56: 606–612.

297. Lappe RW, Todt JA, Wendt RL. Effects of atrial natriuretic factor on the vasoconstrictor actions of the renin-angiotensin system in conscious rats. *Circ Res.* 1987; 61: 134–140.

298. Haass M, Kopin IJ, Goldstein DS, et al. Differential inhibition of alpha adrenoceptor-mediated pressor responses by rat atrial natriuretic peptide in the pithed rat. *J Pharmacol Exp Ther.* 1985; 235: 122–127.

299. Dillingham MA, Anderson RJ. Inhibition of vasopressin action by atrial natriuretic factor. *Science.* 1986; 231: 1572–1573.

300. Kohno M, Yasunari K, Yokokawa K, et al. Inhibition by atrial and brain natriuretic peptides of endothelin-1 secretion after stimulation with angiotensin II and thrombin of cultured human endothelial cells. *J Clin Invest.* 1991; 87: 1999–2004.

301. Huang CL, Lewicki J, Johnson LK, et al. Renal mechanism of action of rat atrial natriuretic factor. *J Clin Invest.* 1985; 75: 769–773.

302. Aalkjaer C, Mulvany MJ, Nyborg NC. Atrial natriuretic factor causes specific relaxation of rat renal arcuate arteries. *Br J Pharmacol.* 1985; 86: 447–453.

303. Veldkamp PJ, Carmines PK, Inscho EW, et al. Direct evaluation of the microvascular actions of ANP in juxtamedullary nephrons. *Am J Physiol.* 1988; 254: F440–F444.

304. Loutzenhiser R, Hayashi K, Epstein M. Atrial natriuretic peptide reverses afferent arteriolar vasoconstriction and potentiates efferent arteriolar vasoconstriction in the isolated perfused rat kidney. *J Pharmacol Exp Ther.* 1988; 246: 522–528.

305. Lanese DM, Yuan BH, Falk SA, et al. Effects of atriopeptin III on isolated rat afferent and efferent arterioles. *Am J Physiol.* 1991; 261: F1102–F1109.

306. Sudoh T, Kangawa K, Minamino N, et al. A new natriuretic peptide in porcine brain. *Nature.* 1988; 332: 78–81.

307. Minamino N, Aburaya M, Ueda S, et al. The presence of brain natriuretic peptide of 12,000 daltons in porcine heart. *Biochem Biophys Res Commun.* 1988; 155: 740–746.

308. Koglin J, Pehlivanli S, Schwaiblmair M, et al. Role of brain natriuretic peptide in risk stratification of patients with congestive heart failure. *J Am Coll Cardiol.* 2001; 38: 1934–1941.

309. Conger JD, Falk SA, Yuan BH, et al. Atrial natriuretic peptide and dopamine in a rat model of ischemic acute renal failure. *Kidney Int.* 1989; 35: 1126–1132.

310. Endlich K, Steinhausen M. Natriuretic peptide receptors mediate different responses in rat renal microvessels. *Kidney Int.* 1997; 52: 202–207.

311. Shaw SG, Weidmann P, Hodler J, et al. Atrial natriuretic factor peptide protects against acute ischemic renal failure in the rat. *J Clin Invest.* 1987; 80: 1232–1237.

312. Lieberthal W, Sheridan AM, Valeri CR. Protective effect of atrial natriuretic factor and mannitol following renal ischemia. *Am J Physiol.* 1990; 258: F1266–F1272.

313. Allgren RL, Marbury TC, Rahman SN, et al. Anaritide in acute tubular necrosis. *N Engl J Med.* 1997; 336: 828–834.

314. Lewis J, Salem MM, Chertow GM, et al. Atrial natriuretic factor in oliguric acute renal failure. Anaritide Acute Renal Failure Study Group. *Am J Kidney Dis.* 2000; 36: 767–774.

315. Malis CD, Cheung JY, Leaf A, et al. Effects of verapamil in models of ischemic acute renal failure in the rat. *Am J Physiol.* 1983; 245: F735–F742.

316. Wagner K, Schultze G, Molzahn M, et al. The influence of long-term infusion of the calcium antagonist diltiazem on postischemic acute renal failure in conscious dogs. *Klin Wochenschr.* 1986; 64: 135–140.

317. Garthoff B, Hirth C, Federmann A, et al. Renal effects of 1,4-dihydropyridines in animal models of hypertension and renal failure. *J Cardiovasc Pharmacol.* 1987; 9(suppl 1): S8–S13.

318. Deray G, Dubois M, Beaufils H, et al. Effects of nifedipine on cisplatinum-induced nephrotoxicity in rats. *Clin Nephrol.* 1988; 30: 146–150.

319. Lee SM, Michael UF. The protective effect of nitrendipine on gentamicin acute renal failure in rats. *Exp Mol Pathol.* 1985; 43: 107–114.

320. Watson AJ, Gimenez LF, Klassen DK, et al. Calcium channel blockade in experimental aminoglycoside nephrotoxicity. *J Clin Pharmacol.* 1987; 27: 625–627.

321. Dobyan DC, Bulger RE. Partial protection by chlorpromazine in mercuric chloride-induced acute renal failure in rats. *Lab Invest.* 1984; 50: 578–586.

322. Yao K, Sato H, Ina Y, et al. Benidipine inhibits apoptosis during ischaemic acute renal failure in rats. *J Pharm Pharmacol.* 2000; 52: 561–568.

323. Schramm L, Heidbreder E, Lukes M, et al. Endotoxin-induced acute renal failure in the rat: effects of urodilatin and diltiazem on renal function. *Clin Nephrol.* 1996; 46: 117–124.

324. Lumlertgul D, Wongmekiat O, Sirivanichai C, et al. Intrarenal infusion of gallopamil in acute renal failure. A preliminary report. *Drugs.* 1991; 42(suppl 1): 44–50.

325. Wagner K, Albrecht S, Neumayer HH. Prevention of posttransplant acute tubular necrosis by the calcium antagonist diltiazem: a prospective randomized study. *Am J Nephrol.* 1987; 7: 287–291.

326. van Riemsdijk IC, Mulder PG, de Fijter JW, et al. Addition of isradipine (Lomir) results in a better renal function after kidney transplantation: a double-blind, randomized, placebo-controlled, multi-center study. *Transplantation.* 2000; 70: 122–126.

327. Umehara H, Goda S, Imai T, et al. Fractalkine, a CX3C-chemokine, functions predominantly as an adhesion molecule in monocytic cell line THP-1. *Immunol Cell Biol.* 2001; 79: 298–302.

328. Beck GC, Ludwig F, Schulte J, et al. Fractalkine is not a major chemoattractant for the migration of neutrophils across microvascular endothelium. *Scand J Immunol.* 2003; 58: 180–187.

329. Cockwell P, Chakravorty SJ, Girdlestone J, et al. Fractalkine expression in human renal inflammation. *J Pathol.* 2002; 196: 85–90.

330. Oh DJ, Dursun B, He Z, et al. Fractalkine receptor (CX3CR1) inhibition is protective against ischemic acute renal failure in mice. *Am J Physiol Renal Physiol.* 2008; 294: 264–271.

331. Lu L, Oh DJ, Dursun B, et al. Increased macrophage infiltration and fractalkine expression in cisplatin-induced acute renal failure in mice. *J Pharmacol Exp Ther.* 2007; 324: 111–117.

332. Williams RH, Thomas CE, Navar LG, et al. Hemodynamic and single nephron function during the maintenance phase of ischemic acute renal failure in the dog. *Kidney Int.* 1981; 19: 503–515.

333. Conger JD. Prophylaxis and treatment of ARF by vasoactive agents. The facts and the myths. *Kidney Int.* 1998; 53(suppl 64): S23–S26.

334. Adams PL, Adams FF, Bell PD, et al. Impaired renal blood flow autoregulation in ischemic acute renal failure. *Kidney Int.* 1980; 18: 68–76.

335. Conger JD. Does hemodialysis delay recovery from acute renal failure? *Semin Dial.* 1990; 3: 146–147.

336. Knotek M, Rogachev B, Gengaro P, et al. Endotoxemic renal failure in mice: role of tumor necrosis factor indepenent of inducible nitric oxide synthase. *Kidney Int.* 2001; 59: 2243–2249.

337. Thijs A, Thijs LG. Pathogenesis of renal failure in sepsis. *Kidney Int Suppl.* 1998; 66: S34–S37.

338. Ortiz-Arduan A, Danoff TM, Kalluri R, et al. Regulation of Fas and Fas ligand expression in cultured murine renal cells and in the kidney during endotoxemia. *Am J Physiol.* 1996; 271: F1193–F1201.

339. Richman AV, Gerber LI, Balis JU. Peritubular capillaries. A major target site of endotoxin-induced vascular injury in the primate kidney. *Lab Invest.* 1980; 43: 327–332.

340. Hickey MJ, Sharkey KA, Sihota EG, et al. Inducible nitric oxide synthase-deficient mice have enhanced leukocyte-endothelium interactions in endotoxemia. *FASEB J.* 1997; 11: 955–964.

341. Schrier RW, Abraham WT. Hormones and hemodynamics in heart failure. *N Engl J Med.* 1999; 341: 577–585.

342. Schrier RW, Arroyo V, Bernardi M, et al. Peripheral arterial vasodilation hypothesis: a proposal for the initiation of renal sodium and water retention in cirrhosis. *Hepatology.* 1988; 8: 1151–1157.

343. Schrier RW. Pathogenesis of sodium and water retention in high-output and low-output cardiac failure, nephrotic syndrome, cirrhosis, and pregnancy (1). *N Engl J Med.* 1988; 319: 1065–1072.

344. Schrier RW. Pathogenesis of sodium and water retention in high-output and low-output cardiac failure, nephrotic syndrome, cirrhosis, and pregnancy (2). *N Engl J Med.* 1988; 319: 1127–1134.

345. Khan RZ, Badr KF. Endotoxin and renal function: perspectives to the understanding of septic acute renal failure and toxic shock. *Nephrol Dial Transplant.* 1999; 14: 814–818.

346. Schwartz D, Mendoca M, Schwartz Y, et al. Inhibition of constitutive nitric oxide synthase (NOS) by nitric oxide generated by inducible NOS after lipopolysaccharide administration provokes renal dysfunction in rats. *J Clin Invest.* 1997; 100: 439–448.

347. Knotek M, Esson M, Gengaro P, et al. Desensitization of soluble guanylate cyclase in renal cortex during endotoxemia in mice. *J Am Soc Nephrol.* 2000; 11: 2133–2137.

348. Filep JG. Role for endogenous endothelin in the regulation of plasma volume and albumin escape during endotoxin shock in conscious rats. *Br J Pharmacol.* 2000; 129: 975–983.

349. Mitaka C, Hirata Y, Yokoyama K, et al. Improvement of renal dysfunction in dogs with endotoxemia by a nonselective endothelin receptor antagonist. *Crit Care Med.* 1999; 27: 146–153.

350. Lievano G, Nguyen L, Radhakrishnan J, et al. Significance of fractional excretion of sodium and endothelin levels in the early diagnosis of renal

failure in septic neonatal piglets. *J Pediatr Surg.* 1998; 33: 1480–1482.

351. Shindo T, Kurihara H, Kurihara Y, et al. Upregulation of endothelin-1 and adrenomedullin gene expression in the mouse endotoxin shock model. *J Cardiovasc Pharmacol.* 1998; 31(suppl 1): S541–S544.

352. Ruetten H, Thiemermann C, Vane JR. Effects of the endothelin receptor antagonist, SB 209670, on circulatory failure and organ injury in endotoxic shock in the anaesthetized rat. *Br J Pharmacol.* 1996; 118: 198–204.

353. Bonventre JV, Zuk A. Ischemic acute renal failure: an inflammatory disease? *Kidney Int.* 2004; 66: 480–485.

354. Friedwald JJ, Rabb H. Inflammatory cells in ischemic acute renal failure. *Kidney Int.* 2004; 66: 486–491.

355. Heinzelmann M, Mercer-Jones MA, Passmore JC. Neutrophils and renal failure. *Am J Kidney Dis.* 1999; 34: 384–399.

356. Kelly KJ, Williams WW Jr, Colvin RB, et al. Intracellular adhesion molecule-1 deficient mice are protected against ischemic renal injury. *J Clin Invest.* 1996; 97: 1056–1063.

357. Paller MS. Effect of neutrophil depletion on ischemic renal injury in the rat. *J Lab Clin Med.* 1989; 113: 379–386.

358. Thadhani R, Pascual M, Bonventre JV. Medical progress-acute renal failure. *N Engl J Med.* 1996; 334: 1448–1460.

359. Linas SL, Shanley PF, Whittenburg D, et al. Neutrophils accentuate ischemia/reperfusion injury in isolated perfused rat kidneys. *Am J Physiol.* 1988; 255: F725–F733.

360. Linas SL, Whittenburg D, Parsons PE, et al. Mild ischemia activates primed neutrophils to cause acute renal failure. *Kidney Int.* 1992; 42: 610–616.

361. Linas SL, Whittenburg D, Parsons PE, et al. Ischemia increases neutrophil retention and worsens acute renal failure: role of oxygen metabolites and ICAM 1. *Kidnet Int.* 1995; 48: 1584–1591.

362. Linas SL, Whittenburg D, Repine JE. Nitric oxide prevents neutrophil-mediated acute renal failure. *Am J Physiol.* 1996; 272: F48–F54.

363. Klausner JM, Paterson IS, Goldman G, et al. Postischemic renal injury is mediated by neutrophils and leukotrienes. *Am J Physiol.* 1989; 256: F794–F802.

364. Caramelo C, Espinosa G, Manzarbeitia F, et al. Role of endothelium-related mechanisms in the pathophysiology of renal ischemia/reperfusion in normal rabbits. *Circ Res.* 1996; 79: 1031–1038.

365. Kelly KJ, Williams WW Jr, Colvin RB, et al. Antibody to intracellular adhesion molecule-1 protects the kidney against ischemic injury. *Proc Natl Acad Sci U S A.* 1994; 91: 812–816.

366. Rabb H, Postler G. Leucocyte adhesion molecules in ischaemic renal injury: kidney specific paradigms? *Clin Exp Pharmacol Physiol.* 1998; 25: 286–291.

367. Rabb H, Martin JG. An emerging paradigm shift on the role of leukocyte adhesion molecules [editorial]. *J Clin Invest.* 1997; 100: 2937–2938.

368. Rabb H, O'Meara YM, Maderna P, et al. Leukocytes, cell adhesion molecules and ischemic acute renal failure. *Kidney Int.* 1997; 51: 1463–1468.

369. Takada M, Nadeau KC, Shaw GD, et al. The cytokine-adhesion molecule cascade in ischemia/reperfusion injury of the rat kidney. Inhibition by a soluble P-selectin ligand. *J Clin Invest.* 1997; 99: 2682–2690.

370. Bolisetty S, Agarwal A. Neutrophils in acute kidney injury: not neutral any more. *Kidney Int.* 2009; 75(7): 674–676.

371. Melnikov VY, Faubel SG, Siegmund B, et al. Neutrophil-independent mechanisms of caspase-1- and IL-18-mediated ischemic acute tubular necrosis in mice. *J Clin Invest.* 2002; 110: 1083–1091.

372. Wipke BT, Allen PM. Essential role of neutrophils in the initiation and progression of a murine model of rheumatoid arthritis. *J Immunol.* 2001; 167: 1601–1608.

373. Burne MJ, Daniels F, El Ghandour A, et al. Identification of the CD4(+) T cell as a major pathogenic factor in ischemic acute renal failure. *J Clin Invest.* 2001; 108: 1283–1290.

374. Faubel SG, Ljubanovic D, Poole B, et al. Peripheral CD4 T cell depletion is not sufficient to prevent ischemic acute renal failure. *Transplantation.* 2005; 80: 643–649.

375. Liew FY, McInnes IB. Role of interleukin 15 and interleukin 18 in inflammatory response. *Ann Rheum Dis.* 2002; 61(suppl 2): ii100–ii102.

376. Kanai T, Watanabe M, Okazawa A, et al. Interleukin-18 and Crohn's disease. *Digestion.* 2001; 63(suppl 1): 37–42.

377. Mahida YR. The key role of macrophages in the immunopathogenesis of inflammatory bowel disease. *Inflamm Bowel Dis.* 2000; 6: 21–33.

378. Nakanishi K, Yoshimoto T, Tsutsui H, et al. Interleukin-18 is a unique cytokine that stimulates both Th1 and Th2 responses depending on its cytokine milieu. *Cytokine Growth Factor Rev.* 2001; 12: 53–72.

379. Jose MD, Ikezumi Y, Van Rooijen N, et al. Macrophages act as effectors of tissue damage in acute renal allograft rejection. *Transplantation.* 2003; 76: 1015–1022.

380. Day YJ, Huang L, Ye H, et al. Renal ischemia-reperfusion injury and adenosine 2A receptor-mediated tissue protection: the role of macrophages. *Am J Physiol Renal Physiol.* 2004; 288: F722–F731.

381. Jo SK, Sung SA, Cho WY, et al. Macrophages contribute to the initiation of ischemic acute renal failure in rats. *Nephrol Dial Transplant.* 2006; 21: 1231–1239.

382. Furuichi K, Wada T, Iwata Y, et al. Gene therapy expressing amino-terminal truncated monocyte chemoattractant protein-1 prevents renal ischemia-reperfusion injury. *J Am Soc Nephrol.* 2003; 14: 1066–1071.

383. Cerwenka A, Lanier LL. Natural killer cells, viruses and cancer. *Nat Rev Immunol.* 2001; 1: 41–49.

384. Badgwell B, Parihar R, Magro C, et al. Natural killer cells contribute to the lethality of a murine model of Escherichia coli infection. *Surgery.* 2002; 132: 205–212.

385. Okamura H, Kashiwamura S, Tsutsui H, et al. Regulation of interferon-gamma production by IL-12 and IL-18. *Curr Opin Immunol.* 1998; 10: 259–264.

386. Moretta A. Natural killer cells and dendritic cells: rendezvous in abused tissues. *Nat Rev Immunol.* 2002; 2: 957–964.

387. Kronenberg M, Gapin L. The unconventional lifestyle of NKT cells. *Nat Rev Immunol.* 2002; 2: 557–568.

388. Zhang ZX, Wang S, Huang X, et al. NK cells induce apoptosis in tubular epithelial cells and contribute to renal ischemia-reperfusion injury. *J Immunol.* 2008; 181(11): 7489–7498.

389. Ejaz AA, Mu W, Kang DH, et al. Could uric acid have a role in acute renal failure? *Clin J Am Soc Nephrol: CJASN.* 2007; 2(1): 16–21.

390. Kanellis J, Watanabe S, Li JH, et al. Uric acid stimulates monocyte chemoattractant protein-1 production in vascular smooth muscle cells via mitogen-activated protein kinase and cyclooxygenase-2. *Hypertension.* 2003; 41(6): 1287–1293.

391. Kang DH, Park SK, Lee IK, et al. Uric acid-induced C-reactive protein expression: implication on cell proliferation and nitric oxide production of human vascular cells. *J Am Soc Nephrol.* 2005; 16(12): 3553–3562.

392. Sanchez-Lozada LG, Tapia E, Santamaria J, et al. Mild hyperuricemia induces vasoconstriction and maintains glomerular hypertension in normal and remnant kidney rats. *Kidney Int.* 2005; 67(1): 237–247.

393. Khosla UM, Zharikov S, Finch JL, et al. Hyperuricemia induces endothelial dysfunction. *Kidney Int.* 2005; 67(5): 1739–1742.

394. Lee HT, Xu H, Nasr SH, et al. A1 adenosine receptor knockout mice exhibit increased renal injury following ischemia and reperfusion. *Am J Physiol Renal Physiol.* 2004; 286(2): F298–F306.

395. Castrop H, Huang Y, Hashimoto S, et al. Impairment of tubuloglomerular feedback regulation of GFR in ecto-5′-nucleotidase/CD73-deficient mice.[see comment]. *J Clin Invest.* 2004; 114(5): 634–642.

396. Day YJ, Huang L, McDuffie MJ, et al. Renal protection from ischemia mediated by A2A adenosine receptors on bone marrow-derived cells. *J Clin Invest.* 2003; 112(6): 883–891.

397. Day YJ, Huang L, Ye H, et al. Renal ischemia-reperfusion injury and adenosine 2A receptor-mediated tissue protection: the role of CD4+ T cells and IFN-gamma. *J Immunol.* 2006; 176(5): 3108–3114.

398. Lee HT, Gallos G, Nasr SH, et al. A1 adenosine receptor activation inhibits inflammation, necrosis, and apoptosis after renal ischemia-reperfusion injury in mice. *J Am Soc Nephrol.* 2004; 15(1): 102–111.

399. Grenz A, Osswald H, Eckle T, et al. The reno-vascular A2B adenosine receptor protects the kidney from ischemia. *PLoS Med.* 2008; 5(6): e137.

400. Grenz A, Zhang H, Eckle T, et al. Protective role of ecto-5′-nucleotidase (CD73) in renal ischemia. *J Am Soc Nephrol.* 2007; 18(3): 833–845.

401. Hirschberg R, Ding H. Growth factors and acute renal failure. *Semin Nephrol.* 1998; 18: 191–207.

402. Nigam S, Lieberthal W. Acute renal failure. III. The role of growth factors in the process of renal regeneration and repair. *Am J Physiol Renal Physiol.* 2000; 279: F3–F11.

403. Humes HD, Cieslinki DA, Coimbra TM. Epidermal growth factor enhances renal tubule cell repair and regeneration and accelerates the recovery of failure. *J Clin Invest.* 1989; 84: 1757–1761.

404. Miller SB, Martin DR, Kissane J, et al. Hepatocyte growth factor accelerates recovery from acute ischemic renal injury in rats. *Am J Physiol.* 1994; 266: F129–F134.

405. Miller SB, Martin DR, Kissane J, et al. Insulin like growth factor 1 accelerates recovery from ischemic acute tubular necrosis in the rat. *Proc Natl Acad Sci U S A.* 1992; 89: 11876–11881.

406. Petrinec D, Reilly JM, Sicard GA, et al. Insulin-like growth factor-1 attenuates delayed graft function in a canine renal autotransplantation model. *Surgery.* 1997; 120: 221–225.

407. Gobe G, Zhang XJ, Cuttle L, et al. Bcl-2 genes and growth factors in the pathology of ischaemic acute renal failure. *Immunol Cell Biol.* 1999; 77: 279–286.

408. Hirschberg R, Kopple J, Lipsett P, et al. Multicenter clinical trial of recombinant human insulin-like growth factor I in patients with acute renal failure. *Kidney Int.* 1999; 55: 2423–2432.

409. Togel F, Hu Z, Weiss K, et al. Administered mesenchymal stem cells protect against ischemic acute renal failure through differentiation-independent mechanisms [see comment]. *Am J Physiol Renal Physiol.* 2005; 289: F31–F42.

410. Morigi M, Introna M, Imberti B, et al. Human bone marrow mesenchymal stem cells accelerate recovery of acute renal injury and prolong survival in mice. *Stem Cells.* 2008; 26(8): 2075–2082.

411. Togel F, Cohen A, Zhang P, et al. Autologous and allogeneic marrow stromal cells are safe and effective for the treatment of acute kidney injury. *Stem Cells Dev.* 2009; 18(3): 475–485.

412. Anderson RJ, Linas SL, Berns AS, et al. Nonoliguric acute renal failure. *N Engl J Med.* 1977; 296: 1134–1138.

413. Miller TR, Anderson RJ, Linas SL, et al. Urinary diagnostic indices in acute renal failure: a prospective study. *Ann Intern Med.* 1978; 89: 47–50.

414. Schrier RW, Henderson HS, Tisher CC, et al. Nephropathy associated with heat stress and exercise. *Ann Intern Med.* 1967; 67: 356–376.

415. Stevens LA, Lafayette RA, Perrone RD, et al. Laboratory evaluation of kidney function. In: Schrier RW, ed. *Diseases of the Kidney and Urinary Tract.* 8th ed. Philadelphia: Lippincott, Williams and Wilkins; 2007: 299–336.

416. Moran SM, Myers BD. Course of acute renal failure studied by a model of creatinine kinetics. *Kidney Int.* 1985; 27: 928–937.

417. Star RA. Treatment of acute renal failure. *Kidney Int.* 1998; 54: 1817–1831.

418. Parikh CR, Jani A, Mishra J, et al. Urine NGAL and IL-18 are predictive biomarkers for delayed graft function following kidney transplantation. *Am J Transplant.* 2006; 6: 1639–1645.

419. Parikh CR, Jani A, Melnikov VY, et al. Urinary interleukin-18 is a marker of human acute tubular necrosis. *Am J Kidney Dis*. 2004; 43: 405–414.

420. Parikh CR, Abraham E, Ancukiewicz M, et al. Urine IL-18 is an early diagnostic marker for acute kidney injury and predicts mortality in the ICU. *J Am Soc Nephrol*. 2005; 16: 3046–3052.

421. Washburn KK, Zapitelli M, Arikan AA, et al. Urinary interleukin-18 as an acute kidney injury biomarker in critically ill children. *Nephrol Dial Transplant*. 2008; 23(2): 566–572.

422. Parikh CR, Mishra J, Thiessen-Philbrook H, et al. Urinary IL-18 is an early predictive biomarker of acute kidney injury after cardiac surgery. *Kidney Int*. 2006; 70: 199–203.

423. Ling W, Zhaohui N, Ben H, et al. Urinary IL-18 and NGAL as early predictive biomarkers in contrast-induced nephropathy after coronary angiography. *Nephron*. 2008; 108: c176–c181.

424. Schmidt-Ott KM, Mori K, Li JY, et al. Dual action of neutrophil gelatinase-associated lipocalin. *J Am Soc Nephrol*. 2007; 18: 407–413.

425. Mishra J, Ma Q, Prada A, et al. Identification of neutrophil gelatinase-associated lipocalin as a novel early urinary biomarker for ischemic renal injury. *J Am Soc Nephrol*. 2003; 14: 2534–2543.

426. Mishra J, Mori K, Ma Q, et al. Neutrophil gelatinase-associated lipocalin: a novel early urinary biomarker for cisplatin nephrotoxicity. *Am J Nephrol*. 2004; 24(3): 307–315.

427. Mishra J, Dent C, Tarabishi R, et al. Neutrophil gelatinase-associated lipocalin (NGAL) as a biomarker for acute renal injury after cardiac surgery. *Lancet*. 2005; 365: 1231–1238.

428. Wagener G, Jan M, Kim M, et al. Association between increases in urinary neutrophil gelatinase-associated lipocalin and acute renal dysfunction after adult cardiac surgery. *Anesthesiology*. 2006; 105(3): 485–491.

429. Zapitelli M, Washburn KK, Arikan AA, et al. Urine neutrophil gelatinase-associated lipocalin is an early marker of acute kidney injury in critically ill children: a prospective cohort study. *Crit Care*. 2007; 11: R84.

430. Wheeler DS, Devarajan P, Ma Q, et al. Serum neutrophil gelatinase-associated lipocalin (NGAL) as a marker of acute kidney injury in critically ill children with septic shock. *Crit Care Med*. 2008; 36: 1297–1303.

431. Hirsch R, Dent C, Pfriem H, et al. NGAL is an early predictive biomarker of contrast-induced nephropathy in children. *Pediatr Nephrol*. 2007; 22: 2089–2095.

432. Bachorzewska-Gajewska H, Malyszko J, Sitniewska E, et al. Neutrophil-gelatinase-associated lipocalin and renal function after percutaneous coronary interventions. *Am J Nephrol*. 2006; 26(3): 287–292.

433. Mishra J, Mori K, Ma Q, et al. Amelioration of ischemic acute renal injury by neutrophil gelatinase-associated lipocalin. *J Am Soc Nephrol*. 2004; 15: 3073–3082.

434. Ichimura T, Bonventre JV, Bailly V, et al. Kidney injury molecule-1 (KIM-1), a putative epithelial cell adhesion molecule containing a novel immunoglobulin domain, is up-regulated in renal cells after injury. *J Biol Chem*. 1998; 273: 4135–4142.

435. Vaidya VS, Ramirez V, Ichimura T, et al. Urinary kidney injury molecule-1: a sensitive quantitative biomarker for early detection of kidney tubular injury. *Am J Physiol Renal Physiol*. 2006; 290: F517–F529.

436. Han WK, Bailly V, Abichandani R, et al. Kidney injury molecule-1 (KIM-1): a novel biomarker for human renal proximal tubule injury. *Kidney Int*. 2002; 62: 237–244.

437. van Timmeren MM, Vaidya VS, van Ree RM, et al. High urinary excretion of kidney injury molecule-1 is an independent predictor of graft loss in renal transplant recipients. *Transplantation*. 2007; 84: 1625–1630.

438. Sarvary E, Borka P, Sulyok B, et al. Diagnostic value of urinary enzyme determination in renal transplantation. *Transpl Int*. 1996; 9(suppl 1): S68–S72.

439. Westhuyzen J. Cystatin C: a promising marker and predictor of impaired renal function. *Ann Clin Lab Sci*. 2006; 36(4): 387–394.

440. Herget-Rosenthal S, Marggraf G, Husing J, et al. Early detection of acute renal failure by serum cystatin C. *Kidney Int*. 2004; 66: 1115–1122.

441. Koyner JL, Bennet MR, Worcester EM, et al. Urinary cystatin c as an early biomarker of acute kidney injury following adult cardiothoracic surgery. *Kidney Int*. 2008; 74(8): 1059–1069.

442. Artunc FH, Fischer IU, Risler T, et al. Improved estimation of GFR by serum cystatin C in patients undergoing cardiac catheterization. *Int J Cardiol*. 2005; 102(2): 173–178.

443. Orlando R, Mussap M, Plebani M, et al. Diagnostic value of plasma cystatin C as a glomerular filtration marker in decompensated liver cirrhosis. *Clin Chem*. 2002; 48(6 pt 1): 850–858.

444. Gerbes AL, Gulberg V, Bilzer M, et al. Evaluation of serum cystatin C concentration as a marker of renal function in patients with cirrhosis of the liver. *Gut*. 2002; 50: 106–110.

445. Villa P, Jimenez M, Soriano MC, et al. Serum cystatin C concentration as a marker of acute renal dysfunction in critically ill patients. *Crit Care*. 2005; 9(2): R139–R143.

446. Herrero-Morin JD, Malaga S, Fernandez N, et al. Cystatin C and beta2-microglobulin: markers of glomerular filtration in critically ill children. *Crit Care*. 2007; 11: R59.

447. Spiegel DM, Ullian ME, Zerbe GO, et al. Determinants of survival and recovery in acute renal failure patients dialyzed in intensive-care units. *Am J Nephrol*. 1991; 11: 44–47.

448. Handa SP, Morrin PA. Diagnostic indices in acute renal failure. *Can Med Assoc J*. 1967; 96: 78–82.

449. Vertel RM, Knochel JP. Nonoliguric acute renal failure. *JAMA*. 1967; 200: 598–602.

450. Nickolas TL, O'Rourke MJ, Yang J, et al. Sensitivity and specificity of a single emergency department measurement of urinary neutrophil gelatinase-associated lipocalin for diagnosing acute kidney injury. *Ann Intern Med*. 2008; 148: 810–819.

451. Luft FC, Patel V, Yum MN, et al. Experimental aminoglycoside nephrotoxicity. *J Lab Clin Med.* 1975; 86: 213–220.

452. Fabre J, Rudhardt M, Blanchard P, et al. Persistence of sisomicin and gentamicin in renal cortex and medulla compared with other organs and serum of rats. *Kidney Int.* 1976; 10: 444–449.

453. Molitoris BA. Cell biology of aminoglycoside nephrotoxicity: newer aspects. *Curr Opin Nephrol Hypertens.* 1997; 6: 384–388.

454. Luft FC, Kleit SA. Renal parenchymal accumulation of aminoglycoside antibiotics in rats. *J Infect Dis.* 1974; 130: 656–659.

455. Walker PD, Barri Y, Shah SV. Oxidant mechanisms in gentamicin nephrotoxicity. *Ren Fail.* 1999; 21: 433–442.

456. Kanbay M, Covic A, Coca SG, et al. Sodium bicarbonate for the prevention of contrast-induced nephropathy: a meta-analysis of 17 randomized trials. *Int Urol Nephrol.* 2009; 41(3): 617–627.

457. Heyman SN, Reichman J, Brezis M. Pathophysiology of radiocontrast nephropathy: a role for medullary hypoxia. *Invest Radiol.* 1999; 34: 685–691.

458. Kohan DE. Endothelins in the normal and diseased kidney. *Am J Kidney Dis.* 1997; 29: 2–26.

459. Wang A, Holcslaw T, Bashore TM, et al. Exacerbation of radiocontrast nephrotoxicity by endothelin receptor antagonism. *Kidney Int.* 2000; 57: 1675–1680.

460. Solomon R. Radiocontrast-induced nephropathy. *Semin Nephrol.* 1998; 18: 551–557.

461. Rudnick MR, Berns JS, Cohen RM, et al. Nephrotoxic risks of renal angiography: contrast media-associated nephrotoxicity and atheroembolism—a critical review. *Am J Kidney Dis.* 1994; 24: 713–727.

462. Apelqvist J, Torffvit O, Agardh CD. The effect of the non-ionic contrast medium iohexol on glomerular and tubular function in diabetic patients. *Diabet Med.* 1996; 13: 487–492.

463. Solomon R, Werner C, Mann D, et al. Effects of saline, mannitol, and furosemide to prevent acute decreases in renal function induced by radiocontrast agents. *N Engl J Med.* 1994; 331: 1416–1420.

464. Tepel M, van der GM, Schwarzfeld C, et al. Prevention of radiographic-contrast-agent-induced reductions in renal function by acetylcysteine. *N Engl J Med.* 2000; 343: 180–184.

465. Weisbord SD, Palevsky PM. Intravenous fluid to prevent contrast-induced AKI. *Nat Clin Pract Nephrol.* 2009; 5: 256–257.

466. Navaneethan SD, Singh S, Appasamy S, et al. Sodium bicarbonate therapy for prevention of contrast-induced nephropathy: a systematic review and meta-analysis. *Am J Kidney Dis.* 2009; 53(4): 617–627.

467. Tan SY, Shapiro R, Kish MA. Reversible acute renal failure induced by indomethacin. *JAMA.* 1979; 241: 2732–2733.

468. Katz SM, Capaldo R, Everts EA, et al. Tolmetin. Association with reversible renal failure and acute interstitial nephritis. *JAMA.* 1981; 246: 243–245.

469. Galler M, Folkert VW, Schlondorff D. Reversible acute renal insufficiency and hyperkalemia following indomethacin therapy. *JAMA.* 1981; 246: 154–155.

470. Morales A, Steyn J. Papillary necrosis following phenylbutazone ingestion. *Arch Surg.* 1971; 103: 420–421.

471. Brezin JH, Katz SM, Schwartz AB, et al. Reversible renal failure and nephrotic syndrome associated with nonsteroidal anti-inflammatory drugs. *N Engl J Med.* 1979; 301: 1271–1273.

472. Donker AJ, Arisz L, Brentjens JR, et al. The effect of indomethacin on kidney function and plasma renin activity in man. *Nephron.* 1976; 17: 288–296.

473. Kimberly RP, Bowden RE, Keiser HR, et al. Reduction of renal function by newer nonsteroidal anti-inflammatory drugs. *Am J Med.* 1978; 64: 804–807.

474. Arisz L, Donker AJ, Brentjens JR, et al. The effect of indomethacin on proteinuria and kidney function in the nephrotic syndrome. *Acta Med Scand.* 1976; 199: 121–125.

475. Zipser RD, Hoefs JC, Speckart PF, et al. Prostaglandins: modulators of renal function and pressor resistance in chronic liver disease. *J Clin Endocrinol Metab.* 1979; 48: 895–900.

476. Riley DJ, Weir M, Bakris GL. Renal adaptation to the failing heart. Avoiding a "therapeutic misadventure." *Postgrad Med.* 1994; 95: 153–156.

477. Guan Y, Chang M, Cho W, et al. Cloning, expression, and regulation of rabbit cyclooxygenase-2 in renal medullary interstitial cells. *Am J Physiol.* 1997; 273: F18–F26.

478. Komers R, Anderson S, Epstein M. Renal and cardiovascular effects of selective cyclooxygenase-2 inhibitors. *Am J Kidney Dis.* 2001; 38: 1145–1157.

479. Breyer MD, Harris RC. Cyclooxygenase 2 and the kidney. *Curr Opin Nephrol Hypertens.* 2001; 10: 89–98.

480. Sheikh-Hamad D, Timmins K, Jalali Z. Cisplatin-induced renal toxicity: possible reversal by N-acetylcysteine treatment. *J Am Soc Nephrol.* 1997; 8: 1640–1644.

481. Dentino M, Luft FC, Yum MN, et al. Long term effect of cis-diamminedichloride platinum (CDDP) on renal function and structure in man. *Cancer.* 1978; 41: 1274–1281.

482. Dobyan DC, Levi J, Jacobs C, et al. Mechanism of cis-platinum nephrotoxicity: II. Morphologic observations. *J Pharmacol Exp Ther.* 1980; 213: 551–556.

483. Offerman JJ, Meijer S, Sleijfer DT, et al. Acute effects of cis-diamminedichloroplatinum (CDDP) on renal function. *Cancer Chemother Pharmacol.* 1984; 12: 36–38.

484. Goode HF, Webster NR. Free radicals and antioxidants in sepsis. *Crit Care Med.* 1993; 21: 1770–1776.

485. Liu Y, Sun AM, Dworkin LD. Hepatocyte growth factor protects renal epithelial cells from apoptotic cell death. *Biochem Biophys Res Commun.* 1998; 246: 821–826.

486. Appenroth D, Winnefeld K, Schroter H, et al. Beneficial effect of acetylcysteine on cisplatin nephrotoxicity in rats. *J Appl Toxicol.* 1993; 13: 189–192.

487. Anderson ME, Naganuma A, Meister A. Protection against cisplatin toxicity by administration of glutathione ester. *FASEB J.* 1990; 4: 3251–3255.

488. Knotek M, Rogachev B, Schrier RW. Update on peripheral arterial vasodilation, ascites and hepatorenal syndrome in cirrhosis. *Can J Gastroenterol.* 2000; 14(suppl D): 112D–121D.

489. Salerno F, Gerbes A, Gines P, et al. Diagnosis, prevention and treatment of hepatorenal syndrome in cirrhosis. *Gut.* 2007; 56(9): 1310–1318.

490. Scolari F, Tardanico R, Zani R, et al. Cholesterol crystal embolism: a recognizable cause of renal disease. *Am J Kidney Dis.* 2000; 36: 1089–1109.

491. Modi KS, Rao VK. Atheroembolic renal disease. *J Am Soc Nephrol.* 2001; 12: 1781–1787.

492. Keen RR, McCarthy WJ, Shireman PK, et al. Surgical management of atheroembolization. *J Vasc Surg.* 1995; 21: 773–780.

493. Liu J, Hutzler M, Li C, et al. Thrombotic thrombocytopenic purpura (ttp) and hemolytic uremic syndrome (hus): the new thinking. *J Thromb Thrombolysis.* 2001; 11: 261–272.

494. Markowitz GS. Oral sodium phosphate bowel purgatives and acute phosphate nephropathy. In: De Broe ME, Porter GA, eds. *Clinical Nephrotoxins-Renal Injury from Drugs and Chemicals.* 3rd ed. New York: Springer; 2008: 579–594.

495. Ritskes-Hoitinga J, Lemmens AG, Danse LH, et al. Phosphorus-induced nephrocalcinosis and kidney function in female rats. *J Nutr.* 1989; 119(10): 1423–1431.

496. Zager RA. Hyperphosphatemia: a factor that provokes severe experimental acute renal failure. *J Lab Clin Med.* 1982; 100(2): 230–239.

497. Bhalla V, Grimm PC, Chertow GM, et al. Melamine nephrotoxicity: an emerging epidemic in an era of globalization. *Kidney Int.* 2009; 75(8): 774–779.

498. Hau AK, Kwan TH, Li PK. Melamine toxicity and the kidney. *J Am Soc Nephrol.* 2009; 20: 245–250.

499. McCluskey RT, Klassen J. Immunologically mediated glomerular, tubular and interstitial renal disease. *N Engl J Med.* 1973; 288: 564–570.

500. Sitprija V, Evans H. The kidney in human leptospirosis. *Am J Med.* 1970; 49: 780–788.

501. Baldwin DS, Levine BB, McCluskey RT, et al. Renal failure and interstitial nephritis due to penicillin and methicillin. *N Engl J Med.* 1968; 279: 1245–1252.

502. Rossert J. Drug-induced acute interstitial nephritis. *Kidney Int.* 2001; 60: 804–817.

503. Friedman J, Hoyer JR, Seiler MW. Formation and clearance of tubulointerstitial immune complexes in kidney of rats immunized with heterologous antisera to Tamm-Horsfall protein. *Kidney Int.* 1982; 21: 575–582.

504. Lehman DH, Wilson CB, Dixon FJ. Interstitial nephritis in rats immunized with heterologous tubular basement membrane. *Kidney Int.* 1974; 5: 187–195.

505. Sugisaki T, Kano K, Andres G, et al. Antibodies to tubular basement membrane elicited by stimulation with allogeneic kidney. *Kidney Int.* 1982; 21: 557–564.

506. Husby G, Tung KS, Williams RC Jr. Characterization of renal tissue lymphocytes in patients with interstitial nephritis. *Am J Med.* 1981; 70: 31–38.

507. Andres GA, McCluskey RT. Tubular and interstitial renal disease due to immunologic mechanisms. *Kidney Int.* 1975; 7: 271–289.

508. Wilson CB. Study of the immunopathogenesis of tubulointerstitial nephritis using model systems. *Kidney Int.* 1989; 35: 938–953.

509. Neilson EG. Pathogenesis and therapy of interstitial nephritis. *Kidney Int.* 1989; 35: 1257–1270.

510. Rossert JA, Garrett LA. Regulation of type I collagen synthesis. *Kidney Int.* 1995; (suppl 49): S34–S38.

511. Rao TK. Renal complications in HIV disease. *Med Clin North Am.* 1996; 80: 1437–1451.

512. Valeri A, Neusy AJ. Acute and chronic renal disease in hospitalized AIDS patients. *Clin Nephrol.* 1991; 35: 110–118.

513. Cohen SD, Chawla LS, Kimmel PL. Acute kidney injury in patients with human immunodeficiency virus infection. *Curr Opin Crit Care.* 2008; 14(6): 647–653.

514. Olyaei AJ, deMattos AM, Bennett WM. Renal toxicity of protease inhibitors. *Curr Opin Nephrol Hypertens.* 2000; 9: 473–476.

515. Kimmel PL. The nephropathies of HIV infection: pathogenesis and treatment. *Curr Opin* Nephrol *Hypertens.* 2000; 9: 117–122.

516. Brezis M, Rosen S, Silva P, et al. Transport activity modifies thick ascending limb damage in the isolated perfused kidney. *Kidney Int.* 1984; 25: 65–72.

517. Eneas JF, Schoenfeld PY, Humphreys MH. The effect of infusion of mannitol-sodium bicarbonate on the clinical course of myoglobinuria. *Arch Intern Med.* 1979; 139: 801–805.

518. Ron D, Taitelman U, Michaelson M, et al. Prevention of acute renal failure in traumatic rhabdomyolysis. *Arch Intern Med.* 1984; 144: 277–280.

519. Better OS, Stein JH. Early management of shock and prophylaxis of acute renal failure in traumatic rhabdomyolysis. *N Engl J Med.* 1990; 322: 825–829.

520. Zager RA. Rhabdomyolysis and myohemoglobinuric acute renal failure. *Kidney Int.* 1996; 49: 314–326.

521. Epstein M, Schneider NS, Befeler B. Effect of intrarenal furosemide on renal function and intratenal hemodynamics in acute renal failure. *Am J Med.* 1975; 58: 510–516.

522. Kleinknecht D, Ganeval D, Gonzalez-Duque LA, et al. Furosemide in acute oliguric renal failure. A controlled trial. *Nephron.* 1976; 17: 51–58.

523. Shilliday IR, Quinn KJ, Allison ME. Loop diuretics in the management of acute renal failure: a prospective, double-blind, placebo-controlled, randomized study. *Nephrol Dial Transplant.* 1997; 12: 2592–2596.

524. Mehta RL, Pascual MT, Soroko S, et al. Diuretics, mortality, and nonrecovery of renal function in acute renal failure. *JAMA.* 2002; 288(20): 2547–2553.

525. Leverve X, Barnoud D. Stress metabolism and nutritional support in acute renal failure. *Kidney Int.* 1998; (suppl 66): S62–S66.

526. Moore FA, Moore EE, Jones TN, et al. TEN versus TPN following major abdominal trauma—reduced septic morbidity. *J Trauma*. 1989; 29: 916–922.

527. Feinstein EI, Kopple JD, Silberman H, et al. Total parenteral nutrition with high or low nitrogen intakes in patients with acute renal failure. *Kidney Int*. 1983; (suppl 16): S319–S323.

528. Bellomo R, Seacombe J, Daskalakis M, et al. A prospective comparative study of moderate versus high protein intake for critically ill patients with acute renal failure. *Ren Fail*. 1997; 19: 111–120.

529. Sponsel H, Conger JD. Is parenteral nutrition therapy of value in acute renal failure patients? *Am J Kidney Dis*. 1995; 25: 96–102.

530. Kopple JD. The nutrition management of the patient with acute renal failure. *JPEN J Parenter Enteral Nutr*. 1996; 20: 3–12.

531. Lassnigg A, Donner E, Grubhofer G, et al. Lack of renoprotective effects of dopamine and furosemide during cardiac surgery. *J Am Soc Nephrol*. 2000; 11: 97–104.

532. Kellum JA. Prophylactic fenoldopam for renal protection? No, thank you, not for me—not yet at least. *Crit Care Med*. 2005; 33(11): 2681–2683.

533. Bellomo R, Ronco C. Acute renal failure in the intensive care unit: adequacy of dialysis and the case for continuous therapies. *Nephrol Dial Transplant*. 1996; 11: 424–428.

534. Gettings LG, Reynolds HN, Scalea T. Outcome in post-traumatic acute renal failure when continuous renal replacement therapy is applied early vs. late. *Intensive Care Med*. 1999; 25(8): 805–813.

535. Liu KD, Himmelfarb J, Paganini E, et al. Timing of initiation of dialysis in critically ill patients with acute kidney injury. *Clin J Am Soc Nephrol: CJASN*. 2006; 1: 915–919.

536. Conger JD. A controlled evaluation of prophylactic dialysis in post-traumatic acute renal failure. *J Trauma*. 1975; 15: 1056–1063.

537. Gillum DM, Dixon BS, Yanover MJ, et al. The role of intensive dialysis in acute renal failure. *Clin Nephrol*. 1986; 25: 249–255.

538. Schiffl H, Lang SM, Konig A, et al. Dose of intermittent hemodialysis and outcome of acute renal failure: a prospective randomized study (abstract). *J Am Soc Nephrol*. 1997; 8: 290A.

539. Pastan S, Bailey J. Dialysis therapy. *N Engl J Med*. 1998; 338: 1428–1437.

540. Evanson JA, Ikizler TA, Wingard R, et al. Measurement of the delivery of dialysis in acute renal failure. *Kidney Int*. 1999; 55: 1501–1508.

541. Evanson JA, Himmelfarb J, Wingard R, et al. Prescribed versus delivered dialysis in acute renal failure patients. *Am J Kidney Dis*. 1998; 32: 731–738.

542. Paganini E, Tapolyai M, Goormastic M, et al. Establishing a dialysis therapy/patient outcome link in intensive care unit acute dialysis for patients with acute renal failure. *Am J Kidney Dis*. 1996; 28: S81–S89.

543. Leblanc M, Tapolyai M, Paganini EP. What dialysis dose should be provided in acute renal failure? A review. *Adv Ren Replace Ther*. 1995; 2: 255–264.

544. Ronco C, Bellomo R, Homel P, et al. Effects of different doses in continuous veno-venous haemofiltration on outcomes of acute renal failure: a prospective randomised trial. *Lancet*. 2000; 356: 26–30.

545. Schiffl H, Lang SM, Fischer R. Daily hemodialysis and the outcome of acute renal failure. *N Engl J Med*. 2002; 346: 305–310.

546. Saudan P, Niederberger M, De Seigneux S, et al. Adding a dialysis dose to continuous hemofiltration increases survival in patients with acute renal failure [see comment]. *Kidney Int*. 2006; 70(7): 1312–1317.

547. VA/NIH Acute Renal Failure Trial Network, Palevsky PM, Zhang JH, et al. Intensity of renal support in critically ill patients with acute kidney injury. *N Engl J Med*. 2008; 359(1): 7–20.

548. RENAL Study Investigators, Bellomo R, Cass A, et al. Design and challenges of the Randomized Evaluation of Normal versus Augmented Level Replacement Therapy (RENAL) Trial: high-dose versus standard-dose hemofiltration in acute renal failure. *Blood Purif*. 2008; 26(5): 407–416.

549. Clark WR, Mueller BA, Kraus MA, et al. Solute control by extracorporeal therapies in acute renal failure. *Am J Kid Dis*. 1996; 28: S21–S27.

550. Swartz RD, Messana JM, Orzol S, et al. Comparing continuous hemofiltration with hemodialysis in patients with severe acute renal failure. *Am J Kidney Dis*. 1999; 34: 424–432.

551. Rialp G, Roglan A, Betbese AJ, et al. Prognostic indexes and mortality in critically ill patients with acute renal failure treated with different dialytic techniques. *Ren Fail*. 1996; 18: 667–675.

552. Mehta RL, McDonald B, Gabbai FB, et al. A randomized clinical trial of continuous versus intermittent dialysis for acute renal failure. *Kidney Int*. 2001; 60: 1154–1163.

553. Lins RL, Elseviers MM, Van der NP, et al. Intermittent versus continuous renal replacement therapy for acute kidney injury patients admitted to the intensive care unit: results of a randomized clinical trial. *Nephrol Dial Transplant*. 2009; 24(2): 512–518.

554. Ghahramani N, Shadrou S, Hollenbeak C. A systematic review of continuous renal replacement therapy and intermittent haemodialysis in management of patients with acute renal failure. *Nephrology*. 2008; 13(7): 570–578.

555. Marshall MR, Golper TA, Shaver MJ, et al. Sustained low-efficiency dialysis for critically ill patients requiring renal replacement therapy. *Kidney Int*. 2001; 60: 777–785.

556. Davenport A. Continuous renal replacement therapy in patients with hepatic and acute renal failure. *Am J Kid Dis*. 1996; 28: S62–S66.

557. Hakim RM, Wingard RL, Parker RA. Effect of dialysis membranes in the treatment of patients with acute renal failure. *N Engl J Med*. 1994; 331: 1338–1347.

558. Schiffl H, Lang SM, Konig A, et al. Biocompatible membranes in acute renal failure: prospective case-controlled study. *Lancet*. 1994; 344: 570–572.

559. Himmelfarb J, Tolkoff RN, Chandran P, et al. A multicenter comparison of dialysis membranes in

the treatment of acute renal failure requiring dialysis. *J Am Soc Nephrol*. 1998; 9: 257–266.

560. Kurtal H, von Herrath D, Schaefer K. Is the choice of membrane important for patients with acute renal failure requiring hemodialysis? *Artif Organs*. 1995; 19: 391–394.

561. Jones CH, Goutcher E, Newstead CG, et al. Hemodynamics and survival of patients with acute renal failure treated by continuous dialysis with two synthetic membranes. *Artif Organs*. 1998; 22: 638–643.

562. Jorres A, Gahl GM, Dobis C, et al. Haemodialysis-membrane biocompatibility and mortality of patients with dialysis-dependent acute renal failure: a prospective randomised multicentre trial. International Multicentre Study Group. *Lancet*. 1999; 354: 1337–1341.

563. Gastaldello K, Melot C, Kahn RJ, et al. Comparison of cellulose diacetate and polysulfone membranes in the outcome of acute renal failure. A prospective randomized study. *Nephrol Dial Transplant*. 2000; 15: 224–230.

564. Yalavarthy R, Edelstein CL. Therapeutic and predictive targets of AKI. *Clin Nephrol*. 2008; 70(6): 453–463.

CHAPTER 11

Chronic Kidney Disease: Manifestations and Pathogenesis

MICHEL CHONCHOL AND LAURENCE CHAN

C hronic kidney disease is characterized by a decrease in glomerular filtration rate (GFR) and histologic evidence of a reduction in nephron population. The clinical course is typically one of a progressive and unrelenting loss of nephron function, ultimately leading to end-stage renal disease (ESRD). However, the time between the initial onset of disease and ultimate development of ESRD may vary considerably, not only between different diseases but also in different patients with similar disease processes.

Assessment of Function in Chronic Kidney Disease

Assessment of GFR continues to be the most useful quantitative index of kidney function. Exogenous and endogenous markers have been used for the measurement of GFR. An ideal filtration marker should be freely filtered across the glomerular capillary wall and excreted only by glomerular filtration (1). Inulin fulfills all the criteria for an ideal filtration marker, and its renal clearance has been considered as a standard measure of GFR. However, renal clearance of inulin requires precise regulation of an intravenous infusion of inulin to achieve a steady-state plasma inulin concentration and several timed urine collection with complete emptying of the bladder. Because of the inconvenience, it is only performed in research settings. Renal ^{125}I-iothalamate or ^{51}Cr-EDTA clearance after subcutaneous injection and timed urine collection also has been used as an alternative method (2,3).

van Slyke et al. introduced the concept of clearance in 1929 in their description of urea clearance. The blood urea nitrogen (BUN), however, is a less reliable indicator of kidney function, because factors other than the GFR—including protein intake, state of hydration, antianabolic agents (tetracycline and corticosteroids), blood in the bowel, fever, and infection—all can cause changes in BUN in the absence of changes in kidney function. In contrast, the blood level of creatinine, produced endogenously by the hydrolysis of phosphocreatinine, provides a reasonable index of kidney function. Approximately 1 mg of creatinine is produced daily by the metabolism of 20 g of muscle (4). In addition, about 20% of urinary creatinine is derived from the ingestion of meat. Small quantities of creatinine are secreted by the renal tubules so that the creatinine clearance slightly overestimates true glomerular filtration. As a result, the 24-hour endogenous creatinine clearance generally exceeds inulin clearance, and this difference increases in patients with advanced chronic kidney disease and proteinuria. For clinical purposes, creatinine clearance is a simple and reliable method of estimating GFR and thus the degree of impairment of kidney function. Creatinine clearance (C_{cr}) can be estimated from serum creatinine (SrCr) determinations alone using the Crockcroft and Gault equation (5):

$$C_{cr}(\text{males}) = \frac{(140 - \text{age})(\text{weight kg})}{(72)(\text{SrCr mg/dL})}$$

$$C_{cr}(\text{females}) = \frac{(140 - \text{age})(\text{weight kg})}{(72)(\text{SrCr mg/dL})} \times .85$$

(11.1)

This equation corrects for the major factors that affect GFR, that is, age, sex, and weight. The normal creatinine clearance established by this method is 140+27 mL/min for men and 112 ± 20 mL/min for women.

A more accurate method to estimate GFR from serum creatinine was recommended by the Modification of Diet in Renal Diseases (MDRD) study (6) which included 1,628 patients with diverse characteristics and causes of chronic kidney disease. The equation derived from this study, as shown in the following, predicts GFR by serum creatinine concentration (Pcr), demographic characteristics (age, gender, and ethnicity) as well as other serum measurements (serum urea nitrogen [SUN] and albumin [Alb]):

$$\text{GFR (mL/min/1.73 m}^2) = 170 \times [\text{Pcr (mg/dL)}]^{-0.999} \times [\text{Age(yr)}]^{-0.176}$$
$$\times (0.762 \text{ if female}) \times (1.180 \text{ if African American}) \quad (11.2)$$
$$\times [\text{SUN (mg/dL)}]^{-0.170} \times [\text{Alb (g/dL)}]^{+0.318}$$

This equation has less variability and is more accurate than other commonly used equations. Besides, it could be easily implemented and there is no need for 24-hour urine collections. It, however, is not very accurate with GFR values of 60 mL/min.

The serum creatinine concentration doubles for every 50% reduction in GFR. For example, if a patient has a GFR of 100 mL/min/1.73 m² with a serum creatinine of 1 mg/dL, when the GFR falls to 50 mL/min/1.73 m² serum creatinine increases to 2 mg/dL. With a further fall in function to 25 mL/min/1.73 m², serum creatinine again doubles and is 4 mg/dL. As can be seen in Figure 11.1, changes in serum creatinine become a very sensitive method of estimating further impairment in kidney function when there is already extensive kidney damage, that is, GFR <25 mL/min/1.73 m². A plot of the reciprocal of the serum creatinine against time yields a straight line in many patients with chronic kidney disease. The linear decline in the reciprocal serum creatinine value with time is consistent with a linear loss of glomerular filtration. A change in the slope may indicate the superimposition of some additional factor that accelerates renal functional loss, such as volume depletion or a nephrotoxic agent if the slope is increased. Conversely, a decrease in the slope represents slowing of the rate of decline in function. Irrespective of the underlying kidney disease, progression to ESRD is a common event once the serum creatinine exceeds 1.5 to 2.0 mg/dL. However, the rate of progression to ESRD occurs at a variable rate. When a patient is first seen with chronic kidney disease, it is most important to document the degree of renal impairment and attempt to determine if potentially reversible factors have contributed to the severity of kidney function decline.

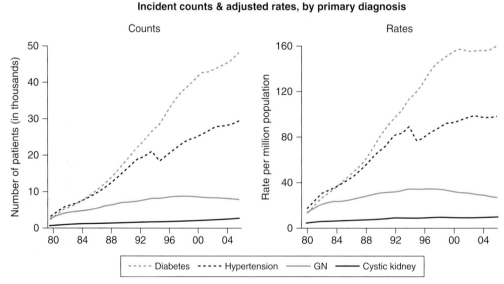

Incident counts & adjusted rates, by primary diagnosis

■ **Figure 11.1** Incident counts & adjusted rates by major etiology for U.S. medicare-treated end-stage renal disease.

Incidence and Prevalence of Chronic Kidney Disease

Chronic kidney disease is defined as the presence of kidney damage or GFR <60 mL/min/1.73 m² for 3 months or longer, irrespective of cause (6). Chronic kidney disease was divided into stages of severity (Table 11.1). The staging of chronic kidney disease is useful because it endorses a model in which primary physicians and specialists share responsibility for the care of patients with kidney disease. This classification also offers a common language for patients and the practitioners involved in the treatment of chronic kidney disease patients. For each stage of chronic kidney disease, the Kidney Disease Outcomes Quality Initiative (K/DOQI) of the National Kidney Foundation (NKF) provides recommendations for a clinical action plan (Table 11.1) (7,8). Importantly, the staging system is based on estimated GFR and not only on the measurement of serum creatinine. The gradual decline of kidney function in patients with chronic kidney disease is initially asymptomatic. The earliest stages of chronic kidney disease are characterized by an apparent preservation of renal function of remaining nephrons. The basal GFR may be normal or even elevated because of hyperfiltration. Measurement of GFR after imposed stresses, such as after a high-protein meal, may reveal the absence of normal renal reserve. A diminution of renal reserve happens when GFR is reduced to 25% of normal. The patient usually has no symptoms, azotemia is present, and the serum creatinine is increased. As GFR falls to <25% of normal, an increasing number and severity of uremic clinical manifestations and biochemical abnormalities supervene. The magnitude of the population with chronic kidney disease is just beginning to be appreciated. Jones et al. (7) analyzed serum creatinine data from the Third National Health and Nutritional Survey (NHANES III), gathered between 1988 and 1994. Among men, the proportion of the population that had serum creatinine levels ≥1.5 mg/dL, ≥1.7 mg/dL, and ≥2.0 mg/dL were 4.98%, 1.87%, and 0.64%, respectively. Among women, the comparable figures were 1.55%, 0.73%, and 0.33%, respectively. On the basis of the population demography, the authors estimated that 6.2 million Americans have serum creatinine levels ≥1.5 mg/dL, 2.5 million have levels of ≥1.7 mg/dL, and 0.8 million have levels of ≥2.0 mg/dL. It is unclear as to what proportion of patients with abnormal serum creatinine progress to ESRD; however, there is increasing evidence that these patients develop irreversible but preventable complications of chronic kidney disease during this phase of renal insufficiency. More recently it was noticed that the prevalence of chronic kidney disease increased from 10.0% in 1988–1994 to 13.1% in 1999–2004, of the U.S. population. This increase was partly explained by the increasing prevalence of diabetes and hypertension (8).

TABLE 11.1 NATIONAL KIDNEY FOUNDATION KIDNEY DISEASE OUTCOMES QUALITY INITIATIVE CLASSIFICATION, PREVALENCE, AND ACTION PLAN FOR STAGES OF CHRONIC KIDNEY DISEASE (7,8)

Stage	Description	GFR, mL/min/1.73 m³	Estimated No of U.S. adults in 2000	Action
—	At increased risk	≥60 (with chronic kidney disease risk factors)	—	Screening: chronic kidney disease risk reduction
1	Kidney damage with normal or increased GFR	≥90	3,600,000	Diagnosis and treatment; treatment of comorbid conditions; slowing progression; CVD risk reduction
2	Kidney damage with slightly decreased GFR	60–89	6,500,000	Estimating progression
3	Moderately decreased GFR	30–59	15,500,000	Evaluating and treating complications
4	Severely decreased GFR	15–29	700,000	Preparation for kidney replacement therapy

The term "ESRD" is used for patients who are on renal replacement therapy (dialysis or transplantation) in order to avoid life-threatening uremia. The incidence of ESRD shows marked geographic variation as determined by the population base with regard to age, race, and sex. The reported incidence of ESRD in the United States in 2006 was 360 per million population (9). The growth of 2.1% over the 2005 rate followed 4 years in which the 1-year change was <1%, and is the highest seen since 1999. The prevalent rate of ESRD, adjusted for age, gender, and race, rose 2.3% between 2005 and 2006 to reach 1,626 per million population. Hence, the incidence and prevalence of ESRD in the United States is increasing. A similar increase in incidence is occurring in most other industrialized countries as well; the reason for this increase in frequency of ESRD is unclear. In the United States, the distribution of patients reported by race most recently shows that 54.7% were white, 38.3% were African American, with the remaining 5.3% Asian/Pacific islanders and Native Americans. Overall, 10.3% of the patients are Hispanic. In the U.S. population, it is clear that chronic kidney disease is more prevalent in the African-American and Native-American populations than in the white population.

Although life for chronic kidney disease patients can be sustained by chronic dialysis and kidney transplantation, neither form of therapy is totally satisfactory. The current yearly mortality rate in the U.S. dialysis population is over 20%. Results with renal transplantation have improved considerably with the advent of improved immunosuppressive therapy (9). The adjusted and averaged 1-year graft survival was over 90% for living related donors and ~85% for cadaveric donor transplants (10,11). With improved transplant outcomes, growth in the number of patients wanting or needing a transplant has outpaced the supply of available organs. Although kidney transplant has become the preferred method of treatment for many ESRD patients, fewer than 20% of patients entering ESRD programs receive kidney transplantation because of age, associated disease, anatomic abnormalities of the urinary tract, the presence of preformed cytotoxic antibodies, or lack of availability of a suitable donor.

The rehabilitation rate of patients on chronic dialysis has been disappointing, and the cost of this treatment has been of increasing concern. Driven predominantly by recent growth in the ESRD patient population, total Medicare expenditures for the ESRD program alone have been increased steadily from $5 billion in 1991 to $23 billion in 2006, 6.4% of the entire Medicare budget (9). The total cost is projected to more than double in the next 10 years. Because of the cost as well as the morbidity and mortality associated with ESRD, every attempt should be made to preserve kidney function as long as possible, ideally preventing any further progression of the underlying renal disease.

Causes of Chronic Kidney Disease

The cause of kidney disease should be established, if possible, because some conditions may result in partial or full functional recovery if corrected. The major causes of chronic kidney disease found in patients entering the ESRD program are shown in Figure 11.2.

GLOMERULAR DISEASES

Diabetes mellitus has become the most common cause of chronic kidney disease. It is estimated that 40% of patients who have type 1 diabetes mellitus for more than 20 years will develop kidney disease. Although the incidence of ESRD in patients with type 2 diabetes may be less than of that found in type 1 diabetes, because of the larger number of patients with type 2 diabetes it is a more frequent cause of ESRD than type 1 diabetes (36.5% versus 7.2%) (11). Of note, in the U.S. at least 80% of diabetic patients with ESRD are type 2 diabetic (9).

Glomerulonephritis represents the third most common cause of ESRD. The most common glomerular diseases are focal and segmental glomerulosclerosis (FSGS) and membranoproliferative and lupus glomerulonephritis. However, it should be noted that the majority of glomerular diseases are unclassified. It is possible that this disease accounts for a relatively large fraction of unclassified glomerular diseases because IgA nephropathy is the most common glomerular disease responsible for ESRD in most other developed countries.

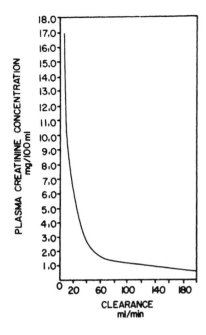

■ **Figure 11.2** Relationship between serum creatinine concentration and creatinine clearance. (From Doolan PD, Alpen EL, Thiel GB. A clinical appraisal of the plasma concentration and endogenous clearance of creatinine. *Am J Med.* 1962;32:65, with permission.)

VASCULAR DISEASE

Hypertension is the second leading reported cause of ESRD. A 15-year follow-up study of 361,659 men with hypertension found that 924 developed ESRD (12). This represented an incidence of 17.12 per 100,000 person-years. The relative risk for development of ESRD for diastolic blood pressure >120 mm Hg versus <70 mm Hg was 30.9. For systolic blood pressure >200 mm Hg versus <120 mm Hg, the relative risk was 48.2. Across the entire range, blood pressure represented an independent risk factor for kidney disease progression. The relative risk for African Americans was 1.99 (12). This increased risk could not be explained by difference in levels of systolic or diastolic pressures or other known risk factors. In general, ESRD secondary to hypertension occurs in African-American patients with a long history of uncontrolled hypertension or almost any patient with a history of malignant or accelerated hypertension (13–15). Although the incidence of chronic kidney disease from hypertension can be markedly attenuated by treatment of accelerated or malignant hypertension (13,16), adequate chronic treatment of milder hypertensive states, especially in the African-American population, may not prevent progression of kidney disease (12,14).

Other less common vascular causes of chronic kidney disease are atheroembolic disease and bilateral renal artery stenosis. Atheroembolic disease should be suspected in any individual who develops progressive decrease in kidney function following a vascular diagnostic procedure or surgery. In contrast to other vascular renal disease, atheroembolic disease may include high-grade proteinuria, eosinophiluria, and decreased serum complement. Diagnosis of atheroembolic disease largely depends on renal biopsy in which the cholesterol clefts are observed. There is no specific treatment for atheroembolic disease. Bilateral renal artery stenosis, as a cause of ischemic nephropathy, is suggested by a further reversible reduction in renal function precipated by converting enzyme inhibitors.

Arteriography usually is required for the diagnosis of renal artery stenosis. As of this time, there is no consistent evidence that kidney function can predictably be improved in patients with bilateral renal artery stenosis by either angioplasty or surgical correction of the lesions. Uncontrolled studies, however, have suggested that these procedures can improve kidney function in some instances.

INTERSTITIAL NEPHRITIS

Interstitial nephritis is a descriptive term implying fibrosis and an inflammatory response in the interstitium of the kidney. The glomeruli are involved only secondarily as a result of the fibrosis and vascular changes. Because of the potential reversibility or prevention of this group of renal diseases, it is important to differentiate interstitial nephritis from glomerulonephritis.

TABLE 11.2 FEATURES DIFFERENTIATING GLOMERULONEPHRITIS AND INTERSTITIAL NEPHRITIS

Feature	Glomerulonephritis	Interstitial nephritis
Proteinuria	>3 g	<1.5 g
Sediment	Numerous cells and red blood cell casts	Few cells and casts
Sodium handling	Normal until late	Sodium wasting
Anemia	Moderate severity until late	Disproportionately severe for degree of renal failure
Hypertension	Common	Less common
Acidosis	Normochloremic	Hyperchloremic
Uric acid	Slightly elevated	Markedly elevated
Urine volume	Normal	Increased

A number of clinical and biochemical features, listed in Table 11.2, tend to separate these two forms of renal disease. Characteristically, patients with interstitial nephritis complain of polyuria and nocturia. Their urine volume is unusually large (3 to 5 L/day) because the kidney's ability to concentrate urine is lost early in the course of kidney disease. The diluting capability in interstitial nephritis is maintained even late in the course of kidney disease; thus, the urine osmolality and specific gravity may be low when determined on a random collection of urine.

A feature of advanced glomerular diseases is high-grade proteinuria, which usually is in excess of 2.5 g/day. Even with advanced interstitial nephritis, the 24-hour urinary protein excretion is usually <1 to 2 g. Furthermore, the urinary protein may be predominantly an α_2- or β-globulin instead of albumin. In interstitial nephritis, serum uric acid is commonly elevated, and in one type of interstitial nephritis—lead nephropathy—clinical gout has been recognized in ~50% of the patients (17,18). The urinary sediment in interstitial nephritis may be totally unremarkable, or there may be a few white blood cells (WBCs) and hyaline casts. Renal salt wasting appears to be more common in patients with interstitial nephritis than in other forms of kidney disease, and salt supplementation sometimes must be given to maintain extracellular fluid (ECF) volume. Finally, hypertension is less common in interstitial nephritis and anemia may be disproportionately more severe for the degree of compromised kidney function than in chronic glomerulonephritis.

As is apparent in Table 11.3, a variety of drugs and toxins can be the etiologic agent responsible for causing interstitial nephritis. In general, with the exception of analgesics, drugs cause an acute interstitial nephritis that is reversible when the drugs are discontinued. The severity and chronicity of other forms of interstitial nephritis are largely related to the amount and duration of exposure to the various nephrotoxins. Interstitial nephritis accounts for 3% of the patients in this country being treated for ESRD. In this group, currently analgesic nephropathy accounts for 0.8% of patients being treated for ESRD. Analgesic nephropathy used to account for up to 20% of ESRD in several countries (19). However, following the removal from the market of analgesics containing the combination of aspirin and phenacetin, the incidence of this disease has markedly decreased worldwide. The typical patient with this disease is a depressed, middle-aged woman who gives a history of years of daily ingestion of analgesics containing caffeine, aspirin, and phenacetin. Usually, the total consumption of analgesics amounts to several kilograms. Patients frequently complain of headaches, backache, or other types of chronic pain and state that the analgesics are consumed to relieve this pain. There is evidence that sometimes the headaches may result from the caffeine or phenacetin ingestion, or both. The headaches may disappear if the patient can be persuaded to discontinue the analgesics. The patient commonly presents with recurrent urinary tract infections, gross hematuria, or symptoms of uremia. However, because papillary necrosis is common, acute kidney injury, and ureteral colic may develop as a result of the passing of necrotic papillae down one or both ureters. In this disease, the kidney has a remarkable capacity to recover even after what would appear to be a terminal state of ESRD (20). With conservative treatment and discontinuation of the analgesics, the patient can achieve significant improvement in kidney function and have a relatively good, long-term survival. Many times, however, it is very difficult to convince the patient to break a long habit of drug abuse.

Uric acid and oxalate nephropathy and cystinosis represent <0.1% each of the ESRD population (11). Chronic kidney disease is uncommon in patients with primary gout, and when it does occur, it is slowly

TABLE 11.3 VARIOUS ETIOLOGIES OF INTERSTITIAL NEPHRITIS

Analgesics

Other drugs
  Sulfonamide
  Penicillin and homologs
  Furosemide, thiazides
  Phenindione
  Phenytoin
  Cimetidine
  Nonsteroidal antiinflammatory drugs

Calcium disorders
  Hyperparathyroidism
  Milk–alkali syndrome
  Sarcoid
  Neoplasms
  Multiple myeloma

Uric acid
  Gouty nephropathy
  Hematologic disorders

Oxalate deposition
  Associated with small-bowel disease
  Hereditary
  Anesthetic agents: methoxyflurane
  Ethylene glycol

Heavy metals
  Lead
  Cadmium
  Uranium
  Copper

Miscellaneous
  Infection
  Idiopathic

progressive and only becomes clinically important late in life (20). However, in some hematologic disorders, particularly in association with the use of chemotherapeutic agents, there may be marked overproduction of uric acid, which may cause acute kidney injury caused by deposition of urate crystals in the tubules.

Another compound capable of inducing a severe interstitial nephritis is oxalate. Besides ethylene glycol intoxication (21), increased urinary excretion of oxalate can occur in association with genetic disorders as well as with a number of acquired conditions. Two enzymatic defects have been described that can result in the accumulation of glyoxylic acid and hyperoxaluria. In the first type, urinary excretion of oxalic acid, glyoxylic acid, and glycolic acid is increased as a result of deficiency of 2-oxoglutarate-glyoxylate carboligase (22). In the second defect, urinary excretion of glycolic acid is normal, but the excretion of L-glyceric acid and oxalate is increased. This condition owes to a deficiency of D-glyceric dehydrogenase (22). Both diseases are characterized by nephrolithiasis, nephrocalcinosis, and ESRD, with few patients living beyond the age of 40 years.

Recently, a number of acquired forms of hyperoxaluria and kidney disease have been described. Methoxyflurane anesthesia can cause hyperoxaluria and azotemia (23). In addition, it has been recognized that patients with distal small-bowel disease may have hyperoxaluria (24). In this group of patients, calcium oxalate stones are common; however, marked oxalate deposition occasionally may occur in the kidney, resulting in interstitial nephritis and loss of kidney function. The mechanism responsible for hyperoxaluria has been shown to be a consequence of increased absorption of dietary oxalate (24). It is felt that this results from calcium and possibly magnesium (which normally binds oxalate in the gut, rendering it insoluble and nonabsorbable) being bound to fatty acids in steatorrheic states, allowing the oxalate to be absorbed. Similarly, this condition has been treated successfully by giving supplemental calcium. Furthermore, cholestyramine also has been shown to be effective in decreasing oxalate absorption from the bowel and thus in decreasing urinary excretion of this compound (24).

All other causes of interstitial nephritis are even less prevalent. Conditions that cause hypercalcemia, hypercalciuria, or both can lead to the deposition of calcium in the kidney, with a resulting interstitial nephritis. Radiographic evidence of nephrocalcinosis is frequently a late finding and even then may be observed only by using the technique of nephrotomography. Thus, radiographic evidence of nephrocalcinosis cannot be relied on to establish the diagnosis even when kidney function is severely impaired. In this condition, if the underlying cause responsible for the disturbance of calcium metabolism such as primary hyperparathyroidism, sarcoid, or milk–alkali syndrome is corrected or treated, further progression of kidney disease can be either slowed or prevented (25,26).

A final group of agents that can produce a chronic interstitial nephritis are some of the heavy metals, including copper, lead, cadmium, and uranium. Lead nephropathy is common in Queensland, Australia (18), and has been reported in some areas of the United States in patients who have consumed moonshine whiskey (27). Lead nephropathy may occur more commonly than previously suspected in this country. Batuman et al. (28) have suggested that patients having the combination of interstitial nephritis and gout should be suspected of having lead nephropathy. This supposition was supported by the finding that ethylenediaminetetraacetic acid (EDTA) mobilized significantly greater amounts of lead in patients with kidney disease and gout than in patients with either gout or chronic kidney disease alone. Cadmium intoxication also can lead to an interstitial nephritis and renal tubular dysfunction. Characteristically, patients present with aminoaciduria, glycosuria, phosphaturia, and severe osteomalacia (29). As a result of industrial contamination with the element, chronic cadmium intoxication is especially prevalent in the people living along the Jinzu River in Japan (29). In Wilson disease, copper is deposited in the proximal tubule cells and may cause a variety of renal functional abnormalities, including Fanconi syndrome, proteinuria, and hematuria; however, it does not appear to progress to ESRD.

Evidence suggests that, in the adult, chronic urinary tract infection without obstruction rarely, if ever, leads to ESRD. However, there are some exceptions in which renal bacterial infections can lead to chronic kidney disease if untreated; among them are tuberculosis, multiple renal abscesses, and bacterial infections associated with papillary necrosis.

Because a number of patients with interstitial nephritis have a potentially preventable or reversible form of kidney disease, a careful history should be obtained relating to medications, small-bowel disease, and possible environmental exposure to some toxin. In addition, serum and urinary uric acid and calcium should be determined. In selected cases, urinary oxalate excretion should be measured and heavy-metal screens performed. The normal values to be used for these screening procedures are given in Table 11.4.

REFLUX NEPHROPATHY

Reflux nephropathy is the second most common kidney disease in children (30). According to the European Dialysis and Transplantation Association, it accounts for 30% of advanced kidney disease in children <16 years. The infant kidney is especially susceptible to intrarenal reflux. Most evidence would suggest that scarring usually occurs by 2 years of age (31) and that new scarring is unusual after age 5 (31–33). Increasing evidence suggests that severe congenital kidney damage already may be present at birth (31). This may represent a disorder in kidney embryogenesis as a result of an abnormal development of the ureteral bud. Recent evidence also suggests that this condition may have a heritable basis with contribution from several genetic foci. Prognosis is largely determined by the extent to which the kidney is scarred and contracted when the patient is initially seen. It has been shown also that the severity of the reflux can be correlated with the degree of kidney damage and that surgical correction of

TABLE 11.4 NORMAL VALUES USED IN SCREENING PATIENTS WITH INTERSTITIAL NEPHRITIS

Substance measured	Plasma	Urine
Calcium	9.5–10.5 mg/dL	<300 mg/d
Oxalate	30 ng/dL	<40 mg/d
Uric acid	5–7 mg/dL	<800 mg/d
Lead	<40 ng/dL	<0.5 mg/d[a]
Cadmium, mercury, and uranium	Normally nondetectable	Normally nondetectable

Note: [a]Following 1 g of ethylenediaminetetraacetic acid.

reflux is associated with eradication of upper urinary tract infection and improvement of renal growth and function. However, a recent study in children suggests that surgical correction of reflux offers no advantage over good medical management (33). Although there are no control trials in adults regarding surgical correction of reflux, most studies suggest that it does not influence the course of kidney disease.

HEREDITARY RENAL DISEASE

Approximately 5% to 8% of patients with chronic kidney disease have an hereditary etiology such as autosomal dominant polycystic kidney disease (ADPKD), Alport syndrome, Fabry disease, congenital nephrotic syndrome, medullary cystic disease, cystinosis, or familial amyloidosis. This is another group of kidney diseases for which specific treatment is not available (34). Through genetic counseling, however, a number of these diseases are potentially preventable. Therefore, the physician has an obligation to advise potential parents of the risk of having children with kidney disease and to determine when possible which family members are at risk or have diagnosable kidney disease. In ADPKD, which is inherited as an autosomal dominant disorder with complete penetrance, a DNA probe has localized the majority of cases (>90%) to a mutation in the short arm of human chromosome 16 (PKD1). This technique has been used to diagnose the disease in utero in a 9-week fetus (35). A mutation of chromosome 4 (PKD2) accounts for ~10% of patients with the disease. The genes for PKD1 and PKD2 have been identified. PKD1 encodes polycystin. An abnormality in polycystin may impair cell–cell and cell–matrix interactions, leading to abnormal epithelial cell differentiation and various phenotypic expressions (36,37). The PKD2 gene encodes for a channel protein. Mutation of the same leads to decrease cellular calcium with increased cyclic AMP that has been known to contribute to cyst formation.

The potential success of genetic counseling for hereditary diseases is demonstrated by a study carried out at the genetic clinic at the Hospital for Sick Children in London. Approximately two-thirds of the families who were informed that the chances were >10% that their children would develop hereditary disease decided to have no more children, whereas three-fourths of families informed that the chances were ≤10% elected to have more children (36).

Risk Factors for Development of End-Stage Renal Disease

The four major risk factors for the development of ESRD are race, age, sex, and family history.

RACE AND ETHNICITY

Male African Americans aged 25 to 44 years are 20 times more likely to develop kidney disease secondary to hypertension than white men (15,38). African Americans also have a very high incidence of idiopathic focal segmental glomerulosclerosis (FSGS) as well as that associated with intravenous drug use and acquired immunodeficiency syndrome (AIDS) (9,39). The attack rate of FSGS in African-American men with AIDS is ~10 times as great as in white men. In fact, FSGS is the most common cause of kidney disease in young adult African-American men. African Americans also have a fourfold greater risk than whites of developing ESRD from type 2 diabetes (11). In contrast, two diseases, ADPKD and especially IgA nephropathy, occur with considerably less frequency in the African-American than in the white population. In Native Americans, diabetes accounts for almost twice as much ESRD (68.2%) as found in the white or African-American population. Hispanics also have a high frequency of diabetic ESRD, with some reports as high as 60% (9).

AGE

Since 2000 the adjusted incident rate of ESRD has increased 11.0% for patients ≥75 years, reaching 1,744 per million population in 2006, while the rate for those age 20 to 44 years has grown 6.1% (9). The incidence of diabetic kidney disease also increases dramatically with age. However, in contrast to the total causes of chronic kidney disease, which continue to increase with advanced age, over 66% of diabetic ESRD occurs before 64 years of age. Before age 40, FSGS, lupus erythematosus, Henoch–Schönlein purpura, AIDS-related nephropathy, and congenital and hereditary disease (e.g., renal agenesis, obstructive nephropathy, Alport syndrome, and reflux nephropathy) are most commonly seen. In the age group 40 to 55 years, ADPKD, membranous glomerulonephritis, membranoproliferative glomerulonephritis, and hemolytic-uremic syndrome are seen with increasing frequency. Goodpasture syndrome, interstitial nephritis, analgesic nephropathy, amyloidosis, multiple myeloma, and Wegener granulomatosis are the most common diseases in the age group >55 years.

SEX

Sex is an additional risk factor for the development and progression of certain types of kidney disease. Overall, the incidence of ESRD is greater in males than females (9). However, there are certain causes of ESRD that occur more frequently in females, such as type 2 diabetes, interstitial nephritis, lupus erythematosus, scleroderma, and hemolytic-uremic syndrome/thrombotic thrombocytopenia purpura.

FAMILY HISTORY

Genetic factors also are important in predisposing individuals to developing ESRD. Patients with diabetes who have a family history of essential hypertension and abnormal lithium–sodium countertransport are at greater risk of developing chronic kidney disease (40,41). Both candidate locus and genome wide strategies have been used to target genes that contribute to the risks for development of these orders. Similarly, there are numerous types of hereditary renal disease such as Alport syndrome and ADPKD, plus a variety of less common and largely recessive or sex-linked hereditary diseases such as Fabry disease, tuberous sclerosis, medullary cystic disease, sickle cell disease, familial Mediterranean fever, type 1 glycogen storage disease, cystinosis, oxalate nephropathy, and infantile PKD (42–44).

Individual variability in the rate of progression to ESRD is a characteristic feature among patients with either inherited or acquired causes of kidney diseases. A number of genetic foci that contribute to the progression of chronic kidney disease have been identified. Most extensively studied has been an insertion/deletion polymorphism of the angiotensin-converting enzyme (ACE) gene. Studies in a variety of disorders have revealed an important contribution of this locus in the progressive deterioration of kidney function. The two different alleles defined by this polymorphism of the ACE gene are associated with corresponding differences in the endogenous activity of the encoded enzyme. The homozygous deletion/deletion (D/D) variant is associated with the highest expression of endogenous activity and a greater risk of progression to ESRD. This group of patients with the DD polymorphism of the ACE gene may also be more likely to have an antiproteinuric response to ACE inhibitors (45–47).

Symptomatology of Chronic Uremia

Early in chronic kidney disease, when the GFR is >25 mL/min/1.73 m^2 (i.e., ~25% of normal), the majority of patients have few symptoms, and the biochemical abnormalities are equally unremarkable. Although a rise in serum uric acid has been reported to occur early in kidney disease, the increment usually is <1 mg/dL (18). Therefore, with the exception of some patients with interstitial nephritis, secondary gout is uncommon in ESRD. Proteinuria is common at this stage and the nephrotic syndrome may be present in some glomerular diseases. In association with high-grade proteinuria, the patient may also lose antithrombin III, with resulting antithrombin III deficiency, a hypercoagulable state, and a predisposition to thromboembolic complications (48). The third major finding in the early stage of kidney disease is hypertension. If the hypertension is not treated, arteriolar nephrosclerosis as well as focal glomerulosclerosis may develop and accelerate the loss of kidney function. Because it is extremely difficult to determine whether the progressive loss of kidney function is a consequence of the underlying kidney disease or the hypertensive state, it is imperative that blood pressure be well controlled.

FLUID AND ELECTROLYTE DISTURBANCES

Disturbances of fluid and electrolytes may occur as the GFR falls below 25 mL/min/1.73 m^2. The interesting aspect is that on a normal diet, even with a GFR of 3 to 5 mL/min/1.73 m^2, there may be only minimal disturbances of plasma electrolytes and the body water content. This is a result of the fact that as GFR falls there is increased fractional clearance of electrolytes, as well as water. This has been termed "the magnification phenomenon" by Bricker et al. (49). This implies that the diseased kidney continues to be under the control of a variety of biologic systems that regulate the excretion of the various electrolytes, and the excretory response per nephron evoked by these systems varies inversely with the number of surviving nephrons. Because of this, the individual with advanced chronic kidney disease is able to excrete the elements and waste products obtained from a normal dietary intake, maintaining reasonable water and electrolyte balance.

However, the range over which the individual can maintain balance is limited with advanced chronic kidney disease. Because of the impaired capacity to dilute or concentrate urine, the patient will develop increasing dehydration and hypernatremia if water intake is restricted; and the degree of azotemia may increase secondary to further impaired excretion of nitrogenous waste products. Conversely, hyponatremia may occur if water intake is excessive.

When placed on a low-sodium diet, the majority of patients with advanced chronic kidney disease are unable to reduce urinary sodium excretion to the level of their sodium intake, or it takes three to four times longer to do so than in a normal person. In a few patients, usually with medullary cystic disease, ADPKD, or interstitial nephritis, an excess sodium intake may be necessary to maintain sodium balance (50). A rare patient may require as much as 10 to 20 g of salt supplementation daily to maintain ECF volume and maximum kidney function. In general, such severe renal salt wasting is very infrequent and occurs in the presence of far-advanced kidney disease.

Hyperkalemia rarely occurs in patients who have a GFR >25 mL/min/1.73 m^2 in the absence of an endogenous or exogenous potassium load. Potassium balance is maintained in the majority of patients by a combination of increased tubular secretion of potassium, which is mediated in part by aldosterone (51,52) and the increased fecal potassium loss (51,52). Because these mechanisms must work to the maximum in advanced kidney disease, there are several circumstances in which hyperkalemia may develop. Competitive inhibition of aldosterone with spironolactone, or inhibitors of distal potassium secretion (e.g., amiloride or triamterene) may induce severe hyperkalemia. A second cause of hyperkalemia is an increased intake of potassium; and third is acute acidosis that caused intracellular potassium to be released into the extracellular pool. A rough clinical estimate of the effect of acidosis on serum potassium concentration is as follows: for every decrease of 0.1 pH unit, serum potassium increases by ~0.6 mEq/L. β-Blockers, nonsteroidal antiinflammatory drugs (NSAIDs), ACE inhibitors, and angiotensin receptor blockers (ARBs) also may interfere with the renin–angiotensin system and lead to hyperkalemia.

Schambelan et al. (53) described an additional cause for the spontaneous occurrence of hyperkalemia in patients with kidney disease. Although all their patients had hyperkalemia in association with chronic kidney disease, the degree of kidney function impairment often was not severe. The majority of their patients had either diabetes mellitus or interstitial nephritis (53). The highlight of the findings in these patients was diminished plasma levels of renin and aldosterone. Studies suggest that the hyperkalemia is a result of hypoaldosteronism, which is attributable to hyporeninemia. The diminished plasma renin activity may in turn result from an autonomic neuropathy or sclerosis of the juxtaglomerular apparatus in the diabetic patients. Sickle cell disease, kidney transplantation, and lupus nephritis also have been associated with hyperkalemia, probably secondary to diminished tubular secretory capacity. Another cause of hyperkalemia occurs in some patients with chronic obstructive uropathy (54). These individuals appear to have a tubular resistance to aldosterone in contrast to the hyporeninemic–hypoaldosterone patients. Thus, these conditions should be considered when hyperkalemia is noted in patients with chronic kidney disease and other causes have been excluded.

Hypokalemia also may occur in patients with chronic kidney disease. A number of factors may be responsible for this finding, including poor dietary intake of potassium, diarrhea, diuretic therapy, metabolic alkalosis with secondary hyperaldosteronism, or specific renal tubular defects such as those found in association with type 1 renal tubular acidosis (RTA) and Fanconi syndrome (type 2 RTA).

Total body burdens of other elements, although not totally corrected by the diseased kidney, are corrected to the extent that the remaining alterations are associated with few, if any, clinical symptomatology until ESRD has occurred. The fractional clearance of phosphorus, magnesium, and calcium all increase as GFR progressively falls. As a result, plasma magnesium and phosphorus are not elevated until GFR falls below 25 mL/min/1.73 m^2 (55). Even then, plasma values rarely increase >1 to 2 mg/dL until GFR falls below 5 mL/min/1.73 m^2. The serum magnesium concentration may be slightly elevated when the patient is ingesting a normal magnesium intake. Magnesium-containing antacids and laxatives should be avoided because such patients have difficulty in excreting large magnesium loads (56).

Although fractional clearance of calcium is increased in kidney disease, absolute excretion is actually decreased. In contrast to other elemental disturbances, there may be major consequences as a result of the altered calcium metabolism associated with the uremic state. Parathyroid hormone (PTH) levels are found to significantly increase when GFR falls to 45% of normal, and 1,25-dihydroxy vitamin D_3 $(1,25[OH]_2D_3)$ levels fall when GFR is 70% to 80% of normal. Hypocalcemia also is a common finding in patients with advanced kidney disease. Hypocalcemia probably results from a combination of factors including low $1,25(OH)_2D_3$ with decreased gastrointestinal absorption of calcium, hyperphosphatemia, and bone resistance to the calcemic effect of PTH.

ACID–BASE DISORDERS

Acidosis is a common disturbance at a more advanced stage of chronic kidney disease. Normally, the kidneys are responsible for excreting 60 to 70 mEq of hydrogen ions daily. Although the urine can be acidified normally in a majority of patients with chronic kidney disease (57), these patients have a reduced ability to produce ammonia. With advanced kidney disease, total daily acid excretion is usually reduced to 30 to 40 mEq; thus, throughout the remainder of their course of chronic kidney disease, many patients may be in a positive hydrogen ion balance of 20 to 40 mEq/day. The retained hydrogen ions probably are buffered by bone salts, although this has not yet been unequivocally proven. On occasion, hyperchloremic renal tubular acidosis with a normal anion gap may occur in the early stage of kidney disease. With more advanced chronic kidney disease, the plasma chloride concentration becomes normal, and a fairly large anion gap may develop. In most patients with chronic kidney disease, the metabolic acidosis is mild, and the pH rarely is <7.35. As with other abnormalities in chronic kidney disease, the primary symptomatic manifestations of the acid–base disturbances occur when the patient receives an excessive endogenous or exogenous acid load or loses excessive alkali (e.g., diarrhea).

The final stage of chronic kidney disease occurs when the GFR falls below 10 mL/min/1.73 m². The deranged metabolic functions present at this stage of kidney disease are responsible for the striking clinical features of uremia.

ANEMIA

The prevalence of anemia increases with progression of kidney disease and 90% of patients with a GFR <25 mL/min/1.73 m² have anemia defined as a hemoglobin <12 g/dL (58). The anemia of chronic kidney disease has been felt to result from a combination of factors, including reduced erythropoietin (EPO) activity, circulating factors that appear to inhibit the bone marrow response to erythropoietin, and shortened erythrocyte life span. Red blood cell (RBC) survival is decreased from 120 to 80 days in chronic kidney disease patients. Both metabolic and mechanical factors contribute to this short life span of RBC. Almost all patients with chronic kidney disease have much lower baseline EPO levels than those of normal subjects at the same degrees of anemia. Patients with ADPKD are the exception and usually have higher EPO levels with less severe anemia. Erythropoietin, a glycosylated, 165 amino-acid protein produced by renal peritubular capillary endothelial cells, acts on erythroid progenitor cells in the bone marrow. With the recent availability of recombinant EPO, it appears that the major cause of anemia has been a failure of EPO production by the diseased kidney, because uremic patients typically respond so well to exogenously administered EPO (58).

Low hemoglobin levels have been associated with increased left ventricular hyperthrophy and cardiovascular outcomes in patients with kidney disease. Therefore, several studies have evaluated whether treatment of anemia results in improved outcomes in chronic kidney disease patients. The United States Normal Hematocrit Trial (59) of chronic hemodialysis patients with cardiac disease randomly assigned patients to a target hematocrit of 42% or 30%. The primary outcome was time to death or nonfatal myocardial infarction. The study was stopped early as the group assigned to the higher hematocrit had an increased risk of mortality that was trending toward statistical significance and a higher rate of adverse vascular access events due to thrombosis. In the Correction of Hemoglobin and Outcomes in Renal Insufficiency (CHOIR) (60) trial, 1,432 patients with moderate and advanced chronic kidney disease and a hemoglobin <11 g/dL were randomized to achieve a target hemoglobin of either 11.3 or 13.5 g/dL.

The CHOIR trial was also terminated early as a significantly higher number of cardiovascular events was observed in the higher hemoglobin group. Of note, the patients in the higher hemoglobin group did not reach the target of 13.5 g/dL, they only reached a mean hemoglobin concentration of 12.6 g/dL and despite randomization, the higher hemoglobin group had more cardiac comorbidities, which could have contributed to the adverse outcomes observed in these patients. Similarly, the Cardiovascular Risk Reduction by Early Anemia Treatment with Epoetin Beta (CREATE) (60) trial randomly assigned 603 patients with moderate and advanced chronic kidney disease and anemia to achieve a target hemoglobin of normal (13 to 15 g/dL) or low normal (10.5 to 11.5 g/dL). After 3 years of follow-up, both groups had a similar risk of achieving the primary endpoint (composite of cardiovascular events) and the higher hemoglobin group had increased quality of life and general health. Treatment of anemia did not have any effect on left ventricular hypertrophy, as the left ventricular mass index remained stable in both groups.

The optimal hemoglobin level remains controversial and the current K/DOQI recommendations are not to exceed a hemoglobin level of 12 g/dL in chronic kidney disease patients (60). The Trial to Reduce Cardiovascular Events with Aranesp Therapy (TREAT) (60) is currently ongoing and has enrolled more patients than the CHOIR and CREATE trials combined. This trial might help answer the question of the value of hemoglobin normalization in patients with kidney disease not requiring renal replacement therapy.

BLEEDING DIATHESIS

Disturbances in the coagulation system also occur with an advanced stage of chronic kidney disease. Approximately 20% of uremic patients have a modest degree of thrombocytopenia, but it is rare to find a platelet count of <50,000. Severe thrombocytopenia may occur in patients with the hemolytic-uremic syndrome as a consequence of disseminated intravascular coagulation. However, this is not a common cause of chronic kidney disease in adults. Platelet factor 3 is reduced and platelet aggregation is decreased (61) in advanced kidney disease. This results in prolongation of the Ivy bleeding time and poor clot retraction. However, platelet function is caused by multiple factors such as the retention of uremic toxins, nitric oxide, anemia, and hyperparathyroidism. The importance of uremic toxins is suggested by the beneficial effect of acute dialysis on platelet dysfunction. How uremic toxins might interfere with platelet function is not completely understood. In vitro studies suggest that a dialyzable factor might interfere with the binding of fibrinogen. Uremia-induced changes in nitric oxide production also may contribute to inhibition of platelet aggregation. Treatment of the uremic state with dialysis improves platelet function in the majority of patients, suggesting some dialyzable factor is responsible for this abnormality. It is of interest that D-deaminoarginine vasopressin (dDAVP) improves the bleeding time without affecting the platelet abnormalities (62). This suggests that an abnormality in factor VIII or von Willebrand factor may play a role in the pathogenesis of the bleeding abnormality in the uremic state (62). Anemia also contributes to the abnormal bleeding time present in uremic patients. A higher hematocrit causes the platelets to skim at the endothelial surface, which is optimal for platelet–endothelium interaction. Such skimming does not occur with hematocrits <25% to 30%.

SEROSITIS

Another complication noted with some frequency in patients with far-advanced chronic kidney disease is involvement of the serous membranes as manifested by pericarditis and pleuritis. The involved membrane is markedly thickened, extremely vascular, and infiltrated with plasma cells and histiocytes (63). Both pleural and pericardial friction rubs may be heard. When pleural and pericardial effusions are present, they are uniformly hemorrhagic and usually contain fewer than 10,000 WBCs/mm^2. Pericardiocentesis, as well as thoracentesis, is occasionally necessary to relieve clinical symptoms. However, if the uremic state is not improved with treatment of reversible factors or hemodialysis, recurrent effusions are common. Rarely, constrictive pericarditis may follow healing of acute uremic pericarditis.

Chronic ascites also may be a manifestation of uremic serositis and advanced kidney disease. This complication arises primarily in patients who have had previous abdominal surgery or peritoneal dialysis. The ascitic fluid is an exudate with the ascitic fluid albumin/plasma albumin concentration ratio of >0.5. Although fluid overload may worsen uremic ascites, fluid removal frequently is not a successful mode of treatment. Renal transplantation or several consecutive days of intensive dialysis has been useful in treating uremic ascites.

GASTROINTESTINAL DISORDERS

Most patients with far-advanced kidney disease have gastrointestinal symptoms that are a major part of their clinical picture (64). Specifically, nausea, vomiting, and anorexia are extremely common. Uremic stomatitis, characterized by dry mucous membranes and multiple, bright-red, small, ulcerative lesions, may occur with advanced uremia. Poor dental hygiene appears to contribute to the development of uremic stomatitis. Because saliva in uremic patients has an increased urea content, it has been suggested that the stomatitis results from high levels of ammonium, which is formed by bacteria ureases from the high levels of salivary urea. Inflammation of salivary glands (e.g., parotitis) also may occur in uremic patients and is usually associated with stomatitis. The salivary glands may become markedly swollen in chronic kidney disease, but characteristically they are not tender or indurated, as might be seen in inflammatory parotitis.

Pancreatic involvement also has been found on postmortem examination in patients who have died from uremia. Typically, on histologic examination of the pancreas, there is dilatation of the acini, flattening of the epithelial cells, and inspissation of the intraacinar secretions. Clinical symptoms of pancreatitis also may occur. It was felt previously that uremia alone, as a result of chronic loss of kidney function and thus the inability to excrete amylase, could significantly elevate the serum amylase concentration, but this has been shown not to be the case (65). Rather, when a high elevation of serum amylase concentration is found in patients with chronic kidney disease, pancreatitis should be considered strongly. In acute kidney injury, however, serum amylase elevations are common but are rarely over twice normal in the absence of clinical evidence of pancreatitis (65). Other findings in the gastrointestinal tract in advanced uremia include erosive gastritis and uremic colitis characterized by submucosal hemorrhages and small mucosal ulcerations. With the exception of anorexia, nausea, and vomiting, the majority of other gastrointestinal complications of uremia are rarely seen in patients with kidney disease now that treatment with dialysis and renal transplantation is possible and initiated relatively early.

NEUROMUSCULAR DISTURBANCES

The neuromuscular disturbances occurring in patients with advanced kidney disease were some of the earliest clinical symptoms described in uremia (66). The initial symptoms are mild and consist of emotional lability, insomnia, and a lack of facility in abstract thinking. If the uremic state is allowed to progress, more striking changes are noted, consisting of increased deep tendon reflexes, clonus, asterixis, and stupor, which progress to coma, convulsions, and death.

Uremic neuropathy is another major and potentially disabling complication of chronic kidney disease. The earliest feature is the restless legs syndrome, in which the patient has a tendency to avoid inactivity of the lower extremities because of a sensation of numbness. This syndrome is followed by a sensory neuropathy characterized by paresthesia and hypalgesia, especially of the feet. In the most severe cases, a motor neuropathy also may occur. Typically, there is symmetrical involvement of the lower extremities, which is more severe distally and usually is manifested initially by bilateral footdrop (66). Uremic neuropathy occasionally can progress rapidly to a state of total quadriplegia. Histologically, the damage in the peripheral nerve occurs in the distal portion of the medullated fibers and involves a loss of myelin. For unknown reasons, the motor neuropathy is much more common in males than in females.

SKELETAL ABNORMALITIES (RENAL OSTEODYSTROPHY)

Other major causes of disability in chronic kidney disease, especially in children, are abnormalities in the skeletal system (Table 11.5). Growth is markedly retarded in children with kidney disease. The reasons are not well understood, but there is evidence that dialysis, especially chronic cyclic peritoneal dialysis, improves the growth rate. A high caloric and protein intake also may be helpful. Even with these measures, however, children on dialysis rarely grow normally. The use of corticosteroids after kidney transplantation also is associated with growth retardation. More recently, recombinant human growth hormone has been used with considerable success to increase height velocity in uremic children and those who have received transplants (67).

TABLE 11.5 CHARACTERISTICS OF RENAL OSTEODYSTROPHY

	High turnover	Low turnover
Parathyroid hormone	Increased	Decreased
Alkaline phosphatase	Increased	Normal
Osteocalcin	Increased	Normal
Calcium	Variable	Can be increased
Phosphorus	Increased	Normal or increased
DFO stimulation test[a]	Normal	Normal (adynamic) Elevated delta (aluminum OM)[a]
Skeletal radiographs	Resorption, sclerosis	Normal
Symptoms	Usually asymptomatic unless very severe disease	Asymptomatic (dynamic) Symptomatic (aluminum OM)

DFO, deferoxamine; OM, osteomalacia.

Severe rickets with resulting deformities and disability can develop in children with advanced chronic kidney disease. The typical radiographic feature of rickets is an irregular and fragmented line that separates the metaphysis from the growth cartilage (Fig. 11.3). The space separating the metaphyseal line and epiphyseal nucleus is widened, and the epiphyseal center appears late. Although this radiographic finding is classic of vitamin D–deficient rickets, uremic children with this finding characteristically show histologic changes of hyperparathyroidism rather than osteomalacia. Nutritional vitamin D and calcium therapy may be effective in correcting this abnormality.

The most common skeletal disturbance found in adults with advanced chronic kidney disease is hyperparathyroid bone disease, which is characterized by increased osteoclastic bone resorption. Bone histomorphometry performed in 60 nondialyzed uremic patients revealed that >80% showed evidence of hyperparathyroid bone disease (68). Only one patient in this series had histologic evidence of osteomalacia, and this patient was an alcoholic with chronic pancreatitis, suggesting an etiology other than uremia. The parathyroid glands may be markedly hyperplastic, and PTH levels are increased. Characteristically, there are few symptoms, and the diagnosis is made by finding the typical radiographic features of subperiosteal resorption. In Figure 11.4 are shown the subperiosteal resorption in the phalanges and the "salt-and-pepper" pattern in the skull of a patient with severe secondary hyperparathyroidism associated with advanced kidney disease. Such patients occasionally develop large osteoclastic tumors (brown cysts) in the skeleton around weight-bearing areas, as shown in Figure 11.5(**A**). In these conditions, parathyroidectomy is indicated, following which there usually is dramatic healing of the cyst

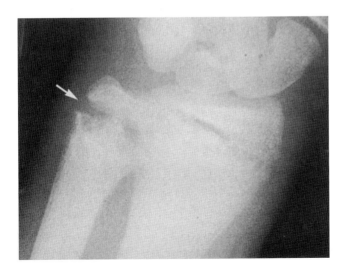

■ **Figure 11.3** Radiographic features of rickets. The metaphysis of the ulna is fragmented and irregular, and the space separating the metaphysis from the epiphyseal nucleus is widened (*arrow*).

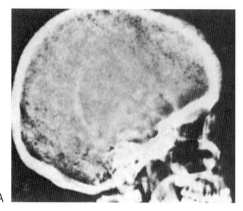
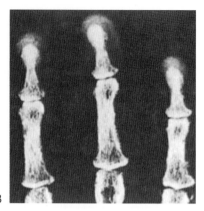

A   B

■ **Figure 11.4 A.** Typical radiographic features of severe secondary hyperparathyroidism involving skull (note *"salt-and-pepper" pattern*). **B.** Phalanges with lacy subperiosteal reabsorption.

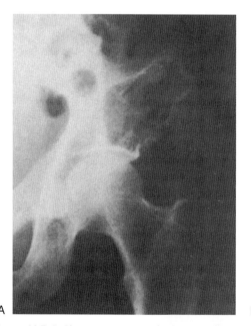
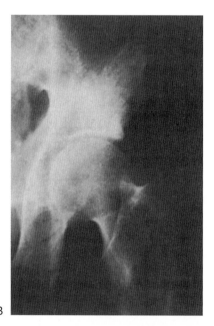

A   B

■ **Figure 11.5 A.** Biopsy-proven osteoclastic tumor (*brown cyst*) in the left ileum. **B.** Appearance 1 year after parathyroid surgery. Healing of the cyst is essentially complete as judged radiologically.

(Fig. 11.5B). The hyperparathyroid state usually resolves following renal transplantation (69). On occasion, however, persistent hypercalcemia that is endangering the integrity of the kidney graft may necessitate parathyroidectomy.

With the advent of chronic hemodialysis, osteomalacia has been noted with increased frequency in uremic patients. This disease is characterized by bone pain, fracturing bone disease, and proximal myopathy. Unlike other types of bone disease, osteomalacia is unresponsive to any vitamin D analogs.

Recently, a third type of bone disease has been described, called adynamic bone disease (70). This is a histologic diagnosis showing lack of bone formation and resorption. There are usually no clinical findings, and there are questions about therapy and the association with vascular calcification (71,72).

METASTATIC CALCIFICATION

A serious complication associated with chronic kidney disease is metastatic calcification. Three distinct types of metastatic calcium–phosphate deposits have been described in uremic patients. The specific mechanisms responsible for the development of these deposits have not been well delineated, and it is possible that all three have different pathogenic mechanisms.

One of the most potentially devastating forms of metastatic calcification is vascular calcification. An example of diffuse calcification in the arterial vessels of the hand of a patient with advanced kidney disease appears in Figure 11.6. This vascular calcification can affect virtually any medium-sized artery in the body and can cause severe vascular insufficiency with the production of gangrene of the extremities (73) and ischemic ulcerations of the skin and gastrointestinal tract. Although improvement occasionally is observed following renal transplantation, in general, this vascular calcification persists after renal transplantation or parathyroidectomy. Histologic evidence of vascular calcification occurs even in young individuals with uremia, and by age 50 years, radiographic evidence of vascular calcification is present in almost 100% of uremic patients (74). It is felt that vascular calcification results from an accelerated aging process of the vessels in the uremic state.

The second variety of calcium–phosphate deposit is felt to result from hyperphosphatemia. This is based on the fact that these deposits can be rapidly mobilized by reducing the serum phosphorus and thus the calcium–phosphate product by dialysis, the use of phosphate-binding antacids, or transplantation (69,75). There is a direct relationship between elevated serum phosphorus levels and increased mortality risk. These may be related to metastatic calcification (precipitation of calcium–phosphate crystals in undamaged soft tissue) as a result of elevated serum phosphorus, and PTH. These deposits occur in three forms. Conjunctival calcification causes a redness and gritty feeling in the eyes. Periarticular calcification occurs over pressure points and around joints (Fig. 11.7). The major symptom associated with these deposits is a limitation of joint movement because of the size of the deposits. The second type of deposit resulting from hyperphosphatemia is acute arthritic episodes secondary to hydroxyapatite crystal deposition in the synovium and joint fluid.

The final type of calcification found in uremic patients is visceral calcification, which occurs in the lung, skeletal muscle, and myocardium. This is an amorphous calcium–phosphate deposit that has markedly different chemical and thermochemical properties from the other two types of calcium–phosphate deposits. The vascular and hyperphosphatemic-induced calcifications appear to consist of

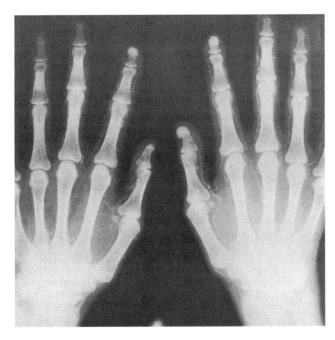

■ **Figure 11.6** Extensive vascular calcification involving the digital arteries.

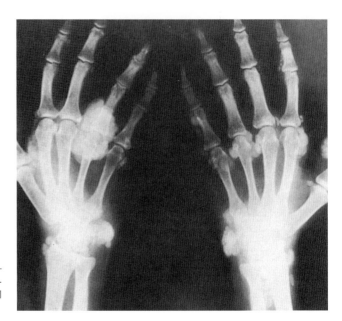

■ **Figure 11.7** Periarticular calcium–phosphate deposits (tumoral calcification) in a patient with advanced renal failure.

hydroxyapatite, whereas visceral calcifications have the thermochemical properties of whitlockite. In cardiac calcification, the deposits occur initially in the conducting system and may cause severe arrhythmias. With far-advanced cardiac calcification, however, there is extensive involvement of the entire myocardium, and death may result from a low cardiac output state. When calcification occurs in the lung, it characteristically causes a fibrous response in the small arteries and alveolar septa (Fig. 11.8). This results in restrictive and diffusion abnormalities and can lead to hypoxemia. The pathogenic mechanism responsible for the development of these visceral calcium–phosphate deposits is not well understood. Furthermore, it is unknown whether once present they can be mobilized by either transplantation or reduction of the plasma calcium or phosphorus level.

Generalized pruritus is an extremely bothersome complication of chronic kidney disease. Some authors have suggested that high skin calcium content may be responsible for it (76,77). However, it is possible that skin calcium content also may be secondarily increased as a result of the scratching. Parathyroidectomy has been used in a few cases as a method of treatment of pruritus. However, the majority of patients can be adequately controlled with less radical forms of treatment such as local lubrication, cyproheptadine (Periactin), and reduction of the serum phosphorus with phosphate-binding gels or intensified dialysis.

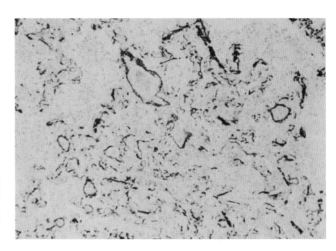

■ **Figure 11.8** Extensive calcification of the lung. The dark-staining material (von Kossa stain) present in the alveolar septa and walls of the small arteries is the calcium–phosphate deposit.

Calciphylaxis

Calciphylaxis is characterized by calcification of small- and medium-sized blood vessels of the skin and subcutaneous tissue. It is a rare but serious disorder that occurs in uremic patients (78,79). It is manifested by painful erythematous subcutaneous nodules and plaques on the trunk, buttocks, or proximal extremity. Lesions finally progress to necrotic ulcer. Septicemia is the primary cause of death. The pathogenesis of calciphylaxis is still unclear. Hyperparathyroidism, vitamin D supplementation, and hyperphosphatemia all are related to calciphylaxis, but none of these factors has been defined as a specific cause. High plasma levels of PTH, phosphate, and calcium are not very helpful with the diagnosis because they may not always be present. The diagnosis can be confirmed by a skin biopsy. Early diagnosis and treatment is important given the high mortality in this condition. Tight control of plasma calcium and phosphorus concentrations, avoidance of trauma, and aggressive wound care are all-important. Parathyroidectomy is suggested in dialysis patients with plasma intact PTH levels higher than 200 pg/mL, but its beneficial role is still controversial (80,81).

IMMUNOLOGIC ALTERATIONS

The immune response also is blunted in the majority of patients with advanced kidney disease, as manifested by depressed delayed hypersensitivity, prolonged survival of skin allografts, and reduced lymphocyte response to phytohemagglutinin (82). The uremic patient also appears to have a poorer immune response to some infections than nonuremic subjects. Perhaps this is best exemplified by the frequent occurrence of positivity for hepatitis B surface antigen (HBsAG) in patients with advanced chronic kidney disease (83). Although these patients usually do not manifest clinical symptoms of hepatitis, they become chronic carriers of the hepatitis-associated antigen. This continuing positivity for HBsAG recently has been related to low interferon levels in uremic patients (84).

Most studies show that humoral immunity is normal otherwise. It has recently been shown that $1,25(OH)_2D_3$ modulates the proliferation, differentiation, and immune function of lymphocytes and monocytes. On the basis of this finding, it has been suggested that part of the compromised immune function in uremia may be a consequence of the low $1,25(OH)_2D_3$ present in this state (85).

OTHER METABOLIC DISTURBANCES

Finally, a variety of generalized metabolic disturbances are present in the uremic patient. As a result of anorexia, nausea, poor dietary intake, and occasional vomiting, many patients with advanced kidney disease present in a chronic state of negative nitrogen balance and protein–calorie malnutrition.

Approximately 70% of uremic patients present with glucose intolerance. In contrast to patients with diabetes mellitus, the fasting blood sugar of uremic patients is normal, but postprandial glucose levels are increased (86). Plasma insulin levels in response to intravenously administered glucose are normal or even accentuated, thus suggesting that the glucose intolerance is a result of peripheral resistance to insulin. There is evidence that this abnormality in glucose metabolism may be improved by hemodialysis. Although glucagon levels are known to be increased in patients with advanced kidney disease, dialysis may improve glucose intolerance without altering glucagon levels.

A number of patients with kidney disease have type IV hyperlipidemia with increased levels of serum triglycerides and reduced HDL cholesterol. Whether this disturbance has any clinical importance has not yet been established, but there is evidence of acceleration of atherosclerosis in patients treated with chronic intermittent hemodialysis. In addition, experimental evidence suggests that abnormal lipid metabolism may contribute to the progression of renal disease. However, there is growing skepticism regarding the benefits of lowering serum cholesterol in the chronic dialysis patient population. This uncertainty is further strengthened by two clinical trials examining the use of statins in dialysis patients. Whereas statins have been consistently shown to reduce cardiovascular death and other cardiovascular events in non–chronic kidney disease patients, neither the Atorvastatin in Patients with Type 2 Diabetes Mellitus Undergoing Hemodialysis (4D) trial (a placebo-controlled randomized trial of atorvastatin in 1,255 maintenance HD patients with type II diabetes) (87) nor the recently published Study to Evaluate the Use of Rosuvastatin in Subjects on Regular Hemodialysis: An Assessment of Survival and Cardiovascular Events (AURORA) trial (a placebo-controlled randomized trial of rosuvastatin in 2,667 patients) (87) showed the anticipated reduction in cardiovascular death, nonfatal myocardial infarction (MI) and nonfatal stroke, despite >40% reductions in serum low-density-lipoprotein cholesterol levels.

Pathogenesis of the Uremic Syndrome

Although the metabolic consequences of uremia have been reasonably well defined, the specific uremia toxins responsible for most of these metabolic alterations have not been identified. It is apparent, however, that certain organic compounds, hormonal alterations, and inorganic substances that are affected by the uremic state may cause a number of defects (Table 11.6).

ORGANIC COMPOUNDS

Most studies of organic compounds have been directed at determining the toxicity of the various nitrogenous waste products, which consist of urea, ammonia, guanidine, guanidinosuccinic acid, and methylguanidine. Because urea is characteristically elevated and can be correlated with the severity of impairment of kidney function, a large number of studies have been directed at determining the role of urea in producing the uremic symptomatology. However, the results of most studies have been disappointing, and at present the only abnormalities that have been suggested as resulting at least in part from urea retention are nausea, anorexia, uremic stomatitis, and possibly uremic colitis.

Guanidine has been found to be increased in the blood of uremic patients. When injected into laboratory animals, guanidine produces muscle twitching, hyperexcitability, paresis, and convulsions. However, recent studies in uremic patients have failed to show a correlation between high guanidine levels and central nervous system symptoms (88).

Another potentially toxic organic compound is myoinositol, a natural constituent of food that also is synthesized in vivo. The concentration of this compound in plasma and cerebrospinal fluid is increased in uremia. Experimentally, myoinositol has been shown to be a neurotoxin, and therefore it has been suggested that this compound might be involved in the pathogenesis of uremic neuropathy (89). Plasma cyclic adenosine monophosphate (cAMP) levels have also been found to be increased in uremic patients (90). Plasma cAMP levels have been found to correlate inversely with platelet aggregation, and cAMP has been shown to inhibit platelet aggregation in vitro (90). Thus, cAMP may be partly responsible for the altered platelet function in uremia.

Possibly the strongest evidence that some of the nitrogenous waste products may be toxic in uremic patients are the studies of Walser et al. (91). In their studies, a number of patients were placed on diets extremely low in nitrogen to reduce the production of nitrogenous waste products. The diets were

TABLE 11.6 COMPOUNDS INCRIMINATED AS "UREMIC TOXINS"

Byproducts of protein and amino acid metabolism
  Urea—80% of total (excreted nitrogen)
  Guanidino compounds
    Guanidines
    Creatinine/creatine
  Other nitrogenous substances
    Polyamines
    Myoinositol
    Phenols
    Benzoates
    Indoles

Advanced glycation end products

Inhibitors of ligand-protein binding

Glucuronoconjugates and aglycones

Inhibitors of somatomedin and insulin action

Middle molecules

Parathyroid hormone

β_2-Microglobulin

supplemented with the ketoanalogs of the essential amino acids. These ketoanalogs were used to supply the carbon skeletons for the essential amino acids and thus to prevent the breakdown of tissue protein. There was marked improvement in the patients' sense of well being and possibly in some other abnormalities associated with the uremic syndrome. These results are deserving of further study, although they are not conclusive in demonstrating that nitrogenous waste products have a role in producing some uremic symptoms.

Another organic toxin recently identified in dialyzed uremic patients is the protein β_2-microglobulin. Normally the kidney is responsible for the elimination of this protein, which has a molecular weight of 11,800 Da. The 150 to 200 mg produced each day are filtered by the glomerulus and catabolized in the proximal tubule. Elimination of this protein is prevented and retained in advanced kidney disease, increasing plasma levels up to 50-fold and causing it to be deposited in tissues. The protein is deposited in tissues as amyloid, with its deposition being present largely in joint capsules, synovial membranes, the carpal tunnel, subchondral bone, tendons, intervertebral discs, and bone marrow (92). Clinical symptomatology from β_2-microglobulin deposition includes carpal tunnel syndrome, bone cysts, destructive spondyloarthropathy, effusive arthritis, scapulohumeral, and periarthritis. These complications usually are seen in dialyzed uremic patients, probably because it requires a minimum of 6 years of almost total loss of kidney function for enough β_2-microglobulin to be deposited to cause any clinical disturbances. Once deposited, it appears that this amyloid is not mobilized, even following reinstitution of kidney function with a successful renal transplant.

HORMONAL ALTERATIONS

Hormonal alterations occur in uremia as a result of four mechanisms. First, the diseased kidney may be unable to produce certain hormones normally, such as EPO and $1,25(OH)_2D_3$ (93). Second, the kidney normally excretes or degrades a variety of hormones: growth hormone, prolactin, luteinizing hormone, gastrin, insulin, glucagon, and PTH. Levels of these hormones may be increased in patients with chronic kidney disease because of lack of ability of the diseased kidney to metabolize or excrete these substances. Third, the diseased kidney may cause increased renin secretion as a result of ischemia, which in turn increases angiotensin and aldosterone production. The final mechanism for hormone alteration in uremia is the *trade-off hypothesis* (94).

The various hormonal alterations present in the uremic state may result in a variety of clinical disturbances (Table 11.7). However, the mere finding of increased levels of immunoreactive hormones does not necessarily mean that they are biologically active. That some of these hormones lack biologic activity is suggested by the fact that gastrin levels are not correlated with basal acid secretion in uremic patients. Studies also suggest that the measured growth hormone and possibly glucagon are not biologically active. Furthermore, it has been shown that the largest fraction of the elevated levels of immunoreactive PTH is the inactive *C*-terminal, which is normally disposed by the kidney.

TABLE 11.7　HORMONAL ALTERATIONS IN UREMIA

Hormone	Potential metabolic consequences
Increased	
Prolactin	Lactation
Luteinizing hormone	Gynecomastia
Gastrin gastritis	
Renin–angiotensin–aldosterone	Hypertension
Glucagon	Glucose intolerance
Growth hormone	
Parathyroid hormone	Osteitis fibrosis
Decreased	
$1,25\text{-}(OH)_2D_3$	Osteitis fibrosa
Erythropoietin	Anemia
Somatomedin	Decreased linear growth
Testosterone	Impotence
Follicle-stimulating hormone	Impotence

Elevated PTH levels have been incriminated in the pathogenesis of numerous abnormalities found in the uremic state, including neuropathy, encephalopathy, anemia, pruritus, impotence, and carbohydrate and lipid alterations (95). Although PTH has been shown in vitro to increase red cell osmotic fragility, decrease erythropoiesis, and decrease myocardial function and in vivo to be associated with increased brain calcium content and electroencephalographic (EEG) alterations, it is still unclear what role PTH plays in the uremic symptomatology found in humans.

Trade-off Hypothesis

Bricker (94) has proposed another conceptual approach to the pathogenesis of uremia, the so-called trade-off hypothesis. This theory suggests that with the progressive destruction of nephrons, a number of adaptive mechanisms are brought into play to allow the remaining nephrons to maintain normal body homeostasis. The adaptive changes that occur to maintain sodium balance in the patient with advanced kidney disease have been used as an illustrative example of the trade-off hypothesis. Approximately 0.5% of the filtered load of sodium is excreted with a normal sodium intake of 120 mEq/day and a normal GFR. However, on a similar sodium intake, when GFR has fallen to 2 mL/min, ~30% of the filtered load of sodium must be excreted to maintain sodium balance. The assumption is made that there is a substance that inhibits the tubular reabsorption of sodium, possibly a natriuretic hormone. It is further suggested that this inhibitor is present in high concentrations in the uremic patient's serum and that it may affect a variety of cellular transport systems and in turn lead to functional changes in other organs and organ systems. The trade-off is that the effects of such a hormone would be beneficial for the kidney and sodium balance but might cause some of the symptoms of uremia by inhibiting transport systems in other organs.

The increased PTH levels found in patients with chronic kidney disease have been suggested to be another example of a trade-off phenomenon. In this instance, it is proposed that phosphate excretion is reduced and serum phosphorus rises as nephrons are lost, even early in the course of kidney disease. The elevated serum phosphorus then causes serum calcium concentration to fall, an effect that leads to increased PTH release. The increased parathyroid activity then is associated with a decrease in tubular reabsorption of phosphorus, which results in increased phosphorus excretion and returns the serum phosphorus to near-normal levels. As more nephrons are lost and the amount of filtered phosphate further decreases, higher serum concentrations of PTH are required to maintain phosphorus balance. The trade-off for the maintenance of phosphorus would be the clinical consequences of secondary hyperparathyroidism on the bony skeleton. More recently, studies suggest that hyperphosphatemia per se can stimulate PTH secretion. However, other factors as well are also probably important in the pathogenesis of the hyperparathyroid state. Studies have shown that there is a reduced number of $1,25(OH)_2D_3$ (calcitriol) receptors on the parathyroid gland in the uremic state (96). Because calcitriol suppresses the synthesis of PTH, the combination of decreased calcitriol receptor number and impaired renal production of $1,25(OH)_2D_3$ markedly decreases this hormone's inhibitor effect on PTH synthesis (97). Bone resistance to PTH in patients with kidney disease may be an additional cause of secondary hyperparathyroidism.

INORGANIC SUBSTANCES

The role of inorganic substances in producing some of the uremic symptomatology has received increasing interest. Brain and peripheral nerve calcium levels have been found to be increased in uremic patients. The elevated calcium levels have been associated with impairment of neurologic function, EEG disturbances (98), and reduced motor nerve conduction velocities (98). The finding that the elevated calcium levels and altered neurologic function can be prevented by parathyroidectomy suggests that PTH is involved in the pathogenesis of these disturbances; however, the observation of increased calcium levels in peripheral nerves awaits confirmation.

Phosphorus represents another inorganic toxin. As stated, phosphorus retention probably is quite important in the pathogenesis of the secondary hyperparathyroidism state in uremic subjects (94). Phosphorus retention also is involved in the pathogenesis of metastatic calcification.

On the basis of strong biochemical and epidemiologic studies, it is now firmly established that aluminum intoxication is responsible for major neurologic and skeletal toxicity in uremic patients (99,100). Although aluminum intoxication initially was felt to result only from aluminum-contaminated dialysate, it is now apparent that toxicity can also result from the orally administered, aluminum-containing phosphate-binding gels commonly given to uremic patients. Aluminum-induced neurologic toxicity is characterized by a distinctive speech disturbance, myoclonus, seizures, and dementia. It is progressive, with death usually occurring 6 to 8 months after the onset of the first symptoms (99). The bone disease associated with aluminum intoxication is fracturing osteomalacia, which is resistant to treatment with vitamin D analogs (100). Studies suggest that both encephalopathy and osteomalacia can be cured by chelation of aluminum with deferoxamine. A microcytic hypochromic anemia also attributed to aluminum intoxication has been found to improve following deferoxamine treatment. Thus, aluminum-containing phosphate-binding gels are not routinely used for the management of hyperphosphatemia.

Although zinc deficiency has been implicated as the cause of impotence and anorexia in uremic patients, zinc replacement has given conflicting results, with some investigators finding improvement in potency, smell, taste, and appetite, whereas others find no effect. There is little evidence that other trace element alterations are responsible for any additional symptomatology found in uremic patients.

Thus, it appears that a variety of toxins are responsible for the array of clinical signs and symptoms of the uremic state and that a number of different pathogenetic mechanisms are involved. However, only a relatively small number of toxins and mechanisms have been identified or defined to explain the wide spectrum of uremic symptomatology.

Progression of Kidney Disease

It has been well documented that when a critical loss of nephron population occurs from a variety of different causes, the remaining renal tissue ultimately is lost, resulting in ESRD. The most classic example of this phenomenon in humans is oligomeganephronia (101). This is a congenital disease in which a child is born with a markedly reduced number of nephrons. The nephrons that are present are greatly hypertrophied. However, these hyperfunctioning nephrons undergo spontaneous destruction over the first few years of life, and the child usually dies of uremia by 3 or 4 years of age. Other examples supporting the concept that secondary or compensatory changes resulting from loss of renal mass may promote further injury are unilateral renal agenesis (102) and severe reflux nephropathy, both of which may develop glomerulosclerosis and progress to ESRD.

The compensatory mechanisms resulting from loss of kidney function that mediate this injury have not been totally defined, although altered intrarenal hemodynamics (103) and systemic hypertension (104) currently are felt to be of major importance. Studies have shown that when renal mass is surgically reduced, glomerular plasma flow, intraglomerular hydraulic pressure, and GFR of the remaining nephrons are markedly increased. These altered intrarenal hemodynamic events may lead to glomerular injury, resulting in glomerular sclerosis and functional deterioration. Any injury or disease that reduces nephron population appears to cause a compensatory afferent arteriolar dilatation, which allows the glomerular capillary bed to be exposed to increased hydraulic pressure with resulting injury. This is supported by the fact that hypertension is especially injurious to the glomeruli of a diseased kidney and that treatment of hypertension markedly reduces the rate and severity of glomerular injury in kidney diseases such as diabetic glomerulosclerosis and experimental glomerulonephritis. The evidence for the harmful effects of altered intrarenal hemodynamics on the diseased kidney is substantial. However, other secondary or compensatory changes, such as compensatory glomerular hypertrophy, may result in glomerular injury (Table 11.8). Similarly, increased intrarenal

TABLE 11.8 SECONDARY FACTORS LEADING TO THE PROGRESSION

Intraglomerular hypertension and glomerular hypertrophy
Proteinuria
Tubulointerstitial disease
Hyperlipidemia
Phosphate retention
Metabolic acidosis
Iron toxicity
Uremic tonxins
Increased prostanoid metabolism

energy requirement (105–108), renal parenchymal calcification, or tubule fluid iron also may be important in promoting tubulointerstitial injury in a diseased kidney (109,110).

Reversible Factors Compromising Kidney Function

Kidney function in chronically diseased kidneys can be further compromised by a number of potentially reversible factors (Table 11.9).

VOLUME DEPLETION

The most common reversible factor that can cause rapid deterioration of kidney function is depletion of the extracellular fluid (ECF) volume. If ECF volume depletion develops in a patient who already has compromised kidney function, a vicious cycle of events may ensue. The diminished kidney function that accompanies ECF volume depletion may cause worsening of the azotemic state. With the increased azotemia, nausea and vomiting may occur, leading to more volume depletion, further compromising GFR, and intensifying the uremia state, thus repeating the cycle. The diagnosis of severe volume depletion usually is obvious, because the patient will demonstrate tachycardia, postural hypotension, a dry furrowed tongue, and loss of skin elasticity. At an earlier stage of volume depletion, however, physical findings may be minimal. A history of overzealous treatment with potent diuretic agents or stringent salt restriction may suggest the diagnosis of modest volume depletion in patients with chronic kidney disease who have had recent deterioration of kidney function. It is frequently necessary to treat the patient with salt supplementation to determine whether kidney function will improve. A weight gain of 1 to 3 kg generally constitutes a reasonable indication of ECF volume expansion.

INFECTION AND OBSTRUCTION

Because many urinary tract infections are asymptomatic, a urine culture should be obtained on the initial evaluation of patients with chronic kidney disease. To prevent the introduction of a bacterial infection, instrumentation and indwelling catheterization of the urinary tract also are best avoided in such patients. Another potentially reversible cause of kidney disease is urinary tract obstruction. Obstruction can be excluded with about 95% confidence by performing ultrasound studies; therefore, retrograde pyelograms are seldom necessary, even when the patient has severely compromised kidney function. Ultrasound also gives valuable information with regard to the presence of two kidneys as well as kidney size. A postvoid residual urine as assessed by a straight catheterization after maximal voiding effort allows exclusion of important bladder–neck obstruction (>50 mL of residual urine). A flat-plate radiograph of the abdomen with nephrotomograms can also help establish kidney size and exclude the presence of radiopaque calculi.

TABLE 11.9 REVERSIBLE FACTORS RESPONSIBLE FOR RENAL FUNCTION DETERIORATION

Infection
Urinary tract obstruction
Extracellular fluid volume depletion
Nephrotoxic agents
Congestive heart failure
Hypertension
Pericardial tamponade
Hypercalcemia
Hyperuricemia >15–20 mg/dL
Hypokalemia

NEPHROTOXIC AGENTS

Nephrotoxic agents are another potential cause of reversible acute kidney injury. The most common are the antimicrobials and antitumor agents, including aminoglycosides, colistin, amphotericin, gallium, and cisplatin. An additional group of agents that can further compromise kidney function in patients with chronic kidney disease is radiocontrast media. Predisposing factors to contrast media-induced kidney injury include diabetes mellitus, advanced age, volume depletion, other nephrotoxic agents such as aminoglycosides, and preexisting kidney disease. Although the use of these agents in patients with chronic kidney disease is not contraindicated, they should be used with the consideration that they can cause permanent as well as reversible changes in kidney function. Because toxicity is somewhat dose dependent, the smallest dose consistent with obtaining an adequate study should be administered. In addition, the patient's volume status should be optimized with saline at the time of the contrast media administration (111).

PHARMACOLOGIC REDUCTION IN FUNCTION

Recently, two other drug classes, ACE inhibitors and cyclooxygenase inhibitors (112,113), have been shown to decrease kidney function acutely and reversibly in patients with underlying kidney disease. NSAIDs cause this effect by inhibiting renal prostaglandins and their vasodilatory effect, which causes a reduction in renal blood flow and GFR. The ACE inhibitors exert their effect by inhibiting angiotensin II constriction of the glomerular efferent arteriole. This causes a reduction in filtration pressure and, in turn, GFR. The effects of these agents on GFR are most commonly seen when renal arterial flow is reduced as a consequence of volume depletion, congestive heart failure, cirrhosis, bilateral renal artery stenosis, where filtration pressure is largely being maintained by angiotensin II–induced efferent arteriolar constriction. The effects of both the cyclooxygenase inhibitors and converting enzyme inhibitors on reducing GFR are rapidly reversed by discontinuing their administration. Therefore, when indicated the use of these drugs in patients with chronic kidney disease is not universally contraindicated.

CARDIOVASCULAR EFFECTS

Congestive heart failure in the uremic patient can result from a variety of causes, such as atherosclerosis, hypertension, and fluid overload. Treatment of congestive heart failure may improve kidney function. Blood pressure should be normalized by fluid removal, antihypertensive agents, or both. Diuresis usually can be accomplished with large doses of furosemide; however, when kidney disease is severe, dialysis may be indicated to remove the excess body fluid. Digoxin dosage has to be modified in patients with compromised kidney function because digoxin is largely excreted by the kidney.

The possibility of uremic pericarditis with associated pericardial effusion and tamponade should be considered in patients with far-advanced kidney disease. The clinical features of this diagnosis consist of increased jugular venous pulsations with a paradoxical inspiratory accentuation (Kussmaul sign), pulsus paradoxus, and a reduction in systemic blood pressure and pulse pressure. A pericardial friction rub may or may not be present. The paradoxical pulse may not be present with an extremely severe cardiac tamponade, and the only finding may be a reduction in blood and pulse pressures. The diagnosis is easily confirmed by ultrasound or blood-pool scanning. Pericardiocentesis may be lifesaving; in addition, by relieving the tamponade, it may improve cardiac output and kidney function. Finally, treatment of severe hypercalcemia, hypokalemia, and hyperuricemia also may lead to improvement in kidney function.

Decreasing Rate of Functional Deterioration

DIABETIC RENAL DISEASE

Diabetic nephropathy is characterized by persistent albuminuria (>300 mg/24 hours), a raised arterial blood pressure, and a relentless decline in GFR (114). Diabetic nephropathy rarely develops before 10 years after the onset of disease in type 1 diabetes, whereas ~3% of newly diagnosed type 2 diabetes patients have overt nephropathy (8). Nephropathy owing to type 2 diabetes accounts for the increasing number of patients with kidney failure in the past decade. Several factors have been identified that might either prevent the development of diabetic renal disease or slow its progression to ESRD.

Metabolic Control

A multicenter study involving 1,441 patients with type 1 diabetes showed that intensive insulin therapy delayed the onset and slowed the progression of diabetic retinopathy, nephropathy, and neuropathy (115). In this Diabetes Control and Complications Trial (DCCT), intensive therapy reduced the occurrence of microalbuminuria by 39% and that of overt albuminuria by 54%. In patients with type 2 diabetes, the UK Prospective Diabetes Study (UKPDS) reported that intensive blood glucose control decreases the risk of microvascular complications, but not macrovascular disease (116). In this study, 3,867 newly diagnosed patients with type 2 diabetes were randomly assigned to intensive treatment with sulfonylureas or insulin, or conventional management with diet. After 12 years of follow-up, there is a decreased rate of doubling serum creatinine with tight blood glucose control.

Further support for the beneficial effect of tight blood glucose control is that transplantation of a kidney in conjunction with a pancreas in patients with ESRD from diabetes has been found to prevent mesangial expansion and thickening of the basement membrane in the transplanted kidney (117,118). These glomerular changes are commonly observed when the kidney alone is transplanted without a pancreas into diabetic patients. As expected, more advanced renal diabetic lesions are not reversible. This raises the possibility of using islet cell transplantation in type 1 diabetes in the absence of diabetic nephropathy (119,120).

Renin–Angiotensin System and Blood Pressure Control

In addition to glycemic control, there also is considerable epidemiologic evidence, suggesting that hypertension plays a significant role in the development and progression of diabetic nephropathy. The long-term antihypertensive treatment in reducing albuminuria and slowing the rate of decline in GFR from 15 to 6 mL/yr in male type 1 diabetic patients with overt nephropathy was first described by Mogensen (121). Parving et al. (122) confirmed these observations and demonstrated that early aggressive antihypertensive treatment with metoprolol, furosemide, and hydralazine reduces albuminuria and the decline in GFR, as well as postponing ESRD in young male and female type 1 diabetic patients with nephropathy. The critical role of the renin–angiotensin system in addition to blood pressure control in slowing the progression of kidney diseases was examined in a multicenter study involving over 400 patients with type 1 diabetes using captopril (123). The study demonstrated that the use of ACE inhibitor protected against deterioration of kidney function independent of blood pressure control. Thus, it is suggested that ACE inhibitors are protective not only as a consequence of blood pressure control but probably more importantly because of their intrarenal effects on decreasing efferent arteriolar constriction, glomerular hydraulic pressure, and reducing proteinuria.

Similar results were also observed with studies in type 2 diabetic patients. The Appropriate Blood Pressure Control in Diabetes trial (ABCD) demonstrated an advantage of an ACE inhibitor over a long-acting calcium channel antagonist with regard to the incidence of myocardial infarction (124–127). The ABCD trial was a prospective randomized study evaluating the effects of intensive diastolic blood pressure control on the progression of diabetic vascular complications. Two groups were studied separately, a normotensive type 2 diabetic population (diastolic blood pressure between 80 and 90 mm Hg) and a hypertensive type 2 diabetic population (diastolic blood pressure $\geq$90 mm Hg). In the hypertensive cohort, at comparable blood pressure, cholesterol, glycohemoglobin levels, myocardial infarctions were decreased with ACE inhibition versus calcium channel blockers as initial therapy. Blood pressure control, either at moderate (mean-138/86 mm Hg) or intensive (mean-132/78 mm Hg) level stabilized kidney function in normoalbuminuric and microalbuminuric patients. Patients with overt diabetic nephropathy however averaged 5 mL/min/1.73 m^2/yr decline, thus they may avoid ESRD until their late seventies. Intensive versus moderate blood pressure control decreased all-cause mortality. In the normotensive cohort, intensive (mean-128/75 mm Hg) and moderate (mean-137/81 mm Hg) blood pressure control stabilized creatinine clearance in normoalbuminuric and microalbuminuric patients. However, there was also 5 mL/min/1.73 m^2/yr decline in creatinine clearance in patients with overt albuminuria. The intensive blood pressure control group also showed an advantage in slowing the progression of normoalbuminuria to mircroalbuminuria, decreasing the progression of diabetic retinopathy, and decreasing the incidence of strokes. Thus, intervention is most effective before overt albuminuria (7,300 mg/24 h) in type 2 diabetes.

The UKPDS study also demonstrated that more tight control of blood pressure decreased stroke, diabetic-related death and microvascular complications including retinopathy and nephropathy (128). A substudy of the Heart Outcome Prevention Evaluation Study, known as MICRO-HOPE, found that ACE inhibition with ramipril provided protection against cardiovascular events and attenuated the increase in proteinuria in diabetic subjects with microalbuminuria (129). Moreover, an analysis by Golan et al. concluded that an ACE inhibitor would be cost effective if it were prescribed for all middle aged patients with type 2 diabetes, irrespective of their base line kidney function (130).

The use of angiotensin-receptor blockers were recently examined in type 2 diabetic patients. Parving et al. (131) used irbesartan in patients with type 2 diabetes and hypertension who had normal GFR, but early kidney damage as manifested by microalbuminuria. The drug was associated with lower levels of microalbuminuria than the placebo. The GFR fell slightly initially, probably because of hemodynamic action of the angiotensin-receptor blocker, but the long-term trend did not differ among the groups. The diminution of albuminuria indicates potential protection from ongoing kidney damage that would translate into preservation of the GFR in the long term. Two other studies, by Brenner et al. (132) and Lewis et al. (133), also used angiotensin-receptor blockers losartan and irbesartan, respectively, to study type 2 diabetic patients with established diabetic nephropathy. In these patients, the use of these drugs resulted in a decrease in the combined endpoint of doubling serum creatinine, progression to ESRD and death in patients receiving the angiotensin-receptor blockers. In both studies, the benefits could not be explained by the effects of the drugs on blood pressure. In both type 1 and 2 diabetic patients, drugs that block the renin–angiotensin–aldosterone system appear to decrease glomerular capillary pressure, reduce fibrogenesis, and attenuate the proliferative actions of angiotensin and aldosterone (134) and thus slowing the progression of chronic kidney disease.

PROTEINURIC KIDNEY DISEASE

In proteinuric kidney disease, evidence is accumulating that suggests that any means of reducing urinary protein excretion (e.g., dietary protein restriction and ACE inhibitors) may exert a protective effect on kidney function. However, a large multicenter trial carried out in 840 patients with chronic kidney disease showed that a very low-protein diet had a minimal effect on slowing the progress of kidney function deterioration (135). In view of this study as well as poor patient acceptance, dietary protein restriction does not appear to be a feasible or effective means of treating patients with chronic kidney disease because of the potential for inducing protein malnutrition and the expense of dietary management and amino acid supplementation. However, there is increasing evidence that ACE inhibitors are effective not only in diabetic kidney disease but also in any proteinuric renal disease (136,137). Furthermore, results from the Modification of Diet in Renal Disease (MDRD) (135) and a ramipril trial (138) are compatible with the importance of the initial antiproteinuric response to antihypertensive therapy. In the MDRD study, for each 1 g/day reduction in protein excretion in the first 4 months, the rate of decline in GFR fell by 0.9 to 1.3 mL/min/yr. The fall in proteinuria was related to the blood pressure, being more prominent in those with more aggressive blood pressure control. In the ramipril trial, the rate of decline in GFR correlated inversely with the degree of proteinuria reduction among patients excreting >3 g protein/day. However, there are studies in which these ACE inhibitors have decreased proteinuria and yet worsened kidney function. Although calcium channel blockers in general do not decrease proteinuria to the degree of ACE inhibitors, some studies using animals have shown protective and additive effects on proteinuria with ACE inhibitors and nondihydropyridine calcium channel blockers (139–141). ACE inhibitors have only been shown to have a protective effect in proteinuric kidney disease. Otherwise, any protection exerted in nonproteinuric kidney disease is probably only a result of blood pressure control. Studies estimate that 10% to 15% of patients may not tolerate these drugs because of their causing chronic coughing or hyperkalemia. To avoid the side effect of coughing, an angiotensin receptor blocker can be used instead. The optimal antiproteinuric effect with therapy is not clear. A target reduction of at least 30% to 40% from baseline urinary protein levels has been recommended because this response appears to correlate with a lowering of intraglomerular pressure in experimental settings.

HYPERTENSION

Increasing evidence also suggests that the control of hypertension can have a major effect on reducing the progression of chronic kidney disease in patients with essential hypertension as well as primary kidney disease. African Americans are especially at risk of ESRD from hypertension (14–17). Initial studies showed that patients with chronic kidney disease and a diastolic pressure <90 mm Hg had better preservation of GFR than hypertensive patients. However, these uncontrolled observations alone do not exclude the possibility that patients with normal blood pressure or easily controlled hypertension have less severe underlying disease. Subsequent clinical trials have confirmed the benefit of antihypertensive therapy, particularly with ACE inhibitors, in patients with nondiabetic chronic kidney disease. Therefore, hypertension should be aggressively controlled in most patients by virtually any agent(s) shown to be effective. The possible exception is patients with proteinuric kidney disease, for whom ACE inhibitors may be the drug of choice for management of hypertension. However, the MDRD trial (135) did not address the potential preferential benefit of ACE inhibitors. This issue has now been addressed in trials involving ramipril (138) and benazepril (142). The later study consisted of almost 600 patients with a variety of chronic kidney diseases. The patients were already in reasonable blood pressure control on a variety of different medications and then were randomized to a benazepril or placebo. Benazepril produced a greater reduction in blood pressure (3.5 to 5.0 versus 0.2 mm Hg reduction in diastolic pressure) than placebo and was associated with 25% reduction in protein excretion. Progression to a primary end point (defined as doubling of the plasma creatinine concentration or progression to dialysis) occurred in 31 of 300 patients treated with benazepril versus 57 of 283 in the placebo group. The risk reduction was 53% in the entire group, 71% in those with a baseline creatinine clearance >45 mL/min/1.73 m^2, and 46% in those with a baseline creatinine clearance <45 mL/min/1.73 m^2. There was clear benefit in patients with chronic glomerular diseases and diabetic nephropathy. A more recent study suggested that there is a lower rate of loss of GFR in patients with essential hypertension who are treated with an ACE inhibitor compared to a β-blocker despite equivalent degrees of blood pressure control. A benefit also was noted in a report from the Ramipril Efficacy in Nephropathy (REIN) trial (138) in which patients with nondiabetic chronic kidney diseases were randomized to ramipril or placebo plus other antihypertensive therapy to attain a diastolic pressure <90 mm Hg. The trial was terminated prematurely among patients excreting >3 g protein/day because of a significant benefit with ACE inhibition in ameliorating the rate of decline of kidney function (0.53 vs 0.88 mL/min/mo for placebo). In a follow-up study of those initially enrolled in the ramipril trial (143,144), the benefits with ramipril continued over time among patients excreting >3 g protein/day. The mean rate of decline of the GFR decreased from 0.44 to 0.10 mL/min/1.73 m^2 for patients originally randomized to ramipril, and from 0.81 to 0.14 mL/min/1.73 m^2 for those not originally given ramipril. Benefits with ramipril also appear to extend to those with lesser degrees of proteinuria. However, the original and follow-up ramipril studies strongly suggest that patients who particularly benefit are those with prominent proteinuria, a finding similar to that noted in the MDRD trial. Additional evidence in support of a preferential benefit with ACE inhibitors has come from two metaanalyses with nondiabetic patients (145,146). Strict control of the blood pressure is beneficial in slowing the rate of progression of nondiabetic chronic kidney disease. ACE inhibitors appear to be more protective than other antihypertensive drugs in chronic glomerular diseases and patients excreting >1 g protein/day. However, hypertensive African Americans' blood pressure responds better to monotherapy with a calcium channel blocker than an ACE inhibitor. Despite this observation, an interim analysis of the African-American Study of Kidney Disease and Hypertension (AASK) (147,148) found that amlodipine was less effective than ramipril in slowing progression of renal disease in African Americans with hypertensive kidney disease. The results of these studies are summarized in Table 11.10.

Overall, the optimal blood pressure in hypertensive patients has not been clearly identified yet. However, the ABCD trial has demonstrated the importance of intensive blood pressure control (124–126). The rate of loss of GFR appears to be more rapid when the mean arterial pressure remains at or >100 mm Hg (which reflects a diastolic pressure of 80 to 85 mm Hg in the absence of systolic hypertension). Thus, a diastolic pressure goal of 80 mm Hg (mean arterial pressure 98 mm Hg in the absence of systolic hypertension) appears reasonable in previously hypertensive patients excreting 1 to 2 g protein/day. A lower diastolic pressure of 75 mm Hg (mean arterial pressure 92 mm Hg) may be appropriate in those patients who are normotensive with heavy proteinuria.

TABLE 11.10 ANTIHYPERTENSIVE THERAPY AND PROGRESSION OF RENAL FAILURE

Trial name	Measures	Results
MDRD, 1994	Aggressive control versus usual BP control in patients with chronic renal diseases	The higher the proteinuria (>3, 1–3, and <1 g/d) the faster the progression of nephropathy and more effective the blood pressure (BP) control became. Blacks may benefit more.
Maschio et al., 1996	Benazepril versus placebo in patients with chronic renal diseases	Better BP control, less proteinuria, slower progression rate of nephropathy with benazepril, especially in patients with glomerular diseases and diabetic nephropathy. Inconclusive results in hypertensive nephrosclerosis. No observed benefit in ADPKD patients.
REIN, 1997 and follow-up, 1998, 1999	Ramipril versus placebo in nondiabetic patients with chronic renal diseases	Ramipril reduced the progression of nephropathy in patients with proteinuria >3 g/day. Sufficient treatment (>3 y) eliminated the need for dialysis. Some patients even showed improved glomerular filtration rate.
UKPDS, 1998	Tight BP control (<150/85 mm Hg) versus moderate control (<180/105 mm Hg) in hypertensive type II diabetes	Tight BP control decreased the incidence of stroke, diabetic related-death, and microvascular complications, including retinopathy and nephropathy.
AASK, 2000	Ramipril versus amlodipine in African Americans with hypertensive renal diseases	Ramipril was more effective than amlodipine in slowing progression of nephropathy in blacks.
Metaanalysis, 2001	ACE inhibitors in nondiabetic nephropathy patients	Patients with angiotensin-converting enzyme (ACE) inhibitor treatment were less likely to develop end-stage renal disease and have slower rate of progression of renal function.
Parving et al., 2001	Irbesartan versus placebo in patients with type II diabetic nephropathy and microalbuminuria	Irbesartan slowed the rate of progression to diabetic nephropathy.
Lewis et al., 2001	Irbesartan versus placebo in patients with nephropathy owing to type II diabetes	Irbesartan protected against the progression of nephrology.
RENAAL, 2001	Losartan versus placebo in patients with nephrology owing to type II diabetes	Less proteinuria and slower progression of nephropathy with losartan treatment
ABCD, 1998–2002	Hypertensive type II diabetic patients	Myocardial infarctions decreased with ACE inhibitors versus calcium channel blockers. BP control stabilized or decreased the rate of decline in renal function. Intensive versus moderate BP control decreased all-cause mortality.
ABCD, 1998–2002	Normotensive type II diabetic patients	BP control stabilized or decreased the rate of decline in renal function. Intensive BP versus moderate control slows progression from normoalbuminuria to microalbuminuria and the progression of diabetic retinopathy and decreased strokes.

AASK, African-American Study of Kidney Disease and Hypertension; ABCD, Appropriate Blood Pressure Control in Diabetes Trial; MDRD, Modification of Diet in Renal Disease; REIN, Ramipril Efficacy in Nephropathy; RENNAL, Reduction of Endpoints in NIDDM with the Angiotensin II Antagonist Losartan; UKPDS, UK Prospective Diabetes Study.

Management of the Uremic State

FLUID AND ELECTROLYTES

Because of the accompanying decrease in tubule processing of the filtrate associated with progressive functional loss, a greater fraction of the filtrate is excreted as urine. As a result, the patient with chronic kidney disease is able to maintain fluid and major elemental balance throughout the course of renal functional deterioration until GFR has fallen to a critical value of <5% of normal. By maintaining a urine volume of ~2 L/day, the patient with advanced kidney disease is able to excrete the normal fluid (2 L), sodium (140 mEq), potassium (70 mEq), osmotic load (600 mOsm), and nitrogen (12 g, equivalent to 72 g protein) present in the average American diet without excreting a concentrated or dilute urine. Therefore, dietary restrictions, which may cause protein–calorie malnutrition, are not required in the majority of uremic patients throughout the entire course of chronic kidney disease up to and including end-stage disease (135). Similarly, dietary sodium and potassium restriction is not required in the majority of patients with chronic kidney disease and actually can be harmful, as described. A high-potassium diet, potassium-sparing diuretics, and high-sodium diet are contraindicated in advanced kidney disease because of hyperkalemia, hypertension, and fluid overload, respectively.

The mild acidosis present in the majority of patients with advanced chronic kidney disease can be treated readily with the administration of 12 mEq (1 g) of sodium bicarbonate given thrice daily. This amount of bicarbonate has minimal effect on blood pressure and ECF volume (149); however, not all nephrologists believe there is a need to treat the mild acidosis of chronic kidney disease.

Chronic kidney disease causes edema by two distinct mechanisms: (a) hypoalbuminemia (serum albumin <2.5 g/dL) secondary to urinary protein loss and (b) when the ingestion of sodium and water exceeds the ability of the diseased kidney to eliminate the ingested loads. In general, development of edema from the latter cause is a consequence of advanced kidney disease and marked reduction in GFR. This frequently necessitates institution of treatment for ESRD (i.e., dialysis or transplantation) because sodium and water restriction with loop diuretics generally is ineffective.

CALCIUM AND PHOSPHATE

Abnormalities in mineral metabolism are well established in chronic kidney disease. As kidney function declines, calcium levels decrease, and PTH and phosphorus levels increase. Numerous observational studies have shown a significant and independent association between elevated serum phosphorus levels and all-cause and cardiovascular mortality in patients with chronic kidney disease (150). Similar findings have been found in chronic kidney disease patients not requiring dialysis. In a study by Kestenbaum et al. (151) of 6,730 patients with chronic kidney disease, serum phosphorus was significantly and independently associated with mortality. For each 1 mg/dL increase in serum phosphorus, the risk for death increased by 23%. Furthermore, after adjustment, serum phosphorus levels >3.5 mg/dL were associated with a significantly increased risk of death and the risk increased linearly with each subsequent 0.5 mg/dL increase in serum phosphorus levels. The mechanism by which serum phosphorus contributes to cardiovascular disease is unclear. It may involve the development of vascular calcification, since serum phosphorus levels have been associated with the presence and extent of coronary artery and aortic calcification in dialysis patients. Elevated serum phosphorus may also contribute to cardiovascular disease by increasing PTH levels. Increased PTH has been associated with left ventricular hypertrophy and an increased risk for cardiovascular and all-cause mortality in dialysis patients. Hence, serum phosphorus appears to be an important predictor of cardiovascular disease. Successful clinical management of hyperphosphatemia consists of several measures including a low-phosphorus diet, adequate dialysis, and effective phosphate-binding therapy. Phosphorus restriction should begin when the GFR is <60 to 70 mg/min. However, it is difficult to balance dietary phosphate restrictions against the need for adequate protein intake (152–155). Low serum albumin has been shown to be a frequent cause of morbidity and mortality. Dialysis does not generally provide adequate phosphorus control because it is difficult to remove significant amount of the total body phosphorus that is in the intracellular compartment. Thus, almost all dialysis patients rely on phosphate binders taken with meals to reduce the absorption of dietary phosphorus and prevent hyperphosphatemia. Those agents include aluminum-, calcium-, other metal-, and other non–metal-based preparations, all of which have limitations. Although extremely efficient, aluminum-containing binders can cause toxic effects such as aluminum bone disease (osteomalacia), dementia, myopathy, and anemia (156–158). This has led to the alternative use of calcium salts. Calcium carbonate and calcium acetate are the most efficacious therapies. Calcium citrate should be avoided because it can increase intestinal absorption of aluminum. Currently, calcium carbonate and calcium acetate are the most widely used phosphate binders (159). To improve their effectiveness and decrease the chance of causing hypercalcemia, these drugs (1 to 2 g) should be given with meals. However, calcium-containing phosphate binders can cause an excess total body calcium load because of significant intestinal calcium absorption. There has been interest in developing calcium- and aluminum-free binders such as magnesium carbonate. A lower dialysate magnesium concentration may be needed to prevent hypermagnesemia. Metal-free binders have also been developed such as sevelamer (RenaGel) and lanthanum. Sevelamer is a nonabsorbable agent that contains neither calcium nor aluminum. This drug is a cationic polymer that binds phosphate through ion exchange. Several studies have reported that this agent is an effective phosphate binder without affecting plasma calcium. It also has the advantage of lowering total cholesterol concentration. Gastrointestinal side effects may limit its use in some patients. Because of its much higher cost, it is primarily reserved for patients with hypercalcemia (160–162).

ANEMIA

Anemia is common in patients with chronic kidney disease. It is well established that hemodynamic changes induced by anemia can precipitate high-output congestive heart failure and ischemic cardiac events (163,164). If treatment is required before ESRD because of associated conditions such as generalized weakness, cardiac or pulmonary disease, EPO, although quite expensive, is effective (165). Before EPO administration, iron stores should be documented to be adequate by the measurement of serum ferritin, iron, and total iron-binding capacity. The initial dosage of EPO should be 75 to 100 U/kg/wk. An adequate response to EPO therapy will result in an increased reticulocyte count within 1 week and rise in hematocrit after 2 to 4 weeks. A potential complication of increasing the hematocrit with EPO is hypertension, which can have an adverse effect on kidney function.

BLEEDING DIATHESIS

The bleeding diathesis present in uremia usually requires no treatment unless the patient requires surgery or experiences a traumatic event. Correction of anemia with either transfusion of packed cells or administration of recombinant human EPO may improve hemostasis. The minimum target hemoglobin should be ~10 g/dL. Fifty to seventy-five percent of uremic patients have improvement or correction of the bleeding time with dDAVP. The usual dosage is 0.3 μg/kg given intravenously, subcutaneously, or intranasally (166–168). It is effective within 1 to 2 hours, with its effect persisting for ~4 hours. Tachyphylaxis can occur within 24 to 48 hours. Conjugated estrogens improve bleeding time in ~80% of the patients. The usual dosage is 0.6 mg/kg daily for 5 consecutive days. The initial effect on bleeding time occurs within 6 hours with peak response in 5 to 7 days, which persists for up to 14 days (169–171). Cryoprecipitate also is effective in controlling the uremic bleeding diathesis. The usual infusion of cryoprecipitate is 10 bags. It affects the bleeding time within 1 hour and persists for 18 hours. Platelet infusions also are effective but are recommended only for life-threatening emergencies.

MISCELLANEOUS DISTURBANCES

In general, other disturbances that occur with chronic kidney disease such as mild glucose intolerance, hypertriglyceridemia, and mild elevation of uric acid require no treatment. However, because of the inability of renal excretion of large loads of magnesium, magnesium-containing antacids, and laxatives should be largely avoided. Similarly, as stated previously, potassium supplementation, even with diuretic administration, potassium sparing diuretics, and salt substitutes, should be avoided unless hypokalemia is present.

Preparation for and Initiation of End-Stage Renal Disease Therapy

Chronic kidney disease progresses at a variable rate because of differences in the clinical course of the underlying diseases and availability of different potential therapeutic interventions. A number of factors have been proposed as possible indicators before development of uremic symptoms (172–176). It is important to note that plasma creatinine reflects not only kidney function but also muscle mass (177,178). Thus, a patient with reduced muscle mass owing to malnutrition has a lower than usual plasma creatinine level and may need to be dialyzed (179,180). It is difficult to assign a certain level of BUN, serum creatinine, or GFR to the need to start dialysis. Nevertheless, the Health Care Financing Administration in the United States has assigned levels of serum creatinine and creatinine clearance to quantify for reimbursement from Medicare for patients receiving dialysis. Serum creatinine must be ≥8.0 mg/dL and the GFR must be ≤10 to 20 mL/min/1.73 m². Symptomatic uremia usually develops when serum creatinine reaches 8 to 10 mg/dL and BUN is >100 mg/dL. Classically, the first manifestations are gastrointestinal symptoms of nausea, anorexia, and possibly vomiting. However, other symptoms and findings of advanced uremia, such as intractable itching, malnutrition, volume overload, protracted hyperkalemia, and impairment of cognitive function represent additional indications for considering ESRD treatment. Serositis (pericarditis and pleuritis) does not respond to conservative measures but usually resolves following initiation of dialysis or transplantation. In addition, uremic motor neuropathy is a progressive and debilitating condition in the uremic state. Its progression can be prevented by adequate dialysis or transplantation.

Data from the U.S. Renal Data System have shown that the majority of patients who began renal replacement therapy, either by dialysis or transplantation, have advanced complications of uremia such as malnutrition, severe anemia, left ventricular hypertrophy, or congestive heart failure (181,182). This suggests the drawbacks of delaying renal replacement therapy for ESRD and possibly inadequate care during the pre-ESRD period (183,184). The processes contributing to cardiovascular disease begin early during the period of kidney disease. Some factors such as hypertension, dyslipidemia, anemia, and hyperparathyroidism are amenable to early intervention.

Consequently, patients with chronic kidney disease should be referred to nephrologists early in the course of their disease. Furthermore, it is important to counsel patients in preparation for optimal renal replacement therapy and to prevent the morbidity and mortality associated with chronic kidney disease. Current clinical practice guidelines (Dialysis Outcomes Quality Initiative Guidelines, NKF-DOQI) in the United States and Canada recommend earlier initiation of dialysis before the overt symptoms and signs of uremia.

REFERENCES

1. Smith HW. *Principles of Renal Physiology.* New York: Oxford University Press, 1956.
2. Brandstrom E, Grzegorczyk A, Jacobsson L, et al. GFR measurement with iohexol and 51Cr-EDTA. A comparison of the two favoured GFR markers in Europe. *Nephrol Dial Transplant.* 1998; 13(5): 1176–1182.
3. Rahn KH, Heidenreich S, Bruckner D. How to assess glomerular function and damage in humans. *J Hypertens.* 1999; 17(3): 309–317.
4. Alleyne GAO, Millward DJ, Scullard GH. Total body potassium, muscle electrolytes, and glycogen in malnourished children. *J Pediatr.* 1970; 76: 75–81.
5. Cockcroft DW, Gault MH. Prediction of creatinine clearance from serum creatinine. *Nephron.* 1976; 16: 31–35.
6. Levey AS, Bosch JP, Lewis JB, et al. A more accurate method to estimate glomerular filtration rate from serum creatinine: a new prediction equation. *Ann Int Med.* 1999; 130: 461–470.
7. Jones CA, McQuillan GM, Kusek JW, et al. Serum creatinine levels in the US population: third National Health and Nutrition Examination Survey. *Am J Kidney Dis.* 1998; 32(6): 992–999.
8. Coresh J, Selvin LA, et al. Prevalence of chronic kidney disease in the United States. *JAMA.* 2007; 298: 2038–2047.
9. US Renal Data System. *USRDS 2008 Annual Report, National Institutes of Health, National Institute of Diabetes, and Digestive and Kidney Diseases.* Bethesda, MD: National Institutes of Health, 2008.
10. Chan L, Wang W, Kam I. Outcomes and complications in Renal Transplantation. In: Schrier RW, ed. *Diseases of the Kidney,* 7th ed. Philadelphia: Lippincott Williams & Wilkins; 2001: 2871–2938.
11. Cowie CC, Port FK, Wolfe RA, et al. Disparities in incidence of diabetic end-stage renal disease according to race and type of diabetes. *N Engl J Med.* 1998; 321: 1074–1079.
12. Klang MJ, Whelton PK, Randall BL, et al. End-stage renal disease in African-American and white men. 16-year MRFIT findings. *JAMA.* 1997; 277(16): 1293–1298.
13. Woods JW, Blythe WB, Huffines WD. Malignant hypertension and renal insufficiency. *N Engl J Med.* 1974; 291: 10–14.
14. Rostand SG, Brown G, Kirk KA, et al. Renal insufficiency in treated essential hypertension. *N Engl J Med.* 1989; 320: 684–688.
15. Rostand SG, Kirk KA, Rutsky EA, et al. Racial differences in the incidence of treatment for end-stage renal disease. *N Engl J Med.* 1982; 306: 1276–1279.
16. Mroczek WJ, Davidson M, Gavrilavich L, et al. The value of aggressive therapy in the hypertensive patient with azotemia. *Circulation.* 1969; 40: 893–904.

17. McPhaul JJ Jr. Hyperuricemia and urate excretion in chronic renal disease. *Metabolism.* 1968; 17: 430–438.

18. Emmerson BT. Chronic lead nephropathy. *Kidney Int.* 1973; 4(1): 1–5.

19. Kincaid-Smith P. Analgesic nephropathy. *Kidney Int.* 1978; 13: 1–8.

20. Talbott JH, Terplan KL. The kidney in gout. *Medicine (Baltimore).* 1990; 39: 405–462.

21. Berman LB, Schreiner GE, Feys J. The nephrotoxic lesion of ethylene glycol. *Ann Intern Med.* 1957; 46: 611–619.

22. Williams HE, Smith LH Jr. Disorders of oxalate metabolism. *Am J Med.* 1968; 45: 715–735.

23. Frascino JA, Vanamee P, Rosen PP. Renal oxalosis and azotemia after methoxyflurane anesthesia. *N Engl J Med.* 1970; 283: 676–679.

24. Stauffer JQ, Humphreys MH, Weir GJ. Acquired hyperoxaluria with regional enteritis after ileal resection. *Ann Intern Med.* 1973; 79: 383–391.

25. Britton DC, Thompson MH, Johnston ID, et al. Renal function following parathyroid surgery in primary hyperparathyroidism. *Lancet.* 1971; 2: 74–75.

26. Burnett CH, Commons RR, Albright F, et al. Hypercalcemia without hypercalciuria or hyperphosphatemia, calcinosis and renal insufficiency: syndrome following prolonged intake of milk and alkali. *N Engl J Med.* 1949; 240: 787–798.

27. Crutcher JC. Clinical manifestations and therapy of acute lead intoxication due to ingestion of illicitly distilled alcohol. *Ann Intern Med.* 1963; 59: 707–715.

28. Batuman V, Maesaka JK, Haddad B, et al. The role of lead in gout nephropathy. *N Engl J Med.* 1981; 304: 520–523.

29. Ui J. Pollution disasters in Japan. *Lakartidningen.* 1972; 69: 2789–2795.

30. Aperia A, Broberger O, Ericson NO, et al. Effect of vesicoureteric reflux on renal function in children with recurrent urinary infections. *Kidney Int.* 1976; 9: 418–423.

31. Smellie M, Edwards D, Hunter N, et al. Vesicoureteric reflux and renal scarring. *Kidney Int.* 1975; 8(suppl 4): S65–S72.

32. Assael BM, Guez S, Marra G, et al. Congenital reflux nephropathy: a follow-up of 108 cases diagnosed perinatally. *Br J Urol.* 1998; 82(2): 252–257.

33. Smellie JM, Tamminen-Mobius T, Olbing C, et al. Five-year study of medical or surgical treatment in children with severe reflux: radiological renal findings. *Pediatr Nephrol.* 1992; 6: 223–230.

34. Perkoff GT. The hereditary renal diseases. *N Engl J Med.* 1967; 277: 79–85.

35. Reeders ST, Zerres K, Gal A, et al. First prenatal diagnosis of autosomal dominant polycystic kidney disease using a DNA probe. *Lancet.* 1986; 2: 6–7.

36. Gabow PA. Autosomal dominant polycystic kidney disease. *N Engl J Med.* 1993; 329: 332.

37. Wilson PD. Polycystin: new aspects of structure, function, and regulation. *J Am Soc Nephrol.* 2001; 12: 834.

38. Martins D, Tareen N, Norris KC. The epidemiology of end-stage renal disease among African Americans. *Am J Med Sci.* 2002; 323(2): 65–71.

39. Pontier PJ, Patel TG. Racial differences in the prevalence and presentation of glomerular disease in adults. *Clin Nephrol.* 1994; 42: 79–84.

40. Solini A, Vestra MD, Saller A, et al. The angiotensin-converting enzyme DD genotype is associated with glomerulopathy lesions in type 2 diabetes. *Diabetes.* 2002; 51(1): 251–255.

41. Krolewski AS, Canessa M, Warram JH, et al. Predisposition to hypertension and susceptibility to renal disease in insulin-dependent diabetes mellitus. *N Engl J Med.* 1988; 318: 140–145.

42. Levy M, Gubler MC, Feingold J. (Contribution of genetics to knowledge and management of hereditary kidney diseases progressing to renal failure). *Arch Pediatr.* 2001; 8(10): 1086–1098.

43. Parvari R, Shnaider A, Basok A, et al. Clinical and genetic characterization of an autosomal dominant nephropathy. *Am J Med Genet.* 2001; 99(3): 204–209.

44. Peters DJ, Breuning MH. Autosomal dominant polycystic kidney disease: modification of disease progression. *Lancet.* 2001; 358(9291): 1439–1444.

45. Phakdeekitcharoen B, Watnik TJ, Germino GG. Mutation analysis of the entire replicated portion of PKD1 using genomic DNA samples. *J Am Soc Nephrol.* 2001; 12(5): 955–963.

46. van Essen GG, Rensma PL, de Zeeuw D, et al. Association between angiotensin-converting-enzyme gene polymorphism and failure of renoprotective therapy. *Lancet.* 1996; 347(8994): 94–95.

47. Yoshida H, Mitarai T, Kawamura T, et al. Role of the deletion of polymorphism of the angiotensin converting enzyme gene in the progression and therapeutic responsiveness of IgA nephropathy. *J Clin Invest.* 1995; 96(5): 2162–2169.

48. Krolewski AS, Canessa M, Warram JH, et al. Predisposition to hypertension and susceptibility to renal disease in insulin-dependent diabetes mellitus. *N Engl J Med.* 1988; 318: 140–145.

49. Bricker NS, Fine LG, Kaplan M, et al. "Magnification" phenomenon in chronic renal disease. *N Engl J Med.* 1978; 299: 1287–1293.

50. Stanbury SW, Mailer RF. Salt-wasting renal disease: metabolic observations on a patient with salt-losing nephritis. *Q J Med.* 1959; 28: 425–477.

51. Schrier RW, Regal EM. Influence of aldosterone on sodium, water, potassium metabolism in chronic renal disease. *Kidney Int.* 1972; 1: 156–168.

52. Hayes CP, McLeod MF, Robinson RR. An extrarenal mechanism for the maintenance of potassium balance in severe chronic renal failure. *Trans Assoc Am Phys.* 1967; 80: 207–216.

53. Schambelan M, Stockist JR, Biglieri EG. Isolated hypoaldosteronism in adults: a rennin-deficiency syndrome. *N Engl J Med.* 1972; 287: 573–578.

54. Battle DC, Arruda JAL, Kurtzman NA. Hyperkalemic distal renal tubular acidosis associated with obstruction. *N Engl J Med.* 1981; 304: 373–379.

55. Bricker NS, Slatopolsky E, Reiss E, et al. Calcium, phosphorus, and bone in renal disease and transplantation. *Arch Intern Med.* 1969; 123: 543–553.

56. Randall RE Jr, Chen MD, Spray CC, et al. Hypermagnesemia in renal failure: etiology and toxic manifestation. *Ann Intern Med.* 1964; 61: 73–88.

57. Seldin DW, Coleman AJ, Carter NW, et al. The effect of Na_2SO_4 on urinary acidification

in chronic renal disease. *J Lab Clin Med.* 1967; 69: 893–903.

58. Kazmi WH, Kausz AT, Khan S, et al. Anemia: an early complication of chronic renal insufficiency. *Am J Kidney Dis.* 2001; 38: 803–812.

59. Besarab A, Bolton WK, Browne JK, et al. The effects of normal as compared with low hematocrit values in patients with cardiac disease who are receiving hemodialysis and epoetin. *N Engl J Med.* 1998; 339: 584–590.

60. Levin A. Understanding recent haemoglobin trials in CKD: methods and lesson learned from CREATE and CHOIR. *Nephrol Dial Transplant.* 2007; 22: 309–312.

61. Castaidi PA, Rozenberg MC, Stewart JH. The bleeding disorder of uremia: a qualitative platelet defect. *Lancet.* 1966; 2: 66–69.

62. Eberst ME, Berkowitz LR. Hemostasis in renal disease: pathophysiology and management. *Am J Med.* 1994; 96: 168–179.

63. Alfrey AC, Goss JE, Ogden DA, et al. Uremic hemopericardium. *Am J Med.* 1968; 45: 391–400.

64. Schreiner GE, Maher JF. *Uremia: Biochemistry, Pathogenesis and Treatment.* Springfield, IL: Charles C Thomas, 1961.

65. Levitt MD, Rapoport M, Cooperband SR. The renal clearance of amylase in renal insufficiency, acute pancreatitis and macroamylasemia. *Ann Intern Med.* 1969; 71: 919–925.

66. Tyler HR. Neurologic disorders in renal failure. *Am J Med.* 1968; 44: 734–748.

67. Rees L, Rigden SPA, Ward GM, et al. Treatment of short stature by recombinant human growth hormone in children with renal disease. *Arch Dis Child.* 1990; 65: 856–862.

68. Dahl E, Nordal KP, Attramadal A, et al. Renal osteodystrophy in predialysis patients without stainable bone aluminum. *Acta Med Scand.* 1988; 224: 157–164.

69. Alfrey AC, Jenkins D, Groth CG, et al. Resolution of hyperparathyroidism, renal osteodystrophy and metastatic calcification after renal homotransplantations. *N Engl J Med.* 1968; 279: 1349–1356.

70. Sherrard DJ, Herez G, Pei Y, et al. The spectrum of bone disease in end-stage renal failure: an evolving disorder. *Kidney Int.* 1993; 43: 436–442.

71. Heaf J. Causes and consequences of adynamic bone disease. *Nephron.* 2001; 88(2): 97–106.

72. Slatopolsky E, Finch J, Clay P, et al. A novel mechanism for skeletal resistance in uremia. *Kidney Int.* 2000; 58(2): 753–761.

73. Massry SG, Coburn JW, Popovtzer MM, et al. Secondary hyperparathyroidism in chronic renal failure. The clinical spectrum in uremia, during hemodialysis, and after renal transplantation. *Arch Intern Med.* 1969; 124(4): 431–441.

74. Meema HE, Oreopoulus DG. Morphology, progression and regression of arterial and periarterial calcification in patients with end-stage renal disease. *Radiology.* 1986; 158: 671–677.

75. Giachelli CM, Jono S, Shioi A, et al. Vascular calcification and inorganic phosphate. *Am J Kidney Dis.* 2001; 38 (4 suppl 1): S34–S37.

76. Hiroshige K, Kuroiwa A. Uremic pruritus. *Int J Artif Organs.* 1996; 19(5): 265–267.

77. Chou FF, Ho JC, Huang SC, et al. A study on pruritus after parathyroidectomy for secondary hyperparathyroidism. *J Am Coll Surg.* 2000; 190(1): 65–70.

78. Hafner J, Keusch G, Wahl C, et al. Uremic small-artery disease with medial calcification and intimal hyperplasia (so-called calciphylaxis): a complication of chronic renal failure and benefit from parathyroidectomy. *J Am Acad Dermatol.* 1995; 33(6): 954–962.

79. Llach F. The evolving pattern of calciphylaxis: therapeutic considerations. *Nephrol Dial Transplant.* 2001; 16(3): 448–451.

80. Coates T, Kirkland GS, Dymock RB, et al. Cutaneous necrosis from calcific uremic arteriolopathy. *Am J Kidney Dis.* 1998; 32(3): 384–391.

81. Kang AS, McCarthy JT, Rowland C, et al. Is calciphylaxis best treated surgically or medically? *Surgery.* 2000; 128(6): 967–971; discussion 971–972.

82. Wilson WEC, Kirkpatrick CH, Talmadge DW. Suppression of immunologic responsiveness in uremia. *Ann Intern Med.* 1965; 62: 1–14.

83. London WT, Di Figlia M, Sutnick A, et al. An epidemic of interferon responses in lymphocytes from patients with uremia. *N Engl J Med.* 1969; 281: 571–578.

84. Sanders CV Jr, Luby JP, Sanford JP, et al. Suppression of interferon responses in lymphocytes from patients with uremia. *J Lab Clin Med.* 1971; 77: 768–776.

85. Manolagas SC, Hustmyer FG, Yu XP. Immunomodulating properties of 1,25-dihydroxyvitamin D_3. *Kidney Int.* 1990; 38(suppl 29): S9–S16.

86. Cerletty JM, Engoring NH. Azotemia and glucose intolerance. *Ann Intern Med.* 1967; 66: 1097–1108.

87. Strippoli GF, Craig JC. Sunset for statins after AURORA? *N Engl J Med.* 2009; 360(14): 1455–1457.

88. Olsen NS, Bassett JW. Blood levels of urea nitrogen, phenol, guanidine and creatinine in uremia. *Am J Med.* 1951; 10: 52–59.

89. Liveson JA, Gardner J, Bernstein MB. Tissue culture studies of possible uremic neurotoxins: myoinositol. *Kidney Int.* 1977; 12: 131–136.

90. Wathem R, Smith M, Keshaviah P, et al. Depressed in vitro aggregation of platelets of chronic hemodialysis patients (CHDP): a role for cyclic AMP. *Trans Am Soc Artif Intern Organs.* 1975; 21: 320–328.

91. Walser M, Coulter AW, Dighe S, et al. The effect of keto-analogs of essential amino acids in severe chronic uremia. *J Clin Invest.* 1973; 52: 678–690.

92. Alfrey AC. Beta$_2$-microglobulin amyloidosis. *AKF Neprhol Letter.* 1989; 6: 27–33.

93. Fraser DR, Kodicek E. Unique biosynthesis by kidney of a biologically active vitamin D metabolite. *Nature.* 1970; 228: 764–766.

94. Bricker NS. On the pathogenesis of the uremic state: an exposition of the "trade-off" hypothesis. *N Engl J Med.* 1972; 286: 1093–1099.

95. Massry SG. Parathyroid hormone as a uremic toxin. In: Massry SG, Glassock RS, eds. *Textbook of Nephrology.* Baltimore: Williams & Wilkins; 2001: 1221–1243.

96. Korkor AB. Reduced binding of (^{3}H) 1,25 dihydroxy vitamin D_3 in patients with renal failure. *N Engl J Med.* 1987; 316: 1573–1577.

97. Silver J, Naveh-Many T, Mayer H, et al. Regulation by vitamin D metabolites of parathyroid gene

transcription in vivo in the rat. *J Clin Invest.* 1986; 78: 1296–1301.

98. Goldstein DA, Chui LA, Massry SG. Effect of parathyroid hormone and uremia on peripheral nerve calcium and motor nerve conduction velocity. *J Clin Invest.* 1978; 62: 88–93.

99. Alfrey AC, LeGendre GR, Kaehny WD. The dialysis encephalopathy syndrome: possible aluminum intoxication. *N Engl J Med.* 1976; 294: 184–188.

100. Ott SM, Maloney NA, Coburn JW, et al. Bone aluminum in renal osteodystrophy: prevalence and relationship to response to 1,25-dihydroxy vitamin D. *N Engl J Med.* 1982; 307: 709–713.

101. Scheinman JL, Abelson HJ. Bilateral renal hypoplasia with oligonephroma. *J Pediatr.* 1970; 76: 389–397.

102. Kiprov DD, Colvin RB, McCluskey RT. Focal and segmental glomerulosclerosis and proteinuria associated with unilateral renal agenesis. *Lab Invest.* 1982; 46: 275–281.

103. Brenner BM, Meyer TW, Hostetter TH. Dietary protein intake and the progressive nature of kidney disease: the role of hemodynamically mediated glomerular injury in the pathogenesis of progressive glomerular sclerosis in aging, renal ablation, and intrinsic renal disease. *N Engl J Med.* 1982; 307: 652–659.

104. Meyer TW, Rennke HG. Progressive glomerular injury after limited renal infarction in the rat. *Am J Physiol.* 1988; 254: F856–F862.

105. Harris DC, Chan L, et al. Remnant kidney hypermetabolism and progression of chronic renal failure. *Am J Physiol.* 1988; 254(2 pt 2): F267–F276.

106. Schrier RW, Harris DC, et al. Tubular hypermetabolism as a factor in the progression of chronic renal failure. *Am J Kidney Dis.* 1988; 12(3): 243–249.

107. Schrier RW, Shapiro JI, et al. Increased nephron oxygen consumption: potential role in progression of chronic renal disease. *Am J Kidney Dis.* 1994; 23(2): 176–182.

108. Shapiro JI, Harris DC, et al. Attenuation of hypermetabolism in the remnant kidney by dietary phosphate restriction in the rat. *Am J Physiol.* 1990; 258(1 pt 2): F183–F188.

109. Alfrey A, Tomford RC. The pathogenesis of progressive renal failure: the case for tubulointerstitial factors. In: Narins RG, ed. *Controversies in Nephrology and Pathophysiology: The Pathogenesis of Progressive Renal Failure.* New York: Churchill Livingstone, 1984: 555.

110. Harris DC, Tay YC, et al. Mechanisms of iron-induced proximal tubule injury in rat remnant kidney. *Am J Physiol.* 1995; 269(2 pt 2): F218–F224.

111. Solomon R, Werner C, Mann D, et al. Effects of saline mannitol and furosemide to prevent decreases in renal function induced by radiocontrast agents. *N Engl J Med.* 1994; 331: 1416–1420.

112. Hricik DE, Browning PJ, Kopelman R, et al. Captopril-induced functional renal insufficiency in patients with bilateral renal-artery stenosis or renal artery stenosis in a solitary kidney. *N Engl J Med.* 1983; 308: 373–376.

113. Kimberly RP, Gill JR Jr, Bowden RE, et al. Elevated urinary prostaglandins and the effect of aspirin on renal function in lupus erythematosus. *Ann Intern Med.* 1978; 89: 336–341.

114. Parving HH, Smidt UM, Friisberg B, et al. A prospective study of glomerular filtration rate and arterial blood pressure in insulin-dependent diabetics with diabetic nephropathy. *Diabetologia.* 1981; 20(4): 457–461.

115. The Diabetes Control and Complications Trial Research Group. The effect of intensive treatment of diabetes on the development and progression of long-term complications in insulin-dependent diabetes mellitus. *N Engl J Med.* 1993; 329: 977–986.

116. UK Prospective Diabetes Study (UKPDS) Group. Intensive blood-glucose control with sulphonylureas or insulin compared with conventional treatment and risk of complications in patients with type 2 diabetes (UKPDS 33). *Lancet.* 1998; 352(9131): 837–853.

117. Bilous RW, Mauer SM, Sutherland DER. The effect of pancreas transplantation on the glomerular structure of renal allografts in patients with insulin dependent diabetes. *N Engl J Med.* 1989; 321: 80–85.

118. Fioretto P, Steffes MW, Sutherland DE, et al. Reversal of lesions of diabetic nephropathy after pancreas transplantation. *N Engl J Med.* 1998; 339(2): 69–75.

119. Robertson RP. Successful islet transplantation for patients with diabetes—fact or fantasy? *N Engl J Med.* 1989; 321: 80–85.

120. Shapiro AM, Lakey JR, Ryan EA, et al. Islet transplantation in seven patients with type 1 diabetes mellitus using a glucocorticoid-free immunosuppressive regimen. *N Engl J Med.* 2000; 343(4): 230–238.

121. Mogensen CE. Long-term antihypertensive treatment inhibiting progression of diabetic nephropathy. *Br Med J (Clin Res Ed).* 1982; 285(6343): 685–688.

122. Parving HH, Smidt UM, Hommel E, et al. Effective antihypertensive treatment postpones renal insufficiency in diabetic nephropathy. *Am J Kidney Dis.* 1993; 22(1): 188–195.

123. Lewis EJ, Hunsicker LG, Bain RP, et al. The effect of angiotensin-converting-enzyme inhibition on diabetic nephropathy. *N Engl J Med.* 1993; 329: 1456–1462.

124. Estacio RO, Jeffers BW, Hiatt WR, et al. The effect of nisoldipine as compared with enalapril on cardiovascular outcomes in patients with non-insulin-dependent diabetes and hypertension. *N Engl J Med.* 1998; 338(10): 645–652.

125. Schrier RW, Estacio RO. Additional follow-up from the ABCD trial in patients with type 2 diabetes and hypertension. *N Engl J Med.* 2000; 343(26): 1969.

126. Estacio RO, Jeffers BW, Gifford N, et al. Effect of blood pressure control on diabetic microvascular complications in patients with hypertension and type 2 diabetes. *Diabetes Care.* 2000; 23(suppl 2): B54–B64.

127. Schrier RW, Estacion R, Esler A, et al. Effects of aggressive blood pressure control in normotensive type II diabetic patients on albuminuria, retinopathy and strokes. *Kidney Int.* 2002; 61: 1086–1097.

128. UK Prospective Diabetes Study Group. Tight blood pressure control and risk of macrovascular and microvascular complications in type 2

diabetes: UKPDS 38. *BMJ*. 1998; 317(7160): 703–713.

129. Heart Outcomes Prevention Evaluation Study Investigators. Effects of ramipril on cardiovascular and microvascular outcomes in people with diabetes mellitus: results of the HOPE study and MICRO-HOPE substudy. *Lancet*. 2000; 355(9200): 253–259.

130. Golan L, Birkmeyer JD, Welch HG. The cost-effectiveness of treating all patients with type 2 diabetes with angiotensin-converting enzyme inhibitors. *Ann Intern Med*. 1999; 131(9): 660–667.

131. Parving HH, Lehnert H, Brochner-Mortensen J, et al. The effect of irbesartan on the development of diabetic nephropathy in patients with type 2 diabetes. *N Engl J Med*. 2001; 345(12): 870–878.

132. Brenner BM, Cooper ME, de Zeeuw D, et al. Effects of losartan on renal and cardiovascular outcomes in patients with type 2 diabetes and nephropathy. *N Engl J Med*. 2001; 345(12): 861–869.

133. Lewis EJ, Hunsicker LG, Clarke WR, et al. Renoprotective effect on the angiotensin-receptor antagonist irbesartan in patients with nephropathy due to type 2 diabetes. *N Engl J Med*. 2001; 345(12): 851–860.

134. Hostetter TH. Prevention of end-stage renal disease due to type 2 diabetes. *N Engl J Med*. 2001; 345(12): 910–912.

135. Klahr S, Levey AS, Beck GJ, et al. The effects of dietary protein restriction and blood pressure control on the progression of chronic renal disease. *N Engl J Med*. 1994; 330: 877–884.

136. Elving LD, Wetzels JF, de Nobel E, et al. Captopril acutely lowers albuminuria in normotensive patients with diabetic nephropathy. *Am J Kidney Dis*. 1992; 20: 559–563.

137. Praga M, Hernandez E, Montoyo C, et al. Long-term effects of angiotensin-converting enzyme inhibitors beneficial in patient with nephrotic syndrome. *Am J Kidney Dis*. 1992; 20: 240–248.

138. The GISEN Group (Gruppo Italiano di Studi Epidemiologici in Nefrologia): randomised placebo-controlled trial of effect of ramipril on decline in glomerular filtration rate and risk of terminal renal failure in proteinuric, non-diabetic nephropathy. *Lancet*. 1997; 349(9069): 1857–1863.

139. Dworkin LD, Benstein JA, Parker M, et al. Calcium antagonists and converting enzyme inhibitors reduce renal injury by different mechanisms. *Kidney Int*. 1993; 43(4): 808–814.

140. Saruta T, Suzuki H. Efficacy of manidipine in the treatment of hypertension with renal impairment: a multicenter trial. *Am Heart J*. 1993; 125(2 pt 2): 630–634.

141. Jarusiripipat C, Chan L, Shapiro JI, et al. Effect of long-acting calcium entry blocker (anipamil) on blood pressure, renal function and survival of uremic rats. *J Pharmacol Exp Ther*. 1992; 260(1): 243–247.

142. Maschio G, Alberti D, Janin G, et al. Effect of the angiotensin-converting-enzyme inhibitor benazepril on the progression of chronic renal insufficiency. The Angiotensin-Converting-Enzyme Inhibition in Progressive Renal Insufficiency Study Group. *N Engl J Med*. 1996; 334(15): 939–945.

143. Ruggenenti P, Perna A, Benini R, et al. In chronic nephropathies prolonged ACE inhibition can reduce remission: dynamics of time-dependent changes in GFR. Investigators of the GISEN Group (Gruppo Italiano Studi Epidemiologici in Nefrologia). *J Am Soc Nephrol*. 1999; 10(5): 997–1006.

144. Ruggenenti P, Perna A, Gherardi G, et al. Renal function and requirement for dialysis in chronic nephropathy patients on long-term ramipril: REIN follow-up trial. Gruppo Italiano di Studi Epidemiologici in Nefrologia (GISEN). Ramipril Efficacy in Nephropathy. *Lancet*. 1998; 352(9136): 1252–1256.

145. Giatras I, Lau J, Levey AS. Effect of angiotensin-converting enzyme inhibitors on the progression of nondiabetic renal disease: a meta-analysis of randomized trials. Angiotensin-Converting-Enzyme Inhibition and Progressive Renal Study Group. *Ann Int Med*. 1997; 127(5): 337–345.

146. Jafar TH, Schmid CH, Landa M, et al. Angiotensin-converting enzyme inhibitors and progression of nondiabetic renal disease: a meta-analysis of patient-level data. *Ann Int Med*. 2001; 135(2): 73–87.

147. Agodoa LY, Appel L, Bakris GL, et al. Effect of ramipril versus amlodipine on renal outcomes in hypertensive nephrosclerosis: a randomized controlled trial. *JAMA*. 2001; 285(21): 2719–2728.

148. Sica DA, Douglas JG. The African American Study of Kidney Disease and Hypertension (AASK): new findings. *J Clin Hypertens (Greenwich)*. 2001; 3(4): 244–251.

149. Husted FC, Nolph KD, Maher JF. NAHCO$_3$ and NaCl tolerance in chronic renal failure. *J Clin Invest*. 1975; 56: 414–419.

150. Block GA, Klassen PS, Lazarus JM, et al. Mineral metabolism, mortality, and morbidity in maintenance hemodialysis. *J Am Soc Nephrol*. 2004; 15(8): 2208–2218.

151. Kestenbaum B, Sampson JN, Rudser KD, et al. Serum phosphate levels and mortality risk among people with chronic kidney disease. *J Am Soc Nephrol*. 2005; 16(2): 520–528.

152. Ibels LS, Alfrey AC, Haut L, et al. Preservation of function in experimental renal disease by dietary restriction of phosphate. *N Engl J Med*. 1978; 298(3): 122–126.

153. Jarusiripipat C, Shapiro JI, Chan L, et al. Reduction of remnant nephron hypermetabolism by protein restriction. *Am J Kidney Dis*. 1991; 18(3): 367–374.

154. Loghman-Adham M. Role of phosphate retention in the progression of renal failure. *J Lab Clin Med*. 1993; 122(1): 16–26.

155. Slatopolsky E, Brown A, Dusso A. Role of phosphorus in the pathogenesis of secondary hyperparathyroidism. *Am J Kidney Dis*. 2001; 37(1 suppl 2): S54–S57.

156. Alfrey AC. Aluminum metabolism and toxicity in uremia. *J Uoeh*. 1987; 9(suppl): 123–132.

157. Alfrey AC. Aluminum toxicity in patients with chronic renal failure. *Ther Drug Monit*. 1993; 15(6): 593–597.

158. Alfrey AC, LeGendre GR, Kaehny WD. The dialysis encephalopathy syndrome. Possible aluminum intoxication. *N Engl J Med*. 1976; 294(4): 184–188.

159. Hsu CH, Patel SR, Young EW. New phosphate binding agents: ferric compounds. *J Am Soc Nephrol*. 1999; 10(6): 1274–1280.

160. Burke SK, Amin NS, Incerti C, et al. Sevelamer hydrochloride (Renagel), a phosphate-binding polymer, does not alter the pharmacokinetics of two commonly used antihypertensives in healthy volunteers. *J Clin Pharmacol*. 2001; 41(2): 199–205.

161. Nagano N, Miyata S, Obana S, et al. Sevelamer hydrochloride (Renagel), a non-calcaemic phosphate binder, arrests parathyroid gland hyperplasia in rats with progressive chronic renal insufficiency. *Nephrol Dial Transplant*. 2001; 16(9): 1870–1878.

162. Ramsdell R. Renagel: a new and different phosphate binder. *Anna J*. 1999; 26(3): 346–347.

163. London GM, Parfrey PS. Cardiac disease in chronic uremia: pathogenesis. *Adv Renal Repl Ther*. 1997; 4: 194–211.

164. Harnett JD, Foley RN, Kent GM, et al. Congestive heart failure in dialysis patients: prevalence, incidence, prognosis and risk factors. *Kidney Int*. 1995; 47(3): 884–890.

165. Lim VERSUS, Kirchner PT, Fangman J, et al. The safety and the efficacy of maintenance therapy of recombinant human erythropoietin in patients with renal insufficiency. *Am J Kidney Dis*. 1989; 14: 496–506.

166. Mannucci PM, Remuzzi G, Pusineri F, et al. Deamino-8-D-arginine vasopressin shortens the bleeding time in uremia. *N Engl J Med*. 1983; 308(1): 8–12.

167. Akpolat T, Eser M, Albayak D, et al. Effect of desmopressin on protein S and antithrombin III in uremia. *Nephron*. 1997; 77(3): 362.

168. Ozen S, Saatci U, Bakkaloglu A, et al. Low-dose intranasal desmopressin (DDAVP) for uremic bleeding. *Nephron*. 1997; 75(1): 119–120.

169. Sloand JA. Long-term therapy for uremic bleeding. *Int J Artif Organs*. 1996; 19(8): 439–440.

170. McCarthy ML, Stoukides CA. Estrogen therapy of uremic bleeding. *Ann Pharmacother*. 1994; 28(1): 60–62.

171. Remuzzi G. Bleeding disorders in uremia: pathophysiology and treatment. *Adv Nephrol Necker Hosp*. 1989; 18: 171–186.

172. Obrador GT, Arora P, Kausz AT, et al. Level of renal function at the initiation of dialysis in the U.S. end-stage renal disease population. *Kidney Int*. 1999; 56(6): 2227–2235.

173. Hakim RM, Lazarus JM. Initiation of dialysis. *J Am Soc Nephrol*. 1995; 6(5): 1319–1328.

174. Lowrie EG, Lew NL. Death risk in hemodialysis patients: the predictive value of commonly measured variables and an evaluation of death rate differences between facilities. *Am J Kidney Dis*. 1990; 15(5): 458–482.

175. Man NK. Initiation of dialysis: when? *Nippon Jinzo Gakkai Shi*. 1992; 34(1): 1–8.

176. Shemesh O, Golbetz H, Kriss JP, et al. Limitations of creatinine as a filtration marker in glomerulopathic patients. *Kidney Int*. 1985; 28(5): 830–838.

177. Levey AS, Berg RL, Gassman JJ, et al. Creatinine filtration, secretion and excretion during progressive renal disease. Modification of Diet in Renal Disease (MDRD) Study Group. *Kidney Int*. 1989; (suppl 27): S73–S80.

178. Acchiardo SR, Moore LW, Latour PA. Malnutrition as the main factor in morbidity and mortality of hemodialysis patients. *Kidney Int*. 1983; (suppl 16): S199–S203.

179. Owen WF Jr, Lew NL, Liu Y, et al. The urea reduction ratio and serum albumin concentration as predictors of mortality in patients undergoing hemodialysis. *N Engl J Med*.1993; 329(14): 1001–1006.

180. Churchill DN, Blake PG, Jindal KK, et al. Clinical practice guidelines for initiation of dialysis. Canadian Society of Nephrology. *J Am Soc Nephrol*. 1999; 10(suppl 13): S289–S291.

181. Levin N, Eknoyan G, Pipp M, et al. National Kidney Foundation: Dialysis Outcome Quality Initiative—development of methodology for clinical practice guidelines. *Nephrol Dial Transplant*. 1997; 12(10): 2060–2063.

182. Eknoyan G, Levin N. NKF-K/DOQI Clinical Practice Guidelines: Update 2000. Foreword. *Am J Kidney Dis*. 2001; 37(1 suppl 1): S5–S6.

183. Eknoyan G, Levin NW. Impact of the new K/DOQI guidelines. *Blood Purif*. 2000; 20(1): 103–108.

184. Pereira BJG. New prospects in chronic renal insufficiency. *Am J Kidney Dis*. 2000; 36(suppl 3): S1–S3.

CHAPTER 12

Obstructive Nephropathy: Pathophysiology and Management

KEVIN P. G. HARRIS

"O bstructive nephropathy," "obstructive uropathy," and "hydronephrosis" are terms commonly used to describe urinary tract obstruction or its consequences. Obstructive nephropathy refers to the renal disease caused by impaired flow of urine or tubular fluid. Such impedance to flow causes high back pressure initially, which has direct and indirect effects on the renal parenchyma. Obstructive uropathy refers to the structural changes of the urinary tract that impair urine outflow and necessitate a rise in proximal pressure to transmit the usual flow through the point of narrowing. Dilatation occurs proximal to the site of obstruction. Hydronephrosis describes this dilatation. Importantly, hydronephrosis is not synonymous with obstructive uropathy as it can occur without functional obstruction to the urinary tract and can be absent in established obstruction. Vesicoureteric reflux, primary megaureter, and diabetes insipidus are examples of nonobstructive causes of ureteral dilatation. Nevertheless, renal parenchymal damage may occur in each of these cases.

Obstructive nephropathy and uropathy frequently coexist, and their effective management requires close collaboration between nephrologists, urologists, and radiologists. Immediately following acute urinary tract obstruction, changes within the kidney are mainly functional, whereas more chronic obstruction will result in irreversible structural damage and scarring. Prompt and effective relief of the obstruction will allow the functional changes to recover, but once structural changes have occurred, the patient will be left with chronic renal impairment. Thus, obstructive nephropathy is different from most of the diseases affecting the kidney in that it is potentially curable (1). However, urinary tract obstruction remains a major cause of chronic kidney disease (CKD) worldwide.

Obstructive uropathy is classified according to the (a) duration, (b) degree, and (c) site of the obstruction. When the obstruction is less than a few days' duration, it is said to be acute and is usually caused by a calculus, blood clot, or sloughed papilla. Obstruction that develops slowly and is long lasting is said to be chronic, as in congenital ureteropelvic or ureterovesical abnormalities and retroperitoneal fibrosis. Obstruction is said to be high grade when it is complete or low grade when it is partial or incomplete. Acute or chronic obstruction is further subdivided into upper and lower urinary tract obstruction. Upper-tract obstruction occurs above the vesicoureteral junction (VUJ) and is usually unilateral. Lower urinary tract obstruction occurs below the VUJ and by definition is bilateral. Complete obstruction of the urinary tract is termed "high grade," whereas partial or incomplete obstruction is termed "low grade."

Unilateral obstruction in a patient with two normal kidneys will not result in significant renal impairment because the contralateral kidney compensates. However, bilateral obstruction or the obstruction of a single functioning kidney will result in renal failure.

Causes of Obstructive Nephropathy

Obstructive uropathy may result from functional or anatomic abnormalities of the urethra, bladder, ureters, or renal pelvis. These abnormalities may be congenital or acquired. Obstructive uropathy also may occur as a result of diseases intrinsic or extrinsic to the urinary tract. The major causes of obstructive uropathy are shown in Table 12.1.

TABLE 12.1 CAUSES OF OBSTRUCTION IN THE URINARY TRACT

Upper Urinary Tract	Lower Urinary Tract
Intrinsic Causes	Phimosis, meatal stenosis, paraphimosis
Intraluminal	Urethra: strictures, stones, diverticulum,
Intratubular deposition of crystals (uric acid, acyclovir)	posterior anterior urethral valves,
Ureter: stones, clots, renal papillae, fungus ball	periurethral abscess, uretheral surgery
Intramural	urethral surgery
Ureteropelvic or ureterovesical junction Dysfunction	Prostate: benign prostatic hyperplasia,
Ureteral valve, polyp, stricture, or tumor	abscess, prostatic carcinoma
Extrinsic Causes	Bladder
Vascular system	Neurogenic bladder: spinal cord defect
Aneurysm: abdominal aorta, iliac vessels	or trauma, diabetes, multiple sclerosis,
Aberrant vessels: ureteropelvic junction	cerbrovascular accidents, Parkinson
Venous: retrocaval ureter, puerperal ovarian	disease
vein thrombophlebitis	Bladder neck dysfunction
Fibrosis following vascular reconstructive surgery	Bladder calculus
Originating in the reproductive system	Bladder cancer
Uterus: pregnancy, prolapse, tumors, endometriosis	Bladder
Ovary: abscess, tumors, ovarian remnants	Trauma
Gartners duct cyst, tuboovarian abscess	Straddle injury
Lesions of the gastrointestinal tract: Crohn disease,	Pelvic fracture
diverticulitis, appendiceal abscess, pancreatic tumor,	
abscess, cyst	
Diseases of the retroperitoneum	
Retroperitoneal fibrosis (idiopathic radiation)	
Inflammatory: tuberculosis, sarcoidosis	
Hematomas	
Primary retroperitoneal tumors (lymphoma, sarcoid, etc.)	
Tumors metastatic to the retroperitoneum	
(cervix, bladder, colon, prostate, etc.)	
Lymphocele	
Pelvic lipomatosis	

CONGENITAL URINARY TRACT OBSTRUCTION

With increased use and improved sensitivity of antenatal scanning, congenital abnormalities of the urinary tract are now frequently identified early, allowing prompt postnatal (and in some cases antenatal) intervention to relieve the obstruction and hence preserve renal function (2). Congenital urinary tract obstruction occurs most frequently in males, most commonly as a result of either posterior urethral valves or pelvic-ureteral junction (PUJ) obstruction. If obstruction occurs early during development, the kidney fails to develop and becomes dysplastic. If the obstruction is bilateral, there is a high mortality rate as a result of severe renal failure. If the obstruction occurs later in gestation and is low grade or unilateral, hydronephrosis and nephron loss will still occur but renal function may be sufficient to allow survival. Such patients may not present until later in life or only be discovered as an incidental finding.

ACQUIRED URINARY TRACT OBSTRUCTION

Acquired urinary tract obstruction may affect either the upper or lower urinary tract and can result from either intrinsic or extrinsic causes. Intrinsic causes of obstruction may be intraluminal or intramural.

Intrinsic Obstruction

Intraluminal Obstruction

Intraluminal obstruction may result from tubular intrarenal obstruction such as the deposition of uric acid crystals in the tubular lumen after treatment of hematologic malignancies (tumor lysis syndrome). It may also occur with the precipitation of Bence–Jones protein in myeloma and with the precipitation or crystal formation of a number of drugs, including sulfonamides, acyclovir, methotrexate, and indinavir.

Extrarenal intraluminal obstruction is most commonly caused by renal calculi, which typically lodge in the calyx, PUJ, or VUJ and at the level of the pelvic brim. Calcium oxalate stones are the most common and typically cause intermittent acute unilateral urinary tract obstruction in young adults, rarely causing significant renal impairment. Less common causes of urinary lithiasis, such as struvite stones, uric acid stones, and cystinuria, are often bilateral and hence more likely to cause long-term renal impairment. Intraluminal obstruction can also result from a sloughed papilla after papillary necrosis or blood clots after macroscopic hematuria (clot colic). Papillary necrosis may occur in diabetes mellitus, sickle cell trait or disease, analgesic nephropathy, renal amyloidosis, and acute pyelonephritis. Clot colic can occur with bleeding from renal tumors or arteriovenous malformations, after renal trauma, and in patients with polycystic kidney disease.

Intramural Obstruction

Intramural obstruction can result from either functional or anatomic changes. Functional disorders include vesicoureteral reflux (VUR), adynamic ureteral segments (usually at the junction of the ureter with the pelvis or bladder), and neurologic disorders. The latter may result in a contracted (hypertonic) bladder or a flaccid (atonic) bladder, depending on whether the lesion affects upper or lower motor neurons, and lead to impaired bladder emptying with VUR. Bladder dysfunction is very common in patients with multiple sclerosis and after spinal cord injury and is also seen in diabetes mellitus and Parkinson disease and after cerebrovascular accidents. Some drugs (anticholinergics, levodopa) can alter neuromuscular activity of the bladder and result in functional obstruction, especially if there is preexisting bladder outflow obstruction (e.g., prostatic hypertrophy). Anatomic causes of intramural obstruction of the upper urinary tract include transitional cell carcinoma of the renal pelvis and ureter and ureteral strictures secondary to radiotherapy or retroperitoneal surgery. Rarely, obstruction may result from ureteral valve malfunction, polyps, or strictures after therapy for tuberculosis. Intramural obstruction of the lower urinary tract can result from urethral strictures, which are usually secondary to chronic instrumentation or previous urethritis, or malignant and benign tumors of the bladder. Infection with *Schistosoma haematobium*, when the ova lodge in the distal ureter and bladder, is a common cause of obstructive uropathy worldwide, with up to 50% of chronically infected patients developing ureteral strictures and fibrosis with contraction of the bladder.

Extrinsic Obstruction

In females the most common cause of extrinsic compression of the urinary tract is pressure from a gravid uterus on the pelvic rim with the right ureter being more commonly affected. It is usually asymptomatic, and the changes resolve rapidly after delivery. Rarely, bilateral obstruction and acute renal failure may occur. Ureteral dilation without functional obstruction is commonly seen in pregnancy as a result of hormonal effects (especially progesterone) on smooth muscle. Direct extension of the tumor to involve the urinary tract occurs in up to 30% of patients with carcinoma of the cervix, and other pelvic pathologies that can cause ureteral compression include benign and malignant uterine and ovarian masses, abscesses, endometriosis, and pelvic inflammatory disease. Inadvertent ureteric ligation is a rare but recognized complication of pelvic surgical procedures.

In males, the most common cause of extrinsic obstruction of the lower urinary tract is benign prostatic hypertrophy. Carcinoma of the prostate can also result in obstruction either from direct tumor extension to the bladder outlet or ureters or from metastases to the ureter or lymph nodes.

Retroperitoneal pathology such are primary or secondary tumors or inflammatory disease may also result in extrinsic obstruction of the ureters. Retroperitoneal fibrosis, in which a thick fibrous tissue extends out from the aorta to encase the ureters and draw them medially, may be idiopathic or result from inflammatory aortic aneurysms, certain drugs (e.g., β-blockers, bromocriptine, and methysergide), previous radiation, trauma or surgery, and granulomatous disease.

Incidence and Prevalence

Obstructive uropathy is a common entity and can occur at all ages. The exact incidence of obstructive uropathy is difficult to ascertain, since obstruction occurs in a variety of diseases that may warrant hospitalization and surgical intervention and may be transient. However, the prevalence of hydronephrosis at autopsy is 3.5% to 3.8% of adults and 2% of children, with about equal distribution between males and females (3).

The frequency and etiology of obstruction vary in both sexes with age. In children younger than 10 years, obstruction is more common in males, with congenital urinary tract anomalies such as urethral valves or PUJ obstruction accounting for most cases. In the United States, obstructive uropathy remains the most common cause of end-stage renal disease (ESRD) in pediatric patients registered for renal transplantation, accounting for 16% of cases. In addition, congenital obstructive uropathy accounts for 0.7% of all patients (median age 31 years) maintained on renal replacement therapy, demonstrating the continued impact of this disease into adult life (4). In young adults (<20 years of age), the frequency of urinary tract obstruction is similar in males and females. Beyond 20 years of age, obstruction becomes more common in females, mainly as a result of pregnancy and gynecologic malignancies. Urolithiasis occurs predominantly in young adults (25 to 45 years old) and is three times more common in men than women. In patients older than 60 years, obstructive uropathy is seen more frequently in men, secondary to benign prostatic hyperplasia and prostatic carcinoma. About 80% of men older than 60 years have some symptoms of bladder outflow obstruction, and up to 10% have hydronephrosis. In Europe, acquired urinary tract obstruction accounts for 3% to 5% of the cases of ESRD in patients older than 65 years, with most resulting from prostatic disease (5). In the United States, the number of patients on renal replacement therapy as a result of acquired obstruction continues to increase, although the rise is not as rapid as with other causes of ESRD (4). Currently about 1.4% of prevalent ESRD patients in the United States have a diagnosis of obstructive nephropathy, with the majority of these patients being >65 years old and male.

Pathophysiolgy of Urinary Tract Obstruction

The profound functional and structural changes that occur within the kidney following obstruction are triggered by the increased pressure that occurs after the onset of ureteral obstruction. This increase in pressure is greatest immediately after the onset of obstruction and tends to fall with time with incomplete obstruction. Damage in the obstructed kidney is potentiated by those conditions that acutely increase ureteral pressure, such as increases in urine flow (i.e., an increase in fluid intake or after administration of diuretics) or augmentation of the degree of obstruction or both.

It is rarely possible to accurately define the time of onset of obstruction in humans or to obtain repetitive measurements of renal function. Therefore our understanding of the consequences of urinary tract obstruction stem mainly from the study of animal models (6). Although many studies have focused on the effects of complete short-term ureteral obstruction in rodents, investigators have also examined models of chronic complete, partial, or reversible obstruction in adult and neonatal animals. Available experimental data show little species-to-species variation in the response to acute obstruction, suggesting similar changes are likely to occur in humans. The effects of obstructive uropathy on the kidney result from a variety of factors with complex interactions that alter both glomerular hemodynamics and tubular function in an interdependent fashion (7). Significant differences exist between the effects of bilateral and unilateral obstruction. Although initially the changes are predominantly functional and potentially reversible, chronic obstruction results in irreversible structural changes, and models of obstruction are often used to examine the pathogenetic mechanisms underlying the development of renal fibrosis from any cause (8).

THE EFFECTS OF ACUTE URETERAL OBSTRUCTION ON GLOMERULAR FUNCTION

The glomerular filtration rate (GFR) falls progressively following the onset of complete ureteral obstruction (9). The maintenance of residual GFR after ureteral ligation is caused by (a) continuous reabsorption of salt and water along the nephron, (b) the ability of the renal tract to dilate, and (c) alterations in renal hemodynamics. Glomerular filtration has four major determinants: (a) the mean difference in hydrostatic pressure between the glomerular capillary lumen and Bowman's space (ΔP); (b) renal plasma flow (Q_A); (c) the ultrafiltration coefficient of the glomerular capillary wall (K_f), which reflects both the total surface area available for filtration and the intrinsic permeability characteristics of the filtering apparatus; and (d) the mean oncotic pressure difference across the glomerular capillary wall ($\Delta\pi$). The manner in which these parameters are affected by ureteral obstruction depends on the duration of the obstruction, the volume status of the animal, and whether or not a contralateral functioning kidney is present.

Changes in Hydrostatic Pressure Gradients

Ligation of the ureter increases ureteral pressure. These changes are instantaneously reflected in changes in proximal tubular pressure, the latter being higher than that in the ureter. The rise in intratubular pressure depends on the degree of hydration of the animal, mean urine flow rate, and whether one or both kidneys are obstructed. Nevertheless, independent of the volume status, intratubular pressure rises within an hour of ureteral obstruction (Fig. 12.1). Concomitantly, there is an increase in glomerular capillary hydrostatic pressure; however, this increase in intraglomerular pressure is not proportional to the rise in intratubular pressure (10). Therefore, the net hydrostatic pressure difference across glomerular capillaries decreases. This results in a decline in GFR. After approximately 5 to 6 hours of ureteral obstruction, proximal intratubular pressure begins to decline (11). After 24 hours, intratubular pressures are lower than (11,12) or equal to (13) values before obstruction in animals with unilateral ureteral obstruction (UUO), but this does not restore an effective filtration pressure, because intraglomerular capillary hydrostatic pressure declines at an even faster rate (11,12) and falls below the levels seen before obstruction. In animals with bilateral ureteral obstruction, proximal intratubular pressures are initially

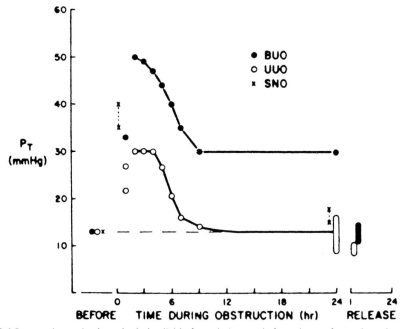

■ **Figure 12.1** Pressure in proximal renal tubules (P_T) before, during, and after release of complete obstruction of one ureter (*UUO*), both ureters (*BUO*), or single nephrons (*SNO*). BUO, bilateral ureteral obstruction; SNO, single-nephron obstruction; UUO, unilateral ureteral obstruction.

twofold higher (11,14) than those seen in rats with UUO (Fig. 12.1). By 24 hours, the levels of in-tratubular pressure have fallen but not back to the baseline (14,15). At this time glomerular capillary pressure is no different from preobstruction values. Thus, in this setting, high intratubular pressures contribute significantly to the decrease in GFR.

Changes in Renal Blood Flow

Ureteral obstruction causes a transient increase in renal blood flow (16). Decreased resistance of the affer-ent arteriole accounts for the increase in blood flow to the unilaterally obstructed kidney (16,17). This phenomenon is observed in both the denervated and the isolated perfused kidney, suggesting that this hy-peremic phase is mediated through an intrarenal mechanism. Measurements of the distribution of blood flow during this phase indicate that inner cortical blood flow is increased (18–20). There is a progressive decrease in blood flow to the inner medulla during ureteral obstruction (21). This increase in renal blood flow may represent a hemodynamic response intended to maintain GFR. The increase in renal blood flow and afferent arteriolar dilatation leads to an increase in glomerular capillary pressure. This response main-tains GFR at approximately 80% of preobstruction values despite the substantial increase in proximal tubular pressure. The mechanism underlying this response involves a signal generated at the single-nephron level because a wax plug placed in the proximal tubule generates an identical hemodynamic re-sponse in a single glomerulus. Tanner (22) suggested that the fall in afferent arteriolar resistance was caused by tubular-glomerular feedback related to interrupting acutely distal delivery of tubular fluid to the macula densa. Ichikawa (23), however, demonstrated that glomerular blood flow does not rise if proximal tubular pressure is maintained in the normal range in the face of tubule blockade, suggesting that the al-tered glomerular hemodynamics are a result of intratubular dynamics rather than cessation of distal deliv-ery of tubule fluid. The transient increase in renal blood flow after ureteral obstruction can be prevented by the administration of inhibitors of prostaglandin synthesis such as indomethacin (24). Thus, vasodila-tor prostaglandins, such as prostaglandin E2 and prostacyclin, may account for this initial vasodilator ef-fect. At this time interval, the renal vascular bed is particularly resistant to vasoconstriction induced by either electrical stimulation of renal nerves or an infusion of catecholamines. In addition, autoregulation of renal blood flow is impaired, suggesting a prominent vasodilating influence following the onset of ureteral obstruction. Usually the increase in blood flow following obstruction peaks at about 2 to 3 hours.

In a second phase, approximately 3 to 5 hours after the onset of obstruction, renal blood flow starts to decline, while ureteral pressure continues to increase. In part this may be a consequence of aug-mented renal resistance owing to increased interstitial pressure. In this phase, ureteral pressure starts to fall toward control values, and renal plasma flow continues to decline, reaching about 30% to 50% of control values by 24 hours (25,26). This vasoconstrictive response of the kidney to UUO results pre-dominantly from an increased resistance of afferent arterioles.

In animals with bilateral ureteral obstruction, the changes in renal hemodynamics are similar to those seen following UUO. There also is an initial hyperemic phase (14,16) that is blocked by cyclooxygenase inhibitors (24), and the decline in GFR thus is secondary to a rise in intratubular pressure. Renal plasma flow falls progressively and is similar at 24 hours to that seen after UUO, although afferent arteriole resis-tance may not increase as much. As a result of the persistently high proximal tubular pressure and decline in renal plasma flow, it would be expected that the decline in GFR would be greater after bilateral ureteral obstruction than after UUO. However, this is not the case and may reflect the effect of a higher intra-glomerular capillary pressure and greater number of filtering nephrons before and after release of obstruc-tion of 24 hours' duration in rats with bilateral ureteral obstruction than in those with UUO (27).

Changes in the Ultrafiltration Coefficient

After ureteral obstruction, GFR falls to a greater extent than renal plasma flow (9). Thus, the filtration fraction decreases. This may reflect preferential constriction of the preglomerular blood vessels because this would lower both blood flow and glomerular capillary pressure, thus resulting in a greater decre-ment in GFR than in blood flow. Alternatively, it is suggested that there is either diversion of blood to nonfiltering areas of the kidney or a reduced area available for filtration per glomerulus. That the latter occurs is suggested by the finding that K_f values in rats with ureteral obstruction are lower than those typically obtained in normal rats (28).

Alterations in Net Oncotic Pressure

There is no information on whether changes in the oncotic pressure difference across the glomerular wall can modify glomerular hemodynamics after ureteral obstruction.

In summary, the fall in single-nephron GFR in obstruction is caused by a decrease in net hydrostatic pressure across the glomerular capillary wall. The fall in net hydrostatic filtration pressure initially is caused by an increase in intratubular pressure. After 24 hours of obstruction, the main mechanism responsible for the decrement in net hydrostatic pressure across the glomerular capillary wall is a fall in intraglomerular pressure. In animals with bilateral ureteral obstruction, both a persistent increase in intratubular pressure and a decrease in intraglomerular pressure contribute to the decrease in net hydrostatic pressure across glomerular capillaries. There also is evidence that K_f is decreased. The greater decrease in total kidney GFR than in single-nephron GFR after 24 hours of obstruction results from the fact that some nephrons cease to function during the period of obstruction.

DIFFERENCES BETWEEN UNILATERAL AND BILATERAL OBSTRUCTION

The precise changes in renal hemodynamics differ according to whether the obstruction is unilateral or bilateral (8,11). After 24 hours of unilateral ureteral ligation, the decrease in single-nephron GFR is almost exclusively a decrease in intraglomerular capillary pressure. However, in rats with bilateral ureteral obstruction, both a decrease in intraglomerular capillary pressure and a persistent elevation of intratubular pressure account for the decrease in net filtration pressure. Furthermore, the number of filtering nephrons after 24 hours of ureteral ligation is greater in animals with bilateral obstruction than in those with unilateral obstruction (27). The causes for these hemodynamic differences between unilateral and bilateral ureteral obstruction have not been elucidated. The levels of circulating atrial natriuretic peptide (ANP), a potent vasodilator, are higher in rats with bilateral ureteral obstruction than in rats with UUO (29). ANP causes preglomerular vasodilatation and postglomerular vasoconstriction and has been demonstrated to increase K_f in the isolated perfused glomerular preparation. In addition, the administration of exogenous ANP increases GFR following release of unilateral or bilateral ureteral obstruction (29,30). Because ANP antagonizes the vasoconstrictive effects of angiotensin II, it is probable that in vivo the elevated levels of endogenous ANP in animals with bilateral ureteral obstruction minimize the renal vasoconstriction that occurs compared with animals with UUO.

THE EFFECTS OF PROLONGED URETERAL OBSTRUCTION ON GLOMERULAR FUNCTION

After complete ureteral obstruction in the rat, GFR reaches 2% of control values by 48 hours and remains at this low level. Renal plasma flow also declines but to a lesser extent (25). The effects of partial chronic obstruction of the ureter depend on both the degree and the duration of the obstruction. Whole-kidney GFR may be reduced to one-third of control values 2 to 4 weeks following partial ureteral obstruction in the rat (31). Single-nephron GFR, however, is reduced by only 20% of control levels, suggesting that the decline in whole-kidney function is a result of a loss in the number of functioning nephrons not accessible to micropuncture, that is, juxtamedullary nephrons (31).

Rats with partial obstruction of 2 to 4 weeks' duration have a 30% decrease in K_f. GFR and single-nephron plasma flow are maintained near normal because of an increase in glomerular capillary pressure secondary to a greater decrease in afferent than efferent arteriolar resistance. This vasodilatation is prostaglandin mediated, and indomethacin administration increases both afferent and efferent arteriolar resistance and causes a decline in single-nephron GFR (32). Changes in the dog are less severe than those in the rat but generally follow a similar pattern (33).

Modulators of Glomerular Function

Two major vasoconstrictors, angiotensin II and thromboxane A2, and several other vasoactive compounds (7) play a role in the changes in plasma flow per nephron and single-nephron GFR seen in obstruction. Inhibition of thromboxane A2 synthesis in rats with ureteral obstruction increases plasma flow per nephron, owing to decreased vasoconstriction of both afferent and efferent arterioles (34). Thromboxane also may decrease K_f through mesangial cell contraction and a decrease in the surface area available for filtration. Although infusion of angiotensin II into normal animals increases net filtration pressure, presumably because of greater vasoconstriction of the efferent than the afferent arteriole, blockade of angiotensin II formation after relief of obstruction increases GFR (34). This increase in GFR may result from a greater filtering surface area, because angiotensin II causes mesangial cell contraction (7) and therefore can reduce the total glomerular capillary area available for filtration. In addition, angiotensin II decreases plasma flow per nephron, which also contributes to the fall in single-nephron GFR. The central and critical role of these two vasoconstrictors in modulating postobstructive renal hemodynamics is illustrated by the fact that rats pretreated with both angiotensin-converting enzyme and thromboxane synthase inhibitors, before obstruction, demonstrate almost normal renal function after release of obstruction (30).

Vasodilator prostaglandins, produced in increased amounts by the obstructed kidney, may prevent further decrements in GFR by antagonizing the vasoconstrictive effects of thromboxane A2 and angiotensin II. Indeed, it has been demonstrated that after release of obstruction in rats, in the setting of prior inhibition of the thromboxane synthase, administration of inhibitors of the cyclooxygenase causes a marked decrease in whole-kidney GFR and renal plasma flow (34).

An interstitial leukocyte infiltrate, predominantly macrophages, is an early event following ureteral obstruction. This begins to increase as early as 4 to 12 hours after ureteral obstruction and continues to increase over the course of days thereafter. By 4 days after left ureteral ligation, there is a 20-fold increment in the renal cortical macrophage number in the obstructed kidney versus either the contralateral unobstructed kidney or normal kidneys from age-matched, sham-operated animals (35). The signal for renal leukocyte recruitment immediately after ureteral obstruction is predominantly macrophage specific because there are few T-lymphocytes noted and an absence of polymorphonuclear leukocytes (35,36). Diamond et al. have noted upregulated expression of monocyte chemoattractant peptide (MCP)-1 (37), osteopontin (38), and intercellular adhesion molecule (ICAM)-1 (39) within the tubular epithelium as early as 12 hours after left ureteral ligation. Thus the proximal tubule is capable of generating macrophage chemoattractants, which participate in a coordinated response to urinary tract obstruction that includes the development of a florid, macrophage-rich interstitial inflammatory infiltrate. This infiltrate plays a key role in the acute functional changes after ureteral obstruction (40) and as in a variety of other organs is implicated in the pathogenesis of the late structural changes that occur after obstruction (41).

Recovery of Glomerular Function After Release of Ureteral Obstruction

The degree of recovery of GFR after release of ureteral obstruction depends on the severity and duration of the obstruction. After release of a 2-week complete ureteral obstruction in the dog, GFR in the postobstructed kidney averages 25% of ipsilateral control values and 16% of concurrent values for the contralateral kidney, the latter having undergone a compensatory increase in GFR (42). Subsequent the GFR of the postobstructed kidney increases, and the GFR of the normal kidney falls, stabilizing at about 2 months after the release of obstruction. However, GFR does not return to normal in the postobstructed kidney, remaining approximately 50% below the value obtained for the contralateral kidney at 2 years. The changes in effective renal plasma flow mirror the changes seen in GFR.

In rats, a permanent decrease in GFR occurs if ureteral obstruction has been present for >72 hours. After obstruction lasting <30 hours, recovery of whole-kidney GFR is complete, although the normalization in GFR may not be a consequence of homogeneous recovery in single-nephron GFR for all nephrons (43). Values for whole-kidney GFR calculated from measurements of surface single-nephron GFR are greater than those obtained from direct whole-kidney clearance measurements (27). Of superficial nephrons (those accessible to micropuncture), 40% do not filter immediately after release of obstruction, whereas only 12% of juxtamedullary nephrons filter, suggesting a selective loss of juxtamedullary nephrons. Subsequent studies revealed that 3 to 6 hours after release of UUO of 24 hours' duration, GFR values were one-sixth of those observed before ligation of the ureter (43). With time the GFR increases such that by 14 and 60 days after the release of obstruction, values in the experimental kidney are comparable to those in the contralateral untouched kidney (43). When single-nephron GFR and the number of filtering nephrons are determined using a modification of Hansen's technique, only 85% of the nephrons filter in the postobstructed kidney

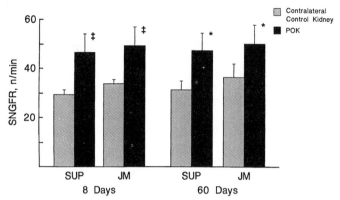

■ **Figure 12.2** SNGFR in SUP and JM nephrons of rats 8 days and 60 days after release of UUO of 24 hours' duration. The SNGFR values for the POK were significantly greater *(asterisk)* than those of the contralateral kidney. JM, juxtamedullary; POK, postobstructed kidney; SNGFR, single-nephron glomerular filtration rate; SUP, superficial; UUO, unilateral ureteral obstruction.

(43), suggesting the normalization of whole-kidney GFR occurs at the expense of hyperfiltration (increase in single-nephron GFR) in the remaining functional nephrons (Fig. 12.2). There appears to be a permanent decrement in the total number of functional nephrons. The mechanism responsible for this loss of nephrons after ureteral obstruction remains to be defined, as does its long-term significance in terms of the development of chronic renal failure following obstructive uropathy.

THE EFFECTS OF URETERAL OBSTRUCTION ON TUBULAR FUNCTION

Abnormalities in tubular function are common in urinary tract obstruction, with major defects located in the distal segments of the nephron. As a result there is altered renal handling of electrolytes and changes in the regulation of water excretion with a decreased ability to concentrate the urine. The degree and nature of the tubular defects after obstruction depend in part on whether the obstruction is bilateral or unilateral. These differences could result from the dissimilar hemodynamic responses, different intrinsic changes within the nephron, differences in extrinsic factors (e.g., volume expansion and accumulation of natriuretic substances in bilateral obstruction) between the two states, or a combination of all three.

Sodium and Water Handling

In spite of a decrease in GFR and hence in the filtered load of sodium, the excretion of sodium by the postobstructed kidney of rats with UUO is similar to that of the contralateral kidney (44). Thus, fractional sodium excretion is greater from the postobstructed than from the contralateral kidney. Similar findings have been reported in the dog and in humans after more prolonged periods of obstruction. These findings indicate significant changes in the tubular reabsorption of sodium and water by the previously obstructed kidney. Changes in intravascular volume may affect the absolute and fractional excretion of salt and water by the postobstructed kidney. Absolute sodium excretion after release of UUO is reduced in rats with volume depletion studied under anesthesia when compared with awake rats. In contrast, expansion of the extracellular fluid (ECF) volume with saline solution increases both absolute and fractional sodium excretion. These increases are greater in the postreleased kidney than in the contralateral untouched kidney.

The release of bilateral ureteral obstruction results in a different quantitative excretion of salt and water than what occurs after release of UUO. There is a dramatic increase in the absolute amount of sodium and water excreted in the urine after release of bilateral ureteral obstruction in humans (45,46) and experimental animals (12,47–49), resulting in the so-called postobstructive diuresis. The differences in salt and water excretion after release of bilateral ureteral obstruction and UUO may be the result of differences in the levels of urea and potential expansion of the ECF volume during the period of bilateral ureteral obstruction compared with UUO. In addition, the circulating levels of ANP are significantly greater in rats with bilateral ureteral obstruction than in those with unilateral obstruction (29).

Urinary Concentration

Patients with partial obstruction of the urinary tract or patients after relief of partial or complete urinary obstruction have impaired renal concentrating capacity (50,51). This may take some months to recover following the release of obstruction. Patients with persistently hypotonic urine and polyuria, which are unresponsive to the administration of vasopressin (52,53), may develop severe dehydration and hypernatremia if fluid intake is inadequate.

The urinary concentrating defect may be explained by both a decreased hypertonicity of the medullary interstitium and a failure of the cortical collecting duct to respond to the action of vasopressin.

After relief of unilateral obstruction of 24 hours' duration in rats, the urine osmolality from the postobstructed kidney seldom exceeds 400 mOsm/kg H_2O compared with approximately 2,000 mOsm/kg H_2O in the contralateral untouched rat kidney. This decrease in urine osmolality is accompanied by a marked decrease in medullary hypertonicity (54,55). There is a decrease in the concentrations of both sodium and urea in the interstitium of the renal medulla. This decrease in the hypertonicity of the renal medullary interstitium may result from a decrease in the reabsorption of sodium chloride in the ascending limb of loop of Henle. Such a decrease in reabsorption would result in a fall in the solute present in the medulla and would lower the tonicity of the medullary interstitium and thus the osmotic driving force for the movement of water from the lumen of the collecting duct into the interstitium. Decreased Na^+/K^+ ATPase activity in the outer medulla of obstructed kidneys may contribute to this defect in sodium reabsorption (56). Increased prostaglandin synthesis may contribute to this defect (57).

Increases in blood flow through the medullary region would remove excessive amounts of both sodium and urea present in the medulla and hence would result in decreased medullary hypertonicity. Although medullary blood flow is decreased during obstruction, a marked overshoot in medullary blood flow is observed following relief of obstruction.

As a result of obstruction there may be a permanent decrease in the number of juxtamedullary nephrons (43). These have the longest loops of Henle and are responsible for the reabsorption of solutes and the creation of a hypertonic medulla. Their loss therefore causes a permanent defect in the concentrating ability of the postobstructed kidney, although this is not as marked as that seen in the acute stages of obstruction (43).

Administration of vasopressin in the setting of partial urinary obstruction does not decrease urine flow and usually does not increase urine osmolality (53). Vasopressin-resistant isotonic urine can be attributed in part to the impaired generation of a hypertonic medullary interstitium. However, because the medullary interstitium is not hypotonic in obstructed kidneys, the presence of hypotonic urine suggests an inability to achieve complete osmotic equilibration between the fluid in the collecting duct and the fluid in the interstitium, caused by a failure of vasopressin to appropriately increase water permeability across the collecting duct (58). Expression of aquaporin-2 (a water channel predominantly found in the collecting duct principal cells [59]) is decreased in the setting of bilateral or unilateral obstruction (60,61) as a result of both cyclooxygenase-2 (62) and angiotensin II (63) mechanisms.

In addition to the mechanisms described above, following release of bilateral ureteral obstruction, the osmotic effect of solutes retained during the period of obstruction contributes to the generation of isotonic urine after relief of bilateral ureteral obstruction.

Urinary Acidification

In humans and experimental animals, acid excretion is impaired after the release of bilateral or UUO (50,64–66). This usually returns to normal after release of obstruction but may take some time (months) to do so. Studies in experimental animal models of urinary tract obstruction (65,66) as well as in patients (50) suggest there is a form of distal renal tubular acidosis with an inability to lower the urine pH to normal minimum values in response to acidemia or acid loading. Bicarbonate titration studies in the rat have shown there is no decrease in proximal reabsorption of bicarbonate after release of UUO (66). Micropuncture experiments also failed to demonstrate decreased bicarbonate reabsorption in proximal or distal segments of surface nephrons. Urine carbon dioxide pressure (P$_{CO_2}$) values remained low after bicarbonate loading. These data suggest that the acidifying defect after release of UUO results from either a decrease in hydrogen ion secretion in the distal tubule and the collecting duct of surface nephrons or alterations in the reabsorption of bicarbonate in juxtamedullary nephrons. A decrease in the number of H$^+$ ATPase pumps in the apical surface of intercalated cells may account for the acidifying defect that occurs with ureteral obstruction. Immunohistochemistry studies have demonstrated a decrease in apical staining of the 31-kDa subunit of the H$^+$ TPase in the collecting duct intercalated cells of rats with ureteral obstruction (67). This returns to normal 3 to 5 days after release of obstruction and is accompanied by a urine pH in the postobstructed kidney similar to that in the contralateral kidney.

Potassium Excretion

Hyperkalemic hyperchloremic acidosis has been described in patients with chronic obstructive uropathy (64). At any given level of GFR, the fractional excretion of potassium is less in patients with obstructive uropathy than in a comparable group of patients with renal insufficiency caused by a variety of renal diseases (Fig. 12.3). The development of hyperkalemic hyperchloremic acidosis in individuals with obstructive uropathy may be explained at least in part by (a) a deficiency of aldosterone secretion probably secondary to diminished production of renin by the kidney (hyporeninemic–hypoaldosteronism), (b) a defect in renal hydrogen ion secretion with an inability to lower pH of the urine maximally in the presence of systemic acidosis and decreased urinary excretion of both ammonium and titratable acid (type 4 distal renal tubular acidosis), (c) a combination of these two defects, or (d) a decreased sensitivity of the distal tubule to the action of aldosterone on potassium secretion. There is also a progressive

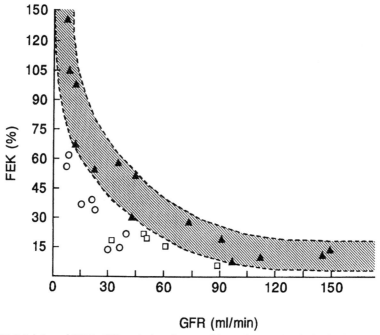

■ **Figure 12.3** Relation of FEK to GFR under baseline conditions. The area inside the broken line depicts the normal adaptive increase in fractional potassium excretion observed with a chronic reduction in GFR. These data were obtained from 14 normokalemic controls (*solid triangles*) with different GFRs. Each patient (*open symbols*) had a baseline FEK lower than that expected for the corresponding GFR. Open circles denote patients with distal renal tubular acidosis (*group I*); open squares represent patients with hyperkalemic metabolic acidosis owing to selective aldosterone deficiencies (*group II*). (From Batlle DC, Arruda JAL, Kurtzman NA. Hyperkalemic distal renal tubular acidosis associated with obstructive uropathy. *N Engl J Med.* 1981; 304: 373–380, with permission.) FEK, fractional excretion of potassium; GFR, glomerular filtration rate.

decrease in in situ turnover of the Na–K pump in intact cortical collecting ducts in rats with UUO (68), which could contribute significantly to the abnormal potassium excretion that accompanies obstructive uropathy.

Excretion of Divalent Cations and Phosphate

The fractional excretion of calcium is decreased after release of unilateral obstruction in both the rat and humans (69,70). However, the mechanisms of altered calcium reabsorption after obstruction have not been determined.

In contrast to calcium, magnesium excretion increases following release of bilateral or UUO and may result in profound hypomagnesaemia. This change is not modified by magnesium restriction in the diet. It is likely that the differences in magnesium and calcium excretion seen after release of UUO in the rat relate to the greater reabsorption of calcium than magnesium in the proximal tubule. Since in the rat a major portion of the magnesium filtered is reabsorbed in the thick ascending limb, a defect in reabsorption in this segment may account for the marked increase in magnesium excretion in the urine.

The reabsorption of phosphate by the postobstructed kidney depends on both the duration of the obstruction and whether the obstruction is bilateral or unilateral (70–72). After release of bilateral ureteral obstruction of 24 hours' duration, phosphate excretion parallels sodium and water excretion and is increased in absolute terms when expressed as a fraction of the filtered load. This increased excretion is not affected by parathyroidectomy and cannot be accounted for by an increase in ECF volume (71). The increase in phosphate excretion, however, can be prevented by phosphate restriction in the diet before bilateral ureteral obstruction, to forestall the rise in serum phosphate that usually occurs. In addition, increasing the phosphate levels of normal rats to concentrations similar to those seen after bilateral ureteral obstruction results in a similar degree of phosphaturia (71). These observations suggest that the filtered load of phosphate is the major determinant of the rate of phosphate excretion after release of bilateral ureteral obstruction. Although no studies have examined the nephron site of impaired phosphate reabsorption, it is assumed that it is in the proximal tubule because of the magnitude of the change involved and the fact that the major site of phosphate reabsorption is in this segment of the nephron.

In contrast, phosphate excretion after release of UUO is decreased in the postobstructed kidney and increased in the contralateral kidney in humans (73), rats (72), and dogs (74). The increase in phosphate excretion by the contralateral kidney in rats with UUO is abolished by parathyroidectomy. The increase in phosphate retention by the postobstructed kidney may result from a decrease in single-nephron GFR and an increase in the phosphate reabsorption by proximal segments. In summary, after release of UUO, altered phosphate excretion results primarily from altered renal hemodynamics, and following release of bilateral ureteral obstruction, phosphate excretion is modulated to a large extent by extrarenal factors, mainly the serum levels of phosphate.

THE EFFECTS OF OBSTRUCTION ON HORMONE RESPONSIVENESS AND RENAL METABOLISM

After release of ureteral obstruction, there is a change in the response of the postobstructed kidney to hormones (75). The consequences of obstructive nephropathy include (a) decreased excretion and altered renal metabolism of hormones produced in extrarenal endocrine organs, (b) altered rates of production of hormones within the kidney, and (c) altered responsiveness and sensitivity of the obstructed kidney to hormones.

Parathyroid Hormone

The obstructed kidney responds to exogenous parathyroid hormone administration with an increase in urine phosphate and cyclic 3'5'-adenosine monophosphate (cAMP) excretion. However, the magnitude of the response is less in the postobstructed kidney than in the contralateral kidney (72). This decrease in response to the hormone is accompanied by decreased generation of cAMP, decreased activation of adenylate cyclase by the hormone in basolateral membranes obtained from the proximal tubule of postobstructed kidneys, and the apparent loss of parathyroid hormone receptors from the same membrane (76).

After relief of bilateral ureteral obstruction, the administration of parathyroid hormone does not further increase the absolute and fractional phosphate excretion (71). However, when the filtered load of phosphate is restored to normal by dietary manipulations, the excretion of phosphate by the postobstructed kidney is normalized as is the response to parathyroid hormone.

Ureteral obstruction blunts the calcemic response of bone to parathyroid hormone, presumably owing to decreased production of 1,25-dihydroxyvitamin D_3 by the obstructed kidney or as a consequence of increased levels of circulating parathyroid hormone.

Angiotensin II

The postobstructed kidney has an increased capacity to release prostaglandins in response to angiotensin II, and those response curves suggest that there is an increase in the number or affinity, or both, of the receptors for the hormone. In addition, the contractile responses of the renal cortex to angiotensin were enhanced in rabbit kidneys that had been obstructed for 8 to 32 days, suggesting that the sensitivity of the postobstructed kidney to angiotensin II is increased. On the other hand, in isolated glomeruli from obstructed kidneys, the eicosanoid production in response to the in vitro addition of angiotensin II is blunted (77).

Antidiuretic Hormone (Vasopressin)

Unresponsiveness of the collecting duct to the effect of antidiuretic hormone (ADH) on water permeability may contribute to the concentrating defect seen after ureteral obstruction. The cAMP response to exogenous ADH is markedly blunted in rats with bilateral ureteral obstruction compared with nonobstructed rats. In addition, ADH-induced osmotic water flow is significantly impaired in cortical collecting tubules isolated from obstructed kidneys of rabbits (58,78).

Renal Metabolism

A variety of changes of renal metabolism have been described following ureteral obstruction (75). The activities of brush-border alkaline phosphatase, of basolateral Na^+/K^+ ATPase, and glucose-6-phosphatase all decrease acutely (within 2 days of ureteral obstruction) and return to normal following the release of obstruction. In contrast, the activities of the enzymes of the pentose shunt pathway increase after ureteral obstruction.

Many of these changes are compatible with the kidney adapting to an anaerobic pattern of metabolism. Anaerobic glycolysis may increase by as much as 10-fold over normal levels with prolonged (10 to 14 days) obstruction (79), and such abnormalities may persist even after release of the obstruction (80). Electron micrographs have shown that ureteral obstruction results in structural changes of mitochondria after 24 hours of ureteral ligation (81). Decreased ammoniagenesis has been demonstrated in cortical slices obtained from postobstructed kidneys (81), which may contribute to the inability to excrete acid following ureteral obstruction.

Experiments using basolateral membranes isolated from renal tubular cells have shown that following obstruction there is a decrease in phospholipid content of the membrane (82). Because the lipid composition, or physical state of the membrane (fluidity), affects the activity of membrane-bound enzymes and water permeability, it is possible that selective changes in the lipid composition of basolateral membranes following obstruction could account for both the altered transport characteristics and the altered response to hormones seen after release of ureteral obstruction.

In addition to changes in enzyme activity, ureteral obstruction also causes changes in gene transcription both in the obstructed kidney and in the contralateral kidney (83).

THE EFFECTS OF URETERAL OBSTRUCTION ON RENAL STRUCTURE

The morphologic alterations of the kidney result from (a) decreased renal blood flow, (b) increased ureteral pressure, (c) invasion by macrophages and lymphocytes, and (d) bacterial infection.

The alterations in renal architecture are similar irrespective of the cause of the obstruction. Following acute complete obstruction initially, there is renal enlargement and edema with pelvicalyceal dilation. Microscopically, tubular dilation develops that predominantly affects the collecting duct and distal tubular segments (84,85), though cellular flattening and atrophy of proximal tubular cells can also occur. Glomerular structures are usually preserved initially, although Bowman's space may be dilated and may contain Tamm–Horsfall protein. Ultimately, some periglomerular fibrosis may develop.

In chronic partial obstruction a grossly hydronephrotic kidney develops with a widely dilated renal pelvis, with the renal papilla either flattened or hollowed out. The first structures to be affected are the ducts of Bellini. Subsequently, other papillary structures are damaged. Ultimately, there is an encroachment on renal cortical tissue, which in advanced cases may be reduced to a thin rim of renal tissue surrounding a large saccular ureteral pelvis.

Prolonged obstruction results in the development of interstitial fibrosis with obliteration of nephrons. There is tubular proliferation and apoptosis, epithelial-mesenchymal transition, (myo)fibroblast accumulation, increased extracellular matrix deposition, and tubular atrophy. Ischemia as a result of the decreased renal blood flow contributes to the parenchymal damage after obstruction, and an important pathologic role for angiotensin II and transforming growth factor-β (TGF-β) has been established (86,87). The increased distance between peritubular capillaries and tubular cells may contribute to the ischemia (88). Invading cells, particularly macrophages, by releasing inflammatory and growth factors, may contribute to interstitial cell proliferation and scarring and widening of the interstitium space. Superimposed bacterial infection (pyelonephritis) may play an additive role in the development of parenchymal fibrosis and in the pathologic changes that are observed (89).

The sequence of events whereby the acute functional and reversible alterations in kidney function following obstruction transform into chronic irreversible structural abnormalities involves a complex interplay between infiltrating and resident cells, the production of hormones, cytokines and growth factors, as well as the modulation of matrix production and degradation. These factors are discussed below and are summarized in Figure 12.4

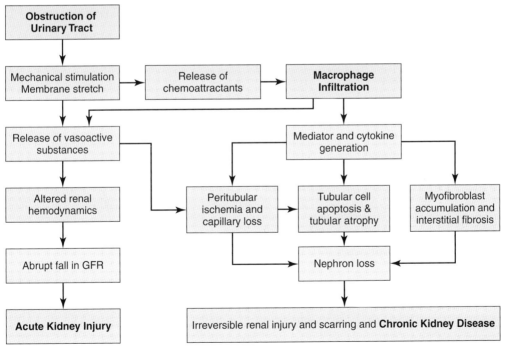

■ **Figure 12.4** The sequence of events whereby the acute functional and reversible alterations in kidney function following obstruction transform into chronic irreversible structural abnormalities. Note the pivotal role of infiltrating macrophages in both modulating acute functional changes and promoting the development of irreversible structural damage and fibrosis.

The Development of Tubulointerstitial Fibrosis

The tubulointerstitium occupies approximately 80% of total kidney volume. Renal interstitial fibrosis is a common consequence of long-standing obstructive uropathy (90,91) and develops because of an imbalance between extracellular matrix synthesis, matrix deposition, and matrix degradation. Rabbits with unilateral ureteral ligation have a widened interstitial space 7 days after the onset of obstruction (90) with a progressive increase in collagen fibers and fibroblasts with time. There is also a mononuclear cell infiltrate and a proliferation of interstitial cells in the renal parenchyma (92). More recently an increase in the renal synthesis of several extracellular matrix components (collagen types I, III, and IV; fibronectin; heparan sulfate proteoglycans) in the renal interstitium of rabbits with ureteral obstruction of 3 and 7 days' duration has been described (91).

Similar observations have been made in the rat following 3 days of UUO in the rat (93), with increased deposition of interstitial collagen (types I and III) and basement membrane collagen (type IV) in the tubulointerstitium. This is associated with an increase in the level of messenger RNA (mRNA) for collagen α_1 (type IV) and TGF-β_1 within the interstitium of the obstructed kidney, suggesting events leading to interstitial fibrosis are initiated promptly after the onset of obstruction.

Renal tubular cells in culture produce collagen types I, III, and IV, and the expression collagen α_1 (type IV) mRNA increases in the tubules of the obstructed kidney. Therefore, renal tubule cells may contribute to the increased production of collagen IV in both tubular basement membrane and the interstitium, which in turn may contribute to alterations in tubular function in the obstructed kidney.

At the same time fibroblasts migrate and proliferate in the interstitium of the obstructed kidney during UUO (90). Several cytokines secreted by infiltrating macrophages and T-lymphocytes act as chemoattractants and stimulate fibroblast proliferation (94). Interstitial fibroblasts produce collagens I, III, and IV, contributing to the increase in the production of collagens in the obstructed kidney of rats with UUO. The substantial increase in collagens I and III in the interstitium of the obstructed kidney at 3 or 5 days after UUO is consistent with the increased cellularity caused by fibroblast proliferation and infiltrating mononuclear cells.

The increased expression of TGF-β_1 mRNA in the obstructed kidney is confined to tubular cells (95). TGF-β_1 has substantial effects on matrix protein production (96). It causes (a) an increase in the mRNA of extracellular matrix components, particularly the collagens; (b) a decrease in proteinases degrading these proteins; and (c) an increase in metalloproteinase inhibitors (Fig. 12.5).

In contrast the amount of glomerular collagens I, III, and IV is unchanged as is mRNA for TGF-β_1 at day 5 after UUO (95), consistent with the finding that glomeruli appear normal by light microscopy through 7 days of obstructive nephropathy (92,93).

Apoptosis

Distinct patterns of cell proliferation and apoptosis have been described for tubular, interstitial, and glomerular cells, as well as infiltrating cells in chronic obstructive nephropathy. The development of interstitial inflammation and fibrosis following prolonged obstruction is accompanied by tissue loss and atrophy of the tubular epithelial cells (97,98). Apoptosis of renal tubular cells in chronic obstructive nephropathy increases rapidly, reaching 30-fold that of controls by 25 days of obstruction (99). This is accompanied by a decrease in the dry weight of the kidney, suggesting apoptosis participates in the tubular atrophy and renal loss observed in prolonged obstructive nephropathy.

Infiltrating Macrophages

Following ureteral obstruction there is an increased synthesis and expression of adhesion proteins and chemoattractants in the kidney, which contribute to monocytic infiltration. MCP-1 mRNA and protein expression is increased within the proximal tubular epithelium of the obstructed but not the contralateral unobstructed kidney (37). The resulting macrophage infiltrate plays a pivotal role in the chronic tissue injury and fibrosis that result from prolonged ureteral obstruction (41,100) by releasing profibrogenic factors such as TGF-β and galectin-3 that promote progressive fibrosis. The critical role for infiltrating macrophages in the pathogenesis of the late structural changes that occur after obstruction is demonstrated by the observation that macrophage depletion markedly limits the development of interstitial fibrosis. In addition to macrophages the cellular infiltrate following obstruction also

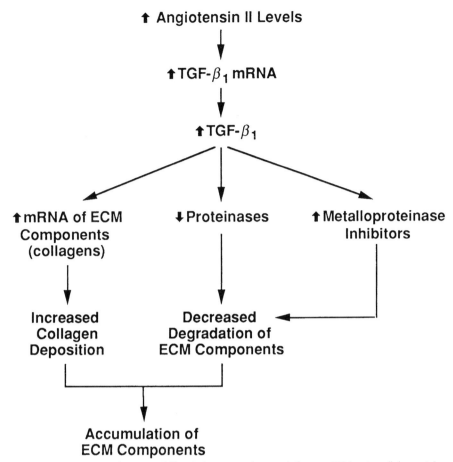

■ **Figure 12.5** Pathogenesis of interstitial fibrosis in progressive renal disease. ECM, extracellular matrix; mRNA, messenger RNA; TGF-β1, transforming growth factor beta-1. (From Klahr S, Ishidoya S, Morrissey J. Role of angiotensin II in the tubulointerstitial fibrosis of obstructive nephropathy. *Am J Kidney Dis.* 1995;26:141–146, with permission.)

contains a number of T cells. The exact way in which the various cell types and complex local cytokine networks interact to modulate the fibrotic response remains to be fully elucidated.

Angiotensin

Local angiotensin II generation can stimulate the production of TGF-β by tubular cells and promote the deposition of the type IV collagen and the development of tubulointerstitial fibrosis within the obstructed kidney (Fig. 12.5).

Angiotensin-converting enzyme (ACE) inhibitors and angiotensin receptor antagonists exert a beneficial effect on the UUO model of experimental hydronephrosis (101). Administration of ACE inhibitors in rats with unilateral obstruction results in a decrease in interstitial volume, a marked decrease in the number of monocytes/macrophages infiltrating the renal parenchyma, a decrease in the expression of TGF-β, and lesser activation of nuclear factor kappa B (NK-$\kappa\beta$) (102). In addition, there is a marked decrease in fibroblast proliferation and myofibroblast phenotype. The administration of ACE inhibitors after 5 days of established UUO prevents the progressive fibrosis that occurred in untreated rats from day 5 to day 10 of ureteral obstruction. Administration of an angiotensin I receptor antagonist has a similar effect, with the exception of the infiltration of the renal parenchyma by monocytes/macrophages and the expression of clusterin, which decreases in the kidney of rats with UUO treated with ACE inhibitors but not in rats treated with angiotensin I receptor antagonist (103). These differences may be explained by the effects of ACE inhibitors on nitric oxide, through the activation of bradykinin (104). Treatment with an angiotensin II receptor antagonist has no effect on interstitial volume, macrophage infiltration, expression of TGF-β, or fibroblast proliferation in rats with UUO (103). However, antagonism of the angiotensin II receptor decreases the appearance of a myofibroblast phenotype and markedly decreases the expression of clusterin, with an intermediate effect on the activation of NF-$\kappa\beta$.

NF-$\kappa\beta$

The activation of a number of genes associated with tissue inflammation is controlled by the NF-$\kappa\beta$ family of transcription factors (105,106). NF-$\kappa\beta$ has been shown to be activated during experimental ureteral obstruction (107). Enalapril, given to rats with ureteral ligation, significantly decreases the ability of proteins extracted from the nucleus to bind to an NF-$\kappa\beta$ consensus oligonucleotide compared with similar extracts obtained from kidneys of untreated animals (108). Thus, ACE inhibitors possess, in addition to their well-known hemodynamic effects, an anti-inflammatory effect, which may be mediated, in part, by decreased activation of NF-$\kappa\beta$ (Fig. 12.6).

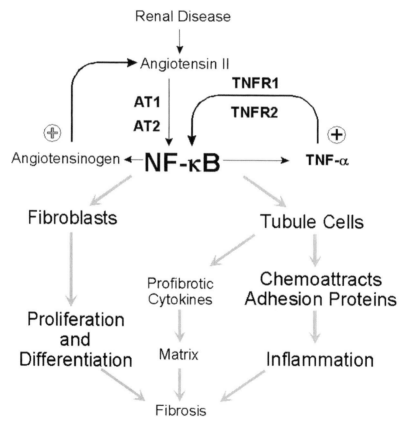

■ Figure 12.6 The regulation of gene expression by angiotensin II occurs through specific receptors that are ultimately linked to changes in the activity of transcription factors within the nucleus of target cells. In particular, members of the NF-$\kappa\beta$ family of transcription factors are activated, which, in turn, fuels at least two autocrine-reinforcing loops that amplify angiotensin II and TNFα formation. (From Klahr S, Morrissey JJ. The role of growth factors, cytokines and vasoactive compounds in obstructive nephropathy. *Semin Nephrol.* 1998; 18: 622–632, with permission.)

REACTIVE OXYGEN SPECIES

A growing body of evidence supports a contributory role of oxidant stress and lipid peroxidation products in a variety of clinical and experimental models of fibrotic disorders (109). Several studies suggest that reactive oxygen metabolites may have an important role in the pathophysiology of renal disease (110), with antioxidant enzymes and reactive oxygen species (ROS) playing an integral role in the development of interstitial fibrosis by inducing extracellular matrix accumulation. ROS also activate ICAM-1 and thus may play a central role in the mediation of inflammatory cell proliferation and extracellular matrix accumulation, which are important events leading to the development of tubulointerstitial fibrosis (111).

In obstructive nephropathy, oxidants generated by infiltrating leukocytes and intrinsic renal cells may account for some of the functional and morphologic changes observed. Probucol, an antioxidant and lipid-lowering agent, improves GFR and renal plasma flow both at 4 hours and 3 days after release of 24 hours of bilateral obstruction (112), whereas lipid lowering with lovastatin, which is devoid of antioxidant properties, has no effect.

A decrease in mRNA and protein expression of cellular antioxidant enzymes and increased generation of ROS may play an integral role in the development of tubulointerstitial injury and fibrosis associated with experimental hydronephrosis. As early as 24 hours after UUO, levels of total cortical mRNA for catalase and Cu-ZnSOD are significantly decreased in the obstructed kidney. Immunohistochemistry showed a decreased staining intensity of Cu-ZnSOD and catalase protein in the cortical tubules of the obstructed kidneys (113). In addition there is an increased generation of ROS within the obstructed kidney cortex. Thus, an increased oxidant burden after obstruction, as well as an impairment of normal antioxidant defense mechanisms, may play an important role in amplifying the proinflammatory state in experimental hydronephrosis, thereby contributing to tubulointerstitial injury and fibrogenesis.

Homeostatic Factors

The majority of studies have investigated the role that the upregulation of hormones and cytokines plays in the development of tubulointerstitial fibrosis. However, a decrease in the production of growth and homeostatic factors, which are normally endogenously produced by the kidney to downregulate the fibrotic process, may also be important in the development of fibrosis. This would offer the prospect that treatment with purified growth and/or homeostatic factors could blunt the progression of disease or possibly reverse the loss of renal function.

The expression of preproepidermal growth factor is suppressed in the kidney with an obstructed ureter in both the neonatal (114) and adult (115) rat. Treatment of both the adult (115) and the neonatal (114) rat with UUO with epidermal growth factor significantly reduces tubule cell apoptosis, blunts tubule atrophy, and preserves renal function where the eventual release of the obstruction is achieved.

Endogenous IGF-1 expression is not changed during UUO in neonatal rats (116), and treatment of neonatal rats with UUO does not affect the suppression of nephrogenesis or tubule cell proliferation seen in UUO. However, treatment with exogenous IGF-1 does significantly blunt tubule cell apoptosis, tubule atrophy, and interstitial collagen deposition (116), suggesting that IGF-1 treatment could offer another means of preserving the capacity of renal function once flow is reestablished.

Hepatocyte growth factor (HGF) has been described as a substance produced by mesenchymal cells that maintains epithelial homeostasis (117). In a mouse model of unilateral obstruction, treatment with recombinant human HGF attenuates apoptosis and TGF-β expression, whereas treatment with an HGF-neutralizing antibody increases TGF-β expression, decreases tubule cell proliferation, and accelerates apoptosis, suggesting that a reduction of endogenous HGF could account for progression of renal fibrosis in tubulointerstitial disease (118).

Bone morphogenetic protein-7 (BMP-7) treatment significantly decreases renal injury in a rat model of UUO when treatment is initiated at the time of injury (119). Subsequent studies suggest that BMP-7 treatment also attenuates renal fibrosis when administered after renal fibrosis has begun (120). Treatment results in a significant improvement in renal function compared to vehicle-treated animals (120).

Tubular epithelial cells are one of the major sites of active vitamin D synthesis. Paricalcitol, a synthetic vitamin D analogue, has been shown to significantly attenuate the development of renal interstitial fibrosis in mouse kidney after ureteral obstruction. It reduces interstitial volume, decreases collagen deposition, and lowers mRNA expression of fibronectin and type I and type III collagens. In addition, paricalcitol suppresses the expression of renal TGF-β1 and its type I receptor and inhibits cell proliferation and apoptosis after obstructive injury. In vitro, paricalcitol was able to block epithelial to mesenchymal transition (EMT). These data suggest that paricalcitol is able to ameliorate renal interstitial fibrosis in obstructive nephropathy, possibly by preserving tubular epithelial integrity through suppression of EMT (121).

Recently heat shock protein (HSP72) has also been shown to ameliorate renal tubulointerstitial fibrosis in obstructive nephropathy by inhibiting both renal tubular epithelial cell apoptosis and EMT (122).

These studies underscore the value of histologic parameters as indicators of renal function and the potential of renal homeostatic factors to beneficially modulate the development of tubulointerstitial inflammation and fibrosis, EMT, and tubular cell apoptosis.

Clinical Consequences of Urinary Tract Obstruction

Obstruction of the urinary tract is a common and potentially reversible cause of acute kidney injury (AKI), and therefore it is important to diagnose and treat it promptly to minimize the chances of long-term chronic damage to the kidney.

Obstruction of the urinary tract can present with a wide range of clinical findings, depending on the site, degree, and duration of obstruction. The clinical manifestations of upper and lower urinary tract obstruction differ. Mechanical obstruction of the urinary tract, causing pain, and lower urinary tract symptoms (protatism) are common presenting complaints. Manifestations can also result from the complex alterations in glomerular and tubular function that may occur in obstructive nephropathy. However, it is important to note that obstructive uropathy and hence obstructive nephropathy can occur without symptoms and with minimal clinical manifestations. Manifestations related to urinary tract infection (and sometimes extrarenal manifestations of the underlying pathologic process responsible for the development of obstructive uropathy) such as tumors or metastases from distal tumors may occur. Obstruction of the urinary tract must be considered in the differential diagnosis of any patient with renal impairment.

SYMPTOMS IN URINARY TRACT OBSTRUCTION

Pain

Pain is a common presenting complaint in patients with obstructive uropathy, particularly in those with ureteral calculi or where the obstruction has developed rapidly. The pain is believed to result from stretching of the collecting system or the renal capsule, with its severity correlating with the degree of distention and not with the degree of dilation of the urinary tract. Occasionally, the location of the pain helps to determine the site of obstruction. With upper ureteral or pelvic obstruction, flank pain and tenderness typically occur, whereas lower ureteral obstruction causes pain that radiates to the groin, the ipsilateral testicle, or the labia. Acute high-grade ureteral obstruction may be accompanied by a steady and severe crescendo flank pain radiating to the labia, the testicles, or the groin ("classic" renal colic). The acute attack may last less than half an hour, or as long as a day. In contrast, pain radiating into the flank during micturition is said to be pathognomonic of VUR. By comparison, patients with a chronic, slowly progressive obstruction may have no pain or minimal pain during the course of their disease. In such patients, any pain that does occur is rarely colicky in nature. In PUJ obstruction, pain may only occur after fluid loading or the use of diuretics to promote a high urine flow rate.

Lower Urinary Tract Symptoms

Obstructive lesions of the bladder neck or bladder pathology may cause a decrease in the force or caliber of the urine stream, intermittency, postmicturition dribbling, hesitancy, or nocturia. Urgency, frequency, and urinary incontinence can result from incomplete bladder emptying. Such symptoms commonly result from prostatic hypertrophy and are frequently referred to as prostatism, but they are not pathognomonic of this condition.

Alterations in Urine Output

Patients with complete bilateral obstruction or obstruction in a single functioning kidney present with anuria and AKI. In contrast partial obstruction may present with polyuria and polydipsia (52,53) as a result of acquired vasopressin resistance. Alternatively, there may be a fluctuating urine output, alternating from oliguria to polyuria. A pattern of alternating oliguria and polyuria or the presence of anuria strongly suggests obstructive uropathy.

Urinary Tract Infection

There is a striking association between urinary tract infection and obstructive uropathy (123). Infection tends to be more common with obstruction of the lower urinary tract, that is, obstruction that is located below the ureterovesical junction, with patients developing cystitis with dysuria and frequency. Two factors may condition the development of infection in the setting of obstruction: (a) the increase of residual urine in the bladder, because urine is an excellent culture medium, and (b) altered properties of the bladder that facilitate bacterial adhesion and growth. Alterations in the glycoprotein composition of epithelial cells of the bladder may explain the greater predisposition to infection in certain patients with urinary tract obstruction than in others. Obstruction of the upper urinary tract is not necessarily accompanied by infection, but when it occurs pyelonephritis with loin pain and systemic symptoms of sepsis, which can be life threatening, may be present.

Further investigation to exclude obstruction should be undertaken following a urinary tract infection in men or young children of either sex, recurrent or persistent infections in women, or infections with unusual organisms, such as Pseudomonas species, with a single attack of acute pyelonephritis. The presence of ongoing obstruction can make the effective eradication of the infection difficult.

Infections of the urinary tract with a urease-producing organism such as *Proteus mirabilis* predispose to stone formation. These organisms generate ammonia, which results in urine alkalinization and favors the development of magnesium ammonium phosphate (struvite) stones. Struvite calculi can fill the entire renal pelvis to form a staghorn calculus that eventually leads to loss of the kidney if untreated. Thus, stone formation and papillary necrosis can also be a consequence of urinary tract obstruction as well as a cause of obstruction.

Hematuria

Calculi may cause trauma to the urinary tract uroepithelium and result in either macroscopic (visible) or microscopic (nonvisible) hematuria. Any neoplastic lesion that obstructs the urinary tract, especially uroepithelial malignancies, may bleed, resulting in macroscopic hematuria. Urinary tract bleeding may also result in obstruction, giving rise to clot colic when in the ureter or clot retention when in the bladder.

Obstruction in Neonates or Infants

Symptoms of obstructive uropathy in neonates and infants are frequently nonspecific and may not be suspected until failure to thrive, voiding difficulties, fever, hematuria, or symptoms of renal failure appear. The advent of routine antenatal scanning has improved the early diagnosis of hydronephrosis and genitourinary abnormalities (124,125). Oligohydramnios at the time of delivery should raise the suspicion of obstructive uropathy, as should the presence of congenital anomalies of the external genitalia. Nonurologic anomalies such as ear deformities, a single umbilical artery, an imperforate anus, or a rectourethral or rectovaginal fistula should prompt investigation for urinary tract obstruction (126). The urinary tract also should be examined in infants born with an imperforate anus or a rectourethral or rectovaginal fistula. The existence of a neurogenic bladder with associated obstructive uropathy should be suspected in infants with neurologic abnormalities.

CLINICAL EXAMINATION IN URINARY TRACT OBSTRUCTION

Physical examination can be completely normal. Some patients with upper urinary tract obstruction may have flank tenderness. Kidney size may increase significantly, particularly in long-standing obstruction. Patients may note increased abdominal girth, and a palpable flank mass may be found. Muscle rigidity over the kidney may be found, and rebound tenderness may be elicited, particularly if acute infection is present. Marked hydronephrosis may present as a flank mass on physical examination, particularly in children with hydronephrosis who are younger than 2 years.

Lower urinary tract obstruction causes a distended, palpable, and occasionally painful bladder. A rectal examination and, in women, a pelvic examination should be performed because they may reveal a local malignancy or prostatic enlargement.

In some cases the finding may be related to the extrarenal manifestations of the underlying pathologic process responsible for the development of obstructive uropathy, such as tumors or metastases from distal tumors.

Hypertension

Hypertension may occur in patients with acute or chronic hydronephrosis, either unilateral or bilateral (127–131). The hypertension could be coincidental or could be related to the hydronephrosis. The mechanisms may relate either to increased ECF volume, owing to decreased sodium excretion, or to an abnormal release of renin and increased generation of angiotensin II. In patients with bilateral hydronephrosis, the increased exchangeable sodium and the usual prompt reversal of the hypertension after catheter drainage and diuresis suggest that the hypertension is caused by abnormal retention of salt and water subsequent to the obstructive process. Thus, these patients appear to have a volume-dependent type of hypertension. In addition, the concentrations of renin in renal venous blood and peripheral venous blood are normal in hypertensive patients with bilaterally hydronephrotic kidneys. After corrective surgery, reversal of the hypertension is associated with an osmotic diuresis and a negative salt and water balance, further suggesting that this type of hypertension is volume dependent.

In contrast, hypertension in patients with UUO may be renin dependent (127,128,130). Elevated values for renal vein renin have been found in unilaterally hydronephrotic kidneys. After appropriate surgery, the hypertension abates and the renin values return to normal (127). Animal studies have demonstrated increased renin release following acute ureteral obstruction (132). In dogs, acute UUO is associated with an increase in blood pressure and a rise in ipsilateral renal vein renin in spite of a concurrent rise in renal blood flow. The causal relation between renin release and the increase in blood pressure is suggested by the fact that pretreatment with desoxycorticosterone acetate (DOCA) and salt abolishes the rise in renin and blood pressure. In contrast, chronic studies in animals have shown that the renin release is not sustained and that the peripheral renin is normal with prolonged unilateral ureteral occlusion. This suggests that chronic, established hypertension in the setting of unilateral obstruction may not be related to increased renin secretion. Because corrective surgery may result in improvement in some of these patients, other abnormalities not related to renin may be important in obstruction. Whether these abnormalities relate to subtle changes in volume or to the lack of release of vasodepressive substances by the obstructed kidney has not been established.

Occasionally, in patients with partial urinary tract obstruction, hypotension occurs as a result of polyuria and volume depletion.

LABORATORY FINDINGS IN URINARY TRACT OBSTRUCTION

Urine Abnormalities

Urinalysis may show hematuria, bacteriuria, pyuria, crystalluria, and low-grade proteinuria, depending on the cause of obstruction. However, urinalysis is commonly completely negative despite advanced obstructive nephropathy. In the acute phase of obstruction, urinary electrolytes are similar to those seen in a "prerenal" state, with a low urinary sodium (<20 mmol/L), a low fractional excretion of sodium (<1%), and a high urinary osmolality (>500 mOsm/kg). However, with more prolonged obstruction, there is a decreased ability to concentrate the urine and an inability to reabsorb sodium and other solutes. These changes are particularly marked after the release of chronic obstruction and give rise to the syndrome commonly referred to as postobstructive diuresis.

Hypernatremia

Children with partial obstructive uropathy and marked polyuria, because of a greater loss of water than sodium, may develop hypernatremia. Thus, the finding of hypernatremia in children should raise the suspicion of partial urinary tract obstruction.

Renal Impairment

Serum electrolytes, urea, and creatinine should be measured. Bilateral obstruction of the urinary tract is one of the many causes of both AKI and CKD. AKI will also occur when a solitary kidney is obstructed. Obstruction should always be considered when AKI presents with complete anuria or if periods of anuria alternate with periods of polyuria.

A number of patients presenting with advanced CKD may have undetected, long-standing urinary tract obstruction. Elderly men can present with advanced CKD and hydronephrosis secondary to bladder outflow obstruction despite remarkably few lower urinary tract symptoms. In patients with retroperitoneal fibrosis in whom the onset of obstruction is slow and progressive, far-advanced CKD may also be the initial presenting finding.

Urinary tract obstruction may also occur in the setting of underlying parenchymal renal disease of another etiology and manifest itself by a change in the rate of progression of renal insufficiency.

Urinary tract obstruction should be considered in patients with CKD and no previous history of renal disease and a relatively benign urinary sediment. Obstruction should also be excluded in patients with known renal disease who develop an abrupt decrease in renal function that is otherwise unexplained.

Hyperkalemic Hyperchloremic Acidosis

In certain patients with obstruction, hyperkalemic hyperchloremic acidosis (renal tubular acidosis type 4) may be a clinical manifestation of partial obstruction of the urinary tract (64,133) (see pathophysiology section of this chapter for the mechanisms).

Polycythemia

Polycythemia has been reported in a few instances of hydronephrosis and is probably related to increased production of erythropoietin by the obstructed kidney. In experimental animals, unilateral hydronephrosis results in elevated plasma levels of erythropoietin that precede the increase in hemoglobin levels.

Diagnosis

Prompt diagnosis of urinary tract obstruction is essential to allow treatment to limit any long-term adverse consequences. Symptoms such as "renal colic" may suggest the diagnosis and prompt appropriate investigation. However, there should be a high index of suspicion of urinary tract obstruction in any patient with unexplained AKI or CKD. The diagnostic approach has to be tailored to the clinical presentation (Fig. 12.7), but a careful history and thorough physical examination are mandatory in all patients.

Certain information is essential when obstructive uropathy is suspected. A history of similar symptoms, the presence or absence of lower urinary tract symptoms or urinary tract infection, and the kinds of drugs ingested should be noted. Review of hospital records may reveal abrupt changes in urine output. Physical examination with particular reference to the flank and abdomen is important. Laboratory analysis of urine and serum as outlined above are mandatory. However, a definitive diagnosis of obstruction requires imaging of the renal tract to confirm the diagnosis, elucidate the cause, and plan treatment.

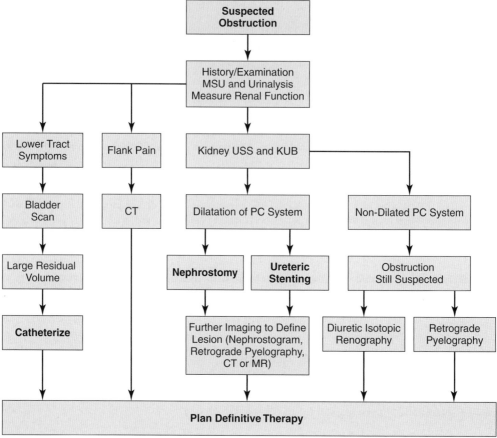

■ **Figure 12.7** Algorithm demonstrating an approach to the investigation and management of suspected urinary tract obstruction. The initial investigations (*boxes*) are dictated by the history and examination. The patient pathway allows rapid relief of the obstruction by nephrostomy or ureteric stenting, while a definitive diagnosis and treatment plan are made. CT, computed tomography; MR, magnetic resonance; USS, ultrasound scan.

DIFFERENTIAL DIAGNOSIS

The entities that should be considered in the differential diagnosis of obstruction vary, depending on the clinical presentation of the obstructive lesion. Patients with anuria and acute renal failure should be evaluated for other potential causes of AKI such as ischemia and nephrotoxins (Chapter YY). The presentation of patients with partial obstruction and polyuria may mimic that of patients with nephrogenic diabetes insipidus. On the basis of low levels of renin and aldosterone secretion, patients with obstruction presenting with hyperchloremic, hyperkalemic metabolic acidosis should be distinguished from patients who have the same syndrome. Renal colic caused by stones may mimic flank pain caused by a gastrointestinal pathologic condition. In children, the manifestations of obstructive uropathy may include gastrointestinal symptoms such as nausea, vomiting, and abdominal pain.

IMAGING TECHNIQUES FOR THE DIAGNOSIS OF URINARY TRACT OBSTRUCTION

As the sites, causes, and consequences of obstruction to the renal tract are so variable, no single imaging investigation is able to diagnose renal tract obstruction with certainty. There have been a number of advances in imaging technology, which have improved diagnostic precision. Computed tomography (CT) scanning and magnetic resonance (MR) urography are increasingly used to diagnose both the site and the cause of obstruction. Both tests can be used to evaluate the urinary tract, each with its own merits. However, there is little consensus on the optimal protocols and appropriate utilization in an era of cost containment and heightened concerns about radiation exposure (134). In addition, the availability and expertise in the use of different imaging techniques varies from center to center, and it is important to remember that older imaging techniques can still be used effectively to evaluate patients with obstructive uropathy.

Generally, the approach to the patient with suspected obstruction may require the complementary use of a number of different imaging techniques, and no single imaging investigation should be relied on to definitively exclude obstruction, especially if the clinical suspicion of obstruction is high.

Several radiologic techniques can be used to infer the presence of upper urinary tract obstruction from the finding of dilatation of the pelvicalyceal system (hydronephrosis). However, it must be remembered that not all dilated collecting systems represent obstruction.

Plain Abdominal X-Ray

A plain abdominal X-ray (or KUB) provides information on renal and bladder morphology, such as size differences between the two kidneys or a large bladder, suggestive of outlet obstruction. It can frequently demonstrate renal calculi, since about 90% of calculi are radioopaque.

Ultrasonography

Ultrasonography is a noninvasive test used as a screening procedure for obstruction. Ultrasonography can define renal size and demonstrate calyceal dilation (135) (Fig. 12.8), but its sensitivity and specificity depend heavily on the expertise of the operator. Ultrasound is rarely able to detect the cause of obstruction, since pathology within the ureter is difficult to demonstrate and tiny stones will not generate acoustic shadows. However, unilateral hydronephrosis suggests obstruction of the upper urinary tract by stones, blood clots, or tumors. Bilateral hydronephrosis is more likely to result from a pelvic problem obstructing both ureters or obstruction of the bladder outlet, in which case the bladder will also be enlarged. Ultrasonography is often combined with a KUB to ensure that ureteral stones or small renal stones are not overlooked.

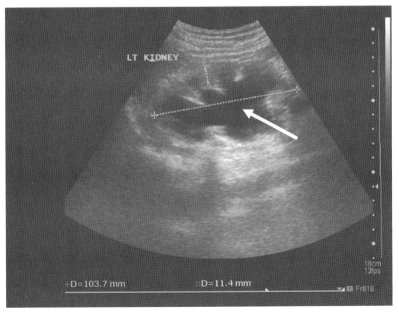

■ **Figure 12.8** Renal ultrasound scan showing a hydronephrotic kidney. There are markers to define renal length and cortical width. There is marked dilation of the pelvicalyceal system with clubbing of the calyces (*arrow*) This is suggestive (but in isolation not diagnostic) of obstruction to the urinary tract.

Ultrasonography produces false-negative results in cases of nondilated obstructive uropathy (135). Immediately after acute obstruction (<24 hours), the relatively noncompliant collecting system may not have dilated such that an ultrasound examination may be normal. Furthermore, if urine flow is low, as in severe dehydration or renal failure, there may be little dilation of the urinary tract. Dilatation may also be absent in slowly progressive obstruction when the ureters are encased by fibrous tissue (as in retroperitoneal fibrosis) or by tumor. The acoustic shadow of a staghorn calculus can also mask dilation of the upper urinary tract. The sensitivity of ultrasound for diagnosing obstruction can be improved by measuring the resistive index using color Doppler sonography. A resistive index >0.7 reflects the increased vascular resistance present in obstruction and effectively discriminates between obstructed and nonobstructed kidneys (135). Such ultrasound techniques avoid the use of ionizing radiation and are particularly useful for pregnant women and children and the follow-up of patients requiring repeated imaging, such as after extracorporeal shock-wave lithotripsy.

Even in experienced hands, ultrasound may have a significant false-positive rate, especially if minimal criteria are adopted to diagnose obstruction. The echogenicity produced by multiple renal cysts may be mistaken for hydronephrosis on ultrasonography, and anatomic variations of the pelvicaliceal system (e.g., extrarenal pelvis) may be interpreted as dilatation of the urinary tract. There are also a number of nonobstructive causes of upper renal tract dilation, for example, vesicoureteric reflux.

Ultrasound scanning can be used at the same time to assess bladder emptying. This should always be undertaken in patients with lower urinary tract symptoms. A large postmicturition residual volume suggests the presence of bladder outflow obstruction, requiring further urologic investigation and treatment.

Intravenous Urography

Historically, intravenous urography (IVU) was the first-line investigation for suspected upper urinary tract obstruction (136). In patients with normal renal function, it can usually define both the site and the cause of the obstruction. However, the excretion of contrast may be poor or delayed in patients with low GFR because of a decreased filtered load of contrast, and films as long as 1 day after radiocontrast injection may be required. In addition the contrast media is potentially nephrotoxic to an already damaged kidney, particularly in patients older than 60 years and those with diabetes mellitus, preexisting CKD, or dehydration.

As such an IVU should no longer be a first-line investigation to diagnose urinary tract obstruction, especially in patients with impaired renal function.

Computed Tomography

Non-contrast-enhanced spiral CT scanning is used increasingly as the primary imaging modality for the evaluation of patients with acute flank pain (137). Stones are easily detected because of their high density, and CT can provide an accurate and rapid diagnosis of an obstructing ureteral calculus (Fig. 12.9). In addition, it provides useful information regarding the site and nature of the obstructing lesion, especially when it is extrinsic to the urinary tract. CT demonstrates retroperitoneal pathology such as para-aortic and paracaval lymphadenopathy, while retroperitoneal fibrosis is evident as increased attenuation within the retroperitoneal fat, with encasement of one or both ureters. Hematomas, primary ureteral tumors, and polyps are also detectable. Enhancements to the technique such as virtual CT pneumoendoscopy have been described, which may provide an important adjunctive diagnostic aid for urologic pathologies, thus avoiding the need for urinary tract endoscopy (138). The diagnostic potential of CT is also enhanced by the use of contrast, but concerns over nephrotoxicity limit its use in patients with renal impairment. The main drawback of CT remains the considerable exposure to ionizing radiation, making it unsuitable when frequent repetitive examinations may be required.

Magnetic Resonance Urography

MR urography (combined with KUB) can diagnose ureteral obstruction due to renal calculi with similar accuracy to spiral CT scanning but without exposure to a contrast medium or ionizing radiation. It is likely to be increasingly utilized in the future.

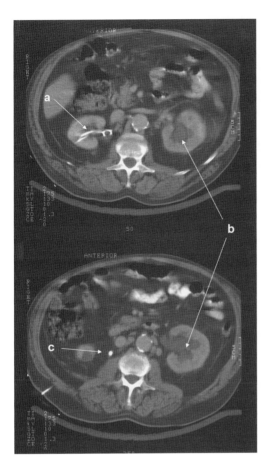

■ **Figure 12.9** Abdominal CT scan of a patient with BUO secondary to renal calculi. In the upper panel, a nephrostome has been inserted into the right kidney **(A)** to decompress the obstruction, while the left kidney remains obstructed and hydronephrotic **(B)**. The lower panel demonstrates a ureteric calculus **(C)**. BUO, bilateral ureteral obstruction; CT, computed tomography.

The technique has less observer variability and is more accurate than CT in detecting indirect evidence of obstruction such as perirenal fluid (139). MR urography can rapidly and accurately depict the morphologic features of dilated urinary tracts and provide information regarding the degree and level of obstruction (140). MR urography also allows functional as well as anatomical parameters of the obstructed kidneys to be determined, as there is an excellent correlation between the GFR determined by MR urography and the isotope GFR (141). However, the possible risk of nephrogenic systemic fibrosis from gadolinium exposure in patients with a GFR <30 mL/min may limit this potential.

MR urography is a particularly attractive imaging modality for the evaluation of hydronephrosis in children as it provides both anatomical and functional data and can indicate whether the hydronephrosis is compensated (symmetrical changes of signal intensity of the nephrogram) or decompensated (142). Signs of decompensation (acute on chronic obstruction) include edema of the renal parenchyma, a delayed and increasingly dense nephrogram, a delayed calyceal transit time, and a >4% difference in the calculated differential renal function.

Retrograde Pyelography

Retrograde pyelography involves the retrograde injection of radiocontrast material and is used to visualize the ureter and the collecting system. This technique may be helpful when nondilated urinary tract obstruction is suspected or when there is a history of allergic reactions to contrast material.

Retrograde pyelography can identify both the site and the cause of the obstruction (143). It is helpful to include a postdrainage film, which is generally obtained 10 minutes after the retrograde injection of the radiocontrast. If the contrast medium does not persist in the collecting system, obstruction is unlikely, although in a patient who is dehydrated, supine, and in the lithotomy position for the performance of the retrograde pyelography, a dilated, but not obstructed, ureter may reveal residual contrast material on a postdrainage film.

Urinary tract infections may occur as a consequence of instrumentation of the urinary tract, and if obstruction is present there is a risk of precipitating overwhelming infection. Hence, if obstruction is diagnosed during retrograde pyelography, it is mandatory to provide adequate drainage of the obstruction to prevent this complication. It may be possible to effectively relieve the obstruction by placing a stent endoscopically in the ureter during the same procedure.

Isotopic Renography (Renal Scintigraphy)

Isotopic renography can be used to determine the functional significance of dilation of the collecting system (144,145). It requires the intravenous injection of the radionuclide technetium-99m mercaptoacetyltriglycine (99mTc-MAG3), combined with intravenous furosemide, administered 20 to 30 minutes after injection of the isotope (diuretic isotopic renography). Normally, there is a rapid washout of the isotope from the kidney. If there is functional dilatation of the collecting system the isotope will be retained in the kidney. However if there is no functional obstruction, the administration of the diuretic should cause a rapid washout of the isotope. Persistence of the isotope suggests that the system is not only dilated but also obstructed. Several tracings are summarized in Figure 12.10. Tracing I is a patient with a normal urinary tract. Tracing II strongly suggests obstruction because the radioisotope is retained in the pelvis and collecting system and there is no excretion following furosemide administration. Tracing III suggests dilatation without obstruction, because after furosemide administration there is rapid disappearance of the isotope. The isotopic renogram is

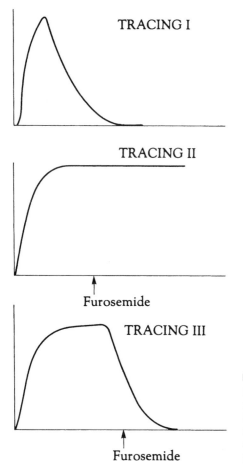

■ Figure 12.10 Pattern of isotopic renography. Tracing 1, normal excretory patter; tracing II, obstruction of the urinary tract; tracing III, stasis of urine with obstruction (From Gonzalez R, Chiou RK. The diagnosis of upper urinary tract obstruction in children: comparison of diuresis renography and pressure flow studies. *J Urol.* 1985; 133: 646–649, with permission.)

relatively noninvasive and can be performed in most hospitals and clinics but is seldom the definitive test. Markedly reduced renal function limits the usefulness of this test because the diuretic response to furosemide may be absent, making interpretation difficult.

Pressure-Flow Studies (Whitaker Test)

Pressure-flow studies may be helpful when upper urinary tract obstruction is difficult to diagnose (146), although with modern imaging it is now rarely required. The collecting system is punctured with a fine-gauge needle, and the bladder is catheterized. Fluid is perfused at a rate of 10 mL/minute. At this perfusion rate, the differential pressure between the bladder and the collecting system should not exceed 15 cm H_2O. A differential pressure >20 cm H_2O indicates obstruction, and a pressure gradient between 15 and 20 cm H_2O is equivocal. The pressure-flow study should be done both with an empty and with a full bladder because sometimes the obstruction is only evident when the bladder is full. An antegrade pyeloureterogram can be performed during pressure-flow studies to define the site of any obstruction, eliminating the need for retrograde pyelography.

Voiding Cystourethrogram

The voiding cystourethrogram is used to investigate the presence of vesicoureteral reflux as a cause of the dilatation of the urinary tract.

Additional Tests to Evaluate Lower Urinary Tract Obstruction

Obstruction of the lower urinary tract may be evaluated by urodynamic studies and cystoscopy. *Cystoscopy* allows visual inspection of the entire urethra and bladder and can usually be carried out under local anesthetic in adults.

Although an IVU with oblique films of the bladder and urethra during voiding (excretory cystogram) and postvoiding can also evaluate the site of lower urinary tract obstruction and the amount of residual urine, this has now largely been superseded by the use of ultrasound, CT, and MR.

Urodynamic tests measuring urine flow rate per unit of time (debimetry) are useful to evaluate bladder outlet obstruction. This test examines the interplay between the expulsive force of the detrusor muscle and urethral resistance (147). The patient voids into a container that has a sensor connected to a recorder that plots micturition time and urine flow rate. From this plot, the urine volume, duration of micturition, average urine flow rate, maximum urine flow, and time required to reach the maximum flow rate can be calculated. The maximum flow rate is useful in assessing bladder outlet obstruction, but the pattern (continuous or intermittent) of flow also is useful. Physiologic filling of the bladder makes this test more reliable. Residual urine may be measured after voiding.

Treatment

GENERAL CONSIDERATIONS

Treatment is dictated by the location of the obstruction, the underlying cause, and the degree of any renal impairment. If renal impairment is present, the treatment of obstruction requires close collaboration between nephrologists and urologists in order to reduce the risks associated with the metabolic and electrolyte consequences of renal failure and to optimize the chances for long-term recovery of renal function. For example, complete bilateral ureteral obstruction presenting as AKI is a medical emergency and requires rapid intervention to salvage renal function. Prompt intervention to relieve the obstruction should result in a rapid improvement in renal function. Dialysis should rarely be required in a patient with AKI secondary to obstruction unless treatment of life-threatening hyperkalemia or severe fluid overload is needed to get the patient fit for intervention. The rapid relief of obstruction will limit permanent renal damage, but renal function may not recover immediately if acute tubular necrosis has occurred as a result of obstruction or any accompanying sepsis.

Surgical intervention can be delayed in patients with low-grade acute obstruction or partial chronic obstruction. However, prompt relief of partial obstruction is indicated when (a) the patient has significant symptoms (flank pain, dysuria, voiding dysfunction), (b) there is urinary retention, (c) there are multiple repeated episodes of urinary tract infection, and (d) there is evidence of progressive renal damage.

MANAGEMENT OF UPPER URINARY TRACT OBSTRUCTION

Calculi

Calculi are a common cause of ureteral obstruction. Their treatment includes relief of pain, elimination of obstruction, and treatment of infection (148). Pain can be relieved by intramuscular injection of a nonsteroidal anti-inflammatory drug (NSAID), which may help dilate the ureter and aid passage of the stone. In some cases a narcotic analgesic may be needed. High fluid intake to increase urine volume to at least 1.5 to 2.0 L daily may also help mobilize the stone. If possible any calculi should be recovered for analysis by straining the urine through a gauze sponge. If the stone is small, the obstruction is partial, there is no infection, and the pain is controlled, expectant management should be followed as many stones will pass spontaneously. Subsequent investigation should be performed to look for metabolic causes for recurrent stone formation and treatment directed accordingly.

Intervention may be required for stones larger than 7 mm, since these usually are not passed spontaneously, or if there is persistent colic, urinary tract infection, complete obstruction, or when the calculus has not moved despite an adequate period of observation and increased fluid intake.

Options for stone removal include:

a.   Open surgery (now rarely required).
b.   Retrograde endoscopic removal using a variety of loops or baskets. This is particularly suitable for calculi located distal to the pelvic brim. This procedure is successful in about 70% of patients. If it fails, dilatation of the ureter or ultrasonic disintegration of the stone can be accomplished using the ureterorendoscope.
c.   Percutaneous nephrolithotomy, where a nephrostome is placed and the track dilated to provide a direct conduit to the kidney for removal of obstructing pelvic and upper ureteral stones. Rigid or flexible endoscopes can be introduced through the nephrostomy tract to remove calculi <1.5 cm in diameter. For larger stones, lithotripter probes that use ultrasonic or electrohydraulic energy to disintegrate calculi have been used under direct visualization. Endourologic methods can be used to treat obstructing stones successfully in about 98% of patients, shortening the hospital stay and the convalescence period.

Extracorporeal shock wave lithotripsy (ESWL) (149) involves the focusing of electrohydraulically or ultrasonically generated shock waves to disintegrate the stone into fragments that then can be easily passed. A ureteral JJ stent is frequently placed to allow the stone fragment to pass more easily and painlessly. The treatment is effective for calculi of 7 to 20 mm, and in 90% of patients, the stone is disintegrated and all particulate matter passes within a 3-month period. It works best for stones located within the kidney and is less successful with ureteric stones. Morbidity is low, and the procedure can be done as an outpatient with rapid return to work. Complications include pain, hematuria, and intrarenal and subcapsular hematoma. Hypertension and worsening CKD have been described, and this may be more common in the elderly with preexisting CKD (150). Damage to surrounding organs is rare.

ESWL should not be performed in the presence of urinary tract sepsis. This requires prompt and aggressive treatment in the face of urinary tract obstruction with the choice of antibiotic depending on appropriate urine culture results and sensitivities. It should be remembered, however, that relief of obstruction is required for antimicrobial therapy to be effective.

Other Specific Therapies

Detailed descriptions of all possible surgical treatments of obstructive uropathy is beyond the scope of this chapter. However the following conditions are commonly encountered in nephrology practice and may be jointly managed with urologists:

a.   *Idiopathic retroperitoneal fibrosis.* In this condition, ureterolysis (in which the ureters are surgically freed from their fibrous encasement) may be beneficial, especially if combined with steroid therapy to prevent recurrence. A recent retrospective study demonstrated the effectiveness of ureteric stent insertion and steroids in idiopathic retroperitoneal fibrosis (151).

b. *Functionally significant PUJ obstruction.* This should be corrected surgically by either an open (Anderson–Hynes pyeloplasty) or laparoscopic approach. The latter results in significantly less morbidity and has good long-term outcomes that are identical to those of the open procedure. Balloon dilation of the abnormal segment of ureter is also possible, but the recurrence rate is high.

c. *Obstruction secondary to neoplastic, inflammatory, or neurologic disease.* This is unlikely to resolve spontaneously, and some form of urinary diversion such as an ileal conduit may be required. Some obstructing neoplastic lesions, such as lymphadenopathy from lymphoma, may respond to chemotherapy.

Nephrostomy

Nephrostomy is the insertion of a tube through the kidney into the renal pelvis to provide urine drainage (152). It is usually undertaken under local anesthetic. Insertion of a nephrostome is generally the appropriate emergency treatment for upper urinary tract obstruction, especially in the setting of AKI. It can be inserted under local anesthetic and should allow rapid recovery of renal function in most patients (>70%), thus avoiding the need for dialysis. Following relief of the obstruction by nephrostomy, the exact site and nature of the obstructing lesion can be determined by infusing X-ray contrast media down the nephrostomy tube (nephrostogram) and time can be taken to plan definitive therapy. Major complications of nephrostomy (abscess, infection, and hematoma) occur in <5% of patients. Bleeding and acute obstruction due to clots may occur, and the tube may become dislodged, requiring immediate replacement.

If both kidneys are obstructed, the nephrostome should initially be placed in the kidney with the most preserved renal parenchyma, though bilateral nephrostomies may be required to maximize the potential for the recovery of renal function. If infection occurs above a ureteral obstruction (pyonephrosis), then drainage of the kidney with nephrostomy tubes can play an important therapeutic role together with appropriate antibiotics.

Nephrostomy can be used to gauge the potential for functional recovery in patients with chronic obstruction. Failure of renal recovery after several weeks of nephrostomy drainage strongly suggests irreversible structural damage, and undertaking a more definitive surgical correction of the obstructing lesion is unlikely to be of benefit. Long-term nephrostomy is increasingly used as a definitive therapy for patients who are unsuitable for major surgical intervention and those with incurable malignant disease.

Cystoscopy and passage of a retrograde ureteral catheter may be considered an alternative to nephrostomy to relieve upper urinary tract obstruction, especially in patients with a bleeding diathesis. However, this may not always be technically possible.

MANAGEMENT OF LOWER URINARY TRACT OBSTRUCTION

Benign prostatic hypertrophy is the most common cause of lower urinary tract obstruction in men and may be mild and nonprogressive. A patient with minimal symptoms, no infection, and a normal upper urinary tract can continue with assessment until he and his physician agree that further treatment is desirable. Medical therapy with either α-adrenergic blockers (e.g., tamsulosin), which relax the smooth muscle of the bladder neck and prostate and decrease urethral pressure and outflow obstruction, or 5α-reductase inhibitors (e.g., finasteride), which inhibit the conversion of testosterone to the active metabolite dihydrotestosterone and reduce prostatic hypertrophy, may be used in patients with moderate symptoms (153). Combination therapy with these agents may be synergistic. Surgical intervention with transurethral resection of the prostate (TURP) is generally required for failed medical treatment, debilitating symptoms, urinary retention, recurrent infection, or evidence of renal parenchymal damage. Holmium laser enucleation of the prostate (HoLEP) is a less invasive alternative to TURP, with good short-term and long-term outcomes (154).

Urethral strictures in men can be treated by dilation or direct-vision internal urethrotomy. The incidence of bladder neck and urethral obstruction in women is low, and treatment is rarely required.

In patients with acute retention of urine, introduction of a urethral catheter is sufficient to relieve symptoms and allow renal function to recover while definitive therapy is planned. If a catheter cannot be passed, a suprapubic cystostomy may be necessary.

Dynamic studies are essential to determine therapy when obstruction is the result of neuropathic bladder function. The main goals of therapy should be (a) to establish the bladder as a urine storage organ, while preventing renal parenchymal injury and (b) to provide a mechanism for bladder emptying that is acceptable to the patient. Two groups of patients are seen: those with atonic bladders secondary to lower motor neuron injury and those with unstable bladder function owing to upper motor neuron disease. In both cases, ureteral reflux and parenchymal damage may develop, although this is more common in patients with a hypertonic bladder. A neurogenic bladder in diabetes mellitus usually is caused by lower motor neuron disease. Voiding at regular intervals achieves satisfactory emptying of the bladder in these patients. The best treatment for patients with significant residual urine and recurrent bouts of urosepsis is the establishment of clean, intermittent catheterization at regular intervals. The goal should be to catheterize four to five times per day such that the amount of urine drained from the bladder does not exceed 400 mL. This useful technique requires patient acceptance and adequate training.

In patients with hypertonic bladder function, the major goal is to improve the storage function of the bladder. The use of anticholinergic agents (e.g., oxybutynin) may be indicated. Occasionally, chronic, clean, intermittent catheterization is necessary.

Chronic indwelling catheters should be avoided, if possible, in all patients with neurogenic bladders. Indwelling catheters usually lead to the formation of bladder stones, urosepsis, urethral erosion, and squamous cell carcinoma of the bladder.

MANAGEMENT OF POSTOBSTRUCTIVE DIURESIS

Postobstructive diuresis refers to the marked polyuria that can occur after relief of obstructive uropathy (45). This polyuria is characterized by the excretion of large amounts of sodium, potassium, magnesium, and other solutes. Although self-limited in duration, the losses of salt and water may result in hypokalemia, hyponatremia or hypernatremia, hypomagnesemia, and/or marked contraction of the ECF volume and peripheral vascular collapse. In many patients, however, a brisk diuresis after relief of obstruction may represent a physiologic response to expansion of the ECF volume occurring during the period of obstruction. This postobstructive diuresis is "appropriate" and does not compromise the volume status of the patient.

Fluid replacement in patients with postobstructive diuresis should be guided by what is excreted. Intravenous and oral fluid replacement is usually required with careful and regular assessment of the patient's fluid balance and serum electrolytes to tailor the fluid replacement regime appropriately. Once the patient is deemed euvolemic, urine losses plus an allowance for insensible losses should be replaced. Urine volume should be measured regularly (hourly), and serum electrolytes should be measured at least daily and as frequently as every 6 hours when there is a massive diuresis. Weighing the patient daily is also helpful. Replacement fluid regimens should include sodium chloride, a source of bicarbonate and potassium. Calcium, phosphate, and magnesium replacement may also be necessary. Orthostatic hypotension and tachycardia are good indicators of when a greater rate of intravenous fluid is required. However, if fluid administration is overzealous, the kidney will not recover its concentrating ability and a continued "driven" diuresis will result. Sometimes to distinguish between a driven diuresis and appropriate excretion of excess fluid, it may be necessary to decrease fluid replacement to levels below those of urine output plus insensible losses and observe the patient carefully for signs of volume depletion.

REFERENCES

1. Klahr S. Nephrology forum: obstructive nephropathy. *Kidney Int.* 1998;54:286–300.
2. Lissauer D, Morris RK, Kilby MD. Fetal lower urinary tract obstruction. *Semin Fetal Neonatal Med.* 2007;12:464–470.
3. Bell ET. *Renal Diseases.* Philadelphia: Lea & Febiger; 1946.
4. U.S. Renal Data System U. *Annual Data Report: Atlas of End-Stage Renal Disease in the United States.* Bethesda, MD: National Institutes of Health, National Institute of Diabetes and Digestive and Kidney Diseases; 2005.
5. Sacks SH, Aparicio SA, Bevan A, et al. Late renal failure due to prostatic outflow obstruction: a preventable disease. *BMJ.* 1989;298:156–159.
6. Harris KPG. Models of obstructive nephropathy. In: Gretz N, Strauch M, eds. *Experimental and*

Genetic Rat Models of Chronic Renal Failure. Basel, Switzerland: Karger; 1993:156–168.

7. Klahr S. New insights into the consequences and the mechanisms of renal impairment in obstructive nephropathy. *Am J Kidney Dis*. 1991;18: 689–699.

8. Chevalier RL, Forbes MS, Thornhill BA. Ureteral obstruction as a model of renal interstitial fibrosis and obstructive nephropathy. *Kidney Int*. 2009; 75(11):1145–1152.

9. Harris RH, Gill JM. Changes in glomerular filtration rate during complete ureteral obstruction in rats. *Kidney Int*. 1981;19:603–608.

10. Dal Canton A, Stanziale R, Corradi A, et al. Effects of acute ureteral obstruction on glomerular hemodynamics in rat kidney. *Kidney Int*. 1977; 12:403–411.

11. Wright FS. Effects of urinary tract obstruction on glomerular filtration rate and renal blood flow. *Semin Nephrol*. 1982;2:5–16.

12. Yarger WE, Aynedjian HS, Bank N. A micropuncture study of postobstructive diuresis in the rat. *J Clin Invest*. 1972;51:625–637.

13. Dal Canton A, Corradi A, Stanziale R, et al. Effects of 24-hour unilateral obstruction on glomerular hemodynamics in rat kidney. *Kidney Int*. 1979;15:457–462.

14. Gaudio KM, Siegel NJ, Hayslett JP, et al. Renal perfusion and intratubular pressure during ureteral occlusion in the rat. *Am J Physiol*. 1980; 238:F205–F209.

15. Dal Canton A, Corradi A, Stanziale, R, et al. Glomerular hemodynamics before and after release of 24-hour bilateral ureteral obstruction. *Kidney Int*. 1980;17:491–496.

16. Moody TE, Vaughan ED Jr, Gillenwater JY. Relationship between renal blood flow and ureteral pressure during 18 hours of total unilateral ureteral occlusion: implications for changing sites of increased renal resistance. *Invest Urol*. 1975; 13:246–251.

17. Moody TE, Vaughan ED Jr, Gillenwater JY. Comparison of the renal hemodynamic response to unilateral and bilateral ureteral occlusion. *Invest Urol*. 1977;14:455–459.

18. Abe Y, Kishimoto T, Yamamoto K, et al. Intrarenal distribution of blood flow during ureteral and venous pressure elevation. *Am J Physiol*. 1973;224: 746–751.

19. Bay WH, Stein JH, Rector JB, et al. Redistribution of renal cortical blood flow during elevated ureteral pressure. *Am J Physiol*. 1972;222:33–37.

20. Edwards GA, Suki WN. Effect of indomethacin on changes of acute ureteral pressure elevation in the dog. *Renal Physiol*. 1978;1:154–165.

21. Solez K, Ponchak S, Buono RA, et al. Inner medullary plasma flow in the kidney with ureteral obstruction. *Am J Physiol*. 1976;231: 1315–1321.

22. Tanner GA. Effects of kidney tubule obstruction on glomerular function in rats. *Am J Physiol*. 1979;237:F379–F385.

23. Ichikawa I. Evidence for altered glomerular hemodynamics during acute nephron obstruction. *Am J Physiol*. 1982;242:F580–F585.

24. Blackshear JL, Edwards BS, Knox FG. Autoregulation of renal blood flow: effects of indomethacin

and ureteral pressure. *Miner Electrolyte Metab*. 1979;2:130–136.

25. Provoost AP, Molenaar JC. Renal function during and after a temporary complete unilateral ureter obstruction in rats. *Invest Urol*. 1981;18: 242–246.

26. Siegel NJ, Feldman RA, Lytton B, et al. Renal cortical blood flow distribution in obstructive nephropathy in rats. *Circ Res*. 1977;40:379–384.

27. Buerkert J, Martin D. Relation of nephron recruitment to detectable filtration and recovery of function after release of ureteral obstruction. *Proc Soc Exp Biol Med*. 1983;173:533–540.

28. Ichikawa I, Purkerson ML, Yates J, et al. Dietary protein intake conditions the degree of renal vasoconstriction in acute renal failure caused by ureteral obstruction. *Am J Physiol*. 1985;249: F54–F61.

29. Purkerson ML, Blaine EH, Stokes TJ, et al. Role of atrial peptide in the natriuresis and diuresis that follows relief of obstruction in rats. *Am J Physiol*. 1989;256:F583–F589.

30. Purkerson ML, Klahr S. Prior inhibition of vasoconstrictors normalizes GFR in postobstructed kidneys. *Kidney Int*. 1989;35:1306–1314.

31. Wilson DR. Micropuncture study of chronic obstructive nephropathy before and after release of obstruction. *Kidney Int*. 1972;2:119–130.

32. Ichikawa I, Brenner BM. Local intrarenal vasoconstrictor-vasodilator interactions in mild partial ureteral obstruction. *Am J Physiol*. 1979;236: F131–F140.

33. Vaughan ED Jr, Sweet RE, Gillenwater JY. Unilateral ureteral occlusion: pattern of nephron repair and compensatory response. *J Urol*. 1973;109: 979–982.

34. Yarger WE, Schocken DD, Harris RH. Obstructive nephropathy in the rat: possible roles for the renin-angiotensin system, prostaglandins, and thromboxanes in postobstructive renal function. *J Clin Invest*. 1980;65:400–412.

35. Schreiner GF, Harris KP, Purkerson ML, et al. Immunological aspects of acute ureteral obstruction: immune cell infiltrate in the kidney. *Kidney Int*. 1988;34:487–493.

36. Rovin BH, Harris KP, Morrison A, et al. Renal cortical release of a specific macrophage chemoattractant in response to ureteral obstruction. *Lab Invest*. 1990;63:213–220.

37. Diamond JR, Kees-Folts D, Ding G, et al. Macrophages, monocyte chemoattractant peptide-1 and transforming growth factor-β in experimental hydronephrosis. *Am J Physiol*. 1994;266: F926–F933.

38. Diamond JR, Kees-Folts D, Ricardo SD, et al. Early and persistent up-regulated expression of renal cortical osteopontin in experimental hydronephrosis. *Am J Pathol*. 1995;146:1455–1466.

39. Ricardo SD, Levinson ME, DeJoseph MR, et al. Expression of adhesion molecules in rat renal cortex during experimental hydronephrosis. *Kidney Int*. 1996;50:2002–2010.

40. Harris KP, Schreiner GF, Klahr S. Effect of leukocyte depletion on the function of the postobstructed kidney in the rat. *Kidney Int*. 1989;36:210–215.

41. Henderson NC, Mackinnon AC, Farnworth SL, et al. Galectin-3 expression and secretion links

macrophages to the promotion of renal fibrosis. *Am J Pathol.* 2008;172:288–298.

42. Kerr WS Jr. Effects of complete ureteral obstruction in dogs on kidney function. *Am J Physiol.* 1956;184:521–526.

43. Bander SJ, Buerkert JE, Martin D, et al. Long-term effects of 24 hour unilateral ureteral obstruction on renal function in the rat. *Kidney Int.* 1985;28:614–620.

44. Buerkert J, Martin D, Head M, et al. Deep nephron function after release of acute unilateral ureteral obstruction in the young rat. *J Clin Invest.* 1978;62:1228–1239.

45. Peterson LJ, Yarger WE, Schocken DD, et al. Postobstructive diuresis: a varied syndrome. *J Urol.* 1975;113:190–194.

46. Vaughan ED Jr, Gillenwater JY. Diagnosis, characterization and management of postobstructive diuresis. *J Urol.* 1973;109:286–292.

47. Buerkert J, Head M, Klahr S. Effects of acute bilateral ureteral obstruction on deep nephron and terminal duct function in the young rat. *J Clin Invest.* 1977;59:1055–1065.

48. Harris RH, Yarger WE. The pathogenesis of postobstructive diuresis: the role of circulating natriuretic and diuretic factors, including urea. *J Clin Invest.* 1975;56:880–887.

49. Sonnenberg H, Wilson DR. The role of medullary collecting ducts in postobstructive diuresis. *J Clin Invest.* 1976;57:1564–1574.

50. Berlyne GM. Distal tubular function in chronic hydronephrosis. *Q J Med.* 1961;30:339–355.

51. McDougal WS, Persky L. Renal functional abnormalities in post-unilateral ureteral obstruction in man: a comparison of these defects to postobstructive diuresis. *J Urol.* 1975;113:601–604.

52. Knowlan D, Corrado M, Schreiner GE, et al. Periureteral fibrosis, with a diabetes insipidus-like syndrome occurring with progressive partial obstruction of a ureter unilaterally. *Am J Med.* 1960;28:22–31.

53. Roussak NJ, Oleesky S. Water-losing nephritis: a syndrome simulating diabetes insipidus. *Q J Med.* 1954;23:147–164.

54. Berlyne GM, Macken A. On the mechanism of renal inability to produce a concentrated urine in chronic hydronephrosis. *Clin Sci.* 1962;22:315–324.

55. Suki WN, Guthrie AG, Martinez-Maldonado M, et al. Effects of ureteral pressure elevation on renal hemodynamics and urine concentration. *Am J Physiol.* 1971;220:38–43.

56. Wilson DR, Knox WH, Sax JA, et al. Postobstructive nephropathy in the rat: relationship between Na-K-ATPase activity and renal function. *Nephron.* 1978;22:55–62.

57. Stokes JB. Effect of prostaglandin E_2 on chloride transport across the rabbit thick ascending limb of Henle: selective inhibition of the medullary portion. *J Clin Invest.* 1979;64:495–502.

58. Campbell HT, Bello-Reuss E, Klahr S. Hydraulic water permeability and transepithelial voltage in the isolated perfused rabbit cortical collecting tubule following acute unilateral ureteral obstruction. *J Clin Invest.* 1985;75:219–225.

59. Fushimi K, Uchida S, Hara Y, et al. Cloning and expression of apical membrane water channel of rat kidney collecting tubule. *Nature.* 1993;361:549–552.

60. Frokiaer J, Marples D, Knepper MA, et al. Bilateral ureteral obstruction downregulates expression of vasopressin-sensitive AQP-2 water channel in rat kidney. *Am J Physiol.* 1996;270:657–658.

61. Frokiaer J, Christensen BM, Marples D, et al. Downregulation of aquaporin-2 parallels changes in renal water excretion in unilateral ureteral obstruction. *Am J Physiol.* 1997;273:F213–F223.

62. Nørregaard R, Jensen BL, Li C, et al. COX-2 inhibition prevents downregulation of key renal water and sodium transport proteins in response to bilateral ureteral obstruction. *Am J Physiol Renal Physiol.* 2005;289:F322–F333.

63. Jensen AM, Li C, Praetorius HA, et al. Angiotensin II mediates downregulation of aquaporin water channels and key renal sodium transporters in response to urinary tract obstruction. *Am J Physiol Renal Physiol.* 2006;291:F1021–F1032.

64. Batlle DC, Arruda JAL, Kurtzman NA. Hyperkalemic distal renal tubular acidosis associated with obstructive uropathy. *N Engl J Med.* 1981;304:373–380.

65. Thirakomen K, Kozlov N, Arruda JAL, et al. Renal hydrogen ion secretion after release of unilateral ureteral obstruction. *Am J Physiol.* 1976;231:1233–1239.

66. Walls J, Buerkert JE, Purkerson ML, et al. Nature of the acidifying defect after the relief of ureteral obstruction. *Kidney Int.* 1975;7:304–316.

67. Purcell H, Bastani B, Harris KPG, et al. Cellular distribution of H^+-ATPase following acute unilateral ureteral obstruction in the rat. *Am J Physiol.* 1991;261:F365–F376.

68. Kimura H, Mujais SK. Cortical collecting duct Na-K pump in obstructive nephropathy. *Am J Physiol.* 1990;258:F1320–F1327.

69. Better OS, Arieff AI, Massry SG, et al. Studies on renal function after relief of complete unilateral ureteral obstruction of three months' duration in man. *Am J Med.* 1973;54:234–240.

70. Purkerson ML, Slatopolsky E, Klahr S. Urinary excretion of magnesium, calcium and phosphate after release of unilateral ureteral obstruction in the rat. *Miner Electrolyte Metab.* 1981;6:182–189.

71. Beck N. Phosphaturia after release of bilateral ureteral obstruction in rats. *Am J Physiol.* 1979;237:F14–F19.

72. Purkerson ML, Rolf DB, Chase LR, et al. Tubular reabsorption of phosphate after release of complete ureteral obstruction in the rat. *Kidney Int.* 1974;5:326–336.

73. Better OS, Tuma S, Kedar S, et al. Enhanced tubular reabsorption of phosphate. *Arch Intern Med.* 1975;135:245–248.

74. Weinreb S, Hruska KA, Klahr S, et al. Uptake of Pi in brush border vesicles after release of unilateral ureteral obstruction. *Am J Physiol.* 1982;243:F29–F35.

75. Kurokawa K, Fine LG, Klahr S. Renal metabolism in obstructive nephropathy. *Semin Nephrol.* 1982;2:31–39.

76. Stokes TJ, Martin KJ, Klahr S. Impaired parathyroid hormone receptor-adenylate cyclase system in

the postobstructed canine kidney. *Endocrinology.* 1985;116:1060–1065.

77. Yanagisawa H, Morrissey J, Morrison AR, et al. Role of ANG II in eicosanoid production by isolated glomeruli from rats with bilateral ureteral obstruction. *Am J Physiol.* 1990;258:F85–F93.

78. Hanley MJ, Davidson K. Isolated nephron segments from rabbit models of obstructive nephropathy. *J Clin Invest.* 1982;69:165–174.

79. Middleton GW, Beamon CR, Panko WB, et al. Effect of ureteral obstruction on the renal metabolism of α-ketoglutarate and other substrates in vivo. *Invest Urol.* 1977;14:255–262.

80. Stecker JF Jr, Vaughan ED Jr, Gillenwater JY. Alteration in renal metabolism occurring in ureteral obstruction in vivo. *Surg Gynecol Obstet.* 1971; 133:846–848.

81. Blondin J, Purkerson ML, Rolf D, et al. Renal function and metabolism after relief of unilateral ureteral obstruction (38976). *Proc Soc Exp Biol Med.* 1975;150:71–76.

82. Morrissey J, Windus D, Schwab S, et al. Ureteral occlusion decreases phospholipid and cholesterol of renal tubular membranes. *Am J Physiol.* 1986; 250:F136–F143.

83. Sawczuk IS, Hoke G, Olsson CA, et al. Gene expression in response to acute unilateral ureteral obstruction. *Kidney Int.* 1989;13:1315–1319.

84. Sheehan HL, Davis JC. Experimental hydronephrosis. *Arch Pathol.* 1959;68:185–225.

85. Shimamura T, Kissane JM, Gyorkey F. Experimental hydronephrosis: nephron dissection and electron microscopy of the kidney following obstruction of the ureter and in recovery from obstruction. *Lab Invest.* 1966;15:629–640.

86. Misseri R, Meldrum KK. Mediators of fibrosis and apoptosis in obstructive uropathies. *Curr Urol Rep.* 2005;6:140–145.

87. Bascands JL, Schanstra JP. Obstructive nephropathy: insights from genetically engineered animals. *Kidney Int.* 2005;68:925–937.

88. Møller JC, Jørgensen TM, Mortensen J. Proximal tubular atrophy: qualitative and quantitative structural changes in chronic obstructive nephropathy in the pig. *Cell Tissue Res.* 1986; 244:479–491.

89. Møller JC, Skriver E. Quantitative ultrastructure of human proximal tubules and cortical interstitium in chronic renal disease (hydronephrosis). *Virchows Arch (A).* 1985;406:389–406.

90. Nagle RB, Bulger RE. Unilateral obstructive nephropathy in the rabbit: II. Late morphologic changes. *Lab Invest.* 1978;38:270–278.

91. Sharma AK, Mauer SM, Kim Y, et al. Interstitial fibrosis in obstructive nephropathy. *Kidney Int.* 1993;44:774–788.

92. Nagle RB, Bulger RE, Cutler RE, et al. Unilateral obstructive nephropathy in the rabbit: I. Early morphologic, physiologic, and histochemical changes. *Lab Invest.* 1973;28:456–467.

93. Kaneto H, Morrissey J, McCracken R, et al. Enalapril reduces collagen type IV synthesis and expansion of the interstitium in the obstructed rat kidney. *Kidney Int.* 1994;45:1637–1647.

94. Kuncio GS, Neilson EG, Haverty T. Mechanisms of tubulointerstitial fibrosis. *Kidney Int.* 1991;39: 550–556.

95. Kaneto H, Morrissey J, Klahr S. Increased expression of TGF-β1 mRNA in the obstructed kidney of rats with unilateral ureteral ligation. *Kidney Int.* 1993;44:313–321.

96. Roberts AB, McCune BK, Sporn MB. TGF-β: regulation of extracellular matrix. *Kidney Int.* 1992; 41:557–559.

97. Lieberthal W, Koh JS, Levine JS. Necrosis and apoptosis in acute renal failure. *Semin Nephrol.* 1998;18:505–518.

98. Chevalier RL. Growth factors and apoptosis in neonatal ureteral obstruction. *J Am Soc Nephrol.* 1996;7:1098–1105.

99. Truong LD, Petrusevska G, Yang G, et al. Cell apoptosis and proliferation in experimental chronic obstructive uropathy. *Kidney Int.* 1996;50: 200–207.

100. Ricardo SD, Diamond JR. The role of macrophages and reactive oxygen species in experimental hydronephrosis. *Semin Nephrol.* 1998; 18:612–621.

101. Ishidoya S, Morrissey J, McCracken R, et al. Angiotensin II receptor antagonist ameliorates renal tubulointerstitial fibrosis caused by unilateral ureteral obstruction. *Kidney Int.* 1995;47: 1285–1294.

102. Klahr S, Morrissey JJ. Comparative study of ACE inhibitors and angiotensin II receptor antagonists in interstitial scarring. *Kidney Int.* 1997;52(suppl 63):S111–S114.

103. Morrissey JJ, Klahr S. Differential effects of ACE and AT1 receptor inhibition on chemoattractant and adhesion molecule synthesis. *Am J Physiol.* 1998;274:F580–F586.

104. Morrissey JJ, Ishidoya S, McCracken R, et al. Nitric oxide generation ameliorates the tubulointerstitial fibrosis of obstructive nephropathy. *J Am Soc Nephrol.* 1996;7:2202–2212.

105. Collins T. Endothelial nuclear factor-kappa B and the initiation of the atherosclerotic lesion. *Lab Invest.* 1993;68:499–508.

106. Baeuerle PA, Henkel T. Function and activation of NF-$k\beta$ in the immune system. *Annu Rev Immunol.* 1994;12:141–179.

107. Wendt T, Zhang YM, Bierhaus A, et al. Tissue factor expression in an animal model of hydronephrosis. *Nephrol Dial Transplant.* 1995;10:1820–1828.

108. Morrissey JJ, Klahr S. Rapid communication. Enalapril decreases nuclear factor kappa B activation in the kidney with ureteral obstruction. *Kidney Int.* 1997;52:926–933.

109. Poli G, Parola M. Oxidative damage and fibrogenesis. *Free Radic Biol Med.* 1997;22:287–305.

110. Shah SV. Role of reactive oxygen metabolites in experimental glomerular disease. *Kidney Int.* 1989;35:1093–1106.

111. Schlondorff D. The role of chemokines in the initiation and progression of renal disease. *Kidney Int.* 1995;47:S44–S47.

112. Modi KS, Morrissey J, Shah SV, et al. Effects of probucol on renal function in rats with bilateral ureteral obstruction. *Kidney Int.* 1990;38: 843–850.

113. Ricardo SD, Ding G, Eufemio M, et al. Antioxidant expression in experimental hydronephrosis: role of mechanical stretch and growth factors. *Am J Physiol.* 1997;272:F789–F789.

114. Chevalier RL, Goyal S, Wolstenholme JT, et al. Obstructive nephropathy in the neonate is attenuated by epidermal growth factor. *Kidney Int.* 1998;54:38–47.

115. Kennedy WA 2nd, Buttyan R, Garcia-Montes E, et al. Epidermal growth factor suppresses renal tubular apoptosis following ureteral obstruction. *Urology.* 1997;49:973–980.

116. Chevalier RL, Goyal S, Kim A, et al. Renal tubulointerstitial injury from ureteral obstruction in the neonatal rat is attenuated by IGF-1. *Kidney Int.* 2000;57:882–890.

117. Kopp JB. Hepatocyte growth factor: mesenchymal signal for epithelial homeostasis. *Kidney Int.* 1998;54:1392–1393.

118. Mizuno S, Matsumoto K, Nakamura T. Hepatocyte growth factor suppresses interstitial fibrosis in a mouse model of obstructive nephropathy. *Kidney Int.* 2001;59:1304–1314.

119. Hruska KA, Guo G, Wozniak M, et al. Osteogenic protein-1 prevents renal fibrogenesis associated with ureteral obstruction. *Am J Physiol Renal Physiol.* 2000;279:F130–F143.

120. Morrissey JJ, Hruska K, Guo G, et al. Bone morphogenetic protein-7 (BMP-7) improves renal fibrosis and accelerates the return of renal function. *J Am Soc Nephrol.* 2002;13:S14–S21.

121. Tan X, Li Y, Liu Y. Paricalcitol attenuates renal interstitial fibrosis in obstructive nephropathy. *J Am Soc Nephrol.* 2006;17:3382–3393.

122. Mao H, Zhou Y, Li Z, et al. HSP72 attenuates renal tubular cell apoptosis and interstitial fibrosis in obstructive nephropathy. *Am J Physiol Renal Physiol.* 2008;295:F202–F214.

123. Santoro J, Kaye D. Recurrent urinary tract infections: pathogenesis and management. *Med Clin North Am.* 1978;62:1005–1020.

124. Crombleholme TM, Harrison MR, Longaker MT, et al. Prenatal diagnosis and management of bilateral hydronephrosis. *Pediatr Nephrol.* 1988;2:334–342.

125. Gray DL, Crane JP. Prenatal diagnosis of urinary tract malformation. *Pediatr Nephrol.* 1988;2:326–333.

126. Coleman BG. Ultrasonography of the upper urinary tract. *Urol Clin North Am.* 1985;12:633–644.

127. Belman AB, Kropp KA, Simon NM. Renal-pressor hypertension secondary to unilateral hydronephrosis. *N Engl J Med.* 1968;278:1133–1136.

128. Nemoy NJ, Fichman MP, Sellers A. Unilateral ureteral obstruction: a cause of reversible high renin content hypertension. *JAMA.* 1973;225:512–513.

129. Palmer JM, Zweiman FG, Assaykeen TA. Renal hypertension due to hydronephrosis with normal plasma renin activity. *N Engl J Med.* 1970;283:1032–1033.

130. Squitieri AP, Ceccarelli FE, Wurster JC. Hypertension with elevated renal vein renins secondary to ureteropelvic junction obstruction. *J Urol.* 1974;111:284–287.

131. Weidmann P, Beretta-Piccoli C, Hirsch D, et al. Curable hypertension with unilateral hydronephrosis: studies of the role of circulating renin. *Ann Intern Med.* 1977;87:437–440.

132. Kaloyanides GJ, Bastron RD, DiBona GF. Effect of ureteral clamping and increased renal arterial pressure on renin release. *Am J Physiol.* 1973;225:95–99.

133. Pelleya R, Oster JR, Perez GO. Hyporeninemic hypoaldosteronism, sodium wasting and mineralocorticoid-resistant hyperkalemia in two patients with obstructive uropathy. *Am J Nephrol.* 1983;3:223–227.

134. Silverman SG, Leyendecker JR, Amis ES Jr. What is the current role of CT urography and MR urography in the evaluation of the urinary tract? *Radiology.* 2009;250:309–323.

135. Mostbeck GH, Zontsich T, Turetschek K. Ultrasound of the kidney: obstruction and medical diseases. *Eur Radiol.* 2001;11:1878–1889.

136. Banner MP, Pollack HM. Evaluation of renal function by excretory urography. *J Urol.* 1980;124:437–443.

137. Pfister SA, Deckart A, Laschke S, et al. Unenhanced helical computed tomography vs intravenous urography in patients with acute flank pain: accuracy and economic impact in a randomized prospective trial. *Eur Radiol.* 2003;13:2513–2520.

138. Croitoru S, Moskovitz B, Nativ O, et al. Diagnostic potential of virtual pneumoendoscopy of the urinary tract. *Abdom Imaging.* 2008;33:717–723.

139. Regan F, Kuszyk B, Bohlman ME, et al. Acute ureteric calculus obstruction: unenhanced spiral CT versus HASTE MR urography and abdominal radiograph. *Br J Radiol.* 2005;78:506–511.

140. Blandino A, Gaeta M, Minutoli F, et al. MR pyelography in 115 patients with a dilated renal collecting system. *Acta Radiol.* 2001;42:532–536.

141. Abou El-Ghar ME, Shokeir AA, Refaie HF, et al. MRI in patients with chronic obstructive uropathy and compromised renal function: a sole method for morphological and functional assessment. *Br J Radiol.* 2008;81:624–629.

142. Grattan-Smith JD, Little SB, Jones RA. MR urography evaluation of obstructive uropathy. *Pediatr Radiol.* 2008;38(suppl 1):S49–S69.

143. McGuire EJ. Retrograde pyelography. In: Rosenfield AT, Glickman MG, Hodson J, eds. *Diagnostic Imaging in Renal Disease.* New York: Appleton-Century-Crofts; 1979:103–112.

144. O'Reilly PH. Diuresis renography 8 years later: an update. *J Urol.* 1986;136:993–999.

145. Powers TA, Grove RB, Baureidel JK, et al. Detection of obstructive uropathy using [99m] technetium diethylenetriaminepentaacetic acid. *J Urol.* 1980;124:588–592.

146. Whitherow RO, Whitaker RH. The predictive accuracy of antegrade pressure flow studies in equivocal upper tract obstruction. *Br J Urol.* 1981;53:496–499.

147. Drach OW, Binard W. Disposable peak urinary flowmeter estimates lower urinary tract obstruction. *J Urol.* 1976;115:175–179.

148. Lemann J Jr, Worcester EM. Nephrolithiasis. In: Massry SO, Glassock RJ, eds. *Textbook of Nephrology.* 2nd ed. Baltimore: Williams & Wilkins; 1989:920–941.

149. Drach GW, Dretler S, Fair W, et al. Report of the United States cooperative study of extracorporeal

shock wave lithotripsy. *J Urol.* 1986;135: 1127–1133.

150. Bataille P, Pruna A, Cardon G, et al. Renal and hypertensive complications of extracorporeal lithotripsy. *Presse Med.* 2000;29:34–38.

151. Fry AC, Singh S, Gunda SS, et al. Successful use of steroids and ureteric stents in 24 patients with idiopathic retroperitoneal fibrosis: a retrospective study. *Nephron Clin Pract.* 2008;108:213–220.

152. Saxton HM. Percutaneous nephrostomy: technique. *Urol Radiol.* 1981;1:131–139.

153. Beckman TJ, Mynderse LA. Evaluation and medical management of benign prostatic hyperplasia. *Mayo Clin Proc.* 2005;80:1356–1362.

154. Suardi N, Gallina A, Salonia A, et al. Holmium laser enucleation of the prostate and holmium laser ablation of the prostate: indications and outcome. *Curr Opin Urol.* 2009;19:38–43.

CHAPTER 13

Renal Physiology and Pathophysiology in Pregnancy

ARUN JEYABALAN AND KIRK P. CONRAD

Renal Physiology

An appreciation of the alterations in renal anatomy and function, as well as volume and osmoregulatory homeostasis during normal gestation, is a prerequisite to complete understanding, proper diagnosis, and management of renal disease and hypertension in gravid women.[1]

ANATOMIC CHANGES

Marked alterations in renal anatomy transpire during normal pregnancy (1). Beginning in the first trimester, overall renal dimensions—length, width, and thickness—increase and peak at 1 cm above prepregnant values during the third trimester (2). This translates into an overall increase in renal volume of ~50% by the end of pregnancy (2) (Fig. 13-1). Both renal parenchymal and pelvicalyceal volumes enlarge, although the latter only starts to increase in the second trimester (Fig. 13-1). Renal parenchymal volume enlarges due to increases in both vascular and interstitial fluid volume; there is little evidence for cellular hyperplasia or hypertrophy (3). There is well-documented dilatation of the upper ureter, renal pelvis, and major and minor calyces, particularly on the right side (see Ref. 1 and citations therein). The causes are disputed but include smooth muscle relaxation by sex steroids and mechanical obstruction of the ureter by dilated arteries and veins as it crosses the pelvic brim, particularly on the right side (1,3), thus causing the "iliac sign," that is, abrupt cutoff of the ureter at the pelvic brim on (IV) pyelography (4). Consequently, urinary stasis and hydronephrosis (with and without calyceal clubbing) are common physiological occurrences in human pregnancy (5) (Fig. 13-2) and usually do not reflect pathologic obstruction. However, urinary stasis may predispose pregnant women to progress from asymptomatic to symptomatic urinary tract infection (UTI) and pyelonephritis (3). Although the more severe signs of this physiological obstruction resolves at least by 6 weeks after delivery, evidence for urinary stasis persists in many women at 12 weeks postpartum (5) (Fig. 13-2).

FUNCTIONAL CHANGES

Renal Hemodynamics and Glomerular Filtration

Several studies of renal function throughout pregnancy in women have been reported over the years (6–11). These investigations are highlighted because of their superior experimental design and meticulous methodologies as previously detailed (1,12). On balance, renal plasma flow (RPF) and glomerular filtration rate (GFR), measured by the renal clearances of para-aminohippurate and inulin, respectively, increase markedly in the first half of pregnancy. Peak levels of approximately 40% to 65% and 50% to

---

[1]Several topics covered in this chapter have been recently reviewed in exhaustive detail by the author(s) elsewhere. Therefore, interested readers are periodically referred to these works for complete renditions and listings of references.

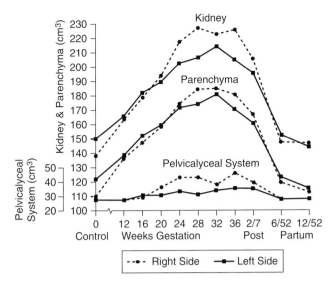

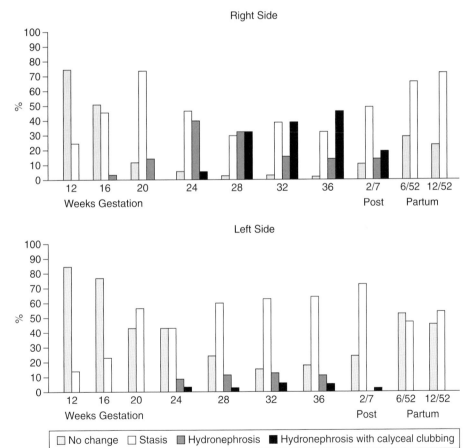

Figure 13.1 Quantitative determination by nephrosonography of total renal and pelvicalyceal volumes, as well as the calculated difference of the two, parenchymal volume, in 34 primigravid women throughout pregnancy and in the postpartum period. The volumes were calculated by the ellipsoid formula, volume = length × width × thickness × 0.5233. 2/7, 6/52, and 12/52 designate day 2, and weeks 6 and 12 postpartum, respectively. (From Cietak KA, Newton JR. Serial quantitative maternal nephrosonography in pregnancy. *Br J Radiol.* 1985;58(689): 405–413, with permission).

Figure 13.2 Qualitative determination by nephrosonography of the right and left upper urinary tracts throughout pregnancy and the postpartum period in the same women as described in Figure 1. No change, absence of visible urine in the renal pelvis seen on both longitudinal and/or transverse planes; urinary stasis, slight separation of the renal pelvis observed on both longitudinal and/or transverse planes; hydronephrosis, marked dilation, and wide separation of the renal pelvis seen on both longitudinal and/or transverse planes; hydronephrosis with calyceal clubbing, dilation of the renal pelvis accompanied by filling and clubbing of the major and minor renal calyces. 2/7, 6/52, and 12/52 designate day 2, and weeks 6 and 12 postpartum, respectively. (From Cietak KA, Newton JR. Serial qualitative maternal nephrosonography in pregnancy. *Br J Radiol.* 1985; 58(689): 399–404, with permission).

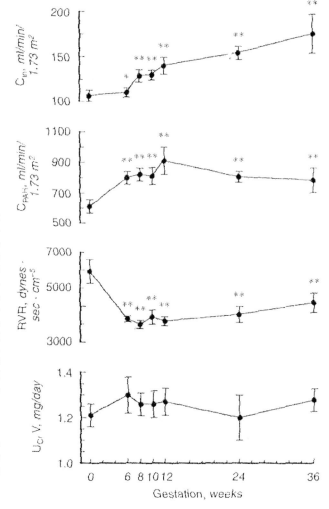

■ Figure 13.3 Renal hemodynamic changes throughout early human pregnancy. Ten women were studied in the mid-follicular phase of the menstrual cycle and weeks 6, 8, 10, 12, 24, and 36 of gestation. RPF and GFR increased significantly in association with a decrease in renal vascular resistance by week 6 gestation. $*p < 0.05$, $**p < 0.001$ versus mid-follicular. Note that authors normalized renal function by body surface area. However, because gestational changes in RPF and glomerular filtration are functional and not anatomical in nature, such normalization will underestimate true values. *Abbreviations:* C_{In}, inulin clearance; C_{PAH}, para-aminohippurate clearance; RVR, renal vascular resistance. (From Chapman AB et al. Temporal relationships between hormonal and hemodynamic changes in early human pregnancy. *Kidney Int.* 1998; 54(6): 2056–2063, with permission).

85% above prepregnant or postpartum values are reached for GFR and RPF, respectively. In general, GFR remains at elevated levels throughout pregnancy, whereas RPF tends to decline in the later stages, but still remains well above the nonpregnant control values. The study of Chapman et al. is particularly comprehensive because it included measurements of renal function before pregnancy in the follicular phase of the menstrual cycle and at several time points during the first trimester (11) (Fig. 13-3). This investigation nicely illustrates that both RPF and GFR increase dramatically in the first trimester, which corroborates an earlier investigation by Davison et al., who also showed a rapid increase in the 24-hour endogenous creatinine clearance during the first trimester (13). As a consequence of the rise in GFR, both serum creatinine and urea concentrations reset to lower values of approximately 0.5 and 9.0 mg/dL, respectively, during normal pregnancy (12).

During late pregnancy, when a pregnant woman is supine, the enlarged uterus can compress the great veins, thereby impeding venous return, cardiac output, and renal perfusion. Thus, RPF and GFR can be reduced depending on the posture, with left lateral recumbency being the least compromising (see Ref. 14 and citations therein). Interestingly, despite compensatory anatomical and functional hypertrophy, the renal allograft and single kidney can adapt even further undergoing gestational hyperfiltration, albeit somewhat subdued compared to normal pregnancy (15,16).

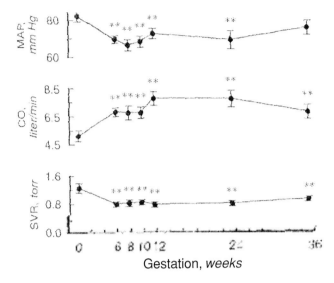

■ **Figure 13.4** Systemic hemodynamic changes throughout early human pregnancy. Ten women were studied in the mid-follicular phase of the menstrual cycle and weeks 6, 8, 10, 12, 24, and 36 of gestation. Systemic vascular resistance (SVR) and mean arterial pressure (MAP) decreased and cardiac output (CO) increased significantly by week 6 of gestation. $*p < 0.05$, $**p < 0.001$ versus mid-follicular. (From Chapman AB et al. Temporal relationships between hormonal and hemodynamic changes in early human pregnancy. *Kidney Int*. 1998; 54(6): 2056–2063, with permission).

The rise in RPF is a consequence of a sharp decline in renal vascular resistance (Fig. 13-3). Indeed, vasodilation of maternal nonreproductive organs, including the kidneys, accounts for the overall decline in systemic vascular resistance and an increase in cardiac output that occurs early in gestation (11,17–19); Fig. 13-4). Both afferent and efferent renal arteriolar resistances decline such that glomerular capillary pressure is unchanged (10,20,21). Thus, the increase in GFR is mainly a consequence of the rise in RPF, although small decreases in plasma oncotic pressure and increases in K_f may contribute (10,20,21).

Interestingly, the renal and systemic hemodynamic changes of pregnancy are anticipated in the luteal phase of the menstrual cycle when RPF, GFR, and cardiac output increase, albeit to a lesser degree (22) (Ref. 12 for review), thus implicating a role for hormones produced by the corpus luteum of the ovary: steroids and/or protein hormones. Estrogen has little or no influence on the renal circulation, although progesterone may increase RPF and GFR, but not to the same extent as observed during pregnancy (see Ref. 12 and citations therein). Relaxin, another hormone secreted by the corpus luteum, circulates during the luteal phase of the menstrual cycle, and then increases dramatically in the first trimester of pregnancy being stimulated primarily by human chorionic gonadotropin (hCG) produced in placental trophoblast cells (23). When administered to conscious rats and humans, relaxin increases RPF, GFR, and cardiac output, thereby mimicking the changes observed during pregnancy (see Ref. 24 and citations therein). Conversely, administration of relaxin-neutralizing antibodies to gravid rats prevents the rise in RPF, GFR and cardiac output at least during mid-gestation (25,26) (Figs. 13-5 and 13-6). Similarly, the rise in GFR during the first trimester as measured by the 24-hour endogenous creatinine clearance is subdued in women with ovarian failure who conceive by egg donation, in vitro fertilization (IVF), and embryo transfer, and who lack a corpus luteum, and thus circulating relaxin (27). Thus, relaxin may be one important hormone that initiates renal and systemic vasodilation during pregnancy.

The vasodilatory responses of relaxin are transduced by its major receptor, the leucine-rich repeat-containing G-protein-coupled receptor, Lgr7 (28,29). The *rapid* vasodilatory responses of relaxin (within minutes) are mediated by a phosphotidylinositol-3 (PI3) kinase/Akt (protein kinase B)-dependent phosphorylation and activation of endothelial nitric oxide synthase (29,30). *Sustained* vasodilatory responses (hours to days) are dependent on vascular placental and/or vascular endothelial growth factors (VEGFs), and an increase in gelatinase(s) activity (12,24,29,31,32). The latter processes big endothelin (ET)-1 at a gly–leu bond to form $ET_{1–32}$, which activates the endothelial ET_B/nitric oxide (NO) vasodilatory pathway (12,24,29) (Fig. 13-7). Notably, blockade of the same molecular intermediates

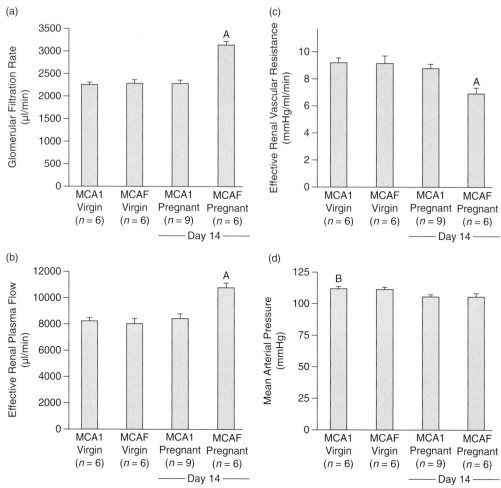

■ **Figure 13.5** Renal function in conscious virgin and day 14 pregnant rats treated with rat relaxin-neutralizing antibody (MCA1) or control antibody (MCAF). (**a**) GFR. (**b**) ERPF. (**c**) ERVR. (**d**) MAP. $^A p < 0.01$ versus other groups; $^B p \leq 0.05$ versus MCA1 and MCAF pregnant. Identical findings were observed on gestation day 11. (From Novak J et al. Relaxin is essential for renal vasodilation during pregnancy in conscious rats. *J Clin Invest*. 2001; 107(11): 1469–1475, with permission).

during pregnancy, that is, gelatinase(s) (33,34), the ET_B receptor (35,36), or NO (36–38), inhibits gestational renal vasodilation, hyperfiltration, and the loss of myogenic reactivity in small renal arteries (another prototypical phenotype of normal pregnancy), thus consistent with the crucial role of relaxin in the renal hemodynamic changes of pregnancy (Fig. 13-5, vide supra).

Another mechanism that contributes to maternal vasodilation of pregnancy is refractoriness to the systemic pressor effects of vasoconstrictors such as angiotensin II (39). Interestingly, renal vasoconstriction to angiotensin II is also blunted during pregnancy in the conscious gravid rat model (37,40), an effect that is mimicked by administering relaxin to nonpregnant animals (41). In addition to nitric oxide (42), vasodilatory prostaglandins have been implicated as mediators of vasodilation in pregnancy; however, with few exceptions, a major role has not been substantiated (see Ref. 12 and citations therein). Finally, volume expansion has also been suggested as initiating the hemodynamic changes of pregnancy. But, the timing of events is not supportive of this hypothesis because the increase in plasma volume lags behind the more rapid increases in RPF, GFR, and cardiac output during early pregnancy (43) (Fig. 13-8). Thus, volume expansion likely abets, but does not initiate the remarkable hyperdynamic circulation of pregnancy.

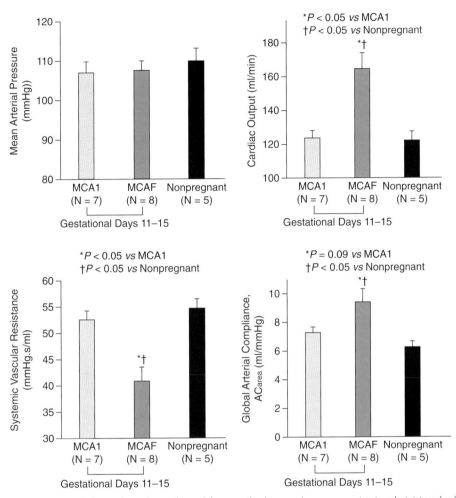

■ Figure 13.6 Systemic hemodynamics and arterial properties in conscious pregnant rats administered relaxin-neutralizing antibody (MCA1) or control antibody (MCAF), and in conscious nonpregnant rats. Pregnant rats were administered daily IV infusions of antibodies beginning on gestational day 8. $*p < 0.05$ versus MCA1, $†p < 0.05$ versus nonpregnant (post hoc Fisher's LSD). There were no differences between phosphate buffered saline (antibody vehicle) and MCAF in midterm pregnant rats. MCA1 did not affect mean arterial pressure, renal hemodynamics, and glomerular filtration in nonpregnant rats (25), nor does relaxin circulate in nonpregnant rats (23). (From Debrah DO et al. Relaxin is essential for systemic vasodilation and increased global arterial compliance during early pregnancy in conscious rats. *Endocrinology.* 2006; 147(11): 5126–5131, with permission.)

Renal Tubular Function

Glucose

Plasma glucose is freely filtered at the glomerulus. Normally, it is reabsorbed in the proximal tubules by a sodium-dependent cotransport mechanism. Thus, only vanishingly small amounts are excreted (44,45). In normal human pregnancy, however, glucosuria is a frequent occurrence (1,46–48). Both the amount and the pattern of excretion throughout the day are variable among women and within the same woman from day to day (46–48). Restoration of glucose excretion to nonpregnant levels occurs within the first postpartum week (46,47).

The renal handling of glucose during pregnancy was investigated thoroughly (49–51). Factors contributing to glucosuria are the increased filtered load by virtue of the rise in GFR, thus overwhelming

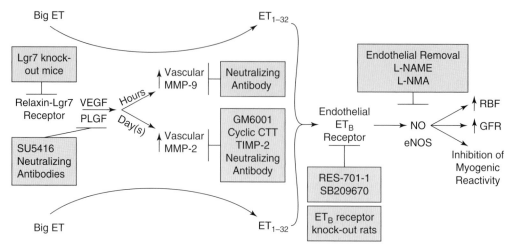

■ **Figure 13.7** Working model for the sustained vasodilatory actions of relaxin. ⊣, indicates inhibitors of relaxin vasodilation; VEGF and PGF, vascular endothelial and placental growth factor activities, respectively; ET, endothelin; MMP, matrix metalloproteinase; RBF, renal blood flow; GFR, glomerular filtration rate; SU5416, an inhibitor of VEGF receptor tyrosine kinase; GM6001, a general MMP inhibitor; cyclic CTT, a specific peptide inhibitor of MMP-2; TIMP-2, tissue inhibitor of metalloproteinase; RES-701-1, a specific ET$_B$ receptor antagonist; SB209670, a mixed ET$_A$ and ET$_B$ receptor antagonist; L-NAME, nitro-L-arginine methyl ester; L-NMA, NG-monomethyl-L-arginine. Note that phosphoramidon (an inhibitor of the classical endothelin-converting enzyme), STT (control peptide for cyclic CTT), heat-inactivated TIMP-2, BQ-123 (a specific ET$_A$ receptor antagonist), D-NAME, and IgGs (control antibodies for MMP-neutralizing antibodies) did not affect the slow vasodilator actions of relaxin.

■ **Figure 13.8** Time course of maternal adaptations to pregnancy. *Abbreviations*: CO, cardiac output; PV, plasma volume; GFR, glomerular filtration rate; PNa, plasma sodium concentration; Posm, plasma osmolality; Ppr, plasma protein concentration; palb, plasma albumin concentration; Pcr, plasma creatinine concentration; SVR, systemic vascular resistance; Purea, plasma urea concentration. (From Davision JM et al. Renal physiology in normal pregnancy. In: Feehally J, Floege J, Johnson RJ, eds. *Comprehensive Clinical Nephrology*. St. Louis, MI: Mosby Inc.; 2004: 475–481, with permission)

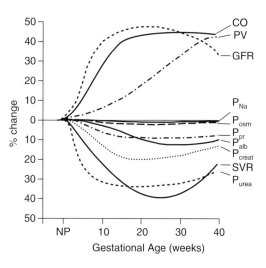

tubular reabsorption in some nephrons, and reduced tubular reabsorption (49–51). In gravid women with excessive amounts of glucosuria (>150 mg/24 h), underlying tubular damage resulting from a prior renal infection may exist (52). Increased urinary excretion of glucose and other nutrients (see later), in concert with the propensity for urinary stasis (vide supra) are likely major predisposing factors for symptomatic UTIs and pyelonephritis in pregnant women (see Renal Pathophysiology section).

Amino Acids

Amino acids are freely filtered at the glomerulus, and subsequently reabsorbed in proximal tubules by several different sodium-dependent cotransporters, each absorbing amino acid(s) belonging to a certain class (44). Thus, normally, only vanishingly small amounts are excreted in the urine. However, urinary excretion of most amino acids increases during pregnancy (1,53). Like glucosuria, aminoaciduria begins early in pregnancy corresponding with the rapid increase in GFR and filtered load. Another parallel is that the tubular reabsorptive capacity is reduced. Although these renal mechanisms contribute to reductions in plasma concentrations of many amino acids during pregnancy, urinary losses are not likely to be clinically relevant except in the face of poor nutritional intake.

Uric Acid

Uric acid is the end product of purine catabolism in humans (54). Purines derive from the diet and are produced endogenously mainly by the liver, the latter being the major source of uric acid. Approximately two-thirds and one-third of uric acid produced is excreted by the kidney and gastrointestinal tract, respectively. Uric acid is freely filtered at the glomerulus except for 5% that is protein bound. The filtered uric acid undergoes both reabsorption and secretion, mainly in the proximal tubule, but overall, net reabsorption occurs from 88% to 93%. Serum concentrations of uric acid decrease by 25% to 30% throughout early pregnancy rising toward nonpregnant levels near term (14,55–58). Of the various factors that could determine serum uric acid levels, renal handling has been investigated the most. Like glucose and amino acids, the renal clearance of uric acid is increased as a consequence of elevated GFR and filtered load, reduced tubular reabsorption, or both. In one study, the restoration in serum uric acid concentration in late pregnancy was associated with the restoration of tubular reabsorption (14,56,58).

Calcium

Approximately 46% of calcium is bound to protein, so that 54% is available for glomerular filtration. The majority, 98% to 99%, is reabsorbed by the kidneys. About 70% of the filtered load is reabsorbed by the proximal tubules, 20% by the medullary thick ascending limb of Henle, and the remainder by more distal nephron segments. The daily urinary excretion of calcium approximately matches net intestinal absorption (59). During normal pregnancy, 24-hour urinary calcium excretion virtually doubles during the first trimester and is maintained throughout pregnancy (1,60–63). Serum-ionized calcium remains constant or may decrease slightly (60,64). Both elevated filtered load by virtue of increasing GFR and reduced tubular reabsorption likely contribute to elevated calcium excretion (60–63). Although the reports of parathyroid hormone concentration are conflicting, investigators who measured the intact, active molecule rather than metabolic fragments report a decrease (65,66), which may contribute to decreased tubular reabsorption. Ultimately, however, the gestational increase in urinary calcium excretion most likely reflects enhanced intestinal uptake. The latter is stimulated by elevated serum 1,25-dihydoxyvitamin D_3 in pregnancy (60,64,67–69), the hormone mainly responsible for intestinal calcium absorption (59). The tissue source of increased circulating 1,25-dihydoxyvitamin D_3 in pregnancy may be the placenta (70). In pregnant women who are vitamin-D deficient, relative hypocalciuria is observed (77 mg/24 h) when compared to nonpregnant (119 mg/24 h) and vitamin D-supplemented pregnant (169 mg/24 h) women (71). Calciuric and calcemic responses to an oral calcium load are augmented in all trimesters, indicating enhanced intestinal absorption, and leading to the concept of the "physiologic absorptive hypercalciuria" of pregnancy (60). The early onset of this physiological adaptation, associated with elevated serum concentrations of 1,25-dihydoxyvitamin D_3 before fetal calcium requirements for skeletal mineralization are much increased, suggests their anticipatory nature. Despite gestational increases in urinary calcium excretion and urinary supersaturations comparable to women with stone disease, pregnancy does not predispose to calcium stones or pathologic crystalluria, possibly due to more abundant glycoprotein inhibitors in the urine of pregnant women (62,72) (see Renal Pathophysiology section).

Proteins

The urinary excretion of various proteins including low-molecular-weight proteins, albumin, and several renal tubular enzymes increases during normal pregnancy, but is not considered to be abnormal unless total protein exceeds 300 mg/24 h (see Ref. 14 and citations therein). The elevated urinary excretion of low-molecular-weight proteins and tubular enzymes supports the concept of a "physiologic impairment of proximal tubular function" in pregnancy, which is consistent with the finding of increased urinary excretion and reduced tubular absorption of glucose, amino acids, uric acid, and calcium (vide supra). In addition to reduced proximal tubular absorption, gestational hyperfiltration and potential alteration in charge, but not in size glomerular permselectivity, likely contribute. To what extent Tamm–Horsefall protein secretion increases, thereby contributing to the relative proteinuria of normal pregnancy, has not been investigated in detail.

Potassium

It is generally accepted that women accumulate approximately 350 mEq of potassium by the end of pregnancy, the majority residing within cells of fetal tissues and maternal reproductive organs (reviewed in Ref. 3). Paradoxically, potassium retention during pregnancy occurs in the face of marked increases in circulating aldosterone. Shedding light on this paradox are the pioneering clinical investigations of Lindheimer et al., which showed that pregnant women are resistant to the combined kaliuretic actions of both exogenous mineralocorticoids and high dietary sodium intake (73). The prevailing view is that the high serum concentrations of progesterone, a mineralocorticoid receptor antagonist, oppose the kaliuretic influence of aldosterone during pregnancy (3,73). Supporting this concept is the rare genetic disorder in which mutation of the mineralocorticoid receptor confers agonist rather than antagonist activity of progesterone. Thus, during pregnancy, heterozygous women manifest sodium retention, potassium wasting, and hypokalemia, as well as hypertension despite undetectable serum aldosterone (74).

Hydrogen Ion

Most likely secondary to the central action of progesterone during pregnancy (75), minute ventilation rises by approximately 40% solely due to an increase in tidal volume without a change in respiratory rate (76). Consequently, PCO_2 falls from approximately 39 Torr in the nonpregnant condition to 31 Torr, resulting in a chronic respiratory alkalosis. The metabolic (renal) compensation for this primary event leads to a decline in plasma bicarbonate from 22 to 26 mEq/L in the nonpregnant state to approximately 18 to 22 mEq/L during pregnancy such that compensated blood pH is typically 7.42 to 7.44 compared with nonpregnant values of 7.38 to 7.40 (76). The decline in plasma bicarbonate is most likely a consequence of slight, but persistent urinary bicarbonate loss beginning at lower plasma bicarbonate concentrations compared with the nonpregnant condition (77). There is no deficit in urinary acidification, or titratable acid and ammonium secretion during normal pregnancy (see Ref. 3 and citations therein).

Osmoregulation and Renal Handling of Water

Plasma osmolality (Posm) decreases by 8 to 10 mOsm/kg H_2O during the first trimester of normal human pregnancy and is sustained until term (78). Although approximately 1.5 mOsm/kg H_2O can be ascribed to the decline in urea, the majority is secondary to a fall in sodium and its attendant anions. One explanation for the gestational decrease in Posm is that the osmotic threshold for stimulation of thirst and of vasopressin release decline concurrently (the so-called "reset osmostat" hypothesis). In fact, according to this hypothesis, the osmotic set-point for both of these changes in parallel, that is, one cannot occur without the other and still maintain reduced Posm (79).

One important factor that may effect resetting of the osmostat, thereby contributing to the gestational decrease in Posm, is the ovarian (corpus luteal) hormone, relaxin. This assertion is supported by several lines of evidence: (i) chronic administration of rhRLX decreases osmolality in rats (41,80,81); (ii) chronic administration of hCG decreases Posm in women but not in men (79), and in sham-ovariectomized but not ovariectomized rats, suggesting the intermediary role of ovarian hormone (82); (iii) Posm declines in the luteal phase of the menstrual cycle (22), when serum relaxin increases (23); (iv) the decline in Posm during the first trimester is subdued in women who conceive by egg donation, IVF, and embryo transfer—these women lack corpora lutea and circulating relaxin, but normal progesterone levels are maintained for luteal support by exogenous administration (27); (v) gravid rats show a reduction in Posm and an increase in water consumption, which is prevented by relaxin-neutralizing antibodies or ovariectomy (while maintaining pregnancy with exogenous estradiol and progesterone in the latter) (25,83); and (vi) Posm does not decline in gravid ewes, a species in which relaxin is not produced due to a stop codon in the gene (83,84).

While the evidence for a role of relaxin in the gestational fall in Posm is compelling, it may not be the only factor in humans (27,83). Also, the hormone causes systemic vasodilation within and outside of pregnancy (vide supra), which can decrease "effective arterial circulating volume" that may also contribute to lowering Posm in pregnancy secondary to nonosmotic release of vasopressin. However, experiments involving head-out water immersion in pregnant women, a maneuver that redistributes body fluid from the caudal regions to the intrathoracic circulation, thereby decreasing the "underfill" stimulus, failed to reverse gestational hyposmolality (79). One caveat to this methodological approach is that by necessity it entails short- but not long-term fluid redistribution, and possibly the latter is required to reverse gestational hypoosmolality. However, this caveat is addressed to some degree by investigations in the gravid rodent model, insofar as chronic elevations in blood volume and pressure achieved by administration of mineralocorticoids and norepinephrine, respectively, also failed to reverse gestational hypoosmolality (85,86). On balance, these experiments in pregnant women and rats fail to support the nonosmotic hypothesis for AVP release in pregnancy. Finally, it is known that relaxin can act directly on the subfornical organ and organ vasculosum of the subfornical organ in the hypothalamus to release AVP and stimulate thirst (83,87), thereby obviating the need to invoke indirect hemodynamic or volume regulatory mechanisms.

More recently, the basal expression of aquaporin-2 mRNA and protein was reported to be increased in the inner medulla of pregnant rats (88). Thus, in addition to central mechanisms, renal alterations may contribute to water retention, and hence hypoosmolality during pregnancy. The mechanism for increasing renal aquaporin-2 expression remains a significant question. However, based on the considerable evidence cited earlier for relaxin's role in the osmoregulatory adaptations of pregnancy, this hormone is a prime suspect (K.P. Conrad and L.J. Parry, unpublished data). Finally, some have argued that an increase in basal expression of aquaporin-2 during pregnancy is not consistent with the finding that gravid women and animals excrete a water load normally (see later). However, this apparent paradox may be resolved, if during the imposition of water loading, the mechanism(s) responsible for the basal increase in aquaporin-2 expression are superseded.

Despite the gestational decline in Posm, gravid women and rats operate more or less normally around the lower osmotic set-point by appropriately diluting and concentrating urine as tested during water loading and fluid restriction, respectively (see Ref. 3 and citations therein). Of clinical relevance is the phenomenon of "transient diabetes insipidus (DI) of pregnancy," which typically presents in the second half of pregnancy and remits postpartum. These women may have partial central DI with sufficient vasopressin reserves to function normally when not pregnant, but become clinically DI during pregnancy secondary to the large increase in vasopressinase produced by the trophoblast cells of the placenta. Alternatively, vasopressinase may be unusually and idiopathically high in otherwise normal pregnant women, or there may be a degree of hepatic dysfunction as in preeclampsia or acute fatty liver of pregnancy that contributes to reduced metabolism of vasopressinase, thereby leading to increased circulating levels (78). The potential clinical danger is profound hypernatremia that must be treated.

What is the purpose of the physiological decline in Posm during pregnancy? Although this mechanism contributes to the increase in plasma volume, which correlates with successful maternal and fetal outcomes, it makes only a minor contribution because the retained "free water" is distributed to the various body fluid compartments in proportion to their original size. Thus, being the largest body fluid compartment, the intracellular water space experiences the greatest absolute increase in volume by this mechanism. Teleologically speaking, this water reserve may have evolved during evolution, being important for survival of the pregnancy during droughts experienced by our predecessors in prehistoric times.

Volume Homeostasis and Renal Handling of Sodium

Total body water increases by approximately 8 L of water during normal human pregnancy. Most of this increase is in the extracellular space, about 6 L. Two compartments of the extracellular space, maternal plasma and interstitial volumes, increase by approximately ~1.5 and ~2.5 L, respectively. The increase in plasma volume begins in the first trimester, accelerating during the second and peaking near 34 gestational weeks, whereas interstitial fluid accumulation is most prominent in the third trimester (reviewed in Ref. 3).

TABLE 13.1 ANTINATRIURETIC AND NATRIURETIC INFLUENCES DURING NORMAL PREGNANCY

Antinatriuretic

Hormonal Factors
- Aldosterone, deoxycorticosterone
- Cortisol
- Angiotensin II
- Renal sympathetic nerve activity
- Increase renal cGMP-specific phosphodiesterase
- Estrogen

Physical Factors
- Maternal vascular shunt (e.g., kidneys, early gestation)
- Uteroplacental shunt (late gestation)
- Supine and standing posture
- Decrease renal interstitial hydrostatic pressure

Natriuretic

Hormonal Factors
- Atrial natriuretic peptide
- Digoxin-like substance
- Renal prostaglandins
- Progesterone
- Relaxin (at least acutely)
- Oxytocin

Physical Factors
- Increase GFR
- Decrease plasma oncotic pressure
- Decrease filtration fraction

Because sodium content is the primary determinant of extracellular volume, the increase in the extracellular space during normal human pregnancy is mainly due to retention of ~950 mEq of sodium and attendant anions. This retention is quite remarkable in light of the marked increase in GFR, and hence, filtered load of sodium, the latter increasing by as much as 10,000 mEq/24 h during pregnancy! There are a number of antinatriuretic and natriuretic factors influencing renal sodium handling during pregnancy as summarized in Table 13.1. Ultimately, however, we do not completely understand the mechanisms for sodium retention and volume expansion during pregnancy, but a few possibilities are highlighted in the following text.

It is certainly attractive to believe that, in the face of the rapid and profound decreases in systemic vascular resistance in early pregnancy due primarily to vasodilation of maternal nonreproductive organs such as the kidneys, an "underfill" condition transpires (i.e., decrease in "effective arterial circulating volume"), which initiates renal sodium and water retention, and increases of extracellular and plasma volume by stimulating sympathetic activity and the renin–angiotensin–aldosterone axis (19,89). Later in gestation, decrease in the uteroplacental vascular resistance contributes to this "underfill" stimulus.

Therefore, in one sense, the nonreproductive organs in early pregnancy act as "arteriovenous" shunts that initiate the marked increase in cardiac output, and consequently, the narrowing of the arterial-mixed venous oxygen content difference as oxygen delivery exceeds metabolic demands (19,90). However, because pregnancy is a physiological condition and an epitome of homeostatic balance, there is tight coupling between the "underfill" stimulus and the compensatory increase in volume such that the two events are contemporaneous and have not been unequivocally dissociated, except perhaps in two studies (17,91). These remarkable maternal adaptations that occur mainly during the first half of pregnancy are apparently anticipatory in nature, that is, in anticipation of the progressively increasing demand for blood flow, and oxygen and nutrient delivery by the fetus and placenta especially in the second half of pregnancy.[2]

---

[2]An agricultural analogy may be used to illustrate the importance of the early increase in cardiac output and consequent plasma volume expansion in early pregnancy, that is, it is more beneficial to construct irrigation canals to water new crops (analogous to the fetal–placental unit) from the Mississippi (equivalent to the gravid circulatory system) rather than the Rio Grande river (nongravid circulation).

Consequently, by many indirect measures, pregnancy is a "normal-fill" condition. For example, gravidae can excrete a water load and dilute their urine as well as nongravidae, and their circulating levels of AVP are comparable to nonpregnant subjects (see Osmoregulation and Renal Handling of Water section). In response to saline infusions, increase in urinary sodium excretion is comparable between pregnant and nonpregnant women (92,93). These observations contrast markedly with the pathophysiological states of cirrhosis and congestive heart failure, in which despite the massive increases in extracellular volume, there is "decreased effective circulatory volume." These patients fail to excrete a water load or dilute their urine adequately, basal levels of AVP are elevated, and sodium excretion is decreased (89). Finally, in gravid rats, tubuloglomerular feedback sensitivity is not suppressed as would be expected in the face of the absolute increase in plasma volume, but is reset around the higher level of single nephron GFR during pregnancy (94). This observation suggests that the volume status of pregnancy is indeed perceived as "normal-fill" by the kidney.

Interestingly, another mechanism for sodium retention in rat pregnancy is increased renal phosphodiesterase-5 activity that, in turn, decreases atrial natriuretic peptide (ANP)-dependent cGMP accumulation, thereby impairing sodium excretion (95,96). However, whether this mechanism pertains to human pregnancy needs to be investigated because there does not appear to be an attenuation of the natriuretic response to ANP (97). Moreover, the fractional excretion of cGMP increases from ~1.0 in the prepregnant (or postpartum) state to ~2.0 during pregnancy suggesting elevated, not reduced nephrogenous cGMP production (98).

Another potential, intriguing mechanism for volume retention during pregnancy relates to renal interstitial hydrostatic pressure (RIHP). Natriuretic and diuretic responses to increases in renal perfusion pressure (RPP) are associated with increases in RIHP (99,100). RIHP is reduced at any given RPP in both midterm and late pregnant rats, which is dictated by an increase in the compliance of the renal capsule and interstitium (101). Indeed, one possible chain of events is that there is a primary increase in the compliance of the renal capsule and interstitium during early pregnancy, which reduces RIHP that, in turn, attenuates natriuresis and diuresis, thereby promoting gestational sodium and water retention (102). This decrease in RIHP may also be abetted by the normal gestational decline in blood pressure. An increase in renal capsular compliance would also accommodate the 50% increase in renal volume that is observed during normal gestation (at least in women—vide supra). In light of relaxin's role in other maternal cardiovascular and renal adaptations to pregnancy including the increases in arterial compliance (vide supra), and its well-known matrix-degrading properties (83,103), this hormone is an attractive candidate molecule for mediating the increase in renal interstitial and capsular compliance during pregnancy.

Renal Pathophysiology

HYPERTENSIVE DISORDERS OF PREGNANCY

Hypertensive disorders of pregnancy consist of a broad spectrum of medical complications including gestational hypertension, preeclampsia, eclampsia, pregestational hypertension, and/or renal disease. The incidence is between 5% and 10% of all pregnancies with an approximate cost of over seven billion dollars in the United States alone (104,105). Preeclampsia and related hypertensive disorders of pregnancy are among the leading causes of maternal mortality worldwide, responsible for approximately 76,000 maternal deaths and 500,000 infant deaths annually (106). Although maternal death due to preeclampsia is less common in developed countries, maternal morbidity remains high and is a major contributor to intensive care unit admissions among pregnant women (107). Approximately 25% of fetal growth restriction (FGR) and 15% of all preterm births are attributable to preeclampsia, and the associated consequences of prematurity are substantial including neonatal death and serious neonatal morbidity (108).

Preeclampsia is a pregnancy-specific disorder that is clinically recognized by new-onset hypertension and proteinuria after 20 weeks of gestation. Vascular dysfunction is central to the systemic maternal manifestations of preeclampsia including increased peripheral vascular resistance, heightened sensitivity to vasopressors, endothelial dysfunction, vasospasm, ischemia, activation of the coagulation cascade, and platelet aggregation leading to multiorgan damage (109–111). The term "eclampsia" is derived from Greek meaning "sudden flashing" or "lightning" and refers to the seizures that can accompany this syndrome. Although the Egyptians and Indians described this disorder over 2,000 years BCE, the only known cure for preeclampsia remains delivery of the fetus and placenta.

DEFINITIONS

The nomenclature for the various hypertensive disorders of pregnancy, including preeclampsia, has changed over time with terms such as "toxemia" and "pregnancy-induced hypertension" now considered outdated (112). Furthermore, the terminology and diagnostic criteria vary geographically across the world. The classification system used in the United States is based on the Working Group Report on High Blood Pressure in Pregnancy (104), which defines four major categories: chronic hypertension, preeclampsia–eclampsia, preeclampsia superimposed on chronic hypertension, and gestational hypertension (Table 13.2).

1. *Chronic hypertension* is defined as hypertension present prior to pregnancy or that is diagnosed before the 20th week of gestation. Persistent blood pressure >140/90 mm Hg is considered hypertension. High blood pressure that persists 6 to 12 weeks postpartum is also classified as chronic hypertension.

TABLE 13.2 CLASSIFICATION OF HYPERTENSIVE DISORDERS OF PREGNANCY

Mild Preeclampsia	• New onset of sustained elevated blood pressure after 20 weeks' gestation in a previously normotensive woman (≥140 mm Hg systolic or ≥90 mm Hg diastolic on at least two occasions 6 hours apart • Proteinuria of at least 1+ on a urine dipstick or ≥300 mg in a 24-hour urine collection after 20 weeks' geatation
Severe Preeclampsia (above criteria plus any of the items listed)	• Blood pressure ≥160 mm Hg systolic or ≥110 mm Hg diastolic • Urine protein excretion of at least 5 g in a 24-hour collection • Neurologic disturbances (visual changes, headache, seizures, coma) • Pulmonary edema • Hepatic dysfunction (elevated liver transaminases2 or epigastric pain) • Renal compromise (oliguria or elevated serum creatinine concentration, ≥1.2 is considered abnormal in women with no history of renal disease) • Thrombocytopenia • Placental abruption, FGR, or oligohydramnios
Eclampsia	• Seizures that occur in a preeclamptic women that can not be attributed to other causes.
Superimposed Preeclampsia	• Sudden and sustained increase in blood pressure with or without substantial increase in proteinuria. • New-onset proteinuria (≥300 mg in a 24-hour protein collection) in a woman with chronic hypertension and no proteinuria prior to 20 weeks' gestation.* • Sudden increase in proteinuria or a sudden increase in blood pressure in a woman with previously well-controlled hypertension in a women with elevated blood pressure and proteinuria prior to 20 weeks of gestation* • Thrombocytopenia, abnormal liver enzymes, or a rapid worsening of renal function • *Precise diagnosis is often challenging and high clinical suspicion is warranted given the increase maternal and fetal/neonatal risks associated with superim posed preeclampsia**
HELLP Syndrome	• Presence of *h*emolysis, *e*levated *l*iver enzymes, and *l*ow *p*latelets. This may or may not occur in the presence of hypertension and is often considered a variant of preeclampsia
Gestational Hypertension	• New onset of sustained elevated blood pressure after 20 weeks' gestation in a previously normotensive woman ≥140 mm Hg systolic or ≥90 mm Hg diastolic on at least 2 occasions 6 hours apart • No proteinuria • Provisional diagnosis (see text)

2. *Preeclampsia* is defined as:

- New onset of sustained elevated blood pressure ($\geq$140 mm Hg systolic or $\geq$90 mm Hg diastolic on at least two occasions 6 hours apart).
- Proteinuria (at least 1+ on a dipstick or $\geq$300 mg in a 24-hour urine collection) first occurring after 20 weeks of gestation.

Blood pressure should be measured in the semi-Fowler's or seated position with an appropriately sized cuff. Disappearance of sounds (Korotkoff phase V) is used to determine diastolic blood pressure. An increase of 30 mm Hg systolic or 15 mm Hg diastolic blood pressure from baseline early pregnancy measurements is no longer used as diagnostic criteria as women with these changes alone are not at increased risk for adverse outcomes (113,114). However, women with these blood pressure changes and proteinuria warrant close observation for the subsequent development of preeclampsia (104). Although edema may raise the clinical suspicion, it is no longer a diagnostic criterion (104). Nondependent edema occurs in 10% to 15% of women who remain normotensive throughout pregnancy (115) and is neither a sensitive nor specific sign of preeclampsia.

Symptoms and signs of preeclampsia occur along a continuum and include a spectrum of disorders. However for the purposes of categorizing and communicating disease status, preeclampsia is often classified as mild or severe. Preeclampsia is considered *severe* when any of the following is present in addition to the defining blood pressure and proteinuria criteria (116):

- Blood pressure $\geq$160 mm Hg systolic or $\geq$110 mm Hg diastolic.
- Urine protein excretion of >5 g in a 24-hour collection.
- Neurologic disturbances (visual changes, headache, seizures, coma, etc.).
- Pulmonary edema.
- Hepatic dysfunction (elevated liver transaminases or epigastric pain).
- Renal compromise (oliguria or elevated serum creatinine concentration; creatinine $\geq$1.2 is considered abnormal in women without a history of renal disease).
- Thrombocytopenia.
- Placental abruption, FGR, or oligohydramnios.

Eclampsia refers to seizures that occur in a preeclamptic woman, which cannot be attributed to other causes.

3. *Superimposed preeclampsia* can develop in women with chronic hypertension. This is characterized by a sudden and sustained increase in blood pressure with or without substantial increase in proteinuria. Diagnosis is often challenging and high clinical suspicion is warranted given the increase in maternal and fetal/neonatal risks. In women with chronic hypertension and no proteinuria prior to 20 weeks' gestation, new-onset proteinuria defined as >300 mg in a 24-hour urine collection strongly supports the diagnosis of superimposed preeclampsia. In a women with elevated blood pressure and proteinuria prior to 20 weeks of gestation, a sudden increase in proteinuria or a sudden increase in blood pressure in a woman with previously well-controlled hypertension defines superimposed preeclampsia. End-organ involvement such as thrombocytopenia, abnormal liver enzymes, or a rapid worsening of renal function may also be features of superimposed disease.

4. *Gestational hypertension* is defined by elevated blood pressure ($\geq$140 mm Hg systolic or $\geq$90 mm Hg diastolic) in a previously normotensive woman. High blood pressure should be sustained with documented elevations on at least two occasions 6 hours apart. Gestational hypertension is a provisional diagnosis during pregnancy and includes women in three major categories: (i) women who will progress to develop preeclampsia, (ii) women with "transient hypertension of pregnancy" who do not develop preeclampsia and revert to having normal blood pressures by 12 weeks postdelivery, and (iii) women who may have previously unrecognized chronic hypertension. Definitive diagnosis is possible only after re-assessment at 6 to 12 weeks postpartum.

HELLP syndrome is defined by the presence of *h*emolysis, *e*levated *l*iver enzymes, and *l*ow *p*latelets. This may or may not occur in the presence of hypertension. It is often considered a variant of preeclampsia (117).

RISK FACTORS

Nulliparity is the biggest risk factor for preeclampsia (118). At least two-thirds of cases occur in the first pregnancy. New paternity also increases the risk of preeclampsia in subsequent pregnancies. Other risk factors are common to both nulliparous and parous women. These can be broadly separated into maternal factors and pregnancy-specific or placental factors. Many of the maternal risk factors for preeclampsia are similar to those for cardiovascular disease. Preexisting hypertension, diabetes, obesity, vascular disorders (e.g., renal disease and connective tissue disorders), and African-American ethnicity are all risk factors for preeclampsia (118). Risk appears to correlate with the severity of the underlying vascular disorder: for example, women with chronic hypertension have a 10% to 25% risk of developing preeclampsia compared to a 3% to 7% risk in the general population; this risk is increased to 31% in women with long-standing chronic hypertension (at least 4 years) (119). Similarly, the risk of developing preeclampsia in women with pregestational diabetes is 21%; however, this ranges from 11% to 12% among women with short duration, White's class B diabetes up to 36% to 54% in women with diabetes-associated microvascular disease (White's class R and F) (120,121). Elevated body mass index is also associated with increased preeclampsia risk. Given the obesity epidemic in the United States, this is one of the largest attributable and potentially modifiable risk factor for preeclampsia (118). Placental factors such as excessive placental size as is seen with hydatidiform moles and multifetal gestation are also associated with the development of preeclampsia. The risk increases with each additional fetus (122). Paradoxically, cigarette smoking during pregnancy is associated with a reduced risk of preeclampsia (123,124), possibly due to modulation of angiogenic factors (125,126).

PREVENTION

A number of different strategies have been tested for the prevention of preeclampsia including but not limited to protein or salt restriction, zinc, magnesium, fish oil, diuretics, antihypertensive medications, heparin, aspirin, calcium, and vitamins. Results from most of these trials have shown little to no benefit. However, it is worth discussing the use of calcium, aspirin, and antioxidant vitamin supplementation. A common theme is that of exciting results from small single-center studies that are followed by larger, well-powered, multicenter trials that fail to demonstrate significant benefit in preventing preeclampsia or associated adverse pregnancy outcomes (127). A meta-analysis of small trials using calcium supplementation indicated a positive effect in preventing preeclampsia (128). This was followed by a multicenter, randomized, controlled trial in the United States, which did not show a benefit of 2 g supplemental calcium during pregnancy for the prevention of preeclampsia in low-risk women (129). A subsequent review of this topic suggested that calcium may be beneficial in preventing preeclampsia if prepregnancy dietary calcium intake was low (130). A World Health Organization trial of calcium supplementation in populations with low calcium intake demonstrated a reduction in adverse pregnancy outcomes such as eclampsia, maternal morbidity, and neonatal mortality but no reduction in the diagnosis of preeclampsia (131). In aggregate, these studies suggest a beneficial effect of calcium supplementation on perinatal outcomes other than preeclampsia in areas of low calcium intake (132).

Aspirin, an antiplatelet agent, was also tested for the prevention of preeclampsia in various low- and high-risk populations. Initial studies revealed a substantial benefit of aspirin therapy (133–135); however, subsequent large randomized trials of high-risk women (136,137) and low-risk women (138,139) did not show a statistically significant benefit. A systematic review as well as Cochrane group meta-analysis of aspirin therapy to prevent preeclampsia in high-risk women demonstrated a modest reduction of preeclampsia, perinatal death, and preterm birth (140,141). In a recent meta-analysis using individual patient data from 32,217 women in 31 randomized trials of antiplatelet therapy for the primary prevention of preeclampsia, there was a lower risk of preeclampsia (RR: 0.90, 95% CI: 0.84–0.97), delivery before 34 weeks' gestation (RR: 0.90, 95% CI: 0.83–0.98), and overall serious adverse pregnancy outcome (RR: 0.90, 95% CI: 0.85–0.96) (142). No single identifiable subgroup benefited preferentially from aspirin therapy. Importantly, however, there were no substantial risks of antiplatelet therapy. Although there is no consensus, low-dose aspirin therapy may be considered in women at moderate-to-high risk for developing preeclampsia.

Oxidative stress has been suggested as a pathogenic factor in preeclampsia (143). As a result, antioxidant vitamins have been proposed for primary prevention of preeclampsia in both low- and high-risk women. Despite promising results from a small study of vitamin C (1,000 mg/day) and E (400 IU/day) in high-risk women (144), a larger, multicenter, randomized, placebo-controlled trial (VIP trial) did not show any benefit (145). In fact, post hoc analyses suggested an increase in gestational hypertension, lower birth weights, and unexplained stillbirth after 24 weeks' gestation in the vitamin group. Three other large trials of antioxidant vitamins C and E for the prevention of preeclampsia in low-risk women did not demonstrate any benefit (146–148). Therefore, antioxidant therapies cannot currently be recommended for the prevention of preeclampsia in either low- or high-risk women.

While these large trials have been mostly disappointing with negative results, the experiences have underscored (i) the importance of appropriately powered, multicenter, randomized trials to guide clinical management and (ii) the concept that preeclampsia is a heterogeneous disorder and therapies may need to be directed at specific underlying causes that warrant further research efforts.

TREATMENT AND MANAGEMENT

The only known cure for preeclampsia is delivery of the fetus and placenta (105). Vaginal delivery is usually appropriate unless other obstetric complications indicate the need for cesarean section. If preeclampsia becomes clinically apparent at term (≥37 weeks' gestation), delivery at that time benefits both the mother and the neonate. In general, this approach results in favorable maternal and neonatal outcomes.

With pregnancies that are preterm, especially those less than 34 weeks of gestation, delivery provides clear maternal benefit but may be disadvantageous to the neonate because of the complications associated with prematurity, such as respiratory distress syndrome, intraventricular hemorrhage, necrotizing enterocolitis, retinopathy of prematurity, and developmental delay. Delaying delivery in early-onset or severe preeclampsia may be acceptable in certain circumstances to improve neonatal outcome, but must be carefully considered so that maternal risks are not excessive (149). The health risk to the mother must be constantly weighed against the potential benefits of delayed delivery for the baby. Close inpatient maternal and fetal surveillance in a tertiary care facility with 24-hour obstetric, neonatology, and anesthesia services is a necessity.

Antepartum Management

A high level of clinical suspicion is important for the prompt diagnosis of preeclampsia. More frequent visits in the third trimester, a part of routine prenatal care, are intended to facilitate timely detection and avoid adverse pregnancy outcomes. Each visit should include assessment of blood pressure, urine dipstick for proteinuria, as well as a careful history for symptoms and signs of maternal end-organ damage. This includes questioning the patient regarding symptoms of headache, visual changes, epigastric or right upper quadrant abdominal pain, nausea/vomiting, difficulty breathing, or decreased urine output. Confirmation of sustained elevated blood pressures and quantification of urinary protein excretion, ideally with a 24-hour timed urine collection should be a part of the initial evaluation if preeclampsia is suspected. Laboratory evaluation is useful in evaluation of possible end-organ involvement—including hemoglobin, platelet count, serum creatinine, and liver transaminases. Uric acid is useful as it may identify a subgroup of hypertensive women at higher risk of premature delivery and small-for-gestational-age infants (150). Fetal well-being should be assessed with ultrasound to evaluate estimated fetal weight, growth, and amniotic fluid index. Nonstress testing and/or biophysical profiles should also be considered. Umbilical artery Doppler velocimetry may be helpful in the setting of FGR.

Intrapartum Management

As delivery is being accomplished, there are four other important considerations that include:

1. Seizure prophylaxis—Most eclamptic seizures occur during the intrapartum and postpartum periods (within 48 hours of delivery). In the Magpie trial of 10,000 preeclamptic women randomized to magnesium sulfate or placebo, magnesium sulfate clearly reduced the risk of eclampsia (151). Magnesium has also been shown to be superior to other prophylactic medications including phenytoin (152,153) and diazepam (154,155) in preventing eclamptic seizures. The usual dose is a 4 g IV loading dose followed by constant infusion of 1 to 2 g IV/h. Patients should be monitored closely for any evidence of toxicity including loss of reflexes and respiratory depression. The infusion dose may need to be reduced in women with renal failure.

2. Antihypertensive therapy—Antihypertensive medications are not routinely given to women with preeclampsia. The primary reason for using antihypertensive drugs is for the treatment of severe maternal blood pressure elevations to reduce cerebrovascular accidents such as stroke and intracranial hemorrhage. There is no evidence that lowering blood pressure might reduce fetal morbidity or prevent seizures. Acute therapy is reserved for systolic blood pressures >160 mm Hg and/or diastolic blood pressures >105 to 110 mm Hg. In contrast to the principles and goals of blood pressure control in nonpregnant adults, the goal with preeclampsia is to avoid maternal cerebrovascular accidents without lowering blood pressure so much that uterine perfusion is compromised leading to iatrogenic fetal distress. IV labetalol and hydralazine are considered first-line agents for acute lowering of blood pressure in preeclamptic women. Table 13.3 summarizes the mechanism of action, dosing, and frequency of commonly used medications. It is worthwhile to comment that angiotensin-converting enzyme (ACE) inhibitors and angiotensin receptor blockers (ARBs) are not recommended for use in pregnancy. These medications have teratogenic potential and their use in the first trimester is associated with a 2.7-fold increase in congenital anomalies, specifically cardiac and central nervous system malformation (156). Use of ACE inhibitors in the second and third trimester is associated with a fetal renal failure and oligohydramnios, which can lead to pulmonary hypoplasia and joint contractures.

TABLE 13.3 DRUGS FOR THE ACUTE MANAGEMENT OF HYPERTENSION

Drug (FDA Category)	Mechanism of Action	Dose	Onset of Action	Maximum Dose	Comments[a]
Labetalol (C)	α- and β-adrenergic antagonist	10–20 mg IV, then 20–80 mg every 10–30 minutes or continuous infusion of 1–2 mg/min[b]	5–10 min	300 mg/24 h	Increasingly preferred as a first-line agent; less risk of tachycardia; avoid in patients with asthma or congestive heart failure
Hydralazine (C)	Arteriolar vasodilator, smooth muscle relaxant	5 mg IV or IM, then 5–10 mg IV every 20–40 min or constant infusion of 0.5–10 mg/h[b]	10–20 min		Frequent administration and/or higher doses may cause maternal or fetal distress secondary to hypotension (more commonly than other drugs); side effects include headache, flushing, nausea, which may mimic preeclamsia
Nifedipine (C)	Calcium channel blocker	10–20 mg orally every 30 min	10–20 min	Max 60 mg in first hour	Side effects include headache, flushing, nausea, which may mimic symptoms of preeclampsia
Sodium Nitroprusside (C)		0.25–20 mcg/kg/min IV[b]	Within seconds		Relatively contraindicated and agent of last resort; longer use associated with cyanide toxicity

[a]All agents are associated with headache, flushing, nausea, and tachycardia (likely due to hypotension and reflex sympathetic activation); these side effects are less with labetalol.

[b]Continuous IV infusions should be used only in an ICU setting.

Fetal skull ossification defects have also been reported (157,158). Diuretics also pose the theoretical risk of reducing intravascular volume that is already reduced in preeclampsia, thus possibly resulting in compromise of uteroplacental perfusion. Management principles and medications used for the management of chronically elevated blood pressures in the preeclamptic woman undergoing expectant management are discussed in the next section.

3. Worsening maternal disease—Preeclamptic women should be monitored closely during the antepartum, intrapartum, and immediate postpartum period for worsening disease. In particular, renal function and urine output should be assessed frequently with attention to fluid management and potential pulmonary edema. In some cases, monitoring may need to be done in the intensive care unit setting with invasive hemodynamic monitoring. Serial laboratory assessments may also be useful in evaluating the progression of disease.

4. Fetal status—Antenatal glucocorticoids [betamethasone 12 mg IM q 24 hours (two doses) or dexamethasone 6 mg IV q 12 hours (four doses)] should be administered, if gestational age is less than 34 weeks. This therapy is associated with reductions in neonatal respiratory distress syndrome, intraventricular hemorrhage, necrotizing enterocolitis, and neonatal death secondary to prematurity. Preeclampsia is associated with placental insufficiency, FGR, and oligohydramnios. Therefore, close fetal surveillance is warranted with ultrasounds to assess fetal growth, nonstress tests, biophysical profiles, and Doppler interrogation of the umbilical artery blood flow, if indicated.

PREECLAMPSIA AND FUTURE CARDIOVASCULAR RISK

Dr. Leon Chesley, a pioneer in the field of preeclampsia, and his co-workers demonstrated that women who had eclampsia in any pregnancy after their first had a mortality risk that was two- to fivefold higher over the next 35 years compared to controls (159). Following this early report, others have also demonstrated an association between preeclampsia and later life cardiovascular disease and related mortality. Irgens et al. reported an eightfold increased risk of cardiovascular disease in a Scandinavian population of healthy nulliparous women who developed preeclampsia severe enough to necessitate a preterm delivery (160). Funai et al. studied a cohort of women who delivered in Jerusalem and found a twofold higher risk of mortality at 24- to 36-year follow-up in women with prior preeclampsia compared with women who did not have this diagnosis. The deaths were largely related to cardiovascular causes (161). The future risk of cardiovascular disease has also been demonstrated in other populations (162,163). Hypertension, dyslipidemia, insulin resistance, endothelial dysfunction, and vascular impairment have all been observed months to years after preeclampsia, further supporting the link between preeclampsia and subsequent cardiovascular disease (refer to Ref. 164 for a detailed review). It remains unresolved as to whether these common risk factors lead to the development of preeclampsia and later life cardiovascular disease or whether preeclampsia itself may contribute to this future risk. Thus, preeclampsia, particularly severe and early-onset disease, should be considered a cardiovascular risk factor requiring attention and close surveillance in later life.

A recent study using birth registry data in Norway demonstrated an association with preeclampsia and increased risk of subsequent end-stage renal disease (ESRD) (165). Among women who had been pregnant and had suffered preeclampsia in the first pregnancy, the relative risk of ESRD was 4.7 (95% CI: 3.6–6.1). This risk was further increased with recurrent preeclampsia and preterm delivery. While this study does not address underlying mechanism, possibilities include (i) common factors that predispose to preeclampsia, ESRD, and cardiovascular disease, such as obesity, metabolic syndrome, and endothelial dysfunction; (ii) exacerbation of previously unrecognized subclinical renal disease by preeclampsia; and (iii) preeclampsia causing later life renal disease.

PATHOPHYSIOLOGY OF PREECLAMPSIA

Preeclampsia can be thought of as a three-stage disease (Fig. 13-9). *Stage I* occurs in early pregnancy and involves impaired trophoblast invasion of uterine spiral arteries, especially within the myometrium. Consequently, uterine spiral arteries fail to be adequately remodeled by trophoblasts cells from small-caliber, high-resistance to large-caliber, low-resistance vessels, thereby impeding uteroplacental blood flow (166). The failure of spiral arteries to convert from resistance- to conduit-sized diameters may also

Pathophysiology of Preeclampsia

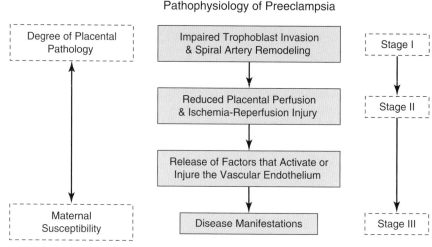

■ **Figure 13.9** Three-stage model of preeclampsia. See text for details.

confer higher blood flow velocities entering the intervillous space, which may further damage placental villi by mechanical forces (167). This structural remodeling of spiral arteries is due primarily to their interaction with invading trophoblast cells and occurs by apoptosis of the spiral artery smooth muscle and endothelial cells, as well as dissolution of extracellular matrix components such as collagen, and the deposition of fibrinoid material in the vascular walls (166,168).

The underlying cause(s) of failed trophoblast invasion in *Stage I* is unknown. Many hormones, growth factors, and cytokines have been shown to facilitate or inhibit trophoblast invasion in vitro. However, which of these are pivotal to trophoblast invasion during normal pregnancy, or underlie defective trophoblast invasion in preeclampsia is difficult to interrogate in vivo. Logically, the impairment of trophoblast invasion in preeclampsia is due to intrinsic defect(s) within the trophoblast cells themselves, in the maternal endometrium and inner myometrium, particularly the spiral arteries which they invade, or both ("seed" and/or "soil"). Thus, abnormalities of maturation in the endometrium and inner myometrium in preparation for placentation prior to and after conception called "predecidualization" and "decidualization," respectively, may be etiological. Alternatively, the optimal complement of uterine immune cells and associated cytokines, or their interaction with the resident decidual and invading trophoblast cells, is deficient. Indeed, a recent pilot report on global gene expression, in chorionic villous tissue containing maternal decidua obtained at 10 to 12 weeks gestation in women who developed preeclampsia 6 months later, prominently featured abnormal expression of genes related to decidualization and immune function (169). As alluded toin the preceding text, it is not inconceivable that in some women, the antecedents of preeclampsia may lie with defective "predecidualization" in the secretory phase of the menstrual cycle (166,169). Because the secretory phase of the menstrual cycle and early pregnancy are primarily under the endocrine control of the corpus luteum of the ovary, the primary etiology may reside with abnormal ovarian function in some women who develop preeclampsia.

Stage II arises as a consequence of *Stage I* and entails inadequate uteroplacental perfusion resulting in placental ischemia–hypoxia (170). In addition, the persistence of uterine spiral artery smooth muscle is postulated to render these blood vessels susceptible to local and circulating vasoconstrictors such as angiotensin II, resulting in vasospasm and hypoxia–reperfusion injury of the placenta. One major consequence of these disturbances in uteroplacental blood flow is upregulation of placental hypoxia–inducible transcription factors (HIF-1α and -2α via hypoxia per se and reactive oxygen species) (171,172). Placental villi also undergo apoptosis and necrosis (173,174). These pathological changes in the placenta herald *Stage III*.

Stage III begins when factors from the damaged placenta are released into the maternal circulation, which cause endothelial activation and injury, thereby producing disease manifestations including hypertension, proteinuria, and glomerular endotheliosis (see later). The identification of these factors linking placental disease with the maternal clinical syndrome has been hotly pursued for many years. There are likely to be a multitude of injurious agents conspiring to produce the florid disease syndrome, the complement of which may vary from patient to patient, and with no one factor alone being responsible. Currently, the leading candidates that link the primary placental injury and resulting maternal disease include inflammatory cytokines, placental microparticles, soluble endoglin, and soluble fms-like tyrosine kinase-1 (sFlt-1 or sVEGFR-1), the latter binding and inactivating VEGF and placental growth factor (PGF) (175,176). Many of these factors begin to increase in the maternal circulation prior to clinical onset, thus reinforcing the concept that they may be cause rather than consequence of the disease.

Some women may be more or less susceptible to these circulating placental factors, thereby necessitating a little or lot of placental pathology, respectively, to precipitate clinical disease, *stage III* (Fig. 13-9). This may be why women with preexisting endothelial dysfunction, for example, as in renal disease, chronic hypertension, or diabetes mellitus are predisposed to preeclampsia. (In these women, preexisting endothelial dysfunction may also affect the uterine vasculature, thereby impairing trophoblast invasion and exacerbating stage II.) Prior to conception, low plasma volume, reduced venous capacitance, and increased sympathetic activation characterize those women destined to recurrent preeeclampsia (177). These findings are remarkably reminiscent of the emerging concept of long-term regulation of arterial pressure by sympathetic activity and peripheral venous (mainly splanchnic) compliance (178). Possibly, circulating factors from the placenta synergize with enhanced sympathetic outflow to exacerbate the reduction in venous compliance, thereby contributing to hypertension in preeclampsia (179,180). This concept would also accommodate the prodromal phase of a hyperdynamic circulation as proposed by Easterling et al. and Bosio et al. (see later). Finally, it should also be noted that circulating deleterious factors in preeclampsia may also derive from other sources besides, or in addition to, the placenta (181–183).

The evidence for the pathological role of elevated sFlt1 levels in preeclampsia represents an important breakthrough in our understanding of the disease, and is unlikely to be a "false start" as is often the case in this field (184). The concept is particularly compelling for several reasons. First, an animal model was employed to provide "proof of principle." That is, adenoviral overexpression of sFlt1 in pregnant (and nonpregnant) rats induced the symptoms of preeclampsia (namely, proteinuria, hypertension, and glomerular endotheliosis, the characteristic renal lesion of preeclampsia) (185,186). Second, a back-to-back publication by Eremina et al. independently showed that targeted knockout of VEGF from glomerular podocytes in mice (thereby depriving glomerular endothelial cells of this essential growth factor) leads to massive proteinuria and glomerular endotheliosis (187), both manifestations of elevated circulating sFlt1 (185) and preeclampsia (186). Third, VEGF-neutralizing antibodies produced hypertension and proteinuria in a clinical trial of metastatic renal cancer (188). Finally, placental hypoxia-inducible factor α (HIFα) proteins and HIFα-regulated genes including membrane-bound Flt1 and sFlt1 are increased in preeclampsia (171,172,179). Thus, sFlt1 is likely to be an important (but certainly not the only) factor emanating from the hypoxic placenta that contributes to endothelial dysfunction in preeclampsia.

Interestingly, sFlt1 also increases in the maternal circulation of normal pregnant women (thus, begging the question of a physiological role for this molecule), but an exaggerated rise occurs in women destined to develop preeclampsia approximately 5 weeks before onset of clinical symptoms (189). This timing places sFlt1 in *Stages II and III* of preeclampsia, being important to disease pathogenesis but unlikely related to etiology (*Stage I*). The additional findings that sFlt1 is not elevated in the maternal circulation during the first half of pregnancy in women destined to develop preeclampsia (189,190), and the lack of evidence for upregulation of hypoxia or oxidative stress regulated genes including Flt-1 in chorionic villous tissue at 10 to 12 weeks of gestation, reinforces the concept that these may be later events in the disease (169).

SYSTEMIC HEMODYNAMICS IN PREECLAMPSIA

An overview of the literature suggests that the systemic hemodynamic pattern in preeclampsia ranges from a high-output–low-resistance to low-output–high-resistance state (191,192). The main controversy has been whether this widely divergent picture results from a wide spectrum of pathophysiology, clinical management, or both. Wallenburg et al. suggested that many studies were conducted after clinical intervention with magnesium sulfate, antihypertensive medications, and IV fluids, all of which can markedly affect systemic hemodynamics (191). Thus, in their own well-controlled, meticulously conducted study using strict definition of preeclampsia, these investigators compared untreated and treated groups of preeclamptic subjects (193). They found a remarkably homogenous pattern of systemic hemodynamics in the untreated group consisting of a low-output–high-resistance state with normal capillary wedge pressure. In contrast, the treated group revealed a varied hemodynamic pattern. Thus the authors concluded: "the [previously] reported extremes of the hemodynamic profile [of preeclampsia] appear to reflect clinical management rather than the pathophysiological state" (193). This conclusion has been substantiated using noninvasive methodologies (194).

Another perspective championed by Easterling et al. (195), and corroborated by Bosio et al. (196), is that a high-output–low-resistance state precedes the clinical onset of preeclampsia when a crossover to low-output–high-resistance state occurs. Interestingly, this argument, by analogy, is consistent with one view of the progression of essential hypertension (197). Possibly, the widely divergent findings of the hemodynamic status of preeclampsia (vide supra) may in fact be due to the timing of the measurements related to the progression of the disease, that is, in relation to the crossover. However, there are a few caveats with the reports of Easterling and Bosio, for example, in the former, the patients were mildly preeclamptic at best, and in both studies, the preeclamptic cohort was much heavier that the normal pregnant control group. Heavier or "obese" women may have higher cardiac output and lower systemic vascular resistance in the nonpregnant condition (198), and therefore this potential confounder may fully account for or contribute to the high-output–low-resistance state reported during early gestation in women destined to develop preeclampsia.

RENAL ALTERATIONS IN PREECLAMPSIA

Renal Hemodynamics and Glomerular Filtration

A review of 23 reports on renal hemodynamics and glomerular filtration in preeclampsia shows that GFR and RPF are reduced, on average by 32% and 24%, respectively, from normal, late gravid levels (14), and citations therein). GFR and RPF may also be reduced in preeclampsia relative to nonpregnant values, but to a lesser extent. Although the criteria used for diagnosing preeclampsia in many of these studies were not presented or failed to live up to modern standards, the investigation of Assali et al. (199) is an exception because rigorous clinical diagnostic criteria were employed. In this work, GFR and RPF were reduced by 29% and 20%, respectively, with respect to normal pregnancy. In the studies by McCartney et al. (200) and Sarles et al. (201), the clinical diagnosis of preeclampsia was corroborated on renal histology showing glomerular endotheliosis. In these publications, GFR and/or RPF were found to be modestly decreased in women with preeclampsia compared to normal pregnant women. Several groups calculated renal segmental vascular resistances. Only the preglomerular arteriolar resistance was increased in preeclampsia, and no alteration in postglomerular arteriolar resistances was noted (reviewed in Ref. 14). Because the decrease in GFR typically exceeded that of RPF and only preglomerular arteriolar resistance was increased, these findings, when taken together, suggest a reduction in the glomerular ultrafiltration coefficient during preeclampsia—a deduction supported by data from Davison et al. (202). Despite persisting structural abnormalities on renal histology, GFR appears to rapidly recover during the first week after delivery; in contrast, RPF may recover more slowly.

The mechanism(s) for impaired GFR and RPF in preeclampsia is unknown, but may be a consequence of the widespread "endothelial dysfunction" believed to account for general vasospasm and organ hypoperfusion in the disease (vide supra). Thus, on this basis, the relaxin vasodilatory pathway that normally signals through the endothelium-derived relaxing factor, NO, to promote renal vasodilation and hyperfiltration during pregnancy may be compromised. On the other hand, in addition to general impairment of NO activity, the selective disruption of discrete renal vasodilatory signaling mechanisms may occur. For example, because local, arterial-derived vascular endothelial and placental growth factors are proximal players in the relaxin renal vasodilatory pathway (29,31,32) (unpublished data), the increased circulating concentrations of soluble VEGF receptor-1 (sflt-1) in preeclampsia may disrupt relaxin mediated renal vasodilation by competing with these angiogenic growth factors. Generally speaking, to promote the processes mediating vasodilation in normal pregnancy is one therapeutic approach to overcome vasoconstriction and organ hypoperfusion that occur in preeclampsia, assuming, of course, that there is no insurmountable block somewhere in the vasodilatory pathway(s), which cannot be either overrun or circumvented. An alternative, but not mutually exclusive approach, is to neutralize the circulating factors injurious to the endothelium. Administration of relaxin as a potential therapeutic for preeclampsia is attractive because it could target both of these endpoints. On the one hand, by augmenting the activity of VEGF and PlGF in arteries, relaxin administration could promote vasodilation and organ perfusion in preeclampsia by reinforcing its own vasodilatory pathway. On the other hand, by increasing arterial VEGF and PlGF activity, relaxin could partly or wholly neutralize the increased, local concentration of sflt-1 that is derived from the systemic circulation, thereby improving endothelial cell health.

Uric Acid

Hyperuricemia is frequently observed in preeclampsia and often in more severe disease (reviewed in Ref. 14). In fact, some researchers include it as a diagnostic criterion because of the strong association between hyperuricemia and the histologic finding of "glomerular endotheliosis" on antepartum percutaneous renal biopsy, which is believed to be a characteristic structural lesion of preeclampsia (203) (see later). Moreover, a strong correlation between the severity of this preeclamptic lesion and the elevation in serum uric acid has been noted (203) (Fig. 13-10). Finally, hyperuricemia manifests relatively early on in gestation frequently antedating preeclampsia manifestations, and is correlated with poor fetal prognosis (204–206).

Abnormal renal handling undoubtedly contributes to hyperuricemia in preeclampsia (see Ref. 14 and citations therein). First and foremost is the impairment of the renal clearance of uric acid, mainly because net tubular reabsorption is pathologically high. When GFR is reduced, the resultant decrease in filtered load of uric acid also contributes to impairment of renal clearance and hyperuricemia. Interestingly, probenecid, which inhibits renal tubular reabsorption of uric acid, restored the renal clearance and plasma levels of uric acid in preeclamptic women to normal pregnancy levels, thus implicating enhanced tubular reabsorption rather than diminished tubular secretion of uric acid as

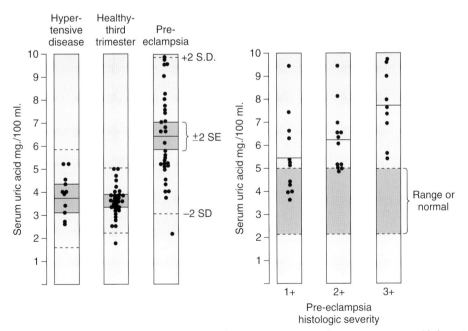

■ **Figure 13.10** (*Left*) Serum uric acid in normal pregnant women and pregnant women with hypertension or preeclampsia. The latter diagnosis was corroborated by the renal histological findings on antepartum percutaneous renal biopsy. (*Right*). Serum uric acid according to the severity of the renal histological findings in women with preeclampsia. See text for details. (From Pollak VE, Nettles JB. The kidney in toxemia of pregnancy: A clinical and pathologic study based on renal biopsies. *Medicine (Baltimore).* 1960; 39: 469–526, with permission)

the underlying cause (207,208). Conflicting with earlier reports (209,210), recent evidence supports the concept that increased metabolic production of uric acid by the fetus, placenta, or maternal tissues may contribute to elevated circulating levels in preeclampsia that, in turn, contribute to disease pathogenesis (211). Finally, renal clearance and plasma concentrations of uric acid are rapidly restored to normal by 5 days after delivery in women who suffered preeclampsia.

The ultimate cause underlying exaggerated renal tubular reabsorption of uric acid in preeclampsia is unknown, but may relate to relative plasma volume depletion that is also a typical early feature of the disease (212,213). Indeed, volume contraction is known to enhance renal reabsorption of sodium (54). Therefore, uric acid reabsorption may be enhanced during preeclampsia because sodium and uric acid are inexorably coupled through a sodium-dependent mechanism in the proximal tubule (54). However, the precise mechanisms are unknown.

Renal Handling of Calcium

Preeclampsia is virtually the polar opposite to normal pregnancy with respect to calcium homeostasis. Marked hypocalciuria occurs in preeclampsia relative to nonpregnant women, normal pregnancy, gestational hypertension, and chronic hypertension (63,214–221). Hypocalciuria is mainly due to enhanced tubular reabsorption because the fractional excretion of calcium is reduced and hypocalciuria is observed even when GFR is not significantly reduced (63,214–221). Serum-ionized calcium is normal or slightly decreased (63,214–221). Although the reports of parathyroid hormone concentration are conflicting, investigators measuring the intact, active molecule rather than metabolic fragments report an increase (217,222,223). Serum 1,25-dihydoxyvitamin D is decreased in most reports (217,218,221–223). Thus, in contrast to normal pregnancy, serum 1,25-dihyroxyvitamin D is decreased in preeclampsia secondary to reduced placental and/or renal production. Consequently, intestinal calcium reabsorption is likely to be reduced (although it has not been rigorously assessed in preeclampsia), and in the face of high maternal and fetal demands, this leads to a state of calcium deficiency. The latter, in turn, slightly decreases serum-ionized calcium as detected in some studies (217), thereby increasing PTH and distal tubular reaborption of calcium.

Proteins

Compared to normal pregnancy, the urinary excretion of total protein, albumin, low-molecular-weight proteins, and several renal tubular enzymes is even further increased during preeclampsia (reviewed in Ref. 14). This additional increase in low-molecular-weight proteins and renal tubular enzymes may indicate pathological impairment of proximal tubular function in the disease. Albuminuria and excretion of other plasma proteins are likely to arise from perturbations of the molecular size constraints and electrostatic properties of the glomerular filter, in addition to compromised proximal tubular reabsorptive capacity. Despite the calculated increase in afferent arteriolar resistance, an increase in glomerular hydrostatic pressure promoting proteinuria cannot be discounted. Further exploration of both the permselective and electrostatic properties of the glomerular filter in preeclampsia is clearly needed. An unresolved paradox is the apparent reduction in reabsorptive capacity for proteins, implicating pathological proximal tubular dysfunction, and the enhanced reabsorptive capacity for uric acid and calcium by the proximal tubule in preeclampsia (see Renal Handling of Uric Acid and Renal Handling of Calcium sections).

With respect to potential molecular underpinnings of proteinuria in preeclampsia, recent investigation indicates that glomerular podocyte secretion of VEGF contributes to the maintenance of glomerular capillary integrity (187). Thus, elevated circulating concentrations of soluble VEGF receptor 1 or sflt-1 in preeclampsia may neutralize VEGF, thereby disrupting the glomerular endothelial barrier (224). Also, see Glomerular Structural Lesion section.

Glomerular Structural Lesion

Swelling and vacuolization of glomerular endothelial cells that can lead to obliteration of the capillary lumens occurs in preeclampsia and is called "glomerular endotheliosis" (Ref. 14 and citations therein; Fig. 13-11). This typical lesion inspired the term "bloodless glomeruli." In addition, endothelial fenestrae disappear and the endothelial swelling can be so severe that the glomerular tuft herniates into

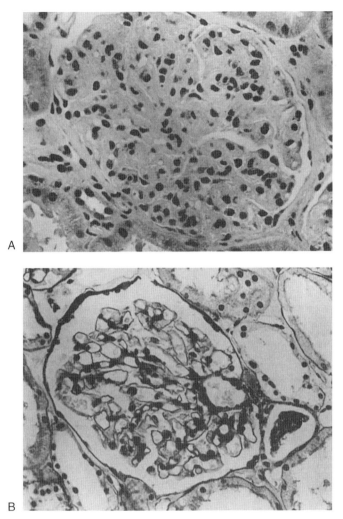

■ **Figure 13.11 A.** Light microscopy of glomerulus demonstrating changes consistent with glomerular endotheliosis. (From Heptinstall RH. Renal disease in pregnancy. In: Heptinstall RH, ed. *Pathology of the Kidney*. 4th ed. Boston: Little, Brown; 1992: 1773, with permission. **B.** Normal glomerulus. (From Venkatachatam MA, Kriz W. Anatomy. In: Heptinstall RH, ed. *Pathology of the Kidney*. 4th ed. Boston: Little, Brown; 1992: 37, with permission.)

the proximal tubule, so-called "pouting." In 1924, Mayer first described glomerular endothelial swelling in eclampsia (225), providing the first clue that endothelial dysfunction may figure prominently in disease pathophysiology.

Perhaps surprisingly, there are no consistent abnormalities noted in the other glomerular structures. That is, the basement membrane, podocyte, and foot processes are usually unaffected and intact, although some have reported swollen mesangial cells and expanded mesangial matrix. Moreover, interstitial and tubular structural abnormalities are absent. Glomerular subendothelial fibrin deposition can be seen particularly in intrapartum biopsies resolving quickly postpartum. Immunoglobulin deposits (IgM and IgG) are infrequent and of low intensity, suggesting nonspecific trapping rather than primary autoimmune disorder. Glomerular endotheliosis is believed to be a renal lesion characteristic of preeclampsia. However, it has also been reported in women with placental abruption (226,227). A recent publication suggests that mild glomerular endotheliosis may be observed in normal pregnancy (228–230), but this claim has been disputed (14). However, if so, it may be related to the physiological elevation of sflt-1 during late pregnancy (189). In this regard, in rats and mice with elevated circulating sflt-1 achieved by infection with adenovirus: sflt-1 expressing constructs, hypertension, proteinuria, and glomerular endotheliosis are observed (185,231).

Comparable glomerular lesions were observed in mutant mice lacking podocyte expression of VEGF (187). Finally, in patients receiving antiangiogenic therapy for cancer, hypertension, proteinuria, and glomerular endotheliosis are not infrequently manifested (224). The overall consensus is that the lesions of preeclampsia resolve completely after delivery, regression seen as early as the first postpartum week (232–235).

CHRONIC HYPERTENSION

Chronic hypertension complicates approximately 0.5% to 5% of all pregnancies (236). The prevalence of chronic hypertension increases with age and is higher in African-American women (237). Perinatal morbidity is increased with chronic hypertension, primarily related to superimposed preeclampsia, FGR, and perinatal death. Superimposed preeclampsia has a prevalence of 20% to 25% in women with mild chronic hypertension, but can be as high as 50% in women with severe prepregnancy hypertension (236). With respect to fetal neonatal outcomes, perinatal death and FGR were significantly more frequent in women with chronic hypertension without superimposed preeclampsia compared with normotensive, pregnant women who served as controls (238). Specifically, the perinatal death frequency was 29/1,000 and FGR 10.5% among uncomplicated chronic hypertensive women. These same investigators reported a relative risk for perinatal death of 3.6 in women with superimposed preeclampsia compared with uncomplicated chronic hypertensive controls. The incidence of FGR was 35% among superimposed preeclamptics (238).

The clinical care is focused on blood pressure management, close monitoring for superimposed preeclampsia, and careful fetal surveillance. In contrast to the clear guidelines for lowering blood pressure and associated benefits for nonpregnant hypertensive individuals (237), the guidelines for pregnant women with chronic hypertension are less clear. As discussed previously, a clear-cut goal of antihypertensive is to prevent maternal cerebrovascular accidents associated with severe elevations in blood pressure. The controversy surrounding "tight control" versus "less tight control" during pregnancy is not yet resolved. Issues include (i) the concern for higher fetal exposure to antihypertensive drugs, which have not been studied well in terms of long-term growth and development, (ii) the theoretical concern that marked lowering of blood pressure could chronically reduce uterine blood flow resulting in reduced delivery of oxygen and nutrients to the feto-placental unit, which may lead to fetal compromise, and (iii) the lack of evidence to support the lowering of blood pressure to prevent superimposed preeclampsia (239). Given these concerns, the focus in pregnancy has been on short-term outcomes and avoiding fetal harm, rather than long-term prevention of cardiovascular risk and end-organ damage. The National High Blood Pressure Education Working Group has recommended initiating therapy when systolic pressures exceed 150 mm Hg and diastolic pressures exceed 95 to 100 mm Hg (104). Exceptions include preexisting renal disease or other evidence of end-organ compromise that may benefit from blood pressure control such as retinopathy and cardiac disease; antihypertensive medications are recommended only if diastolic blood pressure exceeds 90 mm Hg. Additional research is needed to resolve the issue of level of blood pressure control in the chronic hypertensive woman during pregnancy (236).

Frequent outpatient visits and home blood pressure monitoring are helpful in monitoring elevations in blood pressure, which may be the first sign of superimposed preeclampsia. Frequent assessment of urinary protein excretion and educating the patient regarding symptoms of preeclampsia are helpful in early diagnosis of superimposed preeclampsia (see previous discussion on clinical management of preeclampsia). Serial growth ultrasounds, approximately every 3 to 4 weeks, in the third trimester are recommended with nonstress tests and/or biophysical profiles after 32 weeks' gestation, particularly if there is any evidence of FGR. Given the overall increased perinatal morbidity, delivery is recommended at 39 weeks' gestation, or sooner if indicated.

Pharmacologic therapy is guided by safety and efficacy. Medications used for the treatment of chronic hypertension are outlined in Table 13.4. Key issues related to the various medications prescribed for chronic hypertension in pregnancy are discussed in the following text and in Table 13.4; we also recommend referring to a recent, excellent review for further details on the topic (240).

Methyldopa

Methyldopa is a centrally acting antihypertensive, which is reflected in the profile of adverse effects. Methyldopa remains a commonly used drug for long-term control of blood pressure in pregnancy. Methyldopa has been shown to improve fetal outcome when compared to placebo and is not associated with

TABLE 13.4 ANTIHYPERTENSIVE DRUGS USED FOR THE MANAGEMENT OF CHRONIC HYPERTENSION

Drug (FDA Category)	Mechanism of Action	Dose	Maximum Dose	Comments
Methyldopa (B)	Centrally acting $\alpha2$-zeceptor agonist	500–3,000 mg/day in 2–3 divided doses; generally start with 250 mg po twice daily	3 g/day	Preferred agent of National High Blood Pressure Working group; slow onset; side effect profile includes lethargy; best long-term data for children exposed in utero
Labetalol (C)	α- and β-adrenergic antagonist	100–2,400 mg/day in 2–3 divided doses; generally start at 100–200 mg po twice daily	2,400 mg/day	Increasingly preferred as a first-line agent; rapid onset of action; avoid in patients with asthma or congestive heart failure
Nifedipine (C)	Calcium-channel blocker	30–120 mg/day of a slow release preparation	120 mg/day	Side effects include headache, flushing, tachycardia; once a day dosing may improve compliance
Hydrochlorothizide (C)	Thiazide diuretic	12.5–50 mg/day	50 mg/day	Not used as a primary agent in pregnancy; considered an adjunctive agent; theoretical concerns of reduced intravascular volume and decreased uterine blood flow in pregnancy; electrolytes should be monitored
Hydralazine (C)	Vasodilation, smooth muscle relaxant	50–300 mg/day in 2–4 divided doses	300 mg/day	Not used as a primary agent in pregnancy; considered an adjunctive agent; may be used in combination with a sympatholytic agent (e.g., methyldopa or labetalol) to prevent tachycardia

FGR (241). Methyldopa does not appear to have an effect on the uterine or fetal–placental circulations (242,243) or the fetal heart rate (244). There are long-term follow-up data at 7 years, which show no detriment to the offspring of women treated with methyldopa during pregnancy (245). Methyldopa can have a depressant effect on the central nervous system, increasing fatigue and reducing mental acuity. It should be used with caution in women with a history of depression. As the dose of methyldopa increases, the adverse effects, particularly sedation and depression, also increase. Methyldopa-induced hepatitis and Coombs' positive hemolytic anemia are rare side effects (240). Methyldopa is excreted in breast milk, but the amount is too small to be harmful.

Labetalol

Labetalol is a mixed α- and β-adrenergic antagonist that is a well-tolerated antihypertensive, which produces effective reduction in maternal blood pressure without any pronounced fetal effects (246). Labetalol has replaced atenolol as the favored β-blocker in pregnancy as it appears to have a less detrimental effect on fetal growth (247). A small study has found no link between labetalol therapy and altered fetal behavior (248) and there is likewise no apparent association between labetalol administration and abnormalities of fetal heart rate (244). Side effects include fatigue, lethargy, and exercise intolerance. Due to its mode of action labetalol should not be used in patients with asthma or preexisting cardiac disease. Labetalol is safe during breastfeeding.

Nifedipine

Nifedipine is a calcium-channel antagonist, acting on L-type calcium channels that are present in the maternal vasculature and uterine smooth muscle (hence the alternative use in pregnancy as a to-colytic, that is, medication used to inhibit or delay labor). Nifedipine is a potent antihypertensive, and should not be given sublingually as it can cause a precipitate fall in maternal blood pressure, which can lead to fetal distress (249) and has been associated with sudden death in an older cardiac population (250). In contrast, oral long-acting nifedipine does not appear to have any adverse effects on the uteroplacental circulation or fetal heart rate (244). Along with most other calcium-channel blockers, nifedipine does not appear to be teratogenic (251) and is safe for breastfeeding women. Due its effects on cardiac afterload, nifedipine should be avoided in women with advanced aortic stenosis or impaired left ventricular function. The most commonly observed side effects are headache, edema, and palpitations.

Pharmacological Treatments Not Suitable for Administration During Pregnancy

ACE inhibitors and angiotensin receptor blockers are contraindicated in pregnancy as they are feto-toxic leading to fetal renal failure as evidenced by oligohydramnios antenatally and post delivery as oliguria and anuria (157,158). Use of these drugs in the first trimester has been associated with an increased risk of congenital anomalies, specifically malformations of the cardiac and central nervous systems (156).

Diuretics such as furosemide and hydrochlorothiazide are not teratogenic. But, these drugs reduce intravascular volume and preload in opposition to the normal adaptations of pregnancy and, theoretically, can reduce uteroplacental perfusion. Therefore, these drugs are not generally used as single agents in pregnancy.

URINARY TRACT INFECTIONS

UTIs are common in pregnant women and require particular attention because of increased maternal and fetal risk.

Asymptomatic Bacteriuria

Asymptomatic bacteriuria (ASB) is defined as the significant growth of a bacterial uropathogen in the absence of symptoms. ASB occurs in 2% to 10% of pregnant women, an incidence that is similar to the one in sexually active nonpregnant women (252–254). During pregnancy, prompt recognition and treatment of ASB is important since up to 30% of women with untreated ASB will develop pyelonephritis, a serious condition with maternal and fetal morbidity. Early screening and treatment has both maternal and fetal benefits. In a recent Cochrane review of randomized trials of ASB in pregnant women comparing antibiotic therapy with placebo or no treatment, antibiotic treatment was more likely to resolve ASB (OR: 0.07, 95% CI: 0.05–0.10), lower the incidence of pyelonephritis (OR: 0.24, 95% CI: 0.19–0.32), and reduce the rate of preterm delivery or low-birthweight babies (OR: 0.60, 95% CI: 0.45–0.80) (255). Smooth muscle relaxation and ureteral dilation associated with pregnancy likely facilitate bacteria ascending from the bladder to the kidneys. Diagnosis is based on culture results from a freshly voided clean-catch or catheterized urine specimen. For asymptomatic women, bacteriuria is defined as two consecutive voided urine specimens with isolation of the same bacterial strain with more than 100,000 colony-forming units per milliliter or a single catheterized urine specimen with one bacterial species isolated with more than 100 colony-forming units per milliliter (256). In general obstetric practice, a single positive urine culture is often sufficient to initiate treatment given the potential consequences of untreated ASB. Compared to urine culture results, rapid screening tests such as dipstick, enzymatic screen, and interleukin-8 have much lower sensitivity and specificity (257–259); therefore, urine culture remains the gold standard for diagnosis, identification of pathogenic organisms, and targeting antibiotic therapy. The most common bacterial pathogen is *Escherichia coli*. Other common pathogens are bowel commensals including *Klebsiella pneumoniae, Proteus mirabilis*, Group B streptococcus, and enterococci. Antibiotic therapy should be based on bacterial sensitivities as well as on safety during pregnancy. Penicillins and cephalosporins are generally considered safe in pregnancy. Nitrofurantoin is also generally safe in pregnancy but should be avoided in women with glucose-6-phosphatase deficiency due to the risk of hemolytic crisis (260). Trimethoprim/sulfamethoxazole is also commonly used; however, sulfa compounds should be avoided close to delivery as a consequence of the potential risk of kernicterus in the neonate due to competition for bilirubin-binding sites (261–263). Trimethoprim is also usually avoided in the first trimester because of its action as a folic antagonist. Floroquinolones and tetracyclines are contraindicated in pregnancy. Both the Infectious Disease Society of America and the American College of Obstetricians and Gynecologists recommend early screening for bacteriuria by urine culture during pregnancy and prompt treatment if positive (256). The duration of antibiotic therapy should be 3 to 7 days (262,263). Periodic screening for recurrent bacteriuria should be undertaken after therapy and is generally done one week after completion of antibiotics as a test of cure. There are no clear recommendations for or against routine repeated screening of culture-negative women in the later phase of pregnancy. Women with underlying conditions that increase the risk of UTIs, such as sickle cell disease and diabetes, should be screened periodically throughout the pregnancy, at least once a trimester. Suppressive therapy should be considered in women who have two or more recurrent infections. Nitrofurantoin taken daily at bedtime for the duration of pregnancy is most commonly used for suppression.

Acute Cystitis

Symptoms suggestive of a UTI include dysuria, urgency, frequency, nocturia, and/or foul-smelling urine. Many of these symptoms are common in normal pregnant women; therefore, urine culture should be used to confirm the diagnosis. Bacterial pathogens are similar to ASB and pyelonephritis. As with ASB, pregnant women with UTI should be treated with a 3- to 7-day course of antibiotics unless there are additional symptoms concerning for pyelonephritis (264). Although data are limited in pregnant women, there appears to be no difference in outcome between short and long courses of antibiotics (264). Follow-up cultures are recommended 1 to 2 weeks after treatment to ensure that the bacteriuria has been eradicated.

Acute Pyelonephritis

Acute pyelonephritis occurs in 1% to 2% of all pregnant women and is associated with serious maternal and fetal risks (265). In contrast to nonpregnant women with ASB, up to 30% of untreated bacteriuria during pregnancy will result in pyelonephritis. This is reduced by 70% to 80%, if bacteriuria is successfully treated (255). Symptoms of acute pyelonephritis in pregnancy include flank pain, fevers, nausea/vomiting, and costovertebral angle tenderness with or without acute UTI symptoms. Most cases of pyelonephritis occur in the second and third trimesters of pregnancy (79%) (265). The elevated risk of pyelonephritis during pregnancy is attributed to physiologic adaptations of the renal system to pregnancy, specifically ureteral dilation secondary to smooth muscle relaxation, pressure on the ureters and bladder from the enlarging uterus, and possible increased susceptibility to endotoxin-induced tissue damage (266). As with ASB and cystitis, bacteria from the bowel are the primary pathogens. In a prospective study of acute pyelonephritis in the general obstetric population, *E. coli* was isolated in approximately 70% of cases. Other organisms such as *Klebsiella* and *Enterobacter* (3%), *Proteus* (2%), and gram-positive bacteria (10%) including group B streptococcus were isolated in the remaining cases (265).

Major concerns associated with pyelonephritis are septic shock, pulmonary compromise including acute respiratory distress syndrome (ARDS), and preterm contractions/labor. Maternal risk of septic shock syndrome or its variants, including ARDS is estimated to be as high as 20% (265,267–269). Pyelonephritis is also associated with increased uterine contractions (270). Fetal risks include those related to prematurity secondary to preterm labor/delivery and low birthweight (255,270,271). Contrary to these findings, one prospective study suggested no increase in preterm birth compared to the general obstetric population (265). Tocolysis, particularly with β-mimetic agents, has been associated with respiratory compromise (269) and should be avoided with pyelonephritis. If tocolytics are needed, labor-inhibiting agents that have minimal cardiovascular effects, such as indomethacin, should be considered. Other complications of pyelonephritis observed in a prospective study of a general obstetric population included anemia, bacteremia, and renal dysfunction. Anemia may be mediated by bacterial endotoxin-mediated hemolysis (265).

Management of acute pyelonephritis in pregnancy consists of empiric parenteral antibiotic therapy and initial inpatient management to monitor for the above-mentioned complications. Admission to the intensive care unit with close hemodynamic and respiratory monitoring are sometimes warranted due to the potential maternal complications. Symptoms and urine culture are diagnostic; complete blood count, electrolytes, and creatinine evaluation may also help guide management. The utility of routine blood cultures has been questioned (272), as it is unclear whether bacteremia is associated with a longer course or worse prognosis; however, blood cultures are reasonable in women who present with sepsis. Initial antibiotic choice should be guided by local and hospital microbiology and susceptibility information, with directed antibiotics chosen after culture-based sensitivities are available. IV β-lactam antibiotics and/or gentamicin are the preferred antibiotics on the basis of efficacy and safety (273). In general, ceftriaxone 1 g every 24 hours or ampicillin/gentamicin IV is used. Due to the resistance of many bacterial strains to first-generation cephalosporins, these are not used as a single agent for empiric therapy. Some symptomatic improvement is expected in 24 to 48 hours after initiation of antibiotic therapy. If there is no symptomatic relief or improvement in fever curve, urinary tract imaging should be considered to rule out urinary tract pathology such as perirenal abscess, stone, or obstruction. After being afebrile for 24 to 48 hours on IV antibiotics, conversion to oral antibiotics based on microbial sensitivities and completion of a 10- to 14-day course is recommended.

Outpatient management has been studied, but evidence suggests limited utility. For women over 24 weeks' gestation, more than 50% did not qualify for outpatient management based on study criteria or complications precluding early discharge (274). A subgroup that may be appropriate for outpatient management is women with acute pyelonephritis at less than 24 weeks' gestation, who can comply with initial inpatient observation followed by an outpatient visit within 24 hours for a second dose of IV antibiotics and clinical re-assessment. Compliance is a key consideration for outpatient care. Of note, 6 of 120 women ultimately required inpatient management and one developed septic shock during the observation period (275). Recurrent pyelonephritis occurs in 6% to 8% of women during pregnancy; therefore, antimicrobial prophylaxis is recommended for the remainder of pregnancy along with frequent urine culture assessment for infection. Daily doses of nitrofurantoin (50 or 100 mg) or cephalexin (250 or 500 mg) at night are commonly used regimens.

ACUTE RENAL FAILURE IN PREGNANCY

Pregnancy-related acute renal failure (PR-ARF) is a unique and important clinical challenge as there are two patients to consider: the mother and her fetus. A multidisciplinary approach is essential with high-risk obstetricians/maternal–fetal medicine specialists, critical care specialists, nephrologists, and neonatologists participating.

Precise estimation of the incidence of PR-ARF is challenging and imprecise due to the lack of a clear definition. PR-ARF follows a bimodal distribution with one peak in the first trimester largely related to complications of unregulated abortion including sepsis and a second peak in the third trimester related to obstetric complications (276,277). The overall incidence of PR-ARF has decreased since the 1960s from rates of 1/3,000 to current estimates of 1/15,000 to 20,000 (276–278).

This decline has been attributed to two main trends: (i) the legalization and regulation of abortion in many countries resulting in a reduction of abortion-related sepsis and (ii) improved access to prenatal care associated with closer surveillance for preeclampsia and other obstetrical complications. However, there have been no such dramatic changes in mortality rates associated with PR-ARF (0% to 30%) and long-term prognosis remains stable with full renal recovery rates of 60% to 90% (276,277,279,280). Epidemiologic data suggest PR-ARF associated mortality and morbidity remain high in developing countries (281,282) and certain populations within developed countries with limited access to care (283). Early and appropriate management of PR-ARF in the acute care setting are key factors in reducing mortality and improving long-term recovery of renal function in these reproductive-age women.

There are two major categories of PR-ARF: (i) pregnancy-specific diagnoses and (ii) other etiologies relevant to reproductive-age women that may happen to coincide with pregnancy. Therefore, we discuss general diagnostic and therapeutic principles followed by specific etiologies and particular fetal considerations.

DIAGNOSTIC PRINCIPLES

ARF has been broadly defined as "a deterioration of renal function over a period of hours to days, resulting in the failure of the kidney to excrete nitrogenous waste products and to maintain fluid and electrolyte homeostasis" (284). Specific diagnostic criteria for ARF even in the nonpregnant population have been vague and variable, from serum creatinine levels of >0.3 mg/dL to dialysis requirement; thus, comparisons across studies, generalizability of results, and translation of research to clinical management can be problematic. Recent efforts to standardize these definitions such as the Acute Dialysis Quality Initiative are likely to be helpful in the future (285). With pregnancy, these definitions may need to be modified further since normal laboratory parameters are markedly altered due to the anatomic and physiologic changes (Table 13.5; Renal Physiology section) (14,287). Serum levels of blood urea nitrogen and creatinine are markedly reduced due to the increased RPF and GFR; thus, a serum creatinine of 0.9 mg/dL is considered abnormal in pregnancy. Creatinine clearance increases by at least 25% over nonpregnant values over a 24-hour period. The kidney also plays an important role in acid–base homeostasis. The primary acid–base alteration during pregnancy is a respiratory alkalosis (pCO_2 is reduced by approximately 10 mm Hg) secondary to increased minute ventilation. A compensatory metabolic alkalosis occurs with decline in serum bicarbonate concentrations (18 to 20 mEq during pregnancy). These adaptations are beneficial for the fetus by increasing the CO_2 gradient across the placenta, but may reduce maternal acid buffering capacity.

ARF is conventionally and conveniently divided into three main etiologies: prerenal, intrarenal, and postrenal (284). This categorization also provides a useful framework for PR-ARF. Prerenal ARF

TABLE 13.5 NORMAL LABORATORY PARAMETERS IN PREGNANCY*

Variable	Change Compared to Nonpregnant Values	Approximate Normal Value in Pregnancy
Creatinine	↓	0.5 mg/dL
Blood urea nitrogen (BUN)	↓	9.0 mg/dL
GFR	↑	↑ ~40–65% above baseline
Creatinine clearance	↑	↑ ~25% above baseline
Uric acid	↓	2.0–3.0 mg/dL
Urinary protein excretion	Variable to ↑	<300 mg/24 h
Urinary albumin excretion	Variable to ↑	<20 mg/24 h
Sodium retention over pregnancy	↑	900–950 mmol
Plasma osmolality	↓	↓ ~10 mOsm/kg H_2O
PCO_2	↓	↓ ~10 mm Hg below baseline
Serum bicarbonate	↓	18–20 mEq/L
Urinary glucose excretion	Variable to ↑?	Variable

occurs secondary to reduced renal perfusion. Hypovolemia (as with severe hemorrhage or dehydration), hypotension (as in septic shock), or low cardiac output are common reasons for reduced perfusion of the kidneys. If any of the above are severe, prolonged, or uncorrected, the prerenal ARF can lead to intrinsic renal damage and intrarenal ARF (such as with acute tubular necrosis and cortical necrosis). Timely correction of the reduced renal perfection can prevent progression and permanent renal damage. Intrarenal ARF can also be caused by toxins such as nephrotoxic drugs or immune-mediated damage such as glomerulonephritis or lupus nephritis. Postrenal ARF refers to the downstream urinary tract obstruction that can result in renal failure such as urethral obstruction, bilateral ureteral obstruction, or unilateral ureteral obstruction with a nonfunctioning contralateral kidney. While this general classification may be an oversimplification of mechanisms, it is useful in guiding clinical care (288).

Evaluation of a pregnant woman presenting with ARF should begin with a detailed history, physical exam, and laboratory assessment. The etiology of ARF often becomes readily evident based on clinical history, such as severe postpartum hemorrhage; however, in some cases additional diagnostic studies are necessary. Microscopic urinalysis and urinary electrolytes may be helpful in distinguishing prerenal and intrarenal causes of ARF. A functioning kidney with reduced perfusion responds by increasing sodium and water reabsorption and reducing sodium excretion in the urine. In this situation, the urine sodium and fractional excretion of sodium ([(urine sodium $\times$ plasma creatinine)/(plasma sodium $\times$ urine creatinine)] $\times$ 100) would be low, <20 mEq/L and <1%, respectively. With intrarenal etiologies, the tubular function is likely to be impaired, resulting in higher urinary sodium (>40 mEq/L) and percent fractional excretion of sodium (>2%). Urine osmolality would be expected to be low with intrarenal causes and urine microscopy likely to demonstrate granular or cellular casts, and white and red blood cells. Imaging of the urinary tract may be helpful to evaluate for postrenal causes of ARF; ultrasound is used most frequently during pregnancy. Mild-to-moderate hydronephrosis, particularly on the right, is expected during pregnancy.

Renal Biopsy in Pregnancy

In the nonpregnant population, renal biopsy is often helpful in determining precise histologic diagnosis and guiding therapy. The rate of serious complications in this group is low (<1%) (289). Renal biopsy during pregnancy, however, may be associated with higher morbidity and therefore warrants careful consideration.

In most cases of ARF during pregnancy, an empiric diagnosis can be made and treatment instituted accordingly, rendering a smaller role for renal biopsy. However, accurate diagnosis may be useful when there is diagnostic confusion with vastly different treatments. One example is midtrimester renal failure that may be due to causes other than severe or worsening preeclampsia. The only cure for preeclampsia is delivery, and maternal disease including renal function is expected to improve. When the clinical picture is confusing, however, finding renal lesions other than those associated with preeclampsia would allow for directed maternal treatment and avoidance of unnecessary iatrogenic preterm delivery. The clinical decision to biopsy or not to biopsy becomes particularly challenging as the gestational age of neonatal viability approaches (approximately 24 weeks) as well as with the preterm situation.

The risks and benefits of renal biopsy in pregnancy has been a controversial topic with a wide range of safety concerns reported in the literature. Case series from the late 1960s indicated a complication rate of 1.6% to 4.4% including perirenal bleeding requiring nephrectomy, perirenal hematoma, and even maternal death associated with renal biopsy (290,291). In the late 1980s, Packham et al. presented on the safety and utility of renal biopsy during pregnancy on the basis of their case series of 111 renal biopsies in 104 women performed for new-onset hematuria, proteinuria, or impaired renal function in the first or second trimesters of pregnancy (292). These investigators demonstrated a 97% success rate in obtaining tissue with an overall low complication rate (one patient with a serious perirenal hematoma and four with transient hematuria or pain that resolved spontaneously). In 80% of patients, a specific glomerulonephritis was identified. These conflicting safety results were reviewed by experts in the field of renal disease and pregnancy, Drs. Lindheimer and Davison, who suggested that while renal biopsy is overall safe in pregnancy the potential for attendant risks must be taken into account (293). Their recommendations were to limit renal biopsy during pregnancy to situations of sudden deterioration of renal function prior to 32 weeks' gestation and with no obvious cause. Two more recent series using modern techniques such as ultrasound guidance indicate that in a well-selected population of pregnant women, renal histology was helpful in directing clinical management in 66% to 100% of the women. However, the complication rate was noteworthy with perirenal hematoma rates of 0% to 40%, with up to 25% requiring transfusion (294,295). There were no maternal deaths. In aggregate, these studies support the proposal by Lindheimer and Davison that while renal biopsy may have a role in pregnancy management, the potential risks must be factored into the decision making. The gestational age limits at which to consider biopsy may need to be re-evaluated given the improved neonatal outcomes at 28 to 30 weeks' due to antenatal glucocorticoid use and improved neonatal intensive care. Another consideration is empiric medical therapy such as high-dose steroids if a particular diagnosis seems most likely, with continued close monitoring of maternal response to treatment and fetal status. We recommend a multidisciplinary team approach to the decision making with maternal–fetal medicine, nephrology, and neonatology specialists.

THERAPEUTIC GOALS

The general therapeutic goals of PR-ARF are similar to those of ARF in the nonpregnant individual. Important treatment principles are the following: (i) treat the underlying cause, (ii) prevent further renal damage, (iii) continue supportive measures until recovery may occur, and (iv) maternal health comes first, but optimization of fetal status should be considered in the management. Directed treatment for pregnancy-specific etiologies is discussed in the next section. Here we will focus on general medical management including fluid and pharmacologic therapy as well as options for renal replacement therapy (RRT) that may be considered in the setting of pregnancy.

Medical Management

Initial treatment should be directed at correcting the underlying causative factors. This may include stopping renal toxic drugs (e.g., aminoglycosides, radiocontrast agents), treatment of sepsis with appropriate broad-spectrum antibiotics, stopping hemorrhage, and/or delivery in the setting of acute renal deterioration associated with preeclampsia. *By far, the most important aspect of medical management in most PR-ARF is improving and maintaining adequate renal perfusion to limit ongoing renal damage and reverse any preischemic changes.* This may be accomplished by IV administration of isotonic crystalloid solution, colloid solution, or, in many obstetric situations, packed red blood cells and other blood products as indicated. These interventions can be guided by clinical status such as pulmonary function and urine output; however, with complicated cases, invasive hemodynamic assessment with central venous pressure monitoring with or without a pulmonary artery pressure catheter in an intensive care setting may be indicated (284). Maternal intravascular volume and respiratory status are also important considerations for fetal well-being. Once again, we recommend a multidisciplinary team including critical care medicine and maternal–fetal medicine specialists for the acute management.

Pharmacologic therapies can also be considered, but remain secondary in the treatment of PR-ARF. Once thought to improve renal blood flow, low-dose dopamine is no longer used since large trials do not support an improvement in clinical outcome with ARF (296–298). Besides the general risks of vasoactive medications, a pregnancy-specific consideration is the potential effect on uterine blood flow and reducing placental perfusion. The use of loop diuretics in the setting of ARF to improve mortality and prognosis has also been an area of controversy. Loop diuretics increase intratubular flow rates that may decrease renal intratubular obstruction and ameliorate cell damage. In addition, since nonoliguric ARF has a better prognosis than oliguric ARF, it has been proposed that using pharmacologic agents such as furosemide to convert an oliguric state into a nonoliguric condition may be beneficial (284). This topic was recently reviewed by Bagshaw et al. Overall, loop diuretics were not associated with improved mortality or reduced rate of RRT. These authors acknowledge the relative paucity of high-quality data in the setting of ARF and recommend a suitably powered randomized trial (299). The current literature does not support the routine use of diuretics in preventing ARF or improving outcomes once ARF occurs (300).

Downstream effects of ARF, including hyperkalemia, metabolic acidosis, and anemia, must also be evaluated and treated. During pregnancy, hyperkalemia can be treated with polystyrene sulfonate (potassium binding resin) or glucose/insulin (284). Although there is limited data in pregnancy, polystyrene sulfonate's mechanism of action is limited to the intestinal tract and its lack of absorption suggests overall safety for use in pregnancy. Metabolic acidosis during pregnancy can be acutely corrected using bicarbonate; however, the focus should be on treating the underlying cause. The pregnancy-related respiratory alkalosis and compensatory decrease in plasma bicarbonate must be accounted for when considering need for bicarbonate in PR-ARF. Anemia due to ARF is generally secondary to hemolysis and decreased hematopoiesis. In the acute setting, severe anemia should be treated with transfusion during pregnancy. Exogenous erythropoietin may be administered if the process is prolonged. Higher doses may be needed during pregnancy to achieve a good response.

Renal Replacement Therapy

RRT should be considered if the supportive methods discussed previously are inadequate in the setting of PR-ARF. The indications for RRT in pregnancy are similar to those in nonpregnant individuals: (i) volume overload, (ii) hyperkalemia refractory to medical management, (iii) metabolic acidosis, and (iv) symptomatic uremia (mental status changes, pericarditis, neuropathy). The precise timing of RRT initiation (early vs. late) and whether there are long-term benefits remain incompletely resolved. Furthermore, the precise thresholds in pregnancy and whether these should be lower are yet undetermined. Although both hemodialysis and peritoneal dialysis are used during pregnancy (see later discussion in Dialysis in Pregnancy section), hemodialysis is most commonly used in the acute setting particularly because of the ability to remove excessive fluid more efficiently. Intermittent and continuous RRT have been used in the setting of ARF, with some authors suggesting a reduced mortality associated with continuous RRT in severely ill patients. This specific question has not been studied in pregnancy, and decision making should be based on the individual patient.

SPECIFIC ETIOLOGIES OF PR-ARF

Pregnancy-specific etiologies fall into broad categories: hypertensive, thrombotic microangiopathic, infectious, hypovolemia, and obstructive. While these are the most common causes of PR-ARF, particularly during the third trimester, other reasons for ARF that may be coincident with pregnancy must be considered.

HYPERTENSION AND THROMBOTIC MICROANGIOPATHY

Preeclampsia/Eclampsia/HELLP Syndrome

Although it is one of the most common causes of PR-ARF, the majority of preeclamptic patients do not develop renal failure (detailed discussion is presented in Hypertensive Disorders of Pregnancy section). The underlying pathophysiology of preeclampsia may predispose pregnant women to acute kidney injury. In addition to the renal changes of preeclampsia discussed previously, the reduced intravascular volume with resulting decrease in RPF and GFR, endothelial dysfunction, activation of the inflammatory and coagulation cascades, and vasospasm put these women at higher risk for renal failure and slower recovery. A superimposed insult that results in further reductions of intravascular volume, such as hemorrhage associated with abruption or postpartum uterine atony, can lead to acute renal injury. The primary pathology with preeclampsia-related ARF is acute tubular necrosis, with the most severe cases at risk for cortical necrosis (301).

Estimating the precise incidence and morbidity of ARF attributable to preeclampsia is problematic due to the lack of standard definitions, variations in clinical practice, and ability to generalize the results from individual studies. Recent reports indicate a 1.5% to 2% incidence of ARF in preeclampsia (302,303). This incidence is higher in patients with HELLP syndrome (304). Reported maternal mortality rates were 0% to 10%, perinatal mortality 34% to 41%, and short-term RRT rates 10% to 50%. Long-term renal prognosis is largely dependent on the prepregnancy renal and/or hypertensive status (302–304). Forty percent to eighty percent of women with preexisting hypertension or renal disease required long-term dialysis, with several deaths related to ESRD. None of the women who entered the pregnancy with normal blood pressure and renal function required long-term RRT in the average 4-year follow-up.

As with other types of ARF, the focus of preeclampsia-related ARF should be treating the underlying disorder. Preeclampsia is a progressive, multiorgan disease and the only effective treatment strategy to date is delivery of the fetus and placenta. Therefore, delivery is indicated in preeclampsia-related ARF. In addition, supportive care should be instituted including maintenance of intravascular volume, replacement of blood products, and ICU care with or without RRT as needed.

Acute Fatty Liver of Pregnancy

Acute fatty liver of pregnancy (AFLP) is a pregnancy-specific condition characterized by rapidly progressive hepatic failure in late gestation. It affects 1/5,000 to 1/10,000 pregnancies (305,306). The typical clinical presentation is nausea, vomiting, malaise, abdominal pain, and less commonly mental status changes. The diagnosis is based on moderately elevated liver transaminase enzymes, hyperbilirubinemia, elevated ammonia levels, clotting abnormalities, and hypoglycemia (307). Elevated serum creatinine and low antithrombin III are also features of AFLP. The precise diagnosis of AFLP is made after excluding other etiologies such as gall bladder disease and hepatitis. AFLP can occur coincident with preeclampsia and/or HELLP syndrome. Metabolic and laboratory values can help make this distinction (305). Liver biopsy is rarely needed for the diagnosis, and clotting abnormalities must be taken into account when considering the utility of biopsy if the clinical scenario is highly suggestive of AFLP.

An inborn error of mitochondrial fatty acid oxidation, specifically a mutation in the long-chain 3-hydroxyacyl coenzyme A, predisposes both the fetus and the mother to AFLP. It has been suggested that this may explain up to 20% of AFLP worldwide (308). It is hypothesized that this could lead to fatty infiltration of the liver and other organs including the kidney.

The precise etiology of the renal impairment associated with AFLP is unclear. Modest elevations of serum creatinine are frequently observed, with one series reporting a frequent finding of serum creatinine in the 2 to 3 mg/dL range. Fatty infiltration and/or hepatorenal syndrome are proposed etiologies of elevated creatinine. Further renal decline can be exacerbated by hemorrhage and disseminated intravascular coagulation (DIC), which are more common with AFLP. As with preeclampsia, the only curative intervention is delivery. Renal recovery is usually complete in survivors of AFLP (301,305,306). Additional supportive care is critical including correction of coagulopathy and maintenance of intravascular volume. Recovery tends to be more prolonged with AFLP; there are rarely long-term sequelae.

Amniotic Fluid Embolism

Amniotic fluid embolism (AFE) is a dramatic and catastrophic clinical entity that can also cause PR-ARF. The overall incidence is estimated to be 7.7 per 100,000 births (309). AFE is also referred to as "anaphylactoid syndrome of pregnancy." Major clinical findings include the abrupt and fulminant onset of hypoxemia and respiratory failure, cardiogenic shock, and disseminated intravascular coagulation. The maternal mortality has been estimated to be 22% based on a retrospective cohort study of three million birth records; however, other estimates of mortality are >60% (310). Cardiac dysfunction, DIC, and hemorrhage, all features of AFE, can contribute to reduced renal perfusion and PR-ARF; thus, acute kidney injury is a consideration in all survivors and optimal fluid management in an ICU setting is recommended.

Thrombotic Thrombocytopenic Purpura/Hemolytic Uremic Syndrome

Thrombotic thrombocytopenic purpura (TTP) and hemolytic uremic syndrome (HUS) are syndromes characterized by microangiopathic hemolytic anemia, thrombocytopenia, ischemia, and multiple organ involvement. These are not pregnancy-specific conditions, but are often included in the differential diagnosis of preeclamsia/HELLP syndrome and PR-ARF (311–313). Therefore, this discussion will be limited to their relevance in pregnancy.

Briefly, TTP is associated with a pentad of findings: thrombocytopenia, hemolytic anemia, fever, neurologic abnormalities, and renal dysfunction. HUS has similar features, except that renal involvement is more profound and neurologic involvement is infrequent. Women with HUS/TTP develop

TABLE 13.6 GENERAL PRINCIPLES IN THE DIFFERENTIAL DIAGNOSIS OF PREECLAMPSIA, AFLP, TTP, AND HUS[a]

	Preeclampsia/HELLP	Thrombotic Thrombocytopenic Purpura	Hemolytic Uremic Syndrome	Acute Fatty Liver of Pregnancy
Onset	Usually 3rd trimester	Median 23 weeks	Often postpartum	Close to term
Primary/unique	Hypertension and	Neurologic	Renal	Nausea, vomiting,
Clinical manifestation	proteinuria	symptoms	involvement	malaise
Purpura	Absent	Present	Absent	Absent
Fever	Absent	Present	Absent	Absent
Hemolysis	Mild	Severe	Severe	Mild
Coagulation studies	Variable	Normal	Normal	Prolonged abnormal
Hypoglycemia	Absent	Absent	Absent	Present
vWF multimers	Absent	Present	Present	Absent
Primary treatment	Delivery	Plasmapheresis	Plasmapheresis	Delivery

[a]Precise diagnosis can often be made only after delivery. Preeclampsia, HELLP syndrome, and acute fatty liver of pregnancy resolve soon after delivery.

intravascular thrombi associated with consumption of platelets, fragmentation of red blood cells, and resulting ischemia of various organs. Large multimers of von Willebrand's factor are found, and there is evidence that there may be a congenital or acquired deficiency of the plasma protease that cleaves these multimers (314,315). HUS/TTP is more common in women (approximately 70% of cases) and in association with pregnancy (13% of cases) (316). ARF is estimated to occur in two-thirds of these patients. Retrospective reviews have demonstrated that the maternal mortality has decreased over time, with a range of 8% to 44% (311,317,318). In one series, the maternal mortality was low, but long-term morbidity was substantial; the majority of women had hypertension and chronic renal insufficiency, many required dialysis and transplantation, and one died of ESRD (311). As previously mentioned, it is often difficult to differentiate these conditions from the preeclampsia spectrum of disorders (Table 13.6). Proper diagnosis is important as the treatments are different. Delivery is the primary treatment for preeclampsia, whereas plasmaphersis is the mainstay of therapy with TTP/HUS. Often, the diagnosis can only be made by following the disease progression after delivery. Other therapies that are often considered include glucocorticoids and aspirin. Supportive therapy and multidisciplinary medical team are important in the acute phase, particularly until diagnosis is clear.

VOLUME DEPLETION

Obstetric hemorrhage is the most common reason for intravascular volume depletion sufficient to cause ARF during pregnancy. This can occur at any gestational age. First- and second-trimester hemorrhage is largely related to ectopic pregnancies and induced or spontaneous abortions. In the third trimester, placenta previa, abruption, and/or postpartum hemorrhage are major causes of acute blood loss and secondary ARF (319). With placenta previa, the placental implants over the internal os of the cervix place a woman at increased risk of bleeding particularly with labor and cervical dilation. Women may be expectantly managed for minor degrees of bleeding, but delivery by cesarean section is necessary with severe hemorrhage. Placental abruption refers to the separation of the placenta from the uterine wall. This can lead to fetal distress and demise. Massive or complete abruption is often accompanied by excessive blood loss and DIC, major risk factors for ARF. The treatment for abruption consists of stabilizing maternal status and then delivery. Aggressive blood and blood product resuscitation is indicated with massive placental abruptions. There are multiple etiologies for postpartum hemorrhage, with uterine atony being the most common. With poor uterine tone, medical and surgical options to improve uterine tone are employed to reduce bleeding. Hysterectomy is reserved for intractable obstetric hemorrhage. Ongoing volume resuscitation with fluid and blood products is important to avoid ischemic damage to organs including the kidney.

Hyperemesis gravidarum refers to severe nausea and vomiting of pregnancy. While nausea and vomiting accompanies the majority of pregnancies (70% to 85%) particularly in the first trimester, severe symptoms are less common (1% to 2%) (320). Hyperemesis can be managed with oral antiemetics, with a small subset of patients requiring IV hydration and enteral or parenteral nutrition. In rare cases, severe hypovolemia can result in prerenal ischemia and ARF. One case report describes a pregnant woman with severe hyperemesis who required supportive care and short-term RRT with subsequent full recovery of renal function (321).

Postpartum Idiopathic ARF

ARF that develops during the postpartum period without a precise etiology and without fitting into the above-mentioned categories of preeclampsia, HELLP syndrome, AFLP, and TTP/HUS is often placed in this category (301,322). Although poorly defined, it appears that these women fall along the spectrum of thrombotic microangiopathy with renal manifestations. Supportive care is indicated and plasmapheresis may be considered.

INFECTION/SEPSIS

Sepsis can lead to hypotension, intravascular volume depletion, and decreased renal perfusion. This prerenal condition can result in acute kidney injury including sepsis-associated acute tubular necrosis. The most common causes of sepsis in pregnancy are pyelonephritis, chorioamnionitis, and pneumonia. With each of these entities, the mainstay is treatment of the underlying disorder usually with antibiotics and supportive measures, which may include pressor therapy. As previously discussed, pyelonephritis should be promptly diagnosed and treated during pregnancy (see Acute Pyelonephritis section). Chorioamnionitis refers to an intrauterine infection involving the chorion and amniotic membranes. The primary therapy is evacuation of the uterine contents by delivery and concomitant treatment with IV antibiotics. While chorioamnionitis is common (0.5% to 10.5% of all deliveries), bacteremia is observed in only 1% to 5% of these cases, with sepsis being even less frequent (323). Intrauterine infections are most frequently caused by bacterial organisms ascending from the vagina into the cervical canal and uterine cavity. Two-thirds of women have more than one organism identified in amniotic fluid culture. Common organisms include *E. coli,* group B streptococcus, *Gardnerella* species, peptostreptococcus, bacterioides, gram-negative organisms, anaerobes, and enterococci (324). Worldwide, septic abortion is also an important contributor to maternal ARF. Evacuation of the uterus, antibiotic therapy, and supportive measures are key to prevent maternal complications such as acute kidney damage.

OBSTRUCTION

Obstruction of the genitourinary system via compression by the gravid uterus is more common in cases of uterine overdistension such as polyhydramnios, multifetal gestation (particularly higher order multiples), and large fibroids (325–330). Susceptibility to ARF related to obstruction is increased in women with a solitary kidney, genitourinary anomalies, and prior urinary tract surgeries (331). Nephrolithiasis can also cause urinary tract obstruction that could potentially lead to ARF (332). Diagnosis is made using imaging techniques including ultrasound, pyelogram, and CT scan, which are generally safe in pregnancy. Treatment includes cystoscopy and retrograde ureteral stent placement, or percutaneous nephrostomy. Delivery generally ameliorates the obstruction, but needs to be considered in the context of gestational age and response to conservative measures.

OTHER CAUSES OF ACUTE RENAL FAILURE IN PREGNANCY

Although pregnancy-specific causes of ARF are most common particularly in the third trimester, other etiologies that may occur coincident with pregnancy in the reproductive-age population must be considered. Nonsteroidal anti-inflammatory medications and aminoglycosides are nephrotoxins that are commonly used in the obstetric population. These should be stopped in women undergoing a workup for causes of ARF. Autoimmune conditions including renal manifestations such as glomerulonephritis with or without lupus are more common in women of reproductive age and should, therefore, be

TABLE 13.7 FEATURES THAT MAY HELP DIFFERENTIATE PREECLAMPSIA AND ACUTE GLOMERULONEPHRITIS[a]

	Preeclampsia	Acute Glomerulonephritis
Gestational Age	Onset usually in the third trimester (by definition after 20 weeks)	Any
Hypertension Systemic manifestations (may or may not be present)	Present •?Neurologic (headache, scotomata, visual disturbances, seizures) •?Hematologic (low platelets) •?Hepatic involvement (elevated transaminases)	Present •?Collagen-vascular disease (e.g., systemic lupus erythematosus with associated symptoms such as fatigue, arthralgias rash, fevers) •?Preceding infection (e.g., streptococcal infection)
Urine sediment	•?Isolated proteinuria •?Urine microscopy generally benign, may have findings of acute tubular necrosis (brown granular casts, renal tubular cells)	•?Hematuria, RBC casts, oval fat bodies
Proteinuria	>300 mg/24 h (mild), >5 g/24 h (severe)	>2 g/24 h
Complement levels	↔	↓
ANA	↔	↑
Antistreptolysin-O titers	↔	↑
Other autoantibodies	↔	?↑

[a]The diagnosis may be confusing. Presence or absence of above features is not absolute, but may assist in the diagnosis.

included in the differential diagnosis. Differentiating between glomerulonephritis and preeclampsia-related ARF may be challenging. Some of the distinguishing characteristics are summarized in Table 13.7.

FETAL CONSIDERATIONS WITH MATERNAL ARF

With pregnancy, there are two patients to consider—the mother and her fetus. While maternal health comes first, fetal status can be optimized during treatment. The adverse perinatal outcomes associated with PR-ARF are largely associated with the altered uteroplacental hemodynamics. Blood flow to the uterus and placenta are highly dependent on intravascular volume and cardiac function. Therefore, particular attention to fluid management, maternal anemia, safety of medications, and maternal uremia are important fetal considerations with PR-ARF, in addition to treatment of the underlying condition. For viable gestations (>24 weeks' gestation), fetal monitoring is recommended with options including intermittent or continuous fetal heart rate monitoring and/or biophysical profile assessments by ultrasound. The frequency and type of testing can be varied depending on gestational age of the fetus and maternal status. If preterm delivery is indicated for maternal benefit, consideration should be given to administering antenatal glucocorticoids (betamethasone or dexamethasone) to reduce neonatal morbidity related to prematurity. Prematurity and associated complications are the major neonatal issues after birth. Neonatologists and a tertiary neonatal intensive care unit are important in the multidisciplinary team caring for the pregnant woman with ARF.

CHRONIC RENAL DISEASE AND PREGNANCY

Chronic kidney disease (CKD) is estimated to affect at least 4% of women in the reproductive-age group. Retrospective studies have characterized the prevalence of CKD in pregnancy to be 0.03% to 0.12% (333–335). This is likely an underestimate since renal disease is often unrecognized prior to pregnancy and is difficult to diagnose during pregnancy being masked by the normal physiological changes such as increased GFR and lower serum creatinine. Historically, CKD in pregnancy has been associated with significant perinatal morbidity and mortality. A 1975 editorial in the Lancet noted "children of women with renal disease used to be born dangerously or not at all—not at all, if their doctors had their way" (336). An improved understanding of CKD as well as advances in perinatal and neonatal care has contributed to better outcomes in this population. As with many other medical disorders, the two major issues are (i) the effect of maternal renal disease on the progression and outcome of pregnancy, and (ii) the effect of pregnancy on the course of the renal disease.

Before embarking on an evidence-based discussion of pregnancy outcomes with CKD, it is critical to recognize limitations in the published literature (337). Most studies have a small sample size, are conducted at single institutions, and are retrospective without a comparison group. In addition, preconception counseling, pregnancy care, and follow-up are not standardized. Many of the larger studies span long periods in which there have been substantial changes in neonatal care, such as administration of steroids for prematurity, leading to improved outcomes over time. Another major confounder is the inconsistency in the classification of renal disease and the definition of outcomes. For example, some studies use gestational age of less than 37 weeks to define preterm delivery while others use less than 34 weeks. These are just few of the factors that have limited our ability to compare outcomes across studies and generalize the results to other populations. Prepregnancy renal function and hypertension have emerged as the best predictors of adverse perinatal outcome (FGR, preterm delivery, preeclampsia, perinatal death) and decline in renal function. The etiology of the CKD, other than systemic diseases such as lupus, does not appear to be a major factor affecting outcomes.

Classification Systems

The classification of CKD has recently been standardized (Table 13.8a). Preconception classification is useful, since formulas estimating GFR may not accurately represent renal function during pregnancy: formulae such as the Cockroft–Gault use body weight that does not necessarily reflect kidney size, and the Modification of Diet in Renal Disease formula (MDRD) underestimates GFR in pregnancy (261,338). During pregnancy, creatinine clearance and serum creatinine along with the presence or absence of hypertension and proteinuria are helpful in baseline classification. Traditionally, the pregnancy literature has used the mild (serum creatinine <1.4 mg/dL), moderate (serum creatinine 1.4–2.4 mg/dL), and severe (serum Cr ≥2.5 mg/dL) for classification of CKD (Table 13.8b). Stages 3 to 5 correspond to moderate and severe renal disease.

TABLE 13.8a CLASSIFICATION SYSTEMS USED FOR CHRONIC KIDNEY DISEASE

	Stages of Chronic Kidney Disease[a]	
Stage	**Description**	**GFR (mL/min/1.73 m²)**
1	Slight kidney damage with normal or increased GFR	≥90
2	Kidney damage with mildly decreased GFR	60–89
3	Moderately decreased GFR	30–59
4	Severely decreased GFR	15–29
5	Kidney failure	<15 or dialysis

[a]Chronic kidney disease is defined as either kidney damage or GFR <60 mL/min/1.73 m² for ≥3 months. Kidney damage is defined as pathologic abnormalities or markers of damage including abnormalities in the composition of blood or urine or abnormalities on imaging tests. (From The National Kidney Foundation. K/DOQI clinical practice guidelines for chronic kidney disease: Evaluation, classification, and stratification. *Am J Kid Dis.* 39(1 suppl.): S1–S266, 2002, with permission.)

TABLE 13.8b CLASSIFICATION SCHEME THAT HAS BEEN USED FOR WOMEN WITH CHRONIC KIDNEY DISEASE AND PREGNANCY

Level of Renal Impairment	Prepregnancy Serum Creatinine (mg/dL)
Mild	<1.4
Moderate	1.4–2.4 (some use)
Severe	>2.4 (some use >2.8 to indicate severe)
Dialysis	On chronic hemodialysis or peritoneal dialysis

Moderate-to-severe impairment approximates stages 3–5 from Table 13.8a.

IMPACT OF PREGNANCY ON CHRONIC RENAL DISEASE

The precise impact of pregnancy on chronic renal disease has been a controversial topic. It has been proposed that pregnancy-induced hyperfiltration may lead to an acceleration of GFR decline in chronic kidney disease (333,339). However, hyperfiltration in pregnancy appears to be caused primarily by increases in renal blood flow along with vasodilation of the efferent and afferent arterioles, without any marked increase in the intraglomerular pressure that can damage the kidney. Baylis et al. have demonstrated using animal models that glomerular capillary pressure is not increased during pregnancy (340,20). On the other hand, it is not uncommon to observe worsening of proteinuria (~50%) and the development or worsening hypertension (~25%) in pregnancies complicated by CKD (261), which themselves can effect further damage on the kidney (339). For the most part, these changes resolve after delivery. It is very important, therefore, to differentiate between the renal changes that occur during pregnancy and long-term decline in renal function with CKD and pregnancy. Therefore, we will focus our discussion on permanent decline in renal status, which would have long-term implications for the mother.

Mild CKD (Stages 1 and 2)

A permanent decline in renal function is observed in 0% to 10% of women with mild renal disease (341–344) (Table 13.9a). This is comparable to the progression observed in nonpregnant individuals with mild CKD. In one study of 360 women with chronic glomerulonephritis, there was no difference in long-term (up to 25 years) renal function between women who became pregnant and those who did not conceive (343). This and other studies suggest that the progression of mild renal disease is not accelerated by pregnancy (261).

Moderate CKD

Early small-scale studies suggested that >50% of women with moderate renal insufficiency had a permanent decline in renal function after pregnancy. In 1986, Imbasciati et al. were among the first to demonstrate that renal progression was lower than in initial reports and observed long-term renal decline in approximately one-third of mothers with moderate renal disease prior to pregnancy (345). These findings have been corroborated by other studies with larger sample size, essentially demonstrating that women with the worst renal function were at highest risk of accelerated renal decline during pregnancy (344,346–349). Hypertension adds to the risk of progression. Jones et al. studied a total of 87 women with moderate and severe renal disease. Among women with a baseline serum creatinine of 1.5 to 1.9 mg/dL, 40% had a decline in renal function during pregnancy and 2% had permanent progression of renal function. However, among women with a serum creatinine ≥2.0 mg/dL, 65% of women had decline in renal function in the third trimester, which persisted after pregnancy in most women (347). Thirty-five percent had progression to end-stage renal failure.

A recent prospective study of women with CKD stages 3 to 5 assessed progression of renal decline before, during, and after pregnancy (348). Women with a prepregnancy estimated GFR <40 mL/min/1.73 m^2

TABLE 13.9a ESTIMATED IMPACT OF PREGNANCY ON MATERNAL RENAL FUNCTION IN WOMEN WITH CHRONIC KIDNEY DISEASE

Prepregnancy Serum Creatinine	Loss of .25% Renal Function		
	During Pregnancy (%)	Persisting Postdelivery (%)	End-Stage Renal Failure after 1 Year (%)
·< 1.4 mg/dL	2	0	0
1.4–2.0	40	20	2
··· >2.0	70	50	35

From Williams DJ and Davison JM. Renal Disorders. In: Creasy RK, Resnik R, Iams JD, et al., eds. *Creasy and Resnik's Maternal-Fetal Medicine Principles and Practice.* 6th ed. Philadelphia, PA: Elsevier; 2009: 905–926, with permission.

TABLE 13.9b PREGNANCY OUTCOME BASED ON PREPREGNANCY RENAL FUNCTION IN WOMEN WITH CHRONIC KIDNEY DISEASE[a]

Prepregnancy Serum Creatinine	FGR (%)	Preterm Delivery (%)	Preeclampsia (%)	Live Birth (%)
<1.4 mg/dL	16–26	20–24	6–29	95+%
1.4–2.5	31–64	30–79	~40	~92%
>2.5[b]	22–57 (65)	50–86 (>95)	>60–80	Inadequately reported

[a]Ranges are from selected studies 1984–2007 (see text), with pregnancies attaining ≥24 weeks when possible. Not all the studies included provide information in each of these categories.

[b]This category is limited by small numbers. Estimates by Williams and Davison are higher and indicated in parenthesis. (From Williams DJ and Davison JM. In: Creasy RK, Resnik R, Iams JD, et al., eds. *Creasy and Resnik's Maternal-Fetal Medicine Principles and Practice.* 6th ed. Philadelphia, PA: Elsevier; 2009: 905–926, with permission.)

and 24-hour urine protein excretion >1 g, but not either factor alone had accelerated progression of renal function decline after pregnancy compared to before pregnancy. These data may allow for more specific preconception counseling.

With *severe renal impairment* (serum creatinine >3 mg/dL), women are less likely to ovulate, conceive spontaneously, and carry a fetus to term (344,350). However, the same principles likely apply, with the degree of prepregnancy renal impairment associated with worse outcomes.

IMPACT OF CKD ON PREGNANCY OUTCOMES

The major impact of CKD on pregnancy outcomes includes FGR, iatrogenic preterm delivery, preeclampsia, and perinatal death. The rate of live births is >90% in women with mild renal impairment, which is somewhat lower in women with moderate renal insufficiency with good blood pressure control (334,344,350–352). Adverse pregnancy rate is higher with worsening prepregnancy renal status and hypertension (Table 13.9b, adapted from Refs. 261,333,353 and includes studies from Refs. 334,345, 347,348,354–358).

Women with preexisting renal disease are at substantially high risk for developing preeclampsia. Diagnosis is often problematic in women with hypertension and/or proteinuria associated with renal disease. Sudden increases in blood pressure, proteinuria, new onset of preeclampsia symptoms (headache, visual changes, right upper quadrant, or epigastric pain), or other evidence of end-organ disease (drop in platelet count or increase in liver transaminases) supports the diagnosis of preeclampsia.

The incidence of FGR is higher in women with preexisting renal disease (Table 13.9). Careful monitoring of fetal growth and surveillance of fetal well-being are warranted in the third trimester (see Management of Pregnancy in Women with CKD section).

Preterm delivery is most often iatrogenic and related to FGR, preeclampsia, or worsening renal function (Table 13.9). There is marked variability in patient management and criteria for delivery, making comparison across studies problematic. High-risk obstetricians and neonatologists should be involved in the decision-making regarding delivery. Steroids are indicated prior to 34 weeks' gestation to improve neonatal outcomes.

Management of Pregnancy in Women with CKD

These pregnancies should be managed by a high-risk obstetrician/maternal–fetal medicine specialist in conjunction with the multidisciplinary team including nephrologists. Preconception counseling based on the existing evidence is paramount in all reproductive-age women. Effective contraception is recommended until renal function is stable and systemic disease is well controlled. As noted earlier, women with mild and moderate renal disease, particularly with a creatinine <2.0 mg/dL, have a high likelihood of good outcomes. Perinatal morbidities and accelerated decline in renal function after pregnancy are more likely with baseline serum creatinine ≥2.0 mg/dL (347). Baseline laboratory tests should include an assessment of renal function (serum blood urea nitrogen, creatinine, electrolytes including calcium and phosphorus as well as urine for microscopic evaluation, proteinuria, 24-hour collection for creatinine clearance, and total protein excretion). Although random protein to creatinine ratios may be convenient as 24-hour collections are fraught with problems including compliance, the 24-hour collection remains the gold standard during pregnancy particularly for the diagnosis of preeclampsia (104). Baseline complete blood count including platelets and liver transaminases may be useful as these can be altered by preeclampsia. Blood pressure should be assessed and treated with medications considered safe in pregnancy (methyldopa, labetalol, calcium-channel blockers such as nifedipine). In general, one agent is maximized before a second agent is added, partly to minimize fetal exposure to multiple medications. ACE inhibitors and ARBs should be avoided due to their association with birth defects in the first trimester and oligohydramnios and fetal renal failure in the third trimester. Diuretics tend not to be used in pregnancy due to their effect of reducing intravascular volume and potentially blood flow to the uterus. Although the current recommendations are to lower blood pressure <130/80 mm Hg in nonpregnant patients with CKD, this must be balanced against the blood pressure alterations that occur as a part of the normal pregnancy adaptations and the risk of reducing uteroplacental perfusion.

Anemia is common in pregnancy and, if diagnosed with additional studies, appropriate iron, folate, and/or B12 supplementation should be instituted. If the anemia is secondary to renal dysfunction, most commonly with normocytic and normochromic red blood cell indices, then erythropoietin therapy is indicated (261). In addition to the usual prenatal care, renal function should be evaluated approximately once a month. Visits should occur every 2 to 3 weeks and then every week after 28 to 30 weeks to monitor for the development of preeclampsia. Home blood pressure monitoring as well as watchfulness for symptoms of preeclampsia is also useful. The diagnosis of preeclampsia can be confusing, and oftentimes inpatient monitoring is required until the diagnosis becomes more apparent. Fetal surveillance should include an early ultrasound to establish gestational age, detailed anatomic ultrasound survey between 18 and 20 weeks' gestation, and serial ultrasounds to monitor fetal growth. These are usually initiated at 24 to 26 weeks and then performed every 3 to 4 weeks thereafter. The frequency should be increased if there is evidence of FGR. Doppler interrogation of the umbilical arteries can also be useful in the setting of suspected growth restriction. Fetal kick counts should be monitored daily by the mother starting at 28 weeks of pregnancy. Antenatal testing should be initiated between 28 and 32 weeks; this may include nonstress tests one to two times per week and/or biophysical profile testing each week. The frequency of testing should be increased if there are any concerns about fetal wellbeing. Antenatal glucocorticoids should be administered prior to 34 weeks' gestation if delivery is anticipated. The neonatology team should be consulted if a preterm delivery is anticipated. If both mother and baby are doing well, delivery at 39 weeks is recommended. Vaginal route is the preferred mode of delivery, with cesarean section reserved for the usual obstetric indications. Postpartum care should include close monitoring of blood pressure, adjustment of medications, and monitoring of renal function. Physiologic changes of pregnancy generally resolve by 10 to 12 weeks post delivery. Breast feeding is encouraged in women with CKD. Rarely, breastfeeding may be contraindicated based on safety of particular medications.

SPECIFIC RENAL DISORDERS IN PREGNANCY

For most renal disorders, pregnancy outcome and long-term renal function are largely dependent on baseline renal function (serum creatinine) and the presence or absence of hypertension. Systemic lupus erythematosus and diabetes, which are common in reproductive-age women warrant additional discussion. A few other specific disorders will be addressed. Due to space limitations, only key considerations as they apply to pregnancy and renal function are discussed later.

Diabetic Nephropathy

Renal dysfunction secondary to diabetes follows a predictable progression to ESRD if untreated. Rigorous metabolic control, blood pressure treatment, and renoprotection with ACE inhibitors or ARBs are all strategies to prevent and control the progression of diabetic nephropathy. Women with long-standing diabetes often have renal impairment during their reproductive years. Pregnancy does not appear to accelerate renal decline in women with mild renal impairment (serum creatinine <1.5 mg/dL) (359). The data for women with moderate and severe baseline renal disease are more controversial. One report suggested a 40% higher chance of renal deterioration attributable to pregnancy (360). Although these women had good glycemic control, this study suffered from the lack of a control group. Worsening blood pressure over the course of pregnancy, particularly in the third trimester, may contribute to the decline in renal function (361). Larger, well-controlled studies are needed to resolve this issue. To avoid potential renal decline, good glycemic and blood pressure control are recommended during pregnancy. ACE inhibitors and ARBs used for "renoprotection" outside of pregnancy should not be used in pregnancy. There is some evidence to support the use of diltiazem for renal protection (362,363) and it is generally considered safe in pregnancy. While a small study suggests benefit in pregnancy (364), additional data are needed before recommendations can be made for using diltiazem as a renal protective agent during pregnancy.

Systemic Lupus Erythematosus

Systemic lupus erythematosus (SLE) disproportionately affects women and tends to occur during the child-bearing years. It is a systemic autoimmune condition that can affect multiple organs and to varying degrees. The reader is referred to a number of excellent reviews for details on lupus and pregnancy (365–367). Pregnancy planning, effective contraception, and preconception counseling are highly recommended for women with SLE. Renal involvement confers a higher risk on the pregnancy. In women with stable renal disease and well-controlled SLE without flares, pregnancy outcome is based on baseline renal impairment and hypertension. The precise effect of pregnancy on lupus disease activity is unclear; however, women who have been in remission for >1 year are at lower risks for flares during pregnancy. Prepregnancy disease activity appears to be associated with the frequency of exacerbations during pregnancy, ranging from 7% to 33% in women who have been in remission for 6 months, and 61% to 67% in women who have active disease at the time of conception (368,369). Therefore, women with lupus nephritis should be encouraged to delay pregnancy until disease is inactive for approximately 12 months.

Lupus nephritis during pregnancy can be difficult to distinguish from preeclampsia, particularly in the third trimester. Clinical and laboratory features that differentiate the two conditions are listed in Table 13.7. Treatment options for lupus nephritis flares during pregnancy include high-dose steroids and azathioprine. Newer treatments may be considered after weighing risks and benefits. Cyclophosphamide should be avoided if possible during pregnancy. In contrast, the treatment for preeclampsia is delivery; therefore, differentiating between the two conditions is very important.

A multidisciplinary team is ideal for pregnancy care. Close postpartum follow-up is warranted since flares may occur during this time period and symptoms may be difficult to distinguish from the commonly observed postpartum fatigue in new mothers.

Glomerulonephritis

As with other forms of CKD, degree of baseline renal impairment and hypertension are associated with pregnancy outcomes. In general, most pregnancies are successful with stable, mild renal impairment and absence of hypertension (261,370). Several case series indicate that the histological type of glomerulonephritis affects pregnancy outcomes. IgA nephropathy and membranous glomerulonephritis are associated with lowest fetal loss rates (371,372). Membranoproliferative GN type 1 and focal glomerulosclerosis are associated with a higher rate of pregnancy complications including fetal loss rate, growth restriction, and preterm delivery (371). During pregnancy, approximately 20% of women with primary glomerulonephritis will have new-onset hypertension and 10% to 20% of women with preexisting hypertension will have a worsening of blood pressure (352). Jungers et al. performed a large cohort study of primary glomerulonephritis with average patient follow-up of 15 years; pregnancy was not an independent risk factor for permanent renal deterioration among women with normal-to-mild kidney dysfunction (343).

Polycystic Kidney Disease

Adult polycystic kidney disease is an autosomal dominant disorder that usually manifests after the child-bearing years (373). Family history along with ultrasound evaluation of the kidneys is important in early diagnosis. If renal function is normal or mild prior to pregnancy, outcomes are generally favorable. These women are at increased risk of hypertension later in pregnancy, as well as for developing chronic hypertension following pregnancy (373). Genetic counseling should be offered to women with adult polycystic kidney disease or a strong family history of this disorder prior to and during pregnancy. Extrarenal manifestations are observed in 50% of women with polycystic kidney disease, including liver cysts, cerebral aneurysms, cardiac valvular defects, and aortic aneurysms.

Urolithiasis

Urinary tract stones occur in 0.03% to 3% of all pregnancies (261). Pain can be quite severe, often necessitating inpatient management. Calcium oxalate stones are most common. Clinical suspicion, microscopic or gross hematuria, and imaging are the mainstays of diagnosis. Management is with appropriate hydration, pain management, and antibiotics if infection is suspected. Cystoscopic placement of intraureteral stents under local anesthesia or conscious sedation is often used for obstruction and/or severe pain in pregnant women; percutaneous nephrostomy can also be used for these indications.

DIALYSIS IN PREGNANCY

There have been substantial improvements in both fertility and pregnancy rates in women with end-stage renal failure. The incidence of pregnancy among reproductive-age women on dialysis is estimated to be 0.3% to 1.5% per year (349). Improved overall health with dialysis, particularly with the use of erythropoietin, has been associated with an increase in return of menses and ovulation. The first case report of a successful conception and pregnancy while on dialysis was in 1971 (374). A case series published in 1980 reported high rates of preterm birth, low birthweight, and refractory hypertension (375). Although the overall prognosis is improved, pregnancy in women on dialysis is associated with significant perinatal morbidity and mortality. After exclusion of therapeutic abortions, the likelihood of fetal survival is estimated to be 40% to 50% (376). Much of the evidence comes from case reports, case series, surveys, and registries. Based on several large surveys performed since the 1990s in the United States and Belgium, 40% to 52% of pregnancies resulted in a surviving infant (377–379). Outcomes were comparable among women undergoing hemodialysis and peritoneal dialysis. Recent smaller series indicate even higher rates of infant survival (380). Overall, these pregnancies are complicated by preterm delivery (85%), intrauterine growth restriction (90%), polyhydramnios (40%), and hypertension/preeclampsia (70%) (estimates based on review by Williams et al Ref. 261).

Evidence suggests that the overall improvement may be due to the recognition that increased dialysis "dose" may be beneficial. Okundaye et al. noted that an increase in the number of hours of dialysis per week was associated with increased survival and a decrease in the rates of prematurity (379). Similar trends were observed in a national survey of dialysis centers in Belgium where dialysis regimens were adjusted with a goal to attain predialysis urea levels of ≤100 mg/dL (378). A positive correlation was noted between birthweight and additional dialysis hours over nonpregnant recommendations. In addition, maternal uremia increases delivery of urea to the fetus leading to increased fetal solute load and, frequently, fetal diuresis with resulting polyhydramnios and preterm contractions/labor (381–384).

Many experts have suggested using a dialysis protocol that would mimic the physiological changes over the course of pregnancy. Key features of this protocol are outlined in Table 13.9. Important points that are associated with improved outcomes are (i) to increase dialysis time and frequency (often five to seven times per week during pregnancy), (ii) to minimize fluid shifts and hypotension, and (iii) to maintain low maternal serum urea, generally <45 to 60 mg/dL. Weight gain must be monitored closely, and pregnancy-associated weight gains must be taken into account when considering fluid management. Anemia should be managed aggressively during pregnancy with erythropoietin. Although theoretically associated with hypertension, erythropoietin is generally well tolerated in pregnancy. Higher doses are often required during pregnancy. Blood pressure control may be achieved with a combination of pharmacologic therapy (see Table 13.4) and by removing excess intravascular fluid. Vigilant pregnancy management is essential and is similar to that outlined in the previous section on women with chronic kidney disease. A special consideration is the fetal monitoring prior to and post dialysis, particularly in the third trimester, as hypotension and increased contractions associated with dialysis may adversely affect fetal well-being and cause preterm labor, respectively. Importantly, contraception should be addressed in sexually active women who do not desire pregnancy. Preconception consultation is important in the woman on dialysis to review overall concerning prognosis. In conclusion, pregnancy after renal transplant should be a consideration in this population.

Peritoneal Dialysis

Continuous ambulatory peritoneal dialysis is also used in the management of renal failure. Features of peritoneal dialysis that may have theoretical benefit include the lack of abrupt hypotension and fluid shifts observed with hemodialysis, a more constant fluid and electrolyte environment for the fetus, and overall improved blood pressure control. Peritonitis, a potential complication of peritoneal dialysis, may pose a diagnostic problem during pregnancy, since chorioamnionitis and even labor can present with abdominal pain. Overall, there does not appear to be a difference in pregnancy outcomes based on mode of RRT (379,385).

PREGNANCY IN THE RENAL TRANSPLANT RECIPIENT

After renal transplant, renal and endocrine functions as well as fertility return rapidly. It is estimated that 1 in 50 reproductive-age women with a functioning kidney transplant becomes pregnant (261). More than 90% of pregnancies that progress past the first trimester are successful (386–388). As with CKD, FGR, preeclampsia, and preterm delivery are more common. In women with stable renal allograft function, renal function prior to pregnancy is a major predictor of outcome comparable to women with CKD. Maternal and fetal prognosis also depends on a number of other factors including time since transplant, origin of transplant, blood pressure control, and immunosuppressive therapy dosage (389). Most of the data are derived from case series and transplant registries in North America, the United Kingdom, and Europe (353,390–392).

The long-term effect of pregnancy on the renal allograft function has been a major question. The results from a number of small studies have been conflicting (393–395). Rahamimov et al. evaluated long-term outcomes in 39 women with functioning renal allograft who became pregnant and compared them to three matched controls who were not pregnant (395). At the end of the 15-year follow-up period renal function was similar in both groups (72% in pregnant women versus 69% in control subjects). Renal function and overall survival were similar at 1, 5, and 10 years post transplant between the two groups. These extensive, longitudinal data indicate that pregnancy does not accelerate renal decline in women who have undergone renal transplantation.

Preconception Counseling and Pregnancy Management

Given the rapid return of fertility after transplantation, preconception and contraceptive counseling is recommended prior to transplant surgery and preferably in the early planning stages. Current recommendations based on consensus conferences of the American Transplant Society and other experts include the following (261,389,396,397):

1. Wait at least 1 year after transplant before attempting pregnancy. The purpose of this recommendation is to ensure stability of graft function and avoid complications related to rejection. This time frame must be individualized and balanced against the age and fertility of the patient
2. Stable doses of immunosuppressive therapy that are considered safe for pregnancy, ideally prednisone ≤15 mg/day, azathioprine ≤2 mg/kg/day, cyclosporine ≤5mg/kg/day, and tacrolimus ≤0.1 to 0.2 mg/kg/day.
3. No evidence of graft rejection.
4. Optimal and adequate allograft function (preferably serum creatinine <1.5 mg/dL and proteinuria of <500 mg/day).
5. Well-controlled blood pressure.

Immunosuppressive medications should not be stopped during pregnancy since these are important for preventing allograft rejection, maternal health, and the success of the pregnancy. Safety in pregnancy should be considered in the choice of agent. Overall, it becomes a balance of risks and benefits. Prednisone, azathioprine, cyclosporine, and tacrolimus are the most commonly used immunosuppressants in pregnancy. Newer immunosuppressive drugs should be avoided until adequate data are accrued to support their safety in pregnancy. Immunosuppressive medications are an important consideration and we refer the reader to a few excellent reviews on the topic (389,397,398).

Pregnancy care is similar to that outlined previously for women with CKD. However, there are special considerations including changing requirement for immunosuppressant doses, diagnosis of allograft rejection or worsening of function, obstruction or physical damage to the transplanted kidney during pregnancy and delivery, and infections. The dosage of immunosuppressive drugs may need to be adjusted during pregnancy due to the marked volume changes and the increased hepatic metabolism. In general, if graft function is stable on prednisone and azathioprine then dosage can be maintained throughout pregnancy. Cyclosporine and tacrolimus may need to be adjusted to reach therapeutic blood concentrations. With respect to allograft function and rejection, frequent monitoring is recommended as with CKD. In addition, rejection must be kept in the differential diagnosis of abdominal pain, fevers, etc. Although unusual, obstruction of the ureter has been reported secondary to the enlarging uterus. Vaginal delivery is recommended except for the usual obstetric indications. Location of the transplanted kidney should be clearly outlined in the prenatal chart, ideally including the operative report from the transplant surgery. If cesarean section is required, then care must be taken to avoid trauma to the renal allograft. Given the use of immunosuppressive medications, close monitoring for infections with appropriate therapy is recommended. Frequent urine cultures should be obtained and directed antibiotic therapy instituted promptly. Viral and parasitic infections that could affect pregnancy should also be considered including cytomegalovirus, herpes simplex virus, and toxoplasmosis. Primary infections as well as reactivations are more common in women taking immunosuppressive drugs; therefore, serologic assessment is recommended prior to pregnancy. Some authors recommend re-testing each trimester if initial studies are negative. Appropriate counseling and therapy should be instituted if primary infection or reactivation is suspected. In general, breastfeeding is encouraged; however, the safety of some of the immunosuppressive medications remains unclear and recommendations should be made accordingly.

REFERENCES

1. Conrad K. Renal changes in pregnancy. *Urol Ann.* 1992;6:313–340.
2. Cietak KA, Newton JR. Serial quantitative maternal nephrosonography in pregnancy. *Br J Radiol.* 1985;58(689):405–413.
3. Lindheimer MD, Conrad KP, Karamanchi AS. Renal physiology and disease in pregnancy. In: Alpern RJ, Hebert SC, eds. *Seldin and Giebisch's The Kidney Physiology and Pathophysiology.* 4th ed. New York: Elsevier; 2007.
4. Dure-Smith P. Pregnancy dilation of the urinary tract. *Am J Obstet Gynecol.* 1979;135:1066.
5. Cietak KA, Newton JR. Serial qualitative maternal nephrosonography in pregnancy. *Br J Radiol.* 1985;58(689):399–404.
6. Sims EA, Krantz KE. Serial studies of renal function during pregnancy and the puerperium in normal women. *J Clin Invest.* 1958;37(12):1764–1774.
7. De Alvarez RR. Renal glomerulotubular mechanisms during normal pregnancy. I. Glomerular filtration rate, renal plasma flow, and creatinine clearance. *Am J Obstet Gynecol.* 1958;75(5):931–944.
8. Assali NS, Dignam WJ, Dasgupta K. Renal function in human pregnancy. II. Effects of venous pooling on renal hemodynamics and water, electrolyte, and aldosterone excretion during gestation. *J Lab Clin Med.* 1959;54:394–408.
9. Dunlop W. Serial changes in renal hemodynamics during normal human pregnancy. *Br J Obstet Gynaecol.* 1981;88:1–9.
10. Roberts M, Lindheimer MD, Davison JM. Altered glomerular permselectivity to neutral dextrans and heteroporous membrane modeling in human pregnancy. *Am J Physiol.* 1996;270(2 pt 2):F338–F343.
11. Chapman AB, Abraham WT, Zamudio S, et al. Temporal relationships between hormonal and hemodynamic changes in early human pregnancy. *Kidney Int.* 1998;54(6):2056–2063.
12. Conrad KP. Mechanisms of renal vasodilation and hyperfiltration during pregnancy. *J Soc Gynecol Invest.* 2004;11(7):438–448.
13. Davison JM, Noble MC. Serial changes in 24 hour creatinine clearance during normal menstrual cycles and the first trimester of pregnancy. *Br J Obstet Gynaecol.* 1981;88(1):10–17.
14. Conrad KP, Gaber LW, Lindheimer MD. The kidney in normal pregnancy and preeclampsia. In: *Chesley's Hypertensive Disorders in Pregnancy.* 3rd ed. San Diego, CA: Elsevier; 2009:297–333.

15. Davison JM. The effect of pregnancy on kidney function in renal allograft recipients. *Kidney Int.* 1985;27(1):74–79.

16. Davison JM. Changes in renal function in early pregnancy in women with one kidney. *Yale J Biol Med.* 1978;51(3):347–349.

17. Robson SC, Hunter S, Boys RJ, et al. Serial study of factors influencing changes in cardiac output during human pregnancy. *Am J Physiol.* 1989; 256(4 pt 2):H1060–H1065.

18. Slangen BF, Out IC, Verkeste CM, et al. Hemodynamic changes in early pregnancy in chronically instrumented, conscious rats. *Am J Physiol.* 1996;270(5 pt 2):H1779–H1784.

19. Gilson GJ, Mosher MD, Conrad KP. Systemic hemodynamics and oxygen transport during pregnancy in chronically instrumented, conscious rats. *Am J Physiol.* 1992;263(6 pt 2): H1911–H1918.

20. Baylis C. The mechanism of the increase in glomerular filtration rate in the twelve-day pregnant rat. *J Physiol.* 1980;305:405–414.

21. Milne JE, Lindheimer MD, Davison JM. Glomerular heteroporous membrane modeling in third trimester and postpartum before and during amino acid infusion. *Am J Physiol Renal Physiol.* 2002;282(1):F170–F175.

22. Chapman AB, Zamudio S, Woodmansee W, et al. Systemic and renal hemodynamic changes in the luteal phase of the menstrual cycle mimic early pregnancy. *Am J Physiol.* 1997;273(5 pt 2): F777–F782.

23. Sherwood OD. Relaxin. In: Knobil E, Neill JD, Greenwald GS, et al., eds. *The Physiology of Reproduction.* New York: Raven; 1994:861–1009.

24. Jeyabalan A, Shroff SG, Novak J, et al. The vascular actions of relaxin. *Adv Exp Med Biol.* 2007;612:65–87.

25. Novak J, Danielson LA, Kerchner LJ, et al. Relaxin is essential for renal vasodilation during pregnancy in conscious rats. *J Clin Invest.* 2001; 107(11):1469–1475.

26. Debrah DO, Novak J, Matthews JE, et al. Relaxin is essential for systemic vasodilation and increased global arterial compliance during early pregnancy in conscious rats. *Endocrinology.* 2006;147(11):5126–5131.

27. Smith MC, Murdoch AP, Danielson LA, et al. Relaxin has a role in establishing a renal response in pregnancy. *Fertil Steril.* 2006;86(1): 253–255.

28. Debrah JE, Agoulnik A, Conrad KP. Changes in arterial function by chronic relaxin infusion are mediated by the leucine rich repeat G coupled Lgr7 receptor. *Reprod Sci.* 2008;15(1 suppl.): 217A.

29. McGuane JT, Debrah JE, Debrah DO, et al. Role of relaxin in maternal systemic and renal vascular adaptations during gestation. *Ann N Y Acad Sci.* 2009;1160:304–312.

30. Novak J, Rubin JP, Matthews J, et al. Relaxin (Rlx) mediated fast relaxation of arteries through P13 kinase and nitric oxide. *FASEB J.* 2007;21:A1371.

31. Matthews JE, Rubin JP, Novak J, et al. Vascular endothelial growth factor (VEGF) is a new player in the slow relaxin (Rlx) vasodilatory pathway. *Reprod Sci.* 2007;14(1 suppl.): 114A.

32. Debrah JE, McGuane JT, Novak J, et al. *Vascular Endothelial and Placental Growth Factors: New Players in the Slow Relaxin Vasodilatory Pathway.* 5th International Conference on Relaxin and Related Peptides. Hawaii; 2008.

33. Jeyabalan A, Novak J, Danielson LA, et al. Essential role for vascular gelatinase activity in relaxin-induced renal vasodilation, hyperfiltration, and reduced myogenic reactivity of small arteries. *Circ Res.* 2003;93(12): 1249–1257.

34. Jeyabalan A, Novak J, Doty KD, et al. Vascular matrix metalloproteinase-9 mediates the inhibition of myogenic reactivity in small arteries isolated from rats after short-term administration of relaxin. *Endocrinology.* 2007;148(1):189–197.

35. Conrad KP, Gandley RE, Ogawa T, et al. Endothelin mediates renal vasodilation and hyperfiltration during pregnancy in chronically instrumented conscious rats. *Am J Physiol.* 1999;276(5 pt 2): F767–F776.

36. Gandley RE, Conrad KP, McLaughlin MK. Endothelin and nitric oxide mediate reduced myogenic reactivity of small renal arteries from pregnant rats. *Am J Physiol.* 2001;280(1): R1–R7.

37. Danielson LA, Conrad KP. Acute blockade of nitric oxide synthase inhibits renal vasodilation and hyperfiltration during pregnancy in chronically instrumented conscious rats. *J Clin Invest.* 1995;96(1):482–490.

38. Danielson LA, Conrad KP. Prostaglandins maintain renal vasodilation and hyperfiltration during chronic nitric oxide synthase blockade in conscious pregnant rats. *Circ Res.* 1996;79(6): 1161–1166.

39. Gant NF, Daley GL, Chand S, et al. A study of angiotensin II pressor response throughout primigravid pregnancy. *J Clin Invest.* 1973;52(11): 2682–2689.

40. Conrad KP, Colpoys MC. Evidence against the hypothesis that prostaglandins are the vasodepressor agents of pregnancy. Serial studies in chronically instrumented, conscious rats. *J Clin Invest.* 1986;77(1):236–245.

41. Danielson LA, Sherwood OD, Conrad KP. Relaxin is a potent renal vasodilator in conscious rats. *J Clin Invest.* 1999;103(4):525–533.

42. Sladek SM, Magness RR, Conrad KP. Nitric oxide and pregnancy. *Am J Physiol.* 1997;272(2 pt 2): R441–R463.

43. Baylis C, Davison JM. Renal physiology in normal pregnancy. In: Feehally J, Floege J, Johnson RJ, eds. *Comprehensive Clinical Nephrology.* St. Louis, MI: Mosby Inc.; 2004:475–481.

44. Moe OW, Berry CA, Rector FC Jr. Renal transport of glucose, amino acids, sodium, chloride, and water. In: Brenner BM, ed. *Brenner & Rector's The Kidney.* 6th ed. Philadelphia, PA: WB Saunders Company; 2000.

45. Bishop JH, Green R. Glucose handling by distal portions of the nephron during pregnancy in the rat. *J Physiol.* 1983;336:131–142.

46. Davison JM. Renal nutrient excretion with emphasis on glucose. *Clin Obstet Gynecol.* 1975;2:365.

47. Davison JM. The excretion of glucose during normal pregnancy and after delivery. *J Obstet Gynaecol Br Commonw*. 1974;81:30–34.

48. Lind T, Hytten FE. The excretion of glucose during normal pregnancy. *J Obstet Gynaecol Br Commonw*. 1972;79:961–965.

49. Davison JM, Hytten FE. The effect of pregnancy on the renal handling of glucose. *Br J Obstet Gynaecol*. 1975;82(5):374–381.

50. Christensen PJ. Tubular reabsorption of glucose during pregnancy. *Scand J Clin Lab Invest*. 1958;10(4):364–371.

51. Welsh GW 3rd, Sims EA. The mechanisms of renal glucosuria in pregnancy. *Diabetes*. 1960;9:363–369.

52. Davison JM, Sprott MS, Selkon JB. The effect of covert bacteriuria in schoolgirls on renal function at 18 years and during pregnancy. *Lancet*. 1984;2(8404):651–655.

53. Hytten FE, Cheyne GA. The aminoaciduria of pregnancy. *J Obstet Gynaecol Br Commonw*. 1972;79(5):424–432.

54. Sica DA, Schoolwerth AC. Renal handling of organic anions and cations: Excretion of uric acid. In: Brenner BM, ed. *Brenner & Rector's The Kidney*. 6th ed. Philadelphia, PA: WB Saunders Company; 2000.

55. Boyle JA, Campbell S, Duncan AM, et al. Serum uric acid levels in normal pregnancy with observations on the renal excretion of urate in pregnancy. *J Clin Pathol*. 1966;19(5):501–503.

56. Dunlop W, Davison JM. The effect of normal pregnancy upon the renal handling of uric acid. *Br J Obstet Gynaecol*. 1977;84(1):13–21.

57. Lind T, Godfrey KA, Otun H, et al. Changes in serum uric acid concentrations during normal pregnancy. *Br J Obstet Gynaecol*. 1984;91(2):128–132.

58. Semple PF, Carswell W, Boyle JA. Serial studies of the renal clearance of urate and insulin during pregnancy and after the puerperium in normal women. *Clin Sci Mol Med*. 1974;47(6):559–565.

59. Suki WN, Lederer ED, Rouse D. Renal transport of calcium, magnesium, and phosphate. In: Brenner BM, ed. *Brenner & Rector's The Kidney*. 6th ed. Philadelphia, PA: WB Saunders Company; 2000.

60. Gertner JM, Coustan DR, Kliger AS, et al. Pregnancy as state of physiologic absorptive hypercalciuria. *Am J Med*. 1986;81:451–456.

61. Howarth AT, Morgan DB, Payne RB. Urinary excretion of calcium in late pregnancy and its relation to creatinine clearance. *Am J Obstet Gynecol*. 1977;129(5):499–502.

62. Maikranz P, Holley JL, Parks JH, et al. Gestational hypercalciuria causes pathological urine calcium oxalate supersaturations. *Kidney Int*. 1989;36(1):108–113.

63. Pedersen EB, Johannesen P, Kristensen S, et al. Calcium, parathyroid hormone and calcitonin in normal pregnancy and preeclampsia. *Gynecol Obstet Invest*. 1984;18(3):156–164.

64. Pitkin RM. Calcium metabolism in pregnancy and the perinatal period: A review. *Am J Obstet Gynecol*. 1985;151(1):99–109.

65. Davis OK, Hawkins DS, Rubin LP, et al. Serum parathyroid hormone (PTH) in pregnant women determined by an immunoradiometric assay for intact PTH. *J Clin Endocrinol Metab*. 1988;67(4):850–852.

66. Seki K, Makimura N, Mitsui C, et al. Calcium-regulating hormones and osteocalcin levels during pregnancy: A longitudinal study. *Am J Obstet Gynecol*. 1991;164(5 pt 1):1248–1252.

67. Whitehead M, Lane G, Young O, et al. Interrelations of calcium-regulating hormones during normal pregnancy. *Br Med J (Clin Res Ed)*. 1981;283(6283):10–12.

68. Kumar R, Cohen WR, Silva P, et al. Elevated 1,25-dihydroxyvitamin D plasma levels in normal human pregnancy and lactation. *J Clin Invest*. 1979;63(2):342–344.

69. Paulson SK, DeLuca HF. Vitamin D metabolism during pregnancy. *Bone*. 1986;7(5):331–336.

70. Weisman Y, Harell A, Edelstein S, et al. 1 alpha,25-Dihydroxyvitamin D3 and 24,25-dihydroxyvitamin D3 in vitro synthesis by human decidua and placenta. *Nature*. 1979;281(5729):317–319.

71. Marya RK, Rathee S, Manrow M. Urinary calcium excretion in pregnancy. *Gynecol Obstet Invest*. 1987;23(2):141–144.

72. Wabner C, Sirivongs D, Maikranz P, et al. Evidence for increased excretion in pregnancy of nephrocalcin, a urinary inhibitor of calcium oxalate crystal growth. *Kidney Int*. 1987;31:359.

73. Lindheimer MD, Richardson DA, Ehrlich EN, et al. Potassium homeostasis in pregnancy. *J Reprod Med*. 1987;32(7):517–522.

74. Geller DS, Farhi A, Pinkerton N, et al. Activating mineralocorticoid receptor mutation in hypertension exacerbated by pregnancy. *Science*. 2000;289(5476):119–123.

75. Bayliss DA, Millhorn DE, Gallman EA, et al. Progesterone stimulates respiration through a central nervous system steroid receptor-mediated mechanism in cat. *Proc Natl Acad Sci U S A*. 1987;84(21):7788–7792.

76. Weinberger SE, Weiss ST, Cohen WR, et al. Pregnancy and the lung. *Am Rev Respir Dis*. 1980;121(3):559–581.

77. Lim VS, Katz AI, Lindheimer MD. Acid-base regulation in pregnancy. *Am J Physiol*. 1976;231(6):1764–1769.

78. Lindheimer MD, Davison JM. Osmoregulation, the secretion of arginine vasopressin and its metabolism during pregnancy. *Eur J Endocrinol*. 1995;132(2):133–143.

79. Davison JM, Shiells EA, Philips PR, et al. Influence of humoral and volume factors on altered osmoregulation of normal human pregnancy. *Am J Physiol*. 1990;258(4 pt 2):F900–F907.

80. Danielson LA, Kercher LJ, Conrad KP. Impact of gender and endothelin on renal vasodilation and hyperfiltration induced by relaxin in conscious rats. *Am J Physiol*. 2000;279(4):R1298–R1304.

81. Weisinger RS, Burns P, Eddie LW, et al. Relaxin alters the plasma osmolality-arginine vasopressin relationship in the rat. *J Endocrinol*. 1993;137(3):505–510.

82. Danielson LE, Debrah JE, Conrad KP. The role of human chorionic gonadotropin in maternal vasodilation of pregnancy. *Reprod Sci*. 2008;15 (1 suppl.):218A.

83. Sherwood OD. Relaxin's physiological roles and other diverse actions. *Endocr Rev*. 2004;25(2):205–234.

84. Bell RJ, Laurence BM, Meehan PJ, et al. Regulation and function of arginine vasopressin in pregnant sheep. *Am J Physiol.* 1986; 250(5 pt 2):F777–F780.

85. Barron WM, Durr JA, Schrier RW, et al. Role of hemodynamic factors in osmoregulatory alterations of rat pregnancy. *Am J Physiol.* 1989; 257 (4 pt 2):R909–R916.

86. Barron WM, Stamoutsos BA, Lindheimer MD. Role of volume in the regulation of vasopressin secretion during pregnancy in the rat. *J Clin Invest.* 1984;73(4):923–932.

87. Silvertown JD, Fraser R, Poterski RS, et al. Central effects of long-term relaxin expression in the rat. *Ann N Y Acad Sci.* 2005;1041:216–222.

88. Ohara M, Martin PY, Xu DL, et al. Upregulation of aquaporin 2 water channel expression in pregnant rats. *J Clin Invest.* 1998;101(5): 1076–1083.

89. Schrier RW. Pathogenesis of sodium and water retention in high-output and low-output cardiac failure, nephrotic syndrome, cirrhosis, and pregnancy (1). *N Engl J Med.* 1988;16:1065–1072.

90. Spaanderman ME, Meertens M, van Bussel M, et al. Cardiac output increases independently of basal metabolic rate in early human pregnancy. *Am J Physiol Heart Circ Physiol.* 2000;278(5): H1585–H1588.

91. Phippard AF, Horvath JS, Glynn EM, et al. Circulatory adaptation to pregnancy—serial studies of haemodynamics, blood volume, renin and aldosterone in the baboon (*Papio hamadryas*). *J Hypertens.* 1986;4(6):773–779.

92. Chesley LC, Valenti C, Rein H. Excretion of sodium loads by nonpregnant and pregnant normal, hypertensive and pre-eclamptic women. *Metabolism.* 1958;7(5):575–588.

93. Brown MA, Gallery ED, Ross MR, et al. Sodium excretion in normal and hypertensive pregnancy: A prospective study. *Am J Obstet Gynecol.* 1988; 159(2):297–307.

94. Baylis C, Blantz RC. Tubuloglomerular feedback activity in virgin and 12-day-pregnant rats. *Am J Physiol.* 1985;249(1 pt 2):F169–F173.

95. Ni XP, Safai M, Rishi R, et al. Increased activity of cGMP-specific phosphodiesterase (PDE5) contributes to resistance to atrial natriuretic peptide natriuresis in the pregnant rat. *J Am Soc Nephrol.* 2004;15(5):1254–1260.

96. Knight S, Snellen H, Humphreys M, et al. Increased renal phosphodiesterase-5 activity mediates the blunted natriuretic response to ANP in the pregnant rat. *Am J Physiol Renal Physiol.* 2007;292(2):F655–F659.

97. Irons DW, Baylis PH, Davison JM. Effect of atrial natriuretic peptide on renal hemodynamics and sodium excretion during human pregnancy. *Am J Physiol.* 1996;271(1 pt 2):F239–F242.

98. Conrad KP, Kerchner LJ, Mosher MD. Plasma and 24-h NO(x) and cGMP during normal pregnancy and preeclampsia in women on a reduced NO(x) diet. *Am J Physiol.* 1999; 277(1 pt 2):F48–F57.

99. Khraibi AA, Haas JA, Knox FG. Effect of renal perfusion pressure on renal interstitial hydrostatic pressure in rats. *Am J Physiol.* 1989;256(1 pt 2): F165–F170.

100. Garcia-Estan J, Roman RJ. Role of renal interstitial hydrostatic pressure in the pressure diuresis response. *Am J Physiol.* 1989;256(1 pt 2): F63–F70.

101. Khraibi AA. Renal interstitial hydrostatic pressure and pressure natriuresis in pregnant rats. *Am J Physiol Renal Physiol.* 2000;279(2):F353–F357.

102. Khraibi AA, Dobrian AD, Yu T, et al. Role of RIHP and renal tubular sodium transporters in volume retention of pregnant rats. *Am J Hypertens.* 2005; 18(10):1375–1383.

103. Samuel CS, Lekgabe ED, Mookerjee I. The effects of relaxin on extracellular matrix remodeling in health and fibrotic disease. *Adv Exp Med Biol.* 2007;612:88–103.

104. Gifford RW, August PA, Cunningham FG, et al. Report of the National High Blood Pressure Working Group on research on hypertension in pregnancy. *Am J Obstet Gynecol.* 2000;183: S1–S22.

105. Lindheimer MD, Roberts JM, Cunningham FG, et al. Introduction, history, controversies, and definitions. In: Lindheimer MD, Roberts JM, Cunningham FG, eds. *Chesley's Hypertensive Disorders in Pregnancy.* 3rd ed. San Diego, CA: Elsevier; 2009:1–24.

106. Duley L. Maternal mortality associated with hypertensive disorders of pregnancy in Africa, Asia, Latin America and the Caribbean (see comment). *Br J Obstet Gynaecol.* 1992;99(7):547–553.

107. Tang LC, Kwok AC, Wong AY, et al. Critical care in obstetrical patients: An eight-year review. *Chin Med J.* 1997;110(12):936–941.

108. Goldenberg RL, Rouse DJ. Prevention of premature birth. *N Engl J Med.* 1998;339(5):313–320.

109. Roberts JM, Taylor RN, Musci TJ, et al. Preeclampsia: An endothelial cell disorder. *Am J Obstet Gynecol.* 1989;161(5):1200–1204.

110. Roberts JM, Taylor RN, Goldfien A. Endothelial cell activation as a pathogenetic factor in preeclampsia. *Semin Perinatol.* 1991;15(1):86–93.

111. Woelkers DA, Roberts JM. The endothelium and pre-eclampsia. In: Rubin PC, ed. *Handbook of Hypertension.* New York: Elsevier; 2000:126–162.

112. Lindheimer M, Roberts J, Cunningham F, et al. Introduction, history, controversies, and definitions. In: Lindheimer M, Roberts J, Cunningham F, eds. *Chesley's Hypertensive Disorders in Pregnancy.* 2nd ed. Stamford, CN: Appleton and Lange; 1999:3–41.

113. North RA, Taylor RS, Schellenberg JC. Evaluation of a definition of pre-eclampsia. *Br J Obstet Gynaecol.* 1999;106(8):767–773.

114. Zhang J, Klebanoff MA, Roberts JM. Prediction of adverse outcomes by common definitions of hypertension in pregnancy. *Obstet Gynecol.* 2001; 97(2):261–267.

115. Thomson AM, Hytten FE, Billewicz WZ. The epidemiology of oedema during pregnancy. *J Obstet Gynaecol Br Commonw.* 1967;74(1):1–10.

116. American College of Obstetricians and Gynecologists (ACOG). Diagnosis and management of preeclampsia and eclampsia. ACOG practice bulletin no 33, January 2002. *Obstet Gynecol.* 2002;99:159–167.

117. Egerman RS, Sibai BM. HELLP syndrome. *Clin Obstet Gynecol.* 1999;42(2):381–389.

118. Ness RB, Roberts JM. Epidemiology of pregnancy-related hypertension. In: Lindheimer MD, Roberts JM, Cunningham FG, eds. *Chesley's Hypertensive Disorders in Pregnancy.* 3rd ed. San Diego,CA: Elsevier; 2009:37.S–50.S

119. Sibai BM, Lindheimer M, Hauth J, et al. Risk factors for preeclampsia, abruptio placentae, and adverse neonatal outcomes among women with chronic hypertension. National Institute of Child Health and Human Development Network of Maternal-Fetal Medicine Units. *N Engl J Med.* 1998;339(10): 667–671.

120. Hanson U, Persson B. Outcome of pregnancies complicated by type 1 insulin-dependent diabetes in Sweden: Acute pregnancy complications, neonatal mortality and morbidity. *Am J Perinatol.* 1993;10(4):330–333.

121. Sibai BM, Caritis S, Hauth J, et al. Risks of preeclampsia and adverse neonatal outcomes among women with pregestational diabetes mellitus. National Institute of Child Health and Human Development Network of Maternal-Fetal Medicine Units. *Am J Obstet Gynecol.* 2000;182(2): 364–369.

122. Day MC, Barton JR, O'Brien JM, et al. The effect of fetal number on the development of hypertensive conditions of pregnancy. *Obstet Gynecol.* 2005;106(5 pt 1):927–931.

123. England L, Zhang J. Smoking and risk of preeclampsia: A systematic review. *Front Biosci.* 2007;12:2471–2483.

124. Conde-Agudelo A, Althabe F, Belizan JM, et al. Cigarette smoking during pregnancy and risk of preeclampsia: A systematic review. *Am J Obstet Gynecol.* 1999;181(4):1026–1035.

125. Jeyabalan A, Powers RW, Durica AR, et al. Cigarette smoke exposure and angiogenic factors in pregnancy and preeclampsia. *Am J Hypertens.* 2008;21(8):943–947.

126. Mehendale R, Hibbard J, Fazleabas A, et al. Placental angiogenesis markers sFlt-1 and PlGF: Response to cigarette smoke. *Am J Obstet Gynecol.* 2007;197(4):363.e1–e5.

127. Sibai BM, Cunningham FG. Prevention of preeclampsia and eclampsia. In: Lindheimer M, Roberts JM, Cunningham FG, eds. *Chesley's Hypertensive Disorders in Pregnancy.* 3rd ed. San Diego, CA: Elsevier (Academic Press); 2009:213–226.

128. Bucher HC, Guyatt GH, Cook RJ, et al. Effect of calcium supplementation on pregnancy-induced hypertension and preeclampsia: A meta-analysis of randomized controlled trials. *JAMA.* 1996; 275(14):1113–1117.

129. Levine RJ, Hauth JC, Curet LB, et al. Trial of calcium to prevent preeclampsia. *N Engl J Med.* 1997;337(2):69–76.

130. Villar J, Belizan JM. Same nutrient, different hypotheses: Disparities in trials of calcium supplementation during pregnancy. *Am J Clin Nutr.* 2000;71(5 suppl.):1375S–1379S.

131. Villar J, Abdel-Aleem H, Merialdi M, et al. World Health Organization randomized trial of calcium supplementation among low calcium intake pregnant women. *Am J Obstet Gynecol.* 2006;194(3): 639–649.

132. Atallah AN, Hofmeyr GJ, Duley L. Calcium supplementation during pregnancy for preventing hypertensive disorders and related problems *Cochrane Database Syst Rev.* 2005;(4). (Update in *Cochrane Database Syst Rev.* 2006;3:CD001059; PMID:16855957. 2005).

133. Beaufils M, Uzan S, Donsimoni R, et al. Prevention of pre-eclampsia by early antiplatelet therapy. *Lancet.* 1985;1(8433):840–842.

134. Schiff E, Peleg E, Goldenberg M, et al. The use of aspirin to prevent pregnancy-induced hypertension and lower the ratio of thromboxane A2 to prostacyclin in relatively high risk pregnancies. *N Engl J Med.* 1989;321(6):351–356.

135. Hauth JC, Goldenberg RL, Parker CR Jr, et al. Low-dose aspirin therapy to prevent preeclampsia. *Am J Obstet Gynecol.* 1993;168(4): 1083–1091.

136. Caritis S, Sibai B, Hauth J, et al. Low-dose aspirin to prevent preeclampsia in women at high risk. *N Engl J Med.* 1998;338(11):701–705.

137. Anonymous. CLASP: A randomised trial of low-dose aspirin for the prevention and treatment of pre-eclampsia among 9364 pregnant women. CLASP (Collaborative Low-dose Aspirin Study in Pregnancy) Collaborative Group. *Lancet.* 1994;343(8898):619–629.

138. Sibai BM, Caritis SN, Thom E, et al. Prevention of preeclampsia with low-dose aspirin in healthy, nulliparous pregnant women. The National Institute of Child Health and Human Development Network of Maternal-Fetal Medicine Units. *N Engl J Med.* 1993;329(17):1213–1218.

139. Subtil D, Goeusse P, Puech F, et al. Aspirin (100 mg) used for prevention of pre-eclampsia in nulliparous women: The Essai Regional Aspirine Mere-Enfant study (Part 1). *Br J Obstet Gynaecol.* 2003;110(5):475–484.

140. Coomarasamy A, Honest H, Papaioannou S, et al. Aspirin for prevention of preeclampsia in women with historical risk factors: A systematic review. *Obstet Gynecol.* 2003;101(6):1319–1332.

141. Duley L, Henderson-Smart DJ, Knight M, et al. Antiplatelet agents for preventing pre-eclampsia and its complications (systematic review). *Cochrane Database Syst Rev.* 2005;(4).

142. Askie LM, Duley L, Henderson-Smart DJ, et al. Antiplatelet agents for prevention of pre-eclampsia: A meta-analysis of individual patient data. *Lancet.* 2007;369(9575):1791–1798.

143. Bilodeau JF, Hubel CA. Current concepts in the use of antioxidants for the treatment of preeclampsia. *J Obstet Gynaecol Can.* 2003;25(9): 742–750.

144. Chappell LC, Seed PT, Briley AL, et al. Effect of antioxidants on the occurrence of pre-eclampsia in women at increased risk: A randomised trial. *Lancet.* 1999;354(9181):810–816.

145. Poston L, Briley AL, Seed PT, et al. Vitamin C and vitamin E in pregnant women at risk for pre-eclampsia (VIP trial): Randomised placebo-controlled trial. *Lancet.* 2006;367(9517): 1145–1154.

146. Rumbold AR, Crowther CA, Haslam RR, et al. Vitamins C and E and the risks of preeclampsia and perinatal complications. *N Engl J Med.* 2006;354(17):1796–1806.

147. Spinnato JAIIMD, Freire SMD, Pinto e Silva JLMD, et al. Antioxidant therapy to prevent preeclampsia: A randomized controlled trial. *Obstet Gynecol.* 2007;110(6):1311–1318.

148. Roberts JM, for the Eunice Kennedy Shriver NIoCHaHDMN. A randomized controlled trial of antioxidant vitamins to prevent serious complications associated with pregnancy related hypertension in low risk, nulliparous women. *Am J Obstet Gynecol.* 2009;199(6A):S8.

149. Sibai BM, Barton JR. Expectant management of severe preeclampsia remote from term: Patient selection, treatment, and delivery indications. *Am J Obstet Gynecol.* 2007;196:514.e1–e9.

150. Roberts JM, Bodnar LM, Lain KY, et al. Uric acid is as important as proteinuria in identifying fetal risk in women with gestational hypertension. *Hypertension.* 2005;46(6):1263–1269.

151. Altman D, Carroli G, Duley L, et al. Do women with pre-eclampsia, and their babies, benefit from magnesium sulphate? The Magpie Trial: A randomised placebo-controlled trial. *Lancet.* 2002;359(9321):1877–1890.

152. Lucas MJ, Leveno KJ, Cunningham FG. A comparison of magnesium sulfate with phenytoin for the prevention of eclampsia. *N Engl J Med.* 1995;333(4):201–205.

153. Duley L, Henderson-Smart D. Magnesium sulphate versus phenytoin for eclampsia. *Cochrane Database Syst Rev.* 2003;(4):CD000128.

154. Anonymous. Which anticonvulsant for women with eclampsia? Evidence from the Collaborative Eclampsia Trial. *Lancet.* 1995;345(8963): 1455–1463.

155. Duley L, Henderson-Smart D. Magnesium sulphate versus diazepam for eclampsia (systematic review). *Cochrane Database Syst Rev.* 2005;(4).

156. Cooper WO, Hernandez-Diaz S, Arbogast PG, et al. Major congenital malformations after first-trimester exposure to ACE inhibitors. *N Engl J Med.* 2006;354(23):2443–2451.

157. Serreau R, Luton D, Macher MA, et al. Developmental toxicity of the angiotensin II type 1 receptor antagonists during human pregnancy: A report of 10 cases. *Br J Obstet Gynaecol.* 2005; 112(6):710–712.

158. Sedman AB, Kershaw DB, Bunchman TE. Recognition and management of angiotensin converting enzyme inhibitor fetopathy. *Pediatr Nephrol.* 1995;9(3):382–385.

159. Chesley SC, Annitto JE, Cosgrove RA, et al. The remote prognosis of eclamptic women. Sixth periodic report. *Am J Obstet Gynecol.* 1976;124(5): 446–459.

160. Irgens HU, Reisaeter L, Irgens LM, et al. Long term mortality of mothers and fathers after preeclampsia: Population based cohort study. *BMJ.* 2001;323(7323):1213–1217.

161. Funai EF, Friedlander Y, Paltiel O, et al. Long-term mortality after preeclampsia. *Epidemiology.* 2005;16(2):206–215.

162. Smith GC, Pell JP, Walsh D. Pregnancy complications and maternal risk of ischaemic heart disease: A retrospective cohort study of 129,290 births. *Lancet.* 2001;357(9273):2002–2006.

163. Sibai BM, Mercer B, Sarinoglu C. Severe preeclampsia in the second trimester: Recurrence risk and long-term prognosis. *Am J Obstet Gynecol.* 1991;165(5 pt 1):1408–1412.

164. McDonald SD, Malinowski A, Zhou Q, et al. Cardiovascular sequelae of preeclampsia/eclampsia: A systematic review and meta-analyses. *Am Heart J.* 2008;156(5):918–930.

165. Vikse BE, Irgens LM, Leivestad T, et al. Preeclampsia and the risk of end-stage renal disease. *N Engl J Med.* 2008;359(8):800–809.

166. Brosens JJ, Pijnenborg R, Brosens IA. The myometrial junctional zone spiral arteries in normal and abnormal pregnancies: A review of the literature. *Am J Obstet Gynecol.* 2002;187(5):1416–1423.

167. Burton GJ, Woods AW, Jauniaux E. The Effects of Physiological Conversion of the Spiral Arteries on Utero-Placental Blood Flow. *Reprod Sci Suppl.* 2009;16(3):95A.

168. Red-Horse K, Rivera J, Schanz A, et al. Cytotrophoblast induction of arterial apoptosis and lymphangiogenesis in an in vivo model of human placentation. *J Clin Invest.* 2006;116(10):2643–2652.

169. Founds SA, Conley YP, Lyons-Weiler JF, et al. Altered global gene expression in first trimester placentas of women destined to develop preeclampsia. *Placenta.* 2009;30(1):15–24.

170. Page EW. The relation between hydatid moles, relative ischemia of the gravid uterus, and the placental origin of eclampsia. *Am J Obstet Gynecol.* 1939;37:291–293.

171. Rajakumar A, Jeyabalan A, Markovic N, et al. Placental HIF-1 alpha, HIF-2 alpha, membrane and soluble VEGF receptor-1 proteins are not increased in normotensive pregnancies complicated by late-onset intrauterine growth restriction. *Am J Physiol.* 2007;293(2):R766–R774.

172. Rajakumar A, Whitelock KA, Weissfeld LA, et al. Selective overexpression of the hypoxia-inducible transcription factor, HIF-2alpha, in placentas from women with preeclampsia. *Biol Reprod.* 2001;64(2):499–506.

173. DiFederico E, Genbacev O, Fisher SJ. Preeclampsia is associated with widespread apoptosis of placental cytotrophoblasts within the uterine wall. *Am J Pathol.* 1999;155(1):293–301.

174. Redman CW, Sargent IL. Microparticles and immunomodulation in pregnancy and pre-eclampsia. *J Reprod Immunol.* 2007;76(1–2):61–67.

175. Redman CW, Sargent IL. Latest advances in understanding preeclampsia. *Science.* 2005; 308(5728):1592–1594.

176. Gammill HS, Roberts JM. Emerging concepts in preeclampsia investigation. *Front Biosci.* 2007;12: 2403–2411.

177. Aardenburg R, Spaanderman ME, van Eijndhoven HW, et al. A low plasma volume in formerly preeclamptic women predisposes to the recurrence of hypertensive complications in the next pregnancy. *J Soc Gynecol Invest.* 2006;13(8): 598–603.

178. Fink GD. Sympathetic activity, vascular capacitance, and long-term regulation of arterial pressure. *Hypertension.* 2009;53(pt 2):307–312.

179. Rajakumar A, Brandon HM, Daftary A, et al. Evidence for the functional activity of hypoxia-inducible transcription factors overexpressed in preeclamptic placentae. *Placenta.* 2004;25(10): 763–769.

180. Manyonda IT, Slater DM, Fenske C, et al. A role for noradrenaline in pre-eclampsia: Towards a unifying hypothesis for the pathophysiology. *Br J Obstet Gynaecol*. 1998;105(6):641–648.

181. Rajakumar A, Michael HM, Rajakumar PA, et al. Extra-placental expression of vascular endothelial growth factor receptor-1, (Flt-1) and soluble Flt-1 (sFlt-1), by peripheral blood mononuclear cells (PBMCs) in normotensive and preeclamptic pregnant women. *Placenta*. 2005;26(7):563–573.

182. Wallukat G, Homuth V, Fischer T, et al. Patients with preeclampsia develop agonistic autoantibodies against the angiotensin AT1 receptor. *J Clin Invest*. 1999;103(7):945–952.

183. Benyo DF, Smarason A, Redman CW, et al. Expression of inflammatory cytokines in placentas from women with preeclampsia. *J Clin Endocrinol Metab*. 2001;86(6):2505–2512.

184. Chesley LC. False starts in the study of preeclampsia-eclampsia. *Obstet Gynecol Annu*. 1976;5:177–187.

185. Maynard SE, Min JY, Merchan J, et al. Excess placental soluble fms-like tyrosine kinase 1 (sFlt1) may contribute to endothelial dysfunction, hypertension, and proteinuria in preeclampsia. *J Clin Invest*. 2003;111(5):649–658.

186. Lain KY, Wilson JW, Crombleholme WR, et al. Smoking during pregnancy is associated with alterations in markers of endothelial function. *Am J Obstet Gynecol*. 2003;189(4):1196–1201.

187. Eremina V, Sood M, Haigh J, et al. Glomerular-specific alterations of VEGF—A expression lead to distinct congenital and acquired renal diseases. *J Clin Invest*. 2003;111(5):707–716.

188. Yang JC, Haworth L, Sherry RM, et al. A randomized trial of bevacizumab, an anti-vascular endothelial growth factor antibody, for metastatic renal cancer. *N Engl J Med*. 2003;349(5):427–434.

189. Levine RJ, Maynard SE, Qian C, et al. Circulating angiogenic factors and the risk of preeclampsia. *N Engl J Med*. 2004;350(7):672–683.

190. Powers RW, Roberts JM, Cooper KM, et al. Maternal serum soluble fms-like tyrosine kinase 1 concentrations are not increased in early pregnancy and decrease more slowly postpartum in women who develop preeclampsia. *Am J Obstet Gynecol*. 2005;193(1):185–191.

191. Wallenburg HCS. Hemodynamics in hypertensive pregnancy. In: Rubin PC, ed. *Handbook of Hypertension*. New York: Elsevier Science Publishers; 1988:66–101.

192. Sibai BM, Mabie WC. Hemodynamics of preeclampsia. *Clin Perinatol*. 1991;18(4):727–747.

193. Visser W, Wallenburg HC. Central hemodynamic observations in untreated preeclamptic patients. *Hypertension*. 1991;17(6 pt 2):1072–1077.

194. Lang RM, Pridjian G, Feldman T, et al. Left ventricular mechanics in preeclampsia. *Am Heart J*. 1991;121(6 pt 1):1768–1775.

195. Easterling TR, Benedetti TJ, Schmucker BC, et al. Maternal hemodynamics in normal and preeclamptic pregnancies: A longitudinal study. *Obstet Gynecol*. 1990;76(6):1061–1069.

196. Bosio PM, McKenna PJ, Conroy R, et al. Maternal central hemodynamics in hypertensive disorders of pregnancy. *Obstet Gynecol*. 1999;6:978–984.

197. Messerli FH, De Carvalho JG, Christie B, et al. Systemic and regional hemodynamics in low, normal and high cardiac output borderline hypertension. *Circulation*. 1978;58(3 pt 1):441–448.

198. Hall JE. Louis K. Dahl Memorial Lecture. Renal and cardiovascular mechanisms of hypertension in obesity. *Hypertension*. 1994;23(3):381–394.

199. Assali NS, Kaplan SA, Fomon SJ, et al. Renal function studies in toxemia of pregnancy; excretion of solutes and renal hemodynamics during osmotic diuresis in hydropenia. *J Clin Invest*. 1953;32(1):44–51.

200. McCartney CP, Spargo B, Lorincz AB, et al. Renal structure and function in pregnant patients with acute hypertension; osmolar concentration. *Am J Obstet Gynecol*. 1964;90:579–592.

201. Sarles HE, Hil SS, LeBlanc AL, et al. Sodium excretion patterns during and following intravenous sodium chloride loads in normal and hypertensive pregnancies. *Am J Obstet Gynecol*. 1968;102(1):1–7.

202. Moran P, Lindheimer MD, Davison JM. The renal response to preeclampsia. *Semin Nephrol*. 2004;24(6):588–595.

203. Pollak VE, Nettles JB. The kidney in toxemia of pregnancy: A clinical and pathologic study based on renal biopsies. *Medicine (Baltimore)*. 1960;39:469–526.

204. Redman CW, Beilin LJ, Bonnar J, et al. Plasma-urate measurements in predicting fetal death in hypertensive pregnancy. *Lancet*. 1976;1(7974):1370–1373.

205. Redman CW, Beilin LJ, Bonnar J. Renal function in preeclampsia. *J Clin Pathol Suppl (R Coll Pathol)*. 1976;10:91–94.

206. Sagen N, Haram K, Nilsen ST. Serum urate as a predictor of fetal outcome in severe pre-eclampsia. *Acta Obstet Gynecol Scand*. 1984;63(1):71–75.

207. Hayashi TT. The effect of benemid on uric acid excretion in normal pregnancy and in pre-eclampsia. *Am J Obstet Gynecol*. 1957;73(1):17–22.

208. Czaczkes WJ, Ullmann TD, Sadowsky E. Plasma uric acid levels, uric acid excretion, and response to probenecid in toxemia of pregnancy. *J Lab Clin Med*. 1958;51(2):224–229.

209. Fadel H, Osman L. Uterine-vein uric acid in EPH-gestosis and normal pregnancy. *Schweiz Z Gynak Geburtsh*. 1970;1:395–398.

210. Hayashi TT, Gillo D, Robbins H, et al. Simultaneous measurement of plasma and erythrocyte oxypurines. I. Normal and toxemic pregnancy. *Gynecol Invest*. 1972;3(5):221–236.

211. Many A, Hubel CA, Roberts JM. Hyperuricemia and xanthine oxidase in preeclampsia, revisited. *Am J Obstet Gynecol*. 1996;174(1 pt 1):288–291.

212. Redman CW. Maternal plasma volume and disorders of pregnancy. *Br Med J (Clin Res Ed)*. 1984;288(6422):955–956.

213. Brown MA, Zammit VC, Mitar DM. Extracellular fluid volumes in pregnancy-induced hypertension. *J Hypertens*. 1992;10(1):61–68.

214. Taufield PA, Ales KL, Resnick LM, et al. Hypocalciuria in preeclampsia. *N Engl J Med*. 1987;316(12):715–718.

215. Frenkel Y, Barkai G, Mashiach S, et al. Hypocalciuria of preeclampsia is independent of parathyroid hormone level. *Obstet Gynecol.* 1991;77(5): 689–691.

216. Sanchez-Ramos L, Sandroni S, Andres FJ, et al. Calcium excretion in preeclampsia. *Obstet Gynecol.* 1991;77(4):510–513.

217. Seely EW, Wood RJ, Brown EM, et al. Lower serum ionized calcium and abnormal calciotropic hormone levels in preeclampsia. *J Clin Endocrinol Metab.* 1992;74(6):1436–1440.

218. August P, Marcaccio B, Gertner JM, et al. Abnormal 1,25-dihydroxyvitamin D metabolism in preeclampsia. *Am J Obstet Gynecol.* 1992;166(4): 1295–1299.

219. Szmidt-Adjide V, Vendittelli F, David S, et al. Calciuria and preeclampsia: A case-control study. *Eur J Obstet Gynecol Reprod Biol.* 2006;125(2):193–198.

220. Ingec M, Nazik H, Kadanali S. Urinary calcium excretion in severe preeclampsia and eclampsia. *Clin Chem Lab Med.* 2006;44(1):51–53.

221. Halhali A, Diaz L, Avila E, et al. Decreased fractional urinary calcium excretion and serum 1, 25-dihydroxyvitamin D and IGF-I levels in preeclampsia. *J Steroid Biochem Mol Biol.* 2006; 103:803–806.

222. Ohara N, Yamasaki M, Morikawa H, et al. Dynamics of calcium metabolism and calcium-regulating hormones in pregnancy-induced hypertension. *Nippon Naibunpi Gakkai Zasshi.* 1986;8:882–896.

223. Seely EW, Graves SW. Calcium homeostasis in normotensive and hypertensive pregnancy. *Compr Ther.* 1993;19(3):124–128.

224. Stillman IE, Karumanchi SA. The glomerular injury of preeclampsia. *J Am Soc Nephrol.* 2007;18(8):2281–2284.

225. Mayer A. Changes in the endothelium during eclampsia and their significance (translation from German). *Klin Wochenzetschrift.* 1924;H27.

226. Robson JS. Proteinuria and the renal lesion in preeclampsia and abruptio placentae. *Perspect Nephrol Hypertens.* 1976;5:61–73.

227. Lopez-Lera M, Rubio G. Severe abruption placentae, toxemia of pregnancy and renal biopsy. *Am J Obstet Gynecol.* 1965;93:1144–1150.

228. Strevens H, Wide-Swensson D, Hansen A, et al. Glomerular endotheliosis in normal pregnancy and pre-eclampsia. *Br J Obstet Gynaecol.* 2003; 110(9):831–836.

229. Strevens H, Wide-Swensson D, Grubb A, et al. Serum cystatin C reflects glomerular endotheliosis in normal, hypertensive and pre-eclamptic pregnancies. *Br J Obstet Gynaecol.* 2003;110(9): 825–830.

230. Wide-Swensson D, Strevens H, Willner J. Antepartum percutaneous renal biopsy. *Int J Gynaecol Obstet.* 2007;98(2):88–92.

231. Lu F, Longo M, Tamayo E, et al. The effect of over-expression of sFlt-1 on blood pressure and the occurrence of other manifestations of preeclampsia in unrestrained conscious pregnant mice. *Am J Obstet Gynecol.* 2007;196(4):396 e1–7; discussion e7.

232. Kincaid-Smith P. The renal lesion of preeclampsia revisited. *Am J Kidney Dis.* 1991;17:144–148.

233. Fadel HE, Sabour MS, Mahran M, et al. Reversibility of the renal lesion and functional impairment in preeclampsia diagnosed by renal biopsy. *Obstet Gynecol.* 1969;33(4):528–534.

234. Oe PL, Ooms EC, Uttendorfsky OT, et al. Postpartum resolution of glomerular changes in edema-proteinuria-hypertension gestosis. *Ren Physiol.* 1980;3(1–6):375–379.

235. Pollak VE, Pirani CL, Kark RM, et al. Reversible glomerular lesions in toxaemia of pregnancy. *Lancet.* 1956;271(6933):59–62.

236. August PA, Lindheimer M. Chronic hypertension and pregnancy. In: Lindheimer M, Roberts JM, Cunningham FG, eds. *Chesley's Hypertensive Disorders in Pregnancy.* San Diego, CA: Elsevier ; 2009:353–368.

237. Chobanian AV, Bakris GL, Black HR, et al. The seventh report of the Joint National Committee on Prevention, Detection, Evaluation, and Treatment of High Blood Pressure. *JAMA.* 2003;289:2560–2572.

238. Rey E, Couturier A. The prognosis of pregnancy in women with chronic hypertension. *Am J Obstet Gynecol.* 1994;171(2):410–416.

239. Podymow T, August P. Update on the use of antihypertensive drugs in pregnancy. *Hypertension.* 2008;51(4):960–969.

240. Umans JG, Abalos EJ, Lindheimer MD. Antihypertensive treatment. In: Lindheimer MD, Roberts JM, Cunningham FG, eds. *Chesley's Hypertensive Disorders in Pregnancy.* 3rd ed. San Diego, CA: Elsevier; 2009:369–388.

241. Redman CW. Fetal outcome in trial of antihypertensive treatment in pregnancy. *Lancet.* 1976; 2(7989):753–756.

242. Montan S, Anandakumar C, Arulkumaran S, et al. Effects of methyldopa on uteroplacental and fetal hemodynamics in pregnancy-induced hypertension. *Am J Obstet Gynecol.* 1993;168(1 pt 1): 152–156.

243. Houlihan DD, Dennedy MC, Ravikumar N, et al. Anti-hypertensive therapy and the feto-placental circulation: Effects on umbilical artery resistance. *J Perinat Med.* 2004;32(4):315–319.

244. Waterman EJ, Magee LA, Lim KI, et al. Do commonly used oral antihypertensives alter fetal or neonatal heart rate characteristics? A systematic review. *Hypertens Pregnancy.* 2004;23(2): 155–169.

245. Cockburn J, Moar VA, Ounsted M, et al. Final report of study on hypertension during pregnancy: The effects of specific treatment on the growth and development of the children. *Lancet.* 1982;1(8273):647–649.

246. Pickles CJ, Symonds EM, Broughton Pipkin F. The fetal outcome in a randomized double-blind controlled trial of labetalol versus placebo in pregnancy-induced hypertension. *Br J Obstet Gynaecol.* 1989;96(1):38–43.

247. Butters L, Kennedy S, Rubin PC. Atenolol in essential hypertension during pregnancy. *BMJ.* 1990;301(6752):587–589.

248. Gazzolo D, Visser GH, Santi F, et al. Behavioural development and Doppler velocimetry in relation to perinatal outcome in small for dates fetuses. *Early Hum Dev.* 1995;43(2):185–195.

249. Impey L. Severe hypotension and fetal distress following sublingual administration of nifedipine to a patient with severe pregnancy induced hypertension at 33 weeks. *Br J Obstet Gynaecol.* 1993;100:959–961.

250. Grossman E, Messerli FH, Grodzicki T, et al. Should a moratorium be placed on sublingual nifedipine capsules given for hypertensive emergencies and pseudoemergencies? (see comment). *JAMA.* (Review). 1996;276(16):1328–1331.

251. Magee LA, Schick B, Donnenfeld AE, et al. The safety of calcium channel blockers in human pregnancy: A prospective, multicenter cohort study. *Am J Obstet Gynecol.* 1996;174(3):823–828.

252. Little PJ. The incidence of urinary tract infection in 5000 pregnant women. *Lancet.* 1966;2: 925–928.

253. Hooton TM, Scholes D, Stapleton AE, et al. A prospective study of asymptomatic bacteriuria in sexually active young women (see comment). *N Engl J Med.* 2000;343(14):992–997.

254. Sheffield JS, Cunningham FG. Urinary tract infection in women. *Obstet Gynecol.* 2005;106(5): 1085–1092.

255. Smaill F. Antibiotics for asymptomatic bacteriuria in pregnancy. *Cochrane Database Syst Rev.* 2001(2):CD000490.

256. Nicolle Lindsay ÂE, Bradley S, Colgan R, et al. Infectious diseases Society of America Guidelines for the Diagnosis and Treatment of Asymptomatic Bacteriuria in Adults. *Clin Infect Dis.* 2005;40(5): 643–654.

257. Millar L, DeBuque L, Leialoha C, et al. Rapid enzymatic urine screening test to detect bacteriuria in pregnancy. *Obstet Gynecol.* 2000;95(4): 601–604.

258. McNair RD, MacDonald SR, Dooley SL, et al. Evaluation of the centrifuged and Gram-stained smear, urinalysis, and reagent strip testing to detect asymptomatic bacteriuria in obstetric patients. *Am J Obstet Gynecol.* 2000;182(5): 1076–1079.

259. Shelton SD, Boggess KA, Kirvan K, et al. Urinary interleukin-8 with asymptomatic bacteriuria in pregnancy. *Obstet Gynecol.* 2001;97(4):583–586.

260. Ben David S, Einarson T, Ben David Y, et al. The safety of nitrofurantoin during the first trimester of pregnancy: Meta-analysis. *Fundam Clin Pharmacol.* 1995;9(5):503–507.

261. Williams DJ, Davison JM. Renal Disorders. In: Creasy RK, Resnik R, Iams JD, et al., eds. *Creasy and Resnik's Maternal-Fetal Medicine Principles and Practice.* 6th ed. Philadelphia, PA: Elsevier; 2009:905–926.

262. Vercaigne LM, Zhanel GG. Recommended treatment for urinary tract infection in pregnancy. *Ann Pharmacother.* 1994;28(2):248–251.

263. Tan JS, File TM Jr. Treatment of bacteriuria in pregnancy. *Drugs.* 1992;44(6):972–980.

264. Patterson TF, Andriole VT, Patterson TF, et al. Detection, significance, and therapy of bacteriuria in pregnancy. Update in the managed health care era. *Infect Dis Clin North Am.* 1997;11(3): 593–608.

265. Hill JB, Sheffield JS, McIntire DD, et al. Acute pyelonephritis in pregnancy. *Obstet Gynecol.* 2005;105(1):18–23.

266. Petersson C, Hedges S, Stenqvist K, et al. Suppressed antibody and interleukin-6 responses to acute pyelonephritis in pregnancy. *Kidney Int.* 1994;45(2):571–577.

267. Cunningham FG, Lucas MJ. Urinary tract infections complicating pregnancy. *Baillieres Clin Obstet Gynaecol.* 1994;8(2):353–373.

268. Cunningham FG, Lucas MJ, Hankins GD, et al. Pulmonary injury complicating antepartum pyelonephritis. *Am J Obstet Gynecol.* 1987;156(4) : 797–807.

269. Towers CV, Kaminskas CM, Garite TJ, et al. Pulmonary injury associated with antepartum pyelonephritis: Can patients at risk be identified? *Am J Obstet Gynecol.* 1991;164(4):974–978.

270. Millar LK, DeBuque L, Wing DA. Uterine contraction frequency during treatment of pyelonephritis in pregnancy and subsequent risk of preterm birth. *J Perinat Med.* 2003;31(1): 41–46.

271. Lang JM, Lieberman E, Cohen A. A comparison of risk factors for preterm labor and term small-for-gestational-age birth. *Epidemiology.* 1996;7(4): 369–376.

272. Wing DA, Park AS, Debuque L, et al. Limited clinical utility of blood and urine cultures in the treatment of acute pyelonephritis during pregnancy. *Am J Obstet Gynecol.* 2000;182(6): 1437–1440.

273. Wing DA, Hendershott CM, Debuque L, et al. A randomized trial of three antibiotic regimens for the treatment of pyelonephritis in pregnancy. *Obstet Gynecol.* 1998;92(2):249–253.

274. Wing DA, Hendershott CM, Debuque L, et al. Outpatient treatment of acute pyelonephritis in pregnancy after 24 weeks. *Obstet Gynecol.* 1999;94(5 pt 1):683–688.

275. Millar LK, Wing DA, Paul RH, et al. Outpatient treatment of pyelonephritis in pregnancy: A randomized controlled trial. *Obstet Gynecol.* 1995;86(4 pt 1):560–564.

276. Stratta P, Canavese C, Dogliani M, et al. Pregnancy-related acute renal failure. *Clin Nephrol.* 1989; 32(1):14–20.

277. Turney J, Ellis C, Parsons F. Obsteric acute renal failure 1956–1987. *Br J Obstet Gynaecol.* 1989;96: 679–687.

278. Grunfeld J, Pertuiset N. Acute renal failure in pregnancy: 1987. *Am J Kidney Dis.* 1987;9(4): 359–362.

279. Stratta P, Besso L, Canavese C, et al. Is pregnancy-related acute renal failure a disappearing clinical entity? *Ren Fail.* 1996;18(4):575–584.

280. Alexopoulos E, Tambakoudis P, Bili H, et al. Acute renal failure in pregnancy. *Ren Fail.* 1993;15(5):609–613.

281. Chugh K, Singhal P, Sharma B. Acute renal failure of obstetric origin. *Obstet Gynecol.* 1976;48: 642–646.

282. Prakash J, Tripati K, Srivastava P. Pregnancy related acute renal failure is still high in India. In: *Proceedings of the 11th International Congress of Nephrologists.* 1990:15A.

283. Nzerue C, Hewan-Lowe K, Nwawka C. Acute renal failure in pregnancy: A review of clinical outcomes at an inner-city hospital from 1986–1996. *J Natl Med Assoc.* 1998;90:486–490.

284. Thadhani R, Pascual M, Bonventre J. Acute renal failure. *N Engl J Med*. 1996;334(22): 1448–1460.

285. Bouman C, Kellum J, Lamiere N, et al. Definition for acute renal failure. 2003 (updated 2003; cited); Available from: www.adqi.net.

286. Asrat T, Nageotte M. Acute renal failure in pregnancy. In: Foley, ed. *Obstetric Intensive Care Manual*. 2nd ed: McGraw-Hill; 2004:184–195.

287. Gammill HS, Jeyabalan A. Acute renal failure in pregnancy. *Crit Care Med*. 2005;33(10 suppl.): S372–S384.

288. Bellomo R. Defining, quantifying, and classifying acute renal failure. *Crit Care Clin*. 2005;21: 223–237.

289. Parrish A. Complications of percutaneous renal biopsy: A review of 37 years' experience. *Clin Nephrol*. 1992;38:135–141.

290. Dennis EJ, McIver FA, Smythe CM. Renal biopsy in pregnancy. *Clin Obstet Gynecol*. 1968;11(2): 473–486.

291. Schewitz L, Friedman I, Pollack V. Bleeding after renal biosy in pregnancy. *Obstet Gynecol*. 1965;26: 295–304.

292. Packham D, Fairley KF. Renal biopsy: Indications and complications in pregnancy. *Br J Obstet Gynaecol*. 1987;94(10):935–939.

293. Lindheimer MD, Davison JM. Renal biopsy during pregnancy: 'To b . . . or not to b . . .?'. *Br J Obstet Gynaecol*. 1987;94(10):932–934.

294. Kuller JA, D'Andrea NM, McMahon MJ. Renal biopsy and pregnancy. *Am J Obstet Gynecol*. 2001;184(6):1093–1096.

295. Chen HH, Lin HC, Yeh JC, et al. Renal biopsy in pregnancies complicated by undetermined renal disease. *Acta Obstet Gynecol Scand*. 2001;80(10): 888–893.

296. Australian and New Zealand Intensive Care Society (ANZICS) Clinical Trials Group. Low-dose dopamine in patients with early renal dysfunction: A placebo-controlled randomised trial. *Lancet*. 2000;356(9248):2139–2143.

297. Marik PE. Low-dose dopamine: A systematic review [review and 68 references]. *Intensive Care Med*. 2002;28(7):877–883.

298. Kellum JAMD, M Decker JRN. Use of dopamine in acute renal failure: A meta-analysis (Article). *Critical Care Med*. 2001;29(8):1526–1531.

299. Bagshaw SM, Delaney A, Haase M, et al. Loop diuretics in the management of acute renal failure: A systematic review and meta-analysis. *Critical Care Resusc*. 2007;9(1):60–68.

300. Venkataraman R, Kellum JA. Prevention of acute renal failure. *Chest*. 2007;131(1):300–308.

301. Pertuiset N, Grunfeld JP. Acute renal failure in pregnancy [review and 86 references]. *Baillieres Clin Obstet Gynaecol*. 1994;8(2):333–351.

302. Drakeley AJ, Le Roux PA, Anthony J, et al. Acute renal failure complicating severe preeclampsia requiring admission to an obstetric intensive care unit. *Am J Obstet Gynecol*. 2002;186(2): 253–256.

303. Sibai BM, Villar MA, Mabie BC. Acute renal failure in hypertensive disorders of pregnancy. Pregnancy outcome and remote prognosis in thirty-one consecutive cases. *Am J Obstet Gynecol*. 1990;162(3):777–783.

304. Sibai BM, Ramadan MK. Acute renal failure in pregnancies complicated by hemolysis, elevated liver enzymes, and low platelets. *Am J Obstet Gynecol*. 1993;168(6 pt 1):1682–1690.

305. Castro MA, Fassett MJ, Reynolds TB, et al. Reversible peripartum liver failure: A new perspective on the diagnosis, treatment, and cause of acute fatty liver of pregnancy, based on 28 consecutive cases (see comment). *Am J Obstet Gynecol*. 1999;181(2):389–395.

306. Usta IM, Barton JR, Amon EA, et al. Acute fatty liver of pregnancy: An experience in the diagnosis and management of fourteen cases. *Am J Obstet Gynecol*. 1994;171(5):1342–1347.

307. Riely CA. Acute fatty liver of pregnancy. *Semin Liver Dis*. 1987;7(1):47–54.

308. Ibdah JA, Bennett MJ, Rinaldo P, et al. A fetal fatty-acid oxidation disorder as a cause of liver disease in pregnant women. *N Engl J Med*. 1999;340(22):1723–1731.

309. Abenhaim HA, Azoulay L, Kramer MS, et al. Incidence and risk factors of amniotic fluid embolisms: A population-based study on 3 million births in the United States. [see comment]. *Am J Obstet Gynecol*. 2008;199(1):49.e1–e8.

310. Clark SL, Hankins GD, Dudley DA, et al. Amniotic fluid embolism: Analysis of the national registry (see comment). *Am J Obstet Gynecol*. 1995;172(4 pt 1):1158–1167.

311. Dashe JS, Ramin SM, Cunningham FG. The long-term consequences of thrombotic microangiopathy (thrombotic thrombocytopenic purpura and hemolytic uremic syndrome) in pregnancy. *Obstet Gynecol*. 1998;91(5 pt 1):662–668.

312. Esplin MSM, Branch DW. Diagnosis and management of thrombotic microangiopathies during pregnancy (article). *Clin Obstet Gynecol Ambul Gynecol*. 1999;42(2):360–367.

313. Elliott MAMD, Nichols WLMD. Thrombotic thrombocytopenic purpura and hemolytic uremic syndrome (review). *Mayo Clinic Proc*. 2001;76(11):1154–1162.

314. Furlan M, Robles R, Galbusera M, et al. von Willebrand factor-cleaving protease in thrombotic thrombocytopenic purpura and the hemolytic-uremic syndrome. *N Engl J Med*. 1998;339(22): 1578–1584.

315. Tsai H-M, Lian EC-Y. Antibodies to von Willebrand factor-cleaving protease in acute thrombotic thrombocytopenic purpura. *N Engl J Med*. 1998;339(22):1585–1594.

316. George JN. The association of pregnancy with thrombotic thrombocytopenic purpura-hemolytic uremic syndrome. *Curr Opin Hematol*. 2003; 10(5):339–344.

317. Weiner C. Thrombotic microangiopathy in pregnancy and the postpartum period. *Semin Hematol*. 1987;24:119–129.

318. Egerman RSMD, Witlin AGDO, Friedman SAMD, et al. Thrombotic thrombocytopenic purpura and hemolytic uremic syndrome in pregnancy: Review of 11 cases (abstract). *Am J Obstet Gynecol*. 1996;175(4):950–956.

319. Francois KE, Foley MR. Antepartum and postpartum hemorrhage. In: Gabbe SG, Niebyl JR, Simpson JL, eds. *Obstetrics Normal and Problem Pregnancies*. 5th ed. Philadelphia, PA: Elsevier; 2007:456–485.

320. Klebanoff MA, Koslowe PA, Kaslow R, et al. Epidemiology of vomiting in early pregnancy. *Obstet Gynecol.* 1985;66(5):612–616.

321. Hill JB, Yost NP, Wendel GD Jr. Acute renal failure in association with severe hyperemesis gravidarum. *Obstet Gynecol.* 2002;100(5 pt 2): 1119–1121.

322. Robson J, Martin A, Ruckley V, et al. Irreversible postpartum renal failure. *Q J Med.* 1968;37: 423–435.

323. Newton ER. Chorioamnionitis and intraamniotic infection. *Clin Obstet Gynecol.* 1993;36(4): 795–808.

324. Sweet R, Gibbs R. Intraamniotic Infection. In: Sweet R, ed. *Infectious Diseases of the Female Genital Tract.* 4th ed. Philadelphia: Lippincott Williams & Wilkins; 2002:516–527.

325. LaPata R, McElin T, Adelson B. Ureteral obstruction due to compression by the gravid uterus. *Am J Obstet Gynecol.* 1970;106(6):941–942.

326. Courban D, Blank S, Harris M, et al. Acute renal failure in the first trimester resulting from uterine leiomyomas. *Am J Obstet Gynecol.* 1997;177: 472–473.

327. Seeds J, Cefalo R, Herbert W, et al. Hydramnios and maternal renal failure: Relief with fetal therapy. *Obstet Gynecol.* 1984;64(3 suppl.): 26S–29S.

328. Vintzileos A, Turner G, Campbell W, et al. Polyhydramnios and obstructive renal failure: A case report and review of the literature. *Am J Obstet Gynecol.* 1985;152(7):883–885.

329. Brandes J, Fritsche C. Obstructive acute renal failure by a gravid uterus: A case report and review. *Am J Kidney Dis.* 1991;18(3):398–401.

330. Chung P, Abramowicz J, Edgar D, et al. Acute maternal obstructive renal failure in a twin gestation despite normal physiological pregnancy-induced urinary tract dilation. *Am J Perinatol.* 1994;11(3): 242–244.

331. Fox J, Katz M, Klein S, et al. Sudden anuria in a pregnant woman with a solitary kidney. *Am J Obstet Gynecol.* 1978;132(5):583–585.

332. Butler E, Cox S, Eberts E, et al. Symptomatic nephrolithiasis complicating pregnancy. *Obstet Gynecol.* 2000;96(5 pt 1):753–756.

333. Fischer MJ. Chronic kidney disease and pregnancy: Maternal and fetal outcomes. *Adv Chronic Kidney Dis.* 2007;14(2):132–145.

334. Fischer MJ, Lehnerz SD, Hebert JR, et al. Kidney disease is an independent risk factor for adverse fetal and maternal outcomes in pregnancy. *Am J Kidney Dis.* 2004;43(3):415–423.

335. Iseki K, Iseki C, Ikemiya Y, et al. Risk of developing end-stage renal disease in a cohort of mass screening. *Kidney Int.* 1996;49(3): 800–805.

336. Anonymous. Pregnancy and renal disease. *Lancet.* 1975;2:801–802.

337. Lindheimer MD, Davison JM. Pregnancy and CKD: Any progress? (comment). *Am J Kidney Dis.* 2007;49(6):729–731.

338. Smith MC, Moran P, Ward MK, et al. Assessment of glomerular filtration rate during pregnancy using the MDRD formula. *BJOG.* 2008;115(1): 109–112.

339. Brenner BM, Meyer TW, Hostetter TH. Dietary protein intake and the progressive nature of

kidney disease: The role of hemodynamically mediated glomerular injury in the pathogenesis of progressive glomerular sclerosis in aging, renal ablation, and intrinsic renal disease. *N Engl J Med.* 1982;307(11):652–659.

340. Baylis C. Impact of pregnancy on underlying renal disease. *Adv Ren Replace Ther.* 2003;10(1): 31–39.

341. Hayslett JP. Interaction of renal disease and pregnancy. *Kidney Int.* 1984;25(3):579–587.

342. Surian M, Imbasciati E, Cosci P, et al. Glomerular disease and pregnancy. A study of 123 pregnancies in patients with primary and secondary glomerular diseases. *Nephron.* 1984;36(2): 101–105.

343. Jungers P, Houillier P, Forget D, et al. Influence of pregnancy on the course of primary chronic glomerulonephritis. *Lancet.* 1995;346(8983): 1122–1124.

344. Hou S. Pregnancy in women with chronic renal disease. *N Engl J Med.* 1985;312(13):836–839.

345. Imbasciati E, Pardi G, Capetta P, et al. Pregnancy in women with chronic renal failure. *Am J Nephrol.* 1986;6(3):193–198.

346. Cunningham FG, Cox SM, Harstad TW, et al. Chronic renal disease and pregnancy outcome. *Am J Obstet Gynecol.* 1990;163(2):453–459.

347. Jones DC, Hayslett JP. Outcome of pregnancy in women with moderate or severe renal insufficiency. *N Engl J Med.* 1996;335(4): 226–232.

348. Imbasciati E, Gregorini G, Cabiddu G, et al. Pregnancy in CKD stages 3 to 5: Fetal and maternal outcomes. *Am J Kidney Dis.* 2007;49(6):753–762.

349. Hou S. Pregnancy in chronic renal insufficiency and end-stage renal disease. *Am J Kidney Dis.* 1999;33(2):235–252.

350. Hayslett JP. Kidney disease and pregnancy. *Kidney Int.* 1999;25:579.

351. Jungers P, Houillier P, Forget D, et al. Specific controversies concerning the natural history of renal disease in pregnancy. *Am J Kidney Dis.* 1991;17(2):116–122.

352. Packham DK, North RA, Fairley KF, et al. Primary glomerulonephritis and pregnancy. *Q J Med.* 1989;71(266):537–553.

353. Vidaeff AC, Yeomans ER, Ramin SM. Pregnancy in women with renal disease. Part I: General principles. *Am J Perinatol.* 2008;25(7):385–97.

354. Jungers P, Chauveau D, Choukroun G, et al. Pregnancy in women with impaired renal function. *Clin Nephrol.* 1997;47(5):281–288.

355. Jungers P, Houillier P, Chauveau D, et al. Pregnancy in women with reflux nephropathy. *Kidney Int.* 1996;50(2):593–599.

356. Trevisan G, Ramos JG, Martins-Costa S, et al. Pregnancy in patients with chronic renal insufficiency at Hospital de Clinicas of Porto Alegre, Brazil. *Ren Fail.* 2004;26(1): 29–34.

357. Abe S. The influence of pregnancy on the long-term renal prognosis of IgA nephropathy. *Clin Nephrol.* 1994;41(2):61–64.

358. Bar J, Ben-Rafael Z, Padoa A, et al. Prediction of pregnancy outcome in subgroups of women with renal disease. *Clin Nephrol.* 2000;53(6): 437–444.

359. Combs CA, Kitzmiller JL. Diabetic nephropathy and pregnancy. *Clin Obstet Gynecol.* 1991;34(3): 505–515.

360. Purdy LP, Hantsch CE, Molitch ME, et al. Effect of pregnancy on renal function in patients with moderate-to-severe diabetic renal insufficiency. *Diabetes Care.* 1996;19(10):1067–1074.

361. Gordon M, Landon MB, Samuels P, et al. Perinatal outcome and long-term follow-up associated with modern management of diabetic nephropathy. *Obstet Gynecol.* 1996;87(3):401–409.

362. Gashti CN, Bakris GL. The role of calcium antagonists in chronic kidney disease. *Curr Opin Nephrol Hypertens.* 2004;13(2):155–161.

363. Bakris GL, Weir MR, Secic M, et al. Differential effects of calcium antagonist subclasses on markers of nephropathy progression. *Kidney Int.* 2004;65(6):1991–2002.

364. Khandelwal M, Kumanova M, Gaughan JP, et al. Role of diltiazem in pregnant women with chronic renal disease. *J Matern Fetal Neonatal Med.* 2002;12(6):408–412.

365. Petri M. The Hopkins Lupus Pregnancy Center: Ten key issues in management. *Rheum Dis Clin North Am.* 2007;33(2):227–235.

366. Dhar JP, Sokol RJ. Lupus and pregnancy: Complex yet manageable. *Clin Med Res.* 2006;4(4): 310–321.

367. Germain S, Nelson-Piercy C. Lupus nephritis and renal disease in pregnancy. *Lupus.* 2006;15(3): 148–155.

368. Bobrie G, Liote F, Houillier P, et al. Pregnancy in lupus nephritis and related disorders. *Am J Kidney Dis.* 1987;9(4):339–343.

369. Hayslett JP. Maternal and fetal complications in pregnant women with systemic lupus erythematosus. *Am J Kidney Dis.* 1991;17(2): 123–126.

370. Vidaeff AC, Yeomans ER, Ramin SM. Pregnancy in women with renal disease. Part II: Specific underlying renal conditions. *Am J Perinatol.* 2008;25(7):399–405.

371. Jungers P, Chauveau D. Pregnancy in renal disease. *Kidney Int.* 1997;52(4):871–885.

372. Katzir Z, Rotmensch S, Boaz M, et al. Pregnancy in membranous glomerulonephritis—Course, treatment and outcome. *Clin Nephrol.* 2004;61(1): 59–62.

373. Chapman AB, Johnson AM, Gabow PA. Pregnancy outcome and its relationship to progression of renal failure in autosomal dominant polycystic kidney disease. *J Am Soc Nephrol.* 1994;5(5): 1178–1185.

374. Confortini P, Galanti G, Ancona G, et al. Full term pregnancy and successful delivery in a patient on chronic haemodialysis. *Proc Eur Dial Transplant Assoc.* 1971;8:74–78.

375. Anonymous. Successful pregnancies in women treated by dialysis and kidney transplantation. Report from the Registration Committee of the European Dialysis and Transplant Association. *Br J Obstet Gynaecol.* 1980;87(10): 839–845.

376. Hou SH. Pregnancy in women on haemodialysis and peritoneal dialysis. *Baillieres Clin Obstet Gynaecol* (review). 1994;8(2):481–500.

377. Hou SH. Frequency and outcome of pregnancy in women on dialysis. *Am J Kidney Dis.* 1994;23(1): 60–63.

378. Bagon JA, Vernaeve H, De Muylder X, et al. Pregnancy and dialysis. *Am J Kidney Dis.* 1998;31(5): 756–765.

379. Okundaye I, Abrinko P, Hou S. Registry of pregnancy in dialysis patients. *Am J Kidney Dis.* 1998;31(5):766–773.

380. Reddy SS, Holley JL. Management of the pregnant chronic dialysis patient. *Adv Chronic Kidney Dis.* 2007;14(2):146–155.

381. Holley JL, Reddy SS. Pregnancy in dialysis patients: A review of outcomes, complications, and management (review and 31 references). *Semin Dial.* 2003;16(5):384–388.

382. Hou S. Modification of dialysis regimens for pregnancy. *Int J Artif Organs.* 2002;25(9): 823–826S.

383. Eroglu D, Lembet A, Ozdemir FN, et al. Pregnancy during hemodialysis: Perinatal outcome in our cases. *Transplant Proc.* 2004;36(1):53–55.

384. Chao AS, Huang JY, Lien R, et al. Pregnancy in women who undergo long-term hemodialysis. *Am J Obstet Gynecol.* 2002;187(1):152–156.

385. Okundaye I, Hou S. Management of pregnancy in women undergoing continuous ambulatory peritoneal dialysis. *Adv Perit Dial.* 1996;12: 151–155.

386. Davison JM. Dialysis, transplantation, and pregnancy. *Am J Kidney Dis.* 1991;17(2): 127–132.

387. Muirhead N, Sabharwal AR, Rieder MJ, et al. The outcome of pregnancy following renal transplantation—The experience of a single center. *Transplantation.* 1992;54(3):429–432.

388. McKay DB, Josephson MA. Pregnancy in recipients of solid organs—effects on mother and child. *N Engl J Med.* 2006;354(12):1281–1293.

389. Josephson MA, McKay DB. Considerations in the medical management of pregnancy in transplant recipients. *Adv Chronic Kidney Dis.* 2007;14(2): 156–167.

390. Coscia LA, Constantinescu S, Moritz MJ, et al. Report from the National Transplantation Pregnancy Registry (NTPR): Outcomes of pregnancy after transplantation. *Clin Transplant.* 2007: 29–42.

391. Morris PJ, Johnson RJ, Fuggle SV, et al. Analysis of factors that affect outcome of primary cadaveric renal transplantation in the UK. HLA Task Force of the Kidney Advisory Group of the United Kingdom Transplant Support Service Authority (UKTSSA) (see comment). *Lancet.* 1999;354(9185):1147–1152.

392. Briggs JD, Jager K. The first year of the new ERA-EDTA Registry. *Nephrol Dial Transplant.* 2001; 16(6):1130–1131.

393. Sturgiss SN, Davison JM. Effect of pregnancy on the long-term function of renal allografts: An update. *Am J Kidney Dis.* 1995;26(1): 54–56.

394. Salmela KT, Kyllonen LE, Holmberg C, et al. Impaired renal function after pregnancy in renal transplant recipients. *Transplantation.* 1993; 56(6):1372–1375.

395. Rahamimov R, Ben-Haroush A, Wittenberg C, et al. Pregnancy in renal transplant recipients: Long-term effect on patient and graft survival. A single-center experience. *Transplantation*. 2006;81(5):660–664.

396. McKay DB, Josephson MA, Armenti VT, et al. Reproduction and transplantation: Report on the AST Consensus Conference on Reproductive Issues and Transplantation. *Am J Transplant*. 2005;5(7):1592–1599.

397. Armenti VT, Constantinescu S, Moritz MJ, et al. Pregnancy after transplantation. *Transplant Rev*. 2008;22(4):223–240.

398. Petri M. Immunosuppressive drug use in pregnancy. *Autoimmunity*. 2003;36(1):51–56.

Proteinuria and Nephrotic Syndrome

BURL R. DON AND GEORGE A. KAYSEN

T he ability of the kidney to retain plasma proteins is essential for life. Normal serum protein concentration is of the order of 80 mg/mL, whereas urine contains ≤150 mg of protein per day. Additionally, only a small fraction of urinary proteins is of serum origin, suggesting that nearly all plasma proteins are either restricted from filtration or effectively reabsorbed by the renal tubules once they pass the glomerular filtration barrier. Detection of abnormal amounts or types of protein in the urine is frequently the first sign of significant renal or systemic disease. The presence of abnormal amounts of protein in the urine may reflect (a) a defect in the glomerular barrier that allows abnormal amounts of proteins of intermediate molecular weight to enter Bowman space (glomerular proteinuria), (b) diseases resulting in the inability of the kidney to reabsorb normally proteins presented to the renal tubules (tubular proteinuria), and (c) the overproduction of plasma proteins capable of passing the normal glomerular basement membrane (GBM) so that they enter tubular fluid in quantities that exceed the capacity of the normal proximal tubule to reabsorb them (overflow proteinuria).

Glomerular Proteinuria

MECHANISMS OF ALTERED GLOMERULAR PERMSELECTIVITY

The glomerular filtration barrier consists of the three layers of the glomerular capillary wall: the fenestrated endothelium, the GBM, and the podocytes, together with a slit diaphragm between the interdigitating foot processes of the podocytes (1). Of the three layers of the glomerular capillary wall, the podocyte slit diaphragm is the major barrier to the filtration of proteins. The slit diaphragm consists of a group of proteins that form a slit-diaphragm protein complex, which is connected to the intracellular actin cytoskeleton of the podocytes (Fig. 14.1). The hereditary proteinuric syndromes have provided insight into our understanding of the structure and function of the glomerular filtration barrier and, specifically, the podocyte slit diaphragm. Nephrin was the first slit-diaphragm protein to be identified and is the gene product of the podocyte. Mutation of the nephrin gene is the cause of congenital nephrotic syndrome of the Finnish type (nephritic syndrome type t [NPHS1]). Expression of this gene also is reduced in acquired nephrotic syndrome (2). Nephrin is composed of a short intracellular domain, seven transmembrane domains, and an extracellular domain that consists of eight distal immunoglobulin G (IgG)-like motifs and one proximal fibronectin type 111–like motif. The length of the extracellular domain of nephrin is approximately 35 nm, and the nephrin molecules from adjacent foot processes interact in the middle of the slit in a homophilic fashion to form the filtering structure (Fig. 14.1).

Other proteins contribute to the slit-diaphragm complex, including Neph1, Neph2, FAT1, FAT2, podocin, and CD2-associated protein. Neph1 and Neph2 are structurally related to nephrin and consist of five extracellular IgG-like motifs. They are transmembrane proteins located in the slit diaphragm and form heterodimers with nephrin. FAT1 and FAT2 are large slit-diaphragm transmembrane proteins containing 34 tandem cadherin-like repeats. Positional cloning in patients with corticosteroid-resistant congenital nephrotic syndrome (NPHS2) led to the discovery of the protein podocin. Podocin is a hairpin-shaped protein component of the podocyte cell membrane that interacts with the intracellular domains of nephrin, NEPH1, and CD2-associated protein. Podocin-knockout mice develop severe proteinuria.

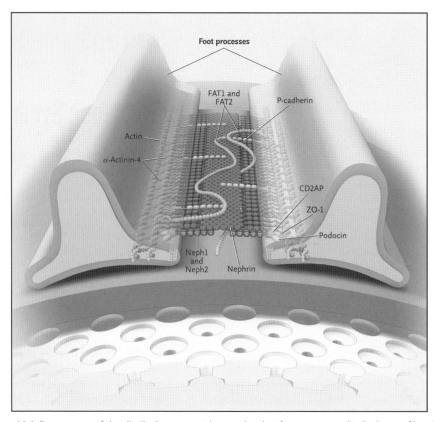

■ **Figure 14.1** Components of the slit-diaphragm protein complex that form a porous slit-diaphragm filter. Nephrin molecules from opposite foot processes interact in the center of the slit, forming a central density with pores on both sides. The zipper-like structure formed by the nephrin molecules probably maintains the width of the slit at about 40 nm. Nephrin could also interact with other proteins in the slit, such as FAT1 and FAT2. The shorter Neph1 and Neph2 molecules may interact with each other, as well as with the proximal part of the nephrin molecules, to stabilize the slit-diaphragm structure. The interactions or role of P-cadherin is unknown. Nephrin and Neph molecules interact with the intracellular podocin and CD2AP. These presumably connect the slit-diaphragm protein complex with ZO-1 and actin strands. The actin strands are joined by α-actinin-4 molecules. The nature of the intracellular interactions of the FAT proteins is unknown. CD2AP, CD2-associated protein. (From Tryggvason K, Patrakka J, Wartiovaara J. Hereditary proteinuria syndromes and mechanisms of proteinuria. *N Eng J Med*. 2006; 354: 1387–1401, with permission.)

The structure of the slit diaphragm is composed of nephrin molecules from adjacent foot processes, interacting in the center of the slit and forming a central density with pores on each side of the central density. This zipper-like structure maintains a constant width of approximately 40 nm. In between the central densities of nephrin are heterogeneously sized pores, which are the diameter of albumin or smaller (Figs. 14.1 and 14.2). The slit-diaphragm protein complex is a true-size selective filter; however, what is not clear is what prevents the pores from becoming clogged during the filtration of middle- and large-molecular-weight proteins. It is speculated that the negative charges on either the GBM or the podocyte cell surface or some other yet unidentified mechanism may repel proteins from the slit diaphragm. Furthermore, the exact locations and function of NEPH1, NEPH2, FAT1, and FAT2 proteins in this slit-diaphragm protein complex are not well understood. What is becoming better appreciated is that the major proteinuric diseases are due to abnormalities of the podocyte and the slit-diaphragm protein complex.

The glomerular filtration barrier is both a size- and charge-selective barrier. It is not possible to directly probe the permeability characteristics of the glomerular filtration barrier by measuring urinary protein excretion alone, because proteins are not only filtered by the glomerulus but also reabsorbed by the renal tubule (3). Neutral and negatively charged dextrans are filtered by the glomerulus but are neither reabsorbed nor catabolized by the renal tubule and thus serve as probes of glomerular size and charge selectivity (4). Neutral dextrans and other nonmetabolized organic molecules are restricted from the urine on the basis of

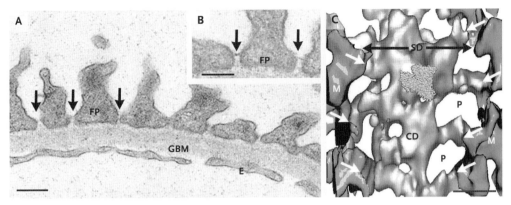

■ **Figure 14.2** Electron-microscopical imaging (**panels A and B**) and electron-tomographic imaging (**panel C**) of the podocyte slit diaphragm. In **panel A**, a cross section of a human glomerular capillary shows filtration slits with slit diaphragms (*arrows*) between the podocyte foot processes (*FPs*). The GBM and an endothelial cell (*E*) are also shown. The scale bar represents 250 nm. **Panel B** shows slit diaphragms (*arrows*) at a higher magnification. The scale bar represents 150 nm. **Panel C** shows a thin, three-dimensional electron tomogram of the mouse slit diaphragm (*SD*) en face. Cross-strands (*arrows*) extend from cross-cut podocyte surface membranes (*M*) to a central density (*CD*), forming lateral pores (*Ps*). The tomogram is a surface-rendered reconstruction. For comparison with the diameter of the pores at the same magnification, a space-filled model of the crystal structure of a serum albumin molecule has been superimposed. The scale bar represents 10 nm. GBM, glomerular basement membrane. (Modified from Wartiovaara J, Ofverstedt LG, Khoshnoodi J, et al. Nephrin strands contribute to a porous slit diaphragm scaffold as revealed by electron tomography. *J Clin Invest* 2004;114:1475–83, with permission.)

size and shape but not of charge (5–7). Negatively charged molecules are more restricted than neutral molecules because of electrostatic interaction with the glomerular filtration barrier (8). Therefore, the normal glomerulus restricts proteins on the basis of both size and charge. The negative charge results from the rich content of heparan sulfate that coats the glomerular filtration barrier (8). The primary site of impedance for filtration of proteins is at the podocyte slit diaphragm (1). Figure 14.3 shows a urine electrophoretic pattern from two patients with glomerular proteinuria. The predominant proteins are of high molecular weight, albumin, transferrin, and, to a lesser extent, IgG. Only small amounts of low-molecular-weight proteins are present.

Figure 14.4 shows the relative renal clearance of neutral dextrans of increasing molecular radius. The curves bearing open symbols represent the clearance of dextrans by the normal human kidney. As the radius of dextrans increase, their clearance relative to inulin, and therefore to water, decreases. One may

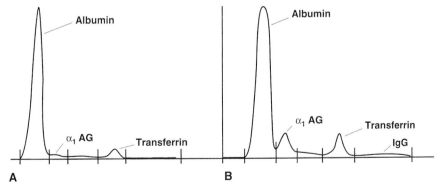

■ **Figure 14.3** Glomerular proteinuria: Scans of electrophoresis of protein from the urine of patients with the nephrotic syndrome. **A:** An example of selective proteinuria. Protein concentration was 63 mg/dL in the urine in **panel A.** Of total urinary protein, albumin was 84.4%, α_1 AG 3.6%, α_2 microglobulin 3.4%, β globulins 5.9%, and γ globulin 2.6%. **B:** An example of nonselective proteinuria. Protein concentration was 680 mg/dL in the urine in **panel B.** Of total urinary protein, albumin was 71.1%, α_1 AG 10.1%, α_2 microglobulin 4.1%, β globulins 9.6%, and γ globulin 5.2%. Albumin is still the predominant protein, but filtration of transferrin, which migrates here as β-globulin, is increased compared with **panel A,** and IgG also is present in greater amounts. Unlike the Ig fragments found in the urine of patients with tubular proteinuria, Igs present in the urine of patients having glomerular proteinuria are full-sized IgG. Ig, immunoglobulin.

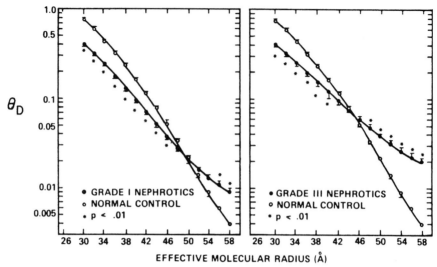

■ **Figure 14.4** Fractional dextran clearances plotted as a function of effective molecular radius. Data from normal subjects are represented by curves bearing open symbols in both panels. Data from patients with nephrotic syndrome are represented by *curves bearing closed symbols*. Dextran-sieving curves from patients with mild renal damage are represented in the **left panel**, and sieving curves from patients with severe glomerular lesions are represented in the **right panel**. All results are expressed as means ± SE. Statistical differences between control and experimental values are connoted by * and reflect a difference at $P < 0.01$. (From Deen WM, Bridges CR, Brenner BM, et al. Heterosporous model of glomerular size selectivity: application to normal and nephrotic humans. *Am J Physiol*. 1985; 249: F374–F389, with permission.)

depict the normal glomerular filtration barrier as being occupied by a series of pores that allow the unrestricted passage of low-molecular-weight solutes and progressively restrict the passage of molecules of greater molecular radius. Figure 14.5 (**left panel**) is a hypothetical representation of the surface of such a filtration barrier. The vast majority of the surface is represented as covered by many pores of similar size, small enough to restrict the passage of large or intermediate-molecular-weight proteins but freely

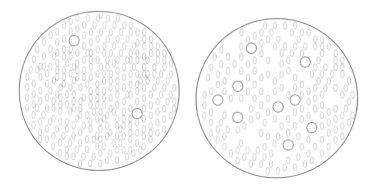

Normal Glomerular
Basement Membrane

"Nephrotic" Glomerular
Basement Membrane

■ **Figure 14.5** Hypothetical representation of the porous surface of a normal GBM (**left panel**) and the GBM from a patient with nephrotic syndrome (**right panel**). The normal GBM is covered predominantly with small pores that are both size and charge selective. They bear a negative charge and exclude anionic proteins more readily than cationic proteins of similar size. Proteinuria results from the development of a separate population of larger pores that allow proteins of intermediate size to pass the GBM, unencumbered. GBM, glomerular basement membrane.

permeable to water and small-molecular-weight peptides and carbohydrate polymers. These pores are estimated to have a radius of between 5.1 and 5.7 nM (6,9,10). A second, much smaller, population of much larger pores also is represented on this hypothetical glomerular filtration barrier. These pores are relatively unselective to molecules of intermediate size and form a shunt pathway that allows proteins to pass into the ultrafiltrate unencumbered (6). Proteinuria results predominantly from the passage of a fraction of glomerular ultrafiltrate through the large nonselective pores.

When the filtration barrier is altered, the total filtration surface is reduced and nephrin gene expression is decreased (2,11,12). Despite thickening of the GBM in the course of a variety of conditions that cause nephrotic syndrome, the diseased glomerulus is far more permeable to proteins than is the normal glomerulus but is less permeable to water and to molecules of lower molecular weight. The reason for this apparent contradiction is that the GBM itself is not the barrier to protein filtration, but instead the greatest impedance to the filtration of proteins is at the glomerular epithelial cell (podocyte) (1). Deen et al. have mathematically modeled the glomerular filtration barrier using data derived from the filtration of neutral dextrans presented in Figure 14.4 (6). They found a reduction in the filtration of low-molecular-weight dextrans. The filtration of low-molecular-weight dextrans is reduced relative to normal in the diseased glomerulus. In contrast, the filtration of high-molecular-weight dextrans is increased in patients with nephrotic syndrome. In the left panel of Figure 14.4 are data derived from patients with less severe renal disease compared to normal subjects. The data in the right panel of Figure 14.4 are derived from patients with more severe renal impairment and less selective proteinuria. The mathematical model proposes that the area of the glomerular filtration barrier covered by small charge- and size-selective pores, and thus available for clearance of water and inulin, is greatly reduced in these patients (Fig. 14.5 [**right panel**]), but the population of larger pores is increased. The larger pores allow proteins such as albumin, transferrin, and IgG to pass the glomerular barrier unrestricted but contribute very little to the total filtration surface and therefore do not offset the surface lost by obliteration of the area covered by smaller pores. High-molecular-weight dextrans pass the glomerular filtration barrier more easily in the abnormal kidney, even though the total filtration surface is reduced, leading to a decline in the glomerular filtration rate (GFR). This phenomenon is responsible for the crossing of the two curves in Figure 14.4. The fractional clearance of low-molecular-weight dextrans is decreased in nephrotic patients, whereas the fractional clearance of high-molecular-weight dextrans is increased. As renal disease progresses, the fraction of GFR passing through the population of large pores increases, whereas the total filtering surface occupied by the normal small pores decreases. The left panel of Figure 14.3 shows the electrophoretic pattern of urinary proteins from a patient with only a mild disruption in glomerular barrier function; the pattern consists predominantly of albumin and 39.5-kDa, highly negatively charged α_1 acid glycoprotein (α_1 AG) and is referred to as a "selective" pattern of glomerular proteinuria. The dextran-sieving pattern from such a patient would be expected to be similar to that in the left panel of Figure 14.4. In contrast, the right panel in Figure 14.3 is from a patient with a greater loss of glomerular size selectivity and consists of transferrin (79.5 kDa) and IgG (150 kDa) in addition to albumin and α_1 AG. The sieving pattern from such a patient would be similar to that in the right panel of Figure 14.5. The more severe the damage is to the capillary wall, the more the large pores become evident, thus leading to the excretion of both middle-molecular-weight (i.e., albumin) and high-molecular-weight (i.e., Igs) proteins in the urine. Most diseases that cause nephrotic syndrome in man primarily cause a loss of glomerular size selectivity (an increase in glomerular permeability to large, uncharged dextrans) without a loss of charge selectivity (13–16).

HORMONAL FACTORS THAT ALTER GLOMERULAR PERMSELECTIVITY

Although changes in the physical dimensions of the glomerular filtration barrier may be responsible for this altered function, alterations in permselectivity can occur quickly, may be transient (13), and are hemodynamically or hormonally mediated (17–19). It is likely that angiotensin II (Ang II) plays an important role in altering glomerular permselectivity, both in disease states and during physiologic circumstances (19).

Constriction of the renal vein in the rat causes an increase in the filtration of high-molecular-weight dextrans, consistent with an increased fraction of glomerular ultrafiltrate passing through a population of large pores. This occurs in conjunction with a nearly tenfold increase in proteinuria and can be almost entirely prevented by infusion of saralasin, an Ang II antagonist (19). Thromboxane synthesis also may play a role in the development of proteinuria in some forms of renal diseases (20,21). Both cyclooxygenase inhibitors and angiotensin-converting enzyme (ACE) inhibitors reduce proteinuria in patients with nephrotic syndrome, in part by reducing the fraction of glomerular filtrate that passes through the large pores (20). Administration of ACE inhibitors to animals having an experimental model of nephrotic syndrome augments nephrin gene expression (11,22). The fact that products of ACE and cyclooxygenase may contribute to the defective filtration barrier in some proteinuric renal disease provides the basis of pharmacologic means for treating proteinuria in some patients, discussed subsequently.

Nitric oxide (NO) is a potent vasodilator released by vascular endothelial cells and macrophages, is derived from the guanidino group on arginine, and plays a role in the regulation of renal blood flow in normal and pathologic states (21,23). Baylis reported that inhibition of NO caused both glomerular hypertension and proteinuria in normal rats (24). It is not known at this time whether NO modulates proteinuria in nephrotic syndrome in patients.

SELECTIVITY OF GLOMERULAR PROTEINURIA

Urine protein electrophoresis patterns have been used in the past to distinguish between different diseases causing glomerular proteinuria. Minimal-change nephrotic syndrome classically has been regarded as causing "selective" proteinuria characterized by a predominance of albumin in comparison to other proteins of intermediate molecular weight. It was believed that minimal-change nephrotic syndrome resulted from loss of charge selectivity, so highly negatively charged albumin was lost in the urine because albumin was restricted on the basis of charge alone, whereas other larger but more neutrally charged proteins were retained. However, minimal-change nephrotic syndrome also is characterized by altered size selectivity, similar to other diseases that cause nephrotic syndrome (18). Many disease entities that can cause proteinuria may cause selective or nonselective proteinuria. The urinary protein electrophoretic pattern encountered in these diseases is determined by the relative fraction of glomerular ultrafiltrate that passes through these large pores.

Renal biopsy has long replaced measurement of the relative concentrations of different proteins in the urine for determination of glomerular pathology. Urinary protein electrophoresis is useful for distinguishing between tubular proteinuria, overflow proteinuria, and glomerular proteinuria but has little utility for distinguishing between diseases of glomerular origin.

Tubular Proteinuria

Tubular proteinuria results from an inability of the proximal tubule to reabsorb proteins filtered by the normal glomerulus in normal amounts. Ideally, urinary protein resulting from tubular abnormalities should consist of a concentrate of proteins present in normal glomerular ultrafiltrate. The total amount of protein in the urine generally is >150 mg/day and <1.5 g/day. Despite its high molecular weight, albumin is still a major constituent of urinary protein, even when the glomerular barrier is normal. Because this protein is present in such great concentrations in blood, appreciable amounts of albumin enter the urine, even though the filtration fraction is only 1/10,000 that of inulin. In contrast, both transferrin and IgG essentially are absent from the urine, both because of their sieving coefficients, which are less than that of albumin (25), and because of their lower concentration in normal plasma. Many of the proteins found in the urine of patients with pure tubular proteinuria are of low molecular weight, such as β_2-microglobulin (11.6 kDa) and α_1-microglobulin (31 kDa) (26).

In its most severe state proximal tubular dysfunction leads to the Fanconi syndrome (25,27), a syndrome characterized by the inability of the proximal tubule to reabsorb glucose, amino acids, uric acid, phosphate, bicarbonate, and other normal components of proximal tubular fluid, in addition to proteins. As a consequence, Fanconi syndrome causes nonanion gap metabolic acidosis, hypouricemia, hypophosphatemia, aminoaciduria, and glycosuria, in addition to proteinuria. The syndrome generally results from one of several inherited metabolic disorders (25,28,29,30), although it also can be caused by exposure to cadmium (31–32), ingestion of outdated tetracycline (26), multiple myeloma, amyloidosis, and other processes detailed in Table 14.1. It is important to recognize the presence of Fanconi syndrome to identify and

TABLE 14.1 DISORDERS CAUSING DISORDERED RENAL REABSORPTION OF FILTERED PROTEINS AT NORMAL FILTERED LOADS

Congenital Disorders

Fanconi syndrome

Hereditary

Cystinosis
Wilson disease
Heritable fructose intolerance
Oxalosis
Hereditary tyrosinemia (257)
Glycogen storage diseases
Galactosemia
Dent disease
Lowe syndrome

Acquired

Heavy metal poisoning
Outdated tetracycline
Multiple myeloma
Amyloidosis
Vitamin D intoxication
Bartter syndrome
Familial asymptomatic tubular proteinuria
Occulocerebrorenal dystrophy
Renal tubular acidosis
Renal dysplasia
Renal cystic disorders (polycystic kidney disease)

Systemic Disease Hereditary

Galactosemia
Glycogen storage disease

Acquired

Balkan nephropathy
Sarcoidosis
Systemic lupus erythematosus
Acute renal disease
Acute tubular necrosis
Renal infarction
Transplant rejection
Infectious disease
Pyelonephritis
Viral- or bacterial-associated interstitial nephritis

Drugs and Toxins

Acute hypersensitivity interstitial nephritis (penicillins, cephalosporins, sulfonamides)
Aminoglycoside toxicity
Analgesic nephropathy
Cyclosporin toxicity
Cd, Pb, As, Hg, ethylene glycol, CC14
Ifosfamide
Vitamin D intoxication

manage the underlying disease and metabolic acidosis. Proteinuria may participate in causing renal injury and not just serve as a marker of renal damage. Patients with inherited forms of Fanconi syndrome progress to renal failure after many years (29).

Tubular proteinuria also may result from more subtle damage to the proximal tubule. The increased presentation of high-molecular-weight proteins to the proximal tubular cells may even cause an increase in the urinary excretion of low-molecular-weight proteins (33,34). β_2-Microglobulin may appear in the urine early in the course of aminoglycoside toxicity before any decrease in GFR or the appearance of more overt forms of proximal tubular dysfunction (35,36). β_2-Microglobulinuria also may be the first manifestation of cadmium or other heavy-metal intoxication (31,32,37–39), although the level of β_2-microglobulin also increases early in the course of chronic cadmium nephropathy and contributes to the increased appearance of this protein in the urine (31). Heavy-metal intoxication also may cause an increased renal clearance of albumin and IgG, as well as increased excretion of low-molecular-weight proteins (31), thus leading to a "mixed" form of proteinuria. Urinary β_2-microglobulin excretion is monitored in workers exposed to nephrotoxic metals so as to avoid the development of chronic renal disease (31,37–39). As with Fanconi syndrome, the appearance of β_2-microglobulin and other low-molecular-weight proteins in the urine is not injurious in and of itself. However, detection of these proteins is important in the diagnosis of exposure to nephrotoxic agents. Cadmium exposure is a risk factor and likely to be a cause of end-stage renal disease (32), making it significant to identify patients exposed to this toxin.

Tubular proteinuria with the excretion of low-molecular-weight proteins is frequently seen with many glomerular diseases, since there is usually concomitant tubulointerstitial damage. The quantitative measure of urinary excretion of low-molecular-weight proteins like β_2-microglobulin in the setting of glomerular disease is a marker of the degree of tubulointerstitial disease associated with the primary glomerular disorder (40).

Overflow Proteinuria

Park and Maack (33) showed in elegant studies using the isolated, perfused proximal tubule in a rabbit that the absorptive capacity for albumin by the healthy proximal tubule is quite high. Before this observation the low affinity of the renal tubule for albumin predicted that an increase in albuminuria should occur with only a slight increase in its filtered load. An increase in the filtered load of several proteins does result in their appearance in the urine. Subsequently large transmembrane spanning receptors that transport albumin have been identified. Megalin (41) and cubilin (42) are heavily expressed in kidney proximal tubule epithelial cells and are responsible for albumin uptake by the proximal nephron as well as the uptake of other filtered proteins that are catabolized by the proximal tubule. Cubulin plays an important role in the reuptake of filtered vitamin B12–binding protein and high-density lipoprotein (HDL)-associated proteins, including apolipoprotein (apo) A-I, apo A-II, and apo J. (43). Overflow proteinuria occurs when these specific receptors can no longer accommodate the filtered load of proteins normally taken up and metabolized by the proximal nephron. Myeloma light chains are also taken up by both of these receptors (44,45). The most common causes of overflow proteinuria are listed in Table 14.2. The most significant of these are the appearance of Bence–Jones proteins in the urine of patients with multiple myeloma.

TABLE 14.2 CAUSES OF OVERFLOW PROTEINURIA

MGUS
Multiple myeloma
Monocytic and myelomonocytic leukemia
Hemoglobinuria
Myoglobinuria
Systemic inflammatory processes
Trauma
Sepsis
HIV infection

HIV, human immunodeficiency virus; MGUS, monoclonal gammopathy of undetermined significance.

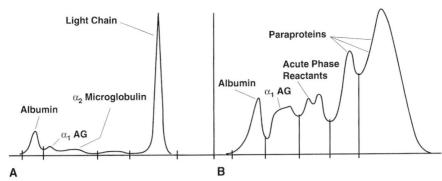

■ Figure 14.6 Overflow proteinuria: Scan of electrophoresis of protein from the urine of a patient with multiple myeloma (**panel A**) and a patient with AIDS (**panel B**). Note the predominance of protein in a single band in the urine of the patient with multiple myeloma. This is caused by the overflow of a homogeneous cationic Ig fragment (*light chains*). In the patient with AIDS, urinary protein is composed of heterogeneous mixtures of acute-phase reactant proteins and polyclonal Ig fragments. Protein concentration was 16 mg/dL in the urine in **panel A**. Of total urinary protein, albumin represented 13.4%, α_1 AG 7.6%, α_2-microglobulin 8.1%, β-globulins 5.3%, and γ-globulin 65.6%. Protein concentration was 220 mg/dL in the urine in **panel B**. Of total urinary protein, albumin represented 7.6%, α_1 AG 11.7%, α_2-microglobulin 13.3%, β-globulins 18.3%, and γ-globulin 49.2%. Ig, immunoglobulin.

Electrophoretic methods used to characterize urinary and serum proteins in clinical laboratories separate them on the basis of charge, not molecular weight. The migration of these proteins in an electorphoretic field is charge dependent, so the distance of migration from the origin is greatest for those having the greatest net positive charge (most cationic).

Figure 14.6 (**left panel**) shows the result of protein electrophoresis of urine from a patient with this disorder. There is a large quantity of light-chain protein in the urine (a so-called "spike"). Some myeloma light-chain proteins are quite nephrotoxic, depending on their isoelectric points (pKi) and other factors. Myeloma light-chain proteins with a pKi of around 5 generally are most toxic, in part because of their reduced solubility in the acid milieu of the renal papilla (46). The continued excretion of these proteins may produce progressive and irreversible renal failure (47). Early treatment of multiple myeloma may prevent the development or progression of renal failure. Maintenance of alkaline diuresis also may be therapeutic. For this reason protein electrophoresis is an important component in the evaluation of any patient with proteinuria, especially in the evaluation of patients over the age of 40.

Ig appearance in the urine, however, does not necessarily indicate malignant disease. Monoclonal gammopathy of undetermined significance (MGUS) may never progress to malignant transformation (48), although the cells responsible for generating this low amount of Ig ultimately may undergo malignant transformation, given sufficient time (49,50), with a rate of onset of frank multiple myeloma of approximately 1% per year (51).

A modest increase in urinary protein excretion can occur in patients during acute inflammatory conditions, such as in patients with human immunodeficiency virus (HIV) infection, after trauma, or as a consequence of severe infection. This is a consequence of increased excretion of a number of low-molecular-weight proteins produced in response to stress, Igs, and acute-phase reactant proteins. Their filtration is increased beyond the tubular capacity for their reabsorption, and they spill into the urine and should be distinguished from glomerular proteinuria, which also can be caused by HIV infection. Figure 14.6 (**right panel**) shows the result of protein electrophoresis of urine from a patient with acquired immunodeficiency syndrome (AIDS) with the overflow pattern of urinary protein excretion. Acute-phase reactant proteins of relatively low molecular weight appear in the urine as well as Ig fragments (paraproteins). These represent the filtration of a variety of polyclonal Ig fragments produced in excess as a result of HIV (52,53) infection and can be distinguished clearly from the monoclonal gammopathy illustrated in the left panel of this figure.

Renal Handling of Proteins

Normally, the major constituent of urinary protein is the Tamm–Horsfall protein, a component of the glycocalyx secreted by renal tubular cells and not of serum origin (54). Because plasma proteins are heterogeneous with respect to size, charge, and shape, different mechanisms have evolved to retain proteins of different classes. Proteins <20 kDa in mass freely pass the glomerular barrier, are reabsorbed, and for the most part are catabolized by proximal tubular cells (55–57) with the amino acids reclaimed. As the molecular radius increases, the fractional sieving coefficient decreases. Norden et al. estimated the sieving coefficients of proteins as a function of molecular radius in patients with a form of Fanconi syndrome (25) (Fig. 14.7) and demonstrated that as the molecular weight of proteins increases above that of β_2-microglobulin, the fractional excretion sharply decreases. The fractional filtration of IgG is estimated to be <0.0001 (25).

The kidney serves as the primary site for catabolism of low-molecular-weight proteins, peptides, hormones (parathyroid hormone, insulin), fragments of Igs (light-chain β_2-microglobulin), and enzymes (lysozyme, amylase, cationic trypsinogen). Because these proteins are freely filtered normally, their appearance in the urine may result from a pathologic increase in their generation so that the capacity of the renal tubule to metabolize them is exceeded. This occurs with the increased production of light chains of Ig in patients with multiple myeloma (47,58). Another cause of proteinuria is a consequence of an intrinsic inability of the proximal tubule to reabsorb filtered proteins (14,25,47,58) as a result of proximal tubular damage. Proteins of intermediate size, between 40 and 150 kDa, corresponding to a Stokes–Einstein radius of between 3.5 and 6 nM are nearly completely restricted from glomerular ultrafiltrate in the absence of disease because of their charge and size, and the small amount of protein filtered is essentially all reabsorbed. These proteins are, however, lost in the greatest quantity when the glomerular barrier is altered (6,59). Proteins typical of this class are albumin, IgG, transferrin,

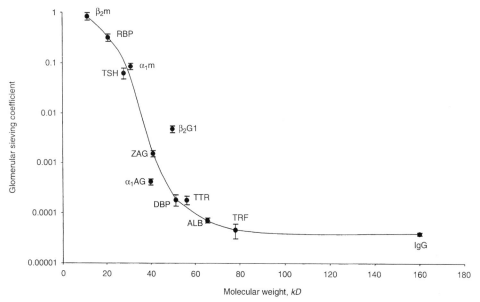

■ **Figure 14.7** Estimated glomerular sieving coefficients for 12 plasma proteins versus molecular weight. Data are mean (±SEM) of five determinations based on results from each of five patients with Dent disease. $\alpha 1$ AG, molecular weight 40 kDa; ALB, molecular weight 65 kDa; $\alpha 1$ M, molecular weight 31 kDa; β_2 GI, molecular weight 50 kDa; β_2 M, molecular weight 11.6 kDa; DPB, molecular weight 51.3 kDa; IgG, molecular weight 160 kDa; RBP, molecular weight 21 kDa; TRF, molecular weight 78 kDa; TSH, molecular weight 28 kDa; TTR, molecular weight 55 kDa; ZAG, molecular weight 41 kDa. $\alpha 1$ AG, $\alpha 1$ acid glycoprotein; ALB, albumin; $\alpha 1$ M, $\alpha 1$ microglobulin; $\beta 2$ M, $\beta 2$ microglobulin; β_2 GI, β_2-glycoprotein I; DPB, vitamin D–binding protein; IgG, immunoglobulin G; RBP, retinol-binding protein; TRF, transferring; TSH, thyroid stimulating hormone; TTR, transthyretin; ZAG, zinc-α_2-globulin. (Reprinted with permission from Norden AGW, Lapsley M, Lee PJ, et al. Glomerular protein sieving and implications for renal failure in Fanconi syndrome. *Kidney Int.* 2001;60:1885–1892, with permission.)

ceruloplasmin, α_1 AG, and HDL. Very large proteins (IgM, α_1 and α_2 macroglobulins, fibrinogen) are completely restricted by the normal glomerulus. Even when glomerular permselectivity is greatly altered, only small quantities of these large proteins pass into the glomerular ultrafiltrate. When they do, the consequences with regard to preservation of renal structure and function are grave (60). The appearance of fibrinogen in Bowman space may be associated with crescent formation (61).

Methods of Measuring Proteinuria

There are several qualitative and quantitative tests available to measure urinary protein excretion. Clinic screening for the presence of proteinuria is generally performed with the use of the urinary dipstick. The reactive portion of the stick is coated with a buffered indicator that changes color in the presence of protein. Urinary dipstick results are semiquantitive and are better utilized as a screening tool for the presence of protein in the urine and a rough guide to urine protein concentration. The standard urinary dipstick measures albumin concentration via a colorimetric reaction between albumin and tetrabromophenol. Use of this dye-binding technique has a number of limitations, such as the indicator is more sensitive to albumin than other plasma proteins and thus is a poor marker for tubular and overflow proteinuria. Moreover, urinary dipsticks usually become positive when protein excretion rates exceed 300 to 500 mg/day; thus it is not a good screening tool for detecting very low-grade proteinuria or microalbuminuria (62,63). False-positive urinary dipstick results have been reported when patients have been administered radiocontrast agents (64).

In contrast to the urinary dipstick, sulfosalicylic acid (SSA) will detect all proteins in the urine and is a useful screening test in a patient suspected of having proteinuria with a negative or trace urinary dipstick protein determination. Measurement of formation of a precipitate by SSA or trichloroacetic acid will detect any type of protein present in urine, although these methods also detect albumin more readily than other proteins (54). Both tests have a lower limit of sensitivity of about 20 mg/L. The classic example of this is a patient with multiple myeloma with overflow proteinuia consisting of light chains not detected by the dipstick but positive by SSA measuring tubidity. This method is nonspecific with regard to protein type. A discordance then between the SSA method and the protein determination by a urinary dipstick is found when proteins other than albumin, that is, Igs, dominate urinary protein content.

The classic method of quantifying the amount of proteinuria is a timed 24-hour urine collection. Because of frequent collection errors and unreliability, this common technique of quantifying urine protein excretion has come under criticism. Random or first-morning single-specimen (spot) collection with measurement of protein to creatinine concentration ratios has been advocated as a more reliable way to assess the degree of proteinuria (65,66). There is a good correlation between the first-morning spot urine specimen measurement of the urine protein to creatinine concentration ratio and timed 24-hour urine collections for protein excretion determination (66). Similarly, a spot urine albumin to creatinine ratio is a useful means of assessing the degree of urinary albumin excretion for a 24-hour period.

The standard method for assessing and quantifying urinary albumin excretion is based on the binding of the pH-sensitive bromcresol green dye by albumin. When bromcresol green is bound to albumin, the dissociation constant of the dye changes so that it is in its ionized form at all physiologic urinary pH values and turns green. This method does not detect other urinary proteins well and is relatively insensitive, the lower limit of detection being slightly <30 mg/dL. If total urine volume is 1 L, urinary albumin excretion will reach the threshold of detection with this method, at slightly <300 mg/day. Because clinically important albuminuria occurs well below this value (>22 mg/day) (13), more sensitive, immunologically based assays using nephelometric methods are employed to detect small amounts of albumin (microalbuminuria) in the urine that may reveal the presence of clinically significant renal diseases, such as diabetic nephropathy, in their early stages and are also a risk factor for cardiovascular disease even in patients without underlying hypertension or diabetes (67,68). As will be discussed later in this chapter, the presence of microalbuminuria is highly predictive of the development of overt proteinuria in patients with diabetes mellitus and also is predictive of subsequent development of hypertension and for cardiovascular events.

In some cases it is important to detect specific proteins that appear in the urine in small amounts as a result of proximal tubular dysfunction. β_2-Microglobulin is efficiently reabsorbed by the normal proximal tubule, but subtle damage to the proximal tubule caused by nephrotoxins results in the urinary loss of this and other proteins in quantities detectable by sensitive immunoassays (69). Electrophoretic methods also are useful in initial evaluation of urinary protein to determine whether the pattern of protein excretion is most compatible with that resulting from a tubular lesion, overflow of abnormal proteins into the urine, or glomerular pathology.

WHY DETECT PROTEINURIA BEFORE THE ONSET OF OVERT RENAL DISEASE?

Some progressive renal diseases, especially diabetes, declare themselves early in their course by the presence of small amounts of albumin in the urine. Mogensen and Christiansen (70) found that patients with microalbuminuria, albuminuria in the range of 15 to 150 μg/min (between 22 and 220 mg/day), were those who developed progressive renal injury with the passage of time. Early treatment of hypertension forestalled the development of renal failure in these patients (71). More recently it has been established that early treatment of diabetic patients with ACE inhibitors (72,73) and Ang II receptor blocking (ARB) drugs (74) prevents the onset of microalbuminuria or the progression of microalbuminuria to clinically overt albuminuria in insulin-dependent diabetic patients. Ang II receptor–blocking drugs and ACEs are similarly effective in preserving renal function in proteinuric diabetic patients (75).

Numerous studies have suggested that, in addition to its relation to renal disease, microalbuminuria is an important risk factor for cardiovascular disease and early cardiovascular mortality in patient with and without diabetes and/or hypertension (67,76–77). The relationship between urinary albumin excretion and cardiovascular disease is more powerfully expressed in diabetic patients but is seen across all populations (78). A number of clinical trials and population studies have demonstrated the presence of microalbuminuria and overt proteinuria as a significant predictor of cardiovascular risk (67,79–81). Inhibition of Ang II reduces cardiovascular risk in this population as well (82). Thus, microalbuminuria is a proxy for vascular injury.

In addition to being a marker of cardiovascular disease, microalbuminuria is highly associated with obesity and the metabolic syndrome, and the degree of microalbuminuria increases with age (83,84). This relationship between albuminuria and adverse cardiovascular events is continuous rather than dichotomous, such that small increases in albumin excretion even within the so-called normal range are associated with subsequent development of hypertension, cardiovascular events, and progressive renal disease (85,86). Although it is not possible to dissociate cause and effect from this relationship, it is likely that the causes of vascular injury also alter glomerular permselectivity so as to cause an increase in the filtered load of plasma proteins, and these plasma proteins appear in the urine as a result of an alteration in renal processing of filtered plasma proteins. Urinary albumin excretion also likely reflects generalized changes in the vascular endothelium, including that encompassing the glomerulus. This abnormality in the endothelium is manifested in the observation that vasodilatation is reduced in older nondiabetic patients with microalbuminuira compared with those without microalbuminuria. This endothelial dysfunction is also present in diabetic patients, and the degree of impaired coronary vasodilatation is greater in patients with microalbuminuria (87,88).

Chronic proteinuria most likely directly causes increased interstitial damage (89–93). Therefore, the early detection of albumin in the urine may permit effective treatment of the underlying condition altering glomerular permselectivity. Reduction of proteinuria also may prevent nephrotoxic effects of filtered proteins (75). Thus, it is possible that aggressive treatment may prevent or delay the eventual development of renal failure (72,73,75).

Overflow proteinuria also may cause acute kidney injury or even chronic kidney disease (47,89–91,94). Renal failure caused by multiple myeloma may be irreversible and shorten survival of patients with this disease. The early detection and treatment of light-chain proteinuria, myoglobinuria, or hemoglobinuria can not only prevent the development of acute or chronic renal failure but also provide diagnostic evidence of treatable diseases in time to alter the course of those diseases. The early detection of myoglobinuria may alert the physician to the presence of a crushed extremity or serious drug toxicity in time to intervene with preventive measures. β_2-Microglobulinuria may herald the onset of renal failure caused by nephrotoxic antibiotics, such as aminoglycosides, so timely discontinuation or dosage adjustment of the drug is possible. β_2-Microglobulinuria also may allow the detection of environmental toxins (38,39).

A very common cause of proteinuria is the so-called transient proteinuria, which is usually low-grade proteinuria (<1 g/24 h) seen on a single urine specimen, which resolves on subsequent urinalysis in almost all patients (95). Transient proteinuria is commonly seen in patients with fevers and urinary tract infection and those who exercise (40,96,97). The cause of transient proteinuria is not well understood but may be due to increases in glomerular permeability induced by Ang II or catecholamines (98).

Another benign cause of proteinuria is orthostatic or postural proteinuria, which is seen more frequently in children and adolescents. This disorder is characterized by an increase in urinary protein excretion with upright posture and normal protein excretion when supine (99). Generally, orthostatic proteinuria is low grade (<1 g/24 h) and is a benign condition without any untoward long-term effect on renal function and resolves over time in most patients (99,100). The etiology of orthostatic proteinuria is not known, but a number of possible causes have been proposed. Upright posture stimulates Ang II, which alters glomerular permeability, leading to low-grade proteinuria. There may be a mild or subtle glomerular disorder such as focal mesangial glomerulonephritis or abnormality in the GBM (101). The diagnosis of orthostatic proteinuria can be made by performing a split urine collection, in which urine protein excretion is assessed in two separate collections during a 24-hour period (upright collection during the daytime and a recumbent nighttime collection). Patients with orthostatic proteinuria will have normal levels of proteinuria during recumbency, with the bulk of proteinuria being noted in the daytime urine collection.

MYOGLOBINURIA

Damage to striated muscle causes the appearance of myoglobin in the blood. This low-molecular-weight protein is freely filtered by the glomerulus and may appear in the urine in large quantities (102). The urine may be turbid or clear but generally is brown. After centrifugation of the urine, the supernatant tests positive for blood using the benzidine test, even in the absence of red blood cells. It is important to identify this entity for two reasons. Most significantly, myoglobinuria is an important cause of acute kidney injury (103–109). The mechanism for the acute kidney injury caused by myoglobinuria is probably multifactorial, including intense renal vasoconstriction, tubular obstruction, and, most importantly, tubular injury. Iron contained in the heme moiety of myoglobin causes direct tubular damage by acting as a Fenton (free radical) reagent (110). Therapies suggested to mitigate or attenuate myoglobin-induced acute kidney injury include vigorous parenteral fluid administration to help accelerate renal clearance of myoglobin and the addition of sodium bicarbonate and mannitol to the parenteral fluids. Alkalinizing the urine with the addition of sodium bicarbonate to parenteral fluids may help prevent the heme moiety separating from the globin component of myoglobin and thus prevent the iron-induced tubular damage (111). The addition of mannitol has a number of theoretical benefits to attenuate acute kidney injury; mannitol is an osmotic diuretic and would accelerate urinary excretion of myoglobin, and it increases renal blood flow and is a scavenger of free radicals (112).

It also is important to identify the cause of rhabdomyolysis. Permanent disability resulting from crush injuries may be avoided by early surgical intervention (104,113). Metabolic disorders, such as hypophosphatemia (114), hyperthermia, and hypokalemia (115), require therapy, whereas inherited disorders (116–117,15,118–120) require both management and genetic counseling.

HEMOGLOBINURIA

Hemoglobinuria results from intravascular hemolysis and occurs when the capacity of haptoglobin to bind free hemoglobin is exceeded. The urine may vary from pink to black in color. Spectroscopic methods may be necessary to distinguish hemoglobinuria from myoglobinuria. It is important to identify this entity because hemoglobinuria also can cause acute renal failure (121). As in the case of myoglobinuria, renal failure caused by hemoglobinuria (122) may be averted by mannitol infusion, hydration, and urinary alkalinization, although this approach remains controversial. Pure hemoglobin has little or no toxic effect when transfused (123), but red cell stroma alone can cause renal failure (124). Therefore, the cause of acute renal failure associated with hemoglobinuria may involve a mechanism other than tubular obstruction by filtered hemoglobin.

Hemoglobinuria may be an initial manifestation of conditions causing acute intravascular hemolysis, which may be life threatening, even in the absence of acute renal failure. These conditions include incompatible blood transfusions (121,122,124); arsine poisoning (125–127); falciparum malaria; red cell enzyme defects; immune hemolytic anemias; and acute hemolysis owing to drugs, chemicals (128), burns, hypophosphatemia (129), infections, eclampsia, or the entrance of hypotonic solutions into the blood, such as hypotonic infusions during prostatectomy. Anemia alone may cause death from many of these entities long before renal failure becomes a clinical problem.

Chronic intravascular hemolysis also may cause hemoglobinuria. Although neither severe, acute anemia nor acute renal failure develops as a consequence of chronic intravascular hemolysis, hemoglobinuria or hemosiderinuria may be the first recognizable symptom of one of several chronic disorders. Diseases responsible for chronic intravascular hemolysis include paroxysmal nocturnal hemoglobinuria (130), paroxysmal cold hemoglobinuria, march hemoglobinuria (131) (resulting from mechanical disruption of red cells during exercise—the pigment excreted also may be myoglobin), and mechanical disruption of red blood cells, owing to prosthetic heart valves (132).

Nephrotic Syndrome

Nephrotic syndrome results from alterations in the permselective characteristics of the GBM that allow increased passage of proteins of intermediate size into the urine and consists of the constellation of heavy proteinuria (≥3.5 g/day), hypoalbuminemia, hyperlipidemia, increased concentration of several high-molecular-weight proteins, and edema formation (133,134). Not all components of this syndrome need be present. It is not known why all manifestations of nephrotic syndrome are expressed in some patients and not in others. Proteinuria >3.5 g/day, however, is predictive of any of several serious renal diseases listed in Table 14.3 and defines nephrotic proteinuria.

It is somewhat surprising that all of these manifestations may result from the loss of the amount of protein in half an egg of a hen. The mean value for proteinuria in a number of studies of nephrotic syndrome is about 8 g/day (135–138), but viewed in the context of normal protein intake, even this external loss is small. Although it is experimentally more difficult to quantitate the losses of tissue protein, continuous massive proteinuria causes marked muscle wasting (139,140), sometimes obscured by edema. How do these extensive metabolic derangements result from a relatively small amount of protein loss? What are the homeostatic adaptations that result from urinary protein loss? Why are urinary protein losses resistant to replacement by dietary protein augmentation? These are questions that are approached in the ensuing sections.

ALBUMIN METABOLISM IN NEPHROTIC SYNDROME

In the absence of external albumin loss, before the onset of albuminuria, a fixed quantity of albumin is synthesized each day and an identical quantity is destroyed by catabolism. Three principal adaptive

---

TABLE 14.3 CAUSES OF GLOMERULAR PROTEINURIA

Diseases Confined to the Kidney
Minimal-change nephrotic syndrome
Membranous nephropathy
Focal segmental glomerulosclerosis
Mesangial proliferative glomerulonephritis
Mesangiocapillary glomerulonephritis
Acute poststreptococcal glomerulonephritis

Systemic Diseases
Diabetes mellitus
Henoch–Schönlein purpura
Systemic lupus erythematosus
Amyloidosis
Goodpasture syndrome
ANCA vasculitis
Hepatitis C and hepatitis B

Hereditary Disorders
Congenital nephrotic syndrome
Hereditary nephritis (Alport syndrome)
Partial lipodystrophy

mechanisms may be brought into play to defend the plasma albumin pool when this steady state is disturbed by the development of albuminuria. The extravascular albumin pool may be mobilized into the intravascular space, the rate of albumin synthesis may be increased, or albumin catabolic rate may be decreased. Of these three adaptive mechanisms, only the last two are capable of reestablishing a steady state such that albumin production is again equal to the sum of external albumin loss plus catabolism.

ALBUMIN CATABOLISM

The bulk of albumin catabolism occurs in a compartment in rapid equilibrium with the vascular compartment and not in any predominant organ (141–144). In the absence of renal disease, approximately 10% to 20% of albumin catabolism takes place in the kidney (144,145), and this represents the amount of albumin filtered by the normal glomerulus (25,59,146,147). When glomerular filtration of albumin is increased, more albumin is presented to the proximal tubular cells and it is possible for the rate of renal albumin catabolism to be increased. However, micropuncture studies in both normal and nephrotic rats suggest that albumin reabsorption by the renal tubules of nephrotic animals might be saturated at near physiologic levels (148–150). Most of the increased albumin filtered by the abnormal glomerulus may in fact be lost in the urine and not catabolized by the renal tubular epithelium. Therefore, urinary albumin excretion is not a gross underestimate of the total albumin lost from the pool in nephrotic syndrome.

The absolute rate of albumin catabolism decreases and the rate of albumin synthesis increases in nephrotic rats almost to an equal extent as albuminuria become progressively severe (151). The fractional rate of albumin catabolism also is increased in nephrotic patients, whereas the absolute rate of albumin catabolism is reduced (139,140). These findings are compatible with a reduced rate of extrarenal albumin catabolism coupled with an increase in intrarenal albumin catabolism.

ALBUMIN SYNTHESIS

Albumin synthesis is predominantly regulated by the availability of adequate dietary protein (152–155) and is suppressed during inflammation (156) and acute metabolic acidosis (157). The rate of albumin synthesis is increased under conditions when plasma π is reduced, such as during nephrotic syndrome. Albumin synthesis is increased as a consequence of increased transcription of the cognate gene (158,159), possibly regulated by the transcription factors early growth response factor-1 (EGRF-1) and hepatocyte nuclear factor-4 (HNF-4) (160). Conditions that cause an increase in plasma π reduce the rate of albumin synthesis in vivo (161–165); however, there is no clear relationship between plasma albumin concentration and albumin synthetic rate in nephrotic patients (57,140,141) or animals (155). Although albumin synthesis increases in direct proportion to albuminuria in both nephrotic patients (136,166–180) and animals (151,158), the response fails to maintain albumin pools or plasma concentration in or near the normal range.

Effect of Dietary Protein on Albumin Synthesis

The rate of albumin synthesis responds rapidly to acute changes in diet (153,156,166). When severely malnourished animals or people are fed, the rate of albumin synthesis increases promptly, although total body protein stores still are severely depleted (167,168). The most important nutritional constituent is dietary protein. The maintenance of a normal plasma albumin concentration and a normal rate of albumin synthesis depends on both total protein availability in the diet and the relative proportion of protein to nonprotein calories. Diets that provide adequate calories but are poor in protein have a more deleterious effect on albumin synthesis and on albumin stores than do diets that contain the same amount of protein but are deficient in calories (169,170). A balanced diet that is inadequate in both protein and calories does not cause hypoalbuminemia. A diet containing adequate calories but insufficient protein results in reduced albumin synthesis, albumin concentration, and total body albumin mass (171), producing kwashiorkor. One would predict that an ideal diet for patients with nephrotic syndrome, a disorder that bears much similarity to protein malnutrition, would contain adequate calories, but above all an adequate or preferably high protein content. Diets containing large excesses of protein, 3 to 4 g/kg body weight, have been prescribed in the past (172), although no data are available demonstrating the effectiveness of these diets in restoring protein pools. Increased

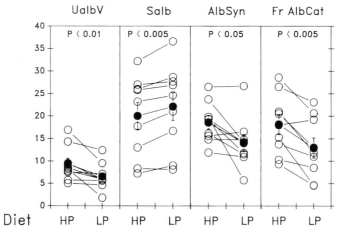

■ **Figure 14.8** Changes in urinary albumin excretion that occurs with isocaloric reduction in dietary protein intake (**first panel**), in albumin concentration (**second panel**), in the rate of albumin synthesis (**third panel**), and in the fractional rate of albumin catabolism (**fourth panel**) in patients with nephrotic syndrome of various etiologies. The fractional albumin catabolic rate is the percentage of the vascular albumin pool catabolized in 24 hours. *Closed circles* represent the mean values for the group. (From Kaysen GA, Kirkpatrick WG, Couser WG. Albumin homeostasis in the nephrotic rat: nutritional considerations. *Am J Physiol*. 1984; 247: F192–F202, with permission.)

dietary protein intake in fact fails to increase either albumin concentration or body albumin pools in patients with nephrotic syndrome (140,143,144,173) (Fig. 14.8) or animals with experimentally induced nephrotic syndrome (155,162,174). Instead, much of the ingested protein is catabolized rather than used for net protein synthesis. Furthermore, the increased albumin synthesis that results from dietary protein augmentation is accompanied by an increased rate of fibrinogen synthesis (175,180). In addition, dietary protein exerts an effect on the kidney, causing a reversible increase in glomerular permeability to large macromolecules (174,175), so most of the additional albumin synthesized is lost in the urine (140,155). Figure 14.9 shows the effect of diets containing either 2 or 0.6 k/kg of protein on the renal clearance of neutral dextrans when fed to nephrotic patients (174). It can be seen clearly that patients clear high-molecular-weight dextrans more easily when fed a high-protein diet. Thus, a change in dietary protein may alter the permselectivity characteristics of the glomerular filtration barrier in these patients.

Virtually every study of the effect of altered dietary protein intake on nephrotic syndrome noted that urinary albumin or protein excretion varied with dietary protein intake (31,140,143,144,149,174–179). The potential adverse consequences of increased dietary protein intake were largely ignored until recently (140,155,177–179). Continued maintenance of a high-protein diet may have the consequence of causing permanent rather than transient changes in the kidney and accelerate the progression of renal diseases (177–180).

The rate of albumin synthesis increases in parallel with urinary protein loss (136,154,158,180) and dietary protein intake (139,175). In nephrotic syndrome the rate of albumin synthesis correlates with that of other proteins, many of which have pathologic consequences. One of these is fibrinogen (Fig. 14.10) (180); another is the atherogenic lipoprotein Lp(a) (Fig. 14.11) (181). Of interest, restriction of dietary protein reduces fibrinogen synthesis in nephrotic patients (175). Fibrinogen levels in nephrotic patients are directly proportional to the rate of synthesis of this protein (180), and because fibrinogen is a powerful cardiovascular risk factor, reducing its rate of synthesis by avoiding a high-protein intake has the potential of reducing this risk factor.

The fractional renal clearance of albumin increases in both the normal rat and the rat with Heymann nephritis (182,183) within only 48 hours of institution of a high-protein diet. Similar reversible changes occur in the human kidney after only a short period of eating a diet rich in protein (139,173). When dietary protein is increased in nephrotic patients, both urinary albumin excretion

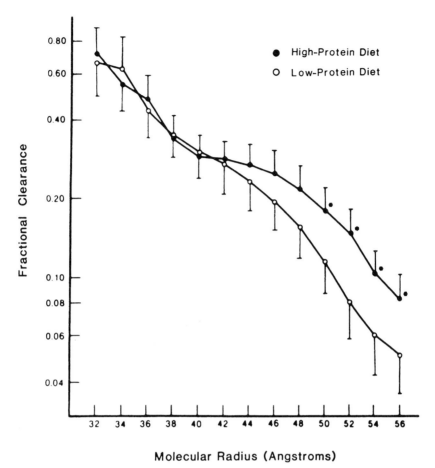

■ Figure 14.9 Effect of a high-protein diet (*solid symbols*) or low-protein diet (*open symbols*) on the fractional renal clearance of neutral dextrans in nephrotic patients. (From Rosenberg ME, Swanson JE, Thomas BL, et al. Glomerular and hormonal responses to dietary protein intake in human renal disease. *Am J Physiol Renal Fluid Electrolyte Physiol.* 1987; 253(22): F1083–F1090, with permission.)

and the rate of albumin catabolism increase (Fig. 14.8). Although augmentation of dietary protein also causes an increase in the rate of albumin synthesis in both animals and patients with nephrotic syndrome, neither protein concentration nor albumin concentration increases as a consequence (136,151,158). The reason lies in the fact that these three processes offset one another, so albumin concentration actually may tend to decrease during consumption of a high-protein diet. If the increase in urinary albumin excretion that follows dietary protein augmentation is prevented by administration of an ACE inhibitor, a high-protein diet will cause an increase in albumin concentration in nephrotic rats (174), although this has yet to be shown in patients. Therefore, the therapeutic approach to maximizing albumin concentration in nephrotic patients primarily should be aimed at reducing urinary albumin excretion.

METABOLISM OF NONALBUMIN SERUM PROTEIN IN NEPHROTIC SYNDROME

Plasma protein composition is greatly altered in nephrotic syndrome (184). Albumin and proteins of similar size are lost in the urine, and their concentration in plasma is decreased. In contrast, the plasma concentration of several proteins of high molecular weight is increased (185). Urinary protein

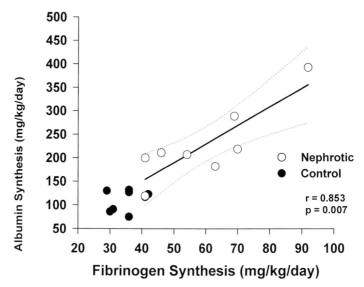

■ **Figure 14.10** Relationship between albumin and fibrinogen synthesis in nephrotic patients (*open symbols*) and control subjects (*closed symbols*) measured as the incorporation of 13C valine. (From de Sain-van der Velden MG, Kaysen GA, de Meer K, et al. Proportionate increase of fibrinogen and albumin synthesis in nephrotic patients: measurements with stable isotopes. *Kidney Int.* 1998; 53: 181–188, with permission.)

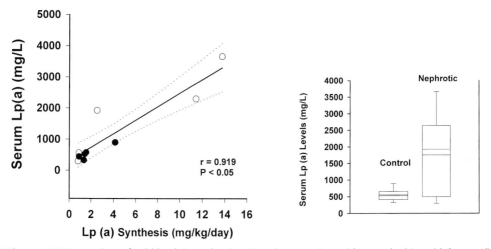

■ **Figure 14.11** Comparison of Lp(a) levels in nephrotic patients in comparison with control subjects (**right panel**) and relationship between plasma Lp(a) levels and Lp(a) synthetic rate in nephrotic patients (**left panel**). Lp(a), atherogenic lipoprotein. (Reprinted from de Sain-van der Velden MG, Jan Reijngoud D, Kaysen GA, et al. Evidence for increased synthesis of Lipoprotein (a) in the nephrotic syndrome. *J Am Soc Nephrol.* 1998; 9: 1474–1481, with permission.)

loss is accompanied by increased synthesis of several proteins secreted by the liver (185). For the most part the compensatory response to urinary protein loss, if indeed the response can be viewed as compensatory, is an increased synthesis of specific proteins secreted by the liver. The response is confined almost, if not entirely, to the liver. For example, the synthesis of both apo A-I and transferrin is increased in the liver in nephrotic syndrome (186), whereas there is no change in synthesis of apo A-I by the gut (187), the other organ that secretes apo A-I, and there is no change in transferrin gene expression by extrahepatic tissues (188). Lipids in the form of oval fat bodies may appear in the urine during nephrotic syndrome when protienuria is extensive. At least part of this phenomena may be explained by failed tubular uptake of filtered proteins, specifically HDL, that are not adequately catabolized by the proximal nephron as a consequence of injury engendered by protein overload. Approximately 25% of HDL catabolism occurs in the kidney following glomerular filtration (189,190). As glomerular protienuria increases, so does the excretion of smaller proteins normally taken up and catabolized most likely as a consequence of secondary injury to the proximal tubule as a result of continued massive proteinuria.

Transferrin Metabolism

Transferrin has a molecular weight of 79.5 kDa and is the principal iron carrier protein in plasma. Each mole of this protein lost in the urine carries potentially 2 moles of iron. Microcytic hypochromic anemia has been described in nephrotic syndrome, although this is uncommon (191–194) and has been attributed to iron loss. Transferrin synthesis is increased in nephrotic syndrome (192,195), and this response is confined to the liver, as in the case of iron deficiency (191). Unlike iron deficiency, however, augmentation in transferrin gene expression cannot be suppressed by administration of even large amounts of iron parenterally, and transferrin synthesis also is increased in hereditary analbuminemia (196), a condition not associated with urinary iron loss. In patients with nephrotic syndrome, transferrin synthesis increases proportionally to that of albumin synthesis (196), suggesting regulation of synthesis of these two proteins is linked in this disorder, similarly to that of other proteins, such as fibrinogen (180) and Lp(a) (181). These findings suggest that augmentation in transferrin synthesis is not proof of iron deficiency. Iron deposited in the renal tubules from reabsorbed transferrin also may play a role in the putative nephrotoxic effects of proteinuria (176,197).

Erythropoietin is synthesized by the kidney and regulates red blood cell levels. This protein also is lost in the urine in both nephrotic patients (198) and rats (199), but synthesis of erythropoietin, like that of other non-liver-derived proteins, is not increased in response, and plasma levels are decreased, as is the hematocrit in nephrotic rats. Erythropoietin deficiency could potentially play a role in the development of anemia in some nephrotic patients, although this has not been established (199). Although urinary iron excretion also increases in nephrotic syndrome as a consequence of urinary transferrin loss (195), the loss of erythropoietin may be a critical factor in development of anemia. No controlled studies have been performed to determine whether administration of either iron or erythropoietin corrects anemia in nephrotic patients so as to test the hypothesis that erythropoietin or iron deficiency is responsible for anemia in some nephrotic patients.

Immunoglobulin Metabolism

Hypogammaglobulinemia has long been recognized as a serious manifestation of nephrotic syndrome (200) and is an important factor in the reduced defenses against bacterial infections (201) in nephrotic patients. In addition to albumin, IgG is lost in the urine when glomerular permselectivity is severely altered (6). The urinary loss of this protein undoubtedly plays a significant role in causing hypogammaglobulinemia in nephrotic syndrome. As glomerular permselectivity is progressively lost, the renal clearance of IgG approaches that of albumin, despite the much larger effective molecular radius of IgG. Like albumin, the fractional catabolic rate of IgG varies directly with concentration in humans and rodents, increasing from 2% during severe hypogammaglobulinemia to as high as 18% when IgG concentration is high (202). As in the case of albumin metabolism, the increased fractional rate of IgG catabolism is inappropriate because of the presence of hypogammaglobulinemia in nephrotic patients (142,203). This phenomenon most likely reflects increased renal catabolism of IgG despite a decrease in IgG catabolism elsewhere in the body.

Although IgG production may be increased in vivo in patients with nephrotic syndrome (204), the rate of IgG production is depressed (205,206) in lymphocytes isolated from patients with nephrotic syndrome of various etiologies when they are exposed to mitogens in culture. This apparent contradiction has not yet been resolved, but it must be remembered that nephrotic syndrome may be the consequence of immunologically mediated disease in some situations, and changes in Ig may reflect the underlying disease and not the physiologic response to urinary protein loss or changed plasma protein composition.

It has been proposed that the urinary losses of IgG cannot alone be an adequate explanation for the low blood levels because the various subclasses of IgG are depressed asymmetrically (207), but it is more likely that IgG levels fall because, unlike the case of liver-derived proteins of the same-size class, there is no compensatory increase in the IgG synthetic rate. When nephrotic syndrome is induced in experimental animals, there is no increase in IgG synthesis, and both plasma levels and total body pools are dramatically reduced (208). Ultimately, at the final steady state, very little IgG is found in the urine because plasma levels are so low.

Of the Igs, IgG is most severely depleted in nephrotic syndrome (209), most likely because it is smallest and its renal clearance greatest. IgA levels also are reduced but less so. In contrast to IgG, IgM levels are increased (210). Although it has been speculated that increased IgM levels might play a role in causing some forms of nephrotic syndrome, such as minimal-change nephrotic syndrome, this is unlikely because the increase in IgM concentration has been reported almost universally. The increase in concentration of this very large, essentially unfilterable protein is similar to the response of many liver-derived proteins (211–213), the metabolism of which is reviewed in the following sections.

Defects in Hormone-Binding Proteins

Thyroid-binding globulin is found in the urine of nephrotic patients (214–217), but the concentration of this protein is reduced only in patients with extremely high urinary protein output. Nephrotic patients are euthyroid, as serum thyrotropin levels are not increased, and thyroid function tests, as assessed by radioactive iodine uptake, are normal. Similarly, although steroid-binding proteins (215) (corticosteroid-binding globulin) are reduced, there is no evidence that this leads to clinically significant reductions in free corticosteroid levels.

Vitamin D–Binding Protein and Hypocalcemia in Nephrotic Syndrome

Hypocalcemia has been long recognized in nephrotic patients (218–220), but it was realized only recently that ionized calcium as well as total calcium are reduced. The urinary loss of vitamin D–binding protein (65 kDa) in nephrotic syndrome (218) may lead to major derangements in calcium metabolism. Therefore, hypocalcemia does not result entirely from a reduction in the fraction of calcium bound to albumin. Vitamin D levels are reduced (221,222), and the decrease in vitamin D concentration correlates with urinary albumin excretion (220). Albumin concentration and vitamin D concentration correlate closely. Vitamin D–binding protein also is identifiable in the urine of nephrotic patients (223,224), and vitamin D levels normalize when proteinuria resolves (222,223). It is not known whether synthesis of vitamin D–binding protein is altered in response to its urinary loss or is modulated by dietary protein intake. Labeled vitamin D appears rapidly in the urine of nephrotic subjects (225). Hypovitaminosis D is not the result of loss of renal mass, because serum vitamin D levels are suppressed in nephrotic patients with normal renal function (220–222). Although it is possible that proteinuria might in some way inhibit vitamin D1-hydroxylase, an enzyme located in the renal proximal tubule, such an explanation seems unwarranted. Hypovitaminosis D of nephrotic syndrome may cause rickets (osteomalacia), especially in children (225,226). Nephrotic patients malabsorb calcium (222,223), a defect that can be corrected with exogenously administered vitamin D (222). Moreover, it has been recognized that vitamin D has pleiotrophic effects beyond its importance in bone mineralization (227). Vitamin D reduces cell proliferation and inflammation and has antineoplastic properties. Vitamin D deficiency has been associated with elevated blood pressure, reduced vascular compliance, impaired wound healing, and increased cancer rates and mortality. Thus, there may be additional morbidity in nephrotic patients related to vitamin D deficiency beyond impaired bone mineralization. However, unlike many of the other manifestations of the nephrotic syndrome, hypovitaminosis D can be managed with replacement therapy.

METABOLISM OF HIGH MOLECULAR WEIGHT

Serum Proteins in Nephrotic Syndrome

The concentration of several proteins that are not lost in the urine or are lost in only limited amounts is increased in plasma because of their increased hepatic synthesis (181,186–188,228,229). It is not known why the liver responds in the way that it does to urinary protein loss (or to reduction in plasma albumin concentration or π), but this seems to be a basic component of nephrotic syndrome both in patients and in experimental models. The increased plasma concentration of several of these proteins (β, α_1, and α_2 macroglobulins) (192,230) causes no readily identifiable clinical effect. In contrast, the increased concentration of lipids or fibrinogen may pose atherogenic risk, as discussed subsequently, and the increased concentration of several large proteins involved in hemostasis contributes to the thrombotic tendency that complicates the nephrotic syndrome.

Thrombosis

Nephrotic syndrome is complicated by venous thrombosis (231). Renal vein thrombosis results from, rather than causes, nephrotic syndrome (232,233). The significant increase in thromboembolic disorders is caused in part by the urinary loss of several proteins that are inhibitors of blood coagulation, specifically antithrombin III (212) and proteins S and C (234,235), and the increased plasma concentration of several high-molecular-weight proteins, including the binding proteins for proteins C and S.

The plasma concentration and the hepatic synthesis of fibrinogen (340 kDa) (181,176,214) are both increased in nephrotic syndrome. Although total proteins C and S may be elevated (212,235) in the nephrotic syndrome, these measurements reflect the total concentration of the proteins. An increased total concentration results from an increment in the plasma concentration of their high-molecular-weight carrier protein, C4b (236). The plasma concentration of the biologically active free form of these intermediate-molecular-weight inhibitors of blood coagulation is decreased as a result of both their increased urinary loss (235,236) and their increased binding in inactive form to C4b. The combination of the increased concentration of high-molecular-weight procoagulants and decreased concentration of intermediate-molecular-weight anticoagulants produces the clotting diathesis that complicates nephrotic syndrome.

HYPERLIPIDEMIA

The characteristic disorder in blood lipid composition in nephrotic patients is an increase in the low-density lipoprotein (LDL), very-low-density lipoprotein (VLDL) (236), and/or intermediate-density lipoprotein (IDL) fractions but no change (237) or a decrease in HDL (237), resulting in an increase in the LDL/HDL cholesterol ratio. Lipoprotein particles rich in phospholipid and esterified and nonesterified cholesterol resembling VLDL remnants (IDL) and chylomicron (CM) remnants accumulate. Apos B and C-III are increased in the serum of nephrotic patients (237), but the concentrations of apos A-I, A-II, and C-II remain unchanged. HDL subtypes found in plasma of nephrotic patients also are abnormally distributed (238). HDL_3 is modestly elevated, whereas HDL_2 is markedly reduced. Because it is primarily the latter subclass of HDL that is protective against atherosclerosis, the combination of reduced HDL_2 in conjunction with increased LDL, VLDL, and IDL cholesterol potentially poses significant risk for cardiovascular disease.

Lp(a) recently has been identified as a prominent risk factor in atherogenesis (239,240). Generally the quantity of this lipoprotein in plasma is genetically determined (241). Lp(a) consists of a molecule of LDL to which one molecule of the apo(a) has been covalently attached to apo B 100. The size of the apo(a) molecule in Lp(a) is genetically determined and distributed in the population in a nonnormal fashion (242). Individuals having the largest apo(a) subtypes are most common and have the lowest plasma concentration of Lp(a) (242). Lp(a) levels are increased in patients with a variety of renal diseases, including nephrotic syndrome (243). Unlike inherited increases in plasma Lp(a) levels, these increases in Lp(a) are acquired and are not associated with increased size of apo(a) (244).

Decreased Lipoprotein Catabolism

Hyperlipidemia in nephrotic syndrome is a consequence of two separate and distinct processes. One of these is an inability to efficiently clear triglyceride (TG)-rich lipoproteins from plasma. These consist primarily of VLDL, CMs, and remnant particles. Although some investigators have shown VLDL synthesis to be increased, this is not the primary cause for increased concentration of these proteins. VLDL apo B 100 synthesis can be increased in patients, whereas the levels of the protein remain quite normal (244). There is no difference between the absolute synthesis rate of apo B 100 in VLDL in nephrotic subjects and controls, and when the subjects with nephrotic syndrome are divided between normal levels of

VLDL Triglycerides vs VLDL apo B FSR   **VLDL Triglycerides vs VLDL apo B ASR**

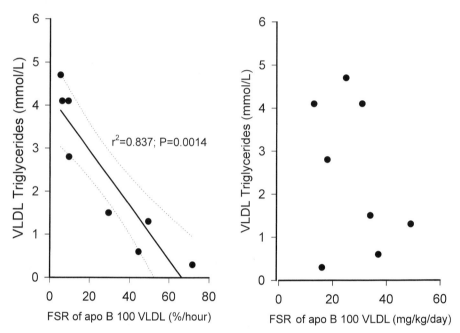

■ **Figure 14.12** Relationship between plasma apo B100 VLDL (mg/L) and the FSR of apo B100 (%/day) in nephrotic patients (left panel). Ninety-five percent confidence limits of the whole group are shown on either side of the regression line. $r^2 = 0.708$, $P = 0.0088$ ($n = 8$). Relationship between plasma apo B100 VLDL (mg/L) and the absolute synthetic rate of apo B100 VLDL (mg/kg/day) for nephrotic patients. $r^2 = 0.25$, $P = 0.21$ ($n = 8$) (right panel). apo, apolipoprotein; FSR, fractional synthetic rate; VLDL, very-low-density lipoprotein. (From de Sain-van der Velden MG, Kaysen GA, Barrett HA, et al. Increased VLDL in nephrotic patients results from a decreased catabolism while increased LDL results from increased synthesis. *Kidney Int.* 1998; 53: 994–1001, with permission.)

TGs (<2.5 mM) and elevated levels, the absolute synthesis rate of apo B 100 in VLDL actually tends to be increased in the patients with lower rather than greater TG levels. By contrast, in Figure 14.12 one can see that although the absolute rate of apo B 100 has no relationship to VLDL TG levels, the fractional rate of apo B 100 synthesis (which is equal to the fractional catabolic rate of VLDL) indeed is inversely related to VLDL TG levels. Thus, it is the catabolic rate and not the synthetic rate that controls VLDL levels in nephrotic patients.

The defect in lipoprotein clearance is a consequence of two separate processes. One is a decreased quantity of lipoprotein lipase bound to the endothelial surface (245,246). This is a result of reduced serum albumin concentration and is found in the absence of albuminuria in the condition of hereditary analbuminemia (247). As an isolated defect, the reduction in lipase leads to, at the most, a small increase in blood lipid levels (Fig. 14.13). The second process involves an alteration in the structure of VLDL, most likely mediated by an interaction with HDL. VLDL incubated with HDL obtained from nephrotic rats is catabolized at a reduced rate in in vitro systems and binds less effectively to lipoprotein lipase (248). The abnormality in the HDL structure has been hypothesized to be a consequence of the urinary loss of lecithin cholesterol transfer protein, an enzyme necessary for HDL maturation (248). In turn, HDL is important for regulating the structure of other lipoproteins.

The abnormality in the lipoprotein structure that leads to its reduced catabolism is a consequence of urinary protein loss and not of hypoalbuminemia. Thus, the two separate components that comprise nephrotic syndrome, proteinuria and hypoalbuminemia, combine in this way to produce this single defect in lipid levels (246–248). The decrease in HDL_2 and increase in HDL_3 are likely to play an important role in causing the defect in lipoprotein catabolism. HDL interacts with other lipoproteins in a number of important ways, but one consists of either acting as a source of apos necessary for their catabolism or binding to receptors or

Binding and Lipolysis in normal rats:

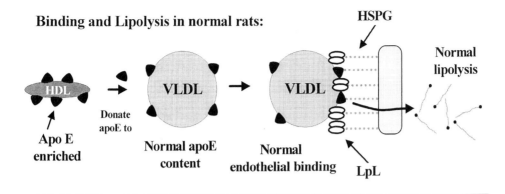

Binding and Lipolysis in analbuminemic rats:

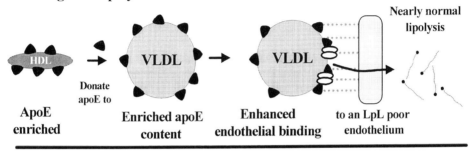

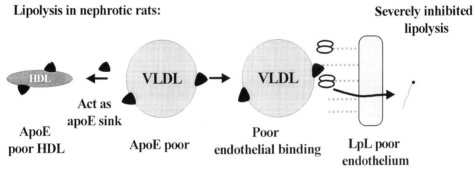

■ **Figure 14.13** Model for defective binding and lipolysis of VLDL mediated by a shift of apo E to HDL in nephrotic syndrome. Hypoalbuminemia leads to reduced amounts of lipoprotein lipase bound to the heparan sulfate on the endothelial surface. This alone leads to a slight decrease in lipoprotein catabolism and a mild increase in triglyceride levels. Proteinuria causes a decrease in apo-bound apo E, a lipoprotein lipase ligand. This combined defect results in a marked reduction in lipoprotein catabolism. apo, apolipoprotein; HDL, high-density lipoprotein; VLDL, very-low-density lipoprotein. (From Shearer GC, Kaysen GA. Proteinuria and plasma compositional changes contribute to defective lipoprotein catabolism in the nephrotic syndrome by separate mechanisms. *Am J Kidney Dis.* 2001; 37(1 suppl 2): S119–S122, with permission.)

ligands. Among these are apo E, a ligand that effects binding both to LPL as well as to several receptors; apo C-II, an activator of LPL; and apo C-III, an inhibitor of LPL. Both VLDL and HDL from nephrotic rats are depleted of apo E (248). It is the larger form of HDL, HDL_2 that effects this transfer most efficiently.

VLDL from nephrotic animals is catabolized by LPL at a reduced rate compared with control (249), but this defect can be repaired by incubation with HDL from normal animals but not following incubation with HDL from nephrotic animals. VLDL obtained from nephrotic rats also binds to LPL, the enzyme necessary for its catabolism, more poorly than does VLDL from control rats or from rats with hereditary analbuminemia (248). Both VLDL and HDL from nephrotic rats are depleted of apo E compared with

TABLE 14.4 LIPOPROTEIN CONTENT

	VLDL	HDL
Ratio	Apo E/Apo B (mol/mol)	Apo E/Apo A1
Control	5.77	0.34
HA	8.81	0.23
NS-Adriamycin	1.57	0.15

Apo composition of VLDL and HDL isolated from normal control Sprague–Dawley rats, rats with HA and rats with NS induced by injection of adriamycin. Because each molecule of VLDL contains 1 mol of apo B, the ratio of apo E/apo B establishes the relative amount of apo E present per mole of VLDL. apo, apolipoprotein; HA, hereditary analbuminemia; LDL, high-density lipoprotein; NS, nephrotic syndrome; VLDL, very-low-density lipoprotein.

control or analbuminemic animals (Table 14.4). Incubation of VLDL from nephrotic animals with HDL from normal animals repairs the binding defect, although incubation of VLDL from normal animals with HDL from nephrotic animals confers a binding defect. Thus, the defect in the VLDL structure and function is a consequence of its interaction with abnormal HDL. Furthermore, injection of normal HDL into nephrotic rats partially repairs the defect in CM clearance in vivo (248). How is this related to other factors in nephrotic syndrome?

Endothelial-bound LPL is greatly reduced both in analbuminemia and in nephrotic syndrome (246,248), yet both VLDL and CM catabolism is not greatly impaired in analbuminemic rats (246). Rats with hereditary analbuminemia have mild hyperlipidemia and only minimal abnormalities in lipoprotein catabolism (246,248) until they develop proteinuria (Fig. 14.14). Thus, urinary protein losses must contribute substantially to the disorder in lipid metabolism. A number of potential substances lost in the urine have been proposed to be responsible, but the most exciting observation was recently published by Vaziri et al. (248). They observed that the enzyme lecithin: cholesterol-acyltransferase (LCAT) was lost in the urine and depleted from plasma. This enzyme is necessary for normal HDL maturation (Fig. 14.14) and its uncompensated urinary loss could well explain the defective structure and function of HDL, which in turn would mediate the cascade of events leading to disordered catabolism of TG-rich lipoproteins.

One function of HDL is to shuttle apo C-II from remnant particles to nascent VLDL and CM (Fig. 14.15). Therefore, normal catabolism of both lipoproteins requires the presence of normally

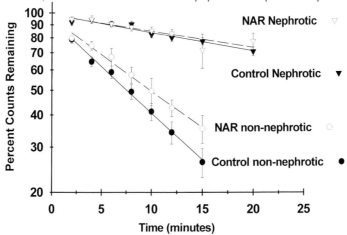

■ **Figure 14.14** CM clearance in normal and nephrotic SD rats and NAR. CM clearance was measured by the disappearance of [³H]-labeled CMs after intravenous injection. NAR, represented by *open symbols* and *broken lines*. SD represented by *solid symbols* and *lines*. Nephrotic rats are represented by *inverted triangles* and nonnephrotic rats by *circles*. The t^{1/2} of each subgroup is indicated in the figure. Nephrotic NAR, N = 7; nephrotic SD, N = 8; normal NAR, N = 6; normal SD, N = 6. CM, chylomicron; NAR, nagase analbuminemic rat; SD, Sprague–Dawley. (From Davies RW, Staprans I, Hutchison FN, et al. Proteinuria, not altered albumin metabolism, effects hyperlipidemia in the nephrotic rat. *J Clin Invest*. 1990; 86: 600–605, with permission.)

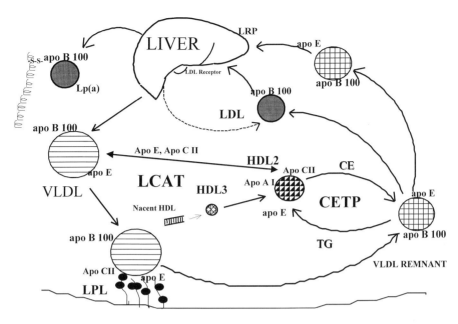

Endothelium

■ **Figure 14.15** Lipoprotein metabolism. VLDL is secreted by the liver and is hydrolyzed on the vascular endothelium by LPL. LDL (*small filled circles*) is bound electrostatically to heparan sulfate and, in the presence of apo C-II hydrolyzes TGs, releasing free fatty acids, monoglycerides, and diglycerides for cellular uptake. Other surface constituents of VLDL, free cholesterol, and phospholipids participate in the formation of nascent HDL. The free cholesterol on the surface of nascent HDL is esterified by the action of LCAT to produce CEs. These sink into the core as nascent HDL is metabolized to the small, dense HDL_3 and finally into the CE-rich HDL_2. The relatively TG-depleted VLDL remnant particle is released from the endothelial surface and then either is taken up by the liver directly via the remnant receptor, which recognizes apo E, or interacts with CE-rich HDL_2. In that interaction, catalyzed by CETP, the CE-rich core of HDL_2 is exchanged for the TG-rich core of the VLDL remnant, yielding a TG-rich HDL molecule (not shown) and LDL, which is then taken up by the LDL receptor in the liver, which recognizes apo B 100, the isoform secreted by the liver. HDL_2 is processed by lipases to HDL_3 to continue the cycle. LDL arises from delipidation of VLDL, but its rate of synthesis in nephrotic syndrome may be greater than that of VLDL, suggesting direct secretion from the liver also may occur. Likewise, Lp(a), which contains a molecule of LDL, has an increased synthetic rate in nephrotic syndrome and also may be secreted directly. VLDL, very-low-density lipoprotein; apo, apolipoprotein; CE, cholesterol ester; CETP, cholesterol ester transfer protein; HDL, high-density lipoprotein; LDL, low-density lipoprotein; LCAT, lecithin: cholesterol-acyltransferase; Lp(a), atherogenic lipoprotein; TG, triglyceride.

functioning HDL. HDL is derived from apos synthesized either in the liver or in the gut and cholesterol and phospholipids released by lipolysis of other lipoproteins (Fig. 14.15). HDL initially appears as discoid nascent HDL, containing little or no cholesterol esters (250). Surface cholesterol is esterified by the enzyme LCAT (221,251). Phospholipids are hydrolyzed; the fatty acid, usually arachidonate, is combined to cholesterol to form cholesterol ester; and a mole of lysolecithin is liberated. As in the case of fatty acid transport, albumin serves to bind liberated lysolecithin and accelerates activity of LCAT, thus facilitating the maturation of HDL (252) (Fig. 14.15). The hydrophobic cholesterol esters formed by the LCAT reaction sink into the core of nascent (discoid) HDL and form a spheroid HDL_3 particle with a molecular weight of about 200 kDa. By further action of LCAT, HDL_3 is converted into the 400-kDa HDL_2 particle, a form of HDL more capable of transporting apo C-II. Without recycling of apo C-II by HDL_2, the action of LPL on CM and VLDL is greatly reduced. The nephrotic syndrome in humans is characterized by reduced HDL_2.

Although this would not explain the increase in LDL and Lp(a), it would nicely close the circle among urinary protein losses, hypoalbuminemia, and decreased lipoprotein catabolism.

Studies in patients with the nephrotic syndrome have not been as detailed as in the rat; however, both species exhibit similar disturbances in lipid metabolism when comparable studies are evaluated. The fractional turnover rate of TGs is reduced in nephrotic subjects compared with controls, and the half-life of TG is prolonged from 4 to 11 hours in VLDL (253). Not only is VLDL catabolism decreased, but the disappearance curve has an unusual shape presumed to result from a delay in the conversion of VLDL to IDL (254). The delay in lipolysis in humans, as in rats, is proposed to result from a decrease in LPL activity. Evidence supporting this hypothesis is that LPL activity is reduced in children with nephrotic syndrome and increases after remission. Furthermore, there is a strong inverse correlation between LPL and the concentration of TGs in the VLDL fraction (255).

When proteinuria is reduced in patients with the nephrotic syndrome, blood lipid levels decrease (256) even if plasma albumin concentration or π is unchanged, suggesting that proteinuria plays a role independently of plasma albumin concentration in nephrotic syndrome in humans as well as in experimental models of nephrotic syndrome in animals.

Increased Lipoprotein Synthesis

The second set of disorders in lipid metabolism, although well characterized with regard to how they affect lipid levels, are less well understood with regard to pathogenesis. Synthesis of both LDL and Lp(a) is increased. Synthesis of the apo B 100 molecule in LDL does not correlate to that of albumin and to the other serum proteins whose rates of synthesis correlate with one another in nephrotic syndrome and is likely regulated by a different mechanism. By contrast, Lp(a) synthesis is greatly increased. Its plasma levels correlate directly with its rate of synthesis, independent of isoform (Fig. 14.11) (181). Unlike VLDL, its fractional rate of catabolism is unchanged, and its levels are controlled entirely by an increase in synthetic rate.

Perhaps of more basic interest is the observation that synthesis of apo B 100 in LDL is greater than that in VLDL in some patients. This is in contradiction with the standard model of lipoprotein production that holds that VLDL is released by the liver and serves as the precursor for LDL (Fig. 14.15). The observations of de Sain suggest that at least some component of the LDL pool bypasses this classic delipidation pathway. Similarly, synthesis of apo(a) and apo B100 in LP(a) occurred at the same rate, suggesting that in the nephrotic syndrome, apo(a) and apo B100 are synthesized simultaneously from the same precursor pools of amino acids, are linked in the liver, and are secreted by a pathway that is independent of the LDL and/or VLDL pathway(s).

Changes in the Activities of Liporegulatory Enzymes and of Lipoprotein: Clinical Implications of Hyperlipidemia in Renal Disease

The changes that occur in blood lipoprotein composition in nephrotic syndrome (238), reduced HDL_2 cholesterol, a relative increase in HDL_3 cholesterol, and the massive increase in total cholesterol, mostly found in the LDL, IDL, and VLDL fractions, should be expected to cause increased risk of atherosclerotic disease. These abnormalities are further complicated by the increase in plasma Lp(a) levels, increased platelet aggregability (257), increased plasma viscosity, increased concentration of highly atherogenic remnants of VLDL, and CM catabolism in plasma. Indeed, accelerated atherosclerosis has been reported in patients with proteinuria and hyperlipidemia and in some studies has been associated with a sharply increased incidence of cardiovascular disease and stroke (258). One study reported an 85-fold increase in the incidence of ischemic heart disease in such patients (259). In another recent retrospective analysis of 142 patients with proteinuria >3.5 g/day, the relative risk of myocardial infarction was found to be 5.5 and the risk of cardiac death 2.8 compared with age-matched, sex-matched controls (260). For this reason, there is no rationale for leaving pronounced hyperlipidemia untreated for prolonged periods of time in a patient with nephrotic syndrome.

Disordered lipid metabolism could also play a role in the cycle of progressive renal failure that occurs following the initiation of renal injury (261), although again this link has by no means been established in humans or in animal models of renal disease that are not associated with substantial increases in cholesterol levels. Although the association between hyperlipidemia and progression of renal disease has not been as yet confirmed in humans, one disorder that causes hypercholesterolemia in humans, hereditary LCAT deficiency, may be linked to progressive mesangial and glomerular sclerosis (262).

Treatment of Hyperlipidemia

It is not indicated to treat the qualitative abnormalities that characterize the lipid disorders of the nephrotic syndrome or to treat hyperlipidemia if the underlying cause of nephrotic syndrome is directly treatable, such as in minimal-change nephrotic syndrome. If, however, the duration of hyperlipidemia is anticipated to be prolonged, it is wise to initiate therapy. The first goal of treatment should be to reduce urinary protein excretion, if possible. Treatment of nephrotic patients with either ACE inhibitors (263) or cyclooxygenase inhibitors (20,264) results in a decline in both proteinuria and blood lipid levels (238,265) even if plasma albumin concentration does not increase (238) or increases only slightly (266). The decline in blood lipid levels include a decrease in total cholesterol, Lp(a), VLDL and LDL cholesterol, and the activities of cholesterol ester transfer protein (CETP) and LCAT (266). The effect of ACE inhibitors is a class effect and appears to be shared by all drugs within this class.

It is probably prudent to restrict dietary cholesterol and saturated lipids in patients with nephrotic syndrome. If conservative therapy (reduction in proteinuria, dietary fat restriction) does not effectively reduce hyperlipidemia, a variety of lipid-lowering drugs, including the 3-hydroxy-3-methyglutaryl coenzyme A reductase (HMG CoA reductase) inhibitors (267), antioxidants (268), and fibric acid derivatives (269), can be useful, but a review of this subject is beyond the scope of this chapter.

Edema Formation: Defenses Against Reduced Plasma π

Capillary hydrostatic pressure serves to force fluid from the vascular compartment into the interstitial space. This hydrostatic force is partially balanced by the difference between plasma π and that exerted by interstitial proteins. Interstitial protein concentration is between 25% and 50% that of plasma protein (270), and the difference between π exerted by plasma and interstitial proteins ($\Delta\overline{\pi}$) serves to retain salt and water in the vascular space. Fluid not reabsorbed by the time blood has reached the venous end of the capillary bed is returned to the vascular space via the lymphatics.

In steady state:

$$\text{Lymph flow} = K_f\,[(\text{Capillary hydrostatic pressure} - \text{tissue hydrostatic pressure}) \\ - (\text{plasma } \pi - \text{tissue } \pi)] = K_f\,(\Delta\overline{P} - \Delta\overline{\pi}) \qquad (14.1)$$

where K_f is capillary hydraulic conductivity (271,272).

When the fall in $\Delta\overline{\pi}$ becomes great enough, the net amount of fluid filtered by the capillaries will exceed maximal lymph flow and edema will inevitably occur. This increased net transport of fluid into the interstitial space should lead to plasma volume contraction. The plasma volume contraction activates the renin–angiotensin–aldosterone axis, the sympathetic nervous system, and other neurohormonal systems, leading to secondary renal sodium retention. This is the so-called "underfill" model of edema formation. However, Meltzer et al. (273) subsequently identified a group of patients with nephrotic syndrome who had a normal or an expanded plasma volume and reduced plasma renin activity despite a profound reduction in π. These patients represented a subset that had nephritic disease as opposed to patients with minimal-change nephrotic syndrome. Some patients with minimal-change nephrotic syndrome also have been found to have an increased plasma and blood volume (274,275).

How is it possible to maintain a normal or even an expanded plasma volume when π is greatly reduced? If it is indeed possible to maintain a normal plasma volume, why does the kidney retain salt and water in nephrotic patients? The answer to the first question lies in part in the fact that interstitial albumin mass is reduced to an even greater extent than is the plasma albumin mass in nephrotic syndrome (144). The mobilization of extravascular albumin is a rapid, hemodynamically mediated response to a decrease in plasma π or to an increase in transcapillary hydrostatic pressure (271–273,276–278). Interstitial albumin concentration decreases in parallel to plasma albumin concentration following the onset of proteinuria in rats with an experimental form of nephrotic syndrome induced by injection of puromycin aminonucleoside (279). Although albumin decreases, $\Delta\bar{\pi}$ decreases little or not at all because interstitial protein is swept into the vascular compartment by increased lymphatic flow. In addition, because the capillary endothelium is far more permeable to water than to protein, when transcapillary hydraulic flux increases, the resulting plasma ultrafiltrate is much poorer in protein than when hydraulic flux is reduced. $\Delta\bar{\pi}$ does not decrease in nephrotic rats until saline is administered resulting in volume expansion.

Edema formation in nephrotic syndrome may involve two parallel processes (Fig. 14.16). Reduced plasma π leads to augmented net flux of fluid across the systemic capillary bed (underfill), but these alterations may be entirely or largely offset by increased lymphatic return from the periphery and reduction in interstitial π so that $\Delta\bar{\pi}$ remains unchanged. Edema formation is not generally obligated to occur until total proteins decrease to around 4 g/dL. The second process results from a primary impaired ability of the nephrotic kidney to excrete a sodium load, either in response to plasma volume expansion (280–282) or in response to atrial natriuretic peptides (ANP) (283–286). This primary renal retention of sodium seen in nephrotic syndrome is sometimes referred to as the "overflow" model of edema formation. A number of mechanisms have been proposed to account for this primary renal sodium retention. First, there may be increased activity of the Na^+/K^+ ATPase pump in the cortical collecting duct (287). The resistance to ANP is mediated at least in part by an increase in cyclic GMP phosphodiesterase activity in the distal nephron (288). This enzyme leads to degradation of the second messenger of ANP, cyclic GMP. Thus, increased activity of phosphodiesterase in the setting of nephritic syndrome will blunt natriuresis. Studies

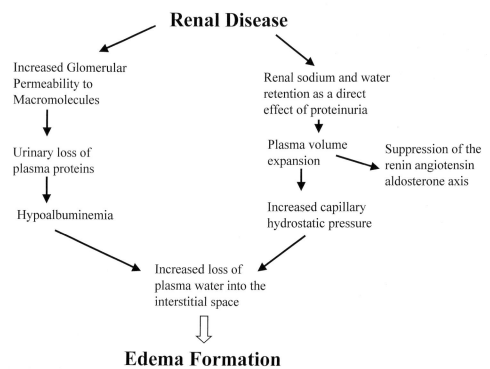

Figure 14.16 Primary renal sodium retention with resultant edema formation. Renal salt and water retention occurs as a result of the renal disease itself and causes plasma volume expansion. This produces increased capillary hydrostatic pressure, which in conjunction with the increased transcapillary flux of fluid resulting from hypoalbuminemia causes edema. Edema formation is not a direct consequence of reduced π alone, nor is renal salt and water retention a consequence of increased transudation of fluid into the interstitial space with resultant activation of the renin–angiotensin–aldosterone axis. (From Kaysen GA, Myers BD, Couser WG, et al. Mechanisms and consequences of proteinuria. *Lab Invest.* 1986; 54: 479–498, with permission.)

using unilateral models of proteinuria most clearly demonstrate that impedance to sodium excretion is intrinsic to the nephrotic kidney and not reflective of plasma volume regulation. In one such study, Perico et al. (284) demonstrated an inability of a proteinuric kidney to excrete fluid or sodium in response to infused ANP, even though ANP increased GFR in both the proteinuric kidney and the normal contralateral kidney equally. Clearly, both the normal contralateral kidney and the proteinuric kidney were exposed to the same π and the same levels of circulating hormones responsible for plasma volume regulation. Proteinuria has been shown to inhibit sodium transporters in the proximal nephron as well (289).

Regardless of the mechanism, the proteinuric kidney avidly reabsorbs filtered salt in the distal nephron (290) even in the presence of plasma volume expansion, and reabsorption of sodium in the proximal nephron is impaired as well. As a consequence of these combined effects, the systemic capillary bed is faced with increased hydrostatic pressure at the very time that defense mechanisms normally employed to counteract edema formation, increased lymphatic flow, and decreased interstitial protein concentration already have been maximized. Edema results from the combined effect of primary renal salt and water retention coupled with reduced defenses against edema formation resulting from the urinary losses of proteins of intermediate weight with the resulting decrease in both and interstitial π. These processes deprive the lymphatic system of the capacity to respond to increased hydrostatic pressure.

Nutritional Recommendations

DIETARY PROTEIN

In patients with nephrotic syndrome, dietary protein augmentation above 1g/kg/day is not of demonstrated benefit and may cause increased urinary albumin losses. These patients' diets should provide between 0.8 to 1.0 g/kg/day of protein and 35 kCal/kg/day of energy. Twenty-four-hour urinary protein excretion should be measured every 2 to 3 months and urinary urea excretion monitored to ensure that patients are eating the quantity of protein recommended and that proteinuria decreases and albumin and protein concentration does not decrease when dietary protein intake is restricted to these levels.

Dietary protein intake can be estimated because in steady state, dietary protein is equal to the protein catabolic rate (PCR). If total body urea pools do not change (blood urea nitrogen, BUN, is neither decreasing nor increasing), it is possible to estimate the amount of protein that has been eaten, by the formula:

$$\text{Protein catabolic rate} = (10.7 + \text{24-hour urinary urea excretion}/0.14) \text{ g/day} + \text{urinary protein excretion}$$

An accurate nutritional history should be obtained and the diet adjusted accordingly if there is variance from the prescribed diet.

In addition to these nutritional recommendations, processes that cause inflammation should be identified and treated, if possible, because these directly suppress albumin synthesis (157,291–293). Obvious hormonal deficiency states, hypoadrenalism, hypothyroidism, or diabetes also should be identified and treated.

DIETARY FAT

Hyperlipidemia is common in nephrotic syndrome and is a consequence of both increased synthesis of lipids and apos (294) and their decreased catabolism (246–248,295,296). The characteristic disorder in blood lipid composition in nephrotic patients is an increase in the LDL, VLDL (237), and/or IDL fractions but no change or decrease in HDL (238), resulting in an increased LDL/HDL cholesterol ratio. The IDL fractions probably arise as VLDL and CM remnants and are atherogenic (297). Lp(a) also increases in patients with nephrotic syndrome (181,244). All of these changes are characteristic of those associated with accelerated atherogenesis in other clinical settings.

Soy or vegan diets have been shown to reduce urinary protein excretion in patients with nephrotic syndrome (298). Although it is claimed that this effect is a consequence of the reduced lipid content of the diets (298), there are no convincing data presented that changes in dietary lipids are responsible for the salutary effects of these diets. Lipids, however, represent a wide variety of substances, including steroids, saturated and unsaturated fatty acids, phospholipids, and other compounds, many of which are either directly biologically active or precursors of important biologically active metabolites. Much attention has been focused on the effect of polyunsaturated fatty acids on renal hemodynamics and on expression or renal injury.

In studies involving human subjects, Gentile et al. (298,299) added 5 g of fish oil per day to the diet of patients with nephrotic syndrome who had been maintained on a soy vegetarian diet, and found no beneficial effect on either proteinuria or on blood lipids compared with patients maintained on the soy diet without fish oil supplementation. In contrast, Hall et al. (300) found that 15 g of fish oil per day caused a decrease in total TGs and in LDL triglycerides with an increase in LDL cholesterol. Donadio et al. (301) treated 55 patients with 12 g of fish oil per day in a prospective randomized placebo-controlled study and found a significant reduction in the rate of progression of renal disease using a 50% increase in serum creatinine concentration as a study end point. At the end of the treatment period, the fish oil–treated group had a lower prevalence of hypertension, elevated serum creatinine, and nephrotic range proteinuria. These studies suggest that although alterations in dietary polyunsaturated fatty acids (PUFA) may alter some manifestations of the nephrotic state; the effects are dependent on the model being investigated and should still be viewed with caution. These agents may be neither predictable nor salutary for all patients with renal disease.

Pharmacologic Means to Reduce Glomerular Proteinuria

ANGIOTENSIN BLOCKADE

ACE inhibitors and ARBs (75) reduce proteinuria in experimental models of nephrotic syndrome and in some nephrotic patients as well. ACE inhibitors may reduce proteinuria by a number of mechanisms. ACE inhibitors decrease the fraction of glomerular ultrafiltrate that passes through the nonselective shunt pathway, described previously, and increases the fraction passing through the normal population of small pores, leading to a reduction in proteinuria. The reduction in the glomerular hydrostatic pressure by ACE inhibitors and ARBs will reduce the glomerular filtration of proteins. Ang is a growth factor; thus, diminishing its production or action may reduce glomerular hypertrophy. Moreover, since Ang II stimulates mesangial matrix formation and fibrosis, in part by enhanced release of transforming growth factor-β and other growth factors, blockade or reduction in Ang II activity may attenuate these profibrotic forces in glomerular disease (302,303). A reduction in mesangial expansion, glomerular hypertrophy, and fibrosis by Ang II blockade may contribute to the reduction in proteinuria. Many glomerular diseases such as diabetes nephropathy are associated with increase podocyte loss and apoptosis and decreased nephrin gene expression. Ang II blockade attenuates these effects on the podocyte (11,304–306).

GFR is generally not reduced by ACE inhibitors or ARBs. Proteinuria is reduced, accompanied by an increase in serum albumin concentration and reduction in blood lipid levels in rats with experimental models of nephrotic syndrome, but it has not yet been definitely established whether reduced albuminuria is accompanied by correction of reduced albumin and hyperlipidemia in nephrotic patients.

The antiproteinuric effect of ACE inhibitors and ARBs seems to be shared by all drugs of these classes studied to date; however, this property is not shared by all other antihypertensive agents. Results obtained with both α antagonists and certain classes of calcium channel blockers have been inconsistent and not sufficiently well documented to warrant clinical use of these agents for control of proteinuria at this time. Dihydropyridine calcium channel blockers may actually increase albuminuria (307).

Recent studies have suggested that combination of ACE inhibitors with ARBs may have a greater antiproteinuric effect than either agent alone, independent of changes in blood pressure (308,309). More definitive trials are currently in progress to determine if combination therapy has better outcomes in patients with proteinuria and chronic kidney disease.

It is important when prescribing an ACE inhibitor or an ARB for the purpose of reducing proteinuria (in contrast to the treatment of hypertension in a nephrotic patient) to monitor the patient closely for a reduction either in blood pressure or in GFR. It also is important to discontinue diuretic therapy for several days preceding initiation of therapy with an ACE inhibitor in order to avoid inhibition of ACE in the presence of a plasma volume–contracted state. If it is possible that the patient is plasma volume contracted, therapy should be initiated with a very low dose (2.5 mg of enalapril or 25 mg of losartan) and the blood pressure checked within 24 hours, with the aim of ultimately reducing mean arterial pressure by about 10 mm Hg. The dose of the ACE inhibitor should be increased every other week to attain that end point. It also is important to obtain measurements of renal function at 1, 2, and 4 weeks, as well as to monitor potassium concentration, especially in individuals who have significant renal insufficiency (creatinine >3 mg/dL), diabetes, or underlying hyperkalemia. ACE inhibitors should be discontinued if potassium concentration remains persistently elevated above 5.5 mEq/L. Urinary protein should be monitored once every month or two to evaluate the clinical response. Decreased urinary protein excretion occurs gradually over 1 or 2 weeks. In some instances neither the blood pressure nor proteinuria responds to rather large doses of ACE inhibitors and therapy with these agents should then be discontinued. Some patients, especially those with renal artery stenosis, may exhibit marked reduction in blood pressure and in GFR with even low doses of ACE inhibitors. It is important to identify these patients as well and discontinue ACE inhibitor therapy if a marked reduction in GFR occurs.

CYCLOOXYGENASE INHIBITORS

Cyclooxygenase inhibitors are another class of drugs that may prove helpful in reducing proteinuria in nephrotic patients, although unlike ACE inhibitors, they generally cause a reduction in GFR. Proteinuria is reduced by a combined effect both to reduce total GFR and also to reduce the fraction of glomerular ultrafiltrate that passes through the large nonselective pores in the GBM (20). The antiproteinuric action of these agents may be potentiated by a low sodium diet and the use of diuretics. Large doses of cyclooxygenase inhibitors, such as 50 mg of indomethacin three times a day, may still be necessary. As with ACE inhibitors, treatment with cyclooxygenase inhibitors may cause hyperkalemia (310), especially in patients with diabetic renal disease and patients with underlying hyperkalemia. The decrease in GFR caused by these agents also may limit their utility. Unlike ACE inhibitors, cyclooxygenase inhibitors are likely to increase renal sodium retention, potentially worsening edema formation or increasing the need for diuretic therapy (311). Treatment of nephrotic patients with an ACE inhibitor and a cyclooxygenase inhibitor simultaneously may be clinically hazardous, resulting in a marked decrease in GFR and hyperkalemia. Other potential risks of cyclooxygenase inhibition include acute renal failure and interstitial nephritis, in addition to gastrointestinal disturbances.

Acknowledgment

This work was supported in part by the research service of the United States Department of Veterans Affairs and in part by a grant from the National Institutes of Health RO1 DK 42297.

REFERENCES

1. Tryggvason K, Patrakka J, Wartiovaara J. Hereditary proteinuria syndromes and mechanisms of proteinuria. *N Eng J Med.* 2006;354:1387–1401.
2. Furness PN, Hall LL, Shaw JA, et al. Glomerular expression of nephrin is decreased in acquired human nephrotic syndrome. *Nephrol Dial Transplant.* 1999;14(5):1234–1237.
3. Maack T, Johnson V, Kau ST, et al. Renal filtration, transport, and metabolism of low-molecular weight proteins: a review. *Kidney Int.* 1979;16: 251–270.
4. Brenner BM, Baylis C, Deen WM. Transport of molecules across renal glomerular capillaries. *Physiol Rev.* 1976;56:502–534.
5. Bohrer MP, Deen WM, Robertson CR, et al. Mechanism of angiotensin II induced proteinuria in the rat. *Am J Physiol Renal Fluid Electrolyte Physiol.* 1977;233(2):F13–F21.
6. Deen WM, Bridges CR, Brenner BM, et al. Heterosporous model of glomerular size selectivity: application to normal and nephrotic humans. *Am J Physiol.* 1985;249:F374–F389.
7. Deen WM, Bridges CR, Brenner BM. Biophysical basis of glomerular permselectivity. *J Membr Biol.* 1983;71:1–10.
8. Kanwar YS. Biophysiology of glomerular filtration and proteinuria. *Lab Invest.* 1984;51:7–21.
9. Daniels BS, Deen WM, Mayer G, et al. Glomerular permeability barrier in the rat. Functional assessment by in vitro methods. *J Clin Invest.* 1993;92: 929–936.

10. Myers BD, Winetz JA, Chui F, et al. Mechanisms of proteinuria in diabetic nephropathy: a study of glomerular barrier function. *Kidney Int.* 1982;21:633–641.

11. Benigni A, Tomasoni S, Gagliardini E, et al. Blocking angiotensin II synthesis/activity preserves glomerular nephrin in rats with severe nephrosis. *J Am Soc Nephrol.* 2001;12(5):941–948.

12. Zhang Z, Zhang Y, Ning G, et al. Combination therapy with AT1 blocker and vitamin D analog markedly ameliorates diabetic nephropathy: blockade of compensatory renin increase. *Proc Natl Acad Sci U S A.* 2008;105:15896–15901.

13. Yoshioka T, Mitarai T, Kon V, et al. Role for angiotensin II in an overt functional proteinuria. *Kidney Int.* 1986;30:538–545.

14. Harrison JF, Cantab MB. Urinary lysozyme, ribonuclease, and low-molecular-weight protein in renal disease. *Lancet.* 1968;1:371–375.

15. Karadimas CL, Greenstein P, Sue CM, et al. Recurrent myoglobinuria due to a nonsense mutation in the COX I gene of mitochondrial DNA. *Neurology.* 2000;55(5):644–649.

16. Hashimoto H, Sibley R, Myers BD. A comparison between the glomerular injuries of minimal change (MCN) and focal/segmental sclerosis (FSGS) in nephrotic humans. *Kidney Int.* 1990;37:507A.

17. Lianos EA, Andres GA, Dunn MJ. Glomerular prostaglandin and thromboxane synthesis in rat nephrotoxic serum nephritis. *J Clin Invest.* 1983;72:1439–1448.

18. Remuzzi G, Imberti L, Rossini M, et al. Increased glomerular thromboxane synthesis as a possible cause of proteinuria in experimental nephrosis. *J Clin Invest.* 1985;75:94–101.

19. Eisenbach GM, Van Liew JB, Boylan JW. Effect of angiotensin on the filtration of protein in the rat kidney. *Kidney Int.* 1975;8:80–87.

20. Goldbetz H, Black V, Shemesh O, et al. Mechanism of the antiproteinuric effect of indomethacin in nephrotic humans. *Am J Physiol Renal Fluid Electrolyte Physiol.* 1989;256(25):F44–F51.

21. Shultz PJ, Tolins JP. Adaptation to increased dietary salt intake in the rat. Role of endogenous nitric oxide. *J Clin Invest.* 1993;91:642–650.

22. Kelly DJ, Aaltonen P, Cox AJ, et al. Expression of the slit-diaphragm protein, nephrin, in experimental diabetic nephropathy: differing effects of anti-proteinuric therapies. *Nephrol Dial Transplant.* 2002;17:1327–1332.

23. Zatz R, De Nucci G. Effects of acute nitric oxide inhibition on rat glomerular inhibition on rat gomerular microcirculation. *Am J Physiol Renal Fluid Electrolyte Physiol.* 1991;261(30): F360–F363.

24. Baylis C, Mitruka B, Deng A. Chronic blockade of nitric oxide synthesis in the rat produces systemic hypertension and glomerular damage. *J Clin Invest.* 1992;90:278–281.

25. Norden AG, Lapsley M, Lee PJ, et al. Glomerular protein sieving and implications for renal failure in Fanconi. *Kidney Int.* 2001;60(5): 1885–1892.

26. Walcynski Z, Rucinski B. Hypersensitivity against tetracycline as caused for Wissler-Fanconi syndrome. *Allerg Asthma (Leipzig).* 1970;16(3): 65–67.

27. DeFronzo RA. Their SO: inherited disorders of renal tubule function. In: Bernner BM, Rector FFC Jr, eds. *The Kidney.* 3rd ed. Philadelphia: WB Saunders; 1985:1297–1339.

28. Morris RC Jr, Sebastian A. Renal tubular acidosis and the Fanconi syndrome. In: Stanbury JB, Wyngaarden JB, Fredrickson DS, et al., eds. *The Metabolic Basis of Inherited Disease.* 5th ed. New York: McGraw-Hill; 1983.

29. Wrong OM, Norden AG, Feest TG. Dent's disease: a familial proximal renal tubular syndrome with low-molecular weight proteinuria, hypercalciuria, nephrocalcinosis, metabolic bone disease, progressive renal failure and a marked male predominance. *Q J Med.* 1994;87:473–493.

30. Low C, Terrey M, MacLachlan E. Organic aciduria, decreased renal ammonia production, hydrophthalmos and mental retardation: a clinical entity. *AMA Am J Dis Child.* 1952;83:164–184.

31. Lauwerys RR, Roels HA, Bucher JP, et al. Investigations on the lung and kidney function in workers exposed to cadmium. *Environ Health Perspect.* 1979;28:137–145.

32. Hellstrom L, Elinder CG, Dahlberg B, et al. Cadmium exposure and end-stage renal disease. *Am J Kidney Dis.* 2001;38(5):1001–1008.

33. Park CH, Maack T. Albumin absorption and catabolism by isolated perfused proximal convoluted tubules of the rabbit. *J Clin Invest.* 1984;73: 767–777.

34. Hutchison FN, Kaysen GA. Albuminuria causes lysozymuria in rats with Heymann nephritis. *Kidney Int.* 1988;33:787–791.

35. Kaye WA, Griffiths WC, Camara PD, et al. The significance of β2-microglobulinuria associated with gentamicin therapy. *Ann Clin Lab Sci.* 1981; 11:530–537.

36. Schentag JJ, Sutfin TA, Plaut ME, et al. Early detection of aminoglycoside nephrotoxicity with urinary β2-microglobulin. *J Med.* 1978;9:201–210.

37. Tsuchiya K, Iwao S, Sugita M, et al. Increased urinary β2-microglobulin in cadmium exposure: dose-effect relationship and biological significance of β2-microglobulin. *Environ Health Perspect.* 1979;28:147–153.

38. Buchet JP, Roels H, Bernard A Jr, et al. Assessment of renal function of workers exposed to inorganic lead, cadmium or mercury vapor. *J Occup Med.* 1980;22:741–750.

39. Kjellstrom T. Exposure and accumulation of cadmium in populations from Japan, the United States, and Sweden. *Environ Health Perspect.* 1979;28:169–197.

40. Poortmans JR. Postexercise proteinuria in humans. Facts and mechanisms. *JAMA.* 1985;253: 236–240.

41. Cui S, Verroust PJ, Moestrup SK, et al. Megalin/ gp330 mediates uptake of albumin in renal proximal tubule. *Am J Physiol.* 1996;271:F900–F907.

42. Birn H, Fyfe JC, Jacobsen C, et al. Cubilin is an albumin binding protein important for renal tubular albumin reabsorption. *J Clin Invest.* 2000;105:1353–1361.

43. Hammad SM, Stefansson S, Twal WO, et al. Cubilin, the endocytic receptor for intrinsic factor-vitamin B(12) complex, mediates high-density lipoprotein holoparticle endocytosis. *Proc Natl Acad Sci U S A.* 1999;96:10158–10163.

44. Li M, Balamuthusamy S, Simon EE, et al. Silencing megalin and cubilin genes inhibits myeloma light chain endocytosis and ameliorates toxicity in human renal proximal tubule epithelial cells. *Am J Physiol Renal Physiol*. 2008;295: F82–F90.

45. Klassen RB, Allen PL, Batuman V, et al. Light chains are a ligand for megalin. *J Appl Physiol*. 2005;98:257–263.

46. Hill GS, Morei-Maroger L, Mercy JP, et al. Renal lesions in multiple myeloma: their relationship to assorted protein abnormalities. *Am J Kidney Dis*. 1983;2:423–438.

47. Kyle R. Multiple myeloma. Review of 869 cases. *Mayo Clin Proc*. 1975;50:29–40.

48. Kyle RA, Gleich GJ. IgG subclasses in monoclonal gammopathy of undetermined significance. *J Lab Clin Med*. 1982;100(5):806–814.

49. Van De Donk N, De Weerdt O, Eurelings M, et al. Malignant transformation of monoclonal gammopathy of undetermined significance: cumulative incidence and prognostic factors. *Leuk Lymphoma*. 2001;42(4):609–618.

50. Gregersen H, Mellemkjar L, Ibsen JS, et al. The impact of M-component type and immunoglobin concentration on the risk of malignant transformation in patients with monoclonal gammopathy of undetermined significance. *Haematologica*. 2001;86(11):1172–1179.

51. Bladé J, Rosiñol L, Cibeira MT, et al. Pathogenesis and progression of monoclonal gammopathy of undetermined significance. *Leukemia*. 2008;22: 1651–1657.

52. Ng VL, Chen KH, Hwang KM, et al. The clinical significance of human immunodeficiency virus type 1-associated paraproteins. *Blood*. 1989;74: 2471–2475.

53. Ng VL, Hwang KM, Reyes GR, et al. High tier anti-HIV antibody reactivity associated with a paraprotein spike in a homosexual male with AIDS related complex. *Blood*. 1988;71:1397–1401.

54. Waller KV, Ward KM, Mahan JD, et al. Current concepts in proteinuria. *Clin Chem*. 1989;35: 755–765.

55. Maack T. Renal handling of low molecular weight proteins. *Am J Med*. 1975;58:57–64.

56. Moglielnicki RP, Waldmann TA, Strober W. Renal handling of low molecular weight proteins: I. L-chain metabolism in experimental renal disease.*J Clin Invest*. 1971;50:901–909.

57. Kaysen GA, Myers BD, Couser WG, et al. Mechanisms and consequences of proteinuria. *Lab Invest*. 1986;54:479–498.

58. Hall CL, Hardwicke J. Low molecular weight proteinuria. *Annu Rev Med*. 1979;30: 199–211.

59. Baldamus CA, Galaske R, Eisenbach GM, et al. Glomerular protein filtration in normal and nephritic rats: a micropuncture study. *Contrib Nephrol*. 1975;1:37–49.

60. Yoshioka K, Takemura T, Akano N, et al. Cellular and non cellular compositions of crescents in human glomerulonephritis. *Kidney Int*. 1987; 32(2):284–291.

61. Kamitsuji H, Whitworth JA, Dowling JP, et al. Urinary crosslinked fibrin degradation products in glomerular disease. *Am J Kidney Dis*. 1986;7: 452–455.

62. Constantiner M, Sehgal AR, Humbert L, et al. A dipstick protein and specific gravity algorithm accurately predicts pathological proteinuria. *Am J Kidney Dis*. 2005;45:833–841.

63. Hillege HL. Can an algortithm based on dipstick urine protein and urine specific gravity accurately predict proteinuria? *Nat Clin Pract Nephrol*. 2006; 2:68–69.

64. Morcos SK, El-Nahas AM, Brown P, et al. Effect of iodinated water soluble contrast media on urinary protein assays. *BMJ*. 1992;305:29.

65. Chitalia VC, Kothari J, Wells EJ, et al. Cost-benefit analysis and prediction of 24-hour proteinuria from the spot urine protein-creatinine ratio. *Clin Nephrol*. 2001;55:436–447.

66. Ginsberg JM, Chang BS, Matarese RA, et al. Use of a single voided urine samples to estimate quantitative proteinuria. *N Engl J Med*. 1983;309: 1543–1546.

67. Gerstein HC, Mann JF, Yi Q, et al. Albuminuria and risk of cardiovascular events, death, and heart failure in diabetic and nondiabetic individuals. *JAMA*. 2001;286(4):421–426.

68. Janssen WM, Hillege H, Pinto-Sietsma SJ, et al. Low levels of urinary albumin excretion are associated with cardiovascular risk factors in the general population. *Clin Chem Lab Med*. 2000;38: 1107–1110.

69. Woo J, Floyd M, Cannon DC. Albumin and β2-microglobulin radioimmunoassay applied to monitoring of renal-allograft function and in differentiating glomerular and tubular diseases. *Clin Chem*. 1981;27:709–713.

70. Mogensen CE, Christiansen CE. Predicting diabetic nephropathy in insulin-dependent patients. *N Engl J Med*. 1984;311:89–93.

71. Mogensen CE. Progression of nephropathy in long-term diabetics with proteinuria and effect of initial anti-hypertensive treatment. *Scand J Clin Lab Invest*. 1976;36:383–386.

72. Viberti G, Mogensen CE, Groop LC, et al. Effect of captopril on progression to clinical proteinuria in patients with insulin-dependent diabetes mellitus and microalbuminuria. European Microalbuminuria Captopril Study Group. *JAMA*. 1994;271: 275–279.

73. Lewis EJ, Hunsicker LG, Bain RP, et al. The effect of angiotensin-converting-enzyme inhibition on diabetic nephropathy. The Collaborative Study Group. *N Engl J Med*. 1993;329:1456–1462.

74. Buter H, Navis G, Dullaart RP, et al. Time course of the antiproteinuric and renal haemodynamic responses to losartan in microalbuminuric IDDM. *Nephrol Dial Transplant*. 2001;16(4): 771–775

75. Brenner BM, Cooper ME, de Zeeuw D, et al. Effects of losartan on renal and cardiovascular outcomes in patients with type 2 diabetes and nephropathy. RENAAL Study Investigators. *N Engl J Med*. 2001;345(12):861–869.

76. Dinneen SF, Gerstein HC. The association of microalbuminuria and mortality in non-insulin-dependent diabetes mellitus. A systemic overview of the literature. *Arch Intern Med*. 1997;157(13): 1413–1418.

77. Weinstock Brown W, Keane WF. Proteinuria and cardiovascular disease. *Am J Kidney Dis*. 2001; 38(4 suppl 1):S8–S13.

78. Spoelstra-De Man AM, Brouwer CB, Stehouwer CD, et al. Rapid progression of albumin excretion is an independent predictor of cardiovascular mortality in patients with type 2 diabetes and microalbuminuria. *Diabetes Care.* 2001;24(12):2097–2101.

79. Wachtell K, Ibsen H, Olsen MH, et al. Albuminuria and cardiovascular risk in hypertensive patients with left ventricular hypertrophy: the LIFE study. *Ann Intern Med.* 2003;139:901–906.

80. Hillege HL, Fidler V, Diercks GF, et al. Urinary albumin excretion predicts cardiovascular and noncardiovascular mortality in general population. *Circulation.* 2002;106:1777–1782.

81. Roest M, Banga JD, Janssen WMT, et al. Excessive urinary albumin levels are associated with future cardiovascular mortality in postmenopausal women. *Circulation.* 2001;103:3057–3061.

82. Asselbergs FW, Diercks GF, Hillege HL, et al. Effects of fosinopril and pravastatin on cardiovascular events in subjects with microalbuminuria. Investigators. *Circulation.* 2004;110:2809–2816.

83. Venkat KK. Proteinuria and microalbuminuiria in adults: significance, evaluation and treatment. *South Med J.* 2004;97:969–979.

84. Pontremoli R, Leoncini G, Viazzi F, et al. Role of microalbuminuria in the assessment of cardiovascular risk in essential hypertension. *J Am Soc Nephrol.* 2005;16(suppl 1):S39–S41.

85. Forman JP, Brenner BM. "Hypertension" and "microalbuminuria": the bell tolls for thee. *Kidney Int.* 2006;69:22–26.

86. Kistorp C, Raymond I, Pedersen F, et al. N-terminal pro-brain natriuretic peptide, C-reactive protein, and urinary albumin levels as predictors of mortality and cardiovascular events in older adults. *JAMA.* 2005;293:1609–1616.

87. Stehouwer CD, Nauta JJ, Zeldenrust GC, et al. Urinary albumin excretion, cardiovascular disease, and endothelial dysfunction in non-insulin-dependent diabetes mellitus. *Lancet.* 1992;340: 319–323.

88. Cosson E, Pham I, Valensi P, et al. Impaired coronary endothelium-dependent vasodilation is associated with microalbuminuria in patients with type 2 diabetes and angiographically normal coronary arteries. *Diabetes Care.* 2006;29: 107–112.

89. Eddy AA. Interstitial nephritis induced by protein-overload proteinuria. *Am J Pathol.* 1989; 135:719–733.

90. Thomas ME, Schreiner GF. Contribution of proteinuria to progressive renal injury: consequences of tubular uptake of fatty acid bearing albumin. *Am J Nephrol.* 1993;13:385–398.

91. Zoja C, Benigni A, Remuzzi G. Protein overload activates proximal tubular cells to release vasoactive and inflammatory mediators. *Exp Nephrol.* 1999;7:420–428.

92. Hill GS, Delahousse M, Nochy D, et al. Proteinuria and tubulointerstitial lesions in lupus nephritis. *Kidney Int.* 2001;60(5):1893–1903.

93. Mezzano SA, Ruiz-Ortega M, Egido J. Angiotensin II and renal fibrosis. *Hypertension.* 2001;38(3 pt 2):635–638.

94. Border WA, Cohen AH. Renal biopsy diagnosis of clinically silent multiple myeloma. *Ann Intern Med.* 1980;93:43–46.

95. Robinson RR. Isolated proteinuria in asymptomatic patients. *Kidney Int.* 1980;18:395–406.

96. Carter JL, Tomson CR, Stevens PE, et al. Does urinary tract infection cause proteinuria or microalbuminuria? A systematic review. *Nephrol Dial Transplant.* 2006;21:3031–3037.

97. Wingo CS, Clapp WL. Proteinuria: potential causes and approach to evaluation. *Am J Med Sci.* 2000;320:188–194.

98. Poortmans JR, Brauman H, Staroukine M, et al. Indirect evidence of glomerular/tubular mixed type postexercise proteinuria in healthy humans. *Am J Physiol.* 1988;254:F277–F283.

99. Springberg PD, Garrett LE Jr, Thompson AL, et al. Fixed and reproducible orthostatic proteinuria: results of a 20-year follow-up study. *Ann Intern Med.* 1982;97:516–519.

100. Rytand DA, Spreiter S. Prognosis in postural (orthostatic proteinuria). Forty to fifty-year follow-up of six patients after diagnosis by Thomas Addis. *N Engl J Med.* 1981;305:618–621.

101. Sinniah R, Law CH, Pwee HS. Glomerular lesions in patients with asymptomatic persistent and orthostatic proteinuria discovered on routine medical examination. *Clin Nephrol.* 1977;7:1–14.

102. Ravnskov U. Low molecular weight proteinuria in association with paroxysmal myoglobinuria. *Clin Nephrol.* 1975;3:65–69.

103. Don BR, Rodriguez RA, Humphreys MH. Acute renal failure associated with pigmenturia or crystal deposits. In: Schrier RW, ed. *Diseases of the Kidney and Urinary Tract.* Vol 8. Philadelphia: Lippincott Williams & Wilkins; 2007:1184–1207.

104. Gabow PA, Kaehny WD, Kelleher SP. The spectrum of rhabdomyolysis. *Medicine.* 1982;61:141–152.

105. Zager RA. Rhabdomyolysis and myohemoglobinuric acute renal failure. *Kidney Int.* 1996;49:314–326.

106. Rice EK, Isbel NM, Becker GJ, et al. Heroin overdose and myoglobinuric acute renal failure. *Clin Nephrol.* 2000;54(6):449–454.

107. Vanholder R, Sever MS, Erek E, et al. Acute renal failure related to the crush syndrome: towards an era of seismo-nephrology? *Nephrol Dial Transplant.* 2000;15(10):1517–1521.

108. Rosen CL, Adler JN, Rabban JT, et al. Early predictors of myoglobinuria and acute renal failure following electrical injury. *J Emerg Med.* 1999; 17(5)783–789.

109. Omar MA, Wilson JP, Cox TS. Rhabdomyolysis and HMG-CoA reductase inhibitors. *Ann Pharmacother.* 2001;35(9):1096–1107.

110. Grisham MB. Myoglobin-catalyzed hydrogen peroxide dependent arachidonic acid peroxidation. *J Free Radic Biol Med.* 1985;1:227–232.

111. Better OS, Stein JH. Early management of shock and prophylaxis of acute renal failure in traumatic rhabdomyolysis. *N Engl J Med.* 1990;322: 825–829.

112. Better OS, Rubinstein I, Winaver J. Recent insights into the pathogenesis and early management of the crush syndrome. *Semin Nephrol.* 1990;12:217–222.

113. Owen CA, Mubarak SJ, Hargens AR, et al. Intramural pressures with limb compression. Clarification of the pathogenesis of drug-induced muscle-compression syndrome. *N Engl J Med.* 1979;300:1169–1172.

114. Knochel JP. Hypophosphatemia in the alcoholic. *Arch Intern Med*. 1980;140:613–615.

115. Knochel JP, Sclein EM. On the mechanism of rhabdomyolysis in potassium depletion. *J Clin Invest*. 1972;51:1750–1758.

116. Bank WJH, DiMauro S, Bonilla E, et al. A disorder of muscle lipid metabolism and myoglobinuria. Absence of carnitine palmityl transferase. *N Engl J Med*. 1975;292:443–449.

117. Cagliani R, Comi GP, Tancredi L, et al. Primary beta-sarcoglycanopathy manifesting as recurrent exercise-induced myoglobinuria. *Neuromuscul Disord*. 2001;11(4):389–394.

118. Roberts MC, Mickelson JR, Patterson EE, et al. Autosomal dominant canine malignant hyperthermia is caused by a mutation in the gene encoding the skeletal muscle calcium release channel (RYR1). *Anesthesiology*. 2001;95(3):716–725.

119. Layzer RB, Rowland LP, Ranney HM. Muscle phosphofructokinase deficiency. *Arch Neurol*. 1967;17:512–523.

120. Paster SB, Adams DF, Hollenberg NK. Acute renal failure in McArdle's disease and myoglobinuric states. *Radiology*. 1979;114:567–570.

121. Todd D. Diagnosis of haemolytic states. *Clin Haematol*. 1975;4:63–81.

122. Goldfinger D. Acute hemolytic transfusion reactions—a fresh look at pathogenesis and considerations regarding therapy. *Transfusion*. 1977;17: 85–98.

123. Relihan M, Litwin MS. Effects of stroma free hemoglobin solution on clearance rate and renal function. *Surgery*. 1972;71:395–399.

124. Schmidt PJ, Holland PV. Pathogenesis of the acute renal failure associated with incompatible transfusion. *Lancet*. 1967;2:1169–1172.

125. Fowler BA, Weissberg JB. Arsine poisoning. *N Engl J Med*. 1974;291:1171–1174.

126. Levinsky WJ, Smalley RV, Hillyer PN, et al. Arsine hemolysis. *Arch Environ Health*. 1970;20:436–440.

127. Pinto SS. Arsine poisoning: evaluation of the acute phase. *J Occup Med*. 1976;18:633–635.

128. Chan TK, Mak LW, Ng RP. Methemoglobinemia, Heinz bodies and acute massive intravascular hemolysis in Lysol poisoning. *Blood*. 1971;38:739–744.

129. Jacob HS, Amsden T. Acute hemolytic anemia with rigid red cells in hypophosphatemia. *N Engl J Med*. 1971;285:1446–1450.

130. Rosse WF. Paroxysmal nocturnal hemoglobinuria—present status and future prospects. *West J Med*. 1980;132:219–228.

131. Davidson RJL. March or exertional haemoglobinuria. *Semin Hematol*. 1969;6:150–161.

132. Crexells C, Aerucgudem N, Bonny Y, et al. Factors influencing hemolysis in valve prostheses. *Am Heart J*. 1972;84:161–170.

133. Earley LE, Farland M. Nephrotic syndrome. In: Strauss MB, Welt LG, eds. *Diseases of the Kidney*. Vol 3. Boston: Little, Brown; 1979:765–813.

134. Earley LE, Havel RJ, Hopper J, et al. Nephrotic syndrome. *Calif Med*. 1971;115:23–41.

135. Jensen H, Rossing N, Anderson SB, et al. Albumin metabolism in the nephrotic syndrome in adults. *Clin Sci*. 1967;33:445–457.

136. Kaysen GA, Gambertoglio J, Jiminez I, et al. Effect of dietary protein intake on albumin homeostasis in nephrotic patients. *Kidney Int*. 1986;29:572–577.

137. Kaitz AL. Albumin metabolism in nephrotic adults. *J Lab Clin Med*. 1959;53:186–194.

138. Gitlin D, Janeway CA, Farr LE. Studies on the metabolism of plasma proteins in nephrotic syndrome: I. Albumin, gamma-globulin and iron-binding globulin. *J Clin Invest*. 1956;35:44–55.

139. Keutmann EH, Bassett SH. Dietary protein in hemorrhagic Bright's disease: II. The effect of diet on serum proteins, proteinuria and tissue proteins. *J Clin Invest*. 1935;14:871–888.

140. Peters JP, Bulger HA. The relation of albuminuria catabolism in the rat. *Arch Intern Med*. 1926;37:153–185.

141. Baynes JW, Thorpe SR. Identification of sites of albumin catabolism in the rat. *Arch Biochem Biophys*. 1981;206:372–379.

142. Waldmann TA. Albumin catabolism. In: Rosemoer M, Oratz M, Rothschild A, eds. *Albumin: Structure, Function and Uses*. New York: Pergamon Press; 1977:255–273.

143. Sellers AL, Katz J, Bonorris G, et al. Determination of extravascular albumin in the rat. *J Lab Clin Med*. 1966;68:177–185.

144. Reeve EB, Chen AY. Regulation of interstitial albumin. In: Rothschild MA, Waldmann T, eds. *Plasma Protein Metabolism, Regulation of Synthesis, Distribution, and Degradation*. New York: Academic Press; 1970.

145. Yedgar S, Carew TE, Pittman RC, et al. Tissue sites of catabolism of albumin in rabbits. *Am J Physiol Endocrinol Metab*. 1983;244(7):E101–E107.

146. Katz J, Rosenfeld S, Sellers AL. Role of the kidney in plasma albumin catabolism. *Am J Physiol*. 1960;198:814–818.

147. Galaske RG, Baldamus CA, Stolte H. Plasma protein handling in the rat kidney: micropuncture experiments in the acute heterologous phase of anti-gbm-nephritis. *Pflugers Arch*. 1978;375:269–277.

148. Landwehr DM, Carvalho JS, Oken DE. Micropuncture studies of the filtration and absorption of albumin by nephrotic rats. *Kidney Int*. 1977;11:9–17.

149. Lewy JE, Pesce A. Micropuncture study of albumin transfer in aminonucleoside nephrosis in the rat. *Pediatr Res*. 1973;7:553–559.

150. Oken DE, Cotes SC, Mende CW. Micropuncture study of tubular transport of albumin in rats with aminonucleoside nephrosis. *Kidney Int*. 1972;1:3–11.

151. Kaysen GA, Kirkpatrick WG, Couser WG. Albumin homeostasis in the nephrotic rat: nutritional considerations. *Am J Physiol Renal Fluid Electrolyte Physiol*. 1984;247(16):F192–F202.

152. Rothschild MA, Oratz M, Evans CD, et al. Albumin synthesis. In: Rosemoer M, Oratz M, Rothschild A, eds. *Albumin Structure, Function and Uses*. New York: Pergamon Press; 1977:227–255.

153. Rothschild MA, Oratz M, Schreiber SS. Albumin synthesis. In: Javitt NB, ed. *Liver and Biliary Tract Physiology: I. International Review of Physiology*. Vol 21. Baltimore: University Park Press; 1980:249–274.

154. Morgan EH, Peters T Jr. The biosynthesis of rat serum albumin. *J Biol Chem.* 1971;246: 3500–3507.

155. Kirsch R, Frith L, Black E, et al. Regulation of albumin synthesis and catabolism by alteration of dietary protein. *Nature.* 1968;217:578–579.

156. Moshage HJ, Janssen JAM, Franssen JH, et al. Study of the molecular mechanisms of decreased liver synthesis of albumin in inflammation. *J Clin Invest.* 1987;79:1635–1641.

157. Ballmer PE, McNurlan MA, Hulter HN, et al. Chronic metabolic acidosis decreases albumin synthesis and induces negative nitrogen balance in humans. *J Clin Invest.* 1995;95(1):39–45.

158. Kaysen GA, Jones H Jr, Martin V, et al. A low protein diet restricts albumin synthesis in nephrotic rats. *J Clin Invest.* 1989;83:1623–1629.

159. Yamauchi A, Imai E, Noguchi T, et al. Albumin gene transcription is enhanced in liver of nephrotic rats. *Am J Physiol Endocrinol Metab.* 1988;254(17):E676–E679.

160. Kang J, Holland M, Jones H, et al. Coordinate augmentation in expression of genes encoding transcription factors and liver secretory proteins in hypo-oncotic states. *Kidney Int.* 1999;56(2): 452–460.

161. Rothschild MA, Oratz M, Franklin EC, et al. The effect of hypergammaglobulinemia on albumin metabolism in hyperimmunized rabbits studied with albumin I131. *J Clin Invest.* 1967;41: 1564–1571.

162. Rothschild MA, Oratz M, Wimer E, et al. Studies on albumin synthesis: the effect of dextran and cortisone on albumin metabolism in rabbits studied with albumin I131. *J Clin Invest.* 1961;40: 545–554.

163. Rothschild MA, Oratz M, Mongelli J, et al. Albumin metabolism in rabbits during gamma globulin infusions. *J Lab Clin Med.* 1965;66:733–740.

164. Rothschild MA, Oratz M, Mongelli J, et al. Effect of albumin concentration on albumin synthesis in the perfused liver. *Am J Physiol.* 1969;216: 1127–1130.

165. Dich J, Hansen SE, Thieden HID. Effect of albumin concentration and colloid osmotic pressure on albumin synthesis in the perfused rat liver. *Acta Physiol Scand.* 1973;89:352–358.

166. Morgan EH, Peters T Jr. The biosynthesis of rat serum albumin. *J Biol Chem.* 1971;246: 3500–3507.

167. Hoffenberg R, Black E, Brock JF. Albumin and gamma-globulin tracer studies in protein depletion states. *J Clin Invest.* 1966;45:143–152.

168. James WP, Hay AM. Albumin metabolism: effect of the nutritional state and the dietary protein intake. *J Clin Invest.* 1968;47:1958–1972.

169. Smith JE, Lunn PG. Albumin-synthesizing capacity of hepatocytes isolated from rats fed diets differing in protein and energy content. *Ann Nutr Metab.* 1984;28:281–287.

170. Lunn PG, Austin S. Excess energy intake promotes the development of hypoalbuminemia in rats fed on low-protein diets. *Br J Nutr.* 1983;49: 9–16.

171. Coward WA, Sawyer MB. Whole-body albumin mass and distribution in rats fed on low-protein diets. *Br J Nutr.* 1977;37:127–134.

172. Blainey JD. High-protein diets in the treatment of the nephrotic syndrome. *Clin Sci.* 1954;13:567–581.

173. Rosenberg ME, Swanson JE, Thomas BL, et al. Glomerular and hormonal responses to dietary protein intake in human renal disease. *Am J Physiol Renal Fluid Electrolyte Physiol.* 1987;253(22):F1083–F1090.

174. Hutchison FN, Schambelan M, Kaysen GA. Modulation of albuminuria by dietary protein and converting enzyme inhibition. *Am J Physiol Renal Fluid Electrolyte Physiol.* 1987;253(22):F719–F725.

175. Giordano M, De Feo P, Lucidi P, et al. Effects of dietary protein restriction on fibrinogen and albumin metabolism in nephrotic patients. *Kidney Int.* 2001;60(1):235–242.

176. Zatz R, Meyer TW, Rennke HG, et al. Predominance of hemodynamic rather than metabolic factors in the pathogenesis of diabetic glomerulopathy. *Proc Natl Acad Sci U S A.* 1985;82: 5963–5967.

177. Brenner BM, Meyer TW, Hostetter TH. Dietary protein intake and the progressive nature of kidney disease: the role of hemodynamically mediated glomerular injury in the pathogenesis of progressive glomerular sclerosis in aging, renal ablation and intrinsic renal disease. *N Engl J Med.* 1982;307:652–659.

178. Klahr S, Buerhert J, Purkerson ML. Role of dietary factors in the progression of chronic renal disease. *Kidney Int.* 1983;24:579–587.

179. Hostetter TH, Olson JL, Rennke HG, et al. Hyperfiltration in remnant nephrons: a potentially adverse response to renal ablation. *Am J Physiol Renal Fluid Electrolyte Physiol.* 1981;241(10):F85–F93.

180. de Sain-van der Velden MG, Kaysen GA, de Meer K, et al. Proportionate increase of fibrinogen and albumin synthesis in nephrotic patients: measurements with stable isotopes. *Kidney Int.* 1998;53:181–188.

181. de Sain-van der Velden MG, Reijngoud DJ, Kaysen GA, et al. Evidence for increased synthesis of lipoprotein(a) in the nephrotic syndrome. *J Am Soc Nephrol.* 1998;9(8):1474–1481.

182. Kaysen GA, Rosenthal C, Hutchison FN. GFR increases before renal mass or ODC activity increase in rats fed high-protein diets. *Kidney Int.* 1989;36:441–446.

183. Hutchison FN, Martin V, Jones H Jr, et al. Differing actions of dietary protein and enalapril on renal function and proteinuria. *Am J Physiol Renal Fluid Electrolyte Physiol.* 1990;258(27): F126–F132.

184. Kaysen GA. Plasma composition in the nephrotic syndrome. *Am J Nephrol.* 1993;13:347–359.

185. Sun X, Martin V, Weiss RH, et al. Selective transcriptional augmentation of hepatic gene expression in the rat with Heymann nephritis. *Am J Physiol.* 1993;264:F441–F447.

186. Sun X, Jones H Jr, Joles JA, et al. Apolipoprotein gene expression in analbuminemic rats and in rats with Heymann nephritis. *Am J Physiol Renal Fluid Electrolyte Physiol.* 1992;262(31):F755–F761.

187. Marshall JF, Apostolopoulos JJ, Brack CM, et al. Regulation of apolipoprotein gene expression and plasma high density lipoprotein composition in experimental nephrosis. *Biochim Biophys Acta.* 1990;1042:271–279.

188. Kaysen GA, Sun X, Jones H Jr, et al. Non-iron mediated alteration in hepatic transferring gene expression in the nephrotic rat. *Kidney Int.* 1995;47:1068–1077.

189. Kaysen GA, Hoye E, Jones H Jr. Apolipoprotein AI levels are increased in part as a consequence of reduced catabolism in nephrotic rats. *Am J Physiol.* 1995;268:F532–F540.

190. Dugué-Pujol S, Rousset X, Château D, et al. Apolipoprotein A-II is catabolized in the kidney as a function of its plasma concentration. *J Lipid Res.* 2007;48:2151–2161.

191. Jensen H, Bro-Jorgensen K, Jarnum S, et al. Transferrin metabolism in the nephrotic syndrome and in protein-losing gastroenteropathy. *Scand J Clin Lab Invest.* 1968;21:293–304.

192. Rifkind D, Kravetz HM, Knight V, et al. Urinary excretion of iron-binding protein in the nephrotic syndrome. *N Engl J Med.* 1961;265:115–118.

193. Ellis D. Anemia in the course of the nephrotic syndrome secondary to transferring depletion. *J Pediatr.* 1977;90:953–955.

194. Hancock DE, Onstad JW, Wolf PL. Transferrin loss into the urine with hypochromic, microcytic anemia. *Am J Clin Pathol.* 1976;65:72–78.

195. Prinsen BH, de Sain-van der Velden MG, Kaysen GA, et al. Transferrin synthesis is increased in nephrotic patients insufficiently to replace urinary losses. *J Am Soc Nephrol.* 2001;12(5): 1017–1025.

196. Esumi H, Sato S, Okui M, et al. Turnover of serum proteins in rats with analbuminemia. *Biochem Biophys Res Commun.* 1979;87: 1191–1199.

197. Alfrey AC, Hammond WS. Renal iron handling in the nephrotic syndrome. *Kidney Int.* 1990;37: 1409–1413.

198. Vaziri ND, Kaupke CJ, Barton CH, et al. Plasma concentration and urinary excretion of erythropoietin in adult nephrotic syndrome. *Am J Med.* 1992;92:35–40.

199. Zhou XJ, Vaziri ND. Erythropoietin metabolism and pharmacokinetics in experimental nephrosis. *Am J Physiol.* 1992;263:F812–F815.

200. Longsworth LG, MacInnes DA. An electrophoretic study of nephrotic sera and urine. *J Exp Med.* 1940;71:77–82.

201. Arneil GC. 164 children with nephrosis. *Lancet.* 1961;2:1103–1110.

202. Rothschild MA, Oratz M, Schreiber SS. Albumin synthesis and albumin degradation. In: Sgouris JT, Rene A, eds. *Proceedings of the Workshop on Albumin.* 1975:57–74.

203. Waldmann TA, Strober W, Mogielnicki RP. The renal handling of low molecular weight proteins: II. Disorders of serum protein catabolism in patients with tubular proteinuria, the nephrotic syndrome or uremia. *J Clin Invest.* 1972;51:2162–2174.

204. Perheentupa J. Serum protein turnover in the congenital nephrotic syndrome. *Ann Paediatr Fenn.* 1966;12:189–233.

205. Heslan JM, Lautie JP, Intrator L, et al. Impaired IgG synthesis in patients with the nephrotic syndrome. *Clin Nephrol.* 1982;18:144–147.

206. Ooi BS, Ooi YM, Hsu A, et al. Diminished synthesis of immunoglobulin by peripheral lymphocytes of patients with idiopathic membranous glomerulonephropathy. *J Clin Invest.* 1980;65:789–797.

207. Bernard DB. Metabolic abnormalities in nephrotic syndrome: pathophysiology and complications. In: Brenner BM, Stein JH, eds. *Contemporary Issues in Nephrology 9: Nephrotic Syndrome.* New York: Churchill Livingstone; 1982:85–120.

208. Al-Bander H, Martin VI, Kaysen GA. Plasma IgG levels are not defended when urinary protein loss occurs. *Am J Physiol.* 1992;262:F333–F337.

209. Giangiacomo J, Cleary TG, Cole BR, et al. Serum immunoglobulins in the nephrotic syndrome. A possible cause of minimal-change nephrotic syndrome. *N Engl J Med.* 1975;293:8–12.

210. Chan MK, Chan KW, Jones B. Immunoglobulins (IgG, IgA, IgM, IgE) and complement components (C3,C4) in nephrotic syndrome due to a minimal change and other forms of glomerulonephritis, a clue for steroid therapy? *Nephron.* 1987;47:125–130.

211. Kauffmann RH, Veltkamp JJ, Van Tilburg NH, et al. Acquired antithrombin III deficiency and thrombosis in the nephrotic syndrome. *Am J Med.* 1978;65:607–613.

212. Rydzewski A, Myslieiec M, Soszka J. Concentration of three thrombin inhibitors in the nephrotic syndrome in adults. *Nephron.* 1986;42:200–203.

213. Girot R, Jaubert F, Leon M, et al. Albumin, fibrinogen prothrombin, and antithrombin III variations in blood, urines and liver in rat nephrotic syndrome (Heymann nephritis). *Thromb Haemost.* 1983;49:13–17.

214. Robbins J, Rall JE, Petermann ML. Thyroxin-binding globulin, thyroxine-binding globulin and total protein in adult males with nephrosis: effect of sex hormones. *J Clin Endocrinol.* 1967;27: 768–774.

215. Musa BU, Seal US, Doe RP. Excretion of corticosteroid-binding globulin, thyroxine-binding globulin and total protein in adult males with nephrosis: effect of sex hormones. *J Clin Endocrinol.* 1967;27:768–744.

216. Gavin LA, McMahon FA, Castle JN, et al. Alterations in serum thyroid hormones and thyroxine-binding globulin in patients with nephrosis. *J Clin Endocrinol Metab.* 1978;46:125–138.

217. Afrasiabi AM, Vaziri ND, Gwinup G, et al. Thyroid function studies in the nephrotic syndrome. *Ann Intern Med.* 1979;90:335–338.

218. Goldstein DA, Haldimann B, Sherman D, et al. Vitamin D metabolites and calcium metabolism in patients with nephrotic syndrome and normal renal function. *J Clin Endocrinol Metab.* 1981;53: 116–121.

219. Salvesen HA, Linder GC. Inorganic bases and phosphates in relation to the protein of blood and other body fluids in Bright's disease and in heart failure. *J Biol Chem.* 1923;58:617–634.

220. Emerson K Jr, Beckman WW. Calcium metabolism in nephrosis: I. A description of an abnormality in calcium metabolism in children with nephrosis. *J Clin Invest.* 1945;24:564–572.

221. Goldstein DA, Oda Y, Kurokawa K, et al. Blood levels of 25-hydroxy-vitamin D in nephrotic syndrome. Studies in 26 patients. *Ann Intern Med.* 1977;87:664–667.

222. Lim P, Jacob E, Chio LF, et al. Serum ionized calcium in nephrotic syndrome. *Q J Med.* 1976; 45:421–426.

223. Haddad JG Jr, Walgate J. Radioimmunoassay of the binding protein for vitamin D and its metabolites in human serum: concentrations in normal subjects and patients with disorders of mineral homeostasis. *J Clin Invest.* 1976;58:1217–1222.

224. Barragry JM, France MW, Carter ND, et al. Vitamin D metabolism in nephrotic syndrome. *Lancet.* 1977;2:629–632.

225. Stickler GB, Rosevear JW, Ulrich JA. Renal tubular dysfunction complicating the nephrotic syndrome: the disturbance in calcium and phosphorus metabolism. *Proc Staff Meet Mayo Clin.* 1962;37:376–387.

226. Stickler GB, Hayles AB, Power MH, et al. Renal tubular dysfunction complicating the nephrotic syndrome. *Pediatrics.* 1960;26:75–85.

227. Holick MF. Vitamin D deficiency. *N Engl J Med.* 2007;357:266–281.

228. de Sain-van der Velden MG, Rabelink TJ, Reijngoud DJ, et al. Plasma alpha 2 macroglobulin is increased in nephrotic patients as a result of increased synthesis alone. *Kidney Int.* 1998;54(2):530–535.

229. Stevenson FT, Greene S, Kaysen GA. Serum alpha 2-macroglobulin and alpha 1-inhibitor 3 concentrations are increased in hypoalbuminemia by post-transcriptional mechanisms. *Kidney Int.* 1998;53(1):67–75.

230. Yssing M, Jensen H, Jarnum S. Albumin metabolism and gastrointestinal protein loss in children with nephrotic syndrome. *Acta Paediatr Scand.* 1969;58:109–115.

231. Llach F. Nephrotic syndrome: hypercoagulability, renal vein thrombosis and other thromboembolic complications. In: Brenner BM, Stein JH, eds. *Contemporary Issues in Nephrology 9: Nephrotic Syndrome.* New York: Churchill Livingstone; 1982:121–144.

232. Llach F, Arieff AI, Massry SG. Renal vein thrombosis and nephrotic syndrome: a prospective study of 36 adult patients. *Ann Intern Med.* 1975;83:8–14.

233. Trew P, Biava C, Jacobs R, et al. Renal vein thrombosis in membranous glomerulonephropathy: incidence and association. *Medicine.* 1978;57: 69–82.

234. D'Angelo S, D'Angelo A, Kaufman CE Jr, et al. Protein S deficiency occurs in the nephrotic syndrome. *Ann Intern Med.* 1987;107: 42–47.

235. Cosio FG, Harker C, Batard MA, et al. Plasma concentrations of the natural anticoagulants protein C and protein S in patients with proteinuria. *J Lab Clin Med.* 1985;106:218–222.

236. Joven J, Villabona C, Vilella E, et al. Abnormalities of lipoprotein metabolism in patients with the nephrotic syndrome. *N Engl J Med.* 1990;323: 579–584.

237. Gherardi E, Rota E, Calandra S, et al. Relationship among the concentrations of serum lipoproteins and changes in their chemical composition in patients with untreated nephrotic syndrome. *Eur J Clin Invest.* 1977;7:563–570.

238. Muls E, Rosseneu M, Daneels R, et al. Lipoprotein distribution and composition in the human nephrotic syndrome. *Atherosclerosis.* 1985;54: 225–237.

239. Kostner GM, Avogaro P, Cazzolato G, et al. Lipoprotein Lp(a) and the risk for myocardial infarction. *Atherosclerosis.* 1981;38:51–61.

240. Utermann G. The mysteries of lipoprotein(a). *Science.* 1989;246:904–910.

241. Boerwinkle E, Menzel HJ, Kraft HG, et al. Genetics of the quantitative Lp(a) lipoprotein trait: III. Contribution of Lp(a) glycoprotein phenotypes to normal lipid variation. *Hum Genet.* 1989;82:73–78.

242. Gavish D, Azrolan N, Breslow J. Plasma Lp(a) concentration is inversely correlated with the ratio of kringle IV/kringle V encoding domains in the apo(a) gene. *J Clin Invest.* 1989;84: 2021–2027.

243. Wanner C, Rader D, Bartens W, et al. Elevated plasma lipoprotein(a) in patients with the nephrotic syndrome. *Ann Intern Med.* 1993;119: 263–269.

244. de Sain-van der Velden MG, Kaysen GA, Barrett HA, et al. Increased VLDL in nephrotic patients results from a decreased catabolism while increased LDL results from increased synthesis. *Kidney Int.* 1998;53(4):994–1001.

245. Davies RW, Staprans I, Hutchison FN, et al. Proteinuria, not altered albumin metabolism, effects hyperlipidemia in the nephrotic rat. *J Clin Invest.* 1990;86:600–605.

246. Shearer GC, Kaysen GA. Proteinuria and plasma compositional changes contribute to defective lipoprotein catabolism in the nephrotic syndrome by separate mechanisms. *Am J Kidney Dis.* 2001;37(1 suppl 2):S119–S122.

247. Shearer GC, Stevenson FT, Atkinson DN, et al. Hypoalbuminemia and proteinuria contribute separately to reduced lipoprotein catabolism in the nephrotic syndrome. *Kidney Int.* 2001;59: 179–189.

248. Vaziri ND, Liang K, Parks JS. Acquired lecithin-cholesterol acyltransferase deficiency in nephrotic syndrome. *Am J Physiol Renal Physiol.* 2001; 280(5):F823–F828.

249. Furukawa S, Hirano T, Mamo JCL, et al. Catabolic defect of triglyceride is associated with abnormal very-low-density lipoprotein in experimental nephrosis. *Metabolism.* 1990;39:101–107.

250. Havel RJ. Lipid transport function of lipoproteins in blood plasma. *Am J Physiol Endocrinol Metab.* 1987;253(16):E1–E5.

251. Eisenberg S. High density lipoprotein metabolism. *J Lipid Res.* 1984;25:1017–1058.

252. Cohen SL, Cramp DG, Lewis AD, et al. The mechanism of hyperlipidemia in nephrotic syndrome: role of low albumin and the LCAT reaction. *Clin Chim Acta.* 1980;104:393–400.

253. Kekki M, Nikkila EA. Plasma triglyceride metabolism in the adult nephrotic syndrome. *Eur J Clin Invest.* 1971;1:345–351.

254. Vega GL, Grundy SM. Lovastatin therapy in nephrotic hyperlipidemia: effects on lipoprotein metabolism. *Kidney Int.* 1988;33:1160–1168.

255. Yamada M, Matsuda I. Lipoprotein lipase in clinical and experimental nephrosis. *Clin Chim Acta.* 1970;30:787–794.

256. Kaysen GA, Don B, Schambelan M. Proteinuria, albumin synthesis and hyperlipidemia in the nephrotic syndrome. *Nephrol Dial Transplant.* 1991;6:141–149.

257. Zwaginga JJ, Koomans HA, Sixma JJ, et al. Thrombus formation and platelet-vessel wall interaction in the nephrotic syndrome under flow conditions. *J Clin Invest*. 1994;93:204–211.

258. Mallick NP, Short CD. The nephrotic syndrome and ischaemic heart disease. *Nephron*. 1981;27: 54–57.

259. Berlyne GM, Mallick NP. Ischemic heart disease as a complication of nephrotic syndrome. *Lancet*. 1969;2:399–400.

260. Ordonez JD, Hiatt RA, Killebrew EJ, et al. The increased risk of coronary heart disease associated with nephrotic syndrome. *Kidney Int*. 1993;44: 638–642.

261. Schmitz PG, Kasiske BL, O'Donnell MP, et al. Lipids and progressive renal injury. *Semin Nephrol*. 1989;9:354–369.

262. Larger DJ, Rosenberg BF, Shapiro H, et al. Lecithin cholesterol acyltransferase deficiency: ultrastructural examination of sequential renal biopsies. *Mod Pathol*. 1991;4:331–335.

263. Don BR, Kaysen GA, Hutchison FN, et al. The effect of angiotensin-converting enzyme inhibition and dietary protein restriction in the treatment of proteinuria. *Am J Kidney Dis*. 1991;17:10–17.

264. Gansevoort RT, Heeg JE, Vriesendorp R, et al. Antiproteinuric drugs in patients with idiopathic membranous glomerulopathy. *Nephrol Dial Transplant*. 1992;7(suppl 1):91–96.

265. Dullaart RP, Gansevoort RT, Dikkeschei BD, et al. Role of elevated lecithin: cholesterol acyltransferase and cholesteryl ester transfer protein activities in abnormal lipoproteins from proteinuric patients. *Kidney Int*. 1993;44:91–97.

266. Keilani T, Schlueter WA, Levin ML, et al. Improvement of lipid abnormalities associated with proteinuria using fosinopril, an angiotensin-converting enzyme inhibitor. *Ann Intern Med*. 1993;118:246–254.

267. Tokoo M, Oguchi H, Terashima M, et al. Effects of pravastatin on serum lipids and apolipoproteins in hyperlipidemia of the nephrotic syndrome. *Nippon Jinzo Gakkai Shi*. 1992;34:397–403.

268. Modi KS, Schreiner GF, Purkerson ML, et al. Effects of probucol in renal function and structure in rats with subtotal kidney ablation. *J Lab Clin Med*. 1992;120:310–317.

269. Groggel GC, Cheung AK, Ellis-Benigni K, et al. Treatment of nephrotic hyperlipoproteinemia with gemfibrozil. *Kidney Int*. 1989;36:266–271.

270. Aukland K, Nicolaysen G. Interstitial fluid volume: local regulatory mechanisms. *Phys Rev*. 1981;61:556–643.

271. Guyton AC, Taylor AE, Granger HJ, eds. *Circulatory Physiology II: Dynamics and Control of Body Fluids*. Philadelphia: WB Saunders;1975:149–165.

272. Taylor AE. Capillary fluid filtration starling forces and lymph flow. *Circ Res*. 1981;49: 557–575.

273. Meltzer JI, Keim HJ, Laragh JH, et al. Nephrotic syndrome: vasoconstriction and hypervolemia types indicated by renin–sodium profiling. *Ann Intern Med*. 1979;67:387–384.

274. Dorhout Mees EJ, Roos JC, Boer P, et al. Observations on edema formation in the nephrotic syndrome in adults with minimal lesions. *Am J Med*. 1979;67:378–384.

275. Geers AB, Koomans HA, Roos JC, et al. Functional relationships in the nephrotic syndrome. *Kidney Int*. 1984;26:324–330.

276. Katz J, Sellers AL, Bonorris G. Plasma albumin metabolism during transient rennin proteinuria. *J Lab Clin Med*. 1964;64:709–716.

277. Garlick DG, Renkin EM. Transport of large molecules from plasma to interstitial fluid and lymph in dogs. *Am J Physiol*. 1970;219: 1595–1605.

278. Fadnes HO, Reed RK, Aukland K. Mechanisms regulating interstitial fluid volume. *Lymphology*. 1978;11:165–257.

279. Aukland K. Autoregulation of interstitial fluid volume: edema-preventing mechanisms. *Scand J Clin Lab Invest*. 1973;31:247–254.

280. Koomans HA, Geers AB, Meiracker AHVD, et al. Effects of plasma volume expansion on renal salt handling in patients with the nephrotic syndrome. *Am J Nephrol*. 1984;4:227–234.

281. Keeler R, Feuchuk D, Wilson N. Atrial peptides and the renal response to hypervolemia in nephrotic rats. *Can J Physiol Pharmacol*. 1987;65:2017–2075.

282. Peterson C, Madsen B, Perlman A, et al. Atrial natriuretic peptide and the renal response to hypervolemia in nephrotic humans. *Kidney Int*. 1988; 34:825–831.

283. Rabelink AJ, Koomans HA, Gaillard CA, et al. Renal response to atrial natriuretic peptide in nephrotic syndrome. *Nephrol Dial Transplant*. 1987;2(6):510–514.

284. Perico N, Delaini F, Lupini C, et al. Blunted excretory response to atrial natriuretic peptide in experimental nephrosis. *Kidney Int*. 1989;36: 57–64.

285. Hildebrandt DA, Banks RO. Effect of atrial natriuretic factor on renal function in rats with nephrotic syndrome. *Am J Physiol Renal Fluid Electrolyte Physiol*. 1988;254(23):F210–F216.

286. Plum J, Mirzaian Y, Grabensee B. Atrial natriuretic peptide, sodium retention, and proteinuria in nephrotic syndrome. *Nephrol Dial Transplant*. 1996;11(6):1034–1042.

287. Féraille E, Vogt B, Rousselot M, et al. Mechanism of enhanced Na-K-ATPase activity in cortical collecting duct from rats with nephrotic syndrome. *J Clin Invest*. 1993;91:1295–1300.

288. Lee EY, Humphreys MH. Phosphodiesterase activity as a mediator of renal resistance to ANP in pathologic salt retention. *Am J Physiol*. 1996;271(1 pt 2):F3–F6.

289. Kastner C, Pohl M, Sendeski M, et al. Effects of receptor-mediated endocytosis and tubular protein composition on volume retention in experimental glomerulonephritis. *Am J Physiol Renal Physiol*. 2009;296:F902–F911.

290. Ichikawa I, Rennke HG, Hoyer JR, et al. Role for intrarenal mechanisms in the impaired salt excretion of experimental nephrotic syndrome. *J Clin Invest*. 1983;71:91–104.

291. Koj A, Gauldie J, Sweeney GD, et al. A simple bioassay for monocyte-derived hepatocyte stimulating factor: Increased synthesis of $\alpha 2$-macroglobulin and reduced synthesis of albumin by cultured rat hepatocytes. *J Immunol Methods*. 1985;76:317–327.

292. Bauer J, Weber W, Tran-Thi T, et al. Murine interleukin 1 stimulates $\alpha 2$- macroglobulin synthesis in rat hepatocyte primary cultures. *FEBS Lett.* 1985;190:271–274.

293. Kaysen GA, Dubin JA, Müller HG, et al. NIDDK Inflammation and reduced albumin synthesis associated with stable decline in serum albumin in hemodialysis patients. *Kidney Int.* 2004;65: 1408–1415.

294. Marsh JB. Lipoprotein metabolism in experimental nephrosis. *J Lipid Res.* 1984;25: 1619–1623.

295. Staprans I, Felts JM, Couser WG. Glycosaminoglycans and chylomicron metabolism in control and nephrotic rats. *Metabolism.* 1987;36:496–501.

296. Garber DW, Gottlieb BA, Marsh JB, et al. Catabolism of very low density lipo-proteins in experimental nephrosis. *J Clin Invest.* 1984;74: 1375–1383.

297. Chung BH, Segrest JP, Smith K, et al. Lipolytic surface remnants of triglyceride-rich lipoproteins are cytotoxic to macrophages but not in the presence of high density lipoprotein. A possible mechanism of atherogenesis? *J Clin Invest.* 1989;83:1363–1374.

298. D'Amico G, Gentile MG, Manna G, et al. Effect of vegetarian soy diet on hyperlipidaemia in nephrotic syndrome. *Lancet.* 1992;339:1131–1134.

299. Gentile MG, Fellin G, Cofano F, et al. Treatment of proteinuric patients with a vegetarian soy diet and fish oil. *Clin Nephrol.* 1993;40:315–320.

300. Hall AV, Parbtani A, Clark WF, et al. Omega-3 fatty acid supplementation in primary nephrotic syndrome: effects on plasma lipids and coagulopathy. *J Am Soc Nephrol.* 1992;3:1321–1329.

301. Donadio JV Jr, Bergstralh EJ, Offord KP, et al. A controlled trial of fish oil in IgA nephropathy. *N Engl J Med.* 1994;331:1194–1199.

302. Wolf G, Neilson EG. Angiotensin II as a renal growth factor. *J Am Soc Nephrol.* 1993;3: 1531–1540.

303. Kagami S, Border W, Miller DE, et al. Angiotensin II stimulates extracellular matrix synthesis through induction of transforming growth factor-ß expression in rat glomerular mesangial cells. *J Clin Invest.* 1994;93:2431.

304. Gross ML, El-Shakmak A, Szabo A, et al. ACE-inhibition but not endothelin receptor blockers prevent podocyte loss in early diabetic nephropathy. *Diabetologia.* 2003;46:856–868.

305. Davis BJ, Cao Z, de Gasparo M, et al. Disparate effects of angiotensin II antagonists and calcium channel blockers on albuminuria in experimental diabetes and hypertension: potentenial role for nephrin. *J Hypertens.* 2003;21:209–216.

306. Benigni A, Gagliardini E, Remuzzi G. Changes in glomerular perm-selectivity induced by angiotensin II imply podocyte dysfunction and slit diaphragm protein rearrangement. *Semin Nephrol.* 2004;24:131–140.

307. Ruggenenti P, Perna A, Benini R, et al. Effects of dihydropyridine calcium channel blockers, angiotensin-converting enzyme inhibition, and blood pressure control on chronic, nondiabetic nephropathies. *J Am Soc Nephrol.* 1998;9(11): 2096–2101.

308. Nakao N, Yoshimura A, Morita H, et al. Combination treatment of angiotensin-II receptor blocker and angiotensin-converting-enzyme inhibitor in non-diabetic renal disease (COOPERATE): a randomized controlled trial. *Lancet.* 2003;361: 117–124.

309. Kunz R, Friedrich C, Wolbers M, et al. Meta-analysis: effect of monotherapy and combination therapy with inhibitors of the renin angiotensin system on proteinuria in renal disease. *Ann Intern Med.* 2008;148:30–48.

310. Tan SY, Shapiro R, Franco R, et al. Indomethacin-induced prostaglandin inhibition with hyperkalemia. *Ann Intern Med.* 1979;90:783–785.

311. Tiggeler RGWL, Koene RAP, Wijdeveld PGAB. Inhibition of frusemide-induced natriuresis by indomethacin in patients with the nephrotic syndrome. *Clin Sci Mol Med.* 1977;52:149–152.

The Glomerulopathies

JOSHUA M. THURMAN AND RYAN GOLDBERG

D isorders affecting the structure and function of the glomeruli (glomerulopathies) are among the most common causes of acute and chronic renal insufficiency. Broadly defined, the glomerulopathies include diseases that may originate in the glomerular capillaries, the glomerular basement membrane (GBM), the mesangium, the podocyte, or outside the glomerular tuft. Such a definition includes diverse diseases such as immune-mediated glomerulonephritis (GN), diabetic kidney disease, and thrombotic microangiopathies. Some of these diseases present as primary diseases of the kidney, and others, such as diabetic nephropathy (DN), represent the renal manifestation of a systemic disorder.

Classification of the glomerular diseases can be complex because the definition of these diseases incorporates etiology, pathogenesis, histologic findings, and clinical syndromes. Disease classification is particularly complex for the different types of glomerulonephritis (Table 15.1). The definition of these diseases relies heavily upon the histologic findings. As more information about the etiology and pathogenesis of glomerular diseases has become available, however, it has enabled more precise subclassification of some disease processes. Patients who previously would have been given the diagnosis of focal segmental glomerulosclerosis (FSGS) or membranoproliferative glomerulonephritis (MPGN) based on the histologic appearance seen on renal biopsy, for example, may now be further subclassified on the basis of genetic factors or infectious etiologies.

It should be emphasized that unique pathogenetic events can give rise to diverse morphologic features and a single morphologic pattern can evolve from several pathogenetic mechanisms. Furthermore, discrete morphologic abnormalities can evoke a spectrum of clinical syndromes. Refining the definition of a disease as new discoveries are made is important insofar as it may offer more accurate prognostic information and may allow us to choose the most appropriate treatment for a given patient. Recent insights into the pathogenesis of MPGN type II, for example, have permitted greater distinction of this disease from MPGN type I, and it is now referred to as Dense Deposit Disease [DDD, (1)]. These diseases originally bore similar names due to their histologic appearance by light-microscopy, but they are caused by distinct immunologic mechanisms. Re-classification of glomerular diseases as new information is gained will likely improve the management of patients with these diseases.

Etiology

Glomerulopathies can arise from the effects of environmental agents (microbial infection, drugs, or toxins) or from endogenous perturbations (altered metabolism, biochemical defects, autoimmunity, or neoplasia). In both instances, underlying genetic factors interact with the environmental agents to generate the morphologic and clinical expression of disease. The etiologic agent responsible for the glomerular disease is well understood in some circumstances [e.g., drug-induced membranous nephropathy (MN)], although the pathogenetic mechanisms responsible for disease production remain unclear or controversial. For others, the etiologic agent remains obscure even though the effector systems engaged in tissue injury are reasonably well known. The search for the etiologic entities involved in the glomerulopathies continues.

TABLE 15.1 TYPES OF GLOMERULONEPHRITIS

Disease	Common Clinical Presentation
IgA nephropathy and Henoch–Schönlein purpura	Microscopic hematuria, subnephrotic proteinuria
Lupus nephritis	Microscopic hematuria, proteinuria, nephritic syndrome, nephrotic syndrome
Membranoproliferative glomerulonephritis	Nephritic syndrome
Dense deposit disease	Nephritic syndrome
Cryoglobulinemia	Nephritic syndrome
Infection associated glomerulonephritis	Nephritic syndrome
Minimal change disease	Nephrotic syndrome
Focal segmental glomerulosclerosis	Nephrotic syndrome
Membranous glomerulonephritis	Nephrotic syndrome
Amyloidosis	Nephrotic syndrome
Fibrillary/immunotactoid glomerulonephritis	Nephrotic syndrome
Wegener's granulomatosis	Rapidly progressive glomerulonephritis
Microscopic polyangiitis	Rapidly progressive glomerulonephritis
Goodpasture disease	Rapidly progressive glomerulonephritis

Clinicopathologic Patterns of Injury

The glomerulus is a highly organized structure, and immunologic glomerular injury generally falls into one of several morphologic patterns. Patients with glomerular disease also tend to present with clinical findings that fit into one of several syndromes. Diseases of varying etiologies may cause glomerular injury with similar morphologic and clinical findings. Conversely, patients with the same underlying disease, such as systemic lupus erythematosus (SLE), may present with different clinical and pathologic patterns of injury. In general, the clinical findings are insufficient to accurately diagnose and treat glomerular diseases and a renal biopsy is necessary. Renal biopsies are processed for evaluation of the tissue by light microscopy, electron microcscopy, and immunofluorescence microscopy in order to fully classify the morphologic features of the disease. Various special stains can also be used to distinguish particular diseases.

The glomerular diseases are associated with several clinical syndromes. The nephrotic syndrome (see also Chapter 14) is usually defined as >3 to 3.5 g of proteinuria per day. Patients with the nephrotic syndrome usually have hypoalbuminemia, edema, and hypercholesterolemia. The urine of patients with the nephrotic syndrome does not typically contain dysmorphic red blood cells or red blood cell casts. Patients with the nephrotic syndrome are at increased risk of venous thrombosis and infection. Diseases causing subnephrotic range proteinuria (<3 g of proteinuria per day) may pose a significant threat to the patient, but they are less likely to develop symptoms of the nephrotic syndrome. The nephritic syndrome often refers to disease presenting with hematuria, proteinuria, and dysmorphic red blood cells or red blood cell casts. Proteinuria is usually present, but can range subnephrotic levels to >10 g per day. Depending upon the extent of glomerular involvement, patients may develop hypertension, edema and/or renal insufficiency. As will be discussed in detail later, there is great heterogeneity in the presentation of the glomerular diseases. Thus, disease etiologies commonly described as presenting with one of these syndromes may present with variable constellations of signs and symptoms.

IMMUNE COMPLEXES

Numerous cellular and molecular mechanisms of glomerular injury have been identified, but immune-complex (IC) mediated injury warrants additional attention since the glomerulus is a common site for IC deposition. The size and charge of ICs is a function of several factors, including the nature of the antigen (which is unknown in most forms of GN), the isotype of the antibodies and their affinity for the antigen, and the relative abundance of antigen and antibody. Circulating ICs may be trapped in the glomerulus, a process that could be enhanced by the large flow of plasma through the kidneys, high intraglomerular pressures, permeable capillary walls, and an anionic basement membrane that can bind cationic antigens (2). These ICs will tend to accumulate in the mesangium and subendothelial space since they are too large to pass through the GBM. ICs may also form in situ when antibodies bind to antigens that are expressed within the glomerulus or that become trapped there. Depending on the antigen in question, these ICs may be located anywhere in the glomerulus. It has recently been reported, for example, that antibodies to the M-type phospholipase A2 receptor (a protein present on podocytes) are present in a substantial portion of patients with idiopathic MN (3). In situ IC formation may lead to deposition between the GBM and the podocytes, and identification of the antigen in various IC-mediated renal diseases will be instrumental in understanding the disease process.

ICs trigger the generation of several pro-inflammatory factors. They activate complement, thereby generating C5a and the membrane attack complex. They also trigger the release of numerous other pathologic factors by resident or infiltrating cells, including chemokines, prostaglandins, platelet-activating factor, procoagulant factors, and adhesion molecules. Many of these molecules are involved in leukocytes trafficking to the site of inflammation, and infiltrating polymorphonuclear neutrophils (PMNs), macrophages, and T cells then release additional factors that also contribute to tissue injury.

- *Mesangial IC deposition—mesangial expansion—hematuria and proteinuria.* Several diseases, such as IgA nephropathy and lupus nephritis, are associated with the deposition of ICs in the mesangium (Fig. 15.1). Mesangial IC deposition is associated with development of hematuria and proteinuria, but nephrotic range proteinuria and significant changes in the glomerular filtration rate (GFR) are not typically seen. Injury of the mesangial cells stimulates the cells to proliferate and to produce extracellular matrix. Over time this can lead to glomerular sclerosis and irreversible renal injury.
- *Subendothelial IC deposition—endovascular proliferation—nephritic syndrome.* In diseases such as lupus, postinfectious GN, and MPGN, ICs deposit in the subendothelial space (Fig. 15.2). The complement activation fragments and inflammatory factors generated at this location have access to the circulation and tend to cause an inflammatory lesion. Subendothelial ICs cause endocapillary proliferation, where the glomerular capillaries appear hypercellular and are filled with inflammatory and

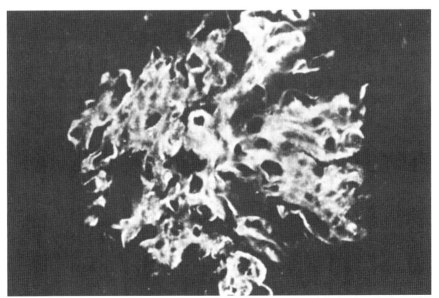

■ **Figure 15.1** Fluorescent-antibody study, showing diffuse, coarse immunoglobulin deposits located predominantly in the glomerular mesangium. This finding is characteristic of a large group of diseases that often demonstrate focal or diffuse mesangial proliferative glomerulonephritis by light microscopy, including IgA nephropathy.

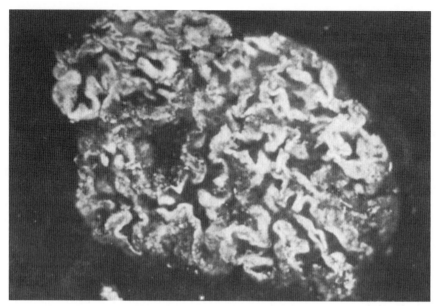

■ **Figure 15.2** Fluorescent-antibody study of the glomerulus, demonstrating discrete granular deposition of immunoglobulin along the basement membrane, which is characteristic of immune complex–mediated glomerulopathies. The immune complexes contained within the granular deposits may have deposited from the circulation *or* formed locally (in situ) as a consequence of interaction of a circulating antibody with a native glomerular capillary wall antigen or an extrinsic antigen planted in the glomerulus because of an affinity for constituents of the capillary wall.

endothelial cells. Clinically, patients with these diseases commonly present with the nephritic syndrome. The extent of glomerular involvement tends to correlate with disease severity (e.g., diffuse involvement causes a greater decline in GFR than focal), but clinical parameters are an unreliable guide to the severity of the underlying lesion.

The endothelial cell is also the primary target in diseases in which ICs are not seen. In small vessel vasculitis, for example, patients may present with a nephritic syndrome. Although they appear "pauci-immune" on biopsy, antibodies probably play a critical role in the pathogenesis of these diseases (vide infra). The thrombotic microangiopathies may also cause endothelial injury and signs of acute GN.

• *Subepithelial IC deposition—Podocyte injury—Nephrotic syndrome.* The podocyte is a highly differentiated cell that forms an important part of the glomerular filtration apparatus. The podocyte has branches that terminate in foot processes that are anchored to the GBM. The foot processes of adjacent cells interdigitate, and they are separated from each other by a slit diaphragm. ICs that form in a subepithelial location (i.e., between the podocyte and the GBM) can injure the podocyte, disrupt the slit diaphragm apparatus, and cause foot process effacement. Clinically, patients with subepithelial ICs present with the nephrotic syndrome (Table 15.2) and with a membranous pattern on biopsy. The inflammatory factors generated by subepithelial ICs are probably excreted in the urine and do not cause leukocyte infiltration or hypercellularity (Fig. 15.3). Consequently, hematuria, pyuria, and cellular casts will typically not be present.

• *Crescentic renal disease—rapidly progressive glomerulonephritis (RPGN).* Glomerular crescents are extra-capillary aggregates that form in Bowman's space and compress the capillary tuft (Fig. 15.4). They are composed of cells (proliferating parietal epithelial cells, infiltrating monocytes, and fibroblasts) and fibrous material. Crescents may be seen in many types of immune-mediated glomerular disease, including anti-GBM disease, IC-mediated GN, and pauci-immune small vessel vasculitis (Table 15.3). It is believed that crescent formation starts with severe inflammatory injury of the capillary wall that allows cells and plasma proteins into Bowman's space. Biopsies in which >25% to 50% of the glomeruli have crescents are often referred to as "crescentic," regardless of the

TABLE 15.2 FREQUENTLY SEEN CLINICOPATHOLOGIC CORRELATIONS IN PATIENTS WITH GLOMERULONEPHRITIS

Pathologic Findings	Syndrome	Diseases
Mesangial immune complexes/mesangial proliferation and expansion	Microscopic hematuria, subnephrotic proteinuria	IgA nephropathy, lupus nephritis
Subendothelial immune complexes/endocapillary proliferation	Nephritic syndrome	MPGN, lupus nephritis
Subepithelial immune complexes/ thickened appearance of glomerular basement membrane	Nephrotic syndrome	Membranous disease, lupus nephritis
Glomerular crescents. May be associated with linear Ig deposited along the GBM, pauci-immune GN, or subendothelial ICs.	Rapidly progressive glomerulonephritis	Goodpasture disease, ANCA associated vasculitis lupus nephritis, MPGN

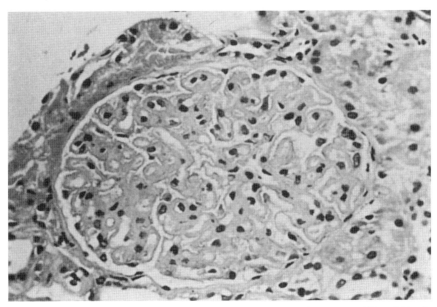

■ **Figure 15.3** Light-microscopic appearance of membranous glomerulonephritis. Note diffuse thickening of the capillary walls without associated inflammatory response.

disease etiology, and this finding is associated with a rapid loss of renal function, oliguria, and signs of acute GN.

TUBULOINTERSTITIAL FIBROSIS

Tubulointerstitial injury is common in disease processes regarded as primarily targeting the glomeruli. Tubulointerstitial injury often correlates better with renal function than the glomerular lesion, and the degree of tubulointerstitial fibrosis is also predictive of the long-term outcome in patients with glomerular disease (4). The glomerular capillaries and the peritubular capillaries are arranged as sequential capillary beds. Glomerular diseases can therefore reduce blood flow to the peritubular capillaries. There is also experimental evidence that altered permselectivity at the glomerulus allows factors into the ultrafiltrate that can harm the downstream tubular epithelial cells, including transferrin and complement proteins. These may be common processes that are important to the progression of glomerular diseases of different etiologies.

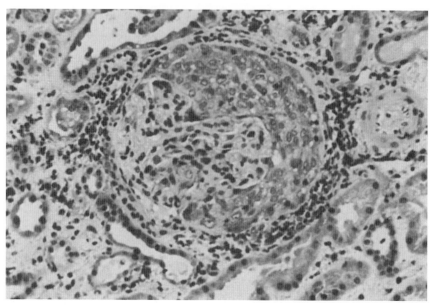

■ **Figure 15.4** Light-microscopic findings characteristic of crescentic glomerulonephritis. Note necrotizing glomerulonephritis with marked extracapillary reaction, including crescent and periglomerular fibrosis.

TABLE 15.3 CAUSES OF CRESCENTIC GLOMERULONEPHRITIS

Primary

Anti-glomerular basement membrane antibody mediated

Immune complex mediated

"Pauci-immune" (antineutrophil cytoplasmic antibody associated)

Membranous glomerulonephritis

Membranoproliferative glomerulonephritis

Dense deposit disease

IgA nephropathy

Secondary

Infectious diseases

  Infective endocarditis, poststreptococcal glomerulonephritis, visceral sepsis, hepatitis B

Multisystem disease

  Systemic lupus erythematosus, Goodpasture disease, Henoch–Schönlein purpura, microscopic polyangiitis, Wegener's granulomatosis, cryoglobulinemia, relapsing polychondritis, malignancy

Drug associated

  Allopurinol, rifampicin, ᴅ-penicillamine

Important Clinical Scenarios

PULMONARY-RENAL SYNDROME

As will be discussed later, diseases such as Goodpasture disease and Wegener's granulomatosis can simultaneously affect the lung and the kidneys. Severe pneumonia can also present with renal failure, and patients with the sepsis syndrome or congestive heart failure frequently have both pulmonary and renal involvement. Given the importance of early treatment for patients with Goodpasture disease or small vessel vasculitis, however, patients presenting with acute disease of the lungs and kidneys should receive close scrutiny. Proteinuria, an active urine sediment, or serologic evidence of vasculitis may be useful for identifying the underlying etiology, but a renal biopsy may be necessary for definitive diagnosis.

GLOMERULAR DISEASE IN THE CANCER PATIENT

Several types of glomerular disease have been associated with underlying tumors. Overall, the incidence of glomerular disease in cancer patients is rare, but cancer may be found relatively frequently in certain groups of patients with glomerular disease. For example, solid tumors may be found in 23% of patients over 60 years old who are diagnosed with MN (5), and basic cancer screening (e.g., chest X-ray, screening for occult blood in the stool, and colonoscopy) is warranted. A high incidence of solid tumors has also been found in older patients with IgA nephropathy (6). Hodgkin disease is associated with minimal change disease (MCD), and non-Hodgkin lymphoma has been associated with several types of glomerular disease including crescentic GN. Monoclonal immunoglobulin deposition diseases of the kidney are frequently caused by underlying lymphoproliferative diseases and are discussed in detail below.

GLOMERULAR DISEASE IN THE PREGNANT PATIENT

The normal pregnancy is associated with several changes in renal physiology (see Chapter 12). Reports have suggested that pregnancy may cause exacerbations of renal disease in patients with chronic GN of several different etiologies. Given the prevalence of lupus nephritis in women of childbearing age, flares of lupus nephritis are relatively common. There are also reports suggesting that pregnancy may cause hypertension or disease flares in patients with pre-existing IgA nephropathy, MPGN, and FSGS. In all of these diseases, however, there is conflicting data as to whether pregnancy actually increases the likelihood of a disease flare or whether these reports simply reflect a coincident worsening of disease during pregnancy. The degree of proteinuria often increases during pregnancy, but this is a result of hemodynamic changes and does not indicate a worsening of the renal disease. Regardless of the disease etiology, pre-existing hypertension or renal insufficiency are risk factors for complications of the pregnancy. Preeclampsia and HELLP (hemolysis, elevated liver enzymes, and low platelets) syndrome are glomerular diseases of pregnancy. These conditions can be difficult to distinguish from the exacerbation of a pre-existing glomerular disease, such as lupus. This distinction is made harder by the fact that pre-existing renal disease is a risk factor for preeclampsia.

General Treatment Strategies

The glomerular diseases share many pathogenetic mechanisms—such as engagement of elements of the innate and adaptive immune systems—and our understanding of the molecular pathogenesis of this diverse group of disorders is constantly growing. Nevertheless, the commonly used therapies usually have broad effects on the overall function of the immune system (Table 15.4). Newer biologic therapies are being developed, however, that offer the possibility of a more targeted approach to the treatment of these diseases. General treatments aimed at controlling the blood pressure and reducing proteinuria are also important for maintaining renal health, even in diseases regarded as being autoimmune in origin.

Primary (Idiopathic) Glomerulopathies

MINIMAL CHANGE DISEASE

MCD, otherwise known as Nil (Nothing-In-Light microscopy) disease or lipoid nephrosis, accounts for 10% to 15% of primary nephrotic syndrome in adults in industrialized countries (7); it is the most common cause of nephrotic syndrome in children. Experts continue to debate whether MCD is its own disease or whether it exists as part of a continuum with FSGS.

In adults, MCD is diagnosed by kidney biopsy. Few if any changes are seen on light microscopy, and immunofluorescence is also usually unremarkable. Electron microscopy shows extensive podocyte foot

TABLE 15.4 DRUGS COMMONLY USED TO TREAT GLOMERULAR DISEASES

Immunomodulatory Agents	Proposed Mechanism of Action
Glucocorticoids	Steroids suppress B-cell and T-cell functions. High doses appear to act in part by inducing the synthesis of IκBa, a protein that traps and thereby inactivates NF-κB thereby decreasing cytokine generation. Steroids may also have cell membrane effects altering the action of membrane bound proteins and receptors.
Cyclophosphamide	An alkylating agent that covalently binds and crosslinks DNA, RNA, and proteins leading to either cell death or altered cellular function. Cyclophosphamide causes neutropenia and lymphopenia.
Mycophenolic acid	Inhibits T and B cell proliferation by blocking purine synthesis via inhibition of inosine monophosphate dehydrogenase.
Cyclosporine/Tacrolimus	Inhibits the phosphatase calcineurin preventing the translocation of nuclear factor of activated T cells (NFAT) leading to reduced transcriptional activation of early cytokine genes. There is evidence that cyclosporine may also stabilize the actin cytoskeleton of podocytes maintaining podocyte function.
Rituximab	Murine/human chimeric anti-CD20 monoclonal antibody that depletes B cells.
Azathioprine	Inhibits T and B cell proliferation by blocking purine synthesis.
Chlorambucil	An alkylating agent that crosslinks DNA. It reduces the number of both B cells and T cells.
Plasma Exchange	Removes large molecular weight substances—autoantibodies, immune complexes, cryoglobulins, myeloma light chains—from the plasma. When replacement fluid is plasma, allows large volumes of plasma to be infused without the risk of intravascular volume overload.
Eculizumab	Monoclonal antibody to the complement protein C5. It blocks cleavage of C5, thereby preventing the formation of C5 and the membrane attack complex.
Nonimmunomodulatory Agents	
ACEI/ARBs	Decrease in intraglomerular pressure. May also have an antifibrotic effect.
Fish oil	Eicosapentaenoic acid (EPA) and docosahexaenoic acid (DHA) serve as substrates for cyclooxygenase and lipoxygenase pathways leading to less potent inflammatory mediators than those produced through the arachidonic acid pathway.
Pentoxifylline	Phosphodiesterase inhibitor that inhibits cell proliferation, inflammation, and extracellular matrix accumulation perhaps through suppressing tumor necrosis factor and other cytokines.

process retraction and effacement. These podocyte changes are not specific for MCD and it is important to exclude other pathologies when making the diagnosis. The lesion of early FSGS may be sparse and usually first appears in deeper glomeruli at the corticomedullary junction. The number of glomeruli obtained by biopsy is important for excluding other diseases. A biopsy with 10 glomeruli has a 35% chance of missing a focal lesion while a biopsy containing 20 glomeruli only has a 12% chance of missing a focal lesion (8). Thus sampling error may miss glomeruli affected by FSGS if <20 cortical glomeruli are obtained. Other rarer disorders may also appear normal by light microscopy, including C1q nephropathy, IgM nephropathy, and idiopathic mesangial proliferative GN. Immunofluorescence typically helps distinguish amongst these diseases.

Pathogenesis

MCD and FSGS are similar clinically and pathologically, and there is debate as to whether they are separate diseases or different ends of a single disease spectrum. Their origins are also, not surprisingly, thought to be similar and likely derive from an immunologic source. A role for T cells in the pathogenesis

TABLE 15.5 SELECTED CAUSES OF SECONDARY MINIMAL CHANGE DISEASE

Neoplasia	Hodgkin disease, non-Hodgkin lymphoma, pancreatic carcinoma, bronchogenic carcinoma, allergic and dysregulated immune responses
Drugs	NSAIDs, antibiotics, lithium, D-penicillamine

of MCD was first suspected in the 1970s, and some evidence has accumulated in recent decades to support this hypothesis. A T cell–derived soluble "permeability" factor, perhaps the Th-2 derived cytokine IL-13 (9), may impair the glomerular capillary wall or slit diaphragm's ability to exclude larger proteins.

Secondary Causes

Most cases of MCD are idiopathic; however, in a small population of patients a secondary cause can be found (Table 15.5). MCD has been associated with a number of drugs, malignancies, infections, environmental allergens, and other glomerular diseases.

Presentation

Adults typically present with mild renal impairment and the sudden onset of nephrotic syndrome, including proteinuria >3.5 g/24 h hypoalbuminemia, hyperlipidemia, and edema. Hypertension is common. Microscopic hematuria is not uncommon. In a recent retrospective review, 20% of patients had acute kidney injury (AKI) at the time of presentation (10).

Prognosis

The prognosis of adult onset MCD is generally good and is related to how patients respond to the initial treatment with steroids (see section on "Treatment"). In current clinical practice all patients are treated at the time of diagnosis; however, there are some older data that suggest a spontaneous remission rate of anywhere from 20% to 65% (11,12). Adults tend to respond to therapy more slowly than children, often requiring over 3 months of therapy before remission is detected (10,12). Over 70% of treated adults have a complete remission (10), but the relapse rate is common with almost 60% to 75% of patients having at least one relapse and 30% to 40% of patients having frequent relapses (10,12). Patients who present with AKI can typically expect to return to their baseline renal function with treatment. Progression to end-stage renal disease (ESRD) is uncommon in MCD but is reported in steroid resistant cases (12); however, subsequent biopsies may demonstrate FSGS that may be from progression of MCD or the original diagnosis that was missed by sampling error.

When children with MCD enter adulthood there is less known about their relapse rate and prognosis. One study found that among steroid sensitive children, young age at onset (<6 years) and more severe disease in childhood, indicated by a greater number of relapses and more frequent use of immunosuppressive drugs, were predictive of the occurrence of MCD relapse in adulthood when evaluated by univariate analysis. By multivariate analysis, only number of relapses during childhood was predictive of adulthood relapses (13).

Severe nephrotic syndrome has nonrenal-related complications as well, including thrombosis and infections (see Chapter 14). Complications arising from these disorders can also impact morbidity and mortality.

Treatment

There are no large, randomized controlled trials on treating adults with MCD. The majority of studies that have helped guide treatment are studies from the pediatric literature. Prednisone is the treatment of choice for adult MCD (14), with the majority of adults experiencing a complete remission by 3 months. Experts have different strategies for dosing prednisone, length of treatment, and tapering. Generally, prednisone is dosed at 1 mg/kg/day or 2 mg/kg every other day and continued for 2 months. If at 2 months complete remission has been obtained, the prednisone is slowly tapered. If at 2 months a remission has not occurred, then the high-dose daily prednisone is continued. If a remission has not been achieved by 4 months the patient is considered to be steroid resistant and other agents are required. Second-line agents typically used include cyclophosphamide, tacrolimus, cyclosporine, mycophenolate mofetil (MMF), and rituximab. Each agent has been shown to be useful in treating steroid dependent and steroid resistant patients; however, there are no adequately powered, randomized studies to help guide practitioners towards one treatment over another.

Relapses of MCD occur frequently. If patients responded well to prednisone during original treatment and there are no contraindications against more prednisone, then a shorter course of high-dose daily prednisone is usually tried. For frequent relapsers low dose prednisone over an extended period of time is a reasonable choice. Again, the second-line agents mentioned earlier have also been employed in treating frequently relapsing disease.

IgM NEPHROPATHY

IgM nephropathy is a rare disease that is characterized by the mesangial deposition of IgM and complement (15). Light microscopy may be normal or may show diffuse proliferation of mesangial cells and accumulation of mesangial matrix with varying degrees of sclerosis (15). Electron microscopy usually shows dense deposits in the mesangium. Experts argue as to whether IgM nephropathy is its own entity, or whether it is a variant of MCD or FSGS and that the IgM deposits are a secondary event. Patients usually present with nephrotic syndrome although patients with hematuria and asymptomatic proteinuria have been described (15). Patients with IgM nephropathy are less likely to respond to immunosuppressive agents when compared to patients with MCD (16).

C1q NEPHROPATHY

C1q nephropathy is another uncommon disorder that can be confused with MCD on light microscopy. By light microscopy, C1q nephropathy can present with no visible lesions, mesangial proliferation, FSGS, or a proliferative GN (17,18). Immunofluorescence demonstrates mesangial staining of C1q in all biopsies and mesangial IgG, IgM, and C3 in the majority of biopsies. IgA and C4 are not uncommon. Electron microscopy can show mesangial, subendothelial, and subepithelial deposits with or without foot process effacement (17). Patients present with the nephrotic syndrome and hematuria. Renal function is usually normal but there have been reports of renal insufficiency at diagnosis. There is debate as to whether C1q nephropathy is its own disease or if it is a variant of MCD or FSGS. Most treatment strategies are based on the histologic lesion. Those with an FSGS pattern of injury are more likely to progress to ESRD.

FOCAL SEGMENTAL GLOMERULOSCLEROSIS

FSGS is one of the most common causes of the nephrotic syndrome in the United States and is the most common primary GN listed as the cause for ESRD (19,20). It shares many features with minimal change disease and experts continue to debate whether the two processes are different diseases or whether FSGS is just a more severe form of minimal change disease. As with other glomerulonephritides, FSGS is a nonspecific pattern of injury diagnosed by renal biopsy. FSGS may be idiopathic or secondary. In order to make a diagnosis of idiopathic FSGS there must not be a history of any other glomerulonephritis, known systemic disease with possible glomerular involvement, or family history of FSGS (21). Secondary FSGS may be due to structural functional adaptations mediated by elevated glomerular pressure, genetic diseases, or as the final common histology of other glomerulonephritides.

FSGS has several morphologic variants that are seen with light microscopy. Generally, FSGS is characterized by the presence of some but not all glomeruli (focal) having segmental mesangial collapse and glomerular sclerosis with partial occlusion of the capillary loops by hyaline material. Hyalinosis, acellular material within the sclerotic area caused by the insudation of plasma proteins, used to be considered a specific histopathologic feature of FSGS but is now not a diagnostic necessity. Mild mesangial hypercellularity may be seen. Tubular atrophy and interstitial fibrosis is frequently present. Immunofluorescence microscopy is nonspecific and may demonstrate entrapment of IgM and C3 in sclerotic regions. Electron microscopy shows foot process effacement, but in secondary forms of FSGS the extent of effacement is usually less than in primary disease (22,23).

Five histologic variants of FSGS have been described: classic FSGS, collapsing variant, tip variant, perihilar variant, and the cellular variant (24). The different lesions have different presentations and responses to therapy. (see "Presentation" and "Prognosis" sections below) The collapsing variant shows segmental or global wrinkling and folding of the GBM with podocyte hypertrophy resembling pseudocrescents (25). The tip variant shows a lesion adjacent to the "tip" of the glomerulus, which is the area next to the proximal tubule (26). The perihilar variant consists of perihilar hyalinosis and sclerosis adjacent to the hilum of the glomerulus (26). This lesion is frequently observed in secondary FSGS thought to be due to increased capillary pressure at the hilum. The cellular variant shows segmental endocapillary hypercellularity that occludes the capillary lumen (21). The cellular lesion is very similar in appearance to the collapsing lesion and many pathologists make no distinction between the two variants (21). In a study examining the recurrence of FSGS in renal allografts, 81% of recurrences occurred in the same pattern as the original disease, giving credence to the different variants proposed (27).

Uninvolved glomeruli in FSGS show no lesions and one segmentally sclerosed glomerulus is sufficient to make the diagnosis of FSGS. Experts have concluded that it takes a biopsy containing 20 glomeruli to decrease the risk of missing glomeruli affected by FSGS by sampling error to approximately 10% (28). FSGS usually starts in the corticomedullary glomeruli so a biopsy should have adequate evaluation of this region.

Pathogenesis

The podocyte appears to be at the focal point of FSGS and injury to this resident renal cell likely initiates the process that leads to the FSGS pattern of injury. In idiopathic FSGS, as in MCD, a circulating permeability factor, perhaps a cytokine, has been implicated to trigger podocyte injury (29). This permeability factor has been blamed for the rapid onset of recurrent FSGS in newly transplanted kidneys.

Recently, the candidate gene *MYH9A*, which encodes a podocyte protein nonmuscle myosin IIA, has been shown to be linked with idiopathic and HIV-associated FSGS and may partly begin to explain the increased incidence of these diseases in African Americans. A number of other genetic forms of FSGS have been identified and are discussed in other sections of this chapter.

Podocyte injury is also likely the inciting event in secondary FSGS and is caused by the compensatory hypertrophy of functional glomeruli that occurs after other glomeruli are lost or injured (22). This hypertrophy causes podocyte connections to the basement membrane and to other podocytes to become diminished; this leads to podocyte detachment and loss. Inflammatory cell infiltration, extracellular matrix accumulation, resident renal cell proliferation, and cytokines then contribute to the sclerotic scar (30).

Secondary Causes

FSGS can occur secondary to a number of different disorders. These can be broken down as structural or functional adaptations, genetic diseases, viral infections, drugs, or as a final pattern of injury after another GN (Table 15.6).

Presentation

FSGS can occur in all age groups. It affects a disproportionate amount of African Americans. Patients with primary FSGS usually present with the acute onset of the nephrotic syndrome—peripheral edema, hypoalbuminemia, and nephrotic range proteinuria. Hypertension is common. Renal function may be

TABLE 15.6 SELECTED CAUSES OF SECONDARY FOCAL SEGMENTAL GLOMERULOSCLEROSIS

Viral	HIV, Parvovirus B19
Drugs	Pamidronate
Structural/functional adaptation to hyperfiltration or reduced renal mass	Reflux nephropathy, papillary necrosis, sickle cell disease, cholesterol embolization, unilateral renal agenesis, obesity, low birth weight
Other glomerular diseases	Minimal change disease, diabetic nephropathy, membranous nephropathy, healing phase of any inflammatory glomerular process

diminished at the time of diagnosis. Microhematuria is not uncommon. Secondary FSGS typically presents with nonnephrotic proteinuria, renal insufficiency, and hypertension.

Of the different variants, the tip and cellular/collapsing lesions frequently have a greater amount of proteinuria (31,32). The cellular/collapsing variants also usually have more severe renal dysfunction at presentation (31).

Prognosis

Untreated FSGS usually follows a progressive course leading to ESRD. Immunosuppressive treatment for idiopathic FSGS has a significant chance of improving outcomes if a partial or complete remission is obtained (33). Higher levels of proteinuria and increased serum creatinine at the time of diagnosis are predictive of lower renal survival. Histologic findings may also predict outcomes, and many experts believe that the "tip" variant is more responsive to therapy and thus more likely to have a favorable prognosis while the collapsing/cellular variant portends a poor prognosis. The amount of interstitial fibrosis, as in other renal diseases, also predicts poor renal survival. Idiopathic FSGS can return in renal allografts.

Treatment

Only patients with idiopathic FSGS should be treated with immunosuppressive medications, and those patients with idiopathic FSGS and nephrotic range proteinuria are almost universally offered aggressive therapy, although discretion should be taken with those patients who have significant renal dysfunction. There are no large, randomized, placebo-controlled trials investigating the best initial treatment for idiopathic FSGS; however, most experts agree that an initial trial of prednisone (1 mg/kg) for at least 16 weeks followed by a taper based on patient response is the best initial strategy (34). Although the criteria can vary, a complete response is often defined as a reduction in proteinuria to <300 mg/day, and a partial response is often defined as at least a 50% reduction in proteinuria. Published reports indicate that close to half of those treated will have at least a partial response to therapy (33). In patients who cannot tolerate high-dose steroids, cyclosporine with low-dose prednisone has been shown to be effective, but the relapse rate is high.

Relapsing FSGS manifested by nephrotic range proteinuria after either a complete or partial remission is often treated with another round of steroids if the side effects were minimal during the first period of treatment. If steroid side effects were significant, cyclosporine and low dose prednisone are recommended. FSGS is considered steroid dependent if a patient relapses while on therapy. Steroid resistant FSGS is defined by little or no reduction in proteinuria after 12 to 16 weeks of adequate prednisone therapy or if the criteria for partial remission are not met.

Experts recommend that both steroid-dependent and steroid-resistant FSGS be treated with cyclosporine combined with low-dose prednisone (35,36). Other agents have been used and reported on for refractory disease; however, the data are sparse and mainly consist of observational reports. For patients who have failed other therapies or who should not be exposed to cyclosporine, MMF has been shown to be effective in the small number of patients who have been studied (37).

Nonimmunosupprisive therapy with renin–angiotensin–aldosterone system (RAAS) inhibitors (e.g., angiotensin-converting enzyme inhibitors or angiotensin receptor blockers) should be used in all patients with idiopathic or secondary FSGS. Blood pressure should be well controlled. Lipids should be managed with statin medications.

MEMBRANOUS NEPHROPATHY

MN is one of the most common causes of the nephrotic syndrome. In the majority of cases the etiology is unknown and is termed "idiopathic." MN is diagnosed by kidney biopsy. The characteristic histologic lesion on light microscopy is diffuse thickening of the GBM, with lesions usually affecting all glomeruli. The glomeruli may appear normal by light microscopy early in the course of the disease. Chronic sclerosing glomerular and tubulointerstitial changes develop as the disease progresses. Immunofluorescence shows a diffuse granular pattern of IgG and C3 staining along the GBM. Electron microscopy demonstrates subepithelial electron dense deposits, effacement of the podocyte foot processes, and expansion of the GBM. Advanced disease may have the presence of "spikes" of membrane interdigitating between immune deposits.

Making a distinction between idiopathic MN and secondary MN can be challenging. There are certain clues on biopsy that can be helpful. In idiopathic MN, electron dense deposits on EM are almost exclusively subepithelial and intramembranous (38). Secondary forms of MN are often associated with mesangial and/or subendothelial deposits, which suggest a circulating IC (38). Tubular basement membrane staining for IgG on immunofluorescence is rare in idiopathic MN, but is common in secondary forms such as SLE (38).

Pathogenesis

MN is an IC-mediated disease as evidenced by the presence of subepithelial ICs visualized by immunofluorescence and electron microscopy. The Heymann model of nephritis induced in rats has led most experts to believe that idiopathic MN is due to the in situ formation of ICs as a consequence of circulating antibody interacting with antigens either planted in the subepithelial compartment or occurring their naturally. The antigen in idiopathic MN is still uncertain, but recent work suggests that it may be the phospholipase A2 receptor (3). Cases have also been reported in which neutral endopeptidase (NEP), an enzyme present on podocyte cell surfaces, has acted as a target antigen for anti-NEP antibodies that crossed the placenta and caused MN in infants (39).

Subepithelial ICs in MN are largely out of the way of direct contact with capillary blood supply, although complement is activated by the ICs. Activation of the classical and alternative pathways of complement causes podocyte injury via the sublytic action of the membrane attack complex (C5b-9) inserted into podocyte membranes. The membrane attack complex stimulates podocytes to produce inflammatory mediators that impair the filtration barrier leading to proteinuria (40).

Secondary Causes

Secondary causes of MN represent 25% to 35% of all patients, with a slightly higher prevalence in children and older adults [Table 15.7, (41)]. In 85% of secondary causes, the etiology can be attributed to infections, neoplasia, or lupus (41). Infections that have been reported to cause MN include hepatitis B, hepatitis C, HIV, syphilis, schistosomiasis, and malaria (38). A minority of older adults with MN have an associated cancer, usually a solid tumor and less frequently a hematologic malignancy (38). The list of medications and toxic agents associated with MN is long and includes penicillamine, gold salts, NSAIDs, captopril, anti-tumor necrosis factor (TNF) agents, mercury, and formaldehyde (38). The mechanisms responsible for drug-induced MN are uncertain. Hematopoietic cell transplantation and graft-versus-host-disease can also cause MN. De novo MN can occur in transplanted kidneys. In addition, there are a number of case reports attributing several other disease states to MN, including sarcoidosis and other autoimmune diseases like Sjögren syndrome and thyroid disease (38).

Presentation

MN affects patients of all ages but has a peak incidence in the fourth to fifth decade. All ethnic groups can be affected. The diagnosis is made in more men than women in a 2:1 ratio (42). Almost 70% of patients present with the nephrotic syndrome as evidenced by severe proteinuria, low albumin, and edema (43). Lipid abnormalities are common. The rest of patients present with subnephrotic range or asymptomatic proteinuria. The onset of clinical symptoms is usually gradual perhaps matching the rate of membranous

TABLE 15.7 SELECTED CAUSES OF SECONDARY MEMBRANOUS DISEASE

Neoplasia	Lung, colon, breast, stomach, bladder, thyroid, prostate, pancreas, kidney, malignant melanoma, Hodgkin disease, non-Hodgkin's lymphoma, CLL
Infection	Hepatitis B, Hepatitis C, HIV, malaria, Schistosomiasis, syphilis, filariasis
Autoimmune disease	Lupus, rheumatoid arthritis, mixed connective tissue disease, Sjøgren disease
Drugs	NSAIDs, gold, penicillamine, captopril, probenicid, clopidogrel, anti-TNF agents
Other systemic disease	Sarcoidosis, sickle cell disease, hematopoietic stem cell transplantation
Other renal diseases	Polycycstic kidney disease

deposit formation. Microscopic hematuria is common but macroscopic hematuria and red blood cell casts are rare (43). Renal function is usually normal at diagnosis. Only a minority of patients have hypertension at the time of diagnosis. Serum complement levels are usually normal. In patients with secondary MN other clinical or laboratory findings may be present that are attributable to the primary disease process. In patients with an underlying malignancy, almost half had a known cancer diagnosis at the time of renal biopsy while the rest had a MN diagnosis before any cancer diagnosis (44). Work up of an adult patient with MN should include age appropriate cancer screens or a direct evaluation of symptoms if present. MN has also been well documented to occur concurrently with other glomerular diseases, including diabetes, IgA, FSGS, and crescentic glomerulonephritis.

Prognosis

Spontaneous complete or partial remission of proteinuria occurs in approximately 50% to 60% of patients within 5 years. The remainder of untreated patients develop progressive renal insufficiency over the next 15 years (45,46). Clinical predictors that signal an increased risk of progressive renal decline include age >50 years, male sex, protein excretion >8 g/24 h, and an increased serum creatinine at presentation (47,48). Histologic findings that may be associated with risk of progression are glomerular scarring and the severity of the tubulointerstitial disease at the time of biopsy (49). Urine excretion ratios of several proteins (IgM, IgG, β-2-microglobulin) have been investigated as a way to predict outcome of MN, but these tests are not widely available. Given the toxicity of available medications used to treat MN and the difficulty in establishing what patient group to treat, the Toronto Glomerulonephritis Registry established a model to help classify patients by risk (47). Patients who present with normal renal function, proteinuria <4 g/24 h, and stable renal function over a 6-month observation period have excellent long-term prognosis and are considered low risk. Patients with normal renal function at diagnosis that remains stable over 6 months but who have between 4 and 8 g /24 h of proteinuria are considered medium risk and have a 55% chance of developing progressive renal insufficiency. Patients with persistent proteinuria >8 g/24 h, independent of renal function, have close to an 80% chance of progressing and are considered high risk. Patients who were never nephrotic or who obtain a complete remission have good long-term renal survival. A partial remission also predicts improved long-term outcome (50).

Treatment

All patients with MN should be on an RAAS inhibitor for both blood pressure and proteinuria control. Lipids should be controlled. As described above, the decision to initiate immunosuppressive therapy treatment for MN should be based on the patient's risk for progressive renal decline. Low-risk patients should have continual monitoring but most experts do not recommend disease specific therapy. Moderate-risk patients who have not improved their degree of proteinuria to <4 g/24 h over the observation period should be started on immunosuppressive therapy. Available options include a cyclophosphamide/steroid regimen and calcineurin/steroid based protocols (46,51,52). The cyclophosphamide/steroid regimen typically consists of 6 months of therapy. Steroids are administered in months 1, 3, and 5, and cyclophosphamide is administered in months 2, 4, and 6. If patients do not respond to the initial therapy, most experts then recommend trying the alternative regimen. High-risk patients are initiated on treatment if there is no improvement in protein excretion after only 3 months or if renal function is reduced and thought secondary to MN. Again, the choices for treatment primarily include a cyclophosphamide/steroid or calcineurin/steroid protocol (46,51–53).

Relapse of MN, as evidenced by an increase in proteinuria after a remission, occurs in approximately 30% of patients treated with cyclophosphamide-based protocols and 40% of those treated with calcineurin inhibitors. There is not a consensus on how to treat relapses, but the decision is generally between retreating the patient with the original protocol versus attempting the other protocol. Decisions are based on how well the patient tolerated the first round and if other side effects can be minimized.

Resistant MN is disease that fails to respond to both cyclophosphamide-based and calcineurin inhibitor-based regimens. Again, there is no clear consensus to what the next step in therapy should be.

Rituximab has been shown to be beneficial in resistant MN (54). Studies using MMF have also been done with varying results (55,56).

In patients with secondary MN, cessation of the offending drug or effective treatment of the underlying disease is usually associated with improvement in the nephrotic syndrome.

MEMBRANOPROLIFERATIVE GLOMERULONEPHRITIS

MPGN is defined by its morphologic characteristics on renal biopsy. Typically there is mesangial expansion and hypercellularity, causing a lobular appearance of the glomerular tuft (57–59). Mesangial interposition into the walls of the capillaries causes the GBM to split, causing reduplication of the GBM and a "double contour" best seen with silver–methanamine–period acid–Schiff stains. Mesangial interposition into the capillary wall and subendothelial IC deposits cause thickening of the capillary wall. C3 deposits in the capillary loops are virtually always seen by immunofluorescence microscopy, and granular deposits of IgG are also usually seen.

Two histologic variants of MPGN have been described in the literature based on electron microscopy. The pathognomonic feature of MPGN type II is the presence of electron-dense deposits in the GBM (60). MPGN type II may have a similar appearance as MPGN type I by light microscopy, but other morphologic patterns are also seen (61). It has been proposed that this disease is distinct from MPGN type I and should be referred to as dense deposit disease [DDD, (1)]. DDD will be discussed separately in the subsequent section of this chapter. A pattern of glomerular injury that is similar to MPGN type I but with abundant subepithelial immune-complex deposits and rupture of the GBM has been termed "MPGN Type III" (62,63). MPGN type III may simply represent a related variant of MPGN type I (62).

Type I MPGN is a rare form of primary GN, and this pattern of glomerular injury may also be caused by IC deposition in patients with chronic infections, cryoglobulinemia, autoimmune disease, malignancy, and sickle cell disease (Table 15.5). This morphologic pattern of injury has also been termed mesangiocapillary glomerulonephritis (64). MPGN typically occurs in children or young adults and accounts for approximately 5% of GN.

Pathogenesis

Circulating ICs are commonly detected in patients with MPGN (65). Immune-complex deposition in the subendothelial space and in the mesangium is probably critical to the development of both the primary and secondary forms of MPGN type I. The ICs activate complement and immunoglobulin receptors (Fc receptors) triggering the recruitment of neutrophils and monocytes. Activated inflammatory cells release reactive oxygen species and proteases. These factors and complement activation fragments can directly damage the capillary wall. Platelets may also accumulate and contribute to glomerular injury by releasing chemotactic factors and growth factors. Patients with MPGN often have low platelet levels and a shortened platelet lifespan, supporting a role of platelets in this disease (66). Cytokines and growth factors may induce proliferation of mesangial cells and the production of mesangial matrix.

Patients with MPGN type I are frequently hypocomplementemic (58). This may reflect consumption of classical pathway components (e.g., C3 and C4) by the ICs. Congenital deficiency of classical pathway components may also predispose patients to IC disease due to impaired solubilization and clearance of ICs (67). An autosomal dominant pattern of transmission of MPGN has been identified in one family (68), and the disease was linked with the area on chromosome 1q, which contains the genes for the complement regulatory proteins. One of these proteins, complement receptor 1, is also critical for IC clearance. Thus, genetic variation in a patient's ability to clear ICs and to regulate complement activation by ICs in the glomerulus likely influences the development of disease.

It seems likely that the mechanisms of glomerular injury in primary and secondary MPGN are similar, but that the antigens are distinct. The identity of the antigen in idiopathic MPGN is not known. The incidence of idiopathic MPGN type I has been decreasing in recent decades (18,69). It is possible that part of the decline of idiopathic MPGN is due to improved diagnosis of secondary causes, such as MPGN caused by hepatitis C and cryoglobulins. Future studies may identify new infectious causes for what is currently considered idiopathic disease. A dysregulated immune response to endogenous antigens may also explain the disease in some patients (70).

TABLE 15.8 SELECTED CAUSES OF SECONDARY MEMBRANOPROLIFERATIVE GLOMERULONEPHRITIS

Autoimmune disease	Lupus, Sjögren syndrome, rheumatoid arthritis, genetic mutations in complement regulatory proteins
Neoplasia	Plasma cell dyscrasias, leukemia, lymphoma, melanoma
Infection	Chronic bacterial infections, Hepatitis C, Hepatitis B, HIV, Coxsackie virus, Epstein–Barr virus

Secondary Factors

As described above, a pattern of injury on light microscopy similar to idiopathic MPGN may be seen in patients with infectious, autoimmune, and malignant disorders (Table 15.8). Many cases that once would have been regarded as "idiopathic" MPGN are now recognized as being caused by Hepatitis C, and many other systemic diseases are associated with this pattern of glomerular injury. In most of these diseases, the glomerular injury is due to persistent IC formation. This may be due to infections that persist in spite of a humoral immune response, autoimmune diseases in which antibodies to endogenous antigens form ICs, or hematologic malignancies.

Presentation

Patients with MPGN can present with a nephritic syndrome, nephrotic syndrome, and sometimes with an RPGN. Patients presenting with nephritic features usually have microscopic hematuria, but episodes of macroscopic hematuria can occur. Idiopathic MPGN is generally a renal limited disease, but patients often have fatigue, anorexia, and weight loss. Hypertension and anemia are also seen in many patients. Complement levels are frequently depressed in patients with MPGN type I. C3 levels are low in approximately 70% of the patients, and C4 levels are also frequently low.

Prognosis

The course and natural history of untreated MPGN are variable. A minority of patients may have spontaneous remissions, but most have persistent proteinuria. The renal function can slowly decline, and there may also be periods of rapid deterioration. Untreated, renal survival is approximately 50% at 10 years (71). Because of the variable course of MPGN type I and the small size of clinical trials, it is difficult to assess whether treatment of the disease significantly improves the outcome. Uncontrolled studies in children, however, suggest that treatment may improve the long-term outcomes, with 10-year renal survival reaching 75% (72). Factors that may predict a worse prognosis include nephrotic range proteinuria, tubulointerstitial fibrosis on biopsy, and renal dysfunction 1 year after diagnosis (73).

Treatment

Patients should receive nonspecific therapies such as control of the blood pressure, and RAAS inhibitors should be used in patients with proteinuria. Complications of the nephrotic syndrome should also be treated. Uncontrolled studies in children suggest that treatment with corticosteroids may improve the outcome of MPGN type I, although not all authors agree that the risks of treatment are justified given the limited efficacy data. Patients can be treated with 40 mg/m^2 of prednisone on alternate days. In patients with severe disease, the high dose can be maintained for 2 years, and then tapered to 20 mg/m^2 and maintained for prolonged periods. There is less evidence for the efficacy of prednisone in adults, but in patients with severe disease, a 6-month course of prednisone (1 mg/kg/day) can be tried. Antiplatelet agents, such as aspirin and dipyridamole, may be of benefit (74). There are not controlled trials to support the use of cytotoxic agents in patients with MPGN. There are several reported cases of steroid-resistant MPGN that were successfully treated with mycophenolate, but no randomized trials of this agent have been performed.

DENSE DEPOSIT DISEASE

Dense deposit disease refers to glomerular disease associated with electron dense deposits in the GBM or electron dense transformation of the GBM (61). Originally DDD was regarded as a variant of MPGN and was referred to as MPGN type II. Accumulating evidence indicates that MPGN is caused by distinct mechanisms (1), however, and kidneys that demonstrate dense deposits by EM (the pathognomonic feature of DDD) do not always have an MPGN pattern by light microscopy (61).

C3 nephritic factor (C3NeF) is an autoantibody that stabilizes the alternative complement pathway C3 convertase, thus amplifying complement activation through this pathway. Greater than 85% of patients with DDD have detectable C3NeF, and >80% of DDD patients with active disease have decreased levels of circulating C3. The pathogenicity of C3NeF is however controversial because C3NeF is not specific to this disease and the titers of C3NeF do not correlate with disease activity or with prognosis (75). Nevertheless, there is now compelling genetic and animal data demonstrating that unregulated activation of the alternative pathway of complement is central to the development of DDD. In some patients, mutations in factor H (a circulating protein that regulates the alternative pathway) are associated with disease. In patients with C3NeF it is possible that the antibody causes uncontrolled activation of the alternative pathway. Elegant work using animal models indicates that the C3b metabolites formed during uncontrolled fluid phase complement activation (iC3b, C3c, C3dg) deposit on the GBM and cause the renal lesion (76). In renal biopsies from patients with DDD the pattern of C3 deposition can vary, but abundant C3 activation fragments are invariably present. In renal biopsies from patients with DDD the pattern of C3 deposition can vary, but C3 activation fragments are invariably present (61).

DDD currently has a very poor prognosis, with >50% of patients progressing to ESRD within 10 years of their diagnosis (1). Therapy for the disease includes plasma exchange, particularly for those patients with mutations in circulating complement regulatory proteins or who are positive for C3NeF, and other nonspecific treatments such as RAAS inhibition (77). Based upon current understanding of the disease pathogenesis, complement inhibitors hold promise as effective therapies for the disease.

IgA NEPHROPATHY

IgA nephropathy (IgAN) is an IC disease that is the most common form of GN in the world. In the United States and Western Europe, IgA accounts for 10% to 30% of GN, while in China, Japan, and Korea IgA causes close to 50% of GNs (78,79).

IgAN is diagnosed by renal biopsy. There have been attempts to use serum and urine markers to predict a diagnosis of IgA, including the serum IgA/C3 ratio (80), urine proteomics (81), and serum galactose deficient IgA levels (82); however, no large scale studies have been performed to determine if these are sufficiently sensitive and/or specific to reliably aid in making the diagnosis of IgAN. IgA nephropathy can have any of the histologic phenotypes of IC-mediated GN (83), including no lesion by light microscopy, mesangioproliferative GN, proliferative GN, crescentic GN, etc. There are several classification systems that have been established to categorize the light microscopy findings, including those developed by Lee and Haas (84,85). A classification system similar to the World Health Organization's (WHO) system for lupus has also been used. It is uncertain whether these classification systems are helpful in predicting prognosis or guiding treatment decisions (86).

The traditional light microscopy histology for IgAN is mesangial proliferation and matrix expansion (83,86). Crescents are not uncommon but full-blown crescentic GN is the exception (83). Immunofluorescence shows staining for IgA (IgA1 predominantly) in the mesangium often accompanied by low intensity staining for IgG and IgM. C3 staining is typically present as well. Electron microscopy shows IC deposition in the mesangium.

IgA deposits have been documented in asymptomatic individuals, primarily in transplant studies (87). The significance of this is unknown. Also, IgA deposits have been reported in other forms of GN, including thin basement membrane nephropathy, lupus nephritis, minimal change disease, Wegener's granulomatosis, and DN. It is possible that these findings are nonspecific and unrelated to the primary disease; however, the true significance and clinical applicability remains largely unknown.

Henoch–Schönlein purpura (HSP) is a systemic vasculitis characterized by the deposition of IgA-containing ICs. It usually presents with a nonthrombocytopenic palpable rash (leukocytoclastic vasculitis), polyarthralgias, abdominal pain, and renal disease. The renal lesion of HSP is indistinguishable from IgAN and the pathogenesis is likely similar to IgAN as well. HSP occurs more often in children than in adults; however, adults and older children are likely to have more severe renal disease (88). HSP resolves spontaneously in the majority of adults and children. However, severe or persistent renal dysfunction often requires specific therapy (see section on "Treatment" below).

Pathogenesis

The initial event in IgAN is the mesangial deposition of IgA, usually polymeric IgA1. The recurrence of IgAN in transplanted kidneys implicates a circulating pool of IgA as opposed to local IgA production. Increased polymeric IgA1 plasma cells are found in the bone marrow and tonsils in IgAN (89,90). A number of studies have shown that patients with IgAN have increased levels of serum IgA, but that increased total levels of IgA are insufficient to cause IgAN. The IgA in patients with IgAN is anionic, overrepresented by λ-light chains, and has an O-glycosylation abnormality with reduced galactosylation of the IgA1 hinge region O-glycans, leading to increased frequency of truncated O-glycans (77). The changes in O-glycosylation only seem to become apparent after antigen encounter and may be linked to B-cell maturation and class switching to IgA1 synthesis (91). The IgA molecule produced in patients with IgAN has low affinity for its antigen, may be poorly cleared, and persists longer in circulation. Aberrantly galactosylated IgA1 molecules also have an increased tendency to self-aggregate and form antigen–antibody complexes. These complexes are prone to mesangial deposition because of an altered number of sialic acid and galactose units secondary to aberrant O-glycosylation allowing binding to extracellular matrix fibronectin and type IV collagen (77). The glomerular response to IgA deposition is variable and it remains unclear what determines the glomerular reaction. IgAN is not usually associated with a cellular infiltrate, except for in severe or crescentic disease, suggesting that the mesangial cells and complement mediate injury. Mesangial cells undergo a phenotypic transformation to a pro-inflammatory and pro-fibrotic cell up regulating secretion of extracellular matrix components, transforming growth factor (TGF)-β, platelet-activating factor, IL-1β, IL-6, and other cytokines and chemokines (77). IgA can activate both the mannose-binding lectin and alternative pathways of the complement cascade. This ultimately leads to the generation of the membrane attack complex causing further damage.

Secondary Causes

Idiopathic IgAN, including HSP, is far more common than secondary disease. The deposition of IgA has also been associated with a number of other clinical conditions, including cirrhosis, HIV, celiac disease, seronegative arthritis, and malignancies. Most adult patients with IgA deposition in association with other diagnosis are asymptomatic with relatively bland urine findings, except for HIV-associated IgAN, which can present more typically. The etiology of secondary IgA deposition is likely due, in part, to the high-circulating load of polyclonal IgA that has been associated with the above-mentioned conditions.

Presentation

IgA nephropathy can present at any age but typically does so in young adulthood. There is a male predominance with Caucasians and Asians being affected much more commonly than blacks. Patients with IgAN typically present in one of three ways (92). Almost half of patients will present with one or more episodes of gross hematuria often times following an upper respiratory tract infection. These patients may have flank pain during acute episodes reflecting kidney edema and stretching of the renal capsule. Low-grade fever may also be present. Another 30% to 40% of patients will have microscopic hematuria and usually mild proteinuria, which is detected on a routine examination. Gross hematuria may eventually occur in some of these patients. Less than 10% present with either nephrotic syndrome or acute RPGN. It is thought that these patients have had undetected disease for some time.

Rarely, patients present with acute renal failure due to either crescentic IgAN or to heavy glomerular hematuria leading to tubular occlusion and/or damage by red cells. The latter is usually a reversible although incomplete recovery of renal function has been described (93).

Prognosis

IgA nephropathy was initially considered to be a relatively benign disease. Now, with more insight into the disease and with more patient-years of follow up, it has been determined that approximately half of all patients with IgAN will slowly progress to ESRD (94). Patients with >0.5 g/24 h of proteinuria, elevated serum creatinine at diagnosis, and hypertension are at greatest risk for progression in the long term, but risk for progression exists in all manifestations of the disease (95,96). As described above, several different classification schemes have been devised to describe the histology of IgAN, however the degree of glomerulosclerosis and tubulointerstitial disease seem to be most strongly associated with a poor prognosis (95,96). Recently there has been evidence that lack of C4d staining within the mesangium indicates a more benign course (97,98). There is disagreement in the IgA literature about whether genetic factors play a role in disease progression. Histologic recurrence with or without clinical disease can occur in transplanted kidneys.

Treatment

Treatment of IgAN is typically based on disease severity; however, there is a lack of any unified algorithm that is widely accepted amongst experts. Part of this uncertainty is due to the slow progression of IgAN, which is further complicated by the patient specific variability of disease progression.

Most experts agree that patients with isolated hematuria, minimal proteinuria, and normal renal function need frequent reevaluation and no specific treatment other than possibly initiating treatment with RAAS inhibitors. For patients with >0.5 g/24 h of proteinuria, a RAAS inhibitor titrated to a dose that attempts to normalize proteinuria is recommended. Evidence suggests that even obtaining a partial remission of proteinuria dramatically slows down progression of renal function decline (99). There have been both positive and negative studies regarding the use of high-dose fish oil (ω-3-polyunsaturated fatty acids) supplements and their ability to slow down the decrease in GFR. If tolerated, some experts advocate using them when RAAS inhibitors are added.

For patients with progressive disease manifested by increasing serum creatinine or proteinuria, a trial of steroids is usually initiated with the goal of reducing proteinuria and improving renal survival (100–102). Regiments including pulse methylprednisolone with oral prednisone or only oral prednisone are described.

For patients who fail to respond to steroid therapy alone or have severe disease at presentation, daily oral cyclophosphamide and steroids are typically initiated to decrease proteinuria and improve long-term renal function (103). For patients with crescentic GN and a rapidly progressive clinical course, therapy with intravenous pulse glucocorticoids and cyclophosphamide is recommended followed by either mycophenolate or azathioprine (104,105). Other more experimental therapies include tonsillectomy and low antigen diets.

Glomerulopathies Associated with Multisystem Disease

POSTSTREPTOCOCCAL GLOMERULONEPHRITIS

Presentation

Poststreptococcal glomerulonephritis (PSGN) typically presents as an acute nephritic syndrome that starts within several weeks of an infection with β-hemolyitic streptococci. Renal disease may develop after pharyngitis or after streptococcal infections of the skin. Most cases of PSGN are caused by group A streptococci, and certain cell wall proteins (called M and T proteins) have been associated with nephritogenic potential. Cases of poststreptococcal glomerulonphritis can occur sporadically or they can occur in epidemics. In either case it occurs more commonly in children than in adults, and males are affected slightly more commonly than females. The triggering infection in patients with PSGN is not always clinically evident.

Patients usually present with edema, hematuria, and proteinuria (usually subnephrotic). The urinary sediment is almost always "active", and dysmorphic red blood cells may suggest a glomerular etiology. Patients can develop renal failure, some with oliguria. Rapidly progressive renal failure with prominent crescents on biopsy can also occur, but only in a small percentage of patients. Hypertension is common. Patients may develop seizures secondary to the hypertension, but there is evidence that this may also be due to cerebral vasculitis (106).

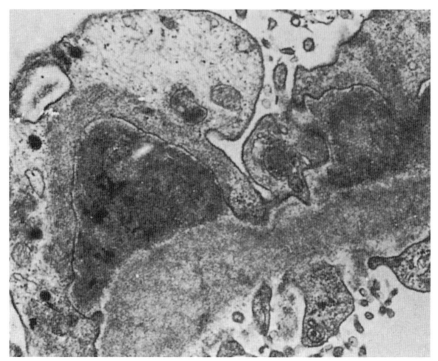

■ **Figure 15.5** Subepithelial deposition of electron-dense material (humps), which may be found in several types of IC glomerulopathies and is characteristic of poststreptococcal diffuse endocapillary proliferative glomerulonephritis.

Patients presenting with PSGN usually have some degree of renal dysfunction. More than 90% of patients with active disease will have a low C3 level (107). The C4 is generally normal, consistent with activation through the alternative pathway. Serologic tests may demonstrate antibodies reactive with streptolysin (ASO), hyaluronidase (AHase), streptokinase (ASKase), nicotinamide-adenine dinucleotidase (anti-NAD), and DNAse B, supporting the diagnosis (108). These antibodies may not however be detectable in patients who have received antibiotics.

On biopsy, PSGN usually causes endocapillary and mesangial proliferation. The lesion is often termed "exudative" because of the presence of abundant PMNs in the glomeruli. Over time, fewer numbers of PMNs are seen but the glomeruli may contain mononuclear cells. Glomeruli may also contain fibrin thrombi and areas of necrosis. Immunofluorescence microscopy often reveals IgG or IgM. C3 is invariably present in the mesangium and in the capillary walls. This can cause a "starry-sky" pattern of fine, scattered deposits, or a "garland" pattern of large deposits in the glomerular tuft (109). Large subepithelial electron dense "humps" are classic for PSGN (Fig. 15.5), and mesangial and subendothelial deposits may also be seen.

Pathogenesis

Two streptococcal molecules have been identified as possibly pathogenic in PSGN: nephritis-associated plasmin receptor (NAPlr) and streptococcal pyrogenic exotoxin B (110). These moieties may directly activate the alternative pathway of complement. They may also provide the antigen for ICs that deposit or form in the capillary wall. Circulating cryoglobulins and rheumatoid factor are also common, suggesting that these antibodies may contribute to the glomerular injury.

Prognosis and Treatment

Even in patients with severe renal dysfunction, PSGN is usually self-limited and renal function returns to normal within a few weeks. Proteinuria and hematuria can however persist for months or even years. The "garland" pattern on biopsy is associated with a greater likelihood of persistent proteinuria. PSGN only rarely causes ESRD, but some patients go on to develop hypertension or chronic renal disease.

Adults are probably more likely than children to develop chronic renal disease. There are no studies to support improved outcomes with corticosteroids or immunosuppressive medications. There are case reports of patients with severe, crescentic disease who appeared to benefit from treatment with corticosteroids, but controlled trials are lacking.

BACTERIAL INFECTION

Bacterial infections can cause acute GN. Well-described causes include bacterial endocarditis (both subacute and acute cases), chronically infected ventricular shunts, abscesses, and bacterial pneumonia. The epidemiology of GN associated with endocarditis has changed in recent years. Improved prevention and treatment of subacute bacterial endocarditis due to organisms such as *Streptococcus viridans* has reduced the incidence of glomerulonephritis associated with this disease, whereas glomerulonephritis caused by acute endocarditis with *Stapholococcus aureus* has risen.

Presentation

Patients with infection associated GN usually develop hematuria and proteinuria. If the glomerular involvement is diffuse, patients may develop the nephrotic syndrome, gross hematuria, or renal insufficiency. Systemic symptoms commonly include fever, purpura and arthralgias. In most instances, the renal injury in infection associated GN is caused by glomerular ICs. The location of the ICs may determine the histologic appearance and the clinical presentation. A proliferative pattern is usually seen by light microscopy, and glomerular ICs are accompanied by C3 deposits by immunofluorescence. Systemic C3 levels are usually depressed during the acute illness, although C3 levels are usually normal in patients with abdominal abscesses or nonendovascular infections with methicillin resistant *Staphylococcus aureas*. Circulating and deposited cryoglobulins are also frequently present in patients with infection associated GN. In early series, chronic bacterial or tubercular infections caused a significant percentage of the cases of AA amyoidosis, but more recent series indicate that infection is now rarely the cause (111).

Prognosis and Treatment

Mildly impaired renal function usually improves with treatment of the underlying infection. Patients with crescentic disease or severe renal impairment, however, may have a progressive decline in renal function in spite of antibiotic therapy. Immunosuppressive drugs and plasmapheresis are of uncertain benefit, and should not be instituted unless the underlying infection has clearly been eradicated.

HIV-RELATED GLOMERULAR DISEASE

HIV-infected patients make up at least 2% of the population with ESRD (112). The prevalence of renal disease related to HIV infection before the highly active antiretroviral therapy (HAART) era is largely unknown; however, a small European autopsy study of primarily Caucasian patients with AIDS found renal pathology in 43% (113). A number of more recent studies in the HAART era have estimated that close to 20% of HIV infected patients have chronic kidney disease (CKD) (114–116). Patients of African descent with HIV are at particularly high risk for progression to ESRD (117).

There are three main classes of HIV glomerulopathies, including HIV-associated nephropathy (HIVAN), HIV immune–mediated GN, and thrombotic microangiopathy secondary to HIV (118). HIVAN and HIV immune–mediated GNs will be discussed here. A discussion of thrombotic microangiopathy can be found elsewhere in this chapter. Other complications of HIV/AIDS including drug-associated renal injury, neoplasms, metabolic abnormalities, and AKI secondary to opportunistic infections can also contribute to renal morbidity and can be found elsewhere in this book.

HIVAN

HIVAN is the most common finding on renal biopsy in patients infected with HIV, with almost 60% of biopsies demonstrating this lesion (119). In the United States, HIVAN is the third most common cause of ESRD among the black population and reports from other countries also report a strong predilection for HIVAN in patients of African descent.

The characteristic histologic findings by light microscopy include collapsing FSGS, podocyte hypertrophy, tubular epithelial atrophy with microcystic dilatation of the tubules, and lymphocytic infiltration. Immunofluorescence is usually nonspecific. Electron microscopy may show endothelial tubuloreticular inclusions related to high plasma interferon levels.

Pathogenesis

The exact pathogenesis of HIVAN is unknown, but it is likely due to viral infection of resident kidney cells, including glomerular endothelial, epithelial, mesangial, and tubular cells. The presence of HIV may also stimulate the release of cytokines, including fibroblast growth factor and TGF-β, which then contribute to the matrix accumulation, fibrosis, and tubular injury seen in HIVAN (120, 121). HIV gene products can directly induce cell-cycle progression, resulting in epithelial cell dedifferentiation and collapse (122).

The increased prevalence of HIVAN in African Americans implies genetic factor involvement as well. Recently it was reported that polymorphisms in the *MYH9* gene, encoding nonmuscle myosin IIA expressed in kidney podocytes, may partially explain this genetic propensity via gene–gene interactions or gene–environment interactions (123).

Presentation

HIVAN can be present in any race but it is typically a disease of patients of African descent. HIVAN classically presents late in the course of HIV/AIDS with low CD4 counts and elevated viral loads. It can, however, also present anytime during the course of HIV with adequate CD4 counts and undetectable viral loads. Patients with HIVAN typically present with heavy proteinuria, hypoalbuminemia, renal dysfunction, and occasionally edema. Microscopic hematuria may also be present. The kidneys often are enlarged and echogenic on ultrasound examination corresponding to the lymphocytic infiltration and tubular dilation seen on biopsy. Blood pressure, surprisingly, is usually normal perhaps related to salt wasting that has been reported in HIVAN. In the HAART era HIVAN has been reported to present with less severe findings.

Prognosis

When HIVAN was first described the prognosis was dismal, with patients progressing to ESRD in months. In the HAART era the rate of progression of HIVAN to ESRD has been reduced by an estimated 40% (117). Some evidence also suggests that HAART may prevent the development of HIVAN (124).

Treatment

HAART is recommended as first line therapy to treat HIVAN even though there are only retrospective and nonrandomized trials demonstrating their effectiveness (125). RAAS inhibitors have been shown in small studies to delay the progression to ESRD and decrease proteinuria and should be used and titrated as tolerated (126). Immunosuppressants including steroids and cyclosporine have also been used in those patients not responding to HAART or RAAS inhibitor therapy (127).

HIV Immune–Mediated Glomerulonephritis

Autopsy and biopsy studies have demonstrated a wide prevalence of immune mediated GN in HIV-infected patients, with anywhere from 10% to 80% being reported (128). IC GN associated with HIV may present with proliferative, lupus-like (immunofluorescence positive for C1q, IgG, IgM, IgA, C3, λ, and κ), mixed proliferative, or sclerotic histology. Membranoproliferative, IgA, membranous, fibrillary, immunotactoid, and postinfectious GN have also been reported (129). The presence of hepatitis C or B co-infection must also be considered, as they are known to cause a number of the histologic patterns of injury mentioned earlier.

Pathogenesis

Infection with HIV may lead to polyclonal hypergammaglobulimemia and to the development of circulating ICs, many of which are composed of HIV peptides and their associated antibody (130,131). Passive trapping of these complexes versus in situ formation of antigen–antibody complexes on glomerular cells can initiate the immune response and trigger IC GN.

Presentation

HIV immune mediated GNs occur more frequently in Caucasians and Asians. Patients usually present with hypertension, an active urine sediment, proteinuria, and renal insufficiency. Low levels of serum complement proteins may be seen. Antinuclear antibody (ANA) and antibodies to double-stranded DNA (anti-dsDNA) are typically negative even in those patients with lupus-like histology. CD4 counts and HIV viral loads do not seem to be predictive of disease type or severity.

Prognosis

The prognosis of HIV immune mediated GNs is largely unknown but is considered to be generally poor in most literature reports. Some studies have demonstrated that renal survival may be predicted in part by the degree of fibrosis at biopsy and by the amount of proteinuria.

Treatment

There is little known about the specific treatments for HIV immune–mediated GNs. Most patients should likely be on an RAAS inhibitor for proteinuria reduction. The data are mixed about whether HAART improves proteinuria or delays progression of disease (132,133). There are case reports involving the use of immunosuppressant drugs with some degree of success (134,135).

HEPATITIS C VIRUS INFECTION AND CRYOGLOBULINEMIA

Chronic infection with hepatitis C virus (HCV) has now been firmly associated with the development of mixed cryoglobulinemia, and >90% of patients with cryoglobulin-associated renal disease are infected with HCV in some series (136). HCV infection has also been linked with the development of glomerular disease in the absence of cryoglobulins.

Presentation

Most patients with cryoglobulin-associated renal disease have proteinuria, hematuria, and an elevated serum creatinine. The presentation can be more fulminant, and some patients present with the full nephritic syndrome and with acute elevations in the serum creatinine. By the time patients present with renal disease, they usually have systemic manifestations of vasculitis. Common extra-renal signs and symptoms include palpable purpura, arthralgias, and weakness. Hypertension is also common. In patients with active disease the serum C4 level is almost always low (136). The cryocrit is quite variable but can usually be detected, and rheumatoid factor is usually present.

HCV infection, even in patients who do not have detectable cryoglobulins, has been linked to the development of MPGN (136,137). HCV has also been linked to MN, although this correlation has not been firmly established. A recent report also suggests that many HCV infected patients with renal involvement may go undetected (138). In this study, 30 patients undergoing liver transplantation for HCV induced cirrhosis underwent renal biopsy at the time of liver transplantation. None of the patients had detectable cryoglobulins, yet all but one had some type of glomerular pathology (138). Of 25 patients with glomerular IC deposits ten had a normal urinalysis, further suggesting that standard screening of patients with HCV infection may underestimate the degree of renal involvement.

Pathophysiolgy

Cryoglobulins are present in the majority of patients with HCV associated glomerular disease (137). Most patients have type II cryoglobulinemia, in which the cryoglobulins contain a monoclonal antibody (usually an IgM) that binds to polyclonal IgG. Studies of biopsy tissue indicate that HCV complexes are present within the glomerular capillary walls (139). Furthermore, the IgM rheumatoid factor present in the cryoglobulins of HCV infected patients can cause GN in mice when passively transferred (140). These findings suggest that cryoglobulins containing HCV cause IC-mediated injury of the glomerulus, perhaps due to the affinity of the IgM component for a glomerular target.

Prognosis and Treatment

Cryoglobulin-associated renal disease has a variable course. Approximately 10% to 15% of patients will enter spontaneous remission, and another 30% will have an indolent course with only a mild degree of renal insufficiency. Some patients, however, will have acute nephritic flares (141). Treatment of the underlying HCV infection with interferon (IFN) α and ribavirin can improve symptoms of cryoglobulinemia (142). There are reports that this treatment reduces proteinuria in patients who achieve a virologic response (143). Acute nephritic flares are not controlled by antiviral therapy. In this setting, aggressive therapy with plasmapheresis, corticosteroids, and cyclophosphamide may be effective at controlling the disease flare (144). Rituximab has also been reported to improve the serologic parameters and the degree of proteinuria (145).

HEPATITIS B VIRUS INFECTION

Chronic infection with hepatitis B virus (HBV) is most common in Asia and Africa, where the prevalence of HBV infection is highest and where there is the highest incidence of vertical transmission. Acute infection with HBV can cause a serum sickness–like syndrome or polyarteritis nodosa (PAN). The latter condition affects small or medium size arteries. The glomeruli may show ischemic changes in patients with PAN, but membranous and proliferative lesions can also occur. Chronic carriers of HBV can develop mesangial, subendothelial, and subepithelial IC deposits, and HBV associated antigens are frequently detectable within the glomerli (146). The mesangial and subendothelial deposits cause MPGN. Subepithelial deposits cause a membranous pattern of disease and nephrotic syndrome, although concurrent mesangial and subendothelial deposits are also frequently present in these patients. HBV infection is also associated with the development of IgA nephropathy. Treatment of the HBV infection with IFN probably ameliorates the renal disease in some patients (147), and treatment with lamivudine has improved the renal disease in some case reports. Treatment with immunosuppressive medications is not recommended since the risk of exacerbating the liver disease outweighs potential improvement of the renal disease.

CHRONIC PARASITIC INFECTIONS

Glomerular disease may be seen in patients infected with several types of parasites. Acute IC–mediated GN may be seen in patients with malaria, including a chronic proliferative GN in patients infected with *Plasmodium malariae* (148). *Schistosoma mansoni* infections may cause IC-mediated GN and amyloidosis. Several other parasitic infections have also been associated with IC-mediated GN, presenting with proliferative or membranous patterns by light-microscopy.

LUPUS NEPHRITIS

SLE is an autoimmune disease that can affect multiple different organs, including the skin, joints, lungs, and kidneys. Up to 60% of adults and 80% of children who are diagnosed with lupus will develop renal abnormalities at some point (149), but there is great patient-to-patient variation in the nature of the renal disease. Aggressive immunosuppressive therapy has greatly improved the outcome in patients with lupus nephritis over the past several decades, and the impact of newer therapies on the overall prognosis is not yet known. Nevertheless, >15% of patients with renal involvement may go on to ESRD (150) and overall patient survival is worse in those with renal involvement (151). One of the great challenges in treating patients with lupus, therefore, is to identify those patients who will most benefit from aggressive immunosuppression while also minimizing the toxicities of therapy.

Pathogenesis

The pathogenesis of lupus itself remains uncertain, but it likely involves genetic defects that cause a loss of tolerance to self-antigens. Patients with lupus frequently develop high-affinity autoantibodies to nuclear antigens, cytoplasmic antigens, platelets, and erythrocytes. Antibodies to dsDNA, other nuclear components, and α-actinin are associated with renal disease, and there is evidence that these antibodies are pathogenic (152). The autoantibodies in lupus may cause renal injury due to deposition of ICs within the glomerulus, but the antibodies may also cross react with renal structures. Antibodies to C1q are also commonly seen in the kidneys of patients with lupus nephritis, and these antibodies may exacerbate renal injury (153).

In patients with lupus nephritis, ICs may be found in mesangial, subendothelial, and/or subepithelial locations. ICs cause tissue inflammation by activating complement and through their interaction with Fc receptors on immune cells. The location of the ICs correlates with the light microscopic changes and with the clinical presentation. Mesangial ICs may cause mesangial expansion and hypercellularity, and patients typically have microscopic hematuria and subnephrotic range proteinuria. Subendothelial ICs cause an exudative lesion in the glomerulus. There is leukocyte infiltration and endocapillary proliferation. Subepithelial ICs tend to cause proteinuria and a membranous pattern of glomerular injury. IC deposition and inflammatory cells can also damage the tubules and blood vessels. Some patients develop renal injury caused by antiphospholipid antibody mediated glomerular thrombosis.

Secondary Factors

Some drugs are associated with the development of a lupus-like syndrome. These patients develop ANA and antihistone antibodies, but anti-dsDNA antibodies and renal involvement are rare. Commonly implicated drugs include procainamide and hydralazine.

Presentation

Depending on the severity of the renal disease, patients may present with proteinuria (subnephrotic or nephrotic), hematuria (microscopic or gross), red blood cell casts, hypertension, edema, and an elevation in serum creatinine. Patients can present with a pulmonary-renal syndrome, and some patients develop an RPGN. Although the clinical presentation may correlate with the histologic pattern (e.g., a nephritic pattern of disease with subendothelial deposits and endocapillary proliferation), the clinical findings do not accurately predict the histology or the prognosis.

Serologic Findings

Virtually all patients with lupus nephritis have a positive ANA. As mentioned above, anti-dsDNA antibodies may be pathogenic in lupus nephritis and are very specific. C3 and C4 levels are frequently depressed in patients with active disease. In some patients serologic changes may predict disease flares (154). Persistently high anti-dsDNA antibodies or low C3 levels are also associated with a greater risk of disease flare and disease progression (155–157), but these tests do not reliably predict disease flares. Thus, although perturbations in the levels of these factors may prompt closer monitoring or even a repeat renal biopsy, there is no evidence to support altering treatment in an effort to normalize the levels of these factors.

Histologic Patterns

Because the clinical course of lupus nephritis is so variable and the medications used to treat the disease have many potential side-effects, great effort has been made to identify which patients benefit from aggressive immunosuppression. The WHO classification scheme was first proposed in 1982 (158), and has been modified several times since then (159). This scheme includes six classes of glomerular involvement, with several different subclasses (Table 15.9). Several series have established the importance of the WHO classification for predicting patients' long-term outcomes (160, 161). Equally important, this classification scheme has been used as a criterion for the selection of patients in most large clinical trials. To determine whether clinical trials apply to a particular patient, therefore, the patient's histologic class must be established. Other factors on the biopsy that may help identify which patients are at a high risk of progression include activity and chronicity indices (162). Over time, the histologic pattern of disease can change (163). For this reason, repeat biopsies are often necessary for optimal assessment of disease activity (164,165).

TABLE 15.9 MAJOR HISTOLOGIC CLASSES OF LUPUS NEPHRITIS

Class	Description
Class I	Normal light microscopy, mesangial immune deposits.
Class II	Mesangial hypercellularity or matrix expansion. Mesangial immune deposits.
Class III	Focal lupus nephritis. Active or inactive focal, segmental or global endocapillary or extracapillary glomerulonephritis involving <50% of all glomeruli, typically with focal subendothelial immune deposits, with or without mesangial alterations.
Class IV	Diffuse lupus nephritis. Active or inactive diffuse, segmental or global endocapillary or extracapillary glomerulonephritis involving >50% of all glomeruli, typically with diffuse subendothelial immune deposits, with or without mesangial alterations.
Class V	Membranous lupus nephritis. Global or segmental subepithelial immune deposits or their morphologic sequelae by light microscopy and by immunofluorescence or electron microscopy, with or without mesangial alterations. Class V lupus nephritis may occur in combination with class III or IV in which case both will be diagnosed.
Class VI	Advanced sclerosis (>90% of glomeruli globally sclerosed)

(From Weening JJ, D'Agati VD, Schwartz MM, et al. The classification of glomerulonephritis in systemic lupus erythematosus revisited. *J Am Soc Nephrol.* 2004;15:241–250, with permission.)

Prognosis

The course of lupus nephritis has improved in recent decades, but lupus is still a significant cause of CKD and of ESRD. Important prognostic factors include the WHO histologic classification and disease activity and chronicity. In some reports patients with WHO class IV disease were more likely to respond to treatment than those with WHO class III disease (166), perhaps due to different mechanisms of glomerular injury (167). Of patients with severe proliferative disease, those who achieve and maintain remission with therapy have better long-term outcomes (166). A lower serum creatinine and lower urine protein excretion predict a response to therapy, and those patients who enter remission tend to show marked improvement within 4 weeks of initiating therapy. Several series have reported that black patients are less likely than white patients to respond to therapy (166,168). Patients who have flares of their renal disease, particularly nephritic flares, have a worse long-term outcome (169).

Treatment

Because of the variable course of lupus nephritis, the decision to treat an individual patient is based upon the overall risk of progression. In general, immunosuppressive treatment is instituted in patients with proliferative GN (classes III and IV) and in some patients with membranous GN (class V). Patients with mesangial disease are not usually treated with immunosuppressive drugs due to the benign long-term prognosis, and patients with advanced sclerosis are not treated due to the low likelihood of responding to therapy.

Several large randomized trials have demonstrated the efficacy of cyclophosphamide combined with corticosteroids for the treatment of proliferative lupus nephritis (170,171). Aggressive induction therapy with combined cyclophosphamide and corticosteroids effectively controls renal inflammation and induces remission. Patients who are subsequently maintained with quarterly intravenous pulses of cyclophosphamide have fewer relapses and a lower likelihood of progressing in long-term follow-up (170). On the basis of these early studies, for many years the standard treatment of patients with WHO class III or IV lupus nephritis included induction with 6 monthly intravenous pulses of cyclophosphamide ($0.5–1.0 \text{ g/m}^2$) and glucocorticoids (e.g., prednisone started at 1 mg/kg/day). Shorter induction protocols have also been effectively used in patients with mild disease (172).

Not all patients can tolerate cyclophosphamide due to its toxicities, and not all patients will respond, even to aggressive induction protocols. Consequently, an effort has been made to identify alternative therapies. Several randomized controlled trials have now demonstrated that MMF is as effective, or possibly even superior to cyclophosphamide for treatment of proliferative lupus nephritis. Chan et al. first demonstrated that induction therapy with 1 g of MMF twice daily was as effective as oral cyclophosphamide for patients from Hong Kong (173). A multicenter randomized controlled trial in the United States also demonstrated that MMF was as effective as cyclophosphamide for treatment of patients with proliferative disease (the dose in this study was escalated to 1.5 g twice daily) (174). MMF is also an effective agent for maintenance therapy in patients with proliferative disease who have achieved remission. Because of the limited number of patients included in the MMF trials and the limited follow-up, patients with severe disease (e.g., histologic activity or chronicity, crescents, fibrinoid necrosis, a reduced GFR, or rapid progression) should probably be treated with cyclophosphamide as induction therapy.

After induction therapy, patients with proliferative GN should be switched to maintenance therapy protocols. The rationale for this is that disease flares are associated with a worse long-term prognosis (169,175). Initial studies demonstrated that patients maintained with pulses of cyclophosphamide every 3 months had fewer disease flares and better long-term renal function than those who did not receive maintenance therapy (170). Regimens containing azathioprine, mycophenolate, and cyclosporine have also been tried as maintenance therapy. In a randomized trial comparing MMF with cyclophosphamide for maintenance therapy, MMF was more efficacious than cyclophosphamide (176). On the basis of these results, many patients are now maintained on MMF for 18 to 24 months after completing their induction protocol. The MMF may be administered in doses of 1 to 2 g/day and tapered to 0.5 to 1 g/day in the third year of treatment. Low-dose prednisone is typically continued during the maintenance period (176).

Several alternative therapies may be of benefit in patients who do not respond to induction therapy or who have relapses. Several small nonrandomized studies have demonstrated that rituximab can induce complete or partial remissions in a substantial number of patients who have relapsed or failed to respond to conventional therapy (177). It has been reported, however, that a randomized controlled trial examining whether the addition of rituximab improves the outcome of patients with proliferative lupus nephritis who are induced with mycophenolate (referred to as the LUNAR study) failed to meet its primary endpoint. The results of this study have not yet been published. Cyclosporine has also been reported to induce remission in patients who either fail induction therapy or who relapse (178). Therapy in resistant or relapsing patients can be changed (e.g., treatment with cyclophosphamide and corticosteroids can be changed to mycophenolate and corticosteroid) or rituximab can be added to their regimen.

Approximately 10% to 15% of patients with lupus nephritis have a pure membranous lesion (WHO class V), and the optimal therapy for this subgroup is not clearly defined. Most treatment studies for these patients have either been uncontrolled, or the studies have combined patients with proliferative and membranous patterns of disease. The newer classification system more clearly defines patients whose biopsies display both proliferative and membranous patterns, and most authors agree that the treatment of patients with combined lesions should be based on the proliferative component of their disease. For patients with a pure membranous lesion, the results of a prospective study, comparing three different immunosuppressive regimens, was recently reported (179). This study demonstrated that IV cyclophosphamide and oral cyclosporine were effective at inducing remission in 60% and 83% of the patients, respectively. Both therapies were superior to alternate day prednisone, but there was a high rate of relapse in the cyclosporine group after therapy was stopped. Retrospective studies indicate that corticosteroids in combination with cyclosporine, azathioprine, cyclophosphamide, or mycophenolate may be effective. The long-term benefit of these therapies on patient outcomes is still unclear, but immunosuppressive treatment may be warranted in patients with severe disease (177).

ANCA ASSOCIATED VASCULITIS

Vasculitis may involve vessels of any size. Small vessel vasculitis commonly involves the arterioles of the kidney and the glomerular capillaries, but these diseases can affect any vessel in the body. Small vessel vasculitis can be caused by IC deposition in the vessel wall in patients with diseases such as lupus and HSP. Vasculitis without IC deposition on tissue biopsy (termed "pauci-immune") is usually associated with circulating antineutrophil cytoplasmic antibodies (ANCA). The ANCA associated vasculitides (AAV) include Wegener's granulomatosis, microscopic polyangiitis, Churg–Strauss disease, and renal limited vasculitis. AAV involving the kidney often causes rapid deterioration of renal function, and the glomerular lesion is commonly necrotizing and crescentic (180). The terms "crescentic GN" or "RPGN" are sometimes used interchangeably with the ANCA associated diseases. However, IC-mediated vasculitides can also cause these clinical and morphologic presentations.

Pathogenesis

ANCA may be identified by indirect immunofluorescence with ethanol fixed neutrophils. Antibodies in the serum from ANCA-positive patients will react with the neutrophils in either a cytoplasmic (C-ANCA) or perinuclear (P-ANCA) pattern. The C-ANCA pattern is usually caused by antibodies directed against proteinase-3 (PR-3), and the P-ANCA pattern is usually caused by antibodies specific to myeloperoxidase (MPO) (181). PR-3 and MPO are proteins contained in the granules of neutrophils and the lysosomes of monocytes. Autoantibodies to lysosomal membrane protein-2 (LAMP-2), a protein present on neutrophils and endothelial cells, have also been identified in patients with AAV (182).

Although the diseases are referred to as pauci-immune, there is strong evidence that the ANCAs are pathogenic in AAV. In vitro studies have demonstrated that ANCAs bind to primed neutrophils and trigger activation of the cells (183), and passive transfer of anti-MPO antibodies in mice has been found to induce a crescentic, pauci-immune GN (184). Autoantibodies to LAMP-2 can also induce crescentic GN in rats when passively transferred or induced by immunization of the rats with LAMP-2 protein (182). The passive transfer of anti-MPO antibodies from mother to newborn has also been reported to cause a pulmonary-renal syndrome in the child (185). ANCAs probably contribute to the development of vasculitis through direct effects on circulating neutrophils or by causing endothelial damage (182,186). Genetic and environmental (drugs, infections, chemicals) factors may also contribute to the development of AAV (187).

Presentation

All patients suspected of having AAV should undergo testing for ANCA with both indirect immunofluorescence and enzyme-linked immunosorbent assays (ELISAs) specific for PR-3 and MPO. The diseases that cause AAV are defined on the basis of the organs involved, their ANCA associations, and the presence or absence of granulomas on the tissue biopsy (Table 15.10). These criteria are not absolute, so there is some overlap in the disease definitions. Other inflammatory and infectious diseases, such as bacterial endocarditis, are associated with the development of ANCA and should be considered in the differential diagnosis. Patients with AAV involving the kidney typically present with hematuria, subnephrotic range proteinuria, and a rapid rise in the serum creatinine. Patients frequently have a nephritic presentation with diffuse necrosis and crescents on biopsy. C3 and C4 levels are usually normal or elevated. The other organ systems that are commonly involved upon presentation include the lungs and upper airways, ears, nose, throat, skin, neurologic system, and gastrointestinal tract. In addition to the involvement of these specific organs, patients with AAV often also have systemic symptoms such as weight loss and fevers. Patients with Churg–Strauss syndrome invariably have a history of asthma, and often present with eosinophilia.

TABLE 15.10 CLINICAL AND MORPHOLOGIC FEATURES OF THE ANCA ASSOCIATED VASCULITIDES

Disease	ANCA PR3-ANCA	ANCA MPO-ANCA	ANCA negative	Other Organs Commonly Involved	Biopsy Findings
Microscopic polyangiitis	40%	50%	10%	Skin, lungs, musculoskeletal, GI	Necrotizing glomerulonephritis and vasculitis. Pulmonary capillaritis.
Wegener's disease	75%	20%	5%	Skin, lungs, musculoskeletal, neurologic, GI	Necrotizing glomerulonephritis. Granulomas in respiratory tract and kidneys.
Churg–Strauss syndrome	10%	60%	30%	Skin, lungs, musculoskeletal, neurologic, GI	Necrotizing glomerulonephritis. Eosinophil rich and granulomatous inflammation in respiratory tract.
Renal limited vasculitis	20%	70%	10%		Necrotizing glomerulonephritis.

GI, gastrointestinal.
(From Nachman PH, Jennette JC, and Falk RJ. Vasculitic diseases of the kidney. In: Schrier RW, ed. *Diseases of the Kidney and Urinary Tract*, 8th ed, Philadelphia: Saunders; 2007, with permission.)

Prognosis

Untreated, the 2-year survival for patients with AAV may be below 20%, and the prognosis for these diseases has been significantly improved by aggressive immunosuppressive protocols (162). With treatment, the long-term survival is now approximately 50% to 80% (162). In one report, 77% of those treated achieved at least partial remission, but 30% of those patients experienced a relapse during the 18 months after entering remission (188).

Treatment

Due to the poor prognosis of untreated disease, virtually all patients with AAV are treated with induction and maintenance protocols of immunosuppressive drugs, and the treatment protocols are similar for all of the diseases discussed above. Patients who present with GN are initially treated with cyclophosphamide and corticosteroids. The exact regimens vary and can include either intravenous or oral cyclophosphamide (187). Patients may be treated with three daily pulses of methylprednisolone and are then usually treated with oral prednisone during the induction period. Plasma exchange may also benefit patients with severe disease, particularly those who are on dialysis at the time of diagnosis (189). Several pilot studies suggest that drugs that block TNF-α and anti-B cell therapies, such as rituximab, may be effective treatments for AAV (189). Steroids are usually tapered off after patients achieve remission, and cyclophosphamide is continued for another 6 to 12 months. Azathioprine can be used to maintain patients in remission (190). MMF may also be effective at inducing and maintaining remission (191,192), but randomized trials are lacking.

ANTI-GLOMERULAR BASEMENT MEMBRANE DISEASE

Anti-glomerular basement membrane (anti-GBM) disease, or Goodpasture disease, is an autoimmune disease caused by the development of autoantibodies directed against the GBM and the alveolar basement membrane. Goodpasture disease commonly presents as an RPGN and may be accompanied by pulmonary hemorrhage (pulmonary-renal syndrome).

Pathogenesis

Goodpasture disease is caused by antibodies (usually IgG, but occasionally IgA or IgM) with high affinity for two specific epitopes in the noncollagenous (NC1) domain of type IV collagen. These epitopes are usually sequestered within the collagen structure. Goodpasture disease is associated with environmental factors such as hydrocarbons and tobacco smoke, and it is believed that these insults may damage the GBM and expose the epitopes. Certain major histocompatibility complex alleles are associated with a greater risk of developing disease, and a loss of T-cell tolerance is probably also necessary for the development of the antibody response. In animal models disease can be caused by the passive transfer of either the antibodies or T cells, both of which can trigger an inflammatory response in the glomerulus.

Presentation

In 1919 Ernest W. Goodpasture reported a patient who presented with renal failure and pulmonary hemorrhage, and the name Goodpasture syndrome was later coined for patients who present with RPGN and pulmonary hemorrhage (193). Diseases causing systemic vasculitis (such as lupus and AAV) can also cause Goodpasture syndrome, and anti-GBM antibodies cause only about 30% of the same. Furthermore, patients with Goodpasture disease (e.g., pulmonary or renal disease specifically caused by anti-GBM antibodies) may present with isolated pulmonary or renal failure. Nevertheless, Goodpasture disease usually manifests with the acute onset of hemoptysis and a nephritic syndrome. The disease is most common in men in their 20s and 30s, and a second peak incidence is seen in people in their 60s. Urinalysis reveals erythrocytes, red cell casts, and subnephrotic range proteinuria, and chest X-rays may reveal diffuse alveolar hemorrhage. Patients with Goodpasture syndrome also usually have anemia.

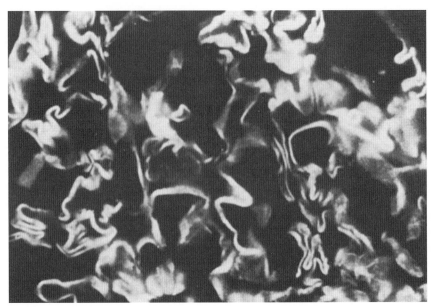

■ **Figure 15.6** Fluorescent-antibody study of the glomerulus, showing discrete linear deposition of immunoglobulin, which is characteristic of anti-GBM mediated glomerulopathies and Goodpasture disease. The immunoglobulin deposits represent autoantibody that has reacted with a native glycoprotein (noncollagen) constituent of the GBM.

Anti-GBM antibodies in the serum of patients with Goodpasture disease can be detected by ELISA, although the assay can be negative in patients with low antibody titers or with isolated pulmonary disease (194). On biopsy, Goodpasture disease usually causes a proliferative GN with crescents and areas of necrosis by light microscopy, similar to the appearance of AAV. In most cases immunofluorescence microscopy reveals the linear deposition of immunoglobulin along the GBM (Fig. 15.6).

Prognosis and Treatment

There is some reported variability in the rate at which Goodpasture disease progresses, but in general it is a fulminant disease that must be identified and treated promptly. Indeed, patients with mild or atypical symptoms may fare worse due to delayed treatment. Before the development of effective treatment the patient and renal survival was dismal (195). Current therapy of patients with Goodpasture disease involves plasma exchange to remove circulating anti-GBM antibodies, cyclophosphamide to prevent new antibody formation, and corticosteroids to dampen tissue inflammation. The titer of anti-GBM antibodies correlates with disease progression, and plasma exchange should be continued while the antibodies remain detectable. Rituximab has been reported to help patients refractory to conventional therapies. Infection is a major cause of mortality in patients with Goodpasture disease, so patients receiving cyclophosphamide should receive *Pneumocystis carinii* pneumonia prophylaxis (e.g., Bactrim) and neutrophil counts should be monitored.

THROMBOTIC MICROANGIOPATHY

"Thrombotic microangiopathy (TMA)" is a descriptive term for a morphologic lesion characterized by platelet thrombi occluding the microvasculature of various organs. Various diverse disorders share this common pathology, including thrombocytopenic purpura (TTP), diarrhea-associated and atypical hemolytic uremic syndrome (d/aHUS), and scleroderma renal crisis. TMAs are thought to be triggered by microvascular endothelial cell injury that then leads to platelet and fibrin thrombi.

On light microscopy, the glomeruli frequently have platelet and fibrin clots. These clots can extend into the arterioles and even occasionally into larger vessels that can show necrosis with intimal swelling, mucoid change, and intimal proliferation. Mesangiolysis can occur. Glomeruli may only show evidence of ischemia with corrugation of the GBM and retraction and collapse of the glomerular tuft. Segmental glomerular necrosis may be seen. Secondary changes late in the course of the disease include reduplication of the GBM often similar in appearance to an MPGN pattern of injury. Immunofluorescence studies show no immunoglobulin deposits. Electron microscopy shows swollen endothelial cells that frequently appear to have detached from their basement membranes.

Pathogenesis

Idiopathic TTP is often secondary to a deficiency in ADAMTS13 (A Disintegrin-like and Metalloprotease with ThromboSpondin type 1 repeats). ADAMTS13 is synthesized primarily by the liver and endothelial cells. Its main function is to cleave ultra-large von Willebrand factor (vWF) multimers that are released from endothelial cells. vWF supports platelet adhesion and aggregation at sites of shear stress. ADAMTS13 deficiency allows circulating ultra-large vWF to persist causing platelet aggregation and clumping leading to TTP. Congenital ADAMTS13 deficiency has been described and is the result of an inactivating mutation. Acquired deficiency is due to inhibitory antibodies, which are found in 50% to 94% of patients with undetectable ADAMTS13 (196). Noninhibitory antibodies that may play a role in increased clearance or endothelial cell binding are now being detected with newer technologies (197).

Diarrhea associated HUS is most commonly caused by shiga toxin producing *Eschrechia coli* O157:H7. The shiga toxin binds the glycolipid cell surface receptor Gb3, is endocytosed, and subsequently binds to the 60S subunit of ribosomes inhibiting protein synthesis and injuring cells. This endothelial cell injury exposes the underlying basement membrane causing activation of platelets and the coagulation cascade (198). In atypical HUS mutations in complement regulatory proteins and activating proteins lead to uncontrolled complement activation and subsequent cell injury (199). The secondary causes of TTP–HUS likely lead to a final common pathologic pathway via endothelial cell injury.

Secondary Causes

TMAs have been associated with a number of different medications, including cyclosporine, tacrolimus, sirolimus, quinine, OKT3, mitomycin C, cisplatin, bleomycin, gemcitabine, cyclophosphamide, antivascular endothelial growth factor (VEGF) antibodies, valacyclovir, oral contraceptives, ticlodipine, and clopidogrel. A syndrome now known as hematopoietic stem cell transplantation thrombotic microangiopathy has been described. TTP–HUS associated with pregnancy is also well described, occurring either in isolation or with severe pre-eclampsia/HELLP syndrome. TMAs can also occur with HIV, malignant hypertension, the antiphospholipid antibody syndrome, lupus, scleroderma, pneumococcal infection, and malignancies.

Presentation

The Oklahoma TTP–HUS registry reports the incidence of suspected TTP at 11 cases/million population per year. Incidence is greater for women and blacks (200). TMAs share a number of clinical and serologic features; all have microangiopathic hemolytic anemia—demonstrated by elevated lactate dehydrogenase levels (also from tissue ischemia), decreased haptoglobin, and elevated indirect bilirubin—thrombocytopenia, and secondary organ involvement. The classic pentad for TTP had been fever, microangiopathic hemolytic anemia, thrombocytopenic purpura, renal failure, and central nervous system involvement. This severe stage of the disease is rarely seen anymore, however, as treatment is usually initiated much earlier. Traditionally HUS is thought of as having more severe renal failure and less severe CNS manifestations than TTP, but significant overlap occurs between the two disorders. Idiopathic TTP can be associated with decreased ADAMTS13 levels, usually with an associated antibody.

Diarrhea associated HUS occurs most commonly in children and presents with bloody diarrhea. *E. coli* O157:H7 accounts for over 60% of cases. Atypical HUS is associated with a number of different mutations in complement related proteins that can be detected by specific assays, including factor H, membrane cofactor protein (CD46), factor I, C3, and factor B. In atypical HUS the serum C3 level is often low.

Prognosis

Diarrhea associated HUS is usually a self-limited disease with a good prognosis. Idiopathic TTP that is treated promptly has a good prognosis, but relapse rates are high with almost 50% having at least one recurrence. Young age and low ADAMTS13 activity are risk factors for recurrence, while there is disagreement in the literature about the significance of persistent anti-ADAMTS13 antibody (201). Atypical HUS has a poor prognosis with many patients reaching ESRD. Kidney transplantation offers little hope except for patients with CD46 mutations since the donor kidney will correct the genetic defect. There has been recent success with liver–kidney transplants (202).

Treatment

Suspected TTP–HUS should be treated with plasma exchange performed daily until the platelet count has normalized and hemolysis ceased (203). If plasma exchange is not available, then plasma infusion can be substituted until exchange can be performed. Steroids are not administered unless platelet counts do not improve after several days of treatment or if platelets fall after the discontinuation of plasma exchange. In patients who do not respond to plasma exchange or who have relapsing disease experts recommend increasing exchange therapy to twice daily and adding either rituximab, cyclosporine, or vincristine (204–206). In atypical HUS eculizumab (a monoclonal antibody that prevents the cleavage of C5 during complement activation) has been used experimentally (207,208).

GLOMERULAR INVOLVEMENT IN OTHER MULTISYSTEM DISEASES

Other autoimmune diseases have been associated with the development of glomerular disease. This is not unexpected as one might predict that diseases in which there are high levels of circulating rheumatoid factors and ICs would cause IC deposition in the kidney. Patients with mixed connective tissue disease may develop anti-dsDNA antibodies, and GN may be common in these patients. Rheumatoid arthritis (RA) is associated with the development of secondary amyloidosis, particularly in those who have had poorly controlled disease for prolonged periods (209). Cases of MN, mesangial IC deposition, and even proliferative disease have been reported in patients with RA. In some reports the patients may have had lupus, so the association and overall incidence is uncertain. The treatment of RA with gold or penicillamine, however, has been clearly linked with the development of MN. IC-mediated GN has been reported in patients with Sjögren syndrome disease, ankylosing spondylitis, Behçet disease, and polymyositis.

Monoclonal Immunoglobulin Related Diseases

Plasma cell dyscrasias result from a clonal expansion of malignant plasma cells that secrete a monoclonal immunoglobulin. In healthy adults, plasma cells also synthesize an excess of light chains that then get freely filtered by the glomerulus and catabolized by proximal tubular cells. The uptake of light chains is constant and occurs via binding to the megalin–cubilin complex followed by the endosomal/lysosomal degradation of the proteins, ultimately leading to the return of the free amino acids to the circulation (210–214). Despite this process, small amounts of polyclonal free light chains do make their way into the urine at a concentration of about 2.5 μg/mL. In multiple myeloma and other plasma cell dyscrasias, the amount of light chains produced and filtered exceeds the maximal reabsorptive capacity of the proximal tubular cells and make their way into the urine at much higher concentrations, where they are also referred to as Bence–Jones proteins.

The toxicity of light chain proteinuria depends upon the specific characteristics of the light chain. Certain toxic light chains are able to self-aggregate forming high molecular weight polymers that are then able to deposit in tissue or form tubular casts after binding to Tamm–Horsfall proteins (215) while some have toxicity based on the variable region of the light chain molecule.

Light chains are known to cause a number of different kidney diseases, some affecting the tubulo-interstitium (see myeloma cast nephropathy, proximal tubule dysfunction, insterstitial nephritis in the appropriate chapters) and others the glomerular compartment.

AMYLOID

The amyloidoses are a collection of both acquired and hereditary protein folding disorders in which deposits of abnormally folded proteins form fibrils and lead to tissue destruction and disease progression. Inherent in all of the amyloid proteins is the β-pleated sheet secondary structure.

The most common type of amyloid in the western world is primary amyloidosis (AL) where the amyloid fibril is derived from an immunoglobulin light chain. Immunoglobulin heavy chain amyloid (AH) is much less common. AL and AH are typically associated with plasma cell dyscrasias. Secondary amyloidosis (AA) is more common in the developing world and occurs in patients with chronic inflammatory conditions, most commonly RA and other connective tissue diseases, familial Mediterranean fever, inflammatory bowel disease, and chronic infections. Its precursor protein, the apolipoprotein serum amyloid A (SAA), is an acute phase reactant. In the hereditary amyloidoses, an inherited gene mutation creates an amyloidigenic protein that triggers the disease. The kidney is one of the most frequent sites of both AL and AA amyloid fibril deposition with slightly less frequent involvement in hereditary amyloid (216).

The light microscopy findings of amyloid appear as amorphous acellular, pale eosinophilic material in the mesangium and capillary loops. Amyloid stains positive with Congo red with apple green birefringence under polarized light. Immunofluorescence usually shows positivity in the affected areas when staining for the responsible light chain; however, false negatives may occur in close to 30% of patients (217). Immunohistochemistry can be used for specific amyloidogenic proteins, such as AA. Electron microscopy shows randomly arranged fibrils 10 to 12 nm in size (218).

Pathogenesis

The pathogenesis of AL amyloid involves the formation of insoluble fibrils from a monoclonal immunoglobulin light chain produced by a modestly infiltrated bone marrow plasma cell clone. The λ-light chain isotype is prevalent in AL. It is postulated that certain germ-line genes for λ-light chains have enhanced propensity to aggregate (219). When mutations cause amino acid substitutions the proteins may have less thermodynamic stability and have different hydrophobic and electrostatic interactions, giving them an even greater propensity to form fibrils (219–221). This abnormal λ-light chain is believed to then interact with a phenotypically changed mesangial cell via a receptor-light chain internalization process; the initiation of monoclonal immunoglobulin deposition disease is thought to occur in the same way. Studies indicate, however, that the initial trafficking of light chains isolated from patients with AL versus those with monoclonal immunoglobulin deposition disease are different thus leading to divergent patterns of light chain deposition. The light chains in AL amyloid are transported to lysosomes leading to fibril formation. The fibril deposits slowly replace extracellular matrix through decreased synthesis of mesangial matrix via a lack of TGF-β and its increased degradation mediated by upregulated expression of matrix metalloproteinases without concomitant upregulation of tissue inhibitors of metalloproteinases (222–225).

AA amyloid develops after a lengthy inflammatory response with overproduction of SAA by proinflammatory cytokines. SSA is proteolytically processed to AA protein in macrophages, which then release the carboxyterminal end of the now amyloidogenic protein into the extracellular space where it is thought to interact with mesangial cells ultimately forming fibrils and disease.

Presentation

Renal AL/AH and AA amyloid typically presents with varying degrees of proteinuria and renal insufficiency, depending on the extent of renal involvement. Hematuria is not uncommon. Other organ systems are typically involved.

Race and sex do not appear to be a factor, with most patients presenting in their sixth decade. The majority of patients with AL amyloid will have monoclonal light chains found in the urine and blood. Approximately 10% of those with AL amyloid will have multiple myeloma.

Prognosis

AL amyloidosis has a poor long-term prognosis without treatment, and the median survival is only 4 to 6 months. Factors that influence the renal response to therapy are the degree of baseline proteinuria, with low baseline proteinuria levels predicting a more favorable renal response. AA amyloid has a better prognosis with the 10-year survival being close to 20%. Mortality is affected by the progression to ESRD, infections, and other organ system involvement.

Treatment

Elimination of the monoclonal protein and the plasma cell clone is the goal of treatment for AL amyloid. Those patients eligible for hematopoietic cell transplantation (HCT) are typically offered such treatment. Those patients not eligible for HCT are treated with various regimens of melphalan and steroids. The process of following response to therapy has been simplified with the advent of the serum-free light chain assay that has a significantly higher sensitivity than serum protein electrophoresis and immunofixation.

AA amyloid is treated with an emphasis at reducing the ongoing underlying inflammatory state. Colchicine has been used to treat AA amyloid associated with familial Mediterranean fever and it has been demonstrated that treatment decreases systemic symptoms and stabilizes renal function. Colchicine has also been used anecdotally in AA amyloid associated with other chronic inflammatory conditions. Anticytokine biologic therapy is currently under investigation.

MONOCLONAL IMMUNOGLOBULIN DEPOSITION DISEASE

In patients with plasma cell dyscrasias the glomerulus is in continual contact with abnormal free light chains. One consequence of light chain proteinuria is the development of the monoclonal immunoglobulin deposition diseases (MIDD). MIDD are classified as light chain deposition disease (LCDD), light- and heavy-chain deposition disease (LHCDD), and heavy-chain deposition disease (HCDD). Light microscopy demonstrates prominent nodular sclerosing glomerulopathy. Glomeruli can be enlarged with a diffuse and nodular expansion of the mesangial matrix. Basement membrane thickening can be seen, as can membranoproliferative features. Findings of myeloma cast nephropathy and amyloid in addition to MIDD have also been reported (226). Congo red stain is negative in MIDD. By immunofluorescence light and/or heavy chain deposits can be found along the glomerular and tubular basement membranes, in the mesangium, renal vasculature, and interstitium. Electron microscopy shows dense deposits within the glomerular and vascular basement membrane and external to tubular basement membranes (227).

Pathogenesis

The initiation of LCDD begins with the interaction of structurally abnormal light chains, usually κ-I and κ-IV light chains, with the mesangial cell of the glomerulus. Amino acid substitutions within the variable region of light chains change the structure of the molecule often introducing hydrophobic residues and regions now able to be posttranslationally modified (228). These abnormal light chains interact with receptors present on mesangial cells causing them to transform into a myofibroblastic phenotype. Activation of growth factors, cytokines, and alteration in mesangial matrix expression leads to the generation of nodular glomerulosclerosis in a process similar to that described for AL amyloid (224).

The abnormal heavy chain molecules that cause disease are described as having a deletion of the CH1 domain of the heavy chain. Lack of this region prevents the complete construction of the immunoglobulin molecule leading to the secretion of free heavy chains from plasma cells (229). How these molecules lead to disease is not understood.

Presentation

MIDD typically presents with proteinuria, renal insufficiency, and hypertension. Nephrotic range proteinuria and microscopic hematuria are not uncommon. A monoclonal spike can be found in the serum and/or urine protein electrophoresis of most patients. Extrarenal deposition can occur in the liver, heart, and peripheral nervous system. Race and sex do not appear to be important factors. Most patients present in their sixth decade. The majority of patients presenting with MIDD have an underlying multiple myeloma/monoclonal gammopathy of undetermined significance (MGUS) or other lymphoproliferative disease; however, isolated MIDD has been reported (226,230). Of the MIDD, LCDD is by far the most prevalent.

Prognosis

The majority of patients diagnosed with MIDD reach ESRD within 2 to 4 years (226,230). Age and serum creatinine at presentation are the major predictive factors for the development of ESRD (230). MIDD does recur in transplanted kidneys if the primary disorder is not effectively treated.

Treatment

There is no definitive treatment for MIDD. Most treatments are similar to those used to treat multiple myeloma, including regimens of melphalan/prednisone, vincristine/adriamycin/dexamethasone, steroids, and vincristine/cyclophosphamide/melphalan/prednisone (226).

CRYOGLOBULINEMIC GLOMERULONEPHRITIS

Cryglobulins are immunoglobulins that precipitate reversibly when cooled to ≤37°C. Type 1 cryoglobulins are composed of a monoclonal population of immunoglobulins, mainly IgG and are strongly associated with lymphoproliferative diseases like leukemia, lymphoma, and plasma cell dyscrasias. Cryoglobulinemic GN is generally an IC-mediated disease and is usually associated with the membranoproliferative pattern of injury by light microscopy; however, type 1 cryoglobulinemia may produce a less inflammatory renal reaction characterized by thrombosis and hypocellular lesions by light microscopy. Patients typically present with proteinuria, hematuria, and renal insufficiency.

WALDENSTRÖM MACROGLOBULINEMIA

Waldenström macroglobulinemia is associated with glomerular lesions consisting of large aggregates of the IgM paraprotein in glomerular capillary loops resembling thrombi. Acute renal failure may ensue. Amyloidosis may also complicate the picture. Therapy with chlorambucil and prednisone is beneficial.

FIBRILLARY AND IMMUNOTACTOID GLOMERULONEPHRITIS

Fibrillary and immunotactoid glomerulonephridities are uncommon causes of GN occurring in <1% and <0.1% of native renal biopsies, respectively (231). Fibrillary glomerulonephritis (FGN) was first described in 1977 and initially labeled "amyloid like" because of the electron microscopy findings of organized electron-dense randomly deposited fibrils that failed to stain with Congo red (232). Since then it has been characterized pathologically primarily by electron microscopy by the deposition in glomeruli of randomly arranged, nonbranching fibrillar immunoglobulin deposits that generally range in size between 18 and 22 nm. These fibrils stain via immunofluorescence for immunoglobulin, light chains, and C3. The light microscopy findings of FGN are heterogeneous and can show proliferative, membranoproliferative, mesangial proliferative, and even crescentic patterns of injury (233,234). Essential to the diagnosis is the absence of reactivity with Congo red.

Immunotactoid glomerulonephritis (ITG) is similar in many ways to FGN. It is Congo red negative with nondiagnostic light microscopy findings. By electron microscopy, however, ITG has microtubular immunoglobulin deposits >30 nm in size, which are often hollow and arranged in parallel arrays (233,234). Experts argue whether these two morphologically different entities should be considered a single disease process or if they have significant clinical and immunopathologic differences to merit differentiation.

Presentation

Both FGN and ITG typically present with nephrotic range proteinuria, hematuria, and renal insufficiency. More than 90% of patients are white. Some studies indicate that there is a slight female preponderance. The mean age at the time of diagnosis is around 50 years old (231,233,235). Patients with ITG are more likely than those with FGN to have an underlying leukemia, lymphoma, or dysproteinemia. Proponents of the theory that FGN and ITG are indeed a different morphologic expression of the same disorder argue that those patients with underlying dysproteinemias should be excluded from a diagnosis of ITG.

Prognosis

Almost half of all patients with FGN or ITG develop ESRD within 2 to 6 years. The rate of disease progression has been linked to light microscopy findings with patients having severe proliferative disease progressing the fastest and those with a membranous pattern of disease progressing slower (231). Both FGN and ITG have been reported to recur in transplanted kidneys.

Treatment

There is no specific treatment for FGN or ITG. Patients should receive nonspecific treatments such as control of blood pressure and proteinuria with RAS inhibitors. There are reports of the use of cytoxic agents, prednisone, plasmapheresis, and NSAIDs with variable results (234). Some experts advocate directing treatment on the basis of light microscopy findings (231). Rituximab has been reported to be effective in a small number of patients (236). If an underlying lymphoproliferative disorder is found, treatment should be aimed at the primary disorder.

Glomerulopathies Associated with Metabolic, Biochemical, or Heredofamilial Disease

DIABETIC NEPHROPATHY

DN is the most common cause of CKD in the United States. Type 1 diabetes is caused by disorders of pancreatic β-cell destruction while type 2 diabetes is due to insulin resistance. Type 1 diabetes accounts for approximately 10% of patients with diabetes while type 2 accounts for 90% of those with disease.

The interpretation of epidemiologic studies in diabetes is challenging as many earlier studies were done in an era without the aggressive diabetic management used today. That being said, approximately 25% of type 1 diabetic patients will have microalbuminuria (persistent albumin excretion between 30 and 300 mg/24 h) after a mean duration of diabetes of 15 years and approximately 15% will progress to overt nephropathy manifested by proteinuria >300 mg/24 h (237,238). The risk of DN in type 2 diabetic patients is almost equivalent to that of type 1 diabetic patients (239,240). Diabetic patients who have no proteinuria after 20 years of disease have a low risk of developing renal disease. Studies have also demonstrated that DN presenting with impaired renal function can occur in the absence of overt albuminuria, including those with normal levels of urinary protein (241,242).

In the setting of aggressive blood glucose control and blood pressure management, the renal prognosis seems to have improved with <10% of patients with overt proteinuria progressing to ESRD (243,244).

A number of different risk factors have been determined which appear to influence the development of DN. These include poor glycemic control, poor blood pressure control, obesity, and smoking. African Americans and Mexican Americans also develop DN more frequently; however, it is difficult to eliminate confounding factors like socioeconomic status from these studies. Age at the time of diagnosis may also be important. The degree of glomerular hyperfiltration increases the risk of developing DN (245). There also appears to be a genetic component to the development of DN with studies suggesting a role for the angiotensin-converting enzyme genotype, the angiotensin-II type 2 receptor gene, and the aldose reductase gene.

Retinopathy is almost always present in type 1 diabetic patients with DN (246). Type 2 diabetic patients have a less predictable relationship with approximately 50% of patients with DN having retinopathy (246,247).

DN affects all of the compartments of the kidney including the glomeruli, vessels, interstitium, and tubules. The first change in the course of DN is hypertrophy of the glomeruli followed by thickening of the glomerular basement and tubular basement membranes and an increase in the mesangial matrix (248). The nodular lesions of DN, also called Kimmelstiel–Wilson nodules, begin in the center of the mesangial region

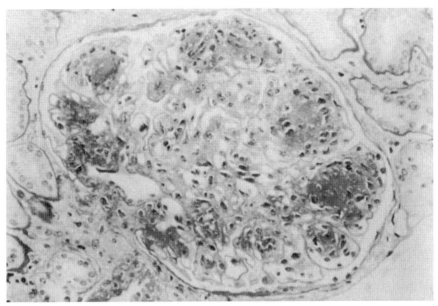

■ **Figure 15.7** Light-microscopic appearance of nodular diabetic glomerulosclerosis. Note the relatively acellular intercapillary nodule and diffuse increase in mesangial matrix. (Courtesy of Dr. Arthur H. Cohen.)

of a segment (Fig. 15.7). Arteriosclerosis is often present as well. Arteriolar hyalinosis at the glomerular hilum typically affects both the afferent and efferent vessel. Atrophic tubules and interstitial fibrosis develop as disease worsens. Electron microscopy shows thickened basement membranes and mesangial expansion.

Pathogenesis

The pathogenesis of DN is a complicated series of events initiated by metabolic factors and then perpetuated by mediator systems. GFR is increased early in the course of diabetes, in part due to increases in glomerular plasma flow, oncotic pressure, transcapillary pressure, and the glomerular ultrafiltration coefficient (249). Other studies have also implicated elevated levels of growth hormone and insulin-like growth factor as having a role in triggering hyperfiltration. Evidence that glomerular hypertension and hyperfiltration are important in DN has also been provided by many studies showing the benefits of blockade of the renin–angiotensin system. Antagonizing the profibrotic effects of angiotensin II may also be a significant factor in benefits observed with these agents (250).

Hyperglycemia stimulates mesangial cell matrix production (251,252) and mesangial cell apoptosis (253). Hyperglycemia also causes glycosylation of proteins and generation of advanced glycosylation end products (AGEs) that further exacerbate disease through collagen cross-linking (254). Hyperglycemia also increases the expression of TGF-β, VEGF, and other cytokines in the glomeruli and matrix proteins that stimulate mesangial matrix accumulation (255,256).

Presentation

DN presents initially with microalbuminuria defined as protein excretion between 30 and 300 mg/ 24 h. Renal function is preserved early on in the course of the disease. Hypertension is common. Microscopic hematuria may be present. Patients who present later in the course of the disease may have the nephrotic syndrome, and renal function may be significantly impaired.

Prognosis

The natural history of DN is a steady decline in GFR ranging from 1 to 24 mL/min/yr associated with an increase in proteinuria and blood pressure (257). With aggressive blood pressure and glucose control this rate of decline can be significantly improved. There is evidence that microalbuminuria can revert back to normal urinary protein excretion with good glucose and blood pressure control as well.

Treatment

The optimal therapy of DN is aggressively being investigated. Goals are to adequately treat blood pressure to a level <130/80 mm Hg, minimize proteinuria with a target goal of 500 to 1,000 mg/day, and control blood glucose. Lipids should be treated to guideline levels.

Blood pressure control and proteinuria reduction should include RAAS inhibition. These medications have been shown to slow the rate of disease progression (237,258). The majority of patients will need additional antihypertensive medications to obtain adequate control in addition to restricted sodium intake; diltiazem or verapamil can produce a further reduction in protein excretion, which may correlate with further protection against progression of the renal disease, while a loop diuretic is typically required in patients with edema or renal insufficiency. Experts continue to debate whether ACE inhibitors and ARBs should be used concurrently in order to maximize RAAS blockade.

ALPORT SYNDROME

Alport syndrome (or hereditary nephritis) is an inherited progressive form of glomerular disease often associated with sensorineural hearing loss and ocular lesions. The prevalence of the disease is estimated at approximately 1 in 50,000 live births. Alport syndrome develops in the setting of defects in type IV collagen, the primary structural component of the GBM. Six different genes have been identified on three different chromosomes; the translated gene products—type IV collagen molecules—interact with each other in complex mechanisms forming a network within basement membranes (259). When an abnormal protein is present it disrupts the orchestrated development of basement membranes and leads to the Alport syndrome phenotype.

The genetics of Alport syndrome are heterogeneous (259). Over 80% of cases are X-linked and arise from mutations in the COL4A5 gene on the X chromosome. Autosomal recessive Alport syndrome accounts for 15% of cases and results from homozygous or compound heterozygous mutations in the COL4A3 or COL3A4 genes. Approximately 5% of Alport syndrome cases display autosomal dominant inheritance and arise from heterozygous mutations in the COL4A3 or COL4A4 genes. It is unclear why some patients with heterozygous mutations develop Alport syndrome, while others develop the usually benign thin basement membrane disease.

The renal manifestations of Alport syndrome include either microscopic or gross hematuria, proteinuria, hypertension, and progression towards ESRD in males with X-linked disease and males and females with either autosomal recessive or dominant disease. Women with X-linked Alport syndrome are carriers for the disease and most have hematuria. Rarely more progressive disease can occur. Diagnosis of Alport syndrome is made by skin or renal biopsy, however often times a positive family history makes tissue diagnosis unnecessary. In a renal biopsy specimen the light microscopy is usually normal in the early course of the disease; however, at later stages glomerulosclerosis and interstitial fibrosis may be present. Immunofluorescence is usually nonspecific unless special studies for type IV collagen are done. Electron microscopy shows irregular thinned and thickened areas of the GBM with splitting and an irregular, multilaminated appearance of the lamina densa (Fig. 15.8). A skin biopsy for the diagnosis of X-linked Alport syndrome is done using a monoclonal antibody against the collagen α-5 (IV) chain, the protein product of COL4A5 (260). If the protein is absent in a male or is clearly mosaic in a female, a diagnosis of Alport syndrome can be made without further testing. If the protein is present then a diagnosis of autosomal recessive Alport syndrome is possible or a mutation in COL4A5 may be present that allows deposition of a functionally abnormal but antigenically normal α-5 (IV) chain. The possibility of another disorder must also be considered.

Treatment of Alport syndrome is supportive. In patients with hypertension or proteinuria RAAS inhibitors are recommended. There are some reports on the use of cyclosporine; however, most experts do not use cyclosporine at this time (261). Alport syndrome does not recur in transplanted kidneys, but de novo anti-GBM antibody disease develops in approximately 3% of transplanted males with antibodies directed against the newly introduced type IV collagen molecule (262).

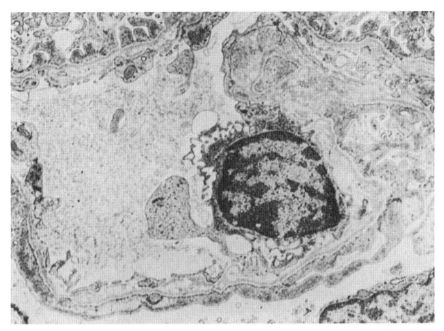

■ Figure 15.8 Electron-microscopic appearance of the lesion in Alport syndrome. Note the thin, altered, glomerular basement membrane.

THIN BASEMENT MEMBRANE NEPHROPATHY

Thin basement membrane nephropathy (TBMN) is an autosomal dominant disorder that frequently results from mutations in two of the genes encoding type IV collagen, *COL4A3* or *COL4A4* on chromosome 2 (259). Its prevalence is estimated to be between 5% and 10% (263). It is frequently familial, with a family history of hematuria reported in almost half of all cases. Patients with TBMN are carriers of autosomal recessive Alport syndrome.

TBMN develops secondary to abnormal collagen that interferes with the normal architecture of GBM. Light and immunofluorescence microscopy are usually normal. Electron microscopy shows diffuse thinning of the GBM.

TBMD is characterized by persistent or recurrent hematuria that frequently begins in childhood. Proteinuria and hypertension are uncommon. The majority of patients have a benign course and a good prognosis; however, there are reports of secondary focal and segmental glomerulosclerosis developing (263). In patients who develop proteinuria, RAAS inhibitors are recommended.

FABRY DISEASE

Fabry disease is an X-linked lysosomal storage disease caused by a deficiency of α-galactosidase A. The incidence of Fabry disease is estimated at 1 in 40,000 to 1 in 117,000 worldwide (264). There does not seem to be any ethnic predisposition. Usual symptom onset is in childhood and life-threatening complications can develop by middle age in untreated patients. Untreated men have a life expectancy that is 20 years shorter than the general population. Women can develop symptoms but generally at a later age.

Deficiency of α-galactosidase A leads to storage of neutral glycosphingolipids in many tissues. The accumulation of these lipids leads to organ dysfunction. Vascular endothelial cells become enlarged by the storage of glycosphingolipids, which then leads to vascular occlusion and ischemia (264). Symptoms develop in a step-wise fashion usually following an age-specific pattern. Initially neuropathic pain, ophthalmologic complications, and gastrointestinal symptoms predominate. School difficulties are common. The first renal manifestations are typically proteinuria and isosthenuria that appear in the second or third decade. Most men usually progress to ESRD. The cardiac and cerebrovascular systems are also frequently involved.

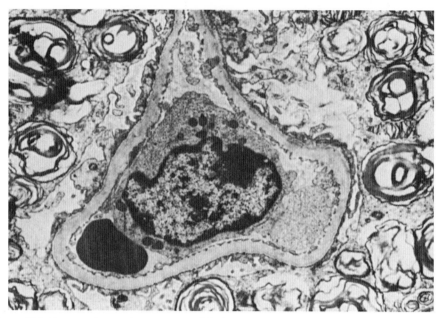

■ **Figure 15.9** Electron-microscopic appearance of the lesion in Fabry disease. Note the whorled "myelin" figures in the epithelial cells. (Courtesy of Dr. Arthur H. Cohen.)

Kidney biopsies demonstrate glycolipid accumulation throughout the kidney. Light microscopy shows vacuolization of podocytes and distal tubular epithelial cells. Deposits can later be seen in the parietal epithelial, mesangial, and glomerular endothelial cells. Glomerulosclerosis and tubulointerstitial fibrosis are seen with more advanced disease. Immunofluorescence is nonspecific. Electron microscopy shows deposits of glycosphingolipids within lysosomes as lamellated membrane structures called myeloid or zebra bodies (Fig. 15.9). These structures are a consistent finding in glycolipid storage diseases (265).

Treatment of Fabry disease is enzyme replacement. RAAS inhibitors should be used for proteinuria control.

NAIL-PATELLA SYNDROME

Nail-patella syndrome (NPS) is an autosomal dominant disorder due to mutations in the gene LMX1B, a transcription factor important for the development of podocytes (266). The incidence of NPS is estimated to be 1 in 50,000, but this might be too high based on the number of detected cases. The classic manifestations reflect dysplasia of structures derived from the dorsal mesenchyme, including hypoplastic nails, hypoplastic patellae, elbow dysplasia, and iliac horns. Kidney disease occurs in approximately half of patients with NPS and is manifested by proteinuria, hematuria, and hypertension. Isothenuria can be seen as well. ESRD develops in approximately 30% of cases by the third decade (266).

Light microscopy in patients with renal manifestations may show basement membrane thickening and nonspecific lesions of focal and segmental glomerulosclerosis. Immunofluorescence is nonspecific. Electron microscopy shows irregular thickening of the GBM, including deposits of bundles of striated type III collagen fibers. Foot process may be focally effaced (266).

There is no specific treatment for NPS. RAAS inhibitors have been used to treat proteinuria. Experts also have postulated that cyclosporine may play a role in treatment. NPS does not recur in transplantation (266).

CONGENITAL NEPHROTIC SYNDROME

Nephrotic syndrome that presents at birth or within the three first months of life is defined as congenital nephrotic syndrome. Most of the children with congenital nephrotic syndrome have a genetic basis for the renal disease.

Recently a number of different gene mutations have been found as a cause for the majority of cases of congenital nephrotic syndrome. A majority of mutations are of NPHS1 and NPHS2. NPHS1 is the gene responsible for nephrin, an integral part of the slit diaphragm, and is responsible for the Finnish-type congenital nephrotic syndrome. NPHS2 encodes podocin, a protein also important at the slit diaphragm, and is responsible for familial focal glomerulosclerosis (267).

Less common mutations are of WT1, which encodes the transcription tumor suppressor and is responsible for the Denys–Drash syndrome, LAMB2 which encodes laminin β-2 and is responsible for the Pierson syndrome, and PLCE1 which encodes phospholipase C epsilon, and is responsible for the early-onset of isolated diffuse mesangial sclerosis (267).

The congenital nephrotic syndromes are resistant to treatment and have a poor prognosis.

LECITHIN–CHOLESTEROL ACYLTRANSFERASE DEFICIENCY

Lecithin–cholesterol acyltransferase (LCAT) deficiency is an autosomal recessive disorder due to the mutation of LCAT gene. The enzyme product is responsible for cholesterol esterification. It is characterized by hyperlipidemia, accelerated atherosclerosis, anemia, corneal opacities, and proteinuria. ESRD may result in patients with LCAT deficiency.

COLLAGENOFIBROTIC GLOMERULOPATHY

Collagenofibrotic glomerulopathy, also called collagen type III glomerulopathy, is an autosomal recessive nephropathy characterized by the accumulation of atypical type III collagen fibrils in the mesangium and subendothelial space. Light microscopy reveals findings consistent with membranoproliferative glomerulonephritis. The fibrils are Congo red negative (nonamyloid) but possess the typical cross striations of mature collagen. A definitive diagnosis requires electron microscopy, which reveals fibers with a transverse band structure and a distinctive periodicity of approximately 60 nm (268).

It tends to cause disease in childhood, and may be a familial disorder. Patients often have hypertension, hemolytic anemia, and some patients have had pulmonary disease.

The pathogenesis and treatment are unknown.

LIPOPROTEIN GLOMERULOPATHY

Lipoprotein glomerulopathy is characterized by the deposition of apolipoprotein E (apoE) within glomerular structures (269). Apparently it is the result of mutations in the apoE gene. Nephrotic syndrome and progressive renal failure are common. Theoretically, lipid apheresis could be of benefit, and protein A immunoadsorption was associated with a resolution of the histologic findings and a reduction in proteinuria in an uncontrolled trial (270).

FIBRONECTIN GLOMERULOPATHY

Fibronectin glomerulopathy is an autosomal dominant disorder associated with the deposition of fibronectin. By EM, fibrillar electron dense deposits are seen in the subendothelial and mesangial spaces (271). Patients may present with proteinuria and microscopic hematuria. Patients with fibronectin glomerulopathy can develop renal insufficiency, and some patients progress to ESRD.

REFERENCES

1. Smith RJ, Alexander J, Barlow PN, et al. New approaches to the treatment of dense deposit disease. *J Am Soc Nephrol.* 2007; 18:2447–2456.
2. Nangaku M, Couser WG. Mechanisms of immune-deposit formation and the mediation of immune renal injury. *Clin Exp Nephrol.* 2005; 9:183–191.
3. Beck L, Bonegio R, Lambeau G, et al. Discovery of the phospholipase A2 receptor as the target antigen in idiopathic membranous nephropathy.
4. Bohle A, Wehrmann M, Bogenschutz O, et al. The long-term prognosis of the primary glomerulonephritides. A morphological and clinical analysis of 1747 cases. *Pathol Res Pract.* 1992; 188:908–924.
5. Zech P, Colon S, Pointet P, et al. The nephrotic syndrome in adults aged over 60: etiology, evolution and treatment of 76 cases. *Clin Nephrol.* 1982; 17:232–236.

6. Mustonen J, Pasternack A, Helin H. IgA mesangial nephropathy in neoplastic diseases. *Contrib Nephrol.* 1984; 40:283–291.

7. Korbet SM, Genchi RM, Borok RZ, et al. The racial prevalence of glomerular lesions in nephrotic adults. *Am J Kidney Dis.* 1996; 27: 647–651.

8. Fogo A, Glick AD, Horn SL, et al. Is focal segmental glomerulosclerosis really focal? Distribution of lesions in adults and children. *Kidney Int.* 1995; 47:1690–1696.

9. Lai KW, Wei CL, Tan LK, et al. Overexpression of interleukin-13 induces minimal-change-like nephropathy in rats. *J Am Soc Nephrol.* 2007; 18:1476–1485.

10. Waldman M, Crew RJ, Valeri A, et al. Adult minimal-change disease: clinical characteristics, treatment, and outcomes. *Clin J Am Soc Nephrol.* 2007; 2:445–453.

11. Black DA, Rose G, Brewer DB. Controlled trial of prednisone in adult patients with the nephrotic syndrome. *Br Med J.* 1970; 3:421–426.

12. Nakayama M, Katafuchi R, Yanase T, et al. Steroid responsiveness and frequency of relapse in adult-onset minimal change nephrotic syndrome. *Am J Kidney Dis.* 2002; 39:503–512.

13. Fakhouri F, Bocquet N, Taupin P, et al. Steroid-sensitive nephrotic syndrome: from childhood to adulthood. *Am J Kidney Dis.* 2003; 41:550–557.

14. Palmer SC, Nand K, Strippoli GF. Interventions for minimal change disease in adults with nephrotic syndrome. *Cochrane Database Syst Rev.* 2008; CD001537.

15. Myllymaki J, Saha H, Mustonen J, et al. IgM nephropathy: clinical picture and long-term prognosis. *Am J Kidney Dis.* 2003; 41:343–350.

16. Border WA. Distinguishing minimal-change disease from mesangial disorders. *Kidney Int.* 1988; 34:419–434.

17. Vizjak A, Ferluga D, Rozic M, et al. Pathology, clinical presentations, and outcomes of C1q nephropathy. *J Am Soc Nephrol.* 2008; 19:2237–2244.

18. Jennette JC, Hipp CG. C1q nephropathy: a distinct pathologic entity usually causing nephrotic syndrome. *Am J Kidney Dis.* 1985; 6:103–110.

19. Haas M, Meehan SM, Karrison TG, et al. Changing etiologies of unexplained adult nephrotic syndrome: a comparison of renal biopsy findings from 1976–1979 and 1995–1997. *Am J Kidney Dis.* 1997; 30:621–631.

20. Kitiyakara C, Eggers P, Kopp JB. Twenty-one-year trend in ESRD due to focal segmental glomerulosclerosis in the United States. *Am J Kidney Dis.* 2004; 44:815–825.

21. Schwartz MM. Focal Segmental Glomerulosclerosis. In: Jennette JC, Olsen JL, Schwarz MM, et al. eds. *Pathology of the Kidney.* Philadelphia: Wolters Kluwer; 2007:155–204.

22. D'Agati VD. Podocyte injury in focal segmental glomerulosclerosis: lessons from animal models (a play in five acts). *Kidney Int.* 2008; 73:399–406.

23. Deegens JK, Dijkman HB, Borm GF, et al. Podocyte foot process effacement as a diagnostic tool in focal segmental glomerulosclerosis. *Kidney Int.* 2008; 74:1568–1576.

24. D'Agati VD, Fogo AB, Bruijn JA, et al. Pathologic classification of focal segmental glomerulosclerosis: a working proposal. *Am J Kidney Dis.* 2004; 43:368–382.

25. Albaqumi M, Barisoni L. Current views on collapsing glomerulopathy. *J Am Soc Nephrol.* 2008; 19:1276–1281.

26. D'Agati V. Pathologic classification of focal segmental glomerulosclerosis. *Semin Nephrol.* 2003; 23:117–134.

27. DH IJ, Farris AB, Goemaere N, et al. Fidelity and evolution of recurrent FSGS in renal allografts. *J Am Soc Nephrol.* 2008; 19:2219–2224.

28. Fogo AB. Minimal change disease and focal segmental glomerulosclerosis. In: Fogo AB, Cohen AH, Jennette JC, et al., eds. *Fundamentals of Renal Pathology.* New York: Springer; 2006:40–52.

29. Sharma M, Sharma R, McCarthy ET, et al. The focal segmental glomerulosclerosis permeability factor: biochemical characteristics and biological effects. *Exp Biol Med (Maywood, N.J).* 2004; 229: 85–98.

30. Floege J, Alpers CE, Burns MW, et al. Glomerular cells, extracellular matrix accumulation, and the development of glomerulosclerosis in the remnant kidney model. *Lab Invest.* 1992; 66:485–497.

31. Schwimmer JA, Markowitz GS, Valeri A, et al. Collapsing glomerulopathy. *Semin Nephrol.* 2003; 23:209–218.

32. Stokes MB, Markowitz GS, Lin J, et al. Glomerular tip lesion: a distinct entity within the minimal change disease/focal segmental glomerulosclerosis spectrum. *Kidney Int.* 2004; 65:1690–1702.

33. Troyanov S, Wall CA, Miller JA, et al. Focal and segmental glomerulosclerosis: definition and relevance of a partial remission. *J Am Soc Nephrol.* 2005; 16:1061–1068.

34. Meyrier A. Nephrotic focal segmental glomerulosclerosis in 2004: an update. *Nephrol Dial Transplant.* 2004; 19:2437–2444.

35. Cattran DC, Appel GB, Hebert LA, et al. A randomized trial of cyclosporine in patients with steroid-resistant focal segmental glomerulosclerosis. North America Nephrotic Syndrome Study Group. *Kidney Int.* 1999; 56: 2220–2226.

36. Ponticelli C, Rizzoni G, Edefonti A, et al. A randomized trial of cyclosporine in steroid-resistant idiopathic nephrotic syndrome. *Kidney Int.* 1993; 43:1377–1384.

37. Cattran DC, Wang MM, Appel G, et al. Mycophenolate mofetil in the treatment of focal segmental glomerulosclerosis. *Clin Nephrol.* 2004; 62:405–411.

38. Schwartz MM. Membranous glomerulonephritis. In: Jennette JC, Olsen JL, Schwarz MM, et al., eds. *Pathology of the Kidney.* Philadelphia: Wolters Kluwer; 2007:205–252.

39. Debiec H, Guigonis V, Mougenot B, et al. Antenatal membranous glomerulonephritis due to anti-neutral endopeptidase antibodies. *N Engl J Med.* 2002; 346:2053–2060.

40. Kerjaschki D. Pathomechanisms and molecular basis of membranous glomerulopathy. *Lancet.* 2004; 364:1194–1196.

41. Glassock RJ. Secondary membranous glomerulonephritis. *Nephrol Dial Transplant.* 1992; 7 (suppl 1):64–71.

42. Hogan SL, Muller KE, Jennette JC, et al. A review of therapeutic studies of idiopathic membranous glomerulopathy. *Am J Kidney Dis.* 1995; 25:862–875.

43. Ponticelli C. Membranous nephropathy. *J Nephrol.* 2007; 20:268–287.

44. Burstein DM, Korbet SM, Schwartz MM. Membranous glomerulonephritis and malignancy. *Am J Kidney Dis.* 1993; 22:5–10.

45. Ponticelli C, Zucchelli P, Passerini P, et al. A 10-year follow-up of a randomized study with methylprednisolone and chlorambucil in membranous nephropathy. *Kidney Int.* 1995; 48: 1600–1604.

46. Jha V, Ganguli A, Saha TK, et al. A randomized, controlled trial of steroids and cyclophosphamide in adults with nephrotic syndrome caused by idiopathic membranous nephropathy. *J Am Soc Nephrol.* 2007; 18:1899–1904.

47. Pei Y, Cattran D, Greenwood C. Predicting chronic renal insufficiency in idiopathic membranous glomerulonephritis. *Kidney Int.* 1992; 42: 960–966.

48. Glassock RJ. Diagnosis and natural course of membranous nephropathy. *Semin Nephrol.* 2003; 23:324–332.

49. Wu Q, Jinde K, Nishina M, et al. Analysis of prognostic predictors in idiopathic membranous nephropathy. *Am J Kidney Dis.* 2001; 37:380–387.

50. Troyanov S, Wall CA, Miller JA, et al. Idiopathic membranous nephropathy: definition and relevance of a partial remission. *Kidney Int.* 2004; 66:1199–1205.

51. Cattran DC, Appel GB, Hebert LA, et al. Cyclosporine in patients with steroid-resistant membranous nephropathy: a randomized trial. *Kidney Int.* 2001; 59:1484–1490.

52. Praga M, Barrio V, Juarez GF, et al. Tacrolimus monotherapy in membranous nephropathy: a randomized controlled trial. *Kidney Int.* 2007; 71:924–930.

53. Cattran DC, Greenwood C, Ritchie S, et al. A controlled trial of cyclosporine in patients with progressive membranous nephropathy. Canadian Glomerulonephritis Study Group. *Kidney Int.* 1995; 47:1130–1135.

54. Fervenza FC, Cosio FG, Erickson SB, et al. Rituximab treatment of idiopathic membranous nephropathy. *Kidney Int.* 2008; 73:117–125.

55. Branten AJ, du Buf-Vereijken PW, Vervloet M, et al. Mycophenolate mofetil in idiopathic membranous nephropathy: a clinical trial with comparison to a historic control group treated with cyclophosphamide. *Am J Kidney Dis.* 2007; 50: 248–256.

56. Miller G, Zimmerman R 3rd, Radhakrishnan J, et al. Use of mycophenolate mofetil in resistant membranous nephropathy. *Am J Kidney Dis.* 2000; 36:250–256.

57. Bohle A, Gartner HV, Fischbach H, et al. The morphological and clinical features of membranoproliferative glomerulonephritis in adults. *Virchows Arch A Pathol Anat Histol.* 1974; 363: 213–224.

58. Cameron JS, Turner DR, Heaton J, et al. Idiopathic mesangiocapillary glomerulonephritis. Comparison of types I and II in children and adults and long-term prognosis. *Am J Med.* 1983; 74:175–192.

59. Donadio JV Jr, Slack TK, Holley KE, et al. Idiopathic membranoproliferative (mesangiocapillary) glomerulonephritis: a clinicopathologic study. *Mayo Clin Proc.* 1979; 54:141–150.

60. Berger J, Galle P. [Dense Deposits within the Basal Membranes of the Kidney. Optical and Electron Microscopic Study.]. *Presse Med.* 1963; 71:2351–2354.

61. Walker PD, Ferrario F, Joh K, et al. Dense deposit disease is not a membranoproliferative glomerulonephritis. *Mod Pathol.* 2007; 20:605–616.

62. Jackson EC, McAdams AJ, Strife CF, et al. Differences between membranoproliferative glomerulonephritis types I and III in clinical presentation, glomerular morphology, and complement perturbation. *Am J Kidney Dis.* 1987; 9:115–120.

63. Strife CF, McEnery PT, McAdams AJ, et al. Membranoproliferative glomerulonephritis with disruption of the glomerular basement membrane. *Clin Nephrol.* 1977; 7:65–72.

64. Cameron JS. Mesangiocapillary glomerulonephritis and persistent hypocomplementemia. In: Kincaid-Smith P, Mathew TH, Becker EL, eds. *Glomerulonephritis: Morphology, Natural History and Treatment.* New York: John Wiley & Sons; 1973:541.

65. Davis CA, Marder H, West CD. Circulating immune complexes in membranoproliferative glomerulonephritis. *Kidney Int.* 1981; 20: 728–732.

66. Donadio JV Jr, Anderson CF, Mitchell JC 3rd, et al. Membranoproliferative glomerulonephritis. A prospective clinical trial of platelet-inhibitor therapy. *N Engl J Med.* 1984; 310:1421–1426.

67. West C. Complement and glomerular disease. In: Volanakis JE, Frank MM, eds. *The Human Complement System in Health and Disease.* New York: Marcel Dekker, Inc.; 1998:571–596.

68. Neary JJ, Conlon PJ, Croke D, et al. Linkage of a gene causing familial membranoproliferative glomerulonephritis type III to chromosome 1. *J Am Soc Nephrol.* 2002; 13:2052–2057.

69. Barbiano di Belgiojoso G, Baroni M, Pagliari B, et al. Is membranoproliferative glomerulonephritis really decreasing? A multicentre study of 1,548 cases of primary glomerulonephritis. *Nephron.* 1985; 40:380–381.

70. Johnson RJ, Hurtado A, Merszei J, et al. Hypothesis: dysregulation of immunologic balance resulting from hygiene and socioeconomic factors may influence the epidemiology and cause of glomerulonephritis worldwide. *Am J Kidney Dis.* 2003; 42:575–581.

71. Swainson CP, Robson JS, Thomson D, et al. Mesangiocapillary glomerulonephritis: a long-term study of 40 cases. *J Pathol.* 1983; 141:449–468.

72. McEnery PT. Membranoproliferative glomerulonephritis: the Cincinnati experience—cumulative renal survival from 1957 to 1989. *J Pediatr.* 1990; 116:S109–S114.

73. Cansick JC, Lennon R, Cummins CL, et al. Prognosis, treatment and outcome of childhood

mesangiocapillary (membranoproliferative) glomerulonephritis. *Nephrol Dial Transplant*. 2004; 19:2769–2777.

74. Zauner I, Bohler J, Braun N, et al. Effect of aspirin and dipyridamole on proteinuria in idiopathic membranoproliferative glomerulonephritis: a multicentre prospective clinical trial. Collaborative Glomerulonephritis Therapy Study Group (CGTS). *Nephrol Dial Transplant*. 1994; 9:619–622.

75. Schwertz R, Rother U, Anders D, et al. Complement analysis in children with idiopathic membranoproliferative glomerulonephritis: a long-term follow-up. *Pediatr Allergy Immunol*. 2001; 12:166–172.

76. Pickering MC, Cook HT. Translational minireview series on complement factor H: renal diseases associated with complement factor H: novel insights from humans and animals. *Clin Exp Immunol*. 2008; 151:210–230.

77. Barratt J, Smith AC, Molyneux K, et al. Immunopathogenesis of IgAN. *Semin Immunopathol*. 2007; 29:427–443.

78. Galla JH. IgA nephropathy. *Kidney Int*. 1995; 47:377–387.

79. Li LS, Liu ZH. Epidemiologic data of renal diseases from a single unit in China: analysis based on 13,519 renal biopsies. *Kidney Int*. 2004; 66: 920–923.

80. Nakayama K, Ohsawa I, Maeda-Ohtani A, et al. Prediction of diagnosis of immunoglobulin A nephropathy prior to renal biopsy and correlation with urinary sediment findings and prognostic grading. *J Clin Lab Anal*. 2008; 22:114–118.

81. Haubitz M, Wittke S, Weissinger EM, et al. Urine protein patterns can serve as diagnostic tools in patients with IgA nephropathy. *Kidney Int*. 2005; 67:2313–2320.

82. Gharavi AG, Moldoveanu Z, Wyatt RJ, et al. Aberrant IgA1 glycosylation is inherited in familial and sporadic IgA nephropathy. *J Am Soc Nephrol*. 2008; 19:1008–1014.

83. Jennette JC. Immunoglobulin A nephropathy and Henoch-Schonlein purpura. In: Fogo AB, Cohen AH, Jennette JC, et al., eds. *Fundamentals of Renal Pathology*. New York: Springer; 2006:61–69.

84. Haas M. Histologic subclassification of IgA nephropathy: a clinicopathologic study of 244 cases. *Am J Kidney Dis*. 1997; 29:829–842.

85. Lee HS, Lee MS, Lee SM, et al. Histological grading of IgA nephropathy predicting renal outcome: revisiting H. S. Lee's glomerular grading system. *Nephrol Dial Transplant*. 2005; 20:342–348.

86. Tumlin JA, Madaio MP, Hennigar R. Idiopathic IgA nephropathy: pathogenesis, histopathology, and therapeutic options. *Clin J Am Soc Nephrol*. 2007; 2:1054–1061.

87. Suzuki K, Honda K, Tanabe K, et al. Incidence of latent mesangial IgA deposition in renal allograft donors in Japan. *Kidney Int*. 2003; 63:2286–2294.

88. Kellerman PS. Henoch-Schonlein purpura in adults. *Am J Kidney Dis*. 2006; 48:1009–1016.

89. Harper SJ, Allen AC, Bene MC, et al. Increased dimeric IgA-producing B cells in tonsils in IgA nephropathy determined by in situ hybridization for J chain mRNA. *Clin Exp Immunol*. 1995; 101: 442–448.

90. Harper SJ, Allen AC, Pringle JH, et al. Increased dimeric IgA producing B cells in the bone marrow

in IgA nephropathy determined by in situ hybridisation for J chain mRNA. *J Clin Pathol*. 1996; 49:38–42.

91. Smith AC, Molyneux K, Feehally J, et al. O-glycosylation of serum IgA1 antibodies against mucosal and systemic antigens in IgA nephropathy. *J Am Soc Nephrol*. 2006; 17:3520–3528.

92. Donadio JV, Grande JP. IgA nephropathy. *N Engl J Med*. 2002; 347:738–748.

93. Gutierrez E, Gonzalez E, Hernandez E, et al. Factors that determine an incomplete recovery of renal function in macrohematuria-induced acute renal failure of IgA nephropathy. *Clin J Am Soc Nephrol*. 2007; 2:51–57.

94. Geddes CC, Rauta V, Gronhagen-Riska C, et al. A tricontinental view of IgA nephropathy. *Nephrol Dial Transplant*. 2003; 18:1541–1548.

95. D'Amico G. Natural history of idiopathic IgA nephropathy: role of clinical and histological prognostic factors. *Am J Kidney Dis*. 2000; 36:227–237.

96. Manno C, Strippoli GF, D'Altri C, et al. A novel simpler histological classification for renal survival in IgA nephropathy: a retrospective study. *Am J Kidney Dis*. 2007; 49:763–775.

97. Espinosa M, Ortega R, Gomez-Carrasco JM, et al. Mesangial C4d deposition: a new prognostic factor in IgA nephropathy. *Nephrol Dial Transplant*. 2009; 24:886–891.

98. Roos A, Rastaldi MP, Calvaresi N, et al. Glomerular activation of the lectin pathway of complement in IgA nephropathy is associated with more severe renal disease. *J Am Soc Nephrol*. 2006; 17:1724–1734.

99. Reich HN, Troyanov S, Scholey JW, et al. Remission of proteinuria improves prognosis in IgA nephropathy. *J Am Soc Nephrol*. 2007; 18:3177–3183.

100. Katafuchi R, Ikeda K, Mizumasa T, et al. Controlled, prospective trial of steroid treatment in IgA nephropathy: a limitation of low-dose prednisolone therapy. *Am J Kidney Dis*. 2003; 41:972–983.

101. Pozzi C, Andrulli S, Del Vecchio L, et al. Corticosteroid effectiveness in IgA nephropathy: long-term results of a randomized, controlled trial. *J Am Soc Nephrol*. 2004; 15:157–163.

102. Pozzi C, Bolasco PG, Fogazzi GB, et al. Corticosteroids in IgA nephropathy: a randomised controlled trial. *Lancet*. 1999; 353:883–887.

103. Ballardie FW, Roberts IS. Controlled prospective trial of prednisolone and cytotoxics in progressive IgA nephropathy. *J Am Soc Nephrol*. 2002; 13: 142–148.

104. Roccatello D, Ferro M, Coppo R, et al. Report on intensive treatment of extracapillary glomerulonephritis with focus on crescentic IgA nephropathy. *Nephrol Dial Transplant*. 1995; 10:2054–2059.

105. Tumlin JA, Lohavichan V, Hennigar R. Crescentic, proliferative IgA nephropathy: clinical and histological response to methylprednisolone and intravenous cyclophosphamide. *Nephrol Dial Transplant*. 2003; 18:1321–1329.

106. Rovang RD, Zawada ET Jr, Santella RN, et al. Cerebral vasculitis associated with acute post-streptococcal glomerulonephritis. *Am J Nephrol*. 1997; 17:89–92.

107. Lewis EJ, Carpenter CB, Schur PH. Serum complement component levels in human glomerulonephritis. *Ann Intern Med*. 1971; 75:555–560.

108. Kobrin S, Madaio MP. Acute poststreptococcal glomerulonephritis and other bacterial infection-related glomerulonephritis. In: Schrier RW, ed. *Diseases of the Kidney and Urinary Tract*. Philadelphia: Lippincott Williams & Wilkins; 2007: 1464–1476.

109. Sorger K. Postinfectious glomerulonephritis. Subtypes, clinico-pathological correlations, and follow-up studies. *Veroff Pathol*. 1986; 125:1–105.

110. Rodriguez-Iturbe B, Musser JM. The current state of poststreptococcal glomerulonephritis. *J Am Soc Nephrol*. 2008; 19:1855–1864.

111. Gillmore JD, Lovat LB, Persey MR, et al. Amyloid load and clinical outcome in AA amyloidosis in relation to circulating concentration of serum amyloid A protein. *Lancet*. 2001; 358:24–29.

112. Weiner NJ, Goodman JW, Kimmel PL. The HIV-associated renal diseases: current insight into pathogenesis and treatment. *Kidney Int*. 2003; 63:1618–1631.

113. Hailemariam S, Walder M, Burger HR, et al. Renal pathology and premortem clinical presentation of Caucasian patients with AIDS: an autopsy study from the era prior to antiretroviral therapy. *Swiss Med Wkly*. 2001; 131:412–417.

114. Cheung CY, Wong KM, Lee MP, et al. Prevalence of chronic kidney disease in Chinese HIV-infected patients. *Nephrol Dial Transplant*. 2007; 22:3186–3190.

115. Fernando SK, Finkelstein FO, Moore BA, et al. Prevalence of chronic kidney disease in an urban HIV infected population. *Am J Med Sci*. 2008; 335:89–94.

116. Wyatt CM, Winston JA, Malvestutto CD, et al. Chronic kidney disease in HIV infection: an urban epidemic. *AIDS*. 2007; 21:2101–2103.

117. Schwartz EJ, Szczech LA, Ross MJ, et al. Highly active antiretroviral therapy and the epidemic of HIV+ end-stage renal disease. *J Am Soc Nephrol*. 2005; 16:2412–2420.

118. Kimmel PL. The nephropathies of HIV infection: pathogenesis and treatment. *Curr Opin Nephrol Hypertens*. 2000; 9:117–122.

119. Ross MJ, Klotman PE. Recent progress in HIV-associated nephropathy. *J Am Soc Nephrol*. 2002; 13:2997–3004.

120. Ray PE, Bruggeman LA, Weeks BS, et al. bFGF and its low affinity receptors in the pathogenesis of HIV-associated nephropathy in transgenic mice. *Kidney Int*. 1994; 46:759–772.

121. Yamamoto T, Noble NA, Miller DE, et al. Increased levels of transforming growth factor-beta in HIV-associated nephropathy. *Kidney Int*. 1999; 55:579–592.

122. Gherardi D, D'Agati V, Chu TH, et al. Reversal of collapsing glomerulopathy in mice with the cyclin-dependent kinase inhibitor CYC202. *J Am Soc Nephrol*. 2004; 15:1212–1222.

123. Kopp JB, Smith MW, Nelson GW, et al. MYH9 is a major-effect risk gene for focal segmental glomerulosclerosis. *Nat Genet*. 2008; 40:1175–1184.

124. Lucas GM, Eustace JA, Sozio S, et al. Highly active antiretroviral therapy and the incidence of HIV-1-associated nephropathy: a 12-year cohort study. *AIDS*. 2004; 18:541–546.

125. Gupta SK, Eustace JA, Winston JA, et al. Guidelines for the management of chronic kidney disease in HIV-infected patients: recommendations of the HIV Medicine Association of the Infectious Diseases Society of America. *Clin Infect Dis*. 2005; 40:1559–1585.

126. Wei A, Burns GC, Williams BA, et al. Long-term renal survival in HIV-associated nephropathy with angiotensin-converting enzyme inhibition. *Kidney Int*. 2003; 64:1462–1471.

127. Eustace JA, Nuermberger E, Choi M, et al. Cohort study of the treatment of severe HIV-associated nephropathy with corticosteroids. *Kidney Int*. 2000; 58:1253–1260.

128. Kimmel PL, Barisoni L, Kopp JB. Pathogenesis and treatment of HIV-associated renal diseases: lessons from clinical and animal studies, molecular pathologic correlations, and genetic investigations. *Ann Intern Med*. 2003; 139:214–226.

129. Cohen SD, Kimmel PL. Immune complex renal disease and human immunodeficiency virus infection. *Semin Nephrol*. 2008; 28:535–544.

130. Kimmel PL, Phillips TM, Ferreira-Centeno A, et al. HIV-associated immune-mediated renal disease. *Kidney Int*. 1993; 44:1327–1340.

131. Nishanian P, Huskins KR, Stehn S, et al. A simple method for improved assay demonstrates that HIV p24 antigen is present as immune complexes in most sera from HIV-infected individuals. *J Infect Dis*. 1990; 162:21–28.

132. Dellow E, Unwin R, Miller R, et al. Protease inhibitor therapy for HIV infection: the effect on HIV-associated nephrotic syndrome. *Nephrol Dial Transplant*. 1999; 14:744–747.

133. Szczech LA, Gupta SK, Habash R, et al. The clinical epidemiology and course of the spectrum of renal diseases associated with HIV infection. *Kidney Int*. 2004; 66:1145–1152.

134. Haas M, Kaul S, Eustace JA. HIV-associated immune complex glomerulonephritis with "lupus-like" features: a clinicopathologic study of 14 cases. *Kidney Int*. 2005; 67:1381–1390.

135. Mattana J, Siegal FP, Schwarzwald E, et al. AIDS-associated membranous nephropathy with advanced renal failure: response to prednisone. *Am J Kidney Dis*. 1997; 30:116–119.

136. Misiani R, Bellavita P, Fenili D, et al. Hepatitis C virus infection in patients with essential mixed cryoglobulinemia. *Ann Intern Med*. 1992; 117: 573–577.

137. Johnson RJ, Gretch DR, Yamabe H, et al. Membranoproliferative glomerulonephritis associated with hepatitis C virus infection. *N Engl J Med*. 1993; 328:465–470.

138. McGuire BM, Julian BA, Bynon JS Jr, et al. Brief communication: Glomerulonephritis in patients with hepatitis C cirrhosis undergoing liver transplantation. *Ann Intern Med*. 2006; 144: 735–741.

139. Sansonno D, Gesualdo L, Manno C, et al. Hepatitis C virus-related proteins in kidney tissue from hepatitis C virus-infected patients with cryoglobulinemic membranoproliferative glomerulonephritis. *Hepatology*. 1997; 25:1237–1244.

140. Fornasieri A, Li M, Armelloni S, et al. Glomerulonephritis induced by human IgMK-IgG cryoglobulins in mice. *Lab Invest*. 1993; 69:531–540.

141. Tarantino A, Campise M, Banfi G, et al. Long-term predictors of survival in essential mixed

cryoglobulinemic glomerulonephritis. *Kidney Int.* 1995; 47:618–623.

142. Zuckerman E, Keren D, Slobodin G, et al. Treatment of refractory, symptomatic, hepatitis C virus related mixed cryoglobulinemia with ribavirin and interferon-alpha. *J Rheumatol.* 2000; 27:2172–2178.

143. Alric L, Plaisier E, Thebault S, et al. Influence of antiviral therapy in hepatitis C virus-associated cryoglobulinemic MPGN. *Am J Kidney Dis.* 2004; 43:617–623.

144. Kamar N, Rostaing L, Alric L. Treatment of hepatitis C-virus-related glomerulonephritis. *Kidney Int.* 2006; 69:436–439.

145. Roccatello D, Baldovino S, Rossi D, et al. Long-term effects of anti-CD20 monoclonal antibody treatment of cryoglobulinaemic glomerulonephritis. *Nephrol Dial Transplant.* 2004; 19:3054–3061.

146. Lai FM, Lai KN, Tam JS, et al. Primary glomerulonephritis with detectable glomerular hepatitis B virus antigens. *Am J Surg Pathol.* 1994; 18:175–186.

147. Lin CY. Treatment of hepatitis B virus-associated membranous nephropathy with recombinant alpha-interferon. *Kidney Int.* 1995; 47:225–230.

148. Elsheikha HM, Sheashaa HA. Epidemiology, pathophysiology, management and outcome of renal dysfunction associated with plasmodia infection. *Parasitol Res.* 2007; 101:1183–1190.

149. Cameron JS. Clinical manifestations of lupus nephritis. In: Lewis EJ, Schwartz MM, Korbet SM, eds. *Lupus Nephritis.* Oxford: Oxford University Press; 1999:159–184.

150. Bono L, Cameron JS, Hicks JA. The very long-term prognosis and complications of lupus nephritis and its treatment. *QJM.* 1999; 92: 211–218.

151. Cervera R, Khamashta MA, Font J, et al. Morbidity and mortality in systemic lupus erythematosus during a 10-year period: a comparison of early and late manifestations in a cohort of 1,000 patients. *Medicine (Baltimore).* 2003; 82:299–308.

152. Rahman A, Isenberg DA. Systemic lupus erythematosus. *N Engl J Med.* 2008; 358:929–939.

153. Trouw LA, Groeneveld TW, Seelen MA, et al. Anti-C1q autoantibodies deposit in glomeruli but are only pathogenic in combination with glomerular C1q-containing immune complexes. *J Clin Invest.* 2004; 114:679–688.

154. ter Borg EJ, Horst G, Hummel EJ, et al. Measurement of increases in anti-double-stranded DNA antibody levels as a predictor of disease exacerbation in systemic lupus erythematosus. A long-term, prospective study. *Arthritis Rheum.* 1990; 33:634–643.

155. Austin HA 3rd, Boumpas DT, Vaughan EM, et al. Predicting renal outcomes in severe lupus nephritis: contributions of clinical and histologic data. *Kidney Int.* 1994; 45:544–550.

156. Pillemer SR, Austin HA 3rd, Tsokos GC, et al. Lupus nephritis: association between serology and renal biopsy measures. *J Rheumatol.* 1988; 15:284–288.

157. Laitman RS, Glicklich D, Sablay LB, et al. Effect of long-term normalization of serum complement levels on the course of lupus nephritis. *Am J Med.* 1989; 87:132–138.

158. Churg J, Sobin LH. Lupus nephritis. In: *Renal Disease: Classification and Atlas of Glomerular Disease.* New York: Igaku-Shoin; 1982:127–149.

159. Weening JJ, D'Agati VD, Schwartz MM, et al. The classification of glomerulonephritis in systemic lupus erythematosus revisited. *J Am Soc Nephrol.* 2004; 15:241–250.

160. Appel GB, Cohen DJ, Pirani CL, et al. Long-term follow-up of patients with lupus nephritis. A study based on the classification of the World Health Organization. *Am J Med.* 1987; 83:877–885.

161. McLaughlin J, Gladman DD, Urowitz MB, et al. Kidney biopsy in systemic lupus erythematosus. II. Survival analyses according to biopsy results. *Arthritis Rheum.* 1991; 34:1268–1273.

162. Parikh C, Gibney E, Thurman J. The long term outcome of glomerular diseases. In: Schrier RW, ed. *Diseases of the Kidney and Urinary Tract.* 8th ed. Philadelphia: Lippincott Williams & Wilkins; 2006:1811–1859.

163. Ginzler EM, Nicastri AD, Chen CK, et al. Progression of mesangial and focal to diffuse lupus nephritis. *N Engl J Med.* 1974; 291:693–696.

164. Morel-Maroger L, Mery JP, Droz D, et al. The course of lupus nephritis: contribution of serial renal biopsies. *Adv Nephrol Necker Hosp.* 1976; 6:79–118.

165. Kuhn K, Menninger H. Is renal biopsy overused in patients with systemic lupus erythematosus? *Contrib Nephrol.* 1984; 43:45–50.

166. Korbet SM, Lewis EJ, Schwartz MM, et al. Factors predictive of outcome in severe lupus nephritis. Lupus Nephritis Collaborative Study Group. *Am J Kidney Dis.* 2000; 35:904–914.

167. Hill GS, Delahousse M, Nochy D, et al. Class IV-S versus class IV-G lupus nephritis: clinical and morphologic differences suggesting different pathogenesis. *Kidney Int.* 2005; 68:2288–2297.

168. Dooley MA, Hogan S, Jennette C, et al. Cyclophosphamide therapy for lupus nephritis: poor renal survival in black Americans. Glomerular Disease Collaborative Network. *Kidney Int.* 1997; 51:1188–1195.

169. Moroni G, Quaglini S, Maccario M, et al. "Nephritic flares" are predictors of bad long-term renal outcome in lupus nephritis. *Kidney Int.* 1996; 50:2047–2053.

170. Boumpas DT, Austin HA 3rd, Vaughn EM, et al. Controlled trial of pulse methylprednisolone versus two regimens of pulse cyclophosphamide in severe lupus nephritis. *Lancet.* 1992; 340:741–745.

171. Gourley MF, Austin HA 3rd, Scott D, et al. Methylprednisolone and cyclophosphamide, alone or in combination, in patients with lupus nephritis. A randomized, controlled trial. *Ann Intern Med.* 1996; 125:549–557.

172. Houssiau FA, Vasconcelos C, D'Cruz D, et al. Immunosuppressive therapy in lupus nephritis: the Euro-Lupus Nephritis Trial, a randomized trial of low-dose versus high-dose intravenous cyclophosphamide. *Arthritis Rheum.* 2002; 46:2121–2131.

173. Chan TM, Li FK, Tang CS, et al. Efficacy of mycophenolate mofetil in patients with diffuse proliferative lupus nephritis. Hong Kong-Guangzhou Nephrology Study Group. *N Engl J Med.* 2000; 343:1156–1162.

174. Ginzler EM, Dooley MA, Aranow C, et al. Mycophenolate mofetil or intravenous cyclophosphamide for lupus nephritis. *N Engl J Med.* 2005; 353:2219–2228.

175. Illei GG, Takada K, Parkin D, et al. Renal flares are common in patients with severe proliferative lupus nephritis treated with pulse immunosuppressive therapy: long-term followup of a cohort of 145 patients participating in randomized controlled studies. *Arthritis Rheum.* 2002; 46:995–1002.

176. Contreras G, Pardo V, Leclercq B, et al. Sequential therapies for proliferative lupus nephritis. *N Engl J Med.* 2004; 350:971–980.

177. Bertsias G, Boumpas DT. Update on the management of lupus nephritis: let the treatment fit the patient. *Nat Clin Pract Rheumatol.* 2008; 4: 464–472.

178. Ogawa H, Kameda H, Nagasawa H, et al. Prospective study of low-dose cyclosporine A in patients with refractory lupus nephritis. *Mod Rheumatol.* 2007; 17:92–97.

179. Austin HA, Illei GG, Braun MJ, et al. Randomized, controlled trial of prednisone, cyclophosphamide, and cyclosporine in lupus membranous nephropathy. *J Am Soc Nephrol.* 2009; 20:901–911.

180. Jennette JC, Falk RJ. The pathology of vasculitis involving the kidney. *Am J Kidney Dis.* 1994; 24: 130–141.

181. Jennette JC, Falk RJ. Small-vessel vasculitis. *N Engl J Med.* 1997; 337:1512–1523.

182. Kain R, Exner M, Brandes R, et al. Molecular mimicry in pauci-immune focal necrotizing glomerulonephritis. *Nat Med.* 2008; 14: 1088–1096.

183. Charles LA, Caldas ML, Falk RJ, et al. Antibodies against granule proteins activate neutrophils in vitro. *J Leukoc Biol.* 1991; 50:539–546.

184. Xiao H, Heeringa P, Hu P, et al. Antineutrophil cytoplasmic autoantibodies specific for myeloperoxidase cause glomerulonephritis and vasculitis in mice. *J Clin Invest.* 2002; 110:955–963.

185. Schlieben DJ, Korbet SM, Kimura RE, et al. Pulmonary-renal syndrome in a newborn with placental transmission of ANCAs. *Am J Kidney Dis.* 2005; 45:758–761.

186. Jennette JC, Falk RJ. New insight into the pathogenesis of vasculitis associated with antineutrophil cytoplasmic autoantibodies. *Curr Opin Rheumatol.* 2008; 20:55–60.

187. Morgan MD, Harper L, Williams J, et al. Anti-neutrophil cytoplasm-associated glomerulonephritis. *J Am Soc Nephrol.* 2006; 17:1224– 1234.

188. Nachman PH, Hogan SL, Jennette JC, et al. Treatment response and relapse in antineutrophil cytoplasmic autoantibody-associated microscopic polyangiitis and glomerulonephritis. *J Am Soc Nephrol.* 1996; 7:33–39.

189. Pusey CD, Rees AJ, Evans DJ, et al. Plasma exchange in focal necrotizing glomerulonephritis without anti-GBM antibodies. *Kidney Int.* 1991; 40:757–763.

190. Jayne D, Rasmussen N, Andrassy K, et al. A randomized trial of maintenance therapy for vasculitis associated with antineutrophil cytoplasmic autoantibodies. *N Engl J Med.* 2003; 349:36–44.

191. Stassen PM, Cohen Tervaert JW, Stegeman CA. Induction of remission in active anti-neutrophil cytoplasmic antibody-associated vasculitis with mycophenolate mofetil in patients who cannot be treated with cyclophosphamide. *Ann Rheum Dis.* 2007; 66:798–802.

192. Joy MS, Hogan SL, Jennette JC, et al. A pilot study using mycophenolate mofetil in relapsing or resistant ANCA small vessel vasculitis. *Nephrol Dial Transplant.* 2005; 20:2725–2732.

193. Stanton MC, Tange JD. Goodpasture's syndrome (pulmonary haemorrhage associated with glomerulonephritis). *Australas Ann Med.* 1958; 7:132–144.

194. Serisier DJ, Wong RC, Armstrong JG. Alveolar haemorrhage in anti-glomerular basement membrane disease without detectable antibodies by conventional assays. *Thorax.* 2006; 61:636–639.

195. Wilson CB, Dixon FJ. Anti-glomerular basement membrane antibody-induced glomerulonephritis. *Kidney Int.* 1973; 3:74–89.

196. Rieger M, Mannucci PM, Kremer Hovinga JA, et al. ADAMTS13 autoantibodies in patients with thrombotic microangiopathies and other immuno-mediated diseases. *Blood.* 2005; 106:1262–1267.

197. Scheiflinger F, Knobl P, Trattner B, et al. Nonneutralizing IgM and IgG antibodies to von Willebrand factor-cleaving protease (ADAMTS-13) in a patient with thrombotic thrombocytopenic purpura. *Blood.* 2003; 102:3241–3243.

198. Obrig TG, Del Vecchio PJ, Brown JE, et al. Direct cytotoxic action of Shiga toxin on human vascular endothelial cells. *Infect immun.* 1988; 56:2373–2378.

199. Kavanagh D, Goodship TH. Update on evaluating complement in hemolytic uremic syndrome. *Curr Opin Nephrol Hypertens.* 2007; 16:565–571.

200. George JN, Terrell DR, Swisher KK, et al. Lessons learned from the Oklahoma thrombotic thrombocytopenic purpura-hemolytic uremic syndrome registry. *J Clin Apher.* 2008; 23:129–137.

201. Jin M, Casper TC, Cataland SR, et al. Relationship between ADAMTS13 activity in clinical remission and the risk of TTP relapse. *Br J Haematol.* 2008; 141:651–658.

202. Saland JM, Shneider BL, Bromberg JS, et al. Successful split liver-kidney transplant for factor H associated hemolytic uremic syndrome. *Clin J Am Soc Nephrol.* 2009; 4:201–206.

203. Rock GA, Shumak KH, Buskard NA, et al. Comparison of plasma exchange with plasma infusion in the treatment of thrombotic thrombocytopenic purpura. Canadian Apheresis Study Group. *N Engl J Med.* 1991; 325:393–397.

204. Cataland SR, Jin M, Lin S, et al. Cyclosporin and plasma exchange in thrombotic thrombocytopenic purpura: long-term follow-up with serial analysis of ADAMTS13 activity. *Br J Haematol.* 2007; 139:486–493.

205. George JN, Woodson RD, Kiss JE, et al. Rituximab therapy for thrombotic thrombocytopenic purpura: a proposed study of the Transfusion Medicine/Hemostasis Clinical Trials Network with a systematic review of rituximab therapy for immune-mediated disorders. *J Clin Apher.* 2006; 21:49–56.

206. Ziman A, Mitri M, Klapper E, et al. Combination vincristine and plasma exchange as initial therapy in patients with thrombotic thrombocytopenic purpura: one institution's experience and review of the literature. *Transfusion.* 2005; 45:41–49.

207. Gruppo RA, Rother RP. Eculizumab for congenital atypical hemolytic-uremic syndrome. *N Engl J Med.* 2009; 360:544–546.

208. Nurnberger J, Witzke O, Opazo Saez A, et al. Eculizumab for atypical hemolytic-uremic syndrome. *N Engl J Med.* 2009; 360:542–544.

209. Laakso M, Mutru O, Isomaki H, et al. Mortality from amyloidosis and renal diseases in patients with rheumatoid arthritis. *Ann Rheum Dis.* 1986; 45:663–667.

210. Christensen EI, Birn H. Megalin and cubilin: synergistic endocytic receptors in renal proximal tubule. *Am J Physiol.* 2001; 280:F562–F573.

211. Klassen RB, Allen PL, Batuman V, et al. Light chains are a ligand for megalin. *J Appl Physiol.* 2005; 98:257–263.

212. Merlini G, Pozzi C. Mechanisms of renal damage in plasma cell dyscrasias: an overview. *Contrib Nephrol.* 2007; 153:66–86.

213. Pesce AJ, Clyne DH, Pollak VE, et al. Renal tubular interactions of proteins. *Clin Biochem.* 1980; 13:209–215.

214. Verroust PJ, Birn H, Nielsen R, et al. The tandem endocytic receptors megalin and cubilin are important proteins in renal pathology. *Kidney Int.* 2002; 62:745–756.

215. Myatt EA, Westholm FA, Weiss DT, et al. Pathogenic potential of human monoclonal immunoglobulin light chains: relationship of in vitro aggregation to in vivo organ deposition. *Proc Natl Acad Sci U S A.* 1994; 91:3034–3038.

216. Dember LM. Amyloidosis-associated kidney disease. *J Am Soc Nephrol.* 2006; 17:3458–3471.

217. Novak L, Cook WJ, Herrera GA, et al. AL-amyloidosis is underdiagnosed in renal biopsies. *Nephrol Dial Transplant.* 2004; 19:3050–3053.

218. Cohen AH. Amyloidosis. In: Fogo AB, Cohen AH, Jennette JC, et al., eds. *Fundamentals of Renal Pathology.* New York: Springer; 2006:170–173.

219. Stevens FJ. Four structural risk factors identify most fibril-forming kappa light chains. *Amyloid.* 2000; 7:200–211.

220. Hurle MR, Helms LR, Li L, et al. A role for destabilizing amino acid replacements in light-chain amyloidosis. *Proc Natl Acad Sci U S A.* 1994; 91:5446–5450.

221. Raffen R, Dieckman LJ, Szpunar M, et al. Physicochemical consequences of amino acid variations that contribute to fibril formation by immunoglobulin light chains. *Protein Sci.* 1999; 8:509–517.

222. Isaac J, Kerby JD, Russell WJ, et al. In vitro modulation of AL-amyloid formation by human mesangial cells exposed to amyloidogenic light chains. *Amyloid.* 1998; 5:238–246.

223. Keeling J, Herrera GA. Matrix metalloproteinases and mesangial remodeling in light chain-related glomerular damage. *Kidney Int.* 2005; 68:1590–1603.

224. Keeling J, Herrera GA. The mesangium as a target for glomerulopathic light and heavy chains: pathogenic considerations in light and heavy chain-mediated glomerular damage. *Contrib Nephrol.* 2007; 153:116–134.

225. Teng J, Russell WJ, Gu X, et al. Different types of glomerulopathic light chains interact with mesangial cells using a common receptor but exhibit different intracellular trafficking patterns. *Lab Invest.* 2004; 84:440–451.

226. Lin J, Markowitz GS, Valeri AM, et al. Renal monoclonal immunoglobulin deposition disease: the disease spectrum. *J Am Soc Nephrol.* 2001; 12:1482–1492.

227. Cohen AH. Monoclonal immunoglobulin deposition disease. In: Fogo AB, Cohen AH, Jennette JC, et al., eds. *Fundamentals of Renal Pathology.* New York: Springer; 2006:165–169.

228. Deret S, Chomilier J, Huang DB, et al. Molecular modeling of immunoglobulin light chains implicates hydrophobic residues in non-amyloid light chain deposition disease. *Protein Eng.* 1997; 10:1191–1197.

229. Hendershot L, Bole D, Kohler G, et al. Assembly and secretion of heavy chains that do not associate posttranslationally with immunoglobulin heavy chain-binding protein. *J Cell Biol.* 1987; 104:761–767.

230. Pozzi C, D'Amico M, Fogazzi GB, et al. Light chain deposition disease with renal involvement: clinical characteristics and prognostic factors. *Am J Kidney Dis.* 2003; 42:1154–1163.

231. Rosenstock JL, Markowitz GS, Valeri AM, et al. Fibrillary and immunotactoid glomerulonephritis: Distinct entities with different clinical and pathologic features. *Kidney Int.* 2003; 63:1450–1461.

232. Rosenmann E, Eliakim M. Nephrotic syndrome associated with amyloid-like glomerular deposits. *Nephron.* 1977; 18:301–308.

233. Alpers CE, Kowalewska J. Fibrillary glomerulonephritis and immunotactoid glomerulopathy. *J Am Soc Nephrol.* 2008; 19:34–37.

234. Schwartz MM, Korbet SM, Lewis EJ. Immunotactoid glomerulopathy. *J Am Soc Nephrol.* 2002; 13:1390–1397.

235. Korbet SM, Schwartz MM, Lewis EJ. Immuotactoid glomerulopathy (fibrillary glomerulonephritis). *Clin J Am Soc Nephrol.* 2006; 1:1351–1356.

236. Collins M, Navaneethan SD, Chung M, et al. Rituximab treatment of fibrillary glomerulonephritis. *Am J Kidney Dis.* 2008; 52:1158–1162.

237. Hovind P, Tarnow L, Rossing P, et al. Predictors for the development of microalbuminuria and macroalbuminuria in patients with type 1 diabetes: inception cohort study. *BMJ.* 2004; 328: 1105.

238. Newman DJ, Mattock MB, Dawnay AB, et al. Systematic review on urine albumin testing for early detection of diabetic complications. *Health Technol Assess.* 2005; 9:iii–vi, xiii–163.

239. Adler AI, Stevens RJ, Manley SE, et al. Development and progression of nephropathy in type 2 diabetes: the United Kingdom Prospective Diabetes Study (UKPDS 64). *Kidney Int.* 2003; 63:225–232.

240. Ritz E, Orth SR. Nephropathy in patients with type 2 diabetes mellitus. *N Engl J Med.* 1999; 341:1127–1133.

241. Bash LD, Selvin E, Steffes M, et al. Poor glycemic control in diabetes and the risk of incident chronic kidney disease even in the absence of albuminuria and retinopathy: Atherosclerosis Risk in Communities (ARIC) Study. *Arch Intern Med.* 2008; 168:2440–2447.

242. Perkins BA, Ficociello LH, Ostrander BE, et al. Microalbuminuria and the risk for early progressive renal function decline in type 1 diabetes. *J Am Soc Nephrol.* 2007; 18:1353–1361.

243. Bojestig M, Arnqvist HJ, Hermansson G, et al. Declining incidence of nephropathy in insulin-dependent diabetes mellitus. *N Engl J Med.* 1994; 330:15–18.

244. Finne P, Reunanen A, Stenman S, et al. Incidence of end-stage renal disease in patients with type 1 diabetes. *JAMA.* 2005; 294:1782–1787.

245. Tuttle KR, Bruton JL, Perusek MC, et al. Effect of strict glycemic control on renal hemodynamic response to amino acids and renal enlargement in insulin-dependent diabetes mellitus. *N Engl J Med.* 1991; 324:1626–1632.

246. Orchard TJ, Dorman JS, Maser RE, et al. Prevalence of complications in IDDM by sex and duration. Pittsburgh Epidemiology of Diabetes Complications Study II. *Diabetes.* 1990; 39: 1116–1124.

247. Parving HH, Gall MA, Skott P, et al. Prevalence and causes of albuminuria in non-insulin-dependent diabetic patients. *Kidney Int.* 1992; 41:758–762.

248. Jennette JC. Diabetic nephropathy. In: Fogo AB, Cohen AH, Jennette JC, et al., eds. *Fundamentals of Renal Pathology.* New York: Springer; 2006: 132–142.

249. Hostetter TH, Rennke HG, Brenner BM. The case for intrarenal hypertension in the initiation and progression of diabetic and other glomerulopathies. *Am J Med.* 1982; 72:375–380.

250. Hilgers KF, Veelken R. Type 2 diabetic nephropathy: never too early to treat? *J Am Soc Nephrol.* 2005; 16:574–575.

251. Harris RD, Steffes MW, Bilous RW, et al. Global glomerular sclerosis and glomerular arteriolar hyalinosis in insulin dependent diabetes. *Kidney Int.* 1991; 40:107–114.

252. Heilig CW, Concepcion LA, Riser BL, et al. Overexpression of glucose transporters in rat mesangial cells cultured in a normal glucose milieu mimics the diabetic phenotype. *J Clin Invest.* 1995; 96:1802–1814.

253. Lin CL, Wang JY, Huang YT, et al. Wnt/beta-catenin signaling modulates survival of high glucose-stressed mesangial cells. *J Am Soc Nephrol.* 2006; 17:2812–2820.

254. Singh AK, Mo W, Dunea G, et al. Effect of glycated proteins on the matrix of glomerular epithelial cells. *J Am Soc Nephrol.* 1998; 9:802–810.

255. Hohenstein B, Hausknecht B, Boehmer K, et al. Local VEGF activity but not VEGF expression is tightly regulated during diabetic nephropathy in man. *Kidney Int.* 2006; 69:1654–1661.

256. Sharma K, Ziyadeh FN. Hyperglycemia and diabetic kidney disease. The case for transforming growth factor-beta as a key mediator. *Diabetes.* 1995; 44:1139–1146.

257. Christensen PK, Rossing P, Nielsen FS, et al. Natural course of kidney function in Type 2 diabetic patients with diabetic nephropathy. *Diabet Med.* 1999; 16:388–394.

258. Lewis EJ, Hunsicker LG, Bain RP, et al. The effect of angiotensin-converting-enzyme inhibition on diabetic nephropathy. The Collaborative Study Group. *N Engl J Med.* 1993; 329:1456–1462.

259. Thorner PS. Alport syndrome and thin basement membrane nephropathy. *Nephron Clin Pract.* 2007; 106:c82–c88.

260. van der Loop FT, Heidet L, Timmer ED, et al. Autosomal dominant Alport syndrome caused by a COL4A3 splice site mutation. *Kidney Int.* 2000; 58:1870–1875.

261. Callis L, Vila A, Carrera M, et al. Long-term effects of cyclosporine A in Alport's syndrome. *Kidney Int.* 1999; 55:1051–1056.

262. Byrne MC, Budisavljevic MN, Fan Z, et al. Renal transplant in patients with Alport's syndrome. *Am J Kidney Dis.* 2002; 39:769–775.

263. Cosio FG, Falkenhain ME, Sedmak DD. Association of thin glomerular basement membrane with other glomerulopathies. *Kidney Int.* 1994; 46: 471–474.

264. Zarate YA, Hopkin RJ. Fabry's disease. *Lancet.* 2008; 372:1427–1435.

265. Alroy J, Sabnis S, Kopp JB. Renal pathology in Fabry disease. *J Am Soc Nephrol.* 2002; 13 (suppl 2):S134–S138.

266. Lemley KV. Kidney disease in nail-patella syndrome. *Pediatr Nephrol.* 2008 Jun 6. [Epub ahead of print].

267. Liapis H. Molecular pathology of nephrotic syndrome in childhood: a contemporary approach to diagnosis. *Pediatr Dev Pathol.* 2008; 11:154–163.

268. Alchi B, Nishi S, Narita I, et al. Collagenofibrotic glomerulopathy: clinicopathologic overview of a rare glomerular disease. *Am J Kidney Dis.* 2007; 49:499–506.

269. Saito T, Sato H, Kudo K, et al. Lipoprotein glomerulopathy: glomerular lipoprotein thrombi in a patient with hyperlipoproteinemia. *Am J Kidney Dis.* 1989; 13:148–153.

270. Xin Z, Zhihong L, Shijun L, et al. Successful treatment of patients with lipoprotein glomerulopathy by protein A immunoadsorption: a pilot study. *Nephrol Dial Transplant.* 2009; 24:864–869.

271. Schwartz MM. Gomerular diseases with organized deposits. In: Jennette JC, Olsen JL, Schwarz MM, et al., eds. *Pathology of the Kidney.* Philadelphia: Wolters Kluwer; 2007:911–936.

Index

Page numbers followed by *f* denote figures; those followed by *t* denote tables.